Stress Science: Neuroendocrinology

STRESS SCIENCE: NEUROENDOCRINOLOGY

EDITOR-IN-CHIEF

GEORGE FINK

Professorial Research Fellow (formerly Director)
Mental Health Research Institute of Victoria
Parkville, Melbourne, Victoria
Australia
Formerly Director, MRC Brain Metabolism Unit
Edinburgh, Scotland
UK

ELSEVIER

AMSTERDAM • BOSTON • HEIDELBERG • LONDON • NEW YORK • OXFORD
PARIS • SAN DIEGO • SAN FRANCISCO • SINGAPORE • SYDNEY • TOKYO
Academic Press is an imprint of Elsevier

ACADEMIC PRESS

Academic Press is an imprint of Elsevier
525 B Street, Suite 1900, San Diego, CA 92101-4495, USA
Linacre House, Jordan Hill, Oxford, OX2 8DP, UK

British Library Cataloguing in Publication Data
A catalogue record for this book is available from the British Library

Library of Congress Catalog Number
A catalog record for this book is available from the Library of Congress

ISBN: 9780123750662

For information on all Elsevier publications
visit our website at books.elsevier.com

07 08 09 10 11 10 9 8 7 6 5 4 3 2 1

INTRODUCTION

Stress is not something to be avoided. Indeed, it cannot be avoided, since just staying alive creates some demand for life-maintaining energy. Complete freedom from stress can be expected only after death. *Hans Selye*

"Stress" remains one of the most frequently used but ill-defined words in the English language. Stress is a phenomenon that has quite different meanings at different times and under different circumstances for different individuals. Stress is a function of three main interactive and often interdependent variables: *(i) excitability/arousal; (ii) perceived aversiveness;* and *(iii) uncontrollability*. We all know when we are stressed – e.g. late for an important meeting and stuck in dense traffic or in a plane that shows no sign of push-back for reasons unknown – but find it difficult rationally to define our feelings. The definition proposed by the distinguished Berkeley psychologist, Richard Lazarus, is perhaps apposite for many stressful situations in man – that is, "a condition or feeling experienced when a person perceives that demands exceed the personal and social resources the individual is able to mobilize."

Hans Selye, sometimes called the "father of stress", coined and defined "stress" as "the nonspecific response of the body to any demand." For some, Selye's definition is "too biological" and ignores cognitive and psychological factors, a criticism that seems to stem from the misconception that cognition is not a function of the brain. For others, Selye's definition is too general. However, Selye's publications show that he understood psychological or cognitive stress. Furthermore, the generality of Selye's definition makes it pertinent for the molecular, genotypic and phenotypic analysis of stress and stress responses across all species from bacteria to man.

The contributions of Walter Bradford Cannon, working at Harvard in the 1920's and '30s, are arguably of equal importance for our understanding of the stress response. Thus, Cannon first proposed the term *homeostasis* (from the Greek homoios, or similar, and stasis, or position) for the coordinated physiological processes that enable the organism to cope with the stressful challenge by maintaining or quickly restoring steady state within the organism. Cannon also coined the term "fight or flight" to describe an animal's response to threat. *Homeostasis*, 'stability through constancy', which has dominated physiological and medical thinking since 1859 (Claude Bernard's "milieu intérieur") seems in several circumstances (e.g. work-induced increase in cardiovascular load) to be giving way to *allostasis,* which provides 'stability through change'. *Homeostasis* depends on negative feedback control systems: *allostasis* refers to the dynamic maintenance of *homeostasis* by appropriate central nervous regulation of the cybernetic set points that adjust physiological parameters to meet various stresses/challenges.

The purpose of *Stress Science* and its companion volume *Stress Consequences* is to package key up-to date concepts and information regarding stress and its consequent and/or associated adverse effects on human health into a systematically formatted and reader friendly handbook. The present work is focused on the fundamental neuroendocrine response to stress and its adverse effects on several key somatic systems. The mental, neuropsychological and socioeconomic consequences of stress are covered in the companion volume on *Stress Consequences*. Comprised of a selection of salient articles published recently in the Encyclopedias of Stress and Neuroscience, *Stress Science* will be useful to students, graduates and professionals in a range of areas including health, biomedical science, neuroscience, psychology, sociology and socioeconomics. *Stress Science,* which will prove to be a useful handbook at the laboratory bench as well as in the office, is organized in a series of sections as outlined below.

The neuroendocrine stress response/control system in vertebrates is comprised of two arms; the hypothalamic-pituitary-adrenal axis (HPA) and the autonomic, predominantly sympathetic, nervous system. Both the HPA and the autonomic nervous arms are covered systematically under Sections II to IV, which are preceded by Section I on stress definitions and concepts. The interactions between the HPA and the autonomic nervous system, and the way in which stress neuropeptides such as corticotropin releasing factor-41 (CRF), the urocortins and arginine vasopressin are involved in mounting stress and related behavioral responses are reviewed in Section V – "Integrative aspects of stress response". Section V also includes papers on the blood-brain barrier and the multi drug resistant P glycoprotein, which have physiological and pharmacological relevance for our understanding of the neuroendocrine stress response and the treatment of stress related disorders (see also companion volume, *Stress Consequences*).

The diurnal rhythm of adrenal glucocorticoid plasma concentrations, with a peak at wakening and trough during sleep, is a robust marker of circadian rhythms generated by the body's 'master clock' located in the suprachiasmatic nuclei of the hypothalamus. Driven by the hypothalamic-pituitary system, the circadian glucocorticoid rhythm in turn affects the periodicity of the 'master clock', and is associated with sleep/wake cycles and circadian rhythms in body temperature and metabolism. Seasonal rhythms in glucocorticoids and responses to stress occur in most vertebrate species from elasmobranchs to man. The diurnal glucocorticoid rhythm, genetics of the circadian clock, and diurnal and seasonal changes in the stress response are reviewed in Section VI, as is the evidence for an apparently distinct mechanism that determines feeding rhythm. The special significance of circadian rhythmicity for cardiovascular events, such as myocardial infarction, is covered in Section VIII C ('Cardiovascular System and Disorders').

Stress, adrenal corticosteroid hormones and the monoamines (norepinephrine, dopamine, and serotonin) have been implicated in neuronal plasticity and memory. This field of intensive ongoing endeavor is covered in Section VII.

Stress-induced or related pathology is covered in Section VIII with focus on immune/inflammatory responses (section A), feeding, obesity and the metabolic syndrome (section B), cardiovascular system and disorders (section C) and the effects of stress on reproduction (section D). Heat shock and chaperone proteins that play a key role in the cellular defense against stress in all species from archaea to man are discussed in *Stress Consequences* in relation to neurodegenerative and protein folding disorders.

Biologically, the stress response reflects a set of integrated cascades in the nervous, endocrine, and immune defense systems. As in most areas of biology, molecular genetics has made a significant impact on the precision with which we now understand the physiological and pathological processes of the stress response. This point is illustrated in *Stress Science* by the step advances that have been made in our understanding, for example, of the central and peripheral actions of CRF and urocortin and their receptors; the role of central CRF in the overall control of the mental, behavioral as well as neuroendocrine response to stress; the cardiac peptides; the cytokines and other inflammatory and immune signaling molecules; and the complex neuropeptide regulation of hunger and satiety. Thus, the adage formerly applied to diabetes mellitus may now apply equally to stress: "Understand stress and you will understand medicine."

Note on Terminology of Corticotropin Releasing Factor/Hormone and the Catecholamines

The central nervous regulation of the anterior pituitary gland is mediated by substances, mainly peptides, which are synthesized in the hypothalamus and transported to the gland by the hypophysial portal vessels. Because these compounds are transported by the blood, the term "hormone" or "neurohormone" gained acceptance in the neuroendocrine literature. The major hypothalamic peptide involved in the stress response is the 41-amino acid corticotropin releasing factor (CRF). The Endocrine Society (USA), following convention, adopted the term corticotropin releasing hormone (CRH). However, this nomenclature has been challenged. Hauger et al. (2003), in liaison with the International Union of Pharmacology Committee on Receptor Nomenclature and Drug Classification, argued that the function of CRF extends well beyond the biology of a hormone, and that therefore it should be termed corticotropin releasing factor (CRF) rather than hormone. Since the terminology of CRF versus CRH has yet to be resolved, the two terms and abbreviations are here used interchangeably, depending on author preference.

Adrenaline and *noradrenaline* are catecholamines that play a pivotal role in the stress response. These terms are synonymous with *epinephrine* and *norepinephrine*, respectively. Both sets of terms are used interchangeably in the endocrine, neuroendocrine and stress literature, and this principle has been adopted here. Style has depended on author preference, but wherever possible within-article consistency has been ensured. The adjectival forms, "adrenergic" and "noradrenergic", are used universally.

Hauger, R. L., Grigoriadis, D. E., Dallman, M. F., Plotsky, P. M., Vale, W. W. and Dautzenberg, F. M. (2003). International Union of Pharmacology. XXXVI. Current status of the nomenclature for receptors for corticotropin-releasing factor and their ligands. *Pharmacological Reviews* 55(1), 21–26.

George Fink

ACKNOWLEDGEMENT

I should much like to thank Mica Haley, Neuroscience Acquisitions Editor for Elsevier, for proposing this exciting project and facilitating its efficient production.

To Ann, my wife, go my best thanks for enduring and enabling yet another frenetic stress adventure.

George Fink
May 11, 2009

CONTRIBUTORS

R A H Adan
Rudolf Magnus Institute of Neuroscience, University Medical Centre Utrecht, Utrecht, The Netherlands

H Akil
University of Michigan, Ann Arbor, MI, USA

M Alevizaki
Evgenidion Hospital and Alexandra Hospital, Athens University School of Medicine, Athens, Greece

L Altshuler
UCLA Neuropsychiatric Institute and Hospital and West LA Veterans Administration Medical Center, Los Angeles, CA, USA

M C Andresen
Oregon Health & Science University, Portland, OR, USA

M P Antoch
Lerner Research Institute, Cleveland Clinic Foundation, Cleveland, OH, USA

G Aston-Jones
Medical University of South Carolina, Charleston, SC, USA

M Bader
Max-Delbrück-Center for Molecular Medicine, Berlin-Buch, Germany

O Baltatu
Max-Delbrück-Center for Molecular Medicine, Berlin-Buch, Germany, and Sultan Qaboos University, Muscat, Sultanate of Oman

D Barb
Beth Israel Deaconess Medical Center, Boston, MA, USA

T Bartfai
The Scripps Research Institute, CA, USA

M Beato
Centre de Regulació de Genòmica, UPF, Barcelona, Spain

S Bhatnagar
University of Michigan, Ann Arbor, MI, USA

A B Bicknell
University of Reading, Reading, UK

J C Bittencourt
Salk Institute for Biological Studies, La Jolla, CA, USA

B Boari
Vascular Diseases Center, University of Ferrara, Italy

C S Boomershine
The Ohlo State University, Columbus, OH, USA

S R Bornstein
Technical University of Dresden, Dresden, Germany

P-M G Bouloux
Royal Free Hospital and Medical School, London, UK

J C Buckingham
Imperial College School of Medicine, London, UK

A J Bugajski
Jagiellonian University, Krakow, Poland

J Bugajski
Polish Academy of Sciences, Krakow, Poland

R M Buijs
Universidad Nacional Autónoma de México, Mexico City, Mexico

R A Carels
Duke University Medical Center

S Chakravarty
University of Texas Southwestern Medical Center, Dallas, TX, USA

F Chiappelli
UCLA School of Dentistry, Los Angeles, CA, USA

G P Chrousos
Athens University Medical School, Athens, Greece

W C J Chung
Colorado State University, Fort Collins, CO, USA

Iain J Clarke
Monash University, Melbourne, Australia

C Coughlin
Wyeth Research, Collegeville, PA, USA

I W Craig
King's College London, London, UK

M F Dallman
University of California at San Francisco, San Francisco, CA, USA

N A Datson
Leiden University, Leiden, The Netherlands

I S P Davis
Institute of Psychiatry, King's College London, London, UK

H E W Day
University of Michigan, Ann Arbor, MI, USA

F H de Jong
Erasmus University Medical Centre, Rotterdam, The Netherlands

E R de Kloet
Leiden University Medical Center and Leiden University, Leiden, Netherlands

E C M de Lange
Leiden University, Leiden, Netherlands

P J Delves
University College London, London, UK

R H DeRijk
Leiden University Medical Center and Leiden University, Leiden, Netherlands

S D Douglas
Children's Hospital of Philadelphia and University of Pennsylvania Medical School, Philadelphia, PA, USA

C A Dudley
University of Texas Southwestern Medical Center, Dallas, TX, USA

M Durai
Johns Hopkins University School of Medicine, Baltimore, MD, USA

M Eleftheriades
Athens University Medical School, Athens, Greece

T Else
University of Michigan, Ann Arbor, MI, USA

C Escobar
Universidad Nacional Autónoma de México, Mexico City, Mexico

M S Fanselow
University of California, Los Angeles, CA, USA

W P Fehder
New York University, New York, NY, USA

É M Fekete
The Scripps Research Institute, La Jolla, CA, USA

A V Ferguson
Queen's University, Kingston, ON, Canada

M Ferin
Columbia University, New York NY, USA

G Z Feuerstein
Wyeth Research, Collegeville, PA, USA

G Fink
Mental Health Research Institute, Melbourne, Australia

G Flügge
German Primate Center, Göttingen, Germany

H Friedman
University of South Florida College of Medicine, Tampa, FL, USA

E Fuchs
German Primate Center and Medical School, University of Göttingen, Göttingen, Germany

A Gądek-Michalska
Polish Academy of Sciences, Krakow, Poland

P J Gasser
Arizona State University, Tempe, AZ, USA

S Gatti McArthur
F. Hoffmann-LaRoche, Basel, Switzerland

A Gavrila
Beth Israel Deaconess Medical Center, Boston, MA, USA

D S Goldstein
National Institutes of Health, Bethesda, MD, USA

E Gould
Princeton University, Princeton, NJ, USA

T Grandfield
University of Sheffield, Sheffield, UK

D E Grigoriadis
Neurocrine Biosciences, Inc., San Diego, CA, USA

M Gruber
Technical University of Dresden, Dresden, Germany

G D Hammer
University of Michigan, Ann Arbor, MI, USA

R J Handa
Colorado State University, Fort Collins, CO, USA

Belinda A Henry
Monash University, Melbourne, Australia

J P Herman
University of Cincinnati, Cincinnati, OH, USA

J P Hieble
Wayne, PA, USA

J J G Hillebrand
Rudolf Magnus Institute of Neuroscience, University Medical Centre Utrecht, Utrecht, The Netherlands

J P Hinson
Queen Mary, University of London, London, UK

P Hjemdahl
Karolinska Institute and University Hospital, Stockholm, Sweden

W-Z Ho
Children's Hospital of Philadelphia and University of Pennsylvania Medical School, Philadelphia, PA, USA

M O Huising
The Salk Institute for Biological Studies, La Jolla, CA, USA
Department of Animal Physiology, Radboud University Nijmegen, Nijmegen, The Netherlands

T A Jenkins
University of Melbourne, Parkville, Victoria, Australia

J R Jennings
University of Pittsburgh School of Medicine, Pittsburgh, PA, USA

M Joëls
University of Amsterdam, Amsterdam, Netherlands

N J Justice
The Salk Institute, La Jolla, CA, USA

A Kalsbeek
Netherlands Institute for Neuroscience, Amsterdam, The Netherlands

J R Kaplan
Wake Forest University School of Medicine, Winston Salem, NC, USA

H Karst
University of Amsterdam, Amsterdam, Netherlands

N R Keller
Vanderbilt University, Nashville, TN, USA

L Keltikangas-Järvinen
University of Helsinki, Helsinki, Finland

C F Kemp
University of Reading, Reading, UK

J Klug
University of Giessen, Giessen, Germany

S Kollack-Walker
University of Michigan, Ann Arbor, MI, USA

R V Kondratov
Lerner Research Institute, Cleveland Clinic Foundation, Cleveland, OH, USA

G F Koob
The Scripps Research Institute, La Jolla, CA, USA

A Kumar
University of Texas Southwestern Medical Center, Dallas, TX, USA

R Kvetnansky
Slovak Academy of Sciences, Slovak Republic

I Kyrou
Evgenidion Hospital, Athens University Medical School, Athens, Greece

S E La Fleur
Rudolf Magnus Institute of Neuroscience, University Medical Centre Utrecht, Utrecht, The Netherlands

F Laplante
Salk Institute for Biological Studies, La Jolla, CA, USA

K-F Lee
The Salk Institute, La Jolla, CA, USA

M Lee
Columbia University College of Physicians and Surgeons, New York, NY, USA

B E Leonard
University of Maastricht, Maastricht, The Netherlands and National University of Ireland, Galway, Ireland

W R Lovallo
Veterans Affairs Medical Center and University of Oklahoma Health Sciences Center, Oklahoma City, OK, USA

P J Lowry
University of Reading, Reading, UK

S J Lupien
McGill University and Geriatric Institute of Montreal, Montreal, Canada

F S Maheu
National Institute of Mental Health, Bethesda, MD, USA

S N Malaeb
Brown Medical School, Providence, RI, USA

A M Malagoni
Vascular Diseases Center, University of Ferrara, Italy

F Manfredini
Vascular Diseases Center, University of Ferrara, Italy

R Manfredini
Vascular Diseases Center, University of Ferrara, Italy

C S Mantzoros
Beth Israel Deaconess Medical Center, Boston, MA, USA

G D Marshall
University of Mississippi Medical Center, Jackson, MS, USA

L B Martin II
Ohio State University, Columbus, OH, USA

M R Mayford
The Scripps Research Institute, La Jolla, CA, USA

R McCarty
University of Virginia, Charlottesville, VA, USA

R McCarty
Vanderbilt University, Nashville, TN, USA

B S McEwen
Rockefeller University, New York, USA

G U Meduri
University of Tennessee Health Science Center Department of Medicine, Memphis, TN USA

C A Meijas-Aponte
National Institutes of Health, Baltimore, MD, USA

O C Meijer
Leiden University, Leiden, Netherlands

D Mendelowitz
George Washington University, Washington, DC, USA

F A O Mendelsohn
University of Melbourne, Parkville, Victoria, Australia

D Miller
Wyeth Research, Collegeville, PA, USA

M C Morsink
Leiden University, Leiden, The Netherlands

S Moshonov
Weizmann Institute of Science, Rehovot, Israel

R L Moss
University of Texas Southwestern Medical Center, Dallas, TX, USA

K D Moudgil
University of Maryland School of Medicine, Baltimore, MD, USA

A Munck
Dartmouth Medical School, Lebanon, NH, USA

B E P Murphy
McGill University, Montreal, Canada

Z Naor
Tel Aviv University, Tel Aviv, Israel

R J Nelson
Ohio State University, Columbus, OH, USA

R M Nesse
University of Michigan, Ann Arbor, MI, USA

M Orchinik
Arizona State University, Tempe, AZ, USA

K Pacak
National Institute of Neurological Disorders and Stroke and National Institute of Child Health and Human Development, National Institutes of Health, Bethesda, MD, USA

M Palkovits
Semmelweis University, Budapest, Hungary

B E Pearson Murphy
McGill University Health Center, Montreal, PQ, Canada

N Pecoraro
University of California at San Francisco, San Francisco, CA, USA

P Pervanidou
Athens University Medical School, Athens, Greece

D W Pfaff
Rockefeller University, New York, NY, USA

R Plomin
Institute of Psychiatry, King's College London, London, UK

T M Pollard
Durham University, Durham, UK

R Ponnusamy
University of California, Los Angeles, CA, USA

S W Porges
University of Illinois at Chicago, Chicago, IL, USA

P Prolo
UCLA School of Dentistry, Los Angeles, CA, USA

S H Pross
University of South Florida College of Medicine, Tampa, FL, USA

B S Rabin
University of Pittsburgh, Pittsburgh, PA, USA

A C Ribeiro
Rockefeller University, New York, NY, USA

R A Rissman
Salk Institute for Biological Studies, La Jolla, CA, USA

S Rivest
Laval University, Québec City, QC, Canada

D Robertson
Vanderbilt University, Nashville, TN, USA

L M Romero
Tufts University, Medford, MA, USA

R Rosmond
Björndammsterrassen 41, Partille, Sweden

R R Ruffolo
Wyeth Research, Collegeville, PA, USA

R Salmi
Vascular Diseases Center, University of Ferrara, Italy

W K Samson
Saint Louis University School of Medicine, St. Louis, MO, USA

R M Sapolsky
Stanford University, Stanford, CA, USA

P E Sawchenko
Salk Institute for Biological Studies, La Jolla, CA, USA

J R Seckl
Edinburgh University, Edinburgh, UK

A Sherwood
Duke University Medical Center

C A Shively
Wake Forest University School of Medicine, Winston-Salem, NC, USA

J J Sollers III
Department of Psychology, Ohio State University, Columbus, OH, USA

A Solomon
Royal Free Hospital and Medical School, London, UK

C Song
University of Prince Edward Island, Charlottetown, PE, Canada

F K Stephan
Florida State University, Tallahassee, FL, USA

A Steptoe
University College London, London, UK

B S Stonestreet
Brown Medical School, Providence, RI, USA

C M Stoney
National Center for Complementary and Alternative Medicine, National Institutes of Health, Bethesda, MD, USA

C A Stratakis
National Institute of Child and Health and Human Development, National Institutes of Health, Bethesda, MD, USA

R Suri
UCLA Neuropsychiatric Institute and Hospital, Los Angeles, CA, USA

P Tanapat
Princeton University, Princeton, NJ, USA

F Tronche
CNRS, Collège de France, Paris, France

C Tsigos
Evgenidion Hospital, Athens University Medical School, Athens, Greece

F Tuluc
Children's Hospital of Philadelphia, Philadelphia, PA, USA

F W Turek
Northwestern University, Evanston, IL, USA

G Turpin
University of Sheffield, Sheffield, UK

W W Vale
The Salk Institute for Biological Studies, La Jolla, CA, USA

G P Vinson
Queen Mary, University of London, London, UK

M H Vitaterna
Northwestern University, Evanston, IL, USA

J Wang
Wyeth Research, Collegeville, PA, USA

S L Wardlaw
Columbia University College of Physicians and Surgeons, New York, NY, USA

B Waterhouse
Drexel University College of Medicine, Philadelphia, PA, USA

A G Watts
University of Southern California, Los Angeles, CA, USA

W J Welch
Georgetown University, Washington, D.C., USA

M M White
Saint Louis University School of Medicine, St. Louis, MO, USA

B J Whitehouse
King's College London, London, UK

H S Willenberg
University Hospital Duesseldorf, Duesseldorf, Germany

O T Wolf
University of Bielefeld, Bielefeld, Germany

R J Woods
University of Reading, Reading, UK

E A Young
University of Michigan, Ann Arbor, MI, USA

Z F Yuan
Salk Institute for Biological Studies, La Jolla, CA, USA

Y Zhao
The Scripps Research Institute, La Jolla, CA, USA

U Zor
Weizmann Institute of Science, Rehovot, Israel

E P Zorrilla
The Scripps Research Institute, La Jolla, CA, USA

B S Zwilling
The Ohlo State University, Columbus, OH, USA

CONTENTS

V. INTEGRATIVE ASPECTS OF STRESS RESPONSE

VI. CIRCADIAN AND SEASONAL RHYTHMS

VII. NEURONAL PLASTICITY - MEMORY

VIII. STRESS - INDUCED/ RELATED PATHOLOGY

A. IMMUNE/INFLAMMATORY RESPONSES

B. STRESS - FEEDING - OBESITY - METABOLIC SYNDROME

C. CARDIOVASCULAR SYSTEM AND DISORDERS

I. STRESS DEFINITIONS AND CONCEPTS

Stress: Definition and History

G Fink
The Mental Health Research Institute of Victoria, Melbourne, VIC, Australia

Introduction and Historical Outline of Several Stress Concepts

Aristotle, Hippocrates, and the other Ancients were aware of stress and its adverse effects. However, Claude Bernard was the first to formally explain how cells and tissues in multicelled organisms might be protected from stress. One of the world's greatest physiologists, Bernard, working in Paris during the second half of the nineteenth century, first pointed out (1859) that the internal medium of the living organism is not merely a vehicle for carrying nourishment to cells. Rather, "it is the fixity of the *milieu intérieur* which is the condition of free and independent life." That is, cells are surrounded by an internal medium that buffers changes in acid-base, gaseous (O_2 and CO_2), and ion concentrations and other biochemical modalities to minimize changes around biologically determined set points, thereby providing a steady state. Fifty years later, Walter Bradford Cannon, working at Harvard, suggested the designation homeostasis (from the Greek *homoios*, or similar, and *stasis*, or position) for the coordinated physiological processes that maintain most of the steady states in the organism. Cannon popularized the concept of 'homeostasis' in his 1932 book, *Wisdom of the Body.*

Cannon also coined the term fight or flight to describe an animal's response to threat. The concept of fight or flight proposes that animals react to threats with a general discharge of the sympathetic nervous system, priming the animal for fighting or fleeing. This response was later recognized as the first stage (acute stress response) of a general adaptation syndrome (GAS) postulated by Hans Selye to be a universal stress response among vertebrates and other organisms.

Born in Vienna in 1907, Hans Hugo Bruno Selye, also known as the 'father of stress,' began his stress research while still a medical student in 1926. He observed that patients with a variety of illnesses had many of the same 'nonspecific' symptoms that were a common response to stressful stimuli experienced by the body. These clinical observations together with experiments on laboratory rats underpinned Selye's concept of GAS, which led Selye to assert that prolonged exposure to stress resulted in 'diseases of adaptation.' That is, chronic stress, by causing the overproduction of chemicals and hormones, produced gastroduodenal ulcers and high blood pressure. Although the GAS hypothesis was subsequently shown to be incorrect, it did put stress on the map and also highlighted the fact that stress had major effects on the immune system as well as on the adrenal glands.

In addition to providing the first clear definition of stress, Hans Selye was also the first to recognize that homeostasis could not by itself ensure stability of body systems under stress. He coined the term heterostasis (from the Greek *heteros*, or other) as the process by which a new steady state was achieved by treatment with agents that stimulate the physiological adaptive mechanisms. Heterostasis could be regarded as the precursor for the concept of allostasis, first advanced by Peter Sterling and Joseph Eyer in the 1980s. That is, homeostasis, which has dominated physiological and medical thinking since the nineteenth century, is thought to provide 'stability through constancy.' Allostasis, on the other hand, provides 'stability through change' brought about by central nervous regulation of the set points that adjust physiological parameters to meet the stress/challenge.

A different tack, focused on cognition, was taken by Richard Lazarus, the eminent and influential Berkeley University psychologist. At a time when psychology tried to understand human behavior by first understanding simple organisms engaging in simple behaviors learned by associations, rewards, or punishments, Lazarus instead emphasized the importance of studying cognition, which he extended into stress and coping.

Epidemiology has been and remains central to stress studies. Numerous epidemiological studies have tried to define the effects of social, workplace, and lifestyle on stress, health, and well-being. However, of the recent epidemiological studies that have generated new stress concepts, the most important perhaps is that of David Barker, which led to the hypothesis that fetal undernutrition in middle to late gestation programs later coronary heart disease. This concept was soon extended by Hales and Barker in their 'thrifty phenotype hypothesis.' The latter proposes an association between poor fetal and infant growth and the subsequent development of type 2 diabetes and the metabolic syndrome, which afflict communities in epidemic proportions. Poor nutrition in early life, it is postulated, produces permanent changes in glucose-insulin metabolism. These changes include insulin resistance (and possibly defective insulin secretion), which combined with effects of obesity, aging, and physical inactivity are the most important factors in determining type 2 diabetes. Many studies worldwide have confirmed Barker's initial epidemiological evidence, although the strength of the relationships has varied between studies.

With advances in genomics, the concept of susceptibility genes that increase the vulnerability of individuals to stressful life events has attracted considerable research interest. Thus, for example, the work of Avshalom Caspi and associates suggests that a polymorphism in the monoamine oxidase A (MAOA) gene promoter, which reduces MAOA expression, influences vulnerability to environmental stress, and that this biological process can be initiated by childhood abuse. Furthermore, Caspi and associates, working at the Institute of Psychiatry, London, have demonstrated that a polymorphism in the promoter of the serotonin transporter gene can render individuals more susceptible to stressful life events. In addition to their disorder-specific value, these findings have heuristic value for further thinking and research on genetic–environmental interactions that determine the response to stress and the development of mental disorders.

In parallel with these stress concepts, neuroendocrine advances revealed the physiological substrate for homeostasis, allostasis, and the stress response mechanisms. The autonomic nervous and the hypothalamic–pituitary–adrenocortical (HPA) systems subserve the afferent and efferent limbs of the stress response in vertebrates and are also central to maintaining homeostasis and effecting allostasis. The term autonomic nervous system was coined in 1898 by the Cambridge physiologist John Newport Langley, who was also renowned for his development (in parallel with Paul Ehrlich) of receptor theory. Controlled by the brain, and utilizing as neurotransmitters epinephrine and norepinephrine (sympathetic nervous component) or acetylcholine (parasympathetic component), the role of the autonomic nervous system in fight-or-flight and homeostasis (especially cardiovascular) was clearly explained by Walter Cannon.

The story of our understanding of the HPA, and the concept of the neurohumoral hypothesis of anterior pituitary control, is tortuous. The pituitary gland had long been regarded, by luminaries such as the great Harvard neurosurgeon Harvey Cushing, as the autonomous controller of the adrenal cortex, the thyroid, and the gonads. That is, the anterior pituitary gland was considered to be the 'conductor of the endocrine orchestra.' This view was reinforced by the dramatic effects of experimental pituitary removal (hypophysectomy) in rodents made feasible by the parapharyngeal surgical approach to the pituitary developed by PE Smith in approximately 1930. However, at approximately the same time, experiments were in progress that would eventually prove that the anterior pituitary gland is not autonomous; rather, it is controlled by the brain. The first of these experiments, carried out by William Rowan working-alone at $-50\,^{\circ}C$ in Edmonton, Alberta, in the late 1920s, showed that migration in birds was controlled by the gonads, and that gonadal size in birds was increased many-fold by increases in day length. Day length and the effects of other exteroreceptive factors, such as stress, on endocrine function together with the effects of brain tumors and trauma in the human led to an acceptance of the then (1930s) revolutionary concept that the pituitary gland is under central nervous system (CNS) control.

The neural lobe of the pituitary gland is composed of nerve projections from the paraventricular and supraoptic nuclei of the hypothalamus: these projections terminate on systemic blood vessels into which they release the nanopeptide neurohormones, vasopressin and oxytocin. In contrast, the anterior pituitary gland receives no direct innervation from the brain. Rather, the CNS control of the anterior pituitary gland is mediated by neurohormones synthesized and released from hypothalamic neurons and transported to the anterior pituitary gland by the hypophysial portal vessels. Proof of the neurohumoral hypothesis of anterior pituitary control came, first, from the elegant pituitary stalk section and pituitary grafting experiments of Geoffrey Harris and Dora Jacobsohn; second, from the characterization of some of the neurohormones by Andrew Schally and Roger Guillemin, for which they were awarded the 1977 Nobel Prize for physiology and medicine; and third, from the demonstration, first by my group, that these neurohormones were indeed released into hypophysial portal blood. Corticotropin-releasing factor (CRF), a 41-amino-acid peptide that mediates neural control of adrenocorticotropic hormone (ACTH) release from pituitary corticotropes, was isolated and sequenced by Wylie Vale and associates in 1981. A series of physiological studies, including measurements of neurohormone release into hypophysial portal blood *in vivo*, have confirmed earlier views that arginine vasopressin acts synergistically with CRF to control ACTH release.

Finally, no outline of the history of stress concepts would be complete without mention of the characterization of the adrenocortical glucocorticoids and their function. The glucocorticoids are steroid hormones whose secretion by the adrenal cortex is controlled by

ACTH. The hormones of the adrenal cortex were isolated, identified, and synthesized independently by Edward Kendall (at the Mayo Foundation) and Tadeus Reichstein (at Zurich) and their associates. The availability of large amounts of synthetic steroids enabled their physiological effects to be studied. Ultimately, Philip Hench was able to test the glucocorticoid, cortisone, in the human and demonstrate that it is a powerful anti-inflammatory agent. Hench, at the Mayo Foundation, had previously observed that rheumatoid arthritis was sometimes relieved during pregnancy and in some patients with jaundice, leading him to conclude that the pain-alleviating substance was a steroid. Kendall, Hench, and Reichstein were jointly awarded the Nobel Prize for physiology and medicine for 1950, and synthetic glucocorticoids continue to be used to treat arthritis, asthma, autoimmune conditions, and other inflammatory disorders in humans.

Definitions of Stress

Stress has a different meaning for different people under different conditions. The first and most generic definition of stress is that proposed by Hans Selye: "Stress is the nonspecific response of the body to any demand." Selye repeatedly emphasized the fact that the continued use of the word stress as a nonspecific-response to any demand was most appropriate. Selye argued that stress is not identical to emotional arousal or nervous tension since stress can occur under or in response to anesthesia in man and animals, and it can also occur in plants and bacteria that have no nervous system. This point is elaborated later in the context of stress-induced heat shock proteins (Hsps) that play a key role in cytoprotection across all three phylogenetic domains of organisms on Earth. The word stress, as used by Selye, is accepted in all foreign languages, including those in which no such word existed previously.

Stress, Selye underscored,

> is not something to be avoided. Indeed, it cannot be avoided, since just staying alive creates some demand for life-maintaining energy. Even when man is asleep, his heart, respiratory apparatus, digestive tract, nervous system, and other organs must continue to function. Complete freedom from stress can be expected only after death.

There has been much controversy and debate about Selye's concepts and particularly Selye's view that stress is best regarded as a nonspecific response. Because of their heuristic value, these points will be further considered later.

Other definitions, reviewed in detail by Selye in his treatise *Stress in Health and Disease*, include the following:

1. In behavioral sciences, stress is regarded as the "perception of threat, with resulting anxiety discomfort, emotional tension, and difficulty in adjustment."
2. In the group situation, lack of structure or loss of anchor "makes it difficult or impossible for the group to cope with the requirements of the situation, and the problem of leadership and interpersonal behavior becomes one of evolving or supplying a structure or anchor and of supplying the expertness for coping with the demands of the situation."
3. Stress can also be defined in terms of pure neuroendocrinology. Eugene Yates, for example, defined stress as any stimulus that will provoke the release of ACTH and adrenal glucocorticoids. Presumably, the same might apply to the equally powerful sympathetic markers of stress, underscored earlier by Walter Cannon.
4. Finally, Selye also mentions Richard Lazarus, famous for his work in cognitive psychology and focus on the emotions. Lazarus underscores the difficulties of reaching a precise overarching definition of stress by setting out the following different meanings of the term: "In spite of consistent confusion about the precise meaning of the term, stress is widely recognized as a central problem in human life. Scientists of many disciplines have conceptualized stress but each field appears to have something different in mind concerning its meaning. For the sociologist, it is social disequilibrium, that is, disturbances in the social structure within which people live. Engineers conceive of stress as some external force which produces strain in the materials exposed to it. Physiologists deal with the physical stressors that include a wide range of stimulus conditions that are noxious to the body. In the history of psychological stress research, there has been no clear separation between physical stressors which attack biological tissue systems and psychological stressors which produce their effects purely because of their psychological significance."

Selye's Definition of Stress – A Further Consideration

Selye's definition and concept of stress has remained controversial. For some, his definition is too biological and ignores cognitive and psychological factors, a criticism that seems to stem from the mistaken idea that cognition is not a function of the brain (a reversion to Rene Descartes' outmoded doctrine that mind and body are separate). For others, Selye's definition is too general. This section reviews the basis for Selye's definition of stress and considers whether the criticisms leveled at Selye's stress concept are valid. Overall, our observations suggest that Selye fully understood so-called psychological or cognitive stress, and that the generality of Selye's stress definition has facilitated the molecular, genotypic and phenotypic analysis of stress and stress responses across all species from bacteria to man.

General Adaptation Syndrome

Selye first put stress on the map with GAS. In search of a new hormone, Selye injected extracts of cattle ovaries into rats. The injection caused the following characteristic triad:

1. The adrenal cortex became enlarged and discharged lipid secretory granules.
2. The thymus, spleen, lymph nodes, and all other lymphatic structures showed severe involution.
3. Deep bleeding ulcers appeared in the stomach and duodenum.

Selye at first thought that these effects were due to a new hormone in the extracts but soon found that all toxic substances – extracts of kidneys, spleen, and even toxicant not derived from living tissue produced the same syndrome.

Selye surmised that the response to the injection of toxic substance reflected his "classroom concept" of "the syndrome of just being sick." That is, adrenal enlargement, thymicolymphatic involution, and gastrointestinal ulcers were the omnipresent signs of damage to the body when under attack. The three changes thus became (for Selye) the objective indices of stress and the basis for the development of the entire stress concept.

First described in a note to *Nature* in 1936, GAS has three stages: alarm, resistance, and exhaustion. In the alarm stage, the body shows changes characteristic of the first exposure to the stressor; these changes generally coincide with the sympathetic discharge that enables the fight-or-flight phenomenon of Cannon. If the stressor continues and is compatible with adaptation, features of the alarm reaction disappear and resistance develops. Prolonged exposure to the stressor may result in exhaustion and finally death.

One of the most important findings of GAS is the stress-induced thymicolymphatic involution, which highlighted for the first time that stress has a major impact on the immune system. This concept preceded by more than 20 years the discoveries of lymphocyte recirculation by James Gowans and acquired immunological tolerance by MacFarlane Burnet and Peter Medawar. Selye's discovery began the field of neuroimmunomodulation.

Selye soon became aware of the fact that the adrenal enlargement of GAS was associated with increased secretion of glucocorticoids (cortisol or corticosterone) that

> induce glycogenolysis, thereby supplying a readily available source of energy for the adaptive reactions necessary to meet the demands made by the stressors. In addition, they facilitate various other enzymatically regulated adaptive metabolic responses and suppress immune reactions as well as inflammation, assisting the body to coexist with potential pathogens.

Selye asserted that glucocorticoids are needed for adaptation to stress primarily during the alarm reaction. Selye's view that glucocorticoids enhance and mediate the stress response has been upheld with the additional concepts that glucocorticoids play a permissive role that primes the body's stress response systems and also prevent overshoot of the defense systems. Overshoots in the body's defense system are perhaps most dramatically seen in major inflammatory cataclysms called cytokine storms and the consequent systemic inflammatory response syndromes that play a key role in the lethality of avian influenza and have also occurred in response to the injection of certain antibodies. Exogenous synthetic glucocorticoids such as methylprednisolone remain a mainstay of the treatment of cytokine storms.

Although GAS is sometimes manifest in extreme stress, the three components of GAS have not withstood the test of time as indices of stress as Selye had originally proposed. Rather, the main biological markers of stress have long been behavioral observations and tests and measures of sympathetic and HPA activation. In the case of the latter measurements of glucocorticoid concentrations in blood, either alone or in parallel with plasma concentrations of ACTH, have been used as the main biological indices of stress. So, despite its heuristic value, especially for stress-induced neuroimmunomodulation, the concept of GAS has lost scientific currency.

Stressors: Features of and Lack of Stressor Sign

In *Stress in Health and Disease*, Selye underscored the fact that

> stress is part of our daily human experience, but it is associated with a great variety of essentially dissimilar problems, such as surgical trauma, burns, emotional arousal, mental or physical effort, fatigue, pain, fear, the need for concentration, the humiliation of frustration, the loss of blood, intoxication with drugs or environmental pollutants, or even the kind of unexpected

> success that requires an individual to reformulate his lifestyle. Stress is present in the businessman under constant pressure; in the athlete straining to win a race; in the air-traffic controller who bears continuous responsibility for hundreds of lives; in the husband helplessly watching his wife's slow, painful death from cancer; in a race horse, its jockey, and the spectator who bets on them.

Selye went on to argue that "while all these subjects face quite different problems they respond with a stereotyped pattern of biochemical, functional, and structural changes essentially involved in coping with any type of increased demand upon vital activity, particularly adaptation to new situations."

Selye also asserted that stressors have no sign as far as evoking the stress response. That is, the response will be the same "whether the agent or situation being faced is pleasant or unpleasant; all that counts is the intensity of the demand for readjustment or adaptation that it creates." Selye underscored this point with the following poignant example:

> The mother who is suddenly told that her only son died in battle suffers a terrible mental shock; if years later, it turns out that the news was false and the son unexpectedly walks into her room alive and well, she experiences extreme joy. The specific results of the two events, sorrow and joy, are completely different, in fact they are opposite to each other, yet their stressor effect – the nonspecific demand for readjustment to a new situation – is the same.

Nonspecificity of Stress Response

Selye seemed to have been driven to find specificity in the response to different types of stressors. Thus, again in *Stress in Health and Disease* he wrote,

> It is difficult to see at first how such essentially different things as cold, heat, drugs, hormones, sorrow, and joy could provoke an identical biologic reaction. Nevertheless this is the case; it can now be demonstrated by highly objective, quantitative biochemical and morphologic parameters that certain reactions are totally nonspecific and common to all types of agents, whatever their superimposed specific effects may be.

Criticism of Selye's definition of stress has been put to experimental test. Pacak, Palkovits, and associates, for example, demonstrated that different stressors activate different stress biomarkers and different regions of the brain. Thus, low blood glucose concentrations (glucopenia) or hemorrhage activate both sympathetic and HPA systems; hyperthermia, cold, and formalin injection selectively activate the sympathetic system. On the basis of these data, Pacak and Palkovits conclude that each stressor has its own specific neurochemical signature. However, since these stress indices are limited to just two neurohumoral systems, and since for most stressors there is at least some overlap in response, it is not clear that this approach invalidates Selye's definition, "stress is the nonspecific response of the body to any demand," which would probably be unassailable had Selye omitted the term 'nonspecific.'

Heat Shock (Stress) Proteins

Whatever the shortcomings of Selye's definition of stress for the human, it is probably appropriate for the vast majority of living organisms. Living cells are classified into three main evolutionary lines or phylogenetic domains: Bacteria (eubacteria), Archaea (formerly archaebacteria), and Eucarya (eukaryotes, which encompass all plants and animals through to man). The cellular response to stress in all three phylogenetic domains is represented at the molecular level by the stress-induced synthesis of stress or Hsps, of which molecular chaperones and proteases represent two well-characterized families. The heat shock response was discovered in 1962 by Ritossa, who observed a pattern of *Drosophila* salivary gland chromosome puffs that were induced in response to transient exposure to elevated temperatures. Since then, many studies have shown that the heat shock response is ubiquitous and highly conserved in all organisms from bacteria to plants and animals. It is an essential defense mechanism for protection of cells from a wide range of stressors, including heat shock, alcohols, ischemia, inhibitors of energy metabolism, heavy metals, oxidative stress, fever, or inflammation, which depending on amplitude and duration can all cause cell death by apoptosis or necrosis. The heat shock response can protect against stress-induced cell death by way of a cell-protective process known as thermotolerance or cytoprotection, in which exposure of cells to mild stress conditions, sufficient to induce the expression and accumulation of Hsps, protects against a subsequent challenge from another stress that is, by itself, lethal. Although their precise function remains to be determined, the high degree of conservation of these Hsps across species, coupled with their importance in cell survival in various conditions, suggests that Hsps are critical for both normal cellular function and survival after a stress. Several cytoprotective functions have been attributed to Hsps and, in particular, the HSP70 family. These include (1) the folding of proteins in various intracellular compartments, (2) the maintenance of structural proteins, (3) the refolding of misfolded proteins, (4) translocation of proteins across membranes and into various cellular compartments, (5) the prevention of protein aggregation, and (6) the degradation of unstable proteins. Hsps also serve as modulating signals for immune and inflammatory responses, and they may have a role in cytokine production.

So, for the heat shock response to stressful stimuli, Selye's "stress is the nonspecific response of the body [or cell] to any demand" would appear to be appropriate.

Concepts of Stress and Disease

There is a vast literature on the role or possible role of stress in the causation and/or exacerbation of disease in most organ systems of the body. Here, attention is focused on mental disorders. The *Diagnostic and Statistical Manual of Mental Disorders* (DSM-IV) of the American Psychiatric Association recognizes two stress disorders: acute stress disorder and posttraumatic stress disorder (PTSD). For the diagnosis of acute stress disorder, the individual, while experiencing the trauma or after the event, must have at least three of several dissociative symptoms, such as a subjective sense of numbing, detachment, or absence of emotional responsiveness; reduction in awareness of surroundings; depersonalization; or dissociative-amnesia. Following the trauma, the traumatic event is persistently reexperienced, the individual avoids stimuli that may arouse recollections of the traumatic event, and he or she has anxiety or increased arousal. The trauma causes clinically significant distress or impairment in social, occupational, or other important areas of functioning.

PTSD is defined as a condition in which a traumatic event is persistently reexperienced in the form of intrusive recollections, dreams, or dissociative flashback episodes. Cues to the event lead to distress and are avoided, and there are symptoms of increased arousal. To meet the diagnostic criteria of the DSM-IV, the full symptom picture must be present for more than 1 month, and the disturbance must cause clinically significant distress or impairment in social, occupational, or other areas of functioning.

PTSD has only been accepted officially as a mental disorder since 1980, when it was included, amid considerable controversy, in the DSM-III. References to the aftereffects of psychological trauma date back as far as the third century BC; achieved prominence during the early period of the railroad in Britain when rail travel, then precarious and physically traumatic, gave rise to a syndrome called railway spine or postconcussion syndrome; and were regarded as the basis for hysteria at the turn of the nineteenth century by neurologists and psychiatrists such as Jean-Martin Charcot, Pierre Janet, and Sigmund Freud. Long before PTSD was included in any diagnostic system, Charles Dickens wrote *A Tale of Two Cities* (1859), which can be considered as an early case report of PTSD. Interest in PTSD increased dramatically during World War I: Charles Samuel Myers was the first to coin the term and report case histories of 'shell shock,' which described a condition that afflicted many troops who screamed and wept uncontrollably, froze and could not move, became mute and unresponsive, and lost their memory, sensations, and capacity to feel. Pat Barker's monumental trilogy, *Regeneration*, deals poignantly with the psychological traumas of war and the nature of shell shock. The condition occurred again in vast numbers of people as a consequence of World War II. However, it was the psychological trauma experienced by Vietnam veterans and their demand for compensation that led to the inclusion of PTSD in the DSM-III as a condition that occurred both in civilian (e.g., rape trauma syndrome, battered woman syndrome, and abused child syndrome) and in military trauma response syndromes.

Future Developments of Stress Concepts

This brief account of some of the definitions and concepts of stress shows that there is still much to be done in the area of stress research. Thus, with respect to gene–environmental interactions, work on susceptibility genes has just begun, and there is still much room for expanding our knowledge about the role in stress of epigenetic factors and other mechanisms of gene control such as RNA interference. On the basis of previous experience, it seems likely that Barker's 'fetal origins' hypothesis might be honed and revised and may lead to a robust understanding of the metabolic syndrome and diabetes type 2. New powerful computer analysis of brain imaging and electrical recording may help to resolve the many questions that surround consciousness and cognition. The vexed cause-and-effect questions regarding the influence of stress in mental disorders, cancer, and other diseases need to be answered. In the past 25 years, we have witnessed how Selye's cherished and widely accepted axiom that stress is the cause of gastric ulceration (one of the three components of GAS) was undone by the careful observations and courageous perseverance of Barry Marshall and Robin Warren, who demonstrated that, in fact, most gastroduodenal ulcers are caused by a microbe, *Helicobacter pyloris*, that is readily amenable to treatment with antibiotics. And yet, there is evidence that stress does play a role in gastric ulceration, so the stress – *H. pyloris* interaction needs to be worked out. These and other biological questions about stress are likely to be tractable – rational and rigorous biology will almost certainly win the day.

However, the causes of human stress, acute and posttraumatic, are commonly social and sociological, political and irrational (beliefs in religious and racial superiority). Our continuing strife and conflict reflect in part man's innate, often irrational (limbic-brain generated) drive for conquest, territory, acquisition, and reproduction of the species. Perhaps the fact that man is such a smart political animal works against us and could ultimately lead to our stressful self-destruction. It is not clear that anything can protect man from this fate.

See Also the Following Articles

Chronic (Repeated) Stress: Consequences, Adaptations; Corticotropin-Releasing Hormone: Integration of Adaptive Responses to Stress; Stress and Neuronal Plasticity; Stress and Parasympathetic Control; Stress: Homeostasis, Rheostasis, Allostasis and Allostatic Load.

Further Reading

Armitage, J. A., Khan, I. Y., Taylor, P. D., Nathanielsz, P. W. and Poston, L. (2004). Developmental programming of the metabolic syndrome by maternal nutritional imbalance: How strong is the evidence from experimental models in mammals? *Journal of Physiology* **561**, 355–377.

Arnetz, B. B. and Ekman, R. (eds.) (2006). *Stress in Health and Disease.* Weinheim: Wiley–VCH Verlag.

Barker, DJP. (1995). Fetal origins of coronary heart disease. *British Medical Journal* **311**, 171–174.

Cannon, W. B. (1915). *Bodily Changes in Pain, Hunger, Fear and Rage: An Account of Recent Researches into the Function of Emotional Excitement.* New York: Appleton.

Cannon, W. B. (1932). *The Wisdom of the Body.* New York: Norton.

Caspi, A., McClay, J., Moffitt, T. E., et al. (2002). Role of genotype in the cycle of violence in maltreated children. *Science* **297**(5582), 851–854.

Caspi, A. and Moffitt, T. E. (2006). Gene–environment interactions in psychiatry: Joining forces with neuroscience. *Nature Reviews Neuroscience* **7**, 583–590.

Caspi, A., Sudgen, K., Moffit, T. E., et al. (2003). Influence of life stress on depression: Moderation by a polymorphism in the *5-HTT* gene. *Science* **301**, 386–389.

Eriksson, J. G. (2005). The fetal origins hypothesis—10 years on. *British Medical Journal* **330**, 1096–1097.

Fink, G. (ed.) (2007). *Encyclopedia of Stress* (2nd edn.) Oxford: Elsevier.

Fink, G., Smith, J. R. and Tibballs, J. (1971). Corticotrophin releasing factor in hypophysial portal blood of rats. *Nature* **203**, 467–468.

Hales, N. C. and Barker, DJP. (2001). The thrifty phenotype hypothesis. *British Medical Bulletin* **60**, 5–20.

Huber, T. J. and te Wildt, A. T. (2005). Charles Dickens' *A Tale of Two Cities*: A case report of posttraumatic stress disorder. *Psychopathology* **38**(6), 334–337.

Jolly, C. and Morimoto, R. I. (2000). Role of the heat shock response and molecular chaperones in oncogenesis and cell death. *Journal of the National Cancer Institute* **92**, 1564–1572.

Kendler, K. S., Kuhn, J. W., Vittum, J., Prescott, C. A. and Riley, B. (2005). The interaction of stressful life events and a serotonin transporter polymorphism in the prediction of episodes of major depression. *Archives of General Psychiatry* **62**, 529–535.

Kregel, K. C. (2002). Heat shock proteins: Modifying factors in physiological stress responses and acquired thermotolerance. *Journal of Applied Physiology* **92**, 2177–2186.

Lasiuk, G. C. and Hegadoren, K. M. (2006). Posttraumatic stress disorder. Part I: Historical development of the concept. *Perspectives in Psychiatric Care* **42**, 13–20.

Lazarus, R. S. (2000). Toward better research on stress and coping. *American Journal of Psychology* **55**(6), 665–673.

Lazarus, R. S. (2006). Emotions and interpersonal relationships: Toward a person-centered conceptualization of emotions and coping. *Journal of Personality* **74**, 9–46.

Macario, A. J. and Conway De Macario, E. (2007). Molecular Chaperones: Multiple functions, pathologies, and potential applications. *Frontiers in Bioscience* **12**, 2588–2600.

Marmot, M. G. (2005). Social determinants of health inequalities. *The Lancet* **365**, 1099–1104.

McMillen, C. and Robinson, J. S. (2005). Developmental origins of the metabolic syndrome: Prediction, plasticity, and programming. *Physiological Reviews* **85**, 571–633.

Myers, C. S. (1915). A contribution to the study of shell shock. *The Lancet* **1**(February 13), 316–320.

Pacak, K. and Palkovits, M. (2001). Stressor specificity of central neuroendocrine responses: Implications for stress-related disorders. *Endocrine Reviewical* **22**, 502–548.

Schulkin, J. (ed.) (2004). *Allostasis, Homeostasis, and the Costs of Physiological Adaptation.* Cambridge, UK: Cambridge University Press.

Selye, H. (1936). A syndrome produced by diverse nocuous agents. *Nature* **138**, 32.

Selye, H. (1975). Confusion and controversy in the stress field. *Journal of Human Stress* **1**(2), 37–44.

Selye, H. (1976). *Stress in Health and Disease.* Stoneham, MA: Butterworth.

Suntharalingam, G., Perry, M. R., Ward, S., et al. (2006). Cytokine storm in a phase 1 trial of the anti-CD28 monoclonal antibody TGN1412. *New England Journal of Medicine* **355**(10), 1018–1028.

Stress: Homeostasis, Rheostasis, Allostasis and Allostatic Load

B S McEwen
The Rockefeller University, New York, NY, USA

Introduction

The brain mediates adaptation to changes in the physical and social environment through the autonomic, neuroendocrine, and immune systems as well as through behavioral responses that include fighting or fleeing, as well as health-promoting or health-damaging responses. Adaptation to stressful events or environmental changes is an active process that involves the output of mediators such as neurotransmitters and modulators, as well as many hormones and cytokines and chemokines of the immune system. The goal of this adaptation is to maintain homeostasis and promote survival of the organism. However, the process of adaptation also produces an almost inevitable wear and tear on the body and brain, and this wear and tear is exacerbated if there are many stressful events and/or if the mediators that normally promote adaptation are dysregulated, that is, not turned on when needed or not turned off efficiently when no longer needed. The description and analysis of this scenario has entailed the addition of some new terminology, such as allostasis, and the refinement of some classical terminology, such as homeostasis and stress.

Characteristics of Homeostatic Systems

Homeostasis refers to the ability of an organism to maintain the internal environment of the body within limits that allow it to survive. Homeostasis also refers to self-regulating processes that return critical systems of the body to a set point within a narrow range of operation, consistent with survival of the organism.

Homeostasis is highly developed in warm-blooded animals living on land, which must maintain body temperature, fluid balance, blood pH, and oxygen tension within rather narrow limits, while at the same time obtaining nutrition to provide the energy to maintain homeostasis. This is because maintaining homeostasis requires the expenditure of energy. Energy is used for locomotion, as the animal seeks and consumes food and water, for maintaining body temperature via the controlled release of calories from metabolism of food or fat stores, and for sustaining cell membrane function as it resorbs electrolytes in the kidney and intestine and maintains neutral blood pH.

Homeostasis also refers to the body's defensive mechanisms. These include protective reflexes against such things as inhaling matter into the lungs, the vomiting reflex as a protection to expel toxic materials from the esophagus or stomach, the eye blink reflex, and the withdrawal response to hot or otherwise painful skin sensations. There is also the defense against pathogens through innate and acquired immunity.

According to Walter B Cannon,

> Bodily homeostasis ... results in liberating those functions of the nervous systems that adapt the organism to new situations, from the necessity of paying routing attention to the management of the details of bare existence. Without homeostatic devices, we should be in constant danger of disaster, unless we were always on the alert to correct voluntarily what normally is corrected automatically. With homeostatic devices, however, that keep essential body processes steady, we as individuals are free from such slavery – free to enter into agreeable relations with our fellows, free to enjoy beautiful things, to explore and understand the wonders of the world about use, to develop new ideas and interests, and to work and play, untrammeled by the anxieties concerning our bodily affairs. (Cannon, 1929).

The body has a considerable redundancy, or safety margin, when it comes to many of these mechanisms. There are two kidneys and adrenal glands, in case one fails, and the digestive tract is able to function adequately in food absorption, even if intestinal length is shortened. Moreover, individuals are able to survive with one lung. Also, the cardiovascular system has a number of devices to maintain blood pressure after considerable blood loss. Finally, as Cannon notes, the body displays considerable resilience in the face of injury and after surgery, in order to compensate for lost function.

Need for Refocusing of the Concept of Homeostasis and Additional Terminology

Yet, there are paradoxes and problems with the notion of a set point that is always maintained. In discussing obesity, Cannon states "What leads to the storage of fat in large amounts – sometimes in grotesquely large amounts – in some persons, and in slight amounts in others, is not well-understood." This and other aspects of pathophysiology, particularly in response to stress, has forced a re-evaluation of the processes that reestablish homeostasis in the face of a challenge and which, under some circumstances, exacerbate disease. This is one of the reasons why the terms allostasis and allostatic load (see below) have been introduced.

Another problem with 'homeostasis' is that, taken literally, it is a rather static concept, akin to the notion of equilibrium in classical thermodynamics, whereas, in real life, an organism experiences changing set points around which it maintains stability over a finite period of time. Moreover, unlike the closed systems of classical thermodynamics, a living organism is an open system in which energy and matter flow in and out, with equilibrium being replaced by steady state. Cannon recognized this and used the term steady state and even suggested that 'homeodynamics' might be a better term than 'homeostasis.'

The same problem was also recognized by a number of other authors. Nicolaides introduced the term homeorheusis, in which 'stasis' is replaced by 'rheusis,' meaning 'something flowing.' Mrozovsky introduced the term rheostasis to mean "a condition or state in which, at any one instant, homeostatic defenses are still present but over a span of time there is a change in the regulated level, or set point of a system." Mrozovsky considers this concept advantageous in explaining how organisms adjust to changing environments such as seasons of the year by storing body fat or changing reproductive physiology, and he believes that rheostasis allows for the kinds of physiological plasticity that is involved in evolution.

What Is Stress?

Stress may be defined as a real or interpreted threat to the physiological or psychological integrity of an individual that results in physiological and/or behavioral responses. In biomedicine, stress often refers to situations in which the adrenal glucocorticoids and catecholamines are elevated because of an experience. Stress is also a subjective experience that may or may not correspond to physiological responses, and the word stress is widely used in many languages as part of daily discourse. There is 'good stress' and 'bad stress,' and people talk about bad stress as 'being stressed out.'

Stress involves a stressor and a stress response. A stressor may be a physical insult, such as trauma or injury, or physical exertion, particularly when the body is being forced to operate beyond its capacity. Other physical stressors include noise, overcrowding, excessive heat or cold. Stressors also include primarily psychological experiences such as time-pressured tasks, interpersonal conflict, unexpected events, frustration, isolation, and traumatic life events, and all of these types of stressors may produce behavioral responses and evoke physiological consequences such as increased blood pressure, elevated heart rate, increased cortisol levels, impaired cognitive function, and altered metabolism.

Behavioral responses to stressors may decrease risk and get the individual out of trouble or involve health-promoting activities such as a good diet and regular exercise, but they may also include responses that exacerbate the physiological consequences of stress, for example, self-damaging behaviors like smoking, drinking, overeating, or consuming a rich diet, or risk-taking behaviors like driving an automobile recklessly. The physiological stress responses include primarily the activation of the autonomic nervous system and the hypothalamo–pituitary–adrenal (HPA) axis, leading to increased blood and tissue levels of catecholamines and glucocorticoids. It is these physiological responses that have both protective and damaging effects (see the sections on allostasis and allostatic load).

There are two important features of the physiological stress response: the first involves turning it on in amounts that are adequate to the challenge (see the section 'Allostasis'). The second is turning off the response when it is no longer needed. The physiological mediators of the stress response, namely, the catecholamines of the sympathetic nervous system and the glucocorticoids from the adrenal cortex, initiate cellular events that promote adaptive changes in cells and tissues throughout the body, which in turn protect the organism and promote survival. However, too much stress, or inefficient operation of the acute responses to stress, can cause wear and tear and exacerbate disease processes.

There are enormous individual differences in interpreting and responding to what is stressful, as well as individual differences in the susceptibility to diseases, in which stress may play a role. Genetic predispostions exist which increase the risk of certain disorders. In addition, developmental process, such as prenatal stress or nurturing postnatal experiences, contribute to the lifelong responsiveness of the behavioral and physiological responses to stressors. Furthermore, experiences throughout the life course resulting in memories of particularly unpleasant or pleasant situations combine with the genetic and developmental influences to produce large differences among individuals in how they react to stress and what the long-term consequences may be.

Allostasis

Allostasis means 'achieving stability through change'; it was introduced by P Sterling and J Eyer in 1988. Allostasis refers to the process that maintains homeostasis, as defined above, and it recognizes that 'set points' and other boundaries of control may change with environmental conditions. There are primary mediators of allostasis such as, but not confined to, hormones of the HPA axis, catecholamines, and cytokines. Allostasis also clarifies the inherent ambiguity in the term homeostasis and distinguishes between the systems that are essential for life (homeostasis) and those that maintain these systems in balance (allostasis). Allostatic systems enable an organism to respond to its physical state (e.g., awake, asleep, supine, standing, exercising) and to cope with noise, crowding, isolation, hunger, extremes of temperature, physical danger, psychosocial stress, and microbial or parasitic infections. For example, blood pressure rises when we get up in the morning and fluctuates with exercise and other demands of the waking period, and these fluctuations make it possible for the individual to function in response to a changing social and physical environment.

Whether exposed to danger, an infection, a crowded and noisy neighborhood, or having to give a speech in public, the body responds to challenge by turning on an allostatic response, thus initiating a complex pathway for adaptation and coping, and then shutting off this response when the challenge has passed. Two primary allostatic responses involve the sympathetic nervous system and HPA axis. 'Turning on' these systems leads to release of catecholamines from sympathetic nerves and the adrenal medulla and the secretion of adrenocorticotropin (ACTH) from the anterior pituitary gland, which stimulates release of glucocorticoids from the adrenal cortex.

'Turning off' these responses leads to a return to baseline concentrations of cortisol and catecholamines, and this normally happens when the danger is past, the infection contained, the living environment is improved or the talk has been given. As long as the allostatic response is limited to the period of challenge, protection via adaptation predominates over adverse consequences. However, over weeks, months, or even years, exposure to elevated levels of stress hormones (an allostatic state) can result in allostatic load and overload, with resultant pathophysiological consequences.

Allostatic States

An allostatic state refers to the altered and sustained activity levels of the primary mediators, for example, glucocorticoids, that integrate energetic and associated behaviors in response to changing environments, challenges such as social interactions, weather, disease, predators, pollution, etc. An allostatic state results in an imbalance of the primary mediators reflecting excessive production of some and inadequate production of others. Examples are hypertension, a perturbed cortisol rhythm in major depression or after chronic sleep deprivation, chronic elevation of inflammatory cytokines and low cortisol in chronic fatigue syndrome, imbalance of cortisol, corticosteroid-releasing factor (CRF), and cytokines in the Lewis rat that increases risk for autoimmune and inflammatory disorders. Allostatic states can be sustained for limited periods if food intake and/or stored energy, such as fat, can fuel homeostatic mechanisms (e.g., bears and other hibernating animals preparing for the winter). If imbalance continues for longer periods and becomes independent of maintaining adequate energy reserves, then symptoms of allostatic overload appear. Abdominal obesity is an example of this condition.

Allostatic Load and Overload

Allostatic load and allostatic overload refers to the cumulative result of an allostatic state. For example, fat deposition in a bear preparing for the winter, a bird preparing to migrate or a fish preparing to spawn are examples of animals experiencing an allostatic load. This is a largely beneficial and adaptive condition and can be considered the result of the daily and seasonal routines which organisms use to obtain food and survive, and obtain the extra energy needed to migrate, molt, and breed. Within limits, they are adaptive responses to seasonal and other demands. However, if one superimposes on this additional load of unpredictable events in the environment, disease, human disturbance (for animals in the wild), and social interactions, then allostatic load can increase dramatically and become allostatic overload, which can become a pathophysiological condition.

There are two distinctly different outcomes of an allostatic state in terms of allostatic load or overload. First, if energy demands exceed energy income, and also exceeds what can be mobilized from stores, then type 1 allostatic overload occurs. For example, breeding birds use increasing food abundance in spring to reproduce and raise their young. If inclement weather then increases costs of maintaining homeostasis and the allostatic load of breeding, and at the same time reduces food available to fuel that allostatic load, then negative energy balance results in loss of body mass and suppression of reproduction. Another example is the mass movement of seabirds to islands in the face of a severe storm that limit access to food. Second, if energy demands are not exceeded and the organism continues to take in or store as much or even more energy than it needs, perhaps as a result of stress-related food consumption, choice of a fat-rich diet, or metabolic imbalances (prediabetic state) that favor fat deposition, then type 2 allostatic overload occurs. Besides fat deposition, there are other cumulative changes in other systems that can result from repeated stress, for example, neuronal remodeling or loss in hippocampus, atherosclerotic plaques, left ventricular hypertrophy of the heart, glycosylated hemoglobin and other proteins by advanced glycosylation end products as a measure of sustained hyperglycemia, high cholesterol with low high-density lipoprotein (HDL), increased oxidative stress, elevated proinflammatory mediators, and chronic pain and fatigue, for example, in arthritis or psoriasis, associated with imbalance of immune mediators.

Types of Allostatic Overload

Four situations can lead to allostatic overload, resulting in overexposure to stress hormones over time. The first is frequent stress, for example, blood pressure surges can trigger myocardial infarction in susceptible persons, and experiments in primates have shown that repeated blood pressure elevations over weeks and months accelerates atherosclerosis, which increases the risk of myocardial infarction. Thus, the frequency of stressful events determines the degree of this type of allostatic load, leading to increased exposure to hormones and other allostatic mediators.

A second type of allostatic overload is the failure to habituate to repeated challenges, such as in some individuals' cortisol response during a repeated public speaking challenge.

The third type of allostatic overload is caused by an inability to shut off allostatic responses. This pertains to the termination of stress and also to the decline of these same hormones during the natural diurnal cycle. With respect to the stress response, blood pressure in some persons fails to recover after acute mental arithmetic stress, and hypertension accelerates atherosclerosis. Intense athletic training also induces allostatic load in the form of elevated sympathetic and HPA activity, which results in reduced body weight and amenorrhea and the often-related condition of anorexia nervosa. Regarding the diurnal cycle, women with a history of depressive illness have decreased bone mineral density because the allostatic load of chronic, moderately elevated glucocorticoid levels, especially at night, that are associated with depression cause chronic, reduced levels of osteocalcin.

The fourth type of allostatic overload is caused by inadequate allostatic responses that trigger compensatory increases in other allostatic systems. When one system does not respond adequately to a stressful stimulus, the activity of other systems is increased because the underactive system is not providing the usual counter-regulation. For example, if adrenal steroid secretion does not increase appropriately in response to stress, secretion of inflammatory cytokines (which are counter-regulated by adrenal steroids) increases. In Lewis rats, the failure to mount an adequate HPA response results in increased vulnerability to autoimmune and inflammatory disturbances; thus, an infection or wound that causes an inflammation will lead to an increased inflammatory response. Human counterparts of the state of HPA hyporesponsiveness include individuals with fibromyalgia and chronic fatigue syndrome.

Examples of allostatic states leading to allostatic overload include hypertension, reduced parasympathetic activity, increased levels of inflammatory cytokines and oxidative stress, elevated insulin and glucose, and triglycerides. In the brain, the remodeling of neurons in the hippocampus, amygdala, and prefrontal cortex, as a result of chronic stress, are examples of allostatic overload, which impair memory and enhance anxiety and aggression. For the immune system, acute stress enhances immune responses, whereas chronic stress has the opposite effect. Chronic stress is reported to shorten teleomeres and reduce telomerase activity on white blood cells (and possibly other cells, as well).

Early stress and neonatal handling influence the course of aging and age-related cognitive impairment in animals. Early experiences are believed to set the level of responsiveness of the HPA axis and autonomic nervous system. These systems overreact in animals subject to early unpredictable stress and underreact in animals exposed to the neonatal handling procedure. In the former condition, brain aging is accelerated, whereas in the latter, brain aging is reduced. Lifespan is also influenced by early-life differences in HPA reactivity: rats that show increased HPA reactivity as neonates to novelty have shorter life spans compared to rats with lesser HPA reactivity to novelty.

Role of Behavior in Allostatic Overload

Anticipation and worry can also contribute to allostatic overload. Anticipation is involved in the reflex that prevents us from blacking out when we get out of bed in the morning and is also a component of worry, anxiety, and cognitive preparation for a threat. Anticipatory anxiety can drive the output of mediators like ACTH, cortisol, and adrenalin; thus, prolonged anxiety and anticipation is likely to result in allostatic overload. For example, salivary cortisol levels increase within 30 min after waking in individuals who are under considerable psychological stress due to work or family matters. Moreover, intrusive memories from a traumatic event (e.g., in posttraumatic stress disorder) can produce a form of chronic, internal stress and can drive physiological responses.

Allostasis, allostatic states, and allostatic overload are also affected by health-damaging behaviors such as smoking, drinking, excess calorie intake, or, on the opposite side, health-promoting behaviors such as a healthy diet and regular moderate exercise. These behaviors are integral to the overall notion of allostasis – how individuals cope with a challenge – and also contribute to increasing or decreasing allostatic overload by known pathways. For example, a rich diet accelerates atherosclerosis and progression to noninsulin-dependent diabetes by increasing cortisol, leading to fat deposition and insulin resistance; smoking elevates blood pressure and atherogenesis. Yet, regular, moderate exercise protects one against cardiovascular disease, prevents diabetes, and increases attention and other aspects of cognitive function.

See Also the Following Articles

Chronic (Repeated) Stress: Consequences, Adaptations; Stress and Parasympathetic Control; Stress: Definition and History.

Further Reading

Cannon, W. B. (1939). *The Wisdom of the Body.* New York:
W. W. Norton and Co.

Cannon, W. (1929). The Wisdom of the Body. *Physiological Reviews* 9, 399–431.

Cavigelli, S. A. and McClintock, M. K. (2003). Fear of novelty in infant rats predicts adult corticosterone dynamics and an early death. *Proceedings of the National Academy of Sciences of the United States of America* **100**, 16131–16136.

Epel, E. S., Blackburn, E. H., Lin, J., et al. (2004). Accelerated telomere shortening in response to life stress. *Proceedings of the National Academy of Sciences of the United States of America* **101**, 17312–17315.

Kirschbaum, C., Prussner, J. C., Stone, A. A., et al. (1995). Persistent high cortisol responses to repeated psychological stress in a subpopulation of healthy men. *Psychosomatic Medicine* 57, 468–474.

Mason, J. (1959). Psychological influences on the pituitary–adrenal cortical system. In: Pincus, G. (ed.) *Recent Progress in Hormone Research*, pp. 345–389. New York: Academic Press.

McEwen, B. S. (1998). Protective and damaging effects of stress mediators. *New England Journal of Medicine* **33**, 171–179.

McEwen, B. S. and Stellar, E. (1993). Stress and the individual: Mechanisms leading to disease. *Archives of Internal Medicine* **153**, 2093–2101.

McEwen, B. S. and Wingfield, J. C. (2003). The concept of allostasis in biology and biomedicine. *Hormones and Behavior* **4**, 2–15.

Meaney, M., Aitken, D., Berkel, H., Bhatnager, S. and Sapolsky, R. (1988). Effect of neonatal handling of age-related impairments associated with the hippocampus. *Science* **239**, 766–768.

Mrosovsky, N. (1990). *Rheostasis: The Physiology of Change.* New York: Oxford University Press.

Nicolaides, S. (1977). Physiologie du comportement alimentaire. In: Meyer, P. (ed.) *Physiologie Humaine*, ch. 2, pp. 908–922. Paris: Flammarion Medecine-Sciences.

Sapolsky, R. (1992). *Stress, the Aging Brain and the Mechanisms of Neuron Death.* Cambridge: MIT Press.

Schulkin, J., McEwen, B. S. and Gold, P. W. (1994). Allostasis, amygdala, and anticipatory angst. *Neuroscience and Biobehavioral Reviews* **18**, 385–396.

Selye, H. (1936). A syndrome produced by diverse nocuous agents. *Nature* **138**, 32.

Selye, H. (1955). Stress and disease. *Science* **122**, 625–631.

Sterling, P. and Eyer, J. (1988). Allostasis: A new paradigm to explain arousal pathology. In: Fisher, S. & Reason, J. (eds.) *Handbook of Life Stress, Cognition and Health*, pp. 629–649. New York: Wiley.

Control and Stress

A Steptoe
University College London, London, UK

This is a revised version of the article by A Steptoe, Encyclopedia of Stress, First edition, volume 1, pp 526–531, © 2000, Elsevier Inc.

Glossary

Behavioral control (instrumental or objective control)	The situation when the organism has at its disposal a behavioral response that can prevent, reduce, or terminate stressful stimulation.
Cognitive control	A form of psychological coping related to perceived control over one's reactions to aversive events.
Locus of control	A set of generalized control beliefs concerning the extent to which individuals feel that aspects of their lives are determined by their own activities and abilities (internal locus of control) or are governed by external factors.
Perceived control	The belief that one can exert control over stressful events, based on the appraisal of the situation and appropriate perceptions of competence (self-efficacy expectancies) and expectations concerning the outcome of making a response.

Stressors come in many guises, for example, confrontation with a predator, death of a close relative, conflict at work, or living in crowded noisy conditions. When we try to understand what aspects of situations make them more or less threatening, the concept of control emerges as a crucial feature. Stressors differ in the extent to which they can be controlled, and behavioral control is typically associated with a diminution of stress responses. Sometimes the perception of control is sufficient to reduce stress reactions, even though control itself is never actually exercised. For example, studies of people who are anxious about dentistry have shown that telling people they can give a signal that will stop the procedure reduces pain and anxiety, even though they never use the signal. Humans and other animals also seek out information about impending threatening events and ways of coping with the situation. This phenomenon is known as cognitive control and is an important weapon in the armory of psychological coping. Finally, there are control beliefs or the sense of control that people have in specific areas or over their lives and destiny more generally. A sense of control is generally adaptive for health, but the need for control may under some circumstances be maladaptive and lead to an inflexibility in coping with difficult problems. Since control has so many facets, there is a danger that the construct is misused and disguises careless reasoning. In this article, the different aspects of control and stress are described, along with evidence related to physiological responses, well-being, and health. The ways in which control can be enhanced to improve quality of life, ameliorate pain, and promote rehabilitation are also discussed.

Behavioral Control and Physiological Stress Responses

Behavioral control can be defined as having at one's disposal a behavioral response that can prevent, reduce, or terminate stressful stimulation. Natural stressors vary across the entire spectrum of controllability. Some events, such as the unexpected death of a family member, are outside personal control. But in many situations there is an element of behavioral control. People who regularly find themselves stuck in traffic jams on their morning journey to work may feel helpless, but actually have some control; they might choose to use some other form of transport, to start their journey at a different time, to select a different route, to stop and take a break until the traffic clears, and so on.

Study of the impact of behavioral control over stress is complicated by the fact that many of the most aversive life events are uncontrollable. Comparisons between controllable and uncontrollable events may therefore be confounded with the aversiveness of the experience. Experimental studies provide the best opportunity to examine the effects of behavioral control, since aversiveness can be held constant. The yoked design championed by Jay Weiss and later by Martin Seligman and others has served to illustrate the effects of behavioral control most clearly. In this paradigm, a pair of rodents is exposed to identical intermittent aversive stimuli (electric shocks or loud noise). One animal is able to make a behavioral response that either terminates the stimuli or delays their onset, while the second animal has no response available. The amount of aversive stimulation experienced by both depends on the effectiveness of the performance of the one in the behavioral control condition, and any differences in physiological responses or pathology will result from the availability of behavioral control.

Table 1 summarizes some of the many physiological and pathological advantages conferred by control in this design. It can be seen that behavioral control

Table 1 Adverse effects of uncontrollable stress in comparison with exposure to matched controllable aversive stimulation

Decreased food/water consumption
Greater weight loss
Higher plasma corticosterone
Increased gastric lesions
Reduced production of specific antibodies
Reduced lymphocyte reactivity
Decreased cytotoxic activity of natural killer cells
Decreased tumor rejection
Increased susceptibility to malignancy

is associated with amelioration of physiological stress responses and pathological outcomes. These range from reduced levels of neuroendocrine response to slower proliferation of experimentally implanted malignancies. The regions of the brain responsible for these effects have been identified. Uncontrollable stressors appear to sensitize serotonergic neurons in the dorsal raphe nucleus, while this activation is blocked by projects from the central medial prefrontal cortex when stressors are controllable. But not all the biological responses to uncontrollable stress are detrimental. For example, uncontrollable conditions tend to lead to greater stress-induced analgesia than matched controllable conditions, and this mechanism may permit organisms to endure stressful stimulation at a reduced level of physical discomfort.

Research in humans has gone some way toward duplicating these effects, with differences in the magnitude of acute cardiovascular and endocrine responses. However, an important caveat concerns the effort or response cost associated with maintaining behavioral control.

Control and Effort

Effects of the type shown in **Table 1** have generally emerged in studies in which behavioral control is easy to exert. For example, electric shock may be avoided by a lever press on a simple schedule of reinforcement. However, control may require great effort to maintain and can be associated with a degree of uncertainty as to whether it has been successful. Under these circumstances, physiological activation may be greater than that elicited in uncontrollable situations. This was illustrated in the classic human experimental studies carried out by Paul Obrist. Obrist randomized human volunteers to three conditions in a shock avoidance reaction time study. All participants had to respond rapidly to aversive stimuli and were informed that successful performance would lead to avoidance of electric shock. Three criteria were employed: an easy condition in which even slow reaction times would be successful, a hard condition in which participants had to maintain or improve performance over time, and an impossible condition in which the reaction time criterion was too fast for most people. The impossible condition is comparable to uncontrollable stress, while the other two conditions represent easy and effortful behavioral control, respectively. The number of shocks administered was held constant across conditions. It was found that the greatest physiological activation was present not in the impossible or uncontrollable condition, but in the hard condition. This physiological reaction pattern was sustained by selective activation of β-adrenergically mediated sympathetic nervous system responses. Later studies have established that the enhanced physiological reactions associated with control under these circumstances are related to the effort expended, with greater effort being correlated with heightened norepinephrine responses.

Control and Fear

Lack of control over aversive stimuli potentiates fear responses. Using the yoked control design, it has been found that rats subsequently placed in a different environment and given two brief shocks so as to generate conditioned fear showed greater freezing responses if they had previously had no control over shock compared with those that had had control. These effects are long-lasting, but can be blocked by benzodiazepines. Fear responses associated with uncontrollable stress are again related to release of serotonin in the dorsal raphe nucleus and amygdala. Experiments using *in vivo* microdialysis have shown that uncontrollable stress leads to increased levels of extracellular serotonin in both these sites, while animals exposed to controllable stress show no such elevation.

Research on humans also suggests that control is relevant to fear responses. Fear of pain during medical and dental procedures is strongly associated with perceptions of uncontrollability. Fear of social threats (for example, when the individual is threatened with physical or sexual assault) is greater when people believe the situation is uncontrollable.

Control and Work

Control is important to understanding the physiological and health consequences of stressful events in human life. One area in which control has emerged as a key variable is in the study of work stress. Jobs vary on many dimensions of control. Some work is self-paced, while other tasks are externally paced by machines or other people. In some jobs, workers have choice about their posture, when they can take rest breaks, and how the work should be done. Flexibility in work hours, participation in decision making, and autonomy at work are all factors that vary across jobs. In psychophysiological studies, it has been found that cardiovascular and neuroendocrine activation is greater during externally paced than self-paced work, even when the actual pace of work is held constant. The same patterns are present in the real work environment. **Figure 1** illustrates the pattern of ambulatory blood pressure measured every 20 min over the working day in middle-aged men and women divided into low and high job control on a standard questionnaire measure. Ambulatory pressure was greater throughout the day in people working in low-control jobs after controlling statistically for covariates.

Several prospective epidemiological observational studies have evaluated the demand/control model of work stress. They have shown that low control at work, either alone or in combination with high demands, predicts future coronary heart disease in previously healthy adults independently of standard

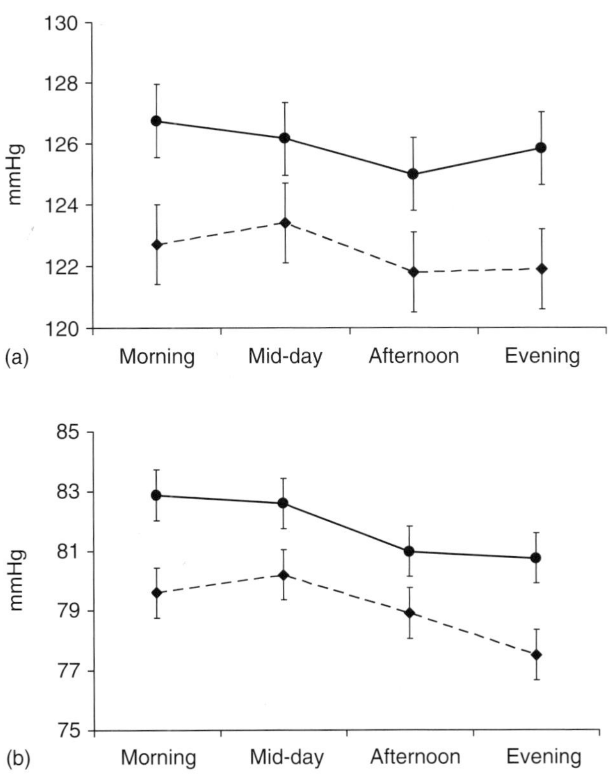

Figure 1 Mean systolic blood pressure (a) and diastolic pressure (b) in the morning, mid-day, afternoon, and evening periods in high (dashed line) and low (solid line) job control groups, adjusted for gender, employment grade, age, body mass index, smoking status, and physical activity. Error bars are standard errors of the mean. From Steptoe and Willemsen (2004). *Journal of Hypertension* **22**, 915–920.

disease risk factors. It has also been found that control over work pace influences health during pregnancy, and that women with lower control jobs may be at greater risk for preeclampsia and low back pain, after statistical adjustment for age, parity, education, smoking, and type of work.

Conversely, greater autonomy and participation at work promote higher levels of self-reported job satisfaction, commitment to work, better performance, and reduced levels of emotional distress, staff turnover, and absenteeism. However, these studies of work illustrate a complication in human research in control, since it is clear that control cannot be seen solely as an objective characteristic of the environment, but depends on subjective perceptions.

Perceived Control

Perceived control is the sense that one has control over aversive events. Objective differences in behavioral control are presumably mediated by perceived control. Thus, the benefits of having control over a particular aspect of work (such as being able to make a personal telephone call if necessary) will be apparent only if the worker realizes that this option is available. Perceived control is the result of a subjective judgment based on the individual's appraisal of the situation. It has two elements. The first is a perception that the situation is potentially controllable, and the second is that the individual can take the correct action. There may be circumstances in which events are perceived as controllable, but no action is taken since people lack (or believe they lack) appropriate behavioral competence. Psychologists such as Albert Bandura have postulated a distinction between outcome expectations and self-efficacy expectations to characterize these two aspects.

It is generally found that distress is associated with a perception that events are uncontrollable, and this phenomenon may operate independently of objective behavioral control. Thus, two individuals may experience the same event, such as the breakdown of an important personal relationship. One may perceive that the event was outside his or her control, due to the callousness of his or her partner, the circumstances in which they lived, or the predatory behavior of a third party. Another person may perceive him- or herself to have been responsible; if the person had not been preoccupied with work or had responded better to the needs of his or her partner, then the relationship might not have floundered. One student who has failed an academic examination may attribute this to lack of preparation and effective revision, while another may blame arbitrary examiners or bad luck in the selection of questions.

Human beings seek to understand their experiences in life by developing explanations for aversive events and often construe events retrospectively as having been controllable (for example, "If I had not stayed later than I planned at that party, and had not decided to walk down that street, I would not have been assaulted"). Such cognitive attributions may be maladaptive in leading to self-blame for occurrences over which one has little control, but also may help to impose sense and order on a world that may otherwise appear cruel and arbitrary.

Sense of Control

Perception of control is not restricted to individual aversive experiences, but also relates to domains of life or even to life in general. The term locus of control is used to describe these generalized control beliefs. This construct was first introduced by Rotter, who argued that people varied in the extent to which they believed that important outcomes were determined by their own internal abilities and activities or by external factors. The idea of locus of control has since been elaborated upon in two important ways. First, locus of control may be domain specific, with different levels of belief in personal control over different aspects of life (health, work, personal relationships, etc.). Thus, people may feel a strong sense of control over their work, but believe that their living environment (traffic, difficult neighbors, etc.) is out of their own control. Second, it may be useful to understand locus of control as consisting of three dimensions: belief in internal control, chance, and powerful others. For example in the domain of health, people can be categorized according to the extent to which they believe that their health is determined by their own actions (internal control), that whether they remain healthy is a matter of fate or luck (belief in chance), and that their health is influenced by the competence of doctors and other health professionals (belief in powerful others). A dimensional perspective implies that people may simultaneously hold strong beliefs about more than one set of influences. They may believe, for instance, that they have quite a lot of control over their health, while at the same time believing that doctors are also very influential.

Sense of control is an individual belief pattern that also has developmental and social determinants. Animal studies indicate that monkeys provided with experiences of controllable (contingent) events early in life are subsequently less reactive to stressful events in adulthood. The experience of a major uncontrollable event in childhood, such as the death of one's mother, is associated with increased likelihood of depression following negative life events in adult life. Differences in sense of control may also relate to social class, with economically more deprived people facing greater external obstacles and fewer opportunities to influence events than the better off. One study assessed sense of mastery (e.g., agreement with the statement "Whether I am able to get what I want is in my own hands") and perceptions of constraints (e.g., "There is little I can do to change many of the important things in my life") in three large population surveys. It was found that sense of mastery was greater in higher than in lower income sectors of the sample, while perceived constraints were less. The financially better off also reported greater life satisfaction and less depression and rated their health as better. However, not all the lower income respondents had low mastery and high constraint ratings. Some individuals in the low-income sectors had high mastery ratings, and they reported greater life satisfaction, less depression, and health levels comparable with those of the high-income group.

Sense of control has cultural and political determinants as well. Surveys in Eastern Europe during the first decade after the collapse of communism identified a profound sense of lack of control over life, as people witnessed the destruction of familiar institutions and ways of life and experienced greater difficulty in fulfilling daily needs. Those years were characterized by a rapid deterioration in health and well-being in many sectors of the population of Russia and several Central-Eastern European countries.

Cognitive Control and Coping

Another closely related phenomenon is cognitive control, which can be defined as the belief that one can control one's reactions to events. It is a common characteristic to seek out information about events even when they cannot be controlled behaviorally. The person who has an abnormal result on a medical test and is scheduled for further examination may try to find out about the test and its consequences from acquaintances, the Internet, or other sources of information. The purpose of this information seeking is not to control the outcome, but to feel in control by reducing uncertainty and increasing the predictability of the situation and to manage reactions to the result by anticipatory coping. This type of control, sometimes known as secondary control, is closely allied with the repertoire of other coping responses that people mobilize in an effort to regulate their responses to aversive experiences. It has important uses in medical settings, where the procedures for psychological preparation for surgery and stressful medical procedures have the effect of increasing cognitive control by providing information and helping patients mobilize a range of coping responses. In the self-regulation model of health developed by Leventhal, control is a key dimension in the cognitive representation of health threats, and variations in controllability influence effective adaptation.

People vary in the extent to which they exert effort to establish control over the situations with which they are confronted, and some individuals appear to have a high need for control. This may be maladaptive in some circumstances. Studies of work stress indicate that when high need for control is blocked by low extrinsic rewards (such as poor pay or promotion prospects), the individual may be placed at increased risk for coronary heart disease. People with a high need for control may find it particularly difficult to come to terms with experiences over which they have no control, such as the injury of a family member in a traffic accident.

Control and Well-Being

Control and Aging

Growing old is associated with a diminution of control. When people retire from work, their economic power is reduced, they have less authority than before, and their social networks shrink. Impaired physical health may increase people's sense of vulnerability, while they are exposed more often to uncontrollable events such as the death of contemporaries. A number of studies have documented the links between aging and the loss of control, though there are exceptions. Successful aging, or the maintenance of well-being and effective functioning despite chronological progression, is coupled with maintenance of beliefs in personal control. People may adapt by lowering their valuation of the importance of areas of life over which they lose control and by investing in social relationships more selectively than before. The impact of increasing sense of control and autonomy on the well-being of elderly population has also been investigated. Randomized trials of increased involvement in decision making in institutionalized elderly groups have demonstrated improvements in mood and activity levels associated with enhanced control.

Control and Pain

The effects on pain of having control over the source of painful stimulation have been studied extensively. These experiments suggest that having behavioral control leads to a reduction in the subjective and physiological impact of the painful stimulus and may also increase pain tolerance. However, the benefits of control depend on the confidence that people have in their response efficacy, so perceptions are again important. It is interesting that the favorable effects of control over acute pain are observed despite the fact that stress-induced analgesia is elicited when there is a lack of control. It is likely that control allows behavioral and cognitive coping methods to be deployed that in turn reduce distress. Brain imaging studies have shown that when pain is perceived to be controllable, there is an attenuation of activation in the anterior cingulated, insular, and secondary somatosensory cortex, areas of the brain that are associated with pain processing. Interestingly, placebo analgesia results in alterations in brain activity in pain-sensitive brain regions, indicating that the control associated with beliefs leads to changes in the experience of pain.

Chronic clinical pain is often accompanied by feelings of helplessness, lack of control, and depression. Some authorities have argued that there may be a progression from feelings of personal helplessness in the early phases of a chronic pain problem to general helplessness (the belief that no one is able to control the pain) in later stages. The impact of chronic pain on well-being is that of a uncontrollable stressor, since by definition a pain that becomes chronic has not been alleviated and so has not been controlled. The generalization of distress about pain to disability and depression mirrors the phenomenon of learned helplessness.

The links between control and pain can be harnessed for patient care. As noted earlier, providing patients with control over sources of potential pain (for example, during dental examinations) can increase tolerance. Patient-controlled analgesia is used in a variety of medical settings with both adults and children and has benefits in terms of both emotional well-being and analgesic use. Several studies have found that when patients can control the level of analgesia, they use less medication than when it is provided by the physician. Rehabilitation programs for patients with chronic pain have a strong element of increasing perceived control by providing patients with greater and more effective coping options.

Control and Illness

Most serious illnesses bring with them strong feelings of loss of control. When people have heart attacks or are diagnosed with cancer, they feel that they are no longer in control of their bodies, and their future plans are put in jeopardy so that they lose a sense of control over their destiny. Loss of control is often accompanied by other facets of helplessness, including hopelessness, distress, and passivity. Similar patterns occur in chronic health problems. For example, high levels of perceived control over asthma are associated with better self-management skills, reduced risk of hospitalization, and less restricted activity, independent of the severity of asthma itself. Some studies have found that recovery from serious illness such as stroke and major fractures is positively correlated with high internal control beliefs.

Many procedures for improving the emotional state of patients have the effect of enhancing perceived control. Thus, the methods used to prepare women for childbirth increase perceived control by providing a repertoire of coping response. Stress management procedures during cardiac rehabilitation enhanced perceived control and patient self-efficacy by increasing confidence in the resumption of normal activities. A particular area in which the issue of control has been contentious surrounds patient choice. To what extent should patients be involved in medical decision making? A number of studies indicate that although patients desire information about issues surrounding medical decisions, they sometimes prefer to delegate responsibility for the decision itself to the doctor. This should not be too surprising, since it is the typical pattern found in any society with specialist roles. While we might want to know all the facts, we would expect the car mechanic to decide how to fix an engine or the chef to use judgment and skill to prepare the complicated dish we have ordered. Patients often wish to be involved in decision making, particularly when there is a genuine choice of more than one effective alternative, but seldom wish to take authority completely away from the physician.

Conclusions

Control has emerged over recent years as a powerful explanatory variable in stress research. It is relevant to a wide variety of settings, from basic experimental research on neuroendocrinology and neurochemistry to the experience of people in different socioeconomic sectors of society. There is a danger that such an attractive integrating notion will be misused and employed as a global explanation for completely unrelated phenomena. However, if care is taken not to confuse the different meanings of control, the construct has considerable value in understanding stress.

Further Reading

Bandura, A. (1997). *Self-efficacy: the exercise of control.* New York: Freeman.

Cockerham, W. C. (1999). *Health and social change in Russia and Eastern Europe.* New York: Routledge.

Guadagnoli, F. and Ward, P. (1998). Patient participation in decision-making. *Social Science and Medicine* **47**, 329–339.

Katouzian, H. D., Cameron, L. D. and Leventhal, H. (eds.) (2002). *The self-regulation of health and illness behaviour.* Taylor & Francis.

Maier, S. F. and Watkins, L. R. (2005). Stressor controllability and learned helplessness: the roles of the dorsal raphe nucleus, serotonin, and corticotropin-releasing factor. *Neuroscience and Biobehavioral Reviews* **29**, 829–841.

Marmot, M. G., Bosma, H., Hemingway, H., Brunner, E. and Stansfeld, S. (1997). Contribution of job control and other risk factors to social variations in coronary heart disease incidence. *Lancet* **350**, 235–239.

Rodin, J. (1986). Aging and health: effects of the sense of control. *Science* **233**, 1271–1276.

Skinner, E. A. (1996). A guide to constructs of control. *Journal of Personal and Social Psychology* **71**, 549–570.

Steenland, K., Fine, L., Belkic, K., et al. (2000). Research findings linking workplace factors to CVD outcomes. *Occupational Medicine* **15**, 7–68.

Steptoe, A. and Appels, A. (eds.) (1989). *Stress, personal control and health.* Chichester, UK: Wiley.

Steptoe, A. and Willemsen, G. (2004). The influence of low job control on ambulatory blood pressure and perceived stress over the working day in men and women from the Whitehall II cohort. *Journal of Hypertension* **22**, 915–920.

Wager, T. D., Rilling, J. K., Smith, E. E., et al. (2004). Placebo-induced changes in FMRI in the anticipation and experience of pain. *Science* **303**, 1162–1167.

Evolutionary Origins and Functions of the Stress Response

R M Nesse, S Bhatnagar and E A Young
University of Michigan, Ann Arbor, MI, USA

This is a revised version of the article by R M Nesse, S Bhatnagar and E A Young, Encyclopedia of Stress, First edition, volume 2, pp 79–83, © 2000, Elsevier Inc.

Glossary

Defense	A trait that is latent until aroused by threatening situations in which it is useful.
Natural selection	The process by which genes that provide a fitness advantage become more common from generation to generation and those that decrease fitness become less common, thus shaping adaptive traits, including defenses.
Phylogeny	The evolutionary history of a trait or a species.
Trade-offs	The fitness costs and benefits of a trait whose net effects yield a selective advantage.

Evolution is the process in which traits such as the capacity for the stress response are shaped by natural selection. Understanding the evolutionary history of a trait, how it gives a selective advantage, and the costs it imposes can help to illuminate its design and regulation and can guide research into its mechanisms and control. The stress response has been shaped by natural selection to increase the ability of organisms to cope with situations that require action or defense. Stress-related mechanisms emerged early in the history of life. Like all traits, they have costs as well as benefits. Because the stress response is so often associated with negative events, its utility has often been neglected. In particular, the release of glucocorticoids, which is often thought to be the hallmark of the stress response, may in fact exist, in part, to protect against other aspects of defensive systems.

Utility of the Stress Response

The vast bulk of research on stress has investigated its causes, mechanisms, and effects. An evolutionary approach instead addresses two very different and relatively neglected questions: (1) How does the stress system give a selective advantage and (2) what is the evolutionary history of the stress system? The answers to these questions provide a foundation in Darwinian medicine for understanding why the stress response is the way it is and why it causes so much suffering and disease. The first and most important contribution of an evolutionary perspective on stress is a clear focus on its utility. The stress system is a complex, sophisticated, and carefully regulated adaptation that has been shaped by natural selection because it gives a selective advantage. That advantage must be substantial in order to outweigh its huge costs. The idea that stress is useful is by no means new. In fact, the very phrase Hans Selye chose to describe it, the general adaptation syndrome, emphasizes its utility. Despite this early emphasis on its benefits, as the idea of stress entered the popular imagination there was a tendency to emphasize its dangers so that the fundamental fact of the utility of the stress response was often forgotten.

Stress and Other Defenses

Other defenses are also often confused with the problems they protect against. The capacities for pain, fever, vomiting, cough, and inflammation are often thought of as medical problems, although a moment's thought reveals that they are useful protective reactions. The ubiquity of the illusion that defenses are abnormalities arises from several sources. First, defenses are often associated with some kind of suffering and therefore seem maladaptive. Unfortunately, however, discomfort is itself probably one aspect of a mechanism that makes it useful. Second, they are reliably associated with disadvantageous situations, so the association bias makes it seem as if they are the problem. Finally, it is possible to use drugs to block the expression of many defenses with very little harm, completing the illusion that defenses are useless. In fact, blocking a defense can be harmful. For instance, suppressing cough in a patient with pneumonia makes it harder to clear the infection and may lead to death, and stopping the diarrhea of a person with a serious intestinal infection may lead to complications. Blocking fever, however, usually has little effect on the speed of recovery from a cold. When blocking a defense is not dangerous, this is because the body has backup protective mechanisms and because the regulation mechanism seems to be set to a hair trigger that expresses the defense at the slightest hint of danger.

Situations in Which Stress Is Useful

Stress, like fever and pain, is useful only in certain situations. Such traits lie latent until aroused by the particular circumstances in which they are useful. This means that the evolutionary explanation for such traits cannot be summarized in a single function. Instead, the inducible defenses give an advantage by changing multiple aspects of the body that increase its ability to cope effectively with the adaptive challenges that arise in a particular situation. One defense may have many aspects that serve many functions. So, the first step in understanding the adaptive value of stress is not to try to specify its function but to understand the exact situations in which the stress response is useful. To do that, we need to go back to the very origins of complex life forms 600 million years ago. If a very primitive organism had only two states, what are they? The answer is quite straightforward: activity and rest. This is a fundamental divide, one that is maintained even in our biochemical and nervous systems. Biochemical pathways are divided into the catabolic, in which energy is used, and the anabolic, in which energy is stored and tissues are repaired. Parallel to this division are the two arms of the autonomic nervous system. The sympathetic system, which is activated as part of the stress response, increases arousal, blood pressure, heart rate, respiratory rate, and physical activity and institutes other endocrine and physiological changes necessary for action. The other half of the autonomic nervous system, the parasympathetic, inhibits muscular activity, stores energy, and shunts blood to digestion and bodily repair. Is stress, then, the same as arousal for action? Not exactly. As soon as a generic state of arousal was well established, natural selection probably began to differentiate it into subtypes to better meet the demands of different kinds of challenges. Here again, the main bifurcation is quite clear. Arousal is useful in two different situations: threats and opportunities. This division is also represented in our nervous systems. As Gray and others have pointed out, the brain seems to have moderately distinct systems for behavioral inhibition and for reward seeking. The corresponding behaviors are said to be defensive or appetitive and are associated with feelings of fear/pain or pleasure. In psychology, the same division is recognized in the distinct cognitive states promotion versus prevention.

Phylogeny of the Stress Response

Cross-Species Comparisons

Comparisons among different species can help to reconstruct the phylogeny of the stress response. All vertebrates have the proopiomelanocortin (POMC) molecule that gives rise not only to adrenocorticotropic hormone (ACTH) but also to opiate-like peptides. It is intriguing to note that these molecules, with their related functions, are derived from the same parent molecule. All vertebrates also make corticosteroids. Peptide sequences very similar to those of human ACTH are found not only in mammals but also in amphibians and reptiles and even in insects, mollusks, and marine worms. Interestingly they are usually associated with immune cells, equivalent to macrophages, where they set defensive processes in motion. ACTH has long been closely associated with other signaling molecules such as corticotropin releasing hormone (CRH), biogenic amines such as epinephrine and norepinephrine, steroids such as cortisol, cytokines such as interleukin-1, and nitric oxide. All these substances are crucial to defensive systems. The remarkable thing is that genetic sequences for these molecules have not only been conserved over hundreds of millions of years but they continue to serve closely related defensive functions. Why have they changed so little? If a single molecule has several essential functions, this creates a strong selective force against mutations that change the sequence. By contrast, mutations that result in the differentiation of different classes of receptors in target tissues can slowly specialize the responses of that tissue to the signal molecule. And they have, judging from the proliferating classes and subclasses of receptors that are now being discovered.

Cost–Benefit Trade-Offs

Why is the stress system not better? It could provide more effective protection against danger – but only at a still greater cost. Drosophila have been bred to resist the stress of food shortage. After 60 generations of such selection, the new strain is 80% more resistant to starvation. However, the larvae are more likely to die, and development is slowed. Similar results have been found for selection of resistance to other stressors and in other species. Like everything else in the body, stress responses are shaped by trade-offs, sometimes with benefits and costs occurring in different parts of the life cycle.

The mechanisms that regulate the responsiveness of the stress system are shaped by the trade-off between the long-term costs and the immediate benefits of a relatively quick or intense or prolonged stress response. It has been hypothesized that the individuals who are most resilient or resistant to the effects of stress on physiology or behavior are the ones least vulnerable to stress-related diseases. However, are these individuals resilient to all stress-related disorders, or are there situations in which resilience to some disorders means vulnerability to others? The answer is not known, but given the large number of physiological systems affected by stress and/or glucocorticoids, it is unlikely that resilience to one stress-related disorder necessarily protects against all.

Another trade-off reflects the benefits and costs of habituation. For instance, rats exposed to some repeated stressors, particularly those that are mild and cognitive in nature, habituate to that stressor. The hypothalamic-pituitary-adrenal (HPA) response is lower to the *n*th exposure than to the first exposure. Such habituation seems adaptive for most situations; if the stressor is known and can be easily coped with, then the HPA response should be moderated. Such habituation would, at the very least, conserve resources. However, it would be maladaptive to habituate to stressors that do present some danger. These trade-offs have shaped the brain mechanisms that regulate habituation.

There are interesting sex differences in the habituation of the stress response, with some evidence indicating that habituation occurs in male but not in female rats. Such findings suggest that the selection forces acting on male and female rats may have differed enough to shape distinctly different patterns of habituation. Research is now addressing whether habituation occurs with some stressors in males but with others in females.

Stress responses in adult animals are profoundly affected by early environmental events such as prenatal stress and variations in maternal care. The effects of variations in maternal care are transmitted across generations, with offspring that experience high maternal care exhibiting lower stress responses and providing high maternal care themselves. Such effects seem adaptive in that offspring are likely to experience an environment similar to that of their parents. So, for example, mothers providing low maternal care have high stress responses and so do their offspring when they become adults. However, when cross-fostered to other mothers, the offspring show patterns of stress responsivity similar to that of their foster mother and not their biological mother. Such results suggest that stress responsivity and maternal care are not simply genetically transmitted but are also regulated by early experiences. Such regulation is seen in other mammals and even plants. Some of such transmission across generations may arise from facultative mechanisms that evolved to adjust the system based on early life experiences, and some may arise from more general learning mechanisms.

Difficulties in Defining Stress

The human mind seems wired to try to make neat categories with sharp boundaries, perhaps because we communicate with words and this requires dividing the world up into categories even when that is unnatural. This leads to a tendency to try to make sharp distinctions between different states that may, in fact, overlap considerably. States of defensive arousal, for instance, are different from states of arousal for seeking food, but there is no reason to expect that the differentiation is complete. For instance, cortisol secretion is aroused by opportunities as well as threats. In fact, cortisol is even involved in reward mechanisms. Thus, any attempt to define the stress response in terms of cortisol arousal is doomed. For that matter, any attempt to define stress or the stress response is liable to be an exercise in frustration for the evolutionary reason that the system does not have sharp boundaries or a single function. The closest we can come to a defining characteristic is the kinds of situations in which stress has given a selective advantage, and those situations are not sharply defined. The stress system was, after all, not designed by an engineer but shaped by a process of tiny tinkering changes. The long unsatisfying history of attempts to define stress and the wish, expressed by many researchers, that the term would go away, arise from this difficulty. Even after defensive arousal was differentiated considerably from appetitive arousal, there were undoubtedly advantages to further differentiating subtypes of stress responses to match specific challenges. Thus, different situations – a predator, a high place, injury, infection, starvation, loss of a status battle, and speaking in public – all seem to have shaped somewhat different defensive responses. These responses are only partially differentiated from a more generic response, so they have overlapping characteristics with functions in common. Attempts to sharply distinguish different kinds of anxiety disorders are as frustrating as attempts to define stress itself and for the same reasons. New attempts to study anxiety disorders in the context of normal anxiety will be helpful.

How Does the Stress Response Help?

Immediate Response

These difficulties notwithstanding, a stress response is a coordinated pattern of changes that is useful in situations in which the organism is faced with possible damage or a loss of resources. The next question is: How is it useful? Even before Selye, Walter Cannon provided some answers. In situations that might require fight or flight, he observed the utility of increased heart rate and contractility to speed circulation, increased rate and depth of breathing to speed gas exchange, sweating to cool the body and make it slippery, increased glucose synthesis to provide energy, shunting of blood from gut and skin to muscles, increased muscle tension to increase strength and endurance, and increased blood clotting in preparation for possible tissue damage. More recently, others have demonstrated faster reaction times and cognitive benefits as a result of sympathetic arousal. These immediate responses are mostly mediated by the sympathetic nervous system and the associated release of epinephrine from the adrenal medulla.

Adrenal Cortical Response

However, the stress system also includes a more delayed-response release of cortisol from the adrenal cortex, although this system does have more rapid effects (such as fast negative feedback) that are probably mediated by putative membrane steroid receptors. This is initiated by neural signals to the hypothalamus, which releases CRH, which in turn results in the secretion of ACTH from the anterior pituitary gland on the bottom of the brain. The ACTH induces cortisol synthesis and release from the adrenal gland. The whole system is called the HPA system because the signal acts via the hypothalamus, the pituitary, and the adrenal glands. Many actions of the HPA system seem, like those of the sympathetic system, well designed for acute action. It changes physiology so the liver breaks down glycogen into glucose, and it alters cells so glucose can get in more readily. Through different populations, CRH not only releases ACTH, but it also directly increases anxiety and arousal and activates cells in the locus coreleus, the brain center where the cell bodies for most noradrenergic neurons are located. All in all, the system seems admirably designed to get the organism ready for action. Indeed, both branches of the system are readily aroused by exercise, and trained athletes, far from having low levels of cortisol, have chronic high levels – just the thing for a person who frequently exerts him- or herself.

Association with Negative Events

So, why should the stress system as a whole be associated so closely with bad events instead of positive ones? To answer that question, we need to understand why the components of the stress system are carefully packaged. If the stress is so useful, why is stress not expressed all the time? There are at least three good reasons why it is not. First, it is expensive in terms of calories. No organism can afford to waste effort. Second, it interferes with other adaptive behaviors. A vigilant organism has less time for finding food and eating, to say nothing of mating. Finally, and most important, some changes that give an advantage in the face of threats may also cause tissue damage. For this reason, they need to be carefully sequestered, except in those few circumstances in which the costs are outweighed by the benefits. This helps to explain why some aspects of the stress response are associated more with negative than positive arousal. The benefits of a stress response that increases the likelihood of catching prey may sometimes be worth it, but if a stress response prevents being caught as prey, this is always worth it, even if substantial damage results from the stress response itself. This helps to explain why the stress response, despite its costs, is so ubiquitous. An optimal regulatory mechanism will express a stress response whenever, on average, it is worth it. Given the uncertainties of environmental cues and the potential life-saving effects of the stress response, there will be many instances where the expression of stress is worthwhile, even though there is only a small chance that danger is actually present. The global conclusion is that the damage caused by stress responses is not necessarily from abnormal stress. Some components of the stress response may be a part of the response specifically because they are too damaging to be expressed except when they protect against great danger. There is every reason to think that normal stress, like every other bodily trait, has costs as well as benefits. This idea is expressed in the concept of allostasis, as proposed by McEwen and colleagues, which emphasizes the short-term benefits and the long-term costs.

That a normal stress response might be crucial for optimal physiological functioning has implications for recent notions about pharmacological therapies for reducing perceived stress. For example, if a drug such as a CRH inhibitor blocks all stress response at the brain level, then how does the body react to what may be real requirements for increases in energy use and how do systems that are generally opposed in functions to those of glucocorticoids, counterregulatory systems such as the regulation of insulin release, stay in check? Furthermore, there are many indications in both human and animal studies of mismatches between perceived stress or behavioral indices of stress and HPA activation. The extreme of an absent stress response is, of course, Addison's disease. Thus, although the cognitive nature of many current human stressors results in costs disproportionate to actual threats, from an evolutionary point of view the general inhibition of stress responses is by no means optimal. It would be ironic as well as tragic if the history of the excessive use of cortisone were to repeat itself with a new generation of drugs that block the stress response.

Cortisol as Protection against Other Aspects of Stress

If some aspects of the stress response cause harm, has selection shaped systems to protect against this damage? In 1984, Munck and colleagues reviewed the actions of cortisol and said, "We propose that stress-induced increases in glucocorticoids levels protect, not against the source of stress itself, but rather against the body's normal reactions to stress, preventing those reactions from overshooting and themselves threatening homeostasis." They noted that many inflammatory diseases had been attributed to overproduction of cortisol until 1941, when adrenal steroids were shown to decrease inflammation. Subsequent demonstrations showed that steroids inhibit the production of cytokines, prostaglandins, and other mediators of the immune response, thus decreasing immune function. This is just the opposite of what would make sense as protection from danger, but it is entirely consistent with a role in protecting against damage from immune system activation induced by other changes. It is now clear that the effects of glucocorticoids on immune function are much more complicated than originally thought. Added to this are recent novel findings regarding the effects of glucocorticoids on the brain versus the body on the regulation of energy balance and fat deposition that suggest that our assumptions about the physiological and neural functions of glucocorticoids will continue to be significantly challenged.

Adaptive Regulation of Stress Responsiveness

The recognition that a moderately responsive stress system is optimal is quickly leading to a consideration of the adaptive significance of variations in stress responsiveness. Several lines of thinking addresses the adaptive significance of innate individual differences in stress responsiveness. The first attempts to explain the growing evidence for a bimodal pattern of stress response in some organisms, with some individuals responding quickly and strongly and others showing a much more restrained response. It has been suggested that these distinct patterns reflect distinct patterns of adaptation,: a hawk pattern that is optimal in crowded situations and a dove pattern that is optimal when population density is low. The different strategies are hypothesized to be the products of frequency-dependent selection. There is also increasing evidence that maternal effects on an offspring's stress responsiveness may be adaptive. Mothers exposed to stressful environments give birth to offspring with especially responsive stress systems that may give them an advantage in harsh environments. The same evolutionary forces may have shaped mechanisms that explain the connection between early abuse or neglect and increased stress vulnerability.

Mismatch between Ancestral and Modern Environments

Much has been made of the differences between our environment and that of our ancestors. In the case of stress, this argument comes in several flavors. Some suggest that life is more stressful now than it was for our predecessors. Special aspects of our environment do cause new kinds of stress. Working in a bureaucracy is tedious and political at best. Driving to work, living in a ghetto, running a corporation, working in a factory – these all arouse the stress system. Despite the amount of stress we experience, however, our ancestors almost certainly experienced more. With no police, no food reserves, no medicine, no laws, rampant infections, and prevalent predators, danger could come at any time. True, social groups were closer, kin networks were stronger, and people spent all their time with one another and none alone reading books. Still, life was hard. Perhaps in that environment, where stressors were more often physical, the stress response was more useful than it is now. Today, we mainly face social and mental threats, so the actions of the HPA system may yield net costs. This is plausible and supports the many efforts to reduce stress and to find drugs that block the stress response. This brings us back to the very concept of stress as a mismatch between the demands made on an individual and that individual's ability to meet those demands. We think of these demands as coming from the outside, and sometimes they do, as when we are attacked by the proverbial tiger. But most stresses in modern life arise not from physical dangers or deficiencies but from our tendency to commit ourselves to personal goals that are too many and too high and to ruminate about them. When our efforts to accomplish these goals are thwarted or when we cannot pursue all the goals at once and must give something up, the stress reaction is expressed. In short, much stress arises, ultimately, not from a mismatch between our abilities and the environment's demands, but from a mismatch between what we desire and what we can have.

Further Reading

Bhatnagar, S., Lee, T. and Vining, C. (2005). Prenatal stress differentially affects habituation to repeated restraint in adult male and female rats. *Hormones and Behavior* 47(4), 430–438.

Cannon, W. B. (1929). *Bodily changes in pain, hunger, fear, and rage: researches into the function of emotional excitement.* New York: Harper and Row.

Charney, D. S. (2004). Psychobiological mechanisms of resilience and vulnerability: implications for successful

adaptation to extreme stress. *American Journal of Psychiatry* **161**(2), 195–216.
Dallman, M. F. (2003). Fast glucocorticoid feedback favors "the munchies." *Trends in Endocrinology and Metabolism* **14**(9), 394–396.
Frankenhauser, M. (1976). The role of peripheral catecholamines in adaptation to understimulation and overstimulation. In: Serban, G. (ed.) *Psychopathology and human adaptation*, pp. 173–191. New York: Plenum.
Gray, J. A. (1987). *Fear and stress* (2nd edn.). Cambridge, UK: Cambridge University Press.
Higgins, E. T. (1997). Beyond pleasure and pain. *American Psychologist* **52**(12), 1280–1300.
Marks, I. M. and Nesse, R. M. (1994). Fear and fitness: an evolutionary analysis of anxiety disorders. *Ethology and Sociobiology* **15**(5–6), 247–261.
McEwen, B. S. (2003). Interacting mediators of allostasis and allostatic load: towards an understanding of resilience in aging. *Metabolism* **10**(supplement 2), 10–16.
Munck, A., Guyre, P. M. and Holbrook, N. J. (1984). Physiological functions of glucocorticoids in stress and their relation to pharmacological actions. *Endocrine Review* **5**(l), 25–44.
Korte, S. M., Koolhaas, J. M., Wingfield, J. C., et al. (2005). The Darwinian concept of stress: benefits of allostasis and costs of allostatic load and the trade-offs in health and disease. *Neuroscience and Biobehavioral Review* **29**, 3–38.
Nesse, R. M. (2005). Natural selection and the regulation of defenses: a signal detection analysis of the smoke detector principle. *Evolution and Human Behavior* **26**, 88–105.
Nesse, R. M. and Williams, G. C. (1994). *Why we get sick: the new science of Darwinian medicine.* New York: Times Books.
Rosen, J. B. and Schulkin, J. (1998). From normal fear to pathological anxiety. *Psychological Review* **105**(2), 325–350.
Young, E. and Vasquez, D. (1996). Hypercortisolemia, hippocampal glucocorticoid receptors, and fast feedback. *Molecular Psychiatry* **1**(2), 149–159.
Zhang, T. Y., Parent, C., Weaver, I., et al. (2004). Maternal programming of individual differences in defensive responses in the rat. *Annals of the New York Academy of Sciences* **1032**, 85–103.

Comparative Anatomy and Physiology

A G Watts
University of Southern California, Los Angeles, CA, USA

This is a revised version of the article by A G Watts, Encyclopedia of Stress, First edition, volume 1, pp 507–511, © 2000, Elsevier Inc.

Glossary

Cyclostome — A member of the order Cyclostomata (class Agnatha): hagfish and lampreys. These primitive vertebrates have relatively rudimentary endocrine and nervous systems that are thought to represent evolutionarily early examples of these functions.

Cytokine — Regulatory proteins secreted by the white blood cells and a variety of other cells in the body. Cytokines can regulate cells of the immune system and modulate immune responses, but act in a relatively local manner.

Elasmobranch — Cartilaginous fish (e.g., sharks, skates, and rays).

Fenestrated capillary — A specialized capillary that has transcellular circular openings in the endothelial walls allowing the passage of large molecules in or out of the capillary. They are particularly prevalent in regions where secretory products are released into the vasculature.

Mesoderm — One of the three principal layers of the mammalian embryo from which the vascular tissues are derived.

Tetrapod — A four-limbed vertebrate.

Stress Responses Defined

Using the simplest and most wide-ranging definition, a stressor can be thought of as any alteration in the animal's environment (internal or external) requiring a response that, if not invoked, could develop into a threat to survival. In some instances, the disturbance might only require a simple avoidance reflex that moves the animal away from an external threat; in others it might invoke an internally directed motor response nullifying a homeostatic disturbance. Considered in this broader manner, stress responses are fundamental characteristics displayed by all living organisms. Protozoans display an avoidance reaction to a detrimental change in the local environment, for example, increased CO_2 concentrations in the water; more complex multicellular organisms such as coelenterates and platyhelminths have sensory-motor networks that allow them to make the appropriate distinction between a threat and a meal. All animals use some sort of avoidance (generally reflexive) reaction that can be considered a stress response to an aversive presence in the environment. However, more complex invertebrates and all vertebrates have also evolved sets of physiological responses that provide the organism with the ability to adapt their metabolic and immune systems to deal with the consequences of stress. In these animals, physiological and neural systems involving learning and memory also provide organisms with anticipatory features allowing them to generate conditioned or habituated responses as well as the capability of dealing with the more extended consequences of stress.

Stress Responses in Invertebrates

Stress responses in invertebrates can be divided into two broad categories: (1) those concerned with abrogating the stressor and (2) adaptive changes invoked to deal with the metabolic consequences of the stressor. In invertebrates, the nervous system generally deals with the first, whereas cellular interactions of a chemical nature (endocrine and immune) generally deal with the second.

Neural

For avoidance responses, sessile invertebrates generally confront a threat by retracting vulnerable body parts into a protective shell or the environmental surroundings, whereas more mobile species have the ability to move away from the threat as fast as possible. In most metazoans, the effector of these responses is the nervous system. Simple invertebrates such as coelenterates have avoidance reactions that may involve little more than invoking the stimulus–response properties of their nerve nets. In more complex invertebrates, these avoidance reactions are neurophysiologically quite complex and involve the regulation of specific neural networks by sensory inputs (e.g., air currents). These networks coordinate the very rapid muscle contraction required for fleeing (e.g., jumping, flying, turning, or running). These responses appear to involve populations of giant interneurons found in the abdominal ganglia that may, because of their fast conduction velocities, bring about the very rapid stimulus–response interactions required for these behaviors. However, the detailed role of these neurons and the wider functioning of this circuitry remains unclear. Although all of these avoidance responses have the characteristics of a reflex, studies from species such as *Aplysia* have shown that contributions from learning and memory mechanisms cannot be overlooked.

Endocrine

Arthropods use hormones to regulate their metabolism in a way that is beneficial during periods of stress. In a manner somewhat analogous to the secretions of the vertebrate chromaffin cell–adrenal medulla system, some insects (e.g., locusts and cockroaches) produce adipokinetic hormones (AKH) in the gland cells of the corpora cardiaca. These hormones increase the heart rate and the carbohydrate and protein metabolism. They also produce hyperglycemia through the breakdown of glycogen to trehalose in the fat bodies and muscles and its facilitated transport into the hemolymph. Starvation, increased activity, and stress all elevate the secretion rate of these hormones.

Complex invertebrates such as annelids, insects, and mollusks possess quite sophisticated immune functions that use interleukin-like signaling molecules and cytotoxic activities derived from natural killer cells. These systems are activated by stressors. Some invertebrates also synthesize corticotropin releasing hormone (CRH) and proopiomelanocortin-(POMC-) derived peptides that are related to their vertebrate homologs. In molluscs, CRH and adrenocorticotropic hormone (ACTH) are capable of releasing biogenic amines from hemocytes (cells that appear to have both endocrine and immune functions), and at least some of the cells that are capable of phagocytosis also exhibit ACTH immunoreactivity. ACTH-like molecules have even been identified in some protozoans, suggesting their great phylogenetic antiquity. Indeed, the existence of those endocrine signals capable of regulating carbohydrate metabolism and immune responses – properties required to generate adaptive responses to stressors – appear to have developed very early in evolution.

Stress Responses in Vertebrates

Not surprisingly, stress responses in vertebrates have more components, variety, and complexity than those found in invertebrates. Although some vertebrate stress responses are similar in principle to those exhibited by invertebrates (e.g., avoidance, endocrine secretions that increase energy substrate availability, and adaptations that restrict reproduction), because of their more complex central nervous systems, vertebrates possess a greater flexibility and adaptative capability.

Comparative Anatomy

The general organization of those parts of the neural and endocrine systems involved with mediating stress responses are remarkably well conserved across all vertebrate classes.

The neurohypophysis The neurohypophysis comprises the median eminence of the tuber cinereum, the infundibular stem, and the neural lobe of the pituitary gland. The median eminence and the neural lobe both contain terminals of neuroendocrine motor neurons. However, neurons that regulate ACTH secretion terminate in the median eminence. With appropriate increases in firing rate, they release releasing factors (CRH and, in some mammals, vasopressin) into the hypophysial portal blood. The neurons that release oxytocin and vasopressin/vasotocin into the general circulation terminate on fenestrated capillaries in the neural lobe. The neural lobe appears to be better developed in tetrapods than in fish, and this may be related to the larger amount of stored hormone required for the increased hydrostatic stresses of terrestrial existence. With a few exceptions (e.g., in cyclostomes, the neurohypophysis is quite poorly developed), the generalized organization of the neurohypophysis is retained across the vertebrate spectrum.

Corticotropes The anterior pituitary of all vertebrates contains cells that synthesize ACTH. In evolutionarily older species (e.g., reptiles and elasmobranchs) there is less intermingling of cell types within the anterior pituitary than is found in more recently evolved species. POMC is cleaved to produce ACTH in the anterior pituitary corticotropes in all vertebrate classes, in which it acts to increase glucocorticoid secretion. Negative glucocorticoid feedback signals also appears to operate in all vertebrate classes examined.

Catecholaminergic and corticosteroidogenic tissues The analog of the adrenal gland is critical to the stress response of all vertebrates. In mammals, it is called the adrenal (or in older literature, the suprarenal) gland because of its position close to the kidneys. In mammals, the adrenal gland has a characteristic cortical and medullary structure – the medulla is neural in origin and synthesizes catecholamines for release into the bloodstream on sympathetic stimulation; the cortex is mesodermal in origin and is the site of glucocorticoid and mineralocorticoid synthesis. Although cells performing these functions are found in all vertebrates, the way they are arranged and their anatomical association vary from class to class. In amphibians, reptiles, and fish, this tissue is found between the renal tissue and is sometimes called the interrenal gland.

All vertebrates possess tissue that can secrete catecholamines into the bloodstream during stress. Catecholamines (usually adrenaline and noradrenaline) universally increase cardiovascular muscle tone, increase heart rate, and can rapidly mobilize fat and carbohydrate stores. There has been a trend during evolution toward a close relationship between catecholamine-synthesizing and steroidogenic tissue. Thus, in the cyclostomes and some elasmobranchs, chromaffin cells are widely scattered along large veins and the dorsal body wall, but steroidogenic tissue has been more difficult to identify. In many vertebrate classes, catecholaminergic tissue is interspersed with steroidogenic tissue. In mammals, however, chromaffin cells are aggregated in the adrenal medulla and are separate from the steroid-synthesizing cells in the adrenal cortex, although a close functional relationship does exist.

Sympathetic branch of the autonomic nervous system Sympathetic motor activation plays an important role in the stress responses in virtually all vertebrates. However, it is poorly developed in cyclostomes, in which there are no sympathetic chains and relatively little sympathetic innervation of the viscera. In teleost fish, catecholamine secretion is regulated by preganglionic sympathetic activation. However, other regulators such as glucocorticoids can also play an important role. It is possible that the chromaffin cell system first evolved to function as the principal regulator of the cardiovascular and energy metabolism under all conditions, not just stress. But as the sympathetic innervation of the cardiovascular system became more sophisticated and was able to regulate visceral organ function under basal conditions, the actions of the chromaffin system during stress became the more important function.

Juxtaglomerular apparatus Renin and the cells that contain juxtaglomular granules are found in all vertebrates other than cyclostomes. In more recently evolved vertebrates, these are aggregated in a specific juxtaglomerular apparatus (juxtaglomerular cells and the macula densa), whereas in others only juxtaglomerular cells are seen. In teleost and more primitive fish species, these are often quite distal from the glomerular apparatus.

Comparative Physiology

Vertebrates invoke sets of stress responses that target three critical physiological systems – those involved with fluid balance, energy metabolism, and tissue damage and immune function. Each set has specific neural and endocrine components.

Impact of stress on the regulation of fluid balance Protecting the fluid compartments of the body is a prime physiological concern, and the physiological systems that contribute to this function are usually activated during stress. Two sets of hormones have evolved to regulate fluid balance; the renin–angiotensin system protects the extracellular fluid compartment, whereas the posterior pituitary lobe hormones regulates the intracellular fluid compartment. In addition, autonomic reflexes are available to regulate cardiovascular and hemodynamic function through the control of vascular tone. Both systems are stimulated by stress.

Renin–angiotensin system The renin–angiotensin system targets vascular smooth muscle, mineralocorticoid-synthesizing tissue in the adrenal cortex, and some circumventricular organs in the brain. Renin is present in all jawed vertebrates, but is absent in the cyclostomes. Its original function may have been to increase blood pressure through vasoconstriction, with its dipsogenic and other effects (e.g., increased release of mineralocorticoids) appearing later.

Vasotocin/vasopressin Maintaining body fluid composition between narrow limits is a requirement for survival for all organisms. This becomes absolute in animals that live in environments of varying temperature or water availability and in animals that move from one major environment to another. Any variation that challenges fluid balance constitutes a stressor that needs to be regulated. The vertebrate brain has evolved a very simple reflex loop to help with this regulation, and such a function has remained reasonably unchanged for the 500 million years since the evolution of the cyclostomes. It involves direct projections from the osmoreceptors to the neuroendocrine neurons that synthesize vasopressin (in mammals) or vasotocin (in birds, reptiles, and most amphibians and fish, including cyclostomes). In this manner, one of the simplest and phylogenetically oldest vertebrate neuroendocrine stress response is probably the reflex release into the circulation of vasopressin/vasotocin that occurs as plasma osmolality increases. The original function of vasotocin (which is still its primary action in some amphibians) may have been a V1 receptor-mediated vasoconstrictive effect that reduces blood flow to the kidney and thereby fluid loss. (In this respect, vasotocin is a more potent vasoconstrictor than its evolutionary descendant, vasopressin). However, during evolution a V2-mediated action on kidney tubules became the predominant action.

Impact of Stress on the Regulation of Energy Metabolism

Glucocorticoids

The stress-induced release of glucocorticoids is found widely throughout vertebrate classes, in which they act to promote gluconeogenesis. Stress-induced hyperglycemia reportedly occurs in all classes of vertebrates that have been investigated, from cyclostomes to mammals, although the contribution of glucocorticoids to this effect is far from clear in more simple vertebrates. It is worth considering that, in many respects, the hypothalamic-pituitary-adrenal (HPA) motor response to stress is a more proactive than a reactive event. Although ACTH and corticosterone secretion are obviously triggered by the stressor, they are not the motor responses that act to remove the immediate consequences of the stress, as occurs with, for example, adrenaline's actions to generate hypoglycemia. The actions of elevated plasma corticosterone levels (mediated in part by interactions with leptin, insulin, and the thyroid hormones) anticipate the possibility that the stressor will lead to a debilitating sequence of events, particularly the catabolic effects of negative energy balance. In those vertebrate classes that have been studied, the principal function of corticosteroids is on the intermediate metabolism, particularly in stimulating proteolysis and then gluconeogenesis.

Catecholamines of chromaffin cell origin

Increased circulating catecholamines lead to hyperglycemia in all vertebrates examined, although noradrenaline and adrenaline show differences in efficacy across different classes. Also, the tissue that is targeted varies; in mammals both muscle and liver are responsive to adrenaline, whereas only liver glycogen is mobilized in cyclostomes. Stress will increase plasma catecholamines in teleost fish and elasmobranchs.

Inhibition of reproduction

A variety of stressors inhibits reproductive function in most vertebrates. The simplest of these is the negative energy balance resulting from food restriction or starvation. Here a mechanism (possibly involving elevated neuropeptide Y synthesis in the hypothalamic arcuate nucleus) leads to the inhibition of reproductive function, ensuring that limited energy supplies are not used to raise offspring in adverse conditions. Related stressors such as social crowding may also restrict reproductive capacity for the same reason, although the neural mechanism responsible for this effect is unclear.

Impact of stress on the regulation of immune function

Immune activation and the consequent increases in circulating interleukins that occur during some stressors provide a marked stimulus to the vertebrate HPA axis. In mammals, this elevates CRH release into the portal vasculature and, hence, ACTH release. Increased glucocorticoid release in response to cytokines has been noted in all the mammals, reptiles, birds, and amphibians that have been investigated. However, it should be noted that in nonmammalian classes, data are very scanty. In turn, corticosteroids have a suppressive effect on immune function. During acute stress, this operates as a dampening effect to restrain any adverse effect of immune stimulation, but in chronic stress this can have a deleterious effect leading to increased infections and mortality. These types of effect have been seen in a wide variety of vertebrates.

Further Reading

Bentley, P. J. (1998). *Comparative vertebrate endocrinology.* Cambridge, UK: Cambridge University Press.

Burrows, M. (1996). *The neurobiology of an insect brain.* Oxford: Oxford University Press.

Dores, R. M. and Lecaude, S. (2005). Trends in the evolution of the proopiomelanocortin gene. *General Comparative Endocrinology* **142**, 81–93.

Flik, G., Klaren, P. H., Van den Burg, E. H., et al. (2006). CRF and stress in fish. *General Comparative Endocrinology* **146**, 36–44.

Highnam, K. C. and Hill, L. (1977). *The comparative endocrinology of the invertebrates* (2nd edn.). Baltimore, MD: University Park Press.

Ottaviani, E. and Franceschi, C. (1996). The neuroimmunology of stress from invertebrates to man. *Progress in Neurobiology* **48**, 421–440.

Wendelaar Bonga, S. E. (1997). The stress response in fish. *Physiological Reviews* 77, 592–625.

Gene–Environment Interactions in Early Development

I S P Davis and R Plomin
Institute of Psychiatry, King's College London, London, UK

Glossary

DNA pooling	A molecular genetic technique that combines DNA from individuals in order to estimate allele frequencies for the group of individuals.
Family chaos	A measure of the family environment derived from the Confusion, Hubbub, and Order Scale.
Genotype–environment correlation (rGE)	Genetic influence on exposure to environments.
Genotype–environment interaction (GxE)	Genetic sensitivity to environments.
Microarray	A technology that allows the genotyping of hundreds of thousands of polymorphisms simultaneously.
Quantitative genetics	The statistical study of the genetic and environmental origins of individual differences in complex traits, using information about the relatedness of individuals; in contrast to molecular genetics, which attempts to identify specific genes.
Quantitative trait locus (QTL)	A genetic polymorphism that plays a role in the etiology of a trait influenced by many such loci.
Single nucleotide polymorphism (SNP)	A genetic polymorphism involving the substitution of a single letter (nucleotide base pair) of the four-letter genetic alphabet.

The interplay between nature and nurture has long been characterized as adversarial; the truth is much more complex, and more interesting. Although there are many ways of thinking about the issue, this article considers genotype–environment (GE) interaction and correlation from a quantitative genetic perspective, where GE interaction refers to genetic sensitivity to environments and GE correlation refers to genetic influence on exposure to environments. Diathesis-stress theories predict that individuals' sensitivity to stressful events and access to social support networks depends on their genotype. Although evidence for such interactions is – as yet – inconclusive, a more convincing case can be made for genetic influence on environmental measures: gene–environment correlations. The ability to detect gene–environment interplay has traditionally relied on the use of specific environmental measures in genetically sensitive designs such as twin or adoption studies. This ability is greatly enhanced by incorporating genotyping for specific genes: new methods for doing this are likely to see future stress research making use of genetic measures as a matter of course.

Quantitative Genetics

Over the past two decades, there has been an increasing tendency to include measures of the environment in quantitative genetic research; without measures of the environment, quantitative genetic designs such as twin and adoption studies cannot contribute much to our understanding of GE interaction and correlation. This section begins with quantitative genetic research on GE interaction and correlation that incorporates measures of the environment and then turns to molecular genetic research that incorporates information from DNA. The effects of stressful environments on learning ability and disability are used as an example of how molecular genetics can contribute to our understanding of gene–environment interplay.

GE Interaction

The great advantage of research with animal models is the ability to manipulate both genes and environment experimentally so that main effects and interaction are assessed directly. That is, genetically different animals such as selected low and high lines or inbred strains can be studied in different environments. Animal models are powerful, but they have been hard-pushed to find GE interaction, especially for learning. The classic example in psychology textbooks is Cooper and Zubek's study of maze-bright and maze-dull rats reared in enriched or deprived environments. However, although it is highly cited, its conclusions are doubtful: Henderson studied GE interaction systematically using inbred strains of mice and found few such effects.

Adoption designs are similar to animal designs, except that they are only quasi-experimental in their separation of genes and environment (**Figure 1**). Parents usually share both genes and environment with their offspring, but adoption separates nature and nurture by creating a distinction between genetic parents whose children are adopted away and environmental parents who adopt these children. Using the phenotype of biological parents as an indicator of genetic risk and the phenotype of adoptive parents as an indicator of environmental risk, we can find genetic effects without environmental effects (**Figure 1a**) and environmental effects without genetic effects (**Figure 1b**). Studies usually reveal both genetic and environmental effects (**Figure 1c**). The adoption design can also identify GE interaction (**Figure 1d**), in which genetic effects depend on environmental effects or vice versa. However, as with animal studies, it has been difficult to find GE interaction, especially for cognitive abilities. Twin studies are much more

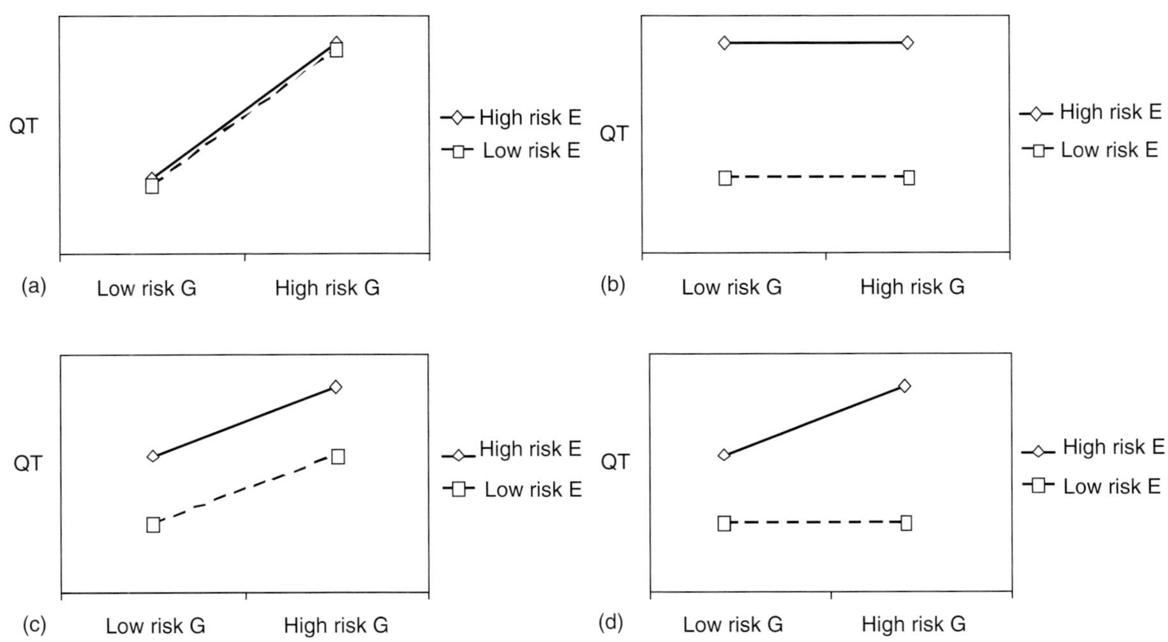

Figure 1 G, E, and GxE in an adoption study. G refers to low or high genetic risk, as indexed by the phenotype (quantitative trait [QT]) of the biological parents. E refers to the environment of the adoptive home. a, A main effect of G, but no effect of E on the phenotype. b, A main effect of E, but no effect of G. Very often, there is a main effect of both G and E, as illustrated in c. d, A main effect of both G and E, and a GxE interaction of the diathesis stress type, in which environmental risk (stress) has a disproportionately large effect on individuals at genetic risk (diathesis).

limited in terms of finding GE interaction because they are essentially constrained to detecting differences in heritability as a function of the environment.

For example, in the Twins Early Development Study (TEDS) of a large twin sample assessed at 2, 3, 4, and 7 years, GE interaction was looked for, but not much evidence for it was found using quantitative genetic methods. Despite this, one promising example of GE interaction is that heritability of verbal ability is significantly higher (about 0.60) in high chaos families and lower (about 0.30) in low chaos families. However, the twin design lacks power to detect even this limited type of GE interaction: about 1000 pairs of each type of twin are needed to detect a heritability difference of 60% versus 40%. As discussed later, the lack of quantitative genetic evidence for GE interaction does not preclude the likelihood that molecular genetic research will find interactions between specific genes and specific environmental stressors.

GE Correlation

In spite of the current interest in GE interaction, it is likely that GE correlation, the nature of nurture, will eventually be seen as more important. Animal models are powerful for investigating GE interaction, but laboratory research has rarely considered GE correlation because it requires a menu of environments from which individuals can choose. The first step in addressing GE correlation is to investigate the extent to which there is genetic influence on environmental measures. This can be done by treating environmental measures as dependent measures in quantitative genetic analyses. Dozens of such twin and adoption studies consistently find genetic influence on environmental measures: nearly all measures of family environment show genetic influence. Most studies that have addressed this question find genetic influence on environmental measures outside the family as well, such as peer groups, life events, and social support, which are of particular relevance to stress.

How can environmental stressors show genetic influence when environments do not have DNA? The answer is that our measures of stress are not independent of us – genetic influence on our behavior is reflected in our experiences. If genetics affects both environmental measures and behavioral measures, then the correlation between environmental measures and behavioral outcomes may be genetically mediated. Life events such as illness and injury have been shown to have a heritability of around 40%, implying that they do not happen capriciously to individuals: they happen, or are perceived to happen, more often to the genetically predisposed. As expected, those life events that the individual is involved in or has control over show more substantial heritability than those that happen to others. Recent research suggests that minor, chronic, daily stressors may be more important in determining outcomes than major life events. New studies are expected to show that these also show genetic influence. In a similar way, social support networks show heritability: studies have demonstrated that although the extensiveness of the network is not heritable, the quality of the relationships is.

The method underlying all these studies is to use multivariate genetic analysis to analyze genetic and environmental sources of covariance between environmental stressors and behavioral outcomes. Studies of this sort consistently show some genetic mediation of the association. In this sense, quantitative genetic research provides much more evidence for GE correlation than for GE interaction. GE correlation suggests an important model of environments that goes beyond the usual passive view in which the environment (and, by extension, stress) is what happens to us. Instead, environments are active: we select, modify, construct and, afterward, reconstruct our experiences partially based on our genetic propensities. From a molecular genetic point of view, GE correlation means that we ought to be able to find specific genes associated with environmental measures.

In summary, quantitative genetic research does not find much evidence for GE interaction, but it finds considerable evidence for GE correlation. This section has not gone into great detail because quantitative genetic results on GE interaction and correlation are not very relevant for future research in this area, which will use specific genes as well as specific environments. The rest of this article considers molecular genetic approaches.

Molecular Genetics

So far, evidence of the existence of interplay between genes and the environment has been considered. Research on GE interaction and correlation will be much more powerful when we are able to include specific genes as well as specific environments, that is, when the G in GE refers to genes in molecular genetic analyses rather than genotypes in quantitative genetic analyses. There have been several replicated linkages and associations, but most people would agree that progress has been slower than expected in terms of finding genes for complex behavioral traits. The problem is that we are looking for needles in a haystack, but we have only had the power to detect very large needles. Very rarely, the effects of a single gene can account for all the variance in a trait. This is the case with phenylketonuria (PKU), in which a mutation in both copies of a single gene results in the inability to metabolize the amino acid phenylalanine. This causes a buildup of toxic products that damage the developing brain. The environmental intervention of a low phenylalanine diet has the effect of preventing mental impairment in children with PKU but has no effect on other children: a dramatic example of a GE interaction.

Despite the slow progress in identifying quantitative trait loci (QTLs) associated with common disorders and complex traits, some evidence has been found for GE interaction using candidate QTLs that affect genetic sensitivity to environments. For example, there are reports that the influence of maltreatment in early life on the development of adult antisocial problems is moderated by a functional polymorphism in the promoter region of the *MAOA* (monoamine oxidase A) gene. Likewise, the influence of stressful life events on depression may be moderated by a functional polymorphism in the promoter region of the *5-HTT* (5-hydroxytryptophan [serotonin] transporter) gene. These examples of GE interaction emerged despite the absence of a main effect for these two genes.

For the vast majority of complex traits, the largest QTL effect is unlikely to account for more than 1% of the variance. Very large samples are needed to attain power to detect such small effects, and even larger samples are needed to detect GE interaction. Rather than just examining a few candidate genes, the trend in molecular genetic research is toward systematic genome-wide scans that require hundreds of thousands of DNA markers. The costs for such genome-wide association scans on very large samples are substantial. One new method that goes some way to solving this problem is genotyping of pooled DNA on microarrays, a method called SNP-MaP (single nucleotide polymorphism microarrays and pooling).

The first application of SNP-MaP involved mild mental impairment (MMI), which can be seen as the low end of general cognitive ability (g). g was assessed in 10 000 children at 7 years, and two independent SNP-MaP studies using a microarray that assessed 10 000 SNPs (the 10K GeneChip) compared high and low g groups. Five SNPs were identified that remained significantly associated with g when individually genotyped for 5000 children. On average, each SNP in the set accounts for just 0.2% of the variance in g. However, as the effects of the SNPs are uncorrelated and additive, it is possible to combine their effects to create a composite SNP set using an additive model in which each SNP is scored 0, 1, or 2, depending on the number of high-g-associated alleles. The SNP set accounts for nearly 1% of the variance of g scores at 7 years. As shown in **Figure 2**, SNP set scores are normally distributed and almost linearly related to g. The difference between those scoring low on the SNP set and those scoring high is about one-third of a standard deviation, or 5 IQ points.

Repeating the analysis using the newly available 500K microarray should find many more SNPs accounting for much more of the variance. It will then be possible to use SNP set scores as genetic risk

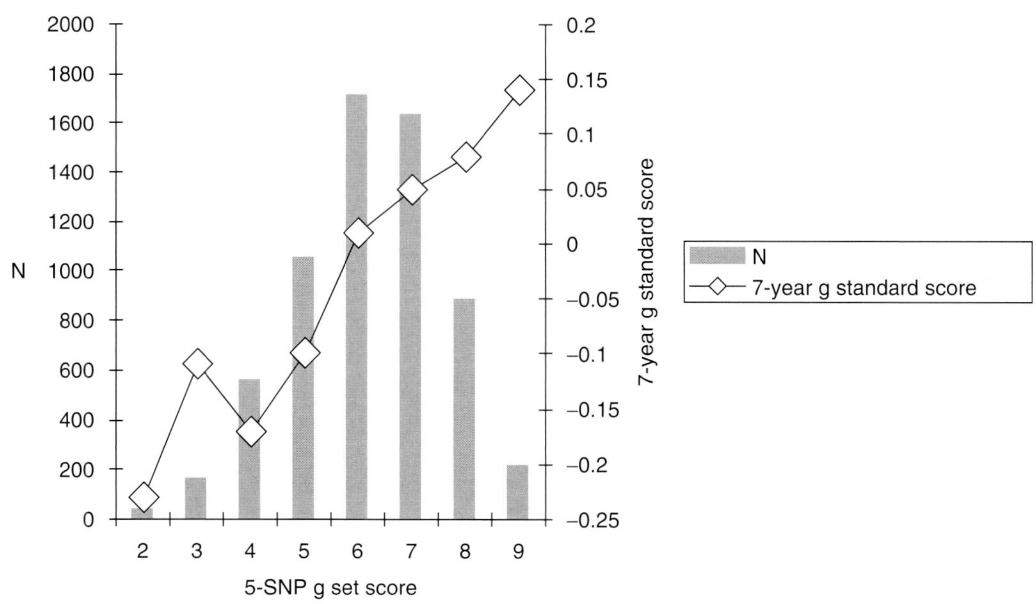

Figure 2 Distribution of 5-SNP g set and association between 5-SNP set and 7-year g. The distribution of scores for the SNP set (derived on the basis of higher scores for high-g-associated alleles) is normal (gray bars). The line represents the means of the 5-SNP set score plotted against means of the g composite score at 7 years.

indicators in research into environmental stressors and to select genotypically for extreme SNP set groups to use in paradigms such as neuroimaging that cannot study large samples.

Behavioral Genomics and GE Interplay

Once genes or QTL sets associated with behavioral dimensions or disorders are found, the next phase of research will investigate the pathways between genes and behavior via the brain, which will represent a paradigm shift in research on GE interplay. The term functional genomics, which has been used to describe this direction for research, usually refers to bottom-up research that begins with understanding the gene product in a cell and works up toward the brain and behavior. However, other levels of analysis can also be useful in understanding pathways between genes and behavior: behavioral genomics refers to a complementary approach that begins with behavior of the individual and works down toward the brain. For example, we can investigate how genetic effects unfold during development or ask multivariate questions about heterogeneity and comorbidity. As the present concern is GE interaction and correlation, the focus will be on behavioral genomic analyses of GE interplay.

To return to the earlier example, the 5-SNP set associated with g at 7 years was used in behavioral genomic analyses of GE interaction and correlation. The environmental measures employed in these analyses included distal environmental measures such as parental occupation or education and proximal measures such as family chaos and discipline in early childhood in those homes. Although GE interaction can be examined in several different ways, the extent to which environmental stressors moderate the SNP set association with g was investigated. Using family chaos as an example, the top panel (a) of **Figure 3** shows a main effect for family chaos (higher g scores for children in families with less chaos) but no statistically significant interaction using linear and nonlinear continuous analyses.

The other three environmental variables shown in **Figure 3** yielded significant but modest GE interaction. For harsh parental discipline (**Figure 3b**), environmental effects are greater at both the high and the low SNP set scores. For high SNP set scores, children with good environments (low harsh discipline) have higher than expected g scores, whereas children with low SNP set scores and harsh parental discipline have lower than expected g scores. In other words, this GE interaction suggests that children with a genetic propensity toward high g profit disproportionately from a good environment, and children with a genetic propensity toward low g suffer disproportionately from a bad environment. A similar sort of GE interaction was found for father occupation (**Figure 3c**): environmental effects were greater at both the high and the low genetic extremes.

We also found a significant GE interaction for the fourth environmental measure, maternal education (**Figure 3d**). However, this GE interaction represents a different sort of interaction, one that is compatible with recent findings from quantitative genetics suggesting that genetic effects on g are weaker for families with lower socioeconomic status. The result for maternal education is compatible with this finding: the association between SNP set and g is weakest for families with the least-educated mothers.

What about GE correlation? As noted earlier, GE correlation refers to the correlation between genes and environment. In contrast to GE interaction, which concerns environmental moderation of the association between the SNP set and g, GE correlation focuses on the extent to which the environment mediates the association between the SNP set and g. Such mediation requires that the environmental measure correlate with the SNP set and also correlate with g. Because the environmental measures were chosen for their correlation with g, the simplest GE correlation analysis was conducted, which was merely to correlate the environmental measures with SNP set scores, rather than conducting more formal mediation analyses. Both proximal measures of the family environment (harsh parental discipline and family chaos) were correlated significantly with the SNP set for g, suggesting GE correlation. It is interesting that the distal measures of family environment (father's occupation and mother's education) showed no GE correlation. Of the three types of GE correlation (passive, evocative, and active), finding GE correlation for distal environmental variables would be most easily characterized as passive GE correlation: the children's family environments would be correlated with their genetic propensities because their parents share the same genes. In contrast, these analyses suggest that GE correlation is stronger for proximal environments, implying evocative (reactive) GE correlation: children evoke reactions based on their genetic propensities.

In summary, there is evidence for both GE interaction and GE correlation in early development. One final caveat is that GE interactions may result from GE correlations under certain circumstances; true GE interaction should remain significant after controlling for GE correlation.

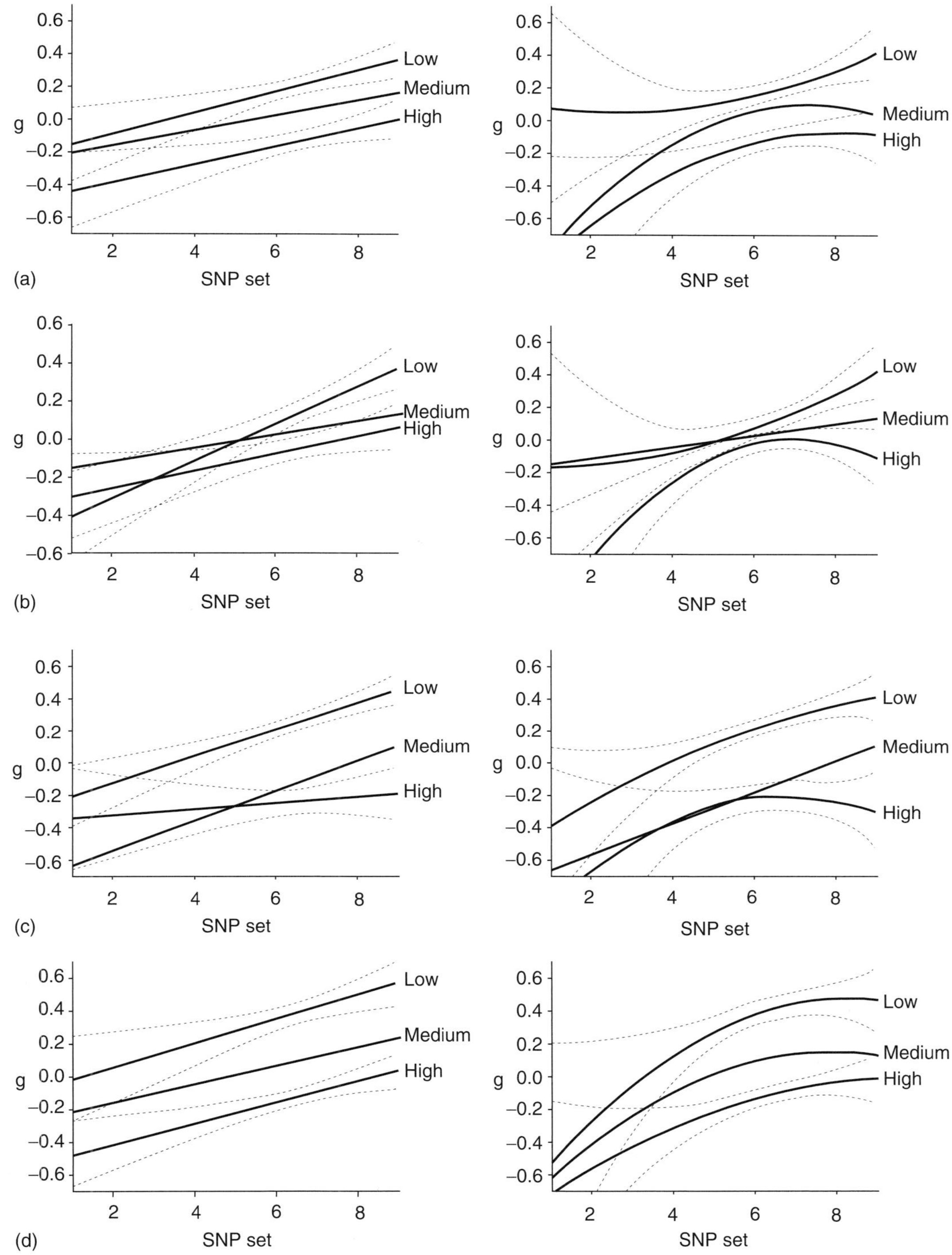

Figure 3 g scores as linear and nonlinear functions of SNP set scores and level (low, medium, and high) of environmental risk for chaos (a), harsh parental discipline (b), father's occupational class (c), and mother's highest qualification (d). Ninety-five percent confidence intervals (dotted lines) are shown for low and high levels of environmental risk.

Future QTL Research on GE Interplay

In addition to using QTLs identified on the basis of their main effect in order to investigate GE interaction and correlation, future research on GE interplay will profit from identifying QTLs that contribute to GE interaction and correlation regardless of their main effect. In the previous example, SNPs were identified based on their association with g (regardless of environment) by comparing SNP allele frequencies for low versus high g groups. **Figure 4** shows a simple

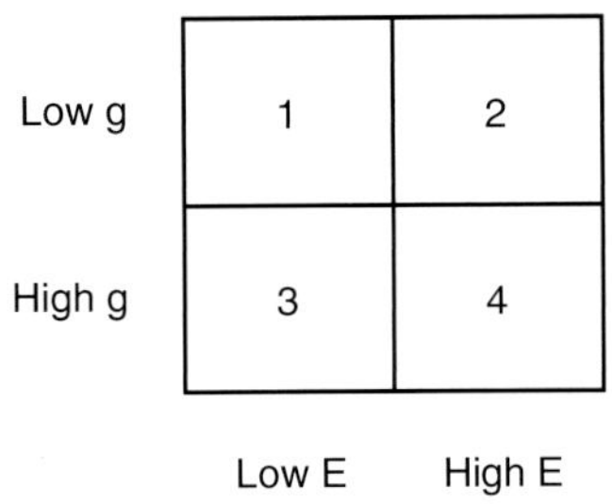

Figure 4 Identifying QTLs on the basis of GE interaction and correlation. Using four, rather than two, DNA pools will facilitate these studies. For example, comparing SNP allele frequencies for pools 1 and 2 versus pools 3 and 4 tests for a main effect for g. Comparing pools 1 and 3 versus 2 and 4 reveals GE correlation, a QTL association with E. Comparing pools 1 and 4 versus 2 and 3 assesses GE interaction, a QTL association for g that depends on E.

two-by-two interaction design in which cases are selected based on low versus high environmental stress as well as on low versus high g. Using DNA pooled separately for the four groups, QTL associations representing the main effect of the QTL on g regardless of environment stressors can be detected by comparing groups 1 and 2 versus groups 3 and 4. The important advantage of this design is that GE correlation and GE interaction can also be detected independent of their contribution to the main effect. GE correlation can be assessed as the main effect of the environment, comparing groups 1 and 3 versus groups 2 and 4, thus identifying QTLs that are associated with low versus high environmental stress. Finally, GE interaction can be detected by comparing the diagonals (groups 1 and 4 versus groups 2 and 3).

The future of research on genotype-environment interaction and correlation looks bright, especially as the G in GE increasingly comes to represent genes in molecular genetic analyses rather than genotypes in quantitative genetic analyses.

Further Reading

Asbury, K., Wachs, T. and Plomin, R. (2005). Environmental moderators of genetic influence on verbal and nonverbal abilities in early childhood. *Intelligence* **33**, 643–661.

Butcher, L. M., Meaburn, E., Liu, L., et al. (2004). Genotyping pooled DNA on microarrays: A systematic genome screen of thousands of SNPs in large samples to detect QTLs for complex traits. *Behavior Genetics* **34**, 549–555.

Butcher, L. M., Meaburn, E., Knight, J., et al. (2005). SNPs, microarrays, and pooled DNA: identification of four loci associated with mild mental impairment in a sample of 6000 children. *Human Molecular Genetics* **14**, 1315–1325.

Caspi, A., McClay, J., Moffitt, T. E., et al. (2002). Role of genotype in the cycle of violence in maltreated children. *Science* **297**, 851–854.

Caspi, A., Sugden, K., Moffitt, T. E., et al. (2003). Influence of life stress on depression: Moderation by a polymorphism in the 5-HTT gene. *Science* **301**, 386–389.

Cooper, R. M. and Zubek, J. P. (1958). Effects of enriched and restricted early environments on the learning ability of bright and dull rats. *Canadian Journal of Psychology* **12**, 159–164.

Harlaar, N., Butcher, L., Meaburn, E., et al. (2005). A behavioural genomic analysis of DNA markers associated with general cognitive ability in 7-year-olds. *Journal of Child Psychology & Psychiatry* **46**, 1097–1107.

Henderson, N. D. (1972). Relative effects of early rearing environment on discrimination learning in housemice. *Journal of Comparative and Psychological Psychology* **72**, 505–511.

Meaburn, E., Butcher, L. M., Liu, L., et al. (2005). Genotyping DNA pools on microarrays: tackling the QTL problem of large samples and large numbers of SNPs. *BMC Genomics* **6**, 52.

Plomin, R. (1977). Genotype–environment interaction and correlation in the analysis of human behavior. *Behavior Genetics* **7**, 83.

Plomin, R. (1994). *Genetics and experience: the interplay between nature and nurture.* Thousand Oaks, CA: Sage Publications Inc.

Plomin, R. and Crabbe, J. C. (2000). DNA. *Psychological Bulletin* **126**, 806–828.

Plomin, R., DeFries, J. C., McClearn, G. E., et al. (2001). *Behavioral genetics* (4th edn.). New York: Worth Publishers.

Rowe, D. (2003). Assessing genotype–environment interactions and correlations in the postgenomic era. In: Plomin, R., DeFries, J. C., Craig, I. W. & McGuffin, P. (eds.) *Behavioral genetics in the postgenomic era*, pp. 71–86. Washington, D.C.: American Psychological Association.

Stress and CNS Arousal: Genomic Contributions

A C Ribeiro and D W Pfaff
Rockefeller University, New York, NY, USA

Glossary

Arousal	The fundamental property of the central nervous system that determines the amplitude of responses to any given stimulus.
Arousal crescent	A group of primitive neurons residing in the ventral and medial edges of the brain stem that have ascending projections that alert the brain.
Arousal-promoting mechanisms	Monoaminergic cell groups (dorsal raphe nuclei, locus coeruleus, substantia nigra and ventral periaqueductal gray, and tuberomammillary nuclei) that have ascending projections to the thalamus, hypothalamus, and cerebral cortex and whose chemical products favor states of behavioral arousal.
Sleep-promoting mechanisms	A small group of neurons residing in the ventrolateral preoptic nucleus that fire predominantly during sleep and send inhibitory projections to the monoaminergic cell groups.

Arousal

Stress responses, whether defined endocrinologically or behaviorally, depend for their expression on the fundamental arousal of the central nervous system (CNS). The relation between stress and arousal is not simple. In terms of a person's psychological feelings, moderate and increasing levels of arousal can be a good thing. However, too much or for too long is both tiring and unpleasant (**Figure 1**).

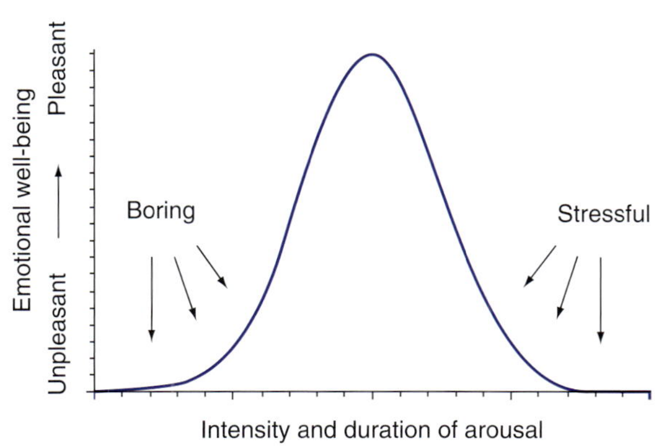

Figure 1 Prolonged arousal can lead to stress.

In the workplace, the relationship between stress and arousal has been defined by occupational psychologists (**Table 1**). Too much demand with too little control can be so stressful as to cause illness. Therefore, it is useful to explore CNS mechanisms underlying the concept of arousal. Here we briefly summarize its operational definition, neuroanatomy, functional genomics, and neurochemistry.

Generalized Arousal

Although intuitively simple to understand, the concept of arousal has not been an easy one to define scientifically. Because all our behaviors and responses to stimuli depend on the underlying state of arousal we are in, it becomes critically important to quantitatively define arousal and to have ways to accurately measure it.

Arousal refers to the degree of stimulation necessary to drive a certain behavior in an animal. The particular stimulus or behavior can vary, but the underlying arousal state determines the magnitude of the response and even if the behavior will occur at all. Another way of envisioning this concept is that arousal is the force or motivation behind a given response, whereas the stimulus dictates what the response modality is.

The overall arousal state of an organism depends on generalized arousal and many specific forms of arousal, such as hunger, thirst, sex, sleep, and fear (**Figure 2**). If we express this concept in the framework of a mathematical equation, then arousal (A) is a function of the general arousal (A_g) state and each individual specific arousal component (A_{s1-n}). Influencing each of these variables is the underlying temperament of the individual, which we express as a constant (K) for each variable (g, 1–n). Because these parameters (thirst, hunger, sex, sleep, fear, etc.) often influence one another, the Arousal Equation can quickly become very complex:

$$A = f(\mathrm{K}_g A_g + \mathrm{K}_{s1} A_{s1} + \mathrm{K}_{s2} A_{s2} + \ldots + \mathrm{K}_{\mathrm{sn}} A_{\mathrm{sn}})$$

Table 1 Relationship between occupational demands and employee's control

		Demand for arousal, alertness, and vigilance	
		High	*Low*
Degree of control by employee	High	Stimulating	Boring
	Low	Stressful	Restful

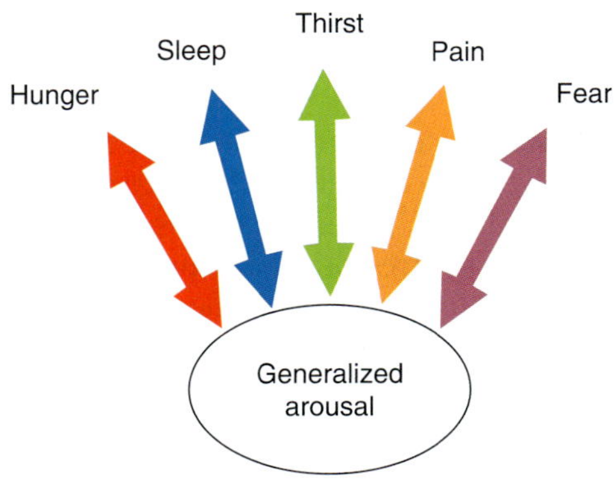

Figure 2 Representation of the arousal equation. Each specific arousal (e.g., pain) depends on the underlying generalized arousal state of the animals, as well as on other specific arousal components (e.g., hunger motivation).

Traditionally, scientists studying arousal often disagreed on a definition of arousal. Some viewed arousal as one large behavioral phenomenon, where others viewed it as a collection of multiple specific components. The concept outlined in the Arousal Equation unifies, for the first time, these two schools of thought and provides a precise, experimentally feasible manner of determining the arousal state of an animal.

Operational Definition and Quantitative Measures of Arousal

Generalized arousal can be experimentally determined and measured. By definition, an animal is considered to be more aroused if it has increased responsiveness to stimuli (S) from the environment (any sensory modality), increased voluntary motor (M) activity, and also increased ability to react emotionally (E). These three components encompass large classes of varied sensory modalities, which invariably give us a better measure of generalized CNS arousal. This is in sharp contrast to classic neuroscience, which sought to characterize the specific responses of an organism to a specific stimulus. Behavioral arousal is produced by select brain pathways and key populations of neurons being activated, eventually leading to changes in gene-expression patterns.

Using a statistical test called principal components analysis has enabled us to screen large amounts of data (e.g., behavioral responses to the three modalities of stimuli – sensory, motor and emotional reactivity – for each mouse) and uncover trends in the data. The use of this mathematical tool has revealed that generalized arousal accounts for approximately one-third (from 29.7 to 45%, depending on the experimental conditions) of all the data in arousal-related activities.

Application of Information Theory to Understanding the Neurobiology of Arousal

Introduced by Claude Shannon in the late 1940s, information theory, also known as Shannon's communication theory, establishes that the probability that an event will occur is inversely proportional to the information carried in that event. Consider, for example, the act of flipping a coin. There is a 50% chance of the coin landing heads up versus tails up; therefore, the possible information carried in this system is maximal – the more uncertain an outcome is, the more information transmittal there is. In contrast, if an event has a very high probability of occurring, there is very little room for doubt and very little information carried by the system. In neurobiological terms, the more unexpected the stimulus, the more dramatic the response (e.g., startle) will be. Likewise, the more nonintellectually stimulating environment, the less alert the animal will be and the less likely it is to respond to a stimulus (i.e., the less aroused it is).

Within the CNS, neuronal firing patterns are also governed by the principles of information theory. At any given time, there is a certain probability that a neuron will fire. The closer this probability is to 0.5 (or 50%), the more aroused the animal will be and the larger the repertoire of possible responses it can mount.

Neuroanatomical and Neurochemical Basis of Arousal

Proper arousal responses are critically important for nearly every aspect of our lives. Given this primal role, it is not surprising that nature has evolved ways to ensure that its regulation is safeguarded. This is accomplished by having multiple, redundant, and independent but cooperative mechanisms contributing to the overall arousal state.

Primordial Arousal-Promoting Neurons in the Arousal Crescent

A population of neurons in the reticular formation plays a key role in the regulation of arousal. These neurons originate in the ventral area of the brain stem, at the junction with the spinal cord, and extend bilaterally in a crescent-shaped form through the brain stem and eventually project ventrally into the thalamus and hypothalamus. This neuronal group is among the most evolutionarily conserved networks in animals, adding support to the hypothesis that it plays a crucial role in modulating arousal. These neurons have a keen ability to sense and respond to a variety of arousing stimuli arising from within the body and the environment, including changes in blood pressure, pain, stress, and hormone levels. These neurons, mostly glutamatergic in nature, have ascending projections to the thalamus, hypothalamus, and basal forebrain, as well as descending projections to the spinal cord. These projections terminate at biologically relevant cell groups that are also involved in arousal control (e.g., the basal forebrain). Projections from this arousal crescent can travel via two routes: a ventral one and a dorsal one. The more ventral one is evolutionarily more primitive and terminates in the cholinergic basal forebrain. The more dorsal route terminates in the thalamus and hypothalamus and is more recent, evolutionarily speaking; it is especially well developed in primates.

Ascending Arousal Activating Pathways

In the 1940s and 1950s, Moruzzi, Magoun, and other neurophysiologists identified a key population of arousal-promoting neurons residing in the brain-stem reticular formation. These cholinergic neurons, found predominantly in the laterodorsal tegmental nucleus and the pedunculopontine tegmental nucleus, have extensive excitatory projections to the thalamus, which in turn project to widespread areas of the cerebral cortex. Acetylcholine release in both the thalamus and the cortex is highest during behaviorally aroused states of wakefulness and rapid eye movement (REM) sleep. In addition to the projections to the thalamus and eventually the cortex, brain-stem reticular neurons also project to the basal forebrain and hypothalamus, which contributes to stabilizing the aroused state.

Monoaminergic nuclei include the serotonergic dorsal raphe nuclei, adrenergic locus coeruleus, and dopaminergic substantia nigra in the brain stem, as well as the histaminergic tuberomammillary nucleus in the posterior hypothalamus. These nuclei all exhibit the highest discharge rates with maximal neurotransmitter release during wakefulness, lower discharge rates in non-REM sleep, and cease firing during REM sleep. The silencing of these neurons, and thus the absence of monoamine neurotransmission, plays a permissive role on REM sleep. These monoaminergic nuclei have ascending projections to the thalamus, hypothalamus, and cerebral cortex that favor states of behavioral arousal (e.g., wakefulness and REM sleep).

Descending Arousal Pathways

In antiphase to these arousal-promoting mechanisms, there are select brain regions that actively promote cortical synchronization, characteristic of non-REM sleep. One such brain nucleus is the hypothalamic ventrolateral preoptic nucleus (VLPO), whose neurons send inhibitory γ-aminobutyric acid (GABA) ergic and galaninergic projections to the monoaminergic cell groups, thus silencing them.

The lateral hypothalamus also contains neurons that are important for vigilance control. Wake-active orexin-producing neurons have been shown to have excitatory projections to monoaminergic cell groups. Significantly, monoaminergic projections to the VLPO express orexin receptors, and the lack of orexin binding at these receptors causes behavioral state instability associated with narcolepsy. In addition, intermingled with these neurons are melanin-concentrating hormone–GABA-containing neurons that are most active during REM sleep.

Neurochemicals Influencing Arousal

Acetylcholine Originally called vagusstoff (in reference to its release after stimulation of the vagus nerve), acetylcholine was the first neurotransmitter to be discovered. It is produced by the enzyme choline acetyltransferase and can bind to two classes of receptors: nicotinic and muscarinic. The major sources of acetylcholine in the CNS are the basal forebrain, pontine reticular formation, and medial septum. Cholinergic neurons from the reticular formation provide a major excitatory input, stimulating cortical activation, and the discharge patterns of these neurons are highest during behavioral aroused states.

Noradrenaline/norepinephrine In the CNS, norepinephrine is primarily produced by the locus ceruleus neurons, and these neurons promote behavioral arousal, primarily via their projections to the forebrain, brain stem, and spinal cord. Like other monoaminergic cell groups in the brain, locus ceruleus neurons discharge maximally during active waking, decrease their firing rates during non-REM sleep, and are silent during REM sleep. Norepinephrine inhibits VLPO sleep-promoting neurons by binding at α_2-adrenoreceptors. Also, significantly, norepinephrine increases the female sexual behavior lordosis by modulating the firing rates of ventromedial hypothalamic neurons, and sexual interactions between mice lead to increased norepinephrine release in the hypothalamus.

Serotonin Produced in the dorsal raphe nuclei of the brain stem, serotonin is a monoaminergic neurotransmitter that, like norepinephrine, promotes arousal. Serotonergic neurons fire maximally during waking (quiet waking), decrease their firing rate during non-REM sleep, and cease firing during REM sleep. Many mood disorders, anxiety, and depression have been linked to deficiencies in serotonergic neurotransmission. Due to the large number of serotonin receptors (14) and their varied functions, studying the pharmacology of serotonin can be quite challenging.

Histamine Produced by tuberomammillary neurons in the posterior hypothalamus, histamine is a biogenic amine involved in vigilance control. With discharge patterns similar to serotonergic and noradrenergic neurons, maximal histamine release occurs during the waking state, and the administration of antihistamines is often accompanied by drowsiness. Like norepinephrine, histamine also increases sexual behavior in female mice by increasing the firing rates of ventromedial hypothalamic neurons. In addition, sleep-promoting VLPO region neurons send inhibitory GABAergic and galaninergic projections to histaminergic neurons, thus establishing a mutually exclusive, reciprocal interaction between the arousal and sleep-promoting brain regions.

Dopamine Neurons containing dopamine in the ventral periaqueductal gray matter have recently been identified as a major dopaminergic input to modulate arousal. These neurons have the highest discharge rates during wakefulness and have extensive projections to brain regions involved in sleep regulation. Dopaminergic neurons from the ventromedial nucleus and the substantia nigra may also contribute to promote arousal.

Orexin/hypocretin The recently discovered neuropeptides orexin/hypocretin are produced by a small population of neurons in the lateral hypothalamus perifornical area. The two peptides have the same precursor protein and, in addition to playing a role in stimulating appetite, they promote wakefulness. Orexinergic neurons have direct excitatory projections to the tuberomammillary nucleus, and a deficiency in either the orexin peptides or the receptors leads to behavioral state instability and narcolepsy.

Prostaglandin D_2 Prostaglandin D synthase catalyzes the isomerization of the common prostanoid precursor prostaglandin H_2 to the endogenous somnogen prostaglandin D_2. The involvement of prostaglandin D_2 in sleep regulation has been studied for the past 25 years. In fact, it was among the first endogenous sleep-promoting substances to be identified. Prostaglandin D_2 is thought to be involved in homeostatic sleep regulatory mechanisms because animals that lack prostaglandin D synthase or prostaglandin D_2 receptor fail to exhibit a sleep rebound in response to sleep deprivation. The somnogenic effects of prostaglandin D_2 are hypothesized to be mediated by the nucleoside adenosine, and infusion of prostaglandin D_2 into the subarachnoid space increases extracellular levels of adenosine.

Adenosine The nucleoside end product of energy metabolism, adenosine, has been shown to accumulate in a wake-dependent manner in the basal forebrain. The sleep-promoting effects of prostaglandin D_2 have been shown to be mediated by adenosine 2A receptors in the VLPO. Adenosine has been shown to disinhibit sleep-active VLPO neurons by blocking inhibitory inputs to these neurons and also by directly exciting these neurons. In addition, adenosine can inhibit wake-active neurons in the tuberomammillary nucleus. Interestingly, the most widely consumed arousal-promoting drug by humans, caffeine, works by blocking adenosine 2A receptors.

Steroid hormones Estrogens are produced by the ovaries and are secreted shortly before ovulation. The major role of estrogen is to prepare the female body for courtship, mating, and, eventually, maternal care. As such, estrogens modulate most of the neurochemicals and pathways mediating arousal to ensure that reproduction occurs. Examples are seen in cholinergic neurotransmission, in which estrogens not only increase the rate of acetylcholine synthesis but also increase the number of cholinergic receptors on target neurons. Similarly, estrogens increase the expression of genes involved in norepinephrine production and enhance the responses of dopamine and histamine. Conversely, the levels of the enzyme that produces the endogenous somnogen prostaglandin D_2 is decreased after estrogen treatment. In addition to the well-established roles of estrogens on sexual behaviors, there are many nonreproductive effects of estrogens on behavior, including anxiety, food intake, learning, memory, mood disorders, and sleep.

Integration of Signals

The neuroanatomical pathways discussed so far refer to mechanisms mediating arousal and sleep–wakefulness induction; there are also underlying circadian and homeostatic forces that determine when sleep can occur. The homeostatic drive for sleep, also known as process S, can be envisioned as an increased pressure that progressively gets larger the longer the animal is kept awake and that eventually reaches threshold levels, which trigger sleep. This mechanism is involved in modulating the day-to-day sleep distribution patterns, as well as sleep rebound in response to extended wakefulness. Homeostatic sleep-regulatory molecules (e.g., prostaglandin D2, adenosine, and nitric oxide) accumulate in a wake-dependent manner and eventually stimulate sleep. Also communicating with these effector pathways is the circadian component, which determines when, along the 24-h light–dark cycle, sleep and arousal are most appropriate. In fact, the suprachiasmatic nucleus, the circadian pacemaker, has many direct and indirect projections to both sleep-promoting and arousal-promoting brain regions and thus contributes to the fine-tuning of arousal.

Amplified States of Arousal

Sex and Fear

Given the elaborate symphony of mechanisms and chemicals underlying arousal regulation, we quickly come to the conclusion that critical biological functions must rely on it. One such function is reproduction. The propagation of the species, our ultimate goal, is intimately dependent on proper levels of arousal at the appropriate times. The primal function that estrogens have is to prepare the body for reproduction. As such, redundant mechanisms have evolved that ensure that, once the hormonal milieu is optimal and ovulation is near, females exhibit the behaviors that attract mates and result in fruitful copulation. Although conceptually ideal, this scenario does not always occur. Imagine, if you will, that the animals are exposed to a stressful stimulus or are in an unfamiliar place; it may not be feasible to invest time and energy in reproduction when they should be worried, really, about survival. This is, in fact, what the literature tells us occurs in rodents. In the protective shelter of a running-wheel cage or a home cage in our arousal-monitoring equipment, after estrogen treatment the animals exhibited increased arousal (e.g., increased running-wheel activity). However, when the animals were tested in an open field or placed in an unfamiliar cage, the arousal behavior was quickly replaced by fear, resulting in lowered responsivity by the animal.

A fine line exists between which estrogen-mediated mechanisms are activated, depending on the environmental circumstances the animal finds itself; therefore, caution must be exercised when analyzing and interpreting such behavioral responses.

Significance of Studying Arousal

Arousal-related disorders affect people of all ages and genders. They comprise a wide spectrum of ailments, ranging from problems of vigilance control (e.g., narcolepsy) to hyperactivity disorders (e.g., attention-deficit hyperactivity disorder) and, in extreme cases, to devastating vegetative states, all of which can have detrimental and costly consequences.

Disorders of Reduced Arousal

Sleep disorders Forty million Americans are chronically affected by sleep disorders, and an additional 20–30 million report episodic sleep problems. Disorders of sleep range from the most common insomnias to sudden infant death syndrome to hypersomnias. Lack of research and adequate public education has led to a rising epidemic of sleep disorders, especially those associated with obesity (e.g., sleep apnea) and also to a chronically sleep-deprived society. Disorders of arousal mechanisms can be disastrous and costly, causing poor job performance, lack of attention in classrooms, and traffic accidents, all resulting from loss of vigilance.

Extreme hypo-arousal states The most extreme and devastating states in which arousal mechanisms are compromised can be seen in patients in vegetative, comatose, and stupurous states. Although the redundancy of neuroanatomical and neurochemical pathways minimize the possibility that this will occur, situations still exist in which the ability to be aroused is compromised. Only by understanding and characterizing these mechanisms can there be hope that someday it may be possible to stimulate certain key elements of this pathway (perhaps neurons in the arousal crescent) to reverse or ameliorate this condition.

Disorders of hyperarousal Cases of excessive arousal can be seen in patients suffering from attention-deficit hyperactivity disorder and posttraumatic stress disorder. Although they do not appear to be as debilitating as disorders of decreased arousal, being too aroused can interfere with a person's ability to function in society, for example, being able to learn in school or to focus at work. Likewise, the inability to repress unwanted detrimental memories in posttraumatic stress disorder can interfere with the healing process and the ability to resume normal activities.

Promising Future Lies Ahead in Arousal Research

Arousal mechanisms underlie all behavioral aspects of our existence. Although nature has done an astonishing job of ensuring that arousal mechanisms function optimally, as can be seen by the many independent but redundant pathways regulating arousal, situations still exist in which this system is compromised. Only by knowing the intricacies of this regulation can researchers develop pharmacological and surgical therapies to reversing these problems.

See Also the Following Articles

Circadian Clock Genes as Modulators of Sensitivity to Genotoxic Stress; Circadian Rhythms, Genetics of; Expression Profiling of Stress Responsive Gene Patterns; Gene-Environment Interactions in Early Development; Genetic Polymorphisms in Stress Response.

Further Reading

Borbely, A. A. (2001). From slow waves to sleep homeostasis: new perspectives. *Archives of Italian Biology* **139** (1–2), 53–61.

Garey, J., Goodwillie, A., Frohlich, J., et al. (2003). Genetic contributions to generalized arousal of brain and behavior. *Proceedings of the National Academy of Sciences USA* **100**(19), 11019–11022.

McEwen, B. S. (2004). *The end of stress as we know it.* Washington, DC: Dana Press/Joseph Henry Press.

Mong, J. A. and Pfaff, D. W. (2004). Hormonal symphony: steroid orchestration of gene modules for sociosexual behaviors. *Molecular Psychiatry* **9**(6), 550–556.

Pfaff, D. W. (2006). *Brain arousal and information theory: neural and genetic mechanisms.* Cambridge, MA: Harvard University Press.

II. HYPOTHALAMIC-PITUITARY – ADRENAL AXIS

A. General

Neuroendocrine Systems

G Fink
Mental Health Research Institute, Melbourne, Australia

This is a revised version of the article by G Fink, Encyclopedia of Stress, First edition, volume 3, pp 14–30, © 2000, Elsevier Inc.

Glossary

Action potentials — Electrical impulses that propagate signals along nerve fibers. The potentials are produced by the flux of ions, in particular sodium and potassium ions, through ion channels along the nerve cell membrane.

Exocytosis — The release of a secretory product, including neurotransmitters, in packets or quanta. The secretory products are packaged by the Golgi apparatus of the cell in membrane-bound vesicles. Exocytosis involves fusion of the vesicular membrane with the cell membrane, resulting in the release of the quantum of product inside the vesicle. This is thought to be the major mechanism of secretion in most secretory cells, including neurons.

Limbic system — The system comprising a number of structures, all interconnected, to form a circuit that is concerned primarily with emotions, memory, olfaction, and neuroendocrine control; gets its name from the fact that it forms a border between the new and old (in evolutionary terms) brains.

Neurohemal junction — A specialized junction between nerve terminals and a plexus of capillaries that facilitates the transport of neurohormones from the nervous system into the bloodstream or *vice versa.*

Neurohormone — A chemical substance released from nerve terminals and transported to its target cells by the bloodstream. Neurohormones are often the same chemical substances as neurotransmitters.

Neurosecretion — The secretion of hormones by nerve cells.

Neurotransmitter — A chemical compound released by nerve cells (at nerve synapses or neuromuscular junctions) that either excites or inhibits a target cell. The target cell may be another nerve cell, glandular cell, or muscle fiber. Chemical neurotransmission is widely used in the nervous system and, because it is capable of analog functions, has a considerable advantage over electrotonic transmission, which is necessarily digital.

Portal vessels — The vessels that transport blood and solutes from one capillary bed to a second capillary bed before joining the systemic circulation. The hypophysial portal vessel system transports neurohormones released from hypothalamic nerve terminals into a primary capillary plexus in the median eminence to a secondary capillary–sinusoidal plexus in the pituitary gland.

Steroid hormones — Molecules composed of a basic fused unit of three 6-membered (cyclohexane) and one 5-membered (cyclopentane) carbon rings with a variety of functional groups attached. The large number of carbon–hydrogen bonds makes steroids nonpolar.

Stimulus secretion coupling — The link between a stimulus, usually membrane depolarization (axon potentials in the case of nerve cells), and the release of a neurotransmitter or neurohormone.

Synapse — A specialized junction between two nerve cells where signaling most commonly occurs by way of the release of neurotransmitters.

Introduction

The human pituitary gland weighs no more than one gram, but it nonetheless controls all the major endocrine systems and is indispensable for life. Located at the base of the brain and closely surrounded by protective dense bone and fibrous membranes, the gland is composed of the neurohypophysis or neural lobe and the adenohypophysis. Derived embryologically from a neural downgrowth, the neural lobe is composed of axons that project from nerve cells in the hypothalamus and terminate on capillaries of the inferior hypophysial artery. This is the site at which arginine vasopressin (AVP) (lysine vasopressin in pigs) and oxytocin are released into the systemic circulation. Synthesized in the supraoptic nucleus (SON) and paraventricular nucleus (PVN), AVP, also called the antidiuretic hormone, controls the volume of body water, whereas oxytocin is concerned mainly with stimulating milk ejection during lactation and contraction of the uterus (womb) during parturition.

The adenohypophysis is derived from an outgrowth of the roof of the mouth and, in subhuman species, is divided into the pars distalis and the pars intermedia. The pars distalis is more commonly called the anterior lobe, whereas the pars intermedia together with the neural lobe or pars nervosa forms the posterior lobe. There is no distinct pars intermedia in the human. The anterior pituitary gland secretes hormones that control the adrenal and thyroid glands, the gonads, body growth, and development of the breast and lactation. The hormones involved in this pituitary control are, respectively, adrenocorticotropic hormone (ACTH), thyrotropin (TSH, thyroid stimulating hormone), the gonadotropins, growth hormone (GH), and prolactin. In addition to being growth promoting (trophic) and stimulating immediate hormonal or cellular events (tropic), these hormones all affect metabolism. The loss of ACTH with the consequent loss of adrenocortical hormone secretion, and perhaps to a lesser degree GH and TSH, makes removal of the gland (hypophysectomy) lethal.

Although ACTH is considered to be the main anterior pituitary stress hormone, GH and prolactin are also released in response to stress and so receive special attention in this article. Thus, for example, insulin-induced hypoglycemia is a potent metabolic stress that, in humans, results in a massive and rapid release of GH. Stress-induced prolactin release may, under certain circumstances, be causally related to infertility.

Anterior pituitary hormone secretion is under central nervous system (CNS) control and is modulated by the feedback of hormones secreted by the pituitary target organs: the adrenal and thyroid glands, the gonads, and, as shown recently, fat tissue by way ofadipokines such as leptin and adiponectin. Neural control of the anterior pituitary hormones is mediated by the hypothalamic-pituitary regulatory neurohormones (formerly termed factors), which are released from the hypothalamus into the hypophysial portal vessels and transported by them to the anterior lobe, where they either stimulate or inhibit the release of the anterior pituitary hormones. The hypothalamic-pituitary regulatory factors are now termed neurohormones because, instead of being released at synapses, they are released and transported to their target cells in the bloodstream.

The hypothalamic-pituitary system is the interface between the CNS and the endocrine system by which external factors, such as stress and day length, and internal factors, such as emotion, trigger endocrine responses. It was therefore termed the neuroendocrine system, and the pituitary gland is said to be under neuroendocrine control. In addition to the hypothalamic-pituitary system, the circumventricular organs also satisfy the criteria of neuroendocrine systems. The term neuroendocrine is also applied to interactions between nerve and endocrine cells in the periphery and especially the viscera, of which the gastrointestinal system and its appendages (especially the pancreas) are the most prominent. Of special relevance to stress is the sympathetic component of the autonomic nervous system and the adrenal medulla. Derived from the embryonic neural crest, the cells of the adrenal medulla are modified postganglionic neurons that secrete their neurotransmitters, mainly adrenaline (epinephrine) and opioids, directly into the bloodstream.

The present article focuses on the principles of neuroendocrine control of the pituitary gland and illustrates how the hypothalamic-pituitary system (1) was used to demonstrate that certain peptides satisfy the criteria of neurotransmitters or neurohormones; (2) played a significant role in our understanding of gene transcription, translation, and posttranslational processing; and (3) could be used as a window to study brain function in the conscious human (neuroendocrine window of the brain). Although only mentioned briefly in this article, neuroendocrinology is also concerned with the effects of pituitary target hormones on the brain-pituitary system, that is, on the way that hormones secreted by the anterior pituitary target glands play an important role in brain differentiation and plasticity; affect central neurotransmission and thereby mood, mental state, and memory; and exert feedback effects on the brain-pituitary system. These hormonal feedback systems constitute the afferent limb of homeostatic regulatory systems, which ensure that the output of pituitary hormones is maintained at a preset and functionally optimal level.

Hypothalamic-Pituitary Axis

Brief History

The central importance of the anterior pituitary gland as conductor of the endocrine orchestra was not understood until the early 1930s when P. E. Smith published his parapharyngeal method for removing the gland (hypophysectomy). The effects of hypophysectomy proved to be so dramatic that for a short period most scientists in the field, including the distinguished neurosurgeon, Harvey Cushing, thought that the pituitary gland was autonomous. However, around the same time, William Rowan, working in Alberta on the annual migration of birds, showed that day length had a potent effect on the growth of the gonads. Rowan's experiments, together with those on seasonal breeding in animals, the effects of stressful stimuli on endocrine organs, and the effects of brain lesions on pituitary hormone secretion led to the concept that the anterior pituitary gland must be under CNS control, a view that Cushing soon adopted. The observational and experimental evidence that supported this concept was summarized by F. H. A. Marshall in his 1936 Croonian lecture.

It had long been known that the pituitary gland and brain were connected by the pituitary stalk, but several lines of evidence suggested that neural control of the anterior pituitary gland was mediated not by nerve fibers in the pituitary stalk but by chemical substances released into the hypophysial portal vessels. These vessels, first described by G. T. Popa and U. Fielding in 1930, surround the pituitary stalk, linking a primary plexus of capillaries at the base of the hypothalamus with a second capillary plexus in the anterior pituitary gland. Throughout the 1930s and 1940s, a debate raged about the direction of blood flow in the hypophysial portal vessels. Based on histological evidence, this debate could have been avoided had someone read the 1935 report by Bernado Houssay and associates that in the living toad blood flowed from the hypothalamus down to the pituitary gland. But Houssay's paper was published in French.

The neurohumoral hypothesis of the control of the anterior pituitary gland was first formally advanced by H. B. Friedgood in 1936 and J. C. Hinsey in 1937. However, it was the elegant pituitary graft experiments of G. W. Harris and Dora Jacobsohn that showed beyond doubt that the anterior pituitary gland was controlled by substances released at nerve terminals in the median eminence at the base of the hypothalamus and transported to the pituitary gland by the hypophysial portal vessels. The characterization of the first three of these substances, thyrotropin-releasing factor (later thyrotropin-releasing hormone, TRH), luteinizing hormone-releasing factor (LRF; later, luteinizing hormone-releasing hormone, LHRH; or gonadotropin-releasing hormone, GnRH), and somatostatin, was to take a further 18–21 years of hard work in the laboratories of Roger Guillemin and Andrew Schally, for which they were awarded the 1977 Nobel Prize for Physiology and Medicine. The sequence of corticotropin releasing factor-41 (CRF-41; later, corticotropin releasing hormone, CRH-41) was determined by Wylie Vale and associates in 1981, a breakthrough that had eluded many workers for more than 25 years.

Soon after its characterization as a decapeptide in 1971, G. Fink and M. Jamieson measured LHRH by radioimmunoassay in hypophysial portal blood of the anesthetized rat and showed that its release could be increased fivefold by a small electrical stimulus applied to the medial preoptic area of the hypothalamus. The neurohumoral hypothesis of neural control of the anterior pituitary control had been proved.

General Anatomy and Development

The pituitary gland is anatomically linked to the hypothalamus at the base of the brain by way of the pituitary stalk (**Figure 1**). The hypothalamus comprises a medial part adjacent to the third cerebral ventricle, in which are located the major hypothalamic nuclei, and a lateral part made up mainly of a large cable of nerve fibers that carries reciprocal fiber tracts between midbrain and forebrain, the medial forebrain bundle (**Figure 2**), in which are embedded aggregations of nerve cell bodies. Axons from nerve cell bodies located in the hypothalamic nuclei project to the median eminence, where they either terminate on the loops of primary capillaries of the hypophysial portal vessels in the external layer of the median eminence or form a cable that passes through the internal layer of the median eminence to form the bulk of the pituitary stalk and then the neural lobe (**Figure 3**). The median eminence, so called because it protrudes as a small dome in the midline from the base of the hypothalamus, forms the floor of the third ventricle and is delineated by the optic chiasm in front, the mamillary bodies behind, and a depression (hypothalamic sulcus) on either side. Arising from the median eminence is the neural stalk, which links the pituitary gland to the brain.

The pituitary gland is located in a fossa in the basisphenoid bone at the base of the skull, the sella turcica (so called because its shape resembles a Turkish saddle). The close proximity of the hypothalamus and pituitary gland to the optic chiasm means that tumors in either the hypothalamus or the pituitary gland may press on, or more rarely invade, the optic chiasm or tracts, thereby leading to visual defects.

The hypothalamic-pituitary axis is divided functionally into two systems (**Figure 4**): the hypothalamo-adenohypophysial axis (the hypothalamus, hypophysial portal vessels, and adenohypophysis) and the hypothalamo-neurohypophysial axis (the hypothalamus, neural stalk, and neural lobe). The neural stalk is made up of numerous nerve fibers that project mainly from the PVN and SON of the hypothalamus to terminate on a capillary bed derived from the inferior hypophysial artery and located in the neural lobe of the pituitary gland. Nerve fibers in the neural lobe (or pars nervosa) are surrounded by pituicytes, the equivalent of glial cells. Also present in the neural stalk are nerve fibers of other types of chemical neurotransmitter (in addition to AVP and oxytocin), such as the endogenous opioids and dopamine, which are present in nerve fibers that project from the arcuate nucleus and innervate the pars intermedia. Because the stalk and median eminence are continuous, these dopaminergic neurons are a continuation of a dense palisade of dopaminergic

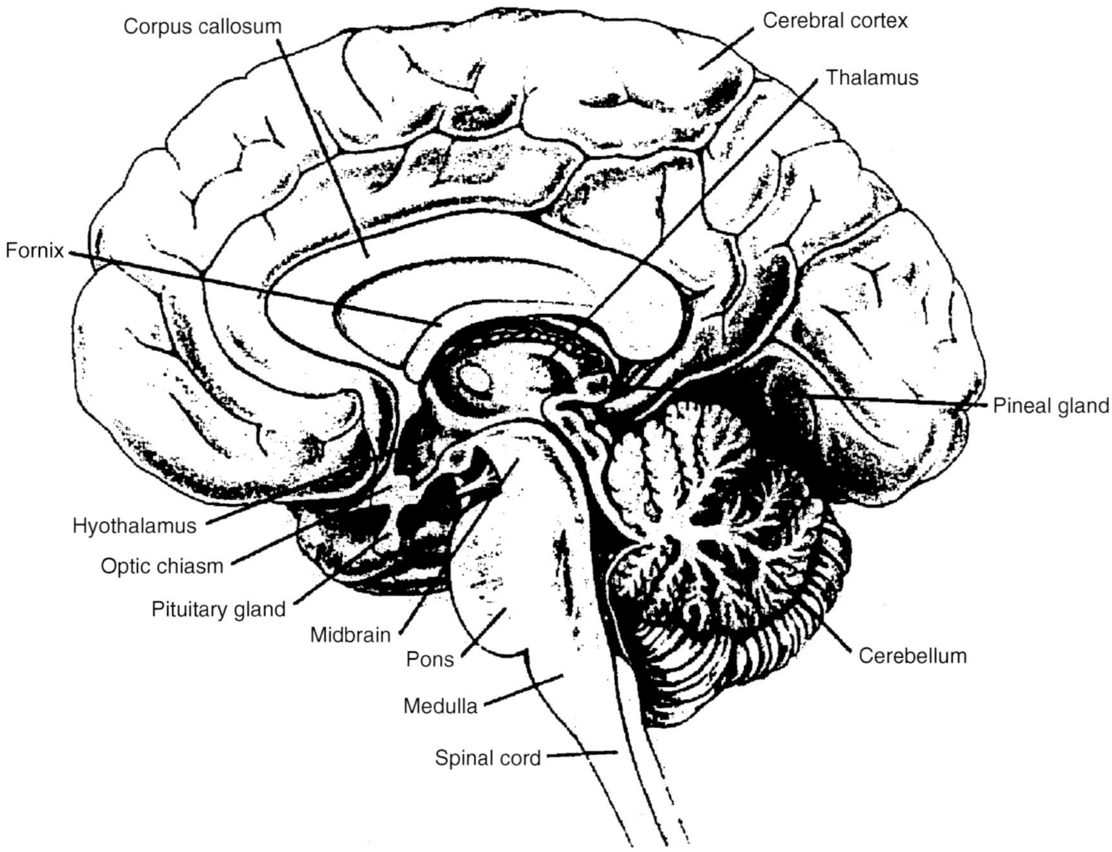

Figure 1 A midsagittal section of the human brain showing the inside (medial) surface. Note the pituitary gland attached by way of the pituitary stalk to the floor of the hypothalamus. The hypothalamus and the thalamus, which lies above it, form the wall of the third cerebral ventricle, at the posterior end of which is the pineal gland.

fibers that also terminate on the primary plexus of the hypophysial portal vessels enmeshed with nerve fibers that contain other neurohormones. The pituitary stalk and median eminence are covered by a single layer of cells termed the pars tuberalis, which is continuous with the pars distalis.

The adenohypophysis develops from an outgrowth of the ectodermal placode, which forms the roof of the embryonic mouth (or stomadeum). This ectodermal outgrowth forms Rathke's pouch and meets the neurohypophysis, which grows down from the floor of the embryonic third ventricle. Rathke's pouch closes and separates from the roof of the mouth. The caudal (rear) part of the pouch remains thin to form the pars intermedia, which becomes tightly juxtaposed to the rostral surface of the neurohypophysis (**Figure 5**). The rostral part of the pouch develops into the pars distalis (**Figure 5**). Vascularization of the median eminence and the pituitary gland begins on approximately day 15 of embryonic life (E15) in the rat, and the hypophysial portal vessels become defined by E18. Nerve terminals in the median eminence with granular vesicles (presumably neurohormones) are first evident on E16 and the first secretory granules appear in pars distalis cells on E17. This sequence of embryonic development suggests that the development of secretory cells in the pars distalis may depend in part on the development of nerve terminals in the median eminence and the anlage of the hypophysial portal vessels.

Neurohemal Junctions and Circumventricular Organs

Neurohemal junctions are the fundamental functional modules of the major central neuroendocrine system, the median eminence. They are composed of nerve terminals and capillaries that are closely juxtaposed and thereby facilitate the transport of chemical messengers from nerve terminals into the bloodstream and *vice versa* (**Figure 6**). Neurohemal junctions are also the fundamental units of the neurohypophysis and of the circumventricular organs, such as the organum vasculosum of the lamina terminalis, the subfornical organ, and the pineal gland, which are located at various sites around the third cerebral ventricle, and the area postrema, located in the floor of the fourth cerebral ventricle. All the circumventricular organs are characterized by the fact that their vessels are fenestrated (**Figure 6**) and that

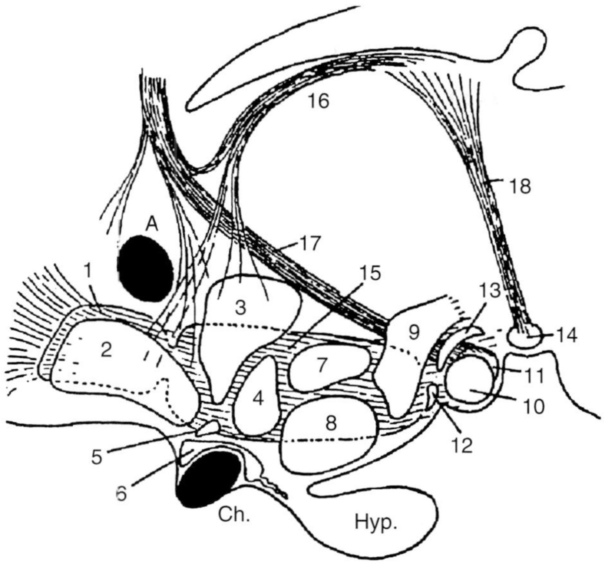

Figure 2 Diagram showing the relative positions in a sagittal plane of hypothalamic nuclei in a typical mammalian brain and their relation to the fornix, stria habenularis, and fasciculus retroflexus. (1) Lateral preoptic nucleus (permeated by the medial forebrain bundle). (2) Medial preoptic nucleus. (3) Paraventricular nucleus. (4) Anterior hypothalamic area. (5) Suprachiasmatic nucleus. (6) Supraoptic nucleus. (7) Dorsomedial hypothalamic nucleus. (8) Ventromedial hypothalamic nucleus. (9) Posterior hypothalamic nucleus. (10) Medial mamillary nucleus. (11) Lateral mamillary nucleus. (12) Premamillary nucleus. (13) Supramamillary nucleus. (14) Interpeduncular nucleus (a mesencephalic element in which the fasciculus retroflexus terminates). (15) Lateral hypothalamic nucleus (permeated by the medial forebrain bundle). (16) Stria habenularis. (17) Fornix. (18) Fasciculus retroflexus of Meynert (habenulopeduncular tract). A, anterior commissure; Ch., optic chiasma; Hyp., hypophysis (pituitary gland).

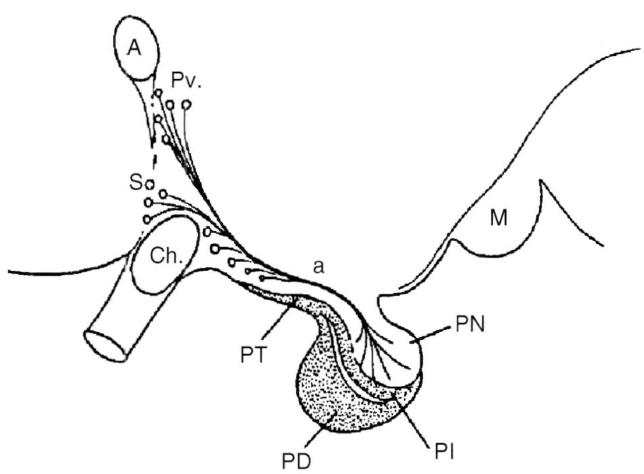

Figure 3 Schematic section of the mammalian hypothalamus and pituitary gland showing the neurohypophysial tract (labeled a) comprised mainly of fibers derived from the paraventricular (Pv.) and supraoptic (So) nuclei. A, anterior commissure; Ch., optic chiasma; M, mamillary bodies; PD, pars distalis; PI, pars intermedia; PN, pars nervosa; PT, pars tuberalis.

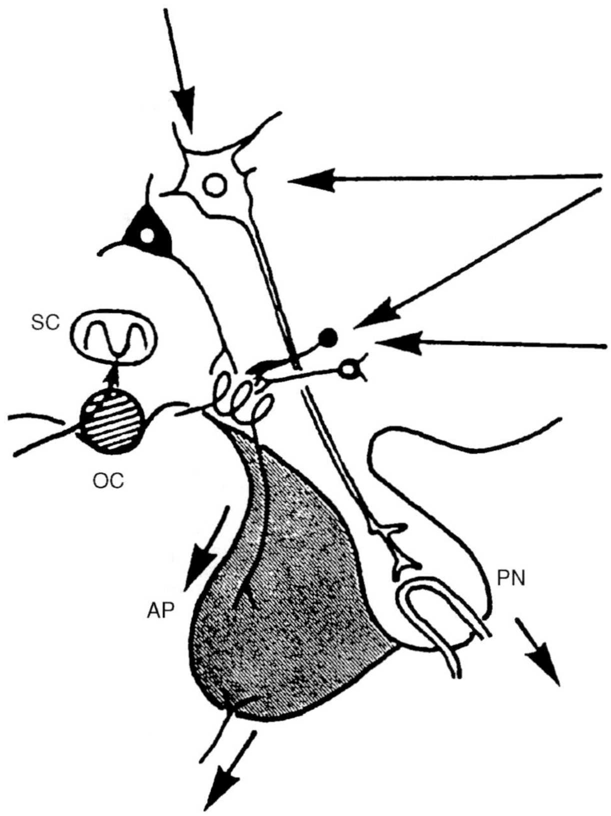

Figure 4 Schematic diagram of the hypothalamic-pituitary system showing the magnocellular (white) projections directly to the systemic capillaries of the pars nervosa (PN) and the parvicellular (black) projections to the primary plexus of the hypophysial portal vessels, which convey neurohormones to the pars distalis of the anterior pituitary gland (AP). Dorsal to the optic chiasm (OC) are suprachiasmatic nuclei (SC), which receive direct projections from the retina and play a key role in the control of circadian rhythms (indicated by the sinusoidal curve). Activity of the intrinsic neurons of the hypothalamus is influenced greatly by projections (arrows) from numerous areas of the forebrain, midbrain, and hindbrain, particularly the limbic system, as well as by hormones, mainly estrogen and progesterone in the case of the hypothalamic-pituitary-gonadal system.

the blood–brain barrier is inoperative at these sites. The neurohemal junctions in the median eminence, neurohypophysis, and pineal gland facilitate the transport of neurohormones from the nerve terminals or nerve cell derivatives (pineal) into the bloodstream, whereas at the other circumventricular organs, neurohemal junctions facilitate the transport of neurohormones from the blood to nerve cells. The latter mechanism has been implicated in the cross-talk between peripheral organs and the brain so that, for example, the hypertensive effect of the peptide, angiotensin, is due in part to its activation of neurons of the subfornical organ, which have a high density of angiotensin receptors. In addition to their importance as sites for the transfer of chemical messengers from nerve terminals into blood vessels, and *vice versa*,

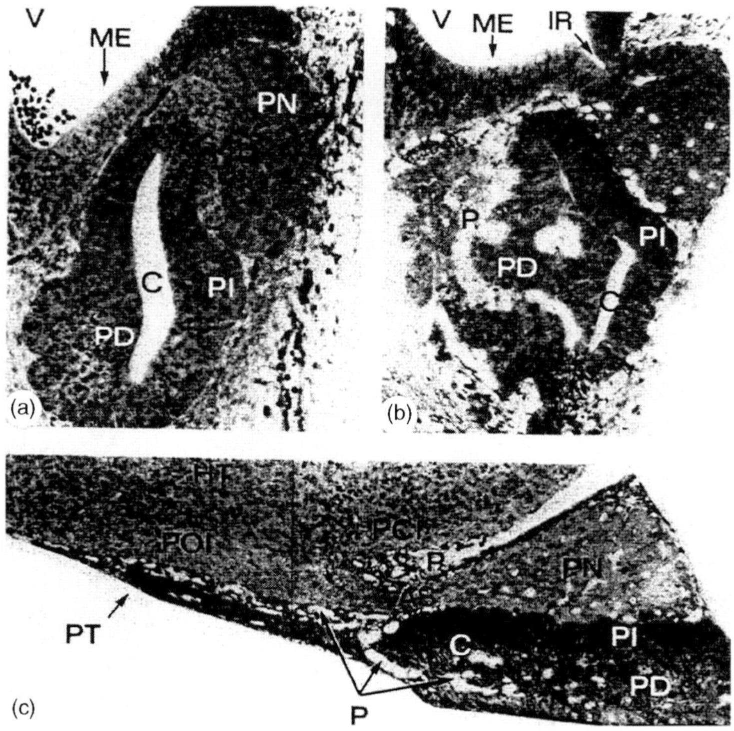

Figure 5 Photomicrographs of midline sagittal sections through the hypothalamic-pituitary complex showing the development of the pituitary gland in the rat. a, On embryonic day 15 (E15; × 120); b, on E17 (× 120); c, on E20 (× 80). In a, the pituitary anlage shortly after closure of Rathke's pouch, which migrates dorsally to meet neurohypophysial downgrowth from the floor of the hypothalamus. Rotation of the pituitary gland caudally through 135° with respect to the base of the diencephalon (hypothalamus) is seen, as is the invasion of the pars distalis (PD) by the leash of portal vessels (P) on E17. AS, anatomical stem; C, hypophysial cleft; HT, hypothalamus; IR, infundibular recess; ME, median eminence; PCI, pars caudalis infundibuli; PI, pars intermedia; PN, pars nervosa; POI, pars oralis infundibuli; PT, pars tuberalis; V, third ventricle. (1-μm Araldite sections, toluidine blue stain.) Reproduced with permission from Fink, G. and Smith, G. C. (1971), Ultrastructural features of the developing hypothalamo-hypophysial axis in the rat, *Zeitschrift für Zellforschung und mikroskopische Anatomie* **119**, 208–226.

the neurohemal junctions of circumventricular organs are also sites at which drugs or toxins, which are normally excluded by the blood–brain barrier, can penetrate the brain and affect brain function.

The Hypothalamo-Adenohypophysial System

Neurohormonal Control of Anterior Pituitary Hormone Secretion

The transmission of signals between the brain and the anterior pituitary gland is mediated by chemical messengers called neurohormones, which are transported by the hypophysial portal vessels from the hypothalamus to the anterior pituitary gland (**Figures 3–5**) where they either stimulate or inhibit the release of anterior pituitary hormones. Synthesized in nerve cells of the hypothalamic nuclei, the neurohormones are released from nerve terminals into the plexus of primary capillaries of the hypophysial portal vessel system. These capillaries are derived from the superior hypophysial arteries and coalesce to form the hypophysial portal veins, which run on the surface or through the pituitary stalk to the anterior pituitary gland, where they form a secondary plexus of vessels called the pituitary sinusoids. Vessels on the surface of the stalk are the long portal vessels, whereas those within the substance of the stalk are the short portal vessels.

Hypophysial Portal Vessels

The portal vessels are so called because they transport chemical messengers from one capillary bed (primary capillaries) to a second capillary bed before entering the general circulation. In principle, this is identical to the hepatic portal system, which transports substances from the primary bed of capillaries in the intestine and its appendages (e.g., the pancreas) to a second bed of capillaries or sinusoids in the liver. Fenestration of the primary and the secondary (sinusoids) plexus of capillaries (**Figure 6**) facilitates the transport of substances across the capillary wall.

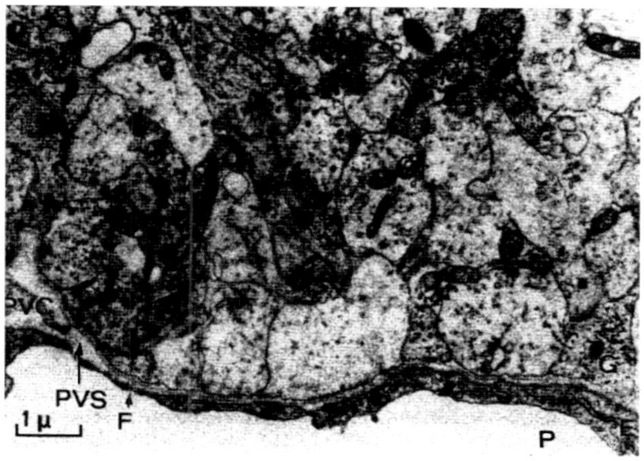

Figure 6 Electromicrograph of the external layer of the median eminence of a rat on the first postnatal day (× 13,200). Note the high density of nerve terminals around part of a primary portal capillary vessel (P), which is fenestrated (F). Note also the large number of agranular and granular vesicles in the nerve terminals. These vesicles contain the packets (quanta) of neurohormone or neurotransmitter that are released on nerve depolarization as a consequence of nerve action potentials. The neurohormones are released into the perivascular space and from there move rapidly into portal vessel blood for transport to the pituitary gland. This arrangement is typical of neurohemal junctions found in the several circumventricular organs of the brain. E, endothelial cell; G, glial process; PVC, perivascular cell; PVS, perivascular space. Reproduced with permission from Fink, G. and Smith, G. C. (1971), Ultrastructural features of the developing hypothalamo-hypophysial axis in the rat, *Zeitschrift für Zellforschung und Mikroskopische Anatomie* **119**, 208–226.

Hormones released from anterior pituitary cells are transported by pituitary veins into the systemic circulation by which they are transported to their major target organs, the gonads and the adrenal and thyroid glands.

Hypothalamic Neurohormones

Outline Most of the neurohormones that mediate the neural control of anterior pituitary hormone secretion are peptides that are synthesized in discrete hypothalamic nuclei. Neurohormone-secreting neurons are the final common pathway neurons for neural control of the anterior pituitary gland, a term borrowed by G. W. Harris from Sherrington's description of the alpha-motor neurons of the spinal cord that innervate and control the contraction of skeletal muscles. Like the alpha-motor neurons, hypothalamic neurons are controlled by inputs to the hypothalamus from the brain stem, midbrain, and higher brain centers. The hypothalamic neuroendocrine neurons are thus connected with many other regions of the nervous system and, in particular, the components of the limbic system, which is involved in higher brain functions, including emotion, olfaction, and memory.

The neural control of all established anterior pituitary hormones is mediated by at least one or more neurohormones. In some cases, two neurohormones may act synergistically, as is the case of ACTH, the release of which is stimulated by both the 41-amino-acid-residue peptide CRH-41 and the nonapeptide AVP. The control of ACTH secretion is further complicated by the fact that urocortins, relatively new members of the CRH-41 family of peptides, act mainly by way of CRH type 2 receptors in the PVN to modulate AVP and CRH-41 synthesis. Hypophysial portal blood and immunoneutralization studies suggest that ACTH secretion may be inhibited by atrial natriuretic peptide (ANP).

In other cases two neurohormones may act antagonistically, as is the case for GH, whose release is stimulated by the 44-amino-acid-residue peptide GH-releasing hormone (GHRH-44) and inhibited by the 14- or 28-residue peptide somatostatin-14 or -28. The neural regulation of pituitary GH secretion is even more complex than originally thought; Bowers and associates discovered in 1981 that a hexapeptide, referred to as GH-releasing peptide-6 (GHRP-6), is a potent GH secretagogue. Subsequent studies showed that GHRP-6 binds to a receptor, GH secretagogue receptor (GHS-R), that is distinct from the GHRH-44 receptor. The endogenous ligand for the GHS-R is ghrelin, a 28-amino-acid-residue peptide secreted mainly by neuroendocrine cells of the gastric mucosa, which also stimulates GH release.

Prolactin seems to be the only anterior pituitary hormone that is predominantly under the inhibitory control of the brain. Evidence for this came first from the studies of Everett and Nikitowitch-Winer, who showed that prolactotrophs were the only cell type that did not undergo atrophy in pituitary grafts underthe kidney capsule, where they are far removed from central neural control. This histological observation was confirmed by the finding that prolactin concentrations in plasma are increased in animals bearing pituitary grafts under the kidney capsule. There is substantial evidence that dopamine, released into hypophysial portal blood from tuberoinfundibular dopaminergic neurons, inhibits prolactin release. Indeed, dopamine agonists such as bromocriptine, cabergoline, and quinagolide are highly effective in treating hyperprolactinemia, a relatively common cause of infertility in women. Dopamine is now regarded as the prolactin inhibitory factor (PIF). Hyperprolactinemia is frequently due to benig tumors (adenomas) of the anterior pituitary gland, and these too can often be controlled by treatment with dopamine agonists. Stress is another common cause of hyperprolactinemia. Indeed, the prolactin response to stress in the human is as sensitive as that of ACTH and adrenal glucocorticoid response to stress.

The search for a prolactin-releasing factor (PRF) has continued for many years. Potential candidates have included TRH, vasoactive intestinal peptide, GnRH-associated peptide (GAP), and two novel, closely related hypothalamic peptides (termed PrRP31 and PrRP20) discovered in 1998 by Hinuma and associates when searching for a ligand for an orphan receptor (hGR3). Recent evidence suggests that the peptides intermedin and adrenomedullin may also release prolactin. However, although all these compounds are capable of stimulating prolactin release from pituitary cells *in vitro*, and in some cases under pharmacological conditions *in vivo*, robust proof that any of these compounds are the physiological PRF remains to be established.

The neural control of the gonadotropins, luteinizing hormone (LH) and follicle-stimulating hormone (FSH), is mediated by one and the same decapeptide, GnRH.

Criteria for neurohormones and neurotransmitters Werman, in 1972, summarized the criteria for classifying a candidate compound as a neurotransmitter or neurohormone thus: "If it can be shown that a substance is released into the extracellular space from presynaptic nerves in quantities consistent with the amount and rate of stimulation and the physiology of transmitter release at that junction, and if it can be shown that the material released acts on postsynaptic membranes by using molecular mechanisms identical with those used by the physiologically evoked transmitter, then that substance is a transmitter." Werman's two principal criteria – endogenous release (collectibility) and exogenous mimicry (identity of action) – should be supplemented by a third criterion invoking the topochemistry of the mechanisms for the synthesis and inactivation of the transmitter.

The technique of collecting hypophysial portal blood in the anesthetized rat (developed by Fink and Worthington in 1966) has made it possible to satisfy these criteria for all the hypothalamic-pituitary neurohormones outlined here, as well to clarify the mechanism and physiological significance of post-translational processing. The measurement of neurohormone release into the hypophysial portal blood has also made it possible to ascertain whether newly discovered hypothalamic compounds could serve as hypothalamic-pituitary regulatory factors. This is exemplified by work in our laboratory, which showed that the concentrations of the cardiac peptide ANP were about four times greater in portal than in systemic blood, a finding that led to immunoneutralization studies that suggest that ANP is an ACTH-inhibiting factor. Studies of hypophysial portal blood can also exclude the neurohormonal role of a candidate neurotransmitter. Thus, for example, although immunohistochemistry suggests that angiotensin and cholecystokinin are both present in the median eminence, their concentrations in portal blood are not greater than in peripheral blood, which makes it unlikely that either plays a role as a neurohormone.

All the hypothalamic-pituitary regulatory neurohormones are present in regions of the nervous system outside the hypothalamus, where Werman's criteria for a neurotransmitter need to be proved by determining whether the neurohormones are released (by push–pull cannulae or dialysis), activate cells (e.g., electophysiologically), and are responsible for a behavioral effect. The functional significance of neurohormone action in areas of the CNS outside the hypothalamus is illustrated poignantly by CRH-41, which is believed to synchronize the endocrine, autonomic, immunological, and behavioral responses to stress.

Neurohormone receptors The hypothalamic neurohormones and their receptors, all members of the G-protein-coupled, seven transmembrane superfamily, underscore the adage that the evolution of hormones is less dependent on structural changes in the hormones than on the uses to which they are put. The latter depends entirely on the receptors and the signal transduction systems that mediate receptor activation, a point illustrated by the receptors that mediate the neurohormone control of ACTH and GH secretion.

The actions of CRH-41 in brain and periphery are mediated by two main receptor subtypes, CRH1 and CRH2, with splice variants CRH2α and CRH2β. A third CRH receptor has recently been discovered in catfish pituitary. cAMP-linked CRH receptors also mediate the action of the urocortins, the mammalian homologs of urotensin in fish, and of sauvagine, a homolog of CRH-41 derived from the South American tree frog. In addition to mediating the neural control of ACTH release, CRH-41 and the urocortins exert actions on the brain and the cardiovascular system. CRH1 receptors (1) are localized predominantly in brain and pituitary, (2) have a high affinity for CRH-41, (3) are expressed by pituitary corticotrophs, and (4) are responsible for mediating the stress-induced CRH-41 stimulation of ACTH release. CRH2 receptors have a greater affinity for the urocortins than for CRH-41 and are present mainly in heart and skeletal muscle. However, the CRH2α splice variant is also present in brain and pituitary gland, where it is expressed by pituitary gonadotrophs, but not corticotrophs, leading to the suggestion that

CRH2α may mediate stress effects on gonadotropin secretion. The ACTH-releasing action of CRH-41 is potentiated by AVP, which binds to the $V_{1\beta}$ receptor. The $V_{1\beta}$ receptor activates the inositol phospholipid cycle. Synergism between CRH-41 and AVP involves calcium-activated cAMP production. ACTH secretion is inhibited by ANP, an action mediated by two guanylyl cyclase-coupled receptor subtypes: A and B.

Human GHRH receptor cDNA was first cloned and sequenced in Mike Thorner's laboratory in 1993 and was found to be a member of a family of receptors that includes secretin, calcitonin, vasoactive intestinal peptide, and parathyroid hormone. The activity of the GHRH receptor (GHRH-R) promoter is enhanced by the pituitary-specific transcription factor POU1FI (formerly Pit-l). The importance of POU1FI, the prototypic POU-homeodomain transcription factor, for the development and activity of the GHRH-R is demonstrated by the fact that the GHRH-R is not present in the pituitary gland of dwarf mice (*dw/dw*) that lack POU1FI. Glucocorticoids stimulate, whereas estrogen inhibits, GHRH-R gene expression, actions that are likely to be mediated by the glucocorticoid and estrogen response elements present in the promoter and that explain in part the physiological effects of glucocorticoids and estrogen on GH secretion. The pituitary expression of GHRH-R mRNA in the rat increases with embryonic development to reach a peak at E19.5 (2 days before parturition), followed by a decline through to postnatal day 12 and then an increase to day 30, followed by a decline with age. If a similar pattern occurs at the corresponding times in humans, then that could be a major factor in the decline in plasma GH concentrations with age in the elderly. The GHRH-R is distinct from the GHS-R whose ligand is the 28-amino-acid-residue gastric peptide ghrelin. Both types of receptor are members of the seven-transmembrane helix, G-protein-coupled receptor family.

There are six receptors for somatostatin (SSTR), encoded by five distinct genes. All six receptors are present in the anterior pituitary gland; SSTR-5 is the most prominent on the somatotrophs, followed by SSTR-2 (which has splice variants A and B). Hypothalamic arcuate neurons that secrete GHRH express SSTR-2 and SSTR-1, supporting the proposition that the action of somatostatin may involve an effect on the release of GHRH. Relatively large amounts of somatostatin are also present in the cerebral cortex and hippocampus, regions that express the SSTR-2A. In the periphery, somatostatin secreted by pancreatic islet cells inhibits the secretion of insulin, glucagon, and a range of gut peptides.

The complexity of the receptors involved in the control of ACTH and GH secretion contrasts with the apparent simplicity of the gonadotropin control system, in which GnRH mediates the neural control of both LH and FSH, and the apparent simplicity of the thyrotropin and prolactin control systems, in which there is evidence, so far, for only one neurohormone each, TRH and the PIF dopamine, respectively. Dopamine inhibition of prolactin release is mediated by the dopamine 2 (D2) receptor. Alternative splicing results in a long and short form of the D2 receptor, and this allows coupling to different types of G-protein. When activated, the D2 receptor inhibits adenylyl cyclase.

Whether the complexity of the neurohormones and receptors involved in the neural control of GH and ACTH release is a consequence of evolutionary convergence of different regulatory systems that are not deleterious and are therefore retained or whether complexity has developed as a consequence of selective pressure to provide flexibility or increase the number of variables that can influence the two systems remains to be determined.

Clinical relevance All the hypothalamic neurohormones have been used extensively as tests of anterior pituitary function, or pituitary responsiveness. In addition, neurohormone agonists and antagonists have been deployed for a variety of diagnostic tests and therapeutic regimes. Thus, analogs of CRH-41 and urocortin have been developed with a view to their possible use in the treatment of depression, anxiety, anorexia nervosa, and stroke. The use of dopamine agonists, such as bromocriptine, cabergoline, and quinagolide, for the treatment of hyperprolactinemia and prolactin-secreting pituitary adenomata has been mentioned previously. GnRH superactive agonists and antagonists are used for chemical castration, as an adjunct treatment of cancer of the breast and prostate gland, for fertility control, and for the treatment of infertility and precocious puberty. Somatostatin, or its potent synthetic analogs such as Octreotride, has been used in the treatment of GH-secreting pituitary adenomas that lead to acromegaly and also ectopic GH-secreting tumors, most commonly small-cell carcinomas of the lung or tumors of the gastrointestinal system. The action of Octreotide in treating GH-secreting tumors can be potentiated by dopamine agonists such as bromocriptine and cabergoline.

Somatostatin and its agonists are also effective in the treatment of pancreatitis. Orally active, nonpeptide mimetics of GHRP-6, such as MK-677, have been developed and these may have therapeutic value in the treatment of children of short stature and adult GH deficiency. GHRH, GHRP-6, and its mimetics are also being explored as useful agents for the treatment of metabolic deficiencies that occur in aging.

Teleology of Neurohormonal Control

The hypothalamic-pituitary axis illustrates the remarkable economy of physiological systems. First, and perhaps most impressive, are the hypophysial portal vessels, which, by transporting the neurohormones from the hypothalamus to the pituitary gland, undiluted by mixture in the systemic circulation, ensure that hypothalamic neurohormones released in very small amounts from the hypothalamus reach the pituitary gland at concentrations several orders of magnitude greater than in the systemic circulation and therefore sufficient to exert their effects. The corollary of this is that relatively little neurohormone needs to be released to exert its effect and that therefore only a small amount of new neurohormone needs to be synthesized. The metabolic economy of the hypophysial portal system is brought into sharp relief by the fact that the hypothalamic concentration and total content of the hypothalamic-anterior pituitary regulatory neurohormones are three or more orders of magnitude lower than those of the neurohypophysial nonapeptides AVP and oxytocin, which reach their peripheral targets by the systemic circulation.

Second, the transport of neurohormones at effective concentrations by the hypophysial portal vessels also protects the body from the potential adverse effects of the high concentrations of neurohormones necessary to stimulate or inhibit pituitary hormone secretion. Thus, for example, the high portal blood concentrations of somatostatin may, in the systemic circulation, have adverse effects on the gut and on insulin secretion by the pancreatic islets. Similarly, as shown by Fink and associates, the portal plasma concentrations of ANP that inhibit ACTH secretion would, in the systemic circulation, cause a lethal drop in blood pressure.

Third, neurohormones in the hypothalamo-adenohypophysial system, by also serving as chemical messengers in several related systems or mechanisms, may serve to orchestrate appropriate physiological responses. Thus, for example, somatostatin, in addition to inhibiting GH secretion is also secreted by pancreatic islets and inhibits the secretion of insulin, glucagon, and a range of gut peptides. As mentioned earlier, CRH-41 is present in higher brain centers and in the periphery, and it has been implicated in stress-related behaviors, cardiovascular control, and the synchronization of the endocrine, autonomic, and immunological components of the stress response.

The Hypothalamo-Neurohypophysial System

Principles and Overview

The neural lobe is the site of release of the nonapeptides oxytocin and AVP into the systemic circulation. Presumably because a considerable distance removes the target cells of these peptides from their site of release in the neural lobe and because there is massive dilution in the systemic circulation, the rate and the amount of synthesis of oxytocin and AVP and their content in the hypothalamus are about three orders of magnitude greater than that of neurohormones concerned in anterior pituitary control. This fact, together with their synthesis in discrete hypothalamic nuclei, their ease of assay, and that both nonapeptides contain disulfide bridges that allow the incorporation of the radioactive tracer [^{35}S]-cysteine, contributed to four important landmarks in neuroendocrinology. First, oxytocin and AVP were the first of the hypothalamic neurohormones to be sequenced (by Du Vigneaud and colleagues). Second, the glycoprotein components of their precursor proteins led to their conspicuous histochemical staining and thereby to the concept of neurosecretion (the Scharrers), a term applied to neurons whose main purpose seemed to be to secrete neurohormones rather than transmit signals by propagated action potentials. Third, the fact that both peptides have disulfide bridges and that synthesis involves the incorporation of cysteine, which can be labeled with the relatively high-energy radionuclide ^{35}S, made them excellent models for the first studies of neuropeptide synthesis and transport (first shown by Sachs and associates). Fourth, oxytocin- and AVP-containing neurons were the first neuroendocrine neurons from which electrophysiological recordings were made (by J. Green and B. Cross in 1959).

The concept of neurosecretion was soon discarded because it was shown that the magnocellular neurons are no different from others – they propagate action potentials and release neurohormones or neurotransmitters. In fact, oxytocin- and AVP-containing neurons facilitate electrophysiological recording because they are large and because their axons terminate in the surgically accessible neural lobe. This makes it relatively easy to locate and verify by antidromic stimulation the identity of the neurons and record from them. Furthermore, the electrophysiological activity of the hypothalamic magnocellular neurons can be correlated with the secretion of AVP and oxytocin.

Finally, because the neural lobe is largely made up of nerve terminals, it proved to be a useful model for the study of exocytosis and stimulus-secretion coupling, the coupling between the cascade of ion fluxes through membrane channels (membrane depolarization) triggered by action potentials and the calcium-dependent release of neurohormones or neurotransmitters. Neurohormones, like all other known neurotransmitters and peptide and protein hormones, are packaged in secretory vesicles (**Figure 6**), which are released in packets or quanta.

Function

AVP (or the antidiuretic hormone) is concerned mainly with the control of body water. As its name implies, AVP also induces vasoconstriction and thereby can increase blood pressure, although this mechanism usually becomes operational only after a substantial loss of blood volume. AVP cells of the SON and PVN respond to osmotic stimuli. An increase in plasma osmolality triggers the release of AVP, which increases water reuptake in the nephron, which as a consequence causes an overall increase in body water with a fall in plasma osmolality. This is a perfect example of a homeostatic regulatory mechanism. In addition to its role in osmoregulation, AVP synthesized in the smaller (parvicellular) neurons of the PVN acts synergistically with CRH-41 to release ACTH.

Oxytocin, concerned mainly with milk ejection during lactation and parturition (the birth process), provides the perfect example of the role of neurohormones in neuroendocrine reflexes. Thus, oxytocin is the neurohormonal component of the milk-ejection reflex whereby suckling at the nipple of lactating mothers triggers volleys of impulses that travel through the mammary nerves to the spinal cord and, by way of a multisynaptic pathway, reach the hypothalamus where they trigger the release of oxytocin. Oxytocin transported by the systemic circulation stimulates the contraction of the myoepithelial cells of the breast, resulting in milk ejection. During parturition, oxytocin coordinates and reinforces uterine contractions. That is, as uterine contractions force the head of the fetus against the cervix, volleys of impulses are triggered that ascend through multisynaptic pathways involving the pelvic nerves and the spinal cord to the hypothalamus to trigger the release of oxytocin, which acts on the smooth muscle cells of the uterus. This is a classical positive feedback system, which is terminated by expulsion of the fetus and placenta.

The Intermediate Lobe of the Pituitary Gland

Model for Posttranslational Processing

The major secretion of the intermediate lobe of the pituitary gland is α-melanocyte-stimulating hormone (α-MSH), a 13-amino-acid-residue peptide that, together with ACTH and β-endorphin, is derived from the precursor proopiomelanocortin (POMC). In addition to α-MSH, the pars intermedia also contains other derivatives of POMC – β-MSH, γ-MSH, corticotropin-like intermediate lobe peptide (CLIP), and β-endorphin – which together with the ACTH make up the melanocortins. The fact that in the pars distalis ACTH is the major hormone derived from posttranslational processing of POMC, whereas in the pars intermedia α-MSH is the major active hormonal product of POMC processing, reflects the presence of different enzymatic processing pathways in the two parts of the gland. The release of α-MSH is inhibited by dopaminergic neurons that originate in the arcuate nucleus and reach the intermediate lobe by way of the neural stalk. Humans are conspicuous among mammals in that the pars intermedia is not defined as a separate lobe of the human pituitary gland.

Melanocortins

Although they are all derived from POMC, melanocortins have diverse physiological functions. α-MSH, first thought to stimulate the growth of melanocytes and pigment formation (melanogenesis), is also involved in fever, inflammation, and the immune response. Indeed, several of the melanocortins, including ACTH, affect cytokine-induced effects on thymocytes, T and B lymphocytes, and neutrophils. The actions of the melanocortins are mediated by five melanocortin receptor subtypes (MC1–5). Although all the melanocortin receptors are seven-transmembrane G-protein-coupled, the tissue distribution of the five receptors is quite distinct. Thus, the MC1 is located on melanocytes and mediates MSH-stimulated melanocyte proliferation and melanogenesis, while the MC2 receptor is located in the adrenal cortex, where it mediates the ACTH-induced secretion of glucocorticoids and mineralocorticoids. The MC3 and MC4 receptors are both located in the brain; the function of MC3 is unknown, but MC4 is involved, together with leptin (a protein produced by adipocytes) and neuropeptide Y, in the regulation of body weight. Studies on mutant *ob/ob* mice show that the action of leptin in regulating body weight is mediated, at least in part, by hypothalamic melanocortin activation, which results in decreased food intake. The importance of hypothalamic melanocortin activity for moderating food intake is illustrated by the agouti peptide, which is a high-affinity antagonist for the MC1 receptor and induces obesity in the mouse. The MC4 receptor is also involved in grooming behavior. The MC5 receptor, whose function remains unknown, is widely distributed in body organs, including the spleen, thymus, skin, and bone marrow. Cutaneous pigmentation is a function of the MC1 receptor, and MC1 gene variants may predispose to red hair and light skin color, which may make the individual susceptible to melanoma.

Pineal Gland: Melatonin and Photoperiodic Control of Circadian Rhythms

The pineal gland is a circumventricular organ (**Figure 1**) that secretes melatonin into the circulation and plays an important role in the photoperiodic control of reproduction in seasonal breeding animals. The gland deserves special mention here because it reinforces the principles of neuroendocrine control. Philosophers (e.g., Descartes, who called this the seat of the soul) and scientists have long been intrigued by the pineal. The secretion of melatonin is exquisitely sensitive to light. Pinealocytes in submammalian species are photoreceptors, and the gland offers an excellent experimental model for studies of the transduction of light into nerve impulses and neurohormone secretion.

The outer segment (sensory pole) of the pinealocyte in fish, amphibia, and reptiles has all the ultrastructural characteristics of a true photoreceptor, but these features are only vestigial in mammals and intermediate forms exist in birds. In fish, amphibia, and reptiles, the effector pole of the pinealocyte synapses with secondary pineal neurons that give rise to the pineal tract, which transmits signals to the CNS. In birds and mammals, however, pinealocytes secrete melatonin directly into the circulation (or cerebrospinal fluid) in a neuroendocrine manner.

Melatonin, a derivative of serotonin, is synthesized within pinealocytes in two steps. First, serotonin is converted by *N*-acetyl-transferase (NAT) to *N*-acetyl serotonin, which is then converted to melatonin by hydroxyindole-*O*-methyltransferase. Because little if any melatonin is stored, the rate of melatonin secretion is tightly linked to its synthesis, which depends on NAT action, which in turn depends on norepinephrine release from the dense sympathetic innervation of the gland. In mammals, the control of melatonin secretion by light is mediated by a multisynaptic pathway that starts in the retina of the eye and successively involves synapses in the suprachiasmatic nuclei, the PVN, the intermediolateral column of the spinal cord, and the neurons of the superior cervical ganglion of the sympathetic nervous system. Sympathetic terminals in the pineal gland release norepinephrine, which stimulates melatonin secretion by an action on adrenoreceptors on pinealocytes. cAMP seems to be the main intracellular second messenger that mediates the action of norepinephrine in this system. The main point of regulation seems to be NAT, which, depending on the species, can be affected at the level of NAT gene expression as well by posttranslational modifications that alter the activity of the enzyme.

The secretion of melatonin starts with the onset of the dark period (night) and stops with the onset of the light period (day). The secretion of melatonin during the dark period is stopped abruptly by exposure to light. In blind people, the secretion of melatonin takes on the typical 25-h free-running period. Taken together, these and other data suggest that the secretion of melatonin is predominantly controlled by light exposure superimposed on the intrinsic rhythm of the major neural clock, the suprachiasmatic nuclei.

An interaction between melatonin and the hypothalamic-pituitary-adrenal stress response system has been suggested; indeed, melatonin has been implicated in glucocorticoid receptor-induced gene expression. However, the precise role of melatonin in the circadian rhythm of ACTH and adrenal corticosteroids, and in the stress response, has yet to be established. This applies equally to the long-researched but unanswered questions as to whether melatonin is a hypnotic or sedative and whether it can resynchronize circadian rhythms that have been disrupted by rapidly crossing time zones (jet lag). Melatonin is a powerful antioxidant, which may explain some of its alleged beneficial effects with respect to aging. So far, the most robust evidence regarding the function of melatonin in mammals relates to its inhibitory actions with respect to reproduction, especially in seasonal breeding animals such as the wallaby, hamster, vole, and sheep.

What is well established is that the suprachiasmatic nuclei constitute the central generator of circadian rhythms of the body, with one notable exception – the daily anticipation of a meal. That is, rats in which the suprachiasmatic nuclei have been lesioned are still able to anticipate one meal per day. This anticipation is associated with an increase in activity, core body temperature, and plasma corticosterone concentrations that occur 2–4 h before access to the meal. The precise nature and location of the feeding-entrained oscillator that presumably determines the daily rhythm of feeding anticipation have yet to be established. However, studies with c-Fos (early immediate gene) activation have implicated the nucleus accumbens and the limbic system. The relative importance of the pineal gland and its precise role in the photoperiodic control of circadian rhythms also wait to be determined. With the discovery of genes that regulate circadian rhythms and melatonin synthesis, the prospects of defining what is likely to be a remarkably elegant and robust molecular control system seem excellent.

Hormonal Effects on the Nervous System

The steroid and thyroid hormones, the secretions of the three major pituitary target organs, exert powerful effects on the brain. These effects may be classified in terms of (1) feedback actions, (2) brain differentiation and neural plasticity, (3) neurotransmission, and (4) membranes and ion channels. Feedback actions of the corticosteroids on the brain and pituitary gland are discussed in detail elsewhere. Many entries also deal with the specific effects of corticosteroids on brain that are mediated by corticosteroid receptors, but that are not necessarily related to the feedback control of ACTH release. For information on the actions of steroids on brain differentiation, neurotransmission, cell membranes, and ion channels, the reader is referred to the Bibilography.

Psychoneuroendocrinology

The recognition that the secretion of pituitary hormones reflects the activity of hypothalamic neurons, which in turn reflects neurotransmitter activity in the brain, provides the basis for the use of pituitary hormone secretion as a marker of disordered central neurotransmission that may underlie or be associated with mental disorders. The development of this discipline, psychoneuroendocrinology, has been impeded by our lack of fundamental knowledge about the precise neurotransmitter regulation of hypothalamic neurons that regulate the anterior pituitary gland. Nonetheless, several robust findings have been made and these provide important clues for further research that might optimally be carried out in conjunction with human genetics and sophisticated brain imaging.

For example, it has long been known that plasma cortisol concentrations are abnormally high in patients with psychosis, especially severe depression. Furthermore, as shown by the groundbreaking work of Carroll and Rubin and their associates, in many psychotic patients it is not possible to suppress these high cortisol concentrations by injecting a glucocorticoid agonist such as dexamethasone (the dexamethasone suppression test). Although it cannot accurately discriminate among the different types of psychoses, the failure of dexamethasone to suppress cortisol levels provides robust biological evidence that a patient is suffering from a severe psychosis. The inability of dexamethasone to suppress cortisol levels in many patients with depressive psychosis points to a significant abnormality in the regulatory mechanism for ACTH release. The elucidation of the precise nature of this abnormality may help explain the central neurotransmitter dysfunction that leads to severe depression or other psychosis.

The growth hormone and prolactin responses to pharmacological challenge are also abnormal in certain psychotic states. In anorexia nervosa, for example, a life-threatening condition that occurs predominantly in young women, the normal GH surge that can be induced by the infusion of L-tryptophan, the precursor for serotonin synthesis, is completely absent. This cannot simply be attributed to a lack of food intake because the GH response to L-tryptophan infusion is enhanced, rather than suppressed, in women of a similar age who have been placed on a low-calorie diet. Again the precise explanation for this phenomenon, first shown by Guy Goodwin and associates, is not established, but points to an abnormality in central serotonin function that may underlie or be associated with anorexia nervosa.

The advantages of the psychoneuroendocrine investigation of mental disorders are that it is relatively inexpensive, only mildly invasive, and can be carried out in severely ill patients. Its power will depend on further fundamental research that may enable us to interpret accurately the neuroendocrine responses to pharmacological challenge.

See Also the Following Articles

Adrenal Medulla; Anti-CRF; Circadian Rhythms, Genetics of; Corticotropin Releasing Factor-Binding Protein; Corticotripin-Releasing Factor Receptors; Corticotropin Releasing Factor Receptor deficiency in Mice; Feedback Systems; Food Shift Effect; Urocortins.

Further Reading

Bale, T. L. and Vale, W. W. (2004). CRF and CRF receptors: role in stress responsivity and other behaviors. *Annual Reviews of Pharmacology and Toxicology* **44**, 525–557.

Balthasar, N., Dalgaard, L. T., Lee, C. E., et al. (2005). Divergence of melanocortin pathways in the control of food intake and energy expenditure. *Cell* **123**(3), 493–505.

Boorse, G. C. and Denver, R. J. (2006). Widespread tissue distribution and diverse functions of corticotropin-releasing factor and related peptides. *General Comparative Endocrinology* **146**(1), 9–18.

Cone, R. D. (2005). Anatomy and regulation of the central melanocortin system. *Nature Neuroscience* **8**(5), 571–578.

Ellacott, K. L., Halatchev, I. G., and Cone, R. D. (2006). Characterization of leptin responsive neurons in the caudal brainstem. *Endocrinology* **147**(7), 3190–3196.

Fink, G. (1988). The G. W. Harris Lecture: Steroid control of brain and pituitary function. *Quarterly Journal of Experimental Physiology* **73**, 257–293.

Fink, G. (1997). Mechanisms of negative and positive feedback of steroids in the hypothalamic-pituitary system. In: Bittar, E. & Bittar, N. (eds.) *Principles of medical biology*, pp. 29–100. Greenwich, CT: JAI.

Fink, G., Dow, R. C., Casley, D., et al. (1992). Atrial natriuretic peptide is involved in the ACTH response to stress and glucocorticoid negative feedback in the rat. *Journal of Endocrinology* **135**, 37–43.

Fink, G. and Smith, G. C. (1971). Ultrastructural features of the developing hypothalamo-hypophysial axis in the rat. *Zeitschrift für Zellforschung und Mikroskopische Anatomie* **119**, 208–226.

Fink, G., Sumner, B., Rosie, R., et al. (1999). Androgen actions on central serotonin neurotransmission: relevance for mood, mental state and memory. *Behavioral Brain Research* **105**, 53–68.

Ganguly, S., Weller, J. L., Ho, A., et al. (2005). Melatonin synthesis: 14-3-3-dependent activation and inhibition of arylalkylamine N-acetyltransferase mediated by phosphoserine-205. *Proceedings of the National Academy of Science USA* **102**(4), 1222–1227.

Getting, S. J. (2006). Targeting melanocortin receptors as potential novel therapeutics. *Pharmacology and Therapeutics* **111**(1), 1–15.

Goodwin, G. M., Shapiro, C. M., Bennie, J., et al. (1989). The neuroendocrine responses and psychological effects of infusion of L-tryptophan in anorexia nervosa. *Psychological Medicine* **19**, 857–864.

Guillermet-Guibert, J., Lahlou, H., Cordelier, P., et al. (2005). Physiology of somatostatin receptors. *Journal of Endocrinological Investigation* **28**(11 supplement), 5–9.

Hauger, R. L., Grigoriadis, D. E., Dallman, M. F., et al. (2003). International Union of Pharmacology. 36: Current status of the nomenclature for receptors for corticotropin-releasing factor and their ligands. *Pharmacological Reviews* **55**(1), 21–26.

Larsen, P. R., Kronenberg, H. M., Melmed, S. and Polonsky, K. S. (eds.) (2003). *Williams textbook of endocrinology* (10th edn.) Philadelphia: Saunders.

Luque, R. M., Kineman, R. D., Park, S., et al. (2004). Homologous and heterologous regulation of pituitary receptors for ghrelin and growth hormone-releasing hormone. *Endocrinology* **145**(7), 3182–3189.

Mayo, K. E., Miller, L. J., Bataille, D., et al. (2003). International Union of Pharmacology. 35: The glucagon receptor family. *Pharmacological Reviews* **55**(1), 167–194.

Mendoza, J., Angeles-Castellanos, M. and Escobar, C. (2005). Entrainment by a palatable meal induces food-anticipatory activity and c-Fos expression in reward-related areas of the brain. *Neuroscience* **133**(1), 293–303.

Schumacher, M., Weill-Engerer, S., Liere, P., et al. (2003). Steroid hormones and neurosteroids in normal and pathological aging of the nervous system. *Progress in Neurobiology* **71**(1), 3–29.

Turek, F. W., Joshu, C., Kohsaka, A., et al. (2005). Obesity and metabolic syndrome in circadian clock mutant mice. *Science* **308**(5724), 1043–1045.

Werman, R. (1972) CNS cellular level: membranes. *Annual Review of Physiology* **34**, 337–374.

Yoo, S. H., Ko, C. H., Lowrey, P. L., et al. (2005). A noncanonical E-box enhancer drives mouse Period2 circadian oscillations in vivo. *Proceedings of the National Academy of Science USA* **102**(7), 2608–2613.

Anatomy of the HPA Axis

A G Watts
University of Southern California, Los Angeles, CA, USA

This is a revised version of the article by A G Watts, Encyclopedia of Stress, First edition, volume 2, pp 477–483, © 2000, Elsevier Inc.

Glossary

Acidophils — Cells that stain with acidic (anionic) histochemical stains.

Basophils — Cells that stain with basic (cationic) histochemical stains.

Chromophobes — Cells that do not stain with either acidic or basic histochemical stains.

Fenestrated capillary — A specialized capillary that has transcellular circular openings in the endothelial walls allowing the passage of large molecules or cells in or out of the capillary. They are particularly prevalent in regions where secretory products are released into the vasculature.

Magnocellular neurons — Neurons of relatively large size.

Mesoderm — A principal layer of the mammalian embryo from which derives the vascular tissue.

Neuroectoderm — A principal layer of the mammalian embryo from which derives the nervous tissue.

Parvicellular neurons	Neurons of relatively small size.
Telencephalon	The part of the forebrain containing the cortical regions, basal ganglia, amygdala, and septal nuclei.

Introduction

The hypothalamic-pituitary-adrenal (HPA) axis is a critical endocrine system that contributes to the maintenance of the daily energy balance and forms a fundamental part of the endocrine stress response. It consists of three serially arranged elements connected by vascular links, whose final motor output depends largely on a feed-forward sequence of humorally directed chemical signals: neuroendocrine (corticotropin releasing hormone, CRH; and in some species arginine vasopressin, AVP) originating from a specific set of neuroendocrine neurons in the hypothalamic paraventricular nucleus (PVN), endocrine (adrenocorticotropic hormone, ACTH, released from the anterior pituitary corticotropes), and adrenal glucocorticoid (generally cortisol or corticosterone, depending on the species). The impact of various neural and humoral inputs on each of these three elements allows for a complex array of interacting regulatory influences including afferent neural control in the brain, a variety of circulating hormones, and local paracrine interactions within the anterior pituitary and adrenal cortex.

Hypothalamus: The Neuroendocrine Paraventricular Nucleus

Location

The hypothalamic paraventricular nucleus (PVN) is a heterogenous collection of neurons that constitutes one of the principal motor output systems of the hypothalamus. It is a bilateral structure located either side of the third ventricle and is an elaboration of the periventricular zone of the hypothalamus. One set of PVN neurons provides extensive projections to the hindbrain and spinal cord and regulates behavioral and autonomic motor activity. The other set is neuroendocrine in nature and has terminals in the neurohypophysis. In turn, these neuroendocrine neurons can be further divided into two groups. The first are magnocellular and are found in the PVN and supraoptic nuclei. They have terminals in the infundibular process (or neural lobe) and release either AVP (or vasotocin in nonmammalian groups) or oxytocin into the general vasculature. The second are parvicellular and are generally located (at least in the rat) more medially than the magnocellular neuroendocrine neurons in the PVN. They have terminals in the median eminence (ME) and release release-regulating hormones into the hypophysial portal vasculature to regulate anterior pituitary function.

Subdivisions

The various subdivisions of the PVN of most species are not easily differentiated into discernible cytoarchitectonic compartments. However, in the rat (in which much of the work on neural compartmentalization has been performed) it is possible to delineate approximately 10 separate subdivisions. Of these, the dorsal aspect of the medial parvicellular (mpd) part contains the CRH neuroendocrine neurons responsible for generating the adrenocortical stress response. CRH stimulates the release of ACTH both *in vivo* and *in vitro*, and lesions of the PVN or its projections to the ME have convincingly demonstrated that these cells are the source of CRH secreted into the hypophysial portal vasculature.

Corticotropin Releasing Hormone Neuroendocrine Motor Neurons

In the rat, there are approximately 2000 CRH neurons on each side of the PVNmpd (**Figure 1a**). The cell bodies of these neurons are typically fusiform and are approximately 10 μm in diameter. They have a rather simple dendritic arbor, usually consisting of two, sometimes three, relatively thick dendrites located in a bipolar arrangement (**Figure 1b**). These dendrites are significantly shorter than those found on neurons with descending projections. The dendrites of CRH neurons generally remain within the nucleus, but in some instances they extend into the magnocellular parts of the PVN. Their axons emerge laterally from the PVN (**Figure 1a**), eventually curving around the dorsal aspect of the fornix, before turning ventrally and then caudally to terminate in the portal capillary plexus located in the external zone of the ME.

In many species, AVP is also an important regulator of ACTH secretion and is released into the hypophysial portal vasculature. In the rat, AVP is synthesized in approximately half of the neuroendocrine CRH neurons in the PVN, which are generally more numerous in the dorsal part of the PVNmpd. AVP appears to play a key role in modulating the actions of CRH on anterior pituitary corticotropes, although the extent of its contribution varies among species. Parvicellular AVP is exquisitely sensitive to corticosterone feedback and is copackaged with CRH in dense core vesicles, but it is regulated differentially from CRH by glucocorticoids and a variety of stressors. Although a number of studies have attempted to

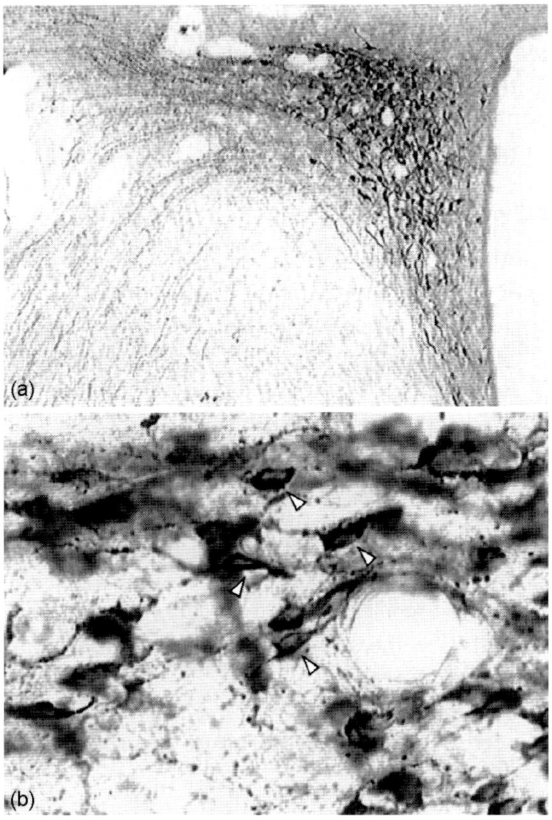

Figure 1 Paraventricular nucleus (PVN) of an adrenalectomized rat and CRH. a, Low-power photomicrograph of PVN stained immunohistochemically for CRH; b, high-power photomicrograph of PVN neuroendocrine CRH neurons. In a, note the densely stained neurons in the medial parvicellular part of the PVN and their axons exiting the nucleus in a lateral direction. The medially located third ventricle is to the right. In b, note the characteristic fusiform cell bodies (white arrowheads) with large unstained nuclei, and the generally bipolar location of the dendrites. Photomicrographs from the author's laboratory.

show that AVP from axons originating in magnocellular cells contribute to ACTH secretogogue release in the external layer of the ME, the precise contribution of this magnocellular system to the regulation of ACTH still remains to be clarified.

Afferent Input

Coordinating the activity of CRH neurons in the PVNmpd in response to stress depends on sets of afferent inputs from many regions of the brain. In general, these inputs can be divided into two groups: those that target PVNmpd neurons directly and those that are channeled through intermediate regions such as the bed nuclei of the stria terminalis (BST) and peri-PVN regions.

Many of the inputs that directly target CRH neurons originate from the hindbrain, some regions of the hypothalamus, and circumventricular organs in the forebrain. Direct catecholaminergic inputs into the PVN from the hindbrain travel in the ventral noradrenergic bundle and play a particularly prominent role in conveying visceral sensory information to neuroendocrine neurons. Noradrenergic innervation to the parvicellular neuroendocrine PVN originates predominantly from the A2 cell group in the medial and commissural divisions of the nucleus of the solitary tract. The A2 cell group receives first-order vagal and glossopharyngeal afferents and therefore can also relay visceral sensory information to the PVN. A minor contribution arises from the A1 and A6 (locus ceruleus) cell groups. Most of the adrenergic fibers (which also contain neuropeptide Y, NPY) arise in the C1 cell groups. The hypothalamic cell groups that project directly into the PVNmpd include the dorsomedial nucleus, some preoptic nuclei, and some peri-PVN regions. The neurochemical nature of these projections is still under investigation, but both γ-aminobutyric acid (GABA) and glutamate are likely to be important transmitters in these projections.

The subfornical organ (SFO) and vascular organ of the lamina terminalis (OVLT) are circumventricular organs that lack a blood–brain barrier and can provide an entry point for humoral factors that are ordinarily excluded from the central nervous system (CNS). Both of these midline structures are located in the forebrain and provide efferent projections directly into the PVN. They are thought to be particularly important for mediating the HPA response to increased circulating angiotensin II (particularly the SFO) and increases in vascular osmolality (the OVLT). In addition, direct projections from a third cell group in the rostral hypothalamus, the median preoptic nucleus, may also contribute in this function.

Information from telencephalic regions, including the amygdala, hippocampus, and lateral septal nuclei, probably play an prominent role in mediating the more cognitive influences on the activity of the HPA axis. However, these particular regions do not provide direct projections into the PVN, and their impact on neuroendocrine CRH neurons and ACTH secretion are thought to be channeled more through projections from a variety of nuclei in the BST. There is evidence that GABA plays an important role in this function.

Neurohypophysis: Median Eminence and Infundibular Stalk

The defining feature of neuroendocrine neurons is that they release their chemical signals into fenestrated capillaries in the neurohypophysis rather than into the characteristic synaptic cleft found in neuron-to-neuron transmission. Once in the vasculature, these signals are then carried to their targets by the blood flow and act on targets that are effectively defined by the presence of specific receptors.

Structure

The neurohypophysis is a midline structure that derives from an outgrowth from the floor of the hypothalamus. It consists of the ME, the infundibular stalk, and the infundibular process (the neural lobe or pars nervosa) of the pituitary gland (**Figure 2**). Of these structures, the ME and infundibular stalk are critical parts of the HPA axis. The ME is where axons from neuroendocrine CRH neurons in the PVNmpd have their terminals adjacent to the primary capillaries of hypophysial portal system. It is a highly complex structure consisting of a looped network of fenestrated capillaries, axon terminals, and tanycytes, which are specialized ependymal cells that have processes extending from the third ventricle to the axon terminals on the capillary plexus. In the case of the CRH neurons that regulate anterior pituitary corticotrope function, secretogogues are released in an activity-dependent manner into the blood flowing through the hypophysial portal vasculature toward the pituitary gland from neuroendocrine terminals in the ME.

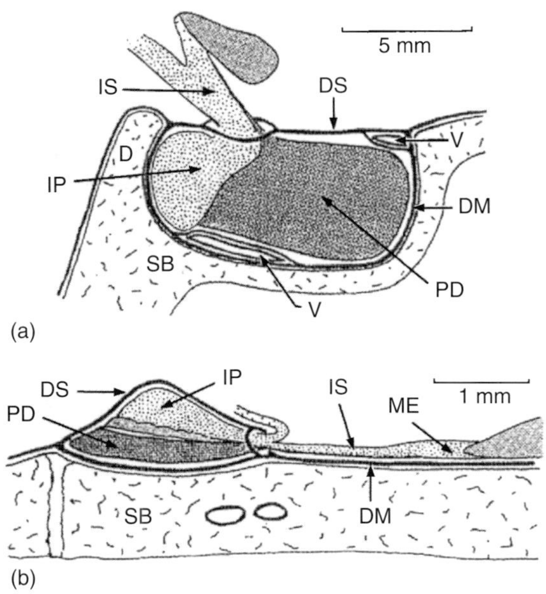

Figure 2 Diagrams based on midsagittal sections of pituitary glands. a, Human; b, rat. Anterior/rostral is to the right. D, dorsum sellae; DM, dura mater; DS, diaphragm dellae; IP, infundibular process of the neurohypophysis; IS, infundibular stem of the neurohypohysis; ME, median eminence of the neurohypophysis; PD, pars distalis; SB, sphenoid bone; V, venous sinus. Adapted from Daniel, P. M. and Pritchard, M. M. L. (1975), Studies of the hypothalamus and the pituitary gland, *Acta Endocrinologia* **30** (supplement 201), p. 45.

Organization of Blood Supply

The organization of the blood supply to the rat pituitary gland is shown in **Figure 3**. The arterial blood supply of the ME and infundibular stalk arises from the internal carotid artery and the circle of Willis, and it flows into the capillary bed of the ME from branches of the anterior hypophysial artery. These vessels form extensive capillary loops in the external part of the ME close to the terminals of the CRH neuroendocrine motor neurons. As they leave the ME, these capillaries drain into the long portal vessels that lie parallel in the infundibular stalk and then course into the pars distalis. On entering the pars distalis, the long portal vessels anastomose, allowing the release-regulating hormones access to its secretory cells. A second capillary bed is found closer the pituitary gland. It is supplied by blood from the artery of the trabecula and produces the short portal vessels, which then enter the pars distalis in parallel to the long portal vessels.

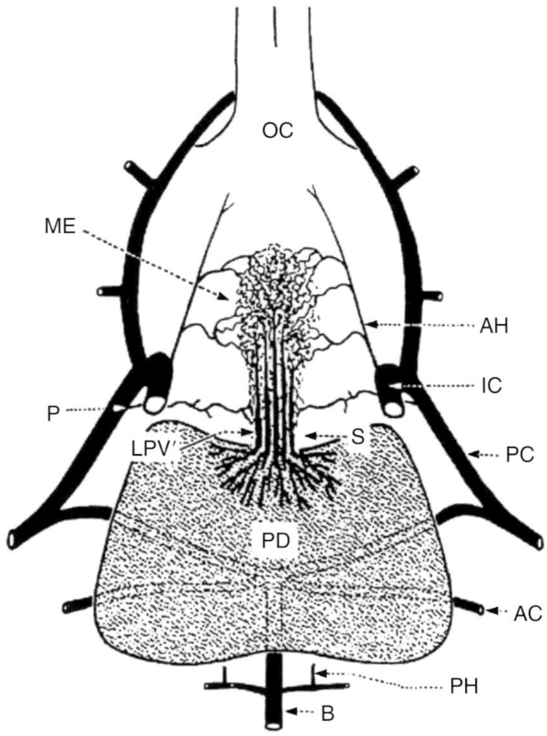

Figure 3 The pituitary gland of the rat showing the main features of the blood supply to its ventral aspect. AC, anterior cerebellar artery; AH, anterior hypophysial artery; B, basilar artery; IC, internal carotid artery; LPV, long portal vessel; ME, median eminence; OC, optic chiasm; P, peduncular artery; PC, posterior communicating artery; PD, pars distalis; PH, posterior hypophysial artery; S, pituitary stalk. Adapted from Daniel, P. M. and Pritchard, M. M. L. (1975), Studies of the hypothalamus and the pituitary gland, *Acta Endocrinologia* **30**(supplement 201, p. 56.)

Adenohypophysis: Corticotropes in the Pars Distalis

The adenohypophysis is nonneural tissue that develops from an ectodermal evagination of the roof of the buccal cavity, Rathke's pouch. It has three parts: pars distalis, tuberalis, and intermedia. The pars tuberalis makes up approximately 75% of the adenohypophysis (**Figure 2**) and contains the corticotropes that synthesize ACTH from its precursor proopiomelanocortin (POMC). Pars distalis cells are arranged in cords or clusters interspersed between capillaries from the hypophysial portal vessels. Corticotropes are separated from one another by thin-walled vascular sinusoids and are supported by a skeleton of reticular tissue. Classically, cells of the pars distalis have been characterized into three groups based on their stainability: acidophils, basophils, and chromophobes. Although these categories are not as clear cut as was originally thought, corticotropes are basophilic and show strong periodic acid Schiff (PAS) staining. CRH and AVP released into the hypophysial portal vasculature eventually bathe corticotropes and stimulate the synthesis and secretion of ACTH. In terms of their response to these secretogogues, there appears to be three type of corticotropes: those responsive to CRH and not AVP; those responsive to CRH or AVP; and those responsive to CRH and AVP. Thus, changes in the CRH/AVP ratio could affect the overall ACTH secretory pattern.

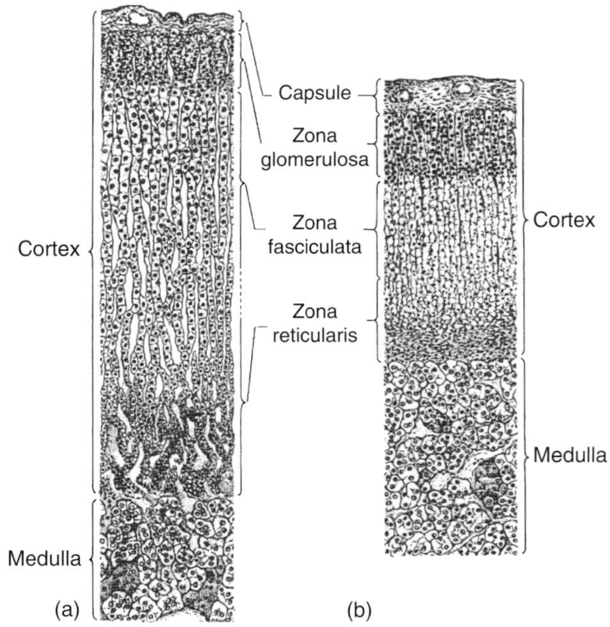

Figure 4 Sections through the adrenal glands of rats. a, Normal rat; b, hypophysectomized rat. Because the functional capacity of the adrenal cortex is maintained by circulating ACTH, hypophysectomy results in tremendous shrinkage of the cortex. The medulla (catecholamine-synthesizing tissue) is not affected by hypophysectomy. Both sections are drawn to scale. Adapted from Turner, C. D. and Bagnara, J. T. (1976), *General endocrinology*, Philadelphia: W. B. Saunders.

Adrenal Cortex: Zona Fasciculata

Structure

The mammalian adrenal glands are bilateral structures located in perirenal adipose tissue found dorsal to the kidney. They each consist of cortical steroid-synthesizing tissue derived from the mesoderm and medullary catecholamine-synthesizing tissue derived from the neuroectoderm (**Figure 4**). The thin outermost part of the adrenal cortex, the zona glomerulosa, is the main site of mineralocorticoid production. Glucocorticoids (either cortisol or corticosterone) are primarily produced by the zona fasciculata in response to circulating ACTH (**Figure 4**), and this constitutes the largest amount of steroid-synthesizing tissue in the adrenal gland. The androgens dehydroepiandrosterone and androstenedione are produced in the innermost zona reticularis. The zona fasciculata consists of long thin cords, each of one or two cells separated by parallel fenestrated venous capillaries. These cells are approximately 20 μm in diameter and contain the large amounts of smooth endoplasmic reticulum, mitochondria, and lipid droplets characteristic of steroid-synthesizing cells. They also possess reasonable amounts of rough endoplasmic reticulum, as well as greater numbers of gap junctions than are found between zona glomerulosa cells.

Blood Supply

The blood supply to the adrenal cortex is ultimately derived from three groups of arteries: the superior (arising from the inferior phrenic artery), the middle (arising from the aorta), and the inferior (arising from the renal artery or aorta) adrenal arteries. These arteries then branch to form a plexus in the adrenal capsule (which constitutes the outside of the gland), from which arises the cortical arteries supplying the three layers of the adrenal cortex. Venous outflow from the cortex enters a number of sinuses in the adrenal medulla and eventually join the adrenal vein. In the human, the left adrenal vein joins the renal vein and the right adrenal vein enters the vena cava.

Innervation

The mammalian adrenal cortex is innervated by postganglionic sympathetic fibers in the greater and lesser splanchnic nerves originating in thoracic regions T8 to T11 of the vertebral column. This postganglionic innervation is most likely derived from pre- and paravertebral ganglia, including the suprarenal ganglion.

Moreover, the cortex also receives input from adrenal medullary ganglion cells, emphasizing the complexity of the local regulation that can occur within the adrenal gland. Nerve terminals have been found adjacent to adrenal parenchyma and blood vessels in rat and human adrenal cortices. Although the function of preganglionic innervation of the cortex is not entirely clear, there are experimental reports documenting that in the rat the splanchnic nerve plays a role in regulating the prefeeding increase in corticosterone secretion. Although vagal sensory innervation of the adrenal is present, parasympathetic motor innervation of the adrenal is not as clearly defined.

See Also the Following Articles

Adrenal Cortex; Neuroendocrine Systems.

Further Reading

Black, V. A. (1988). The adrenal gland. In: Weiss, L. (ed.) *Cell and tissue biology. A textbook of histology*, pp. 1035–1066. Baltimore, MD: Urban & Schwarzenberg.

Daniel, P. M. and Pritchard, M. M. L. (1975). Studies of the hypothalamus and the pituitary gland. *Acta Endocrinologia* **30**(supplement 201), pp. 45, 56.

Halmi, N. S. (1988). The hypophysis. In: Weiss, L. (ed.) *Cell and tissue biology. A textbook of histology*, pp. 973–994. Baltimore, MD: Urban & Schwarzenberg.

Herman, J. P., Figueiredo, H., Mueller, N. K., et al. (2003). Central mechanisms of stress integration: hierarchical circuitry controlling hypothalamo-pituitary-adrenocortical responsiveness. *Frontiers in Neuroendocrinology* **24**, 151–180.

Swanson, L. W. and Sawchenko, P. E. (1983). Hypothalamic integration: organization of the paraventricular and supraoptic nuclei. *Annual Review of Neuroscience* **6**, 275–325.

Turner, C. D. and Bagnara, J. T. (1976). *General endocrinology.* Philadelphia: W. B. Saunders.

Watts, A. G. (2005). Glucocorticoid regulation of peptide genes in neuroendocrine CRH neurons: a complexity beyond negative feedback. *Frontiers in Neuroendocrinology* **26**, 109–130.

Feedback Systems

G Fink
Mental Health Research Institute, Parkville, Victoria, Australia

This is a revised version of the article by G Fink, Encyclopedia of Stress, First edition, volume 2, pp 124–137, © 2000, Elsevier Inc.

Glossary

Allostasis — Maintaining stability (or homeostasis) through change; term introduced by Sterling and Eyer in 1988 to describe cardiovascular adjustments to resting and active states.

Homeostasis — The maintenance of equilibrium, or constant conditions, in a biological system by means of automatic mechanisms (generally feedback systems) that counteract influences (stressors) that tend toward disequilibrium (term introduced by Walter Cannon in 1932).

Hypercortisolemia — Excessively high concentrations of adrenal corticosteroids in plasma.

Hypophysial portal vessels — A group of small venules that connect a primary plexus of capillaries in the median eminence of the hypothalamus (base of the brain) with a secondary plexus of sinusoids in the pituitary gland. Blood flowing in these vessels, which run down the pituitary stalk, transports hypothalamic-pituitary regulatory neurohormones, released at nerve terminals in the median eminence of the hypothalamus, to the anterior pituitary gland, where they stimulate or inhibit the release of anterior pituitary hormones.

Limbic system — An extensive brain region that includes the cingulate and parahippocampal cortex, hippocampus, amygdala, hypothalamus, septal nuclei, and other structures. The precise interaction of the several components of the system is poorly understood, but since the proposal by Papez, the limbic system has been implicated in emotion. The connections between the limbic system and the neocortex, hypothalamus, and the olfactory bulb via the olfactory tract suggest that it serves as an important analyzer-integrator of signals, which it conveys from the neocortex to the hypothalamus. The input of olfactory information to the limbic system has led to its alternative name, the rhinencephalon (olfactory brain), and possibly reflects the strong emotive and signaling effects of smell in many animals. The structure and relative size of the limbic system have remained remarkably constant through evolution; in humans it is overshadowed by the massive development of the neocortex.

Neurohormones Chemical neurotransmitters released from nerve terminals into the hypophysial portal vessels or the systemic circulation at neurohemal junctions and conveyed to their target cells by the blood stream. This contrasts with classical neurotransmitters that reach receptors on target cells by crossing synaptic clefts or neuromuscular junctions.

Suprachiasmatic nuclei Two small hypothalamic nuclei located immediately above (dorsal to) the optic chiasm that are responsible for regulating most circadian rhythms of the body.

Introduction

Feedback control systems are fundamental for the normal physiological functioning of the body. There are two types of feedback, negative and positive, of which the former is the more common. Removal of the main pituitary target glands, the adrenals, gonads, and thyroid, the most reproducible and reproduced experiment in classical endocrinology, demonstrates that the secretion of pituitary adrenocorticotropin (ACTH), gonadotropins, and thyrotropin is controlled by negative feedback exerted by the adrenal corticosteroids, gonadal steroids, and thyroid hormones, respectively. Interruption of the negative feedback loop caused, for example, by surgical or pharmacological adrenalectomy, gonadectomy, or thyroidectomy, or an enzymatic defect in steroid or thyroid hormone biosynthesis, results in massive hypersecretion of pituitary ACTH, gonadotropin, or thyrotropin.

Crucial for homeostasis, negative feedback control mechanisms are composed of a system in which the output moderates the strength of the controller to a predetermined set point level (**Figures 1** and **2**). The set point–stimulator complex contains a comparator (error detector), which compares the strength of the feedback signal with a preset level. An increase in the strength of the feedback signal above the preset level reduces the output of the stimulator, whereas a decrease in the strength of the feedback signal below the preset level results in an increase in output of the feedback signal and corrects the error. Negative feedback control operates widely throughout the body at the molecular (e.g., end product inhibition of enzyme activity), cellular, and whole system/body levels. The mechanisms by which the set point is determined vary between systems: in the case of the hypothalamic-pituitary-adrenocortical (HPA) feedback system, the set point is regulated by the central nervous system. GABAergic and glutamatergic neural projections from the limbic system and other brain regions to the paraventricular nuclei (PVN) of the

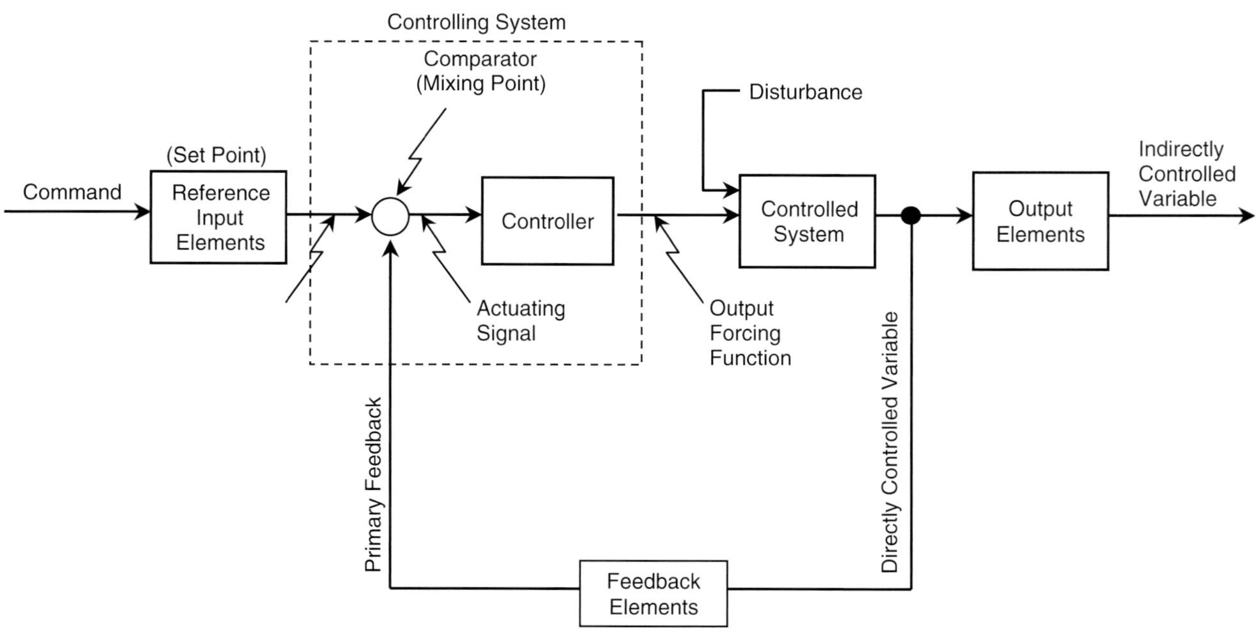

Figure 1 A generalized feedback control system. Modified from Milhorn, H. T. J. (1966). *The application of control theory to physiological systems,* with permission from Saunders, Philadelphia, PA.

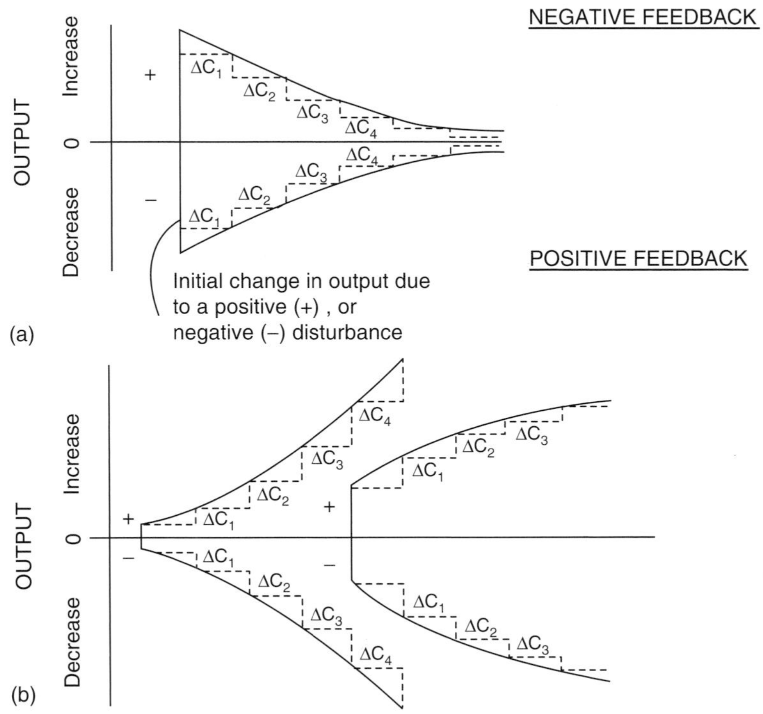

Figure 2 (a) Negative feedback minimizes the disturbance to a regulator, resulting in a system in which the output tends to remain constant. In this case, the ratios of the decrements of the controlled variable C (C_2/C_1, C_3/C_2) are less than unity. (b) In positive feedback (left-hand curves) an initial disturbance results in a continuous increase in output (vicious cycle). The increments of the controlled variable (C_2/C_1, C_3/C_2) are greater than unity. When the response does not result in a vicious cycle, the ratios of C_2/C_1, C_3/C_2, and so on are less than unity (see right-hand curves in B). From Milhorn, H. T. J. (1966). *The application of control theory to physiological systems,* with permission from Saunders, Philadelphia, PA.

hypothalamus may play a key role in HPA set point regulation.

Positive feedback, whereby the output of a system increases the output of the stimulator (gain in the system) (**Figure 2b**), is far less common than negative feedback, possibly because taken to its logical conclusion, a positive feedback system, uncontrolled, will eventually self-destruct. Some systems loosely termed positive feedback are, in fact, servomechanisms. A servomechanism is a closed loop control system, which increases significantly the power of a small signal. Positive feedback is exemplified by (1) estrogen stimulation of gonadotropin secretion, which results in ovulation, and (2) the release of oxytocin induced during parturition by pressure of the fetal head on the uterine cervix. The latter triggers volleys of impulses that, by way of a multisynaptic pathway to the hypothalamus, stimulate oxytocin release. Oxytocin stimulates further contraction of the uterus, which results in a further increase in pressure on the uterine cervix. This vicious cycle is broken only when the fetus is expelled. Servomechanisms are illustrated by the way that, just before ovulation in humans as well as in other spontaneously ovulating mammals, elevated plasma estrogen concentrations increase the responsiveness of the anterior pituitary gland to gonadotropin-releasing hormone (GnRH) by 20- to 50-fold. This estrogen effect, reinforced by the priming effect of GnRH, whereby a small pulse of GnRH further potentiates pituitary responsiveness to itself, ensures the occurrence of a massive ovulatory gonadotropin surge in response to a small surge or increased pulse frequency of GnRH.

This article focuses on the principles of negative feedback control in the HPA system with emphasis on neurohormone and hormone release. While the discussion concentrates on negative feedback maintenance of homeostasis, the same mechanisms are involved in allostasis that is brought about by a change in set point so as to enable the organism to deal with the physiological challenge or stress.

Overview

In the normal state, with the negative feedback loop intact, the set point in the brain-pituitary module maintains the secretion of ACTH within a relatively narrow bandwidth. Within this bandwidth, the basal secretion of ACTH is pulsatile. Plasma ACTH concentrations also show a circadian rhythm, with a peak

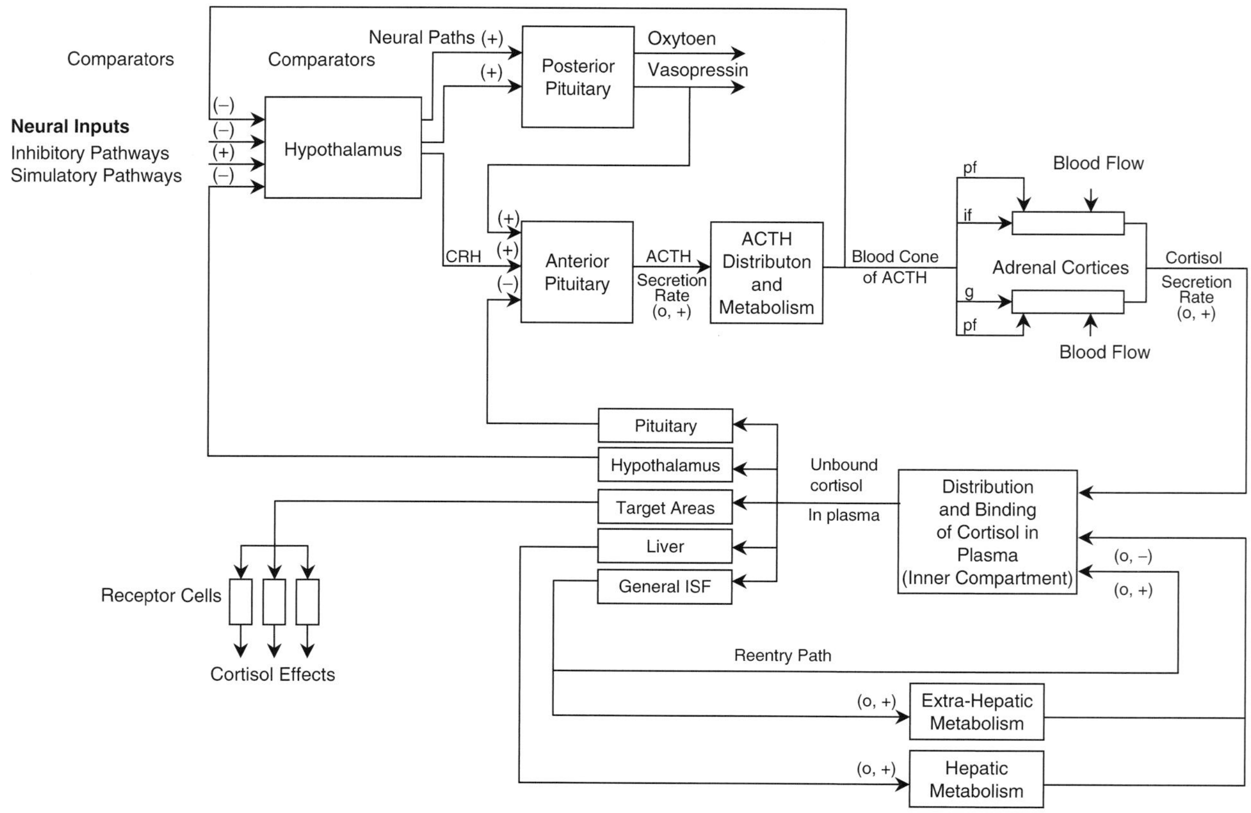

Figure 3 Block diagram of the hypothalamic-pituitary-adrenal glucocorticoid control system. Abbreviations: if, input forcing of adrenal by ACTH; pf, parametric forcing of adrenal (hypertrophic effect) caused by ACTH over a longer time period. The parametric effect of changes in adrenal blood flow is also indicated. The designators 0, + and 0, − indicate that signals in pathways are restricted in values (e.g., there are no negative masses or frequencies, and removal processes or inhibitors are negative in effects). From Yates, F. E. and Maran, J. W. (1975). In: Knobil, E. & Sawyer, W. H. (eds.) *Handbook of physiology* (pp. 367–404). Washington, D.C.: American Physiological Society, with permission.

in the morning and a trough approaching a nadir around midnight. In nocturnal animals, such as rodents, the phase of this rhythm is reversed so that plasma ACTH concentrations reach a peak just before the onset of darkness. The circadian rhythm of ACTH results in a circadian rhythm in the plasma concentrations of adrenal corticosteroids: cortisol in humans and corticosterone in rodents. A key feature in both diurnal and nocturnal animals is that corticosteroid plasma concentrations reach a peak just before the animal is due to wake from sleep; the levels are lowest just before or during sleep.

Glucocorticoids (cortisol in the human; corticosterone in rodents) secreted by the adrenal cortex exert their inhibitory action both on the brain and on the pituitary gland (**Figures** 3 and 4). The PVN of the hypothalamus contain the final common pathway neurons that mediate the neural control of pituitary ACTH synthesis and release. The PVN receive stimulatory and inhibitory neural inputs and an important projection from the suprachiasmatic nuclei (SCN), the key circadian oscillator in brain. PVN drive is mediated by stress neurohormones, corticotropin releasing factor-41 (CRF-41) and arginine vasopressin (AVP), which are released into hypophysial portal vessel blood. ACTH is released into the systemic circulation and stimulates adrenal corticosteroid synthesis and release. In keeping with revised standard nomenclature, CRF-41 will be abbreviated to CRH (corticotropin-releasing hormone).

The release of ACTH is pulsatile in humans and is cleared rapidly from the blood by both metabolic degradation and distribution into several body compartments. The glucocorticoids are bound rapidly by albumin and a specific corticosteroid-binding protein, transcortin, and are metabolized by several organs, especially the liver and kidney (**Figure** 3). Only unbound (free) glucocorticoids inhibit ACTH release, and therefore the degree of glucocorticoid binding and metabolism, as well as the magnitude of adrenal secretion (**Figure** 3), determines the strength of the negative feedback signal. The HPA feedback system might also be influenced by a CRH-binding protein in plasma (first discovered by Orth and

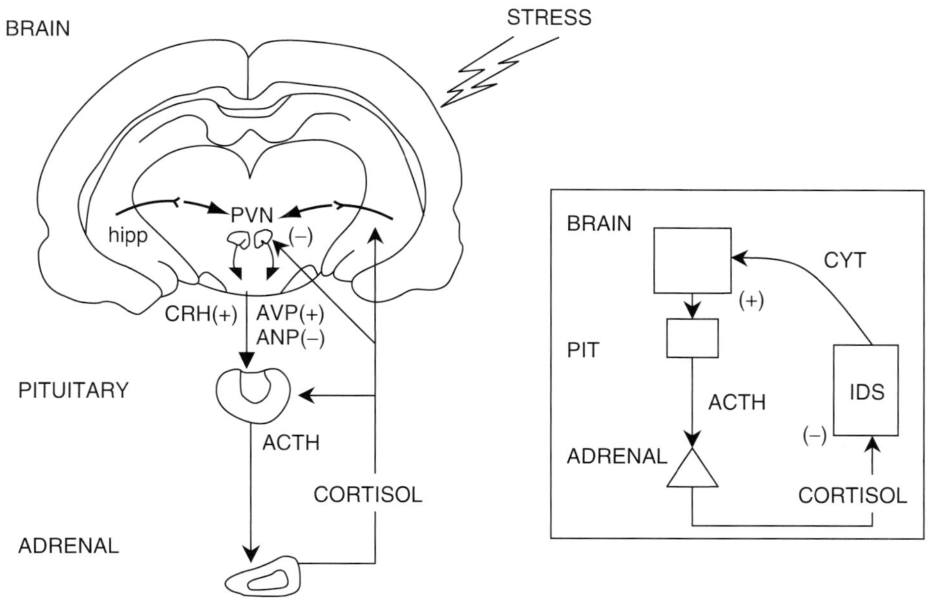

Figure 4 Schematic diagram of the elements involved in glucocorticoid negative feedback. The paraventricular nuclei (PVN) contain the main stress (final common pathway neurons) secreting both CRH and AVP. The negative feedback action of cortisol (corticosterone in rodents) is exerted mainly on the PVN and the pituitary corticotropes. However, long-term effects mediated through the hippocampus (Hipp) and amygdala (not shown) cannot be excluded. There are several possible indirect connections between the hippocampus and PVN. Neural control of ACTH secretion may also be mediated by a corticotropin inhibitory peptide, atrial natriuretic peptide (ANP). The inset shows the important inhibitory action of cortisol on the immune defense system (IDS). The IDS produces cytokines (CYT), which act on the brain to stimulate ACTH secretion. Cytokine secretion is inhibited by the negative feedback effect of glucocorticoids.

Mount in 1987). The physiological role of the CRH-binding (glyco) protein, which is synthesized in the liver, awaits to be determined – in humans, CRH-binding protein concentrations in plasma increase during the third trimester of pregnancy (see **Corticotropin Releasing Factor-Binding Protein**).

Interaction between Negative Feedback and Circadian Rhythm in the HPA System

The circadian rhythm of ACTH and (the consequent) glucocorticoid secretion, which has a peak at the end and a nadir at the beginning of the sleep phase, is driven by a neural mechanism mediated mainly by the stress neurohormones. The twofold increase in the ACTH signal between the nadir and the peak of the circadian rhythm in the rat results in a ninefold increase in corticosterone due to an increase in the responsiveness of the adrenal cortex.

In the unstressed state, the HPA system operates in an approximately linear domain with all the loop variables (**Figure** 3) showing circadian periodicity. Ultradian rhythms in plasma cortisol concentration, independent of ACTH concentration, occur in humans and rhesus monkeys, in which they are highly synchronized between animals with a predominant periodicity of 85–90 min.

The circadian rhythm of ACTH secretion is driven by the SCN. In addition to the diurnal rhythm of corticosterone, the SCN are involved in other key rhythms in the body, such as the sleep–wake cycle, motor activity, thermoregulation, pineal *N*-acetyl transferase activity, and the regular occurrence of ovulation. If any one of these functions is abnormal, then there is a high probability that the others will also be abnormal. The corticosterone rhythm is especially sensitive in that even partial lesions of the SCN, which have no effect on any of the other circadian functions, do disrupt the adrenal rhythm.

The SCN receive afferent projections from (1) the retina (direct as well as indirect after a relay in the ventral lateral geniculate nucleus), (2) the 5-hydroxytryptamine (5-HT) raphe neurons, and (3) the hippocampus by way of the medial corticohypothalamic tract. Each of these inputs to the SCN is likely to affect the periodicity of the pacemaker: the retinal input affects the time of the light–dark cycle; the hippocampal input may be related to the sleep–wake cycle; the raphe input may be related to paradoxical sleep. The raphe input also plays a major role in determining the amplitude of diurnal ACTH oscillations.

Although the central action of glucocorticoids is mainly on the PVN, the 5-HT neurons of the dorsal raphe nuclei, which project to the SCN, have high concentrations of glucocorticoid receptors. The SCN have direct projections to the PVN and may also affect PVN function by way of their projections to the subparaventricular zone. While circadian rhythmicity of the HPA is modulated by glucocorticoids and other factors, the intrinsic rhythmicity of the SCN circadian pacemaker is primarily under genetic control (see **Circadian Rhythms, Genetics of**).

Corticosteroid Feedback on the Hypothalamus and Pituitary Gland: Phase Differences

The seminal modeling studies of Eugene Yates and associates suggested that corticosteroid negative feedback on ACTH release occurs in three phases: a fast and immediate rate-sensitive phase of about 30 min, followed by a level-sensitive phase that occurs 2–3 h after the start of corticosteroid administration, followed by a long-term chronic phase. Fink and associates investigated the effect of corticosteroids on the release of stress neurohormones into hypophysial portal blood (see **Neuroendocrine Systems**) in the intermediate and chronic phase. They found that adrenalectomy induced a three- to fourfold increase in the release of both CRH and AVP into hypophysial portal blood. Administration of the synthetic glucocorticoid dexamethasone 2.5 h before portal blood collection significantly reduced the release of AVP, but not CRH (**Figure 5**), and also blocked the ACTH response to CRH (**Figure 6**). These findings suggest that intermediate-delayed (2–3 h) glucocorticoid feedback is mediated by the blockade of pituitary responsiveness to CRH and a reduction in AVP output into hypophysial portal blood. That is, in this situation AVP is the regulatory or signaling neurohormone, whereas CRH is the permissive neurohormone. In contrast, studies on the long-term effects of corticosterone administered by a subcutaneous pellet suggested that long-term negative glucocorticoid feedback is due to a decreased release of CRH, as well as AVP, into portal blood. That is, both stress neurohormones are sensitive to the long-term effects of corticosteroids.

These findings agree broadly with those of Plotsky and associates, which showed that pharmacological adrenalectomy with metyrapone and aminoglutethimide (which block glucocorticoid biosynthesis) resulted in a significant increase in the release of both CRH and AVP into hypophysial portal blood. The intravenous infusion of corticosterone inhibited nitroprusside-evoked CRH release into portal blood, but had no effect on AVP release.

Data in the rat are complemented by those obtained in the sheep. Thus, the concentrations of CRH and

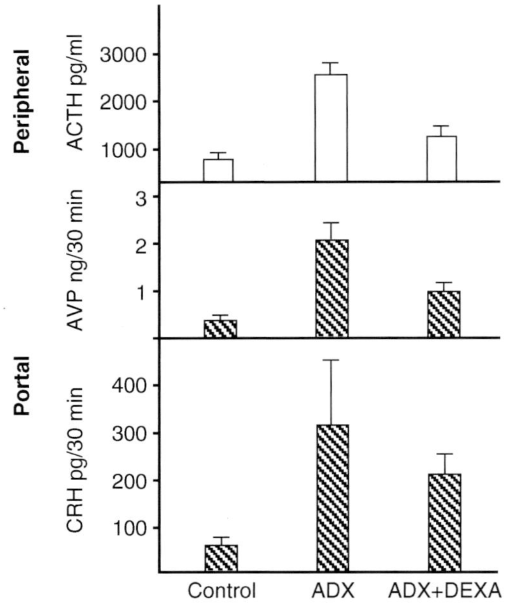

Figure 5 The delayed negative feedback action of glucocorticoid in adult female Wistar rats anesthetized with sodium pentobarbitone. ACTH was measured in plasma taken immediately before sectioning of the pituitary stalk for the collection of hypophysial portal vessel blood. Adrenalectomy (ADX) resulted in a fourfold increase in ACTH concentration and a similar increase in the output of AVP and CRH release relative to that in intact, untreated animals (control). The administration of dexamethasone (DEXA) significantly reduced the levels of ACTH and AVP, but not CRH. Modified from Fink, G., Robinson, I. C. A. F. and Tannahill, L. A. (1988). Effects of adrenalectomy and glucocorticoids on the peptides, CRF-41, AVP and oxytocin in rat hypophysial portal blood. *Journal of Physiology* **401**, 329–345, with permission of the authors and Cambridge University Press.

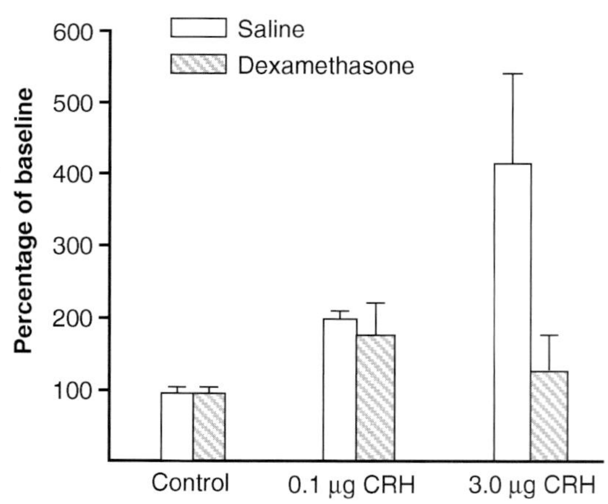

Figure 6 Mean (±SEM, $n = 5$) percentage increase over the basal concentration of ACTH after the injection of saline, 0.1 μg CRH, or 3 μg CRH. Female Wistar rats that had been adrenalectomized 3 weeks earlier were treated with either saline or dexamethasone 3 h before injection of CRH. Note that dexamethasone blocked the ACTH response to 3.0 μg of CRH. From Fink, G., Robinson, I. C. A. F. and Tannahill, L. A. (1988). Effects of adrenalectomy and glucocorticoids on the peptides, CRF-41, AVP and oxytocin in rat hypophysial portal blood. *Journal of Physiology* **401**, 329–345, with permission of the authors and Cambridge University Press.

AVP in hypophysial portal blood collected from conscious sheep were (1) similar to those in the rat, (2) increased by volume depletion, fear-associated audiovisual stimuli, and insulin-induced hypoglycemia, and (3) inhibited by dexamethasone.

Glucocorticoid Feedback Effects on Stress Neurohormone Biosynthesis

Glucocorticoids have potent inhibitory effects on CRH biosynthesis as well as release. Thus, adrenalectomy is followed by a significant increase in CRH mRNA levels in the parvocellular PVN, and this increase can be reduced by either corticosterone or dexamethasone. As assessed by CRH-intron *in situ* hybridization, the stimulation of CRH gene transcription can be detected as early as 15 to 30 min after the injection of the glucocorticoid synthesis inhibitor metyrapone. This increase in CRH gene transcription in the PVN was associated with a coincident increase in c-fos mRNA in the PVN. An increase in the levels of CRH mRNA in the PVN after metyrapone injection was delayed by about 60 min, possibly a function of the high resting levels of CRH mRNA and the time taken to assemble mRNA from the CRH primary transcript.

The effects of corticosterone and dexamethasone are dose dependent and can be demonstrated by systemic administration of the steroid, as well as by implantation of steroid pellets into the brain. This effect of glucocorticoids is cell specific in that the glucocorticoid-induced decrease in CRH mRNA was localized to the dorsomedial parvocellular neurons of the PVN, the major source of CRH fiber projections to the median eminence. In contrast, glucocorticoid increased the levels of CRH mRNA in parvocellular neurons that project to the brain stem and the spinal cord. The implantation of dexamethasone micropellets in cerebral cortex, dorsal hippocampus, ventral subiculum, lateral septum, or amygdala had no effect on CRH mRNA levels in the PVN.

The molecular mechanism by which glucocorticoids regulate CRH gene expression remains unclear. Recent data show that the repressor isoform of cAMP response element modulator (CREM) is involved in CRH gene regulation, and that, *in vivo*, stress-induced glucocorticoids do not limit CRH gene transcription, in spite of the fact that the CRH promoter has a glucocorticoid receptor response element. The inhibitory effect of glucocorticoids on CRH gene transcription may be mediated, at least in part, by GABAergic, glutamatergic, and monoaminergic projections to the PVN from the forebrain and hindbrain limbic system.

The concentration of AVP mRNA in the dorsomedial parvocellular neurons of the PVN paralleled those of CRH mRNA, that is, levels increased after adrenalectomy and decreased after treatment with glucocorticoids. Corticosterone treatment also produced a modest reduction in the levels of enkephalin mRNA in all four regions of the PVN, but glucocorticoid manipulation had no significant effect on the PVN concentrations of the mRNAs for angiotensin, cholecystokinin, preprotachykinin, and tyrosine hydroxylase. There is, therefore, a close correlation between the synthesis and the release of CRH and AVP. Whether this means that synthesis and release are mechanistically coupled is not established.

Data on the release and synthesis of stress neurohormones suggest that even though corticosteroid receptors are present in high concentration in parts of the brain remote from the hypothalamus, including the hippocampus, amygdala, and the monoaminergic nuclei of the hindbrain, central inhibition of CRH and AVP synthesis and release may be due in large part to corticosteroid action mainly at the level of the PVN. Although a role for mineralocorticoid receptors cannot be excluded, glucocorticoid receptors predominate.

Role of Atrial Natriuretic Peptide in Glucocorticoid Inhibition

Fink and associates showed that atrial natriuretic peptide (ANP) is released into hypophysial portal blood and, by immunoneutralization, that ANP is possibly an inhibitor of ACTH release. This suggests that the glucocorticoid inhibition of ACTH release may be mediated in part by ANP. A consensus sequence for the glucocorticoid response element is present in the second intron of the ANP gene, and ANP gene expression in and ANP release from cardiac cells are increased significantly by glucocorticoids. A pathophysiological role for ANP is suggested by multiple trauma and septic shock in humans, where, paradoxically, plasma ACTH concentrations are decreased but plasma cortisol concentrations are increased. These results raise the possibility that under conditions of extreme stress, increased levels of ANP inhibit ACTH release while cortisol secretion is stimulated by a direct action of endothelin-l on the adrenal gland. ANP inhibition of ACTH release might also explain the dissociation between plasma ACTH and CRH in patients who have undergone cardiac surgery or sustained myocardial infarction. Dissociation between plasma concentrations of ACTH and CRH under extreme, and especially cardiopulmonary, stress is relevant to allostatic override of the normal glucocorticoid negative feedback system.

On the basis of all the present *in vivo* and *in vitro* data, Engler and colleagues conclude that studies with ANP have so far provided the most compelling evidence that a neuropeptide may inhibit ACTH release.

Role of Hippocampus and Amygdala in Glucocorticoid Negative Feedback

It has long been assumed that the hippocampus and the amygdala, major components of the forebrain limbic system, play a key role in the stress response. The forebrain limbic system, together with the thalamus and neocortex and brain stem structures, form an analyzer-integrator system involved in neuroendocrine control. The hypothalamus can be considered an intermediate relay station in the reciprocal circuits between the limbic forebrain and brain stem structures, receiving inputs from both. The forebrain limbic system is thought to be involved in stressors that require analysis by higher brain structures (processive stressors), whereas direct brain stem projections to the PVN subserve stressors that pose an immediate physiological threat (systemic stressors).

Projections to the PVN from the hippocampus are mainly multisynaptic, involving (1) the hippocampal fimbria-fornix system involving the lateral septum, bed nucleus of the stria terminalis (BNST), and anterior hypothalamus, which all project to the parvocellular PVN, and (2) the medial corticohypothalamic tract from the anteroventral subiculum to the ventromedial, arcuate, and suprachiasmatic nuclei of the hypothalamus. The PVN also receive direct projections from the amygdala as well as projections that relay in the BNST.

Many, but not all, studies in which HPA activity was assessed by the assay of corticosterone and, less frequently, ACTH suggest that the hippocampus inhibits HPA activity. Hippocampal inhibition of the HPA appears to be due mainly to corticosteroid negative feedback inhibition, although there is also evidence that the hippocampus may exert an inhibitory tone on the HPA independently of corticosteroid feedback. However, the hippocampus is neither the only site nor necessarily the major site of corticosteroid negative feedback, since removal of its input to the hypothalamus reduces, but does not abolish, the efficacy of corticosteroid inhibition. Thus, for example, (1) although electrical stimulation of the PVN resulted in a two- to threefold increase in CRH release into hypophysial portal blood, stimulation of the hippocampus had no effect on the release of CRH, AVP, or oxytocin; (2) transection of the fornix, the major hippocampal-hypothalamic connection, had no significant effect on either basal or stress (nitroprusside-induced hypotension) evoked CRH release into hypophysial portal blood; and (3) implantation of dexamethasone pellets in hippocampus had no effect on CRH synthesis in the PVN. Nevertheless, fornix section did elevate AVP concentrations in portal blood and blocked corticosterone reduction of elevated CRH, but not AVP, levels in portal blood during hypotensive stress.

Further evidence that the hippocampus normally moderates the synthesis of stress neurohormones is suggested by the finding that lateral fimbria-fornix lesions increased CRH mRNA and AVP mRNA in medial parvocellular PVN, and also plasma ACTH concentrations.

Feldman and Weidenfeld showed that, in freely moving male rats, photic and acoustic stimuli depleted the CRH content of the median eminence with a concomitant increase in plasma ACTH and corticosterone levels. This photic/acoustic activation of the HPA was inhibited by the systemic administration of dexamethasone. HPA inhibition by dexamethasone was in turn inhibited by hippocampal implants of glucocorticoid and, to a lesser extent, mineralocorticoid receptor antagonists. These results suggest that in conscious animals the hippocampus does play a role in corticosteroid feedback inhibition of stress-induced ACTH release.

Herman and associates have underscored the role of the BNST as a nucleus that integrates or processes hippocampal and amygdaloid modulation of the HPA. This hypothesis is based, first, on the anatomical connections of the BNST in that the nucleus receives rich projections from the amygdala and hippocampus and projects to the parvocellular PVN. Second, lesion of the anterior BNST resulted in a 30% decrease in CRH mRNA levels in the PVN, whereas lesion of the posterior BNST resulted in a 13% increase in the level of CRH mRNA in the PVN. On the basis of these data, Herman and colleagues inferred that the anterior BNST integrates excitatory inputs mainly from the amygdala, whereas the posterior BNST integrates inhibitory inputs mainly from the hippocampus.

In summary, the hippocampus plays an important role in moderating the HPA both by mediating corticosteroid negative feedback and by exerting an endogenous inhibitory tone on the HPA. Corticosteroid negative feedback is also exerted directly on the PVN and the pituitary gland. The hippocampus is a heterogeneous structure; thus, for example, Dunn and Orr found that electrical stimulation of the CA1 region increased corticosterone levels, whereas stimulation of the CA3, dentate, and subiculum decreased plasma corticosterone concentrations. This heterogeneity will need to be considered in the design of further studies on the role of the hippocampus in negative feedback control of the HPA.

Glucocorticoid Negative Feedback at the Pituitary Level

As well as exerting a central effect, corticosteroids inhibit ACTH synthesis and release by an action at the level of the anterior pituitary gland. As in brain, the inhibitory action of corticosteroids on pituitary corticotropes is mediated by glucocorticoid (type II) receptors.

Studies on dispersed pituitary cells with inhibitors of mRNA and protein synthesis have shown that both the rapid and delayed glucocorticoid inhibition of ACTH release depends upon mRNA and protein synthesis. Glucocorticoids also exert potent inhibitory effects on the expression of the ACTH precursor proopiomelanocortin (POMC) in the anterior lobe of the pituitary gland. In male Sprague-Dawley rats, transcription assays showed that dexamethasone inhibited POMC gene transcription by 10-fold within 30 min of a single injection of the glucocorticoid. Inhibition of POMC transcription was paralleled by a dramatic fall in plasma ACTH concentrations. The same study showed that CRH stimulated POMC transcription by nearly twofold within 15 min, which coincided with a massive increase in ACTH release. The action of dexamethasone is cell specific in that the steroid had no effect on the transcription rate of POMC in primary cultures of neurointermediate lobe cells.

Studies in transgenic mice showed that no more than 769 base pairs of the rat POMC promoter are required for cell-specific expression and glucocorticoid inhibition of the POMC gene in the anterior pituitary gland. A good deal is known about the glucocorticoid response elements in the POMC promoter and the transcription factors involved in POMC expression, but the precise molecular mechanism of glucocorticoid inhibition of POMC transcription remains to be elucidated.

In addition to a direct action on POMC gene expression, which determines the amount of ACTH available for release, glucocorticoids inhibit ACTH release by a mechanism mediated by adenylate cyclase.

Possible Role of 11β-Hydroxysteroid Dehydrogenase

Two types of 11β-hydroxysteroid dehydrogenase play a pivotal role in glucocorticoid synthesis and metabolism. This enzyme is involved in glucocorticoid negative feedback (see **11ß-Hydroxysteroid Dehydrogenases**).

Functional Importance of Glucocorticoid Negative Feedback

Glucocorticoid feedback inhibition of ACTH release protects the organism against the deleterious effects of hypercortisolemia (excessive concentrations of cortisol in blood). Whether due to endocrine disorders, such as Cushing's syndrome, or other causes such as trauma or chronic stress, hypercortisolemia is associated with at least three major deleterious effects. First, it suppresses the immune-inflammatory defense system and so incapacitates the animal's ability to respond to infection by pathogenic microorganisms or to chemical or physical insult. Second, persistent hypercortisolemia has major adverse effects on intermediary metabolism, resulting eventually in all the features of Cushing's syndrome, that is, android obesity, diabetes mellitus, hyperlipidemia, hypertension, and osteoporosis. Third, hypercortisolemia and/or stress are associated with reduction in hippocampal volume (atrophy) in several neuropsychiatric disorders, such as depression and posttraumatic stress disorder, as well as in Cushing's syndrome. In all three disorders, the hippocampal atrophy is associated with explicit memory deficits.

Clinical Manifestations of Disordered Glucocorticoid Feedback Regulation of the HPA System

No attempt is made here to give a detailed account of the clinical effects of disruption of feedback control within the HPA system. Rather, this section considers two clinical examples that underscore the principles of negative feedback and illustrate the consequences of disruption of normal HPA feedback control. The first example is of enzyme defect in the adrenal cortex that results in the absence or deficiency of the afferent glucocorticoid signal of the HPA negative feedback system, whereas the second is probably due to an alteration in the central set point of the negative feedback control system.

Congenital Adrenal Hyperplasia: Failure of Glucocorticoid Negative Feedback

There are several types of inherited enzymatic defects in cortisol synthesis known to result in congenital adrenal hyperplasia (CAH), also known as the adrenogenital syndrome. By far the most common form

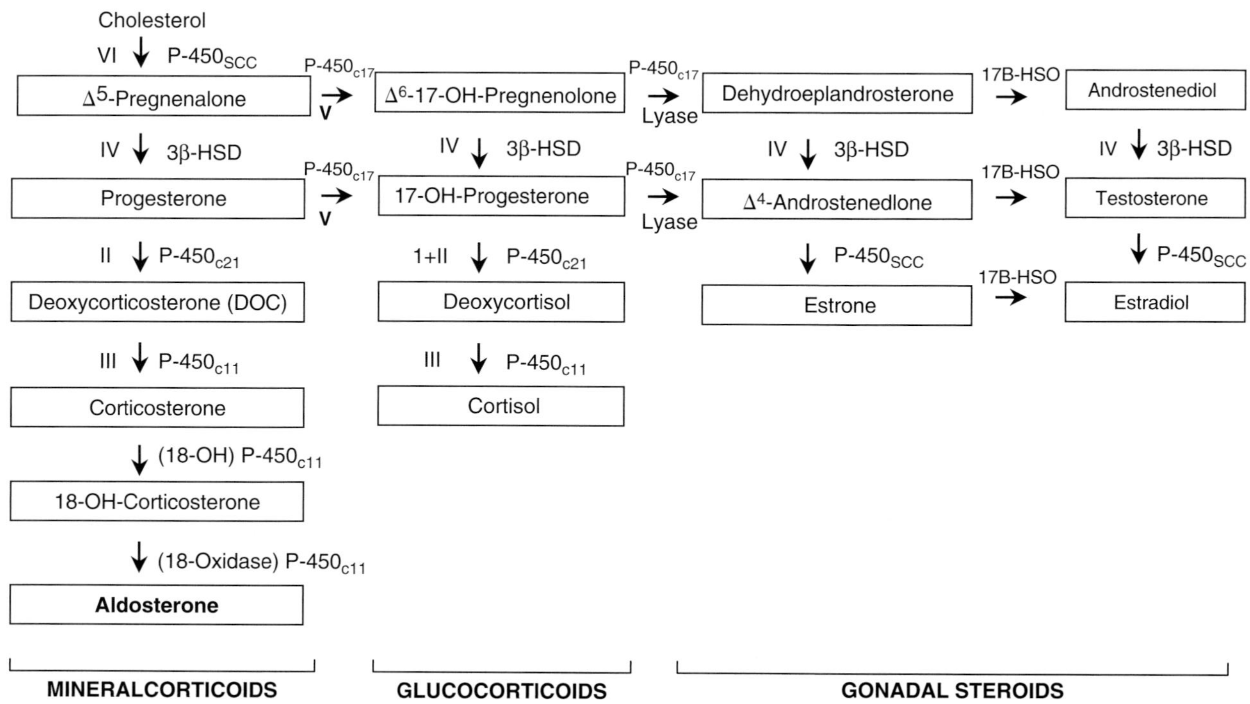

Figure 7 A diagrammatic representation of the steroid biosynthetic pathways in humans. I to VI correspond to numbers for specific biosynthetic defects that result in congenital hyperplasia. $P450_{scc}$, cholesterol side chain cleavage; 3β-HSD, 3β-hydroxysteroid dehydrogenase/$\Delta^{4,5}$-isomerase; $P450_{c21}$, 21-hydroxylase; 17β-HSO,17α-hydroxysteroid oxidoreductase; $P450_{c11}$ catalyzes 11β-hydroxylation, as well as 18-hydroxylation and 18-oxidation; $P450_{cl7}$ catalyzes 17-hydroxylation and 17,20-lyase activity. Subscripts refer to the steroidogenic enzymatic action of the several cytochrome P450 enzymes. From Grumbach, M. M. and Conte, F. A. (1998). Disorders of sexual differentiation. In: Wilson, J. D., Foster, D. W., Kronenberg, H. M. & Larsen, P. R. (eds.) *Williams textbook of endocrinology* (9th edn., pp.1303–1425). Philadelphia, PA: Saunders, with permission.

is due to a deficiency of $P450c_{21}$ (21-hydroxylase; see **Figure** 7), which leads to a deficiency in cortisol biosynthesis. Excessive androgen secretion results from a failure of glucocorticoid negative feedback and consequent, uncontrolled, high ACTH secretion. Excessive androgen levels may lead to virilization of females *in utero*. About two-thirds of patients also have mineralocorticoid deficiency, resulting in salt wasting. If not obvious during the neonatal period, androgen excess may appear in early infancy, resulting in sexual precocity in boys and clitoral enlargement and pubic hair growth in girls. Excess androgen accelerates linear growth and epiphyseal closure, leading ultimately to diminished adult height. In adult women with untreated CAH, reproductive function is impaired due to (1) the disturbance of normal menstrual cycles as a consequence of the high plasma progesterone and androgen concentrations and (2) labial fusion, which prevents successful coitus. The former can be corrected by glucocorticoid replacement therapy, whereas the latter can be treated surgically.

The $P450c_{21}$ deficiency is transmitted as a single gene autosomal recessive trait linked to the major histocompatibility complex locus on the short arm of chromosome 6. An allelic variable of classical 21-hydroxylase deficiency results in a late-onset type, which frequently presents with clinical features similar to those of polycystic ovarian disease.

Deficiency of $P450c_{II}$ (11β-hydroxylase) is a much less common cause of CAH. As in the case of $P450c_{21}$ deficiency, it is transmitted as an autosomal recessive disorder but is not linked to the HLA locus. As in the case of $P450c_{21}$ deficiency, a deficiency in $P450c_{11}$ results in impaired glucocorticoid feedback and a consequent hypersecretion of ACTH and adrenal androgens. The condition is treated with glucocorticoid replacement therapy.

Much more rare forms of CAH are produced by deficiencies of 17α-hydroxylase and 3β-hydroxysteroid dehydrogenase, which result in defective adrenal androgen, as well as glucocorticoid secretion.

Hypercortisolemia in Major Depression: Possibly due to an Altered Set Point in Glucocorticoid Negative Feedback

Major depressive disorder is characterized by a significant increase in plasma cortisol concentrations (hypercortisolemia), which is most prominent at the nadir of the circadian rhythm around midnight. It was first thought that hypercortisolemia and resistance to the suppression of endogenous cortisol secretion by dexamethasone were specific features of major depression, which led to the hope that the dexamethasone suppression test could be used as a specific biological marker of depression. However, extensive studies have shown that hypercortisolemia and resistance to dexamethasone suppression are also associated with other types of psychoses, such as schizoaffective disorder and organic dementia, including Alzheimer's disease.

As shown by Goodwin and associates, hypercortisolemia in major depression is associated with a threefold increase in the mean plasma concentration of β-endorphin. In fact, resistance of β-endorphin to dexamethasone suppression appears to be a more robust marker of major depression than cortisol. Thus, in a study by Young and associates of 73 patients with major depressive disorder, 39 (53%) showed β-endorphin nonsuppression to dexamethasone, while only 8 patients (11%) showed cortisol nonsuppression. These findings suggest that hypercortisolemia in major depression is due to a resistance of the brain-pituitary-ACTH module to glucocorticoid negative feedback, that is, an elevation of the set point for glucocorticoid feedback. The precise mechanism remains to be determined, but decreased responsiveness of the limbic system, PVN, and/or pituitary gland to glucocorticoid negative feedback is a likely explanation. Reduced responsiveness of the PVN could be caused by transynaptic changes triggered by changes in function of the limbic system and frontal cortex. Because the serotonergic raphe neurons determine the amplitude of the circadian excursions of plasma ACTH and corticosterone, it is also conceivable that hypercortisolemia reflects dysregulation of serotonergic function, which seems to occur in major depression.

Allostasis and Allostatic Load

Allostasis and allostatic load are mentioned here to clarify the link between homeostasis and allostasis. The latter refers to maintenance of stability through change or adaptation and is illustrated by the increase in blood pressure on wakening or sex to cope with extra circulatory demands. In normal subjects, the increased blood pressure required to match increase in load does not necessarily reflect all but a transitory override of blood pressure control mechanisms involving baroreceptors (pressure receptors in the carotid sinus) and chemoreceptors (chemical sensors in the carotid body). Rather, there is a shift or adaptation in set point of the blood pressure control system so that it maintains mean arterial blood pressure within narrow limits around the new set point commensurate with the new load. Simply put, this is the same as altering the set point of a thermostat in a room to increase or decrease the mean ambient temperature – the set point has been changed, but the control mechanisms remain the same. The same principle may be applied to the control of plasma cortisol or adrenaline concentrations. The ability to alter the set point of one or more feedback control systems is termed regulation. In the case of the HPA and systemic blood pressure, set point regulation is located within the CNS. The elements that change the controlled variable (e.g., blood pressure, cortisol, adrenaline) toward the new set point are the control mechanisms.

Allostatic load was first introduced and defined by McEwen and Stellar (McEwen 2001) "as the cost of chronic exposure to fluctuating or heightened neural or neuroendocrine response resulting from repeated or chronic environmental challenge that an individual reacts to as being particularly stressful." That is, allostatic load reflects the hidden cost of chronic stresses to the body that act as a predisposing factor for the adverse effects of acute, stressful life events.

Conclusion

The HPA system, together with the sympathetic-medullary system, plays a pivotal role in the neuroendocrine response to stress. Homeostasis within the HPA is maintained by a precise negative feedback system by which the adrenal glucocorticoids (the afferent inhibitory signal), cortisol in humans or corticosterone in rodents, moderate ACTH synthesis and release (efferent output signal). Allostasis – that is, change in HPA activity to cope with increased stress load – is brought about by change in feedback set point. The major sites of negative feedback are the PVN, where glucocorticoids inhibit CRH and AVP synthesis and release, and the pituitary gland, where they block the ACTH response to CRH and inhibit POMC/ACTH synthesis. The limbic system of the brain, especially the hippocampus and amygdala, plays an important role in glucocorticoid negative feedback control.

Disruption of the HPA negative feedback system has serious deleterious effects, a point illustrated by the congenital adrenogenital syndrome and hypercortisolemia associated with serious mental illnesses. The adrenogenital syndrome, due to defective or absent cortisol secretion (loss of the afferent feedback signal) consequent on a congenital enzyme defect in the adrenal cortex, results in massive uncontrolled pituitary ACTH release. The latter induces excessive androgen production that in turn causes precocious puberty in males and masculinization of females. Hypercortisolemia, a prominent feature of major depressive disorder and other psychoses and organic dementias, is probably due to elevation of the set point of the HPA negative feedback system. Elucidation of the precise cause of this change in feedback set point may provide insight into the central disorder in depression. Hypercortisolemia may exert adverse effects by (1) inhibiting immune-inflammatory defense mechanisms, (2) disrupting intermediary metabolism, (3) inducing effects akin to Cushing's syndrome that lead to obesity, diabetes type II, and osteoporosis, and (4) compromising hippocampal structure, neurogenesis, and function that might lead to cognitive impairment.

See Also the Following Articles

11β-Hydroxysteroid Dehydrogenases; Circadian Rhythms, Genetics of; Corticotropin Releasing Factor-Binding Protein; Food Shift Effect; Gleucocorticoid Negative Feedback; Glucocorticoids – Adverse Effects on the Nervous System; Neuroendocrine Systems.

Further Reading

Bremner, J. D. and Vermetten, E. (2004). Neuroanatomical changes associated with pharmacotherapy in posttraumatic stress disorder. *Annals of the New York Academy of Science* **1032**, 154–157.

Christie, J. E., Whalley, L. J., Fink, G., et al. (1986). Raised plasma cortisol concentrations are a feature of drug-free psychotics and not specific for depression. *British Journal of Psychiatry* **148**, 58–65.

Christie, J. E., Whalley, L. J., Fink, G., et al. (1987). Characteristic plasma hormone changes in Alzheimer's disease. *British Journal of Psychiatry* **150**, 674–681.

Copolov, D. L., Rubin, R. T., Stuart, G. W., et al. (1989). Specificity of the salivary cortisol dexamethasone suppression test across psychiatric diagnoses. *Biological Psychiatry* **25**, 879–893.

Engler, D., Redei, E. and Kola, I. (1999). The corticotropin-release inhibitory factor hypothesis: A review of the evidence for the existence of inhibitory as well as stimulatory hypophysiotropic regulation of adrenocorticotropin secretion and biosynthesis. *Endocrine Review* **20**, 460–500.

Feldman, S. and Weidenfeld, J. (1999). Glucocorticoid receptor antagonists in the hippocampus modify the negative feedback following neural stimuli. *Brain Research* **821**, 33–37.

Fink, G. (1979). Feedback actions of target hormones on hypothalamus and pituitary with special reference to gonadal steroids. *Annual Review of Physiology* **41**, 571–585.

Fink, G. (1988). The G. W. Harris Lecture: steroid control of brain and pituitary function. *Quarterly Journal of Experimental Physiology* **73**, 257–293.

Fink, G. (1995). The self-priming effect of LHRH: a unique servomechanism and possible cellular model for memory. *Frontiers in Neuroendocrinology* **16**, 183–190.

Fink, G. (1997). Mechanisms of negative and positive feedback of steroids in the hypothalamic-pituitary system. In: Bittar, E. E. & Bittar, N. (eds.) *Principles of medical biology* (vol. 10A), pp. 29–100. New York: JAI Press.

Fink, G., Robinson, I. C. A. F. and Tannahill, L. A. (1988). Effects of adrenalectomy and glucocorticoids on the peptides, CRF-41, AVP and oxytocin in rat hypophysial portal blood. *Journal of Physiology* **401**, 329–345.

Fink, G., Dow, R. C., Casley, D., et al. (1992). Atrial natriuretic peptide is involved in the ACTH response to stress and glucocorticoid negative feedback in the rat. *Journal of Endocrinology* **135**, 37–43.

Grumbach, M. M. and Conte, F. A. (1998). Disorders of sexual differentiation. In: Wilson, J. D., Foster, D. W., Kronenberg, H. M. & Larsen, P. R. (eds.) *Williams textbook of endocrinology* (9th edn., pp. 1303–1425). Philadelphia, PA: Saunders.

Herman, J. P. and Cullinan, W. E. (1997). Neurocircuitry of stress: central control of the hypothalamo-pituitary-adrenocortical axis. *Trends in Neurosciences* **20**, 78–84.

Malberg, J. E. and Schechter, L. E. (2005). Increasing hippocampal neurogenesis; a novel mechanism for antidepressant drugs. *Current Pharmaceutical Design* **11**, 145–155.

Malkoski, S. P. and Dorin, R. I. (1999). Composite glucocorticoid regulation at a functionally defined negative glucocorticoid response element of the human corticotropin-releasing hormone gene. *Molecular Endocrinology* **13**, 1629–1644.

McEwen, B. S. (2002). Sex, stress and the hippocampus: allostasis, allostatic load and the aging process. *Neurobiology of Aging* **23**, 921–939.

Milhorn, H. T. J. (1966). *The application of control theory to physiological systems*. Philadelphia, PA: Saunders.

Munck, A., Guyre, P. M. and Holbrook, N. J. (1984). Physiological functions of glucocorticoids in stress and their relation to pharmacological actions. *Endocrine Reviews* **5**, 22–44.

Roth-Isigkeit, A., Dibbelt, L., Eichler, W., et al. (2001). Blood levels of atrial natriuretic peptide, endothelin, cortisol and ACTH in patients undergoing coronary artery bypass grafting surgery with cardiopulmonary bypass. *Journal of Endocrinology Investigation* **24**, 777–785.

Sapolsky, R. M., Armanini, M. P., Sutton, S. W., et al. (1989). Elevation of hypophysial portal concentrations of adrenocorticotropin secretagogues after fornix transection. *Endocrinology* **125**, 2881–2887.

Sawchenko, P. E. and Swanson, L. W. (1983). The organization of forebrain afferents to the paraventricular and supraoptic nuclei of the rat. *Journal Comparative Neurology* **218**, 121–144.

Schulkin, J. (ed.) (2004). *Allostasis, homeostasis, and the costs of physiological adaptation*, pp. 1–372. Cambridge: Cambridge University Press.

Shepard, J. D., Liu, Y., Sassone-Corsi, P. and Aguilera, G. (2005). Role of glucocorticoids and cAMP-mediated repression in limiting corticotropin-releasing hormone transcription during stress. *Journal of Neuroscience* **25**, 4073–4081.

Tannahill, L. A., Sheward, W. J., Robinson, I. C. A. F. and Fink, G. (1991). Corticotropin-releasing factor-41, vasopressin and oxytocin release into hypophysial portal blood in the rat; effects of electrical stimulation of the hypothalamus, amygdala and hippocampus. *Journal of Endocrinology* **129**, 99–107.

Watts, A. G., Tanimura, S. and Sanchez-Watts, G. (2004). Corticotropin-releasing hormone and arginine vasopressin gene transcription in the hypothalamic paraventricular nucleus of unstressed rats: daily rhythms and their interactions with corticosterone. *Endocrinology* **145**, 529–540.

Yates, F. E. and Maran, J. W. (1974). Stimulation and inhibition of adrenocorticotropin release. In: Knobil, E. & Sawyer, W.H. (eds.) *Handbook of physiology*, pp. 367–404. Washington, D.C.: American Physiological Society.

Young, D. A., Kotun, J., Haskett, R. F., et al. (1993). Dissociation between pituitary and adrenal supression to dexamethasone in depression. *Archives of General Psychiatry* **50**, 395–403.

Stress Response: Neural and Feedback Regulation of the HPA Axis

J P Herman
University of Cincinnati, Cincinnati, OH, USA

The Hypothalamic–Pituitary–Adrenal Axis

The hypothalamic–pituitary–adrenal (HPA) axis is essential for adaptation to physical or psychological stress. Glucocorticoid hormones, which are the ultimate product of HPA axis activation, act on multiple bodily systems to maintain homeostasis. Many of the effects of glucocorticoids are beneficial for short-term survival but can be counterproductive or even deleterious if prolonged. Therefore, the activation and inhibition of glucocorticoid is a temporally regulated process involving rapid neuronal activation and efficient feedback inhibition.

Stimulation of the HPA axis occurs in reaction to or in anticipation of physiologic challenge. Reactive or 'reflexive' release of glucocorticoids occurs in response to physiological challenges (e.g., blood loss, hemorrhage). This type of response is initiated by stimuli that signal a direct threat to homeostasis or survival and can be triggered without conscious perception. However, it is important to note that organisms also generate 'anticipatory' HPA axis responses to environmental cues associated with threats to survival or homeostasis. Thus, stimuli that predict adversity can generate a glucocorticoid response in the absence of an existing physiologic insult. These responses are generated by comparison of environmental stimuli with either innate programs (e.g., instinctual fear of predators) or memories (e.g., prior experience with a painful or fearful stimulus). The relevance of the anticipatory response hinges on the predicted need for an adaptive hormonal response, with the glucocorticoid secretory process begun in preparation of a survival challenge (prolonged flight, fight, and injury).

Glucocorticoid release is commonly associated with an inferred state of 'stress.' From the perspective of this article, 'stress' can be defined as 'a real or perceived threat to homeostasis or well-being.' There are four somewhat distinct 'stress' responses: behavioral change, activation of the sympathoadrenomedullary system, activation of the HPA axis, and activation of the immune system, roughly in order of threshold and timing. The glucocorticoid stress response addressed in this article is but one component of an integrated set of responses to stress.

The hypothalamic paraventricular nucleus (PVN) is responsible for regulation of HPA axis stress responses (**Figure 1**). Activation of the HPA axis is mediated by neurosecretory neurons localized in the medial parvocellular zone of this nucleus. These neurons project to blood vessels in the external lamina of the median eminence, where they release numerous adrenocorticotropin (ACTH) 'secretagogues,' the most important of which are corticotropin-releasing hormone (CRH) and arginine vasopressin.

The medial parvocellular PVN is in receipt of synaptic innervation from a relatively circumscribed set of central nervous system structures, summarized in **Figure 2**. In general, PVN projection neurons are localized in regions known to receive first- or second-order inputs from somatic nociceptors, visceral afferents,

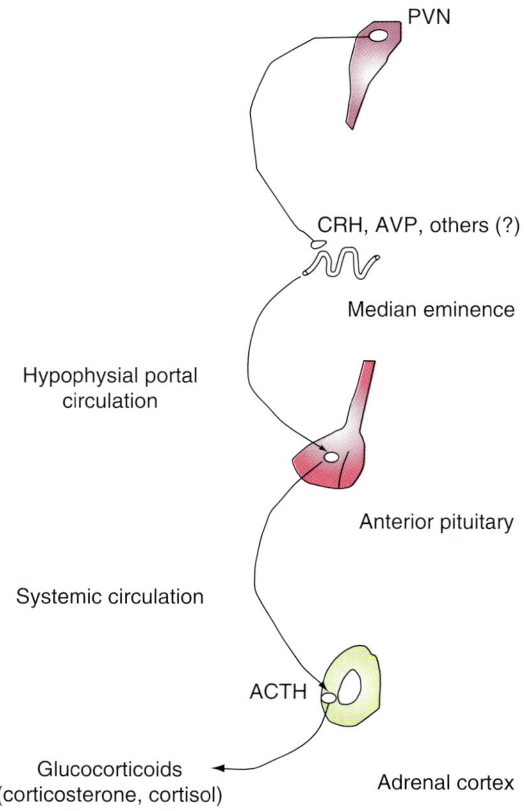

Figure 1 Schematic of the hypothalamic–pituitary–adrenal (HPA) axis. Stress triggers activation of paraventricular hypothalamic nucleus (PVN) neurons, causing release of corticotropin releasing hormone (CRH), and co-secretagogues (such as arginine vasopressin (AVP) in the portal vessels of the median eminence. Secretagogues travel via the portal blood to the anterior pituitary, where they elicit secretion of adrenocorticotrophic hormone (ACTH). ACTH travels via the systemic circulation to the adrenal cortex, causing synthesis and secretion of glucocorticoids.

or humoral sensory pathways. Thus, the majority of PVN-projecting neurons are positioned to evoke rapid, reflexive activation of the HPA axis. These PVN projection neurons can in turn be influenced by inputs from cortical and limbic structures, which are likely to transduce anticipatory activation.

Glucocorticoids released following stress exert classical negative feedback effects on the HPA axis. Feedback effects of glucocorticoids occur in distinct time domains. Fast feedback occurs within minutes and is nongenomic in nature. Fast feedback is sensitive to the rate of change in circulating glucocorticoid levels and is essential for rapid termination of PVN activation and ACTH release normally seen during an acute stress response. The nongenomic mechanism involves membrane glucocorticoid receptors. Delayed feedback occurs over hours to days and involves genomic mechanisms. Delayed feedback is sensitive to the levels of circulating glucocorticoids rather than the rate of rise.

Glucocorticoid negative feedback may be mediated at multiple levels. The nuclear glucocorticoid receptor is though to regulate genomic negative feedback, perhaps in conjunction with permissive actions of the mineralocorticoid receptor, which binds glucocorticoids with high affinity and is extensively bound even under unstressed conditions. The glucocorticoid receptor is abundantly expressed in the pituitary, PVN, and numerous brain regions implicated in HPA axis regulation, all of which may contribute to negative feedback.

It is important that regulation of the HPA axis can be mediated by peripheral feedback factors other than glucocorticoids. For example, ingestion of a caloric load (e.g., sucrose consumption) can inhibit activation of the HPA axis independent of glucocorticoid secretion. The neural mechanism subserving this alternative feedback pathway remains to be determined.

Direct Pathways Controlling HPA Axis Activation

Brain Stem

The PVN receives a large input from noradrenergic and adrenergic neurons of the nucleus tractus solitarius (NTS). Lesions of these neurons or their terminals attenuate HPA axis stress responses to reflexive stressors, whereas direct adrenergic receptor stimulation activates CRH and ACTH secretion, confirming that norepinephrine (and perhaps epinephrine) neurons are necessary and sufficient for stress activation of the HPA axis. However, the influence of NTS norepinephrine–epinephrine on anticipatory stress responses is not observed consistently, suggesting that anticipatory excitation occurs by other mechanisms.

The NTS also contains a noncatecholaminergic PVN-projecting cell population. Many of these cells contain important peptidergic neuromodulators (e.g., glucagon-like peptide-1, neuropeptide Y) that are HPA axis excitatory, and there is evidence that these peptides may participate in generation of both reflexive and anticipatory stress responses.

Serotonergic systems also participate in HPA axis activation by way of projections from the midbrain and pontine raphe nuclei. Serotonergic innervation of the PVN is more circumscribed than that of the NTS, and modulation of extra-PVN serotonin can also have potent actions on HPA axis activity. The relative strengths of direct versus indirect serotonin serotonergic modulation of the stress response remain to be resolved.

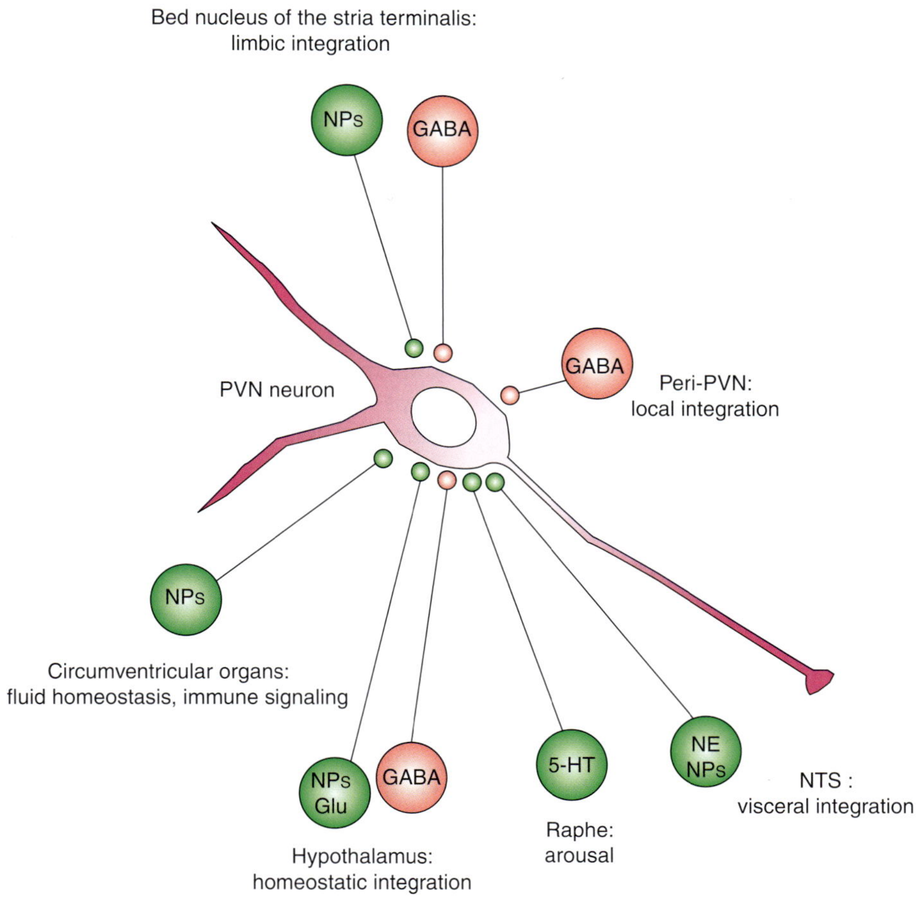

Figure 2 Direct projections to the paraventricular hypothalamic nucleus (PVN). Excitatory inputs are in green, inhibitory in pink. The PVN receives predominantly excitatory inputs from brain stem noradrenergic (NE), neuropeptidergic (NP), and serotonergic (5-hydroxytryptamine; 5-HT) cell groups, as well as from circumventircular structures (such as the subfornical organ). Inputs from the hypothalamus and bed nucleus of the stria terminalis can be excitatory (glutamate (Glu) or NPs) or inhibitory (γ-aminobutyric acid; GABA), depending on location. Neurons in the immediate vicinity of the PVN may serve as local inhibitors of HPA axis activation. NTS, nucleus tractus solitarius.

Lamina Terminalis System

The PVN is in direct receipt of information on fluid and electrolyte status by way of the subfornical organ–lamina terminalis system. Signals are relayed through direct projections of the subfornical organ, median preoptic nucleus, and organum vasculosum of the lamina terminalis to medial parvocellular PVN neurons. These regions are critically involved in control of osmoregulation and drinking behavior, and this pathway may be critical for initiation of HPA responses to thirst or dehydration.

Hypothalamus

The PVN receives massive input from numerous regions of the hypothalamus, a large component of which is γ-aminobutyricacidergic (GABAergic; inhibitory). GABA inputs to the PVN originate in numerous hypothalamic nuclei concerned with homeostatic regulation, including the dorsomedial hypothalamus (autonomic function), preoptic area (thermoregulation), arcuate nucleus (energy balance), and lateral hypothalamus (ingestive behavior).

The PVN also receives input from hypothalamic neuropeptidergic (e.g., corticotrophin releasing factor, melanocortin) and glutamatergic neurons. These inputs are presumably excitatory and may serve to activate the HPA axis in response to homeostatic imbalance. Thus, hypothalamic inputs are sufficient to both excite and inhibit the PVN, consistent with a role in maintenance of homeostasis.

Bed Nucleus of the Stria Terminalis

Direct nonhypothalamic forebrain inputs to the parvocellular PVN are largely confined to discrete subnuclei of the bed nucleus of the stria terminalis (BST). The influence of the BST on HPA function is complex. Posterior regions of the BST inhibit HPA axis responses to stress, whereas ventrolateral PVN projecting neurons provide excitatory input. This complexity may be related to differential limbic inputs to these regions, as noted below.

Thalamus

Neurons in auditory-responsive posterior thalamic nuclei, including the subparafascicular and posterior intralaminar regions, send direct projections to the medial parvocellular PVN and are likely involved in pathways mediating activation of the HPA axis by auditory stimuli.

Local PVN Information Processing

The PVN is well positioned to receive direct input from blood- and CSF-borne factors. The PVN has a dense nonfenestrated capillary plexus that can allow ready access to blood–brain barrier permeable factors, including glucocorticoids. Thus, the PVN is one site of potential glucocorticoid negative feedback regulation of the HPA axis. Brain microvessels may also play a major role in communicating immune (cytokine) signals to the CNS, through activation of prostaglandin biosynthesis. Notably, the medial parvocellular PVN richly expresses prostaglandin receptors, suggesting a capacity for local integration of immune signals within the PVN proper.

Neurons of the PVN have limited dendritic extensions that largely remain within the nucleus proper. This morphological arrangement supports intranuclear communication among different PVN subdivisions (e.g., magnocellular divisions projecting to the neurohypophysis), which may subserve intrinsic modulation of excitability. The restricted dendritic branching scheme also prevents parvocellular PVN neurons from sampling the peri-PVN region, which is richly invested with terminals and axons from limbic structures such as the hippocampus, prefrontal cortex, and lateral septum. This arrangement likely prevents direct modulation of HPA axis function by descending limbic structures.

The peri-PVN region contains large numbers of GABAergic neurons, some of which project into the PVN proper. The peri-PVN region receives rich input from limbic structures, hypothalamic cell groups, and serotonin neurons, suggesting that it may play a role in 'gating' of information coming into the PVN.

Indirect Paths to the PVN

Limbic brain structures modulate anticipatory HPA responses to stress. These structures, including regions such as the hippocampus, prefrontal cortex, amygdala, septum, and midline thalamus, are critical for emotional responses and memory and are logical candidates for modulating pituitary–adrenal secretions with respect to prior experience. These regions have no substantial direct interactions with medial parvocellular PVN neurons, requiring intermediary neurons to relay their influence on ACTH secretagogue release (see **Figure 3**).

Hippocampus

The hippocampus is involved in terminating HPA axis responses to stress. Accumulating evidence indicates that the hippocampus is involved in inhibiting anticipatory but not reflexive stress responses, perhaps consistent with its role in memory and information processing. The observation that hippocampal damage can delay termination of corticosterone release is consistent with a role in glucocorticoid negative feedback inhibition of the HPA axis. This hypothesis is supported by rich localization of glucocorticoid receptors in the hippocampus and by functional studies demonstrating diminished feedback efficacy following hippocampal lesions, local glucocorticoid receptor inactivation, or hippocampal–cortical glucocorticoid receptor gene deletion.

Anatomical tracing studies reveal that the hippocampus can communicate with the PVN by way of relay neurons in the hypothalamus and BST. Given that the output of the hippocampus is largely excitatory, it is likely that inhibition is mediated by activation of inhibitory, PVN-projecting GABAergic neurons in these regions.

Medial Prefrontal Cortex

The medial prefrontal cortex also modulates HPA axis activation, albeit in a more complex fashion. Numerous studies indicate that dorsal components of the medial prefrontal cortex inhibit anticipatory but not reflexive HPA axis responses and may be another site for glucocorticoid negative feedback signaling. Conversely, the more ventral components of the medial prefrontal cortex (e.g., infralimbic cortex) heavily innervate subcortical autonomic sites and may be involved in stress excitation. There is also some evidence that ventral medial prefrontal cortex excitation of the stress response is lateralized in the rat (driven by the right hemisphere).

Anatomical studies indicate that the prefrontal cortex does not innervate the PVN to any substantial degree. Dorsal regions of the medial prefrontal cortex project to regions such as the BST as well as a number of non-PVN projecting regulatory regions, whereas ventral regions (encompassing the infralimbic cortex) innervate autonomic regions such as the ventral BST, central amygdala, and NTS. Thus, like the hippocampus, HPA regulation by the medial prefrontal cortex is indirect.

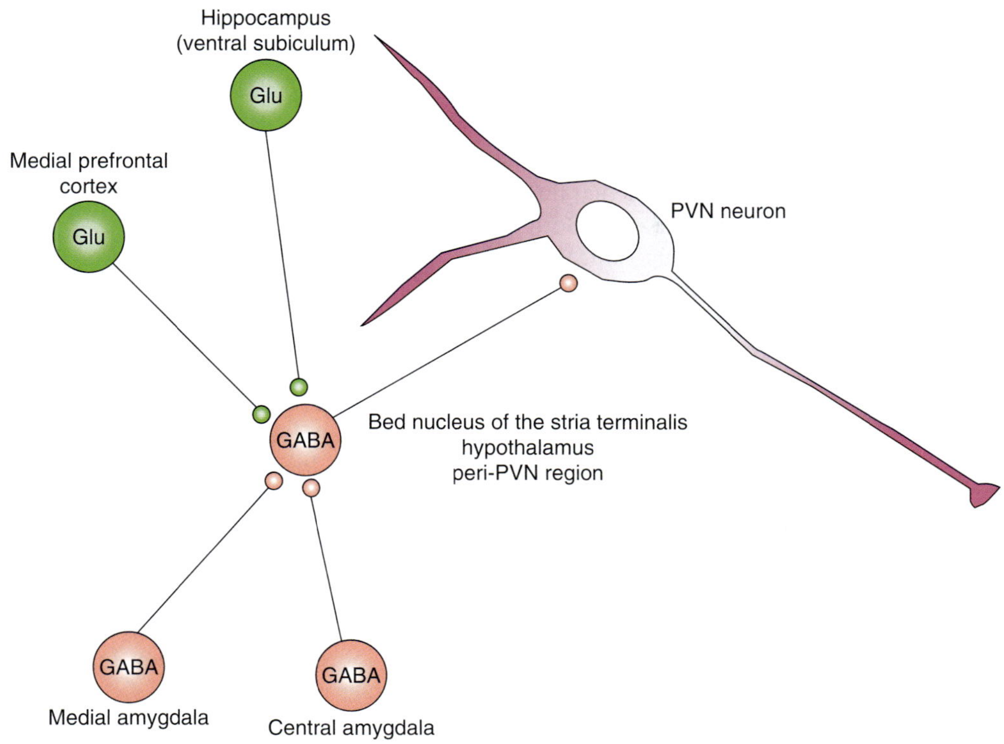

Figure 3 Simplified schematic of possible bisynaptic limbic connections with the paraventricular hypothalamic nucleus (PVN). Regions such as the hippocampus and medial prefrontal cortex inhibit the HPA axis by supplying excitatory glutamatergic innervation of PVN-projecting GABAergic neurons in the bed nucleus of the stria terminalis, hypothalamus, and peri-PVN region (see **Figure 2**). In contrast, amygdalar activation of the HPA axis is likely to occur by disinhibition, involving GABAergic inhibition of GABA projecting PVN neurons. Glu, glutamate.

Amygdala

In contrast with the hippocampus and medial prefrontal cortex, amygdaloid nuclei appear to stimulate the HPA axis. However, there is considerable functional differentiation among individual amygdalar regions. The central amygdaloid nucleus is involved in activation of the HPA axis to reflexive but not anticipatory stressors, whereas the medial amygdala appears to selectively involved in generation of anticipatory responses.

Projection neurons of the central and medial amygdala are primarily GABAergic and do not directly innervate the PVN. However, both regions project heavily to the BST and preoptic area, which contain populations of GABAergic PVN-projecting neurons. Therefore, excitatory effects on HPA axis stress responses are likely mediated by inhibition of GABA neurons in the hypothalamus or BST, effectively resulting in activation by disinhibition.

Lateral Septum

Lateral septal lesions are known to produce a constellation of behavioral and autonomic symptoms consistent with extreme anxiety ('septal rage'). Not surprisingly, this region inhibits HPA axis stress responses. Neurons in this area are activated by a variety of 'anticipatory' stressors but show little induction following activation of the 'reactive' stress pathway, suggesting selective involvement in the former process.

The anatomy of the septal region predicts prominent interactions with hypothalamic and midbrain PVN-projecting regions. As the majority of lateral septal neurons express GABA as their primary transmitter, it is likely that the HPA inhibitory effects of this region are mediated by inhibition of excitatory projections to the PVN.

Thalamus

Several recent reports implicate midline limbic thalamic nuclei in HPA axis regulation. Of the known stress-responsive thalamic nuclei, the paraventricular thalamus appears to play a major role in integrating HPA axis responses to repeated stressors, mediating both stress habituation and sensitization of responses to new stressors. The influence of the paraventicular thalamus is likely to be communicated by way of hypothalamic nuclei (e.g., dorsomedial nucleus).

Hypothalamus

There are several hypothalamic regions that appear able to interact with the PVN through intrahypothalamic relays. Prominent among these is the suprachiasmatic nucleus, which is the major integrator of circadian HPA rhythmicity, and the ventromedial nucleus, which is concerned with energy balance. Both regions interconnect with the PVN through intrahypothalamic relays, including the dorsomedial nucleus and lateral hypothalamus.

Brain Stem

Noradrenergic neurons of the locus coeruleus do not project directly to the medial parvocellular PVN. Nonetheless, lesions of this cell group reduce HPA axis stress responses, implying a transsynaptic excitatory action. This may also be the case for serotonin, as reduction of serotonergic neurotransmission in the amygdala reduces HPA axis responses to stress. In addition, the excitatory action of brain stem acetylcholine on CRH and ACTH release appears to be mediated by norepinephrine neurons of the NTS.

Principles Governing Neurocircuit Regulation of the HPA Axis

The organization of PVN inputs indicates that stress responses are dependent on the overall 'set' of central sensorial input, involving synthesis of homeostatic and cognitive information. Circuits that process reflexive responses have direct access to PVN neurons and tend to be excitatory in nature. These pathways are positioned to communicate sensory information regarding homeostatic imbalance, consistent with a mechanism for rapid adaptation to adversity. \In contrast, anticipatory responses appear to be activated by disinhibition, whereby amygdalar neurons 'turn off' GABAergic projections to the PVN. These GABAergic neurons are strategically positioned in hypothalamic nuclei regulating homeostatic function, providing a possible means for polysensorial cognitive inputs to override ongoing homeostatic regulatory information.

Stress-induced HPA axis activity is temporally limited by inhibitory inputs from the hypothalamus and forebrain. Hypothalamic inputs can directly relay inhibitory information from homeostatic effector pathways. In contrast, forebrain outflow from hippocampus and medial prefrontal cortex mediate inhibition by intermediary synapses, many of which involve hypothalamic homeostatic effector circuits. Thus, as was the case for the amygdala, the impact of hippocampal and cortical circuitry is positioned to act through modulating the ongoing activity of homeostatic pathways to the PVN.

Glucocorticoid negative feedback can be exerted at multiple levels of the neuraxis. Glucocorticoid receptors are present on PVN neurons, and these are involved in rapid as well as sustained feedback inhibition of the HPA axis. However, forebrain glucocorticoid receptors also play a role in inhibition of anticipatory HPA axis stress responses, mediated by effects of glucocorticoids on hippocampal and cortical output circuits.

Overall, regulation of the HPA axis appears to involve hierarchical processing of stressful information and glucocorticoid negative feedback. Reflexive responses represent a first line of defense and are directly wired to rapidly induce ACTH release. Anticipatory responses relay through nuclei that modulate reflexive HPA activation, providing a means by which psychological information can modulate or interact with homeostatic integration. Thus, the reflexive stress response is the default and is subject to modification by prior experience or innate programs. The hierarchical organization of brain stress integration is consistent with theories of brain evolution whereby increasingly complex functions are layered atop simpler reflex pathways.

Control of the HPA axis stress response is of substantial health significance. The impact of gross dysregulation of glucocorticoid secretion on metabolism and cardiovascular function is well known. In addition, more-subtle dysregulation of the HPA axis occurs in stress-related affective disease states, such as depression (hypersecretion) and posttraumatic stress disorder (hyposecretion). The HPA axis pathologies are intimately associated with altered activation or volume of the hippocampus, amygdala, and prefrontal cortices, suggesting that the disease process involves the anticipatory stress response. Thus, appropriate initiation and appropriate cessation of the HPA axis stress responses are a clear priority for both homeostatic balance and adaptation to adversity.

See Also the Following Articles

Hypothalamic–Pituitary–Adrenal (HPA) Axis; Stress: Definition and History; Sympathetic Noradrenergic and Adrenomedullary Hormonal Systems in Stress and Distress.

Further Reading

Boyle, M. P., Brewer, J. A., Funatsu, M., et al. (2005). Acquired deficit of forebrain glucocorticoid receptor produces depression-like changes in adrenal axis regulation and behavior. *Proceedings of the National Academy of Sciences of the United States of America* **102**, 473–478.

Dayas, C. V., Buller, K. M., Crane, J. W., Xu, Y. and Day, T. A. (2001). Stressor categorization: Acute physical and psychological stressors elicit distinctive recruitment patterns in the amygdala and in medullary noradrenergic cell groups. *European Journal of Neuroscience* **14**, 1143–1152.

De Kloet, E. R., Vreugdenhil, E., Oitzl, M. S. and Joels, M. (1998). Brain corticosteroid receptor balance in health and disease. *Endocrine Reviews* **19**, 269–301.
Herman, J. P. and Cullinan, W. E. (1997). Neurocircuitry of stress: Central control of the hypothalamo–pituitary–adrenocortical axis. *Trends in Neuroscience* **20**, 78–83.
Herman, J. P., Figueiredo, H., Mueller, N. K., et al. (2003). Central mechanisms of stress integration: Hierarchical circuitry controlling hypothalamo–pituitary–adrenocortical responsiveness. *Frontiers in Neuroendocrinology* **24**, 151–180.
Herman, J. P., Tasker, J. G., Ziegler, D. R. and Cullinan, W. E. (2002). Local circuit regulation of paraventricular nucleus stress integration: Glutamate-GABA connections. *Pharmacology, Biochemistry, and Behavior* **71**, 457–468.
Keller-Wood, M. and Dallman, M. F. (1984). Corticosteroid inhibition of ACTH secretion. *Endocrine Reviews* **5**, 1–24.
Laugero, K. D., Bell, M. E., Bhatnagar, S., Soriano, L. and Dallman, M. F. (2001). Sucrose ingestion normalizes central expression of corticotropin-releasing-factor messenger ribonucleic acid and energy balance in adrenalectomized rats: A glucocorticoid-metabolic-brain axis? *Endocrinology* **142**, 2796–2804.
McEwen, B. S. and Stellar, E. (1993). Stress and the individual: Mechanisms leading to disease. *Archives of Internal Medicine* **153**, 2093–2101.
Munck, A., Guyre, P. M. and Holbrook, N. J. (1984). Physiological functions of glucocorticoids in stress and their relations to pharmacological actions. *Endocrine Reviews* **5**, 25–44.
Rivest, S. (2001). How circulating cytokines trigger the neural circuits that control the hypothalamic–pituitary–adrenal axis. *Psychoneuroendocrinology* **26**, 761–788.
Sapolsky, R. M. (1994). *Why Zebras Don't Get Ulcers: A Guide to Stress, Stress Related Diseases, and Coping.* New York: Freeman.
Sawchenko, P. E., Li, H. Y. and Ericsson, A. (2000). Circuits and mechanisms governing hypothalamic responses to stress: A tale of two paradigms. *Progress in Brain Research* **122**, 61–78.
Selye, H. (1936). A syndrome produced by diverse nocuous agents. *Nature* **138**, 32.
Selye, H. (1976). *The Stress of Life.* New York: McGraw-Hill.
Whitnall, M. H. (1993). Regulation of the hypothalamic corticotropin-releasing hormone neurosecretory system. *Progress in Neurobiology* **40**, 573–629.

Glucocorticoid Negative Feedback

M F Dallman
University of California, San Francisco, CA, USA

This article is reproduced from Encyclopedia of Stress, First edition, volume 2, pp 224–228, © 2000, Elsevier Inc.

Glossary

Adrenocorticotropic hormone (ACTH) — A hormone made in corticotroph cells of the anterior pituitary; it stimulates the synthesis and secretion of corticosteroids from the adrenal cortex.

Arginine vasopressin (AVP) — A hormone that, when cosecreted with CRH, potentiates ACTH release.

Corticotropin releasing hormone (CRH) — A hormone synthesized in the hypothalamus; it stimulates ACTH synthesis and secretion from anterior pituitary corticotropic cells.

Dexamethasone — A potent synthetic glucocorticoid that does not bind to transcortin (corticosteroid-binding globulin, CBG).

Glucocorticoid receptor (GR) — Low-affinity intracellular corticosteroid receptor that prefers dexamethasone, cortisol, and corticosterone.

Limbic system — A system of neural structures (amygdala, bed nuclei of the stria terminalis, hippocampus, septal nuclei, and hypothalamic and midbrain cell groups) that subserve the emotional and other associative memory, determining overall responsiveness to stressors.

Mineralocorticoid receptor (MR) — High-affinity intracellular corticosteroid receptor that selectively binds aldosterone, corticosterone, and cortisol.

Paraventricular nucleus (PVN) — Hypothalamic site of neuronal synthesis of CRH and AVP, which are secreted from axonal endings in the median eminence to act on pituitary corticotrophs.

Stressors — Stimuli that challenge the physical or psychological stability of the organism and cause the activation of the hypothalamic-pituitary-adrenal axis.

Transcortin (CBG) — A high-affinity binder for cortisol and corticosterone made by the liver; it reversibly binds corticosteroids in the circulation; also called corticosteroid-binding globulin.

Negative feedback inhibition by adrenal glucocorticoids is the means by which the brain is informed that the pituitary ACTH-secreting cells and adrenocortical fasciculata cells have done its bidding. However, a great deal of flexibility is required for an effective feedback system to serve its appropriate function. Thus, there are various time domains and mechanisms by which the glucocorticoids act to inhibit further brain-induced stimulation of the hypothalamic-pituitary-adrenocortical (HPA) axis, the different sites at which the steroids act, and the state-dependent modifications of the brain response to the feedback action of the steroids. The net result of this seeming complexity is a spectacularly functional feedback system that maintains glucocorticoid levels at values appropriate for the physiology of the organism at most times.

Characteristics of Feedback in the Hypothalamic-Pituitary-Adrenocortical Axis

The wide variation in total circulating corticosteroid levels, from the low nanomolar range during the daily circadian trough to the micromolar range during stress, provides a problem for feedback regulation by corticosteroids; the solution is to use two receptors of differing affinities to regulate the brain activation of the adrenocortical system. In addition, there are three temporal domains for the inhibitory effects of corticosteroids and the brain also manages to modify the apparent efficacy of the negative feedback effects of corticosteroids under persistently stressful conditions, thus maintaining an HPA axis that is responsive under conditions in which circulating corticosteroid levels are higher than the usual set point.

Two Receptors Mediate the Feedback Effects of Glucocorticoids

Figure 1 indicates the problem that must be solved by a corticosteroid feedback system in order to control accurately the activity of the HPA axis under circadian and stressful conditions. During the trough of the basal rhythm, total cortisol levels range between 50 and 100 nM. Because at low values ~99% of this represents cortisol bound to CBG, the free cortisol levels that can diffuse from the vascular compartment into the interstitial fluid to bathe cells range between ~0.5 and 1.0 nM. By contrast, at the peak of the circadian rhythm and after stress, total cortisol ranges up to micromolar concentrations and free cortisol levels approach 100–300 nM or even higher. Because receptors characteristically bind hormone over a 100-fold range, it is clear that a single receptor for cortisol cannot control the range of cortisol concentrations required during the normal physiological excursions of the HPA axis. The solution is the use of two receptors of differing affinities to inform the brain of adrenocortical activity.

1. The MR is a high-affinity receptor (K_d 0.5–1 nM) that has roughly equally high affinity for aldosterone, cortisol, and corticosterone. In cells that are selectively responsive to aldosterone, such as the principal cells of the renal nephron, there is an enzyme (11-β-hydroxysteroid dehydrogenase type II) that oxidizes the 11-hydroxyl groups of cortisol and corticosterone to the inactive 11-keto form. Aldosterone exists as an 11-18-hemiketal in solution and is not oxidized by this enzyme; therefore, it can exert its actions selective-

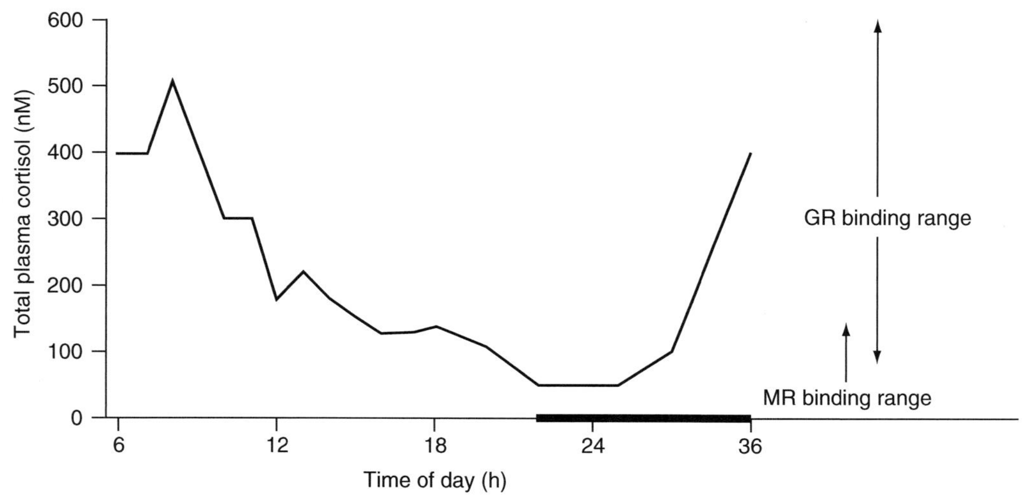

Figure 1 The two-receptor system that provides feedback information to the central HPA axis about adrenocortical performance. A hypothetical normal circadian rhythm in total plasma cortisol (CBG-bound and free) in humans. The dark bar on the abscissa represents the hours of darkness and sleep. The peak occurs just prior to awakening and the beginning of the daily activity cycle. The trough (MR occupancy) occurs early in the hours of sleep and inactivity before values rise again. Stressor-induced increases in cortisol can reach micromolar concentrations. Clearly, if GRs are occupied, MRs are as well. The estimated occupancy of MRs and GRs by free steroid at the various levels of total steroid is shown on the right.

ly in these target cells. Cells that do not contain the enzyme but do have MRs bind all three steroids; however, cortisol and corticosterone circulate in higher concentrations and gain entry to the brain much more easily than aldosterone; therefore, these steroids primarily occupy MRs in the brain. In the brain, MRs have a highly discrete distribution, primarily in neurons in entorhinal cortex, limbic structures, and motor output neurons. There is a very low density of MRs in the neurons of the hypothalamus.

2. The GR is a lower-affinity (K_d 10–30 nM) corticosteroid receptor that prefers dexamethasone $\gg$ cortisol, corticosterone $>$ aldosterone. The GRs are distributed in every cell type in the organism. The distribution of GR in the brain is very widespread in both glial cells and neurons. CRH neurons in hypothalamus are well endowed with GRs, as are the neurons in the limbic system, the monoaminergic systems, and others.

Both occupied MRs and GRs dimerize in the cell nucleus to alter transcriptional rates of tissue-specific genes. In addition, MRs and GRs in the same cell can heterodimerize and act transcriptionally. Moreover, it is increasingly clear that the hormone receptor complexes can function in protein–protein interactions with other transcription factors to alter transcription rates. At this time, the specific effect of occupancy of MRs and GRs on transcription is impossible to predict. Nonetheless, occupancy of MRs and GRs by cortisol or corticosterone serves to inhibit activity in the HPA axis, generally by an action on brain.

Feedback regulation in the animal and its utility Using adrenalectomy and infusion of MR and GR agonists as well as treatment with specific antagonists in intact animals, it is clear that occupancy of the MRs is required to maintain ACTH secretion at low levels during the trough of the circadian rhythm. By contrast, at the circadian peak and during stress, the occupancy of both MR and GR restrains ACTH secretion, maintaining it within the normal limits observed in intact organisms. Because occupied GRs and MRs are powerful modulators of cell function, it is important to maintain their overall concentrations at tightly regulated levels. Many corticosteroid-sensitive end points change their levels and activity when there is slight deviance on either side of the normal daily mean value. In studies of the daily mean of plasma cortisol in humans, values range from 6 to 8 μg dl^{-1} when levels collected over 24 h are averaged. Similarly, in rats, the 24-h mean corticosterone concentration ranges between 4.5 and 7 μg dl^{-1}. Both species have relatively high circulating CBG levels. Above or below these ranges in unstressed humans and rats, untoward metabolic, behavioral, and immunological changes occur.

Temporally Discrete Effects of Corticosteroids on Hypothalamic-Pituitary-Adrenal Axis Function

Feedback inhibition of (CRH, AVP, and) ACTH secretion can be shown to exist in fast, intermediate, and slow time domains when corticosteroids are administered exogenously. Normally these segue smoothly from one to the other, but they can be distinguished mechanistically, and the degree of inhibition increases as the duration and amount of the corticosteroid exposure increases. In all time domains, the magnitude of the effect is strictly proportional to the dose of steroid, between the limits of threshold and saturating quantities.

1. The fast effects occur within milliseconds on neurons and must be exerted by an effect at the cell membrane. A membrane receptor has not yet been characterized. The iontophoresis of corticosteroids onto neurons or bathing tissue slices with corticosteroids shows effects within milliseconds to seconds on membrane function. Similarly, in animals the stimulation of pathways to CRH neurons does not evoke the normal response within minutes of a systemic injection of corticosteroids. At the pituitary corticotroph, CRH-stimulated ACTH secretion is inhibited within a few minutes of the application of corticosteroids; this inhibition is not altered by the inhibition of RNA or protein synthesis, showing that it is not mediated by the usual genomic effects of corticosteroids, although it may be mediated by interference with the generation of adenyl cyclase, the intracellular messenger for CRH. The magnitude of the fast inhibition of ACTH secretion by corticosteroids acting on the corticotroph is small ($\sim$25% of the maximal inhibition possible); thus, fast feedback leaves the organism responsive to further stressors and capable of secreting nearly normal amounts of ACTH.

2. Intermediate feedback has its onset at approximately 30 min after a pulse or continuous exposure to the steroid and lasts for a period of hours. The inhibition of protein synthesis with cyclohexamide blocks this feedback and, although it is powerful and can completely inhibit CRH-induced ACTH secretion in the whole animal, ACTH secretion can usually be stimulated by further treatment with CRH or AVP. This temporal domain of corticosteroid feedback appears to dampen the excitability in the HPA axis without abolishing it (i.e., excitability is returned to prestress levels so that subsequent responsivity is not excessive). At the pituitary, AVP-stimulated ACTH secretion is less sensitive than CRH to corticosteroid inhibition.

3. Slow feedback is found in conditions in which the supraphysiological levels of exogenous corticosteroids have been provided for days or weeks. All components of the HPA axis are unresponsive to stimulation, both by intense stressors and, at the pituitary, by CRH and AVP. The CRH and AVP mRNA expression in the hypothalamus and proopiomelanocorticoid expression in the pituitary is markedly decreased. This condition is most frequently observed in humans with active Cushing disease or after prolonged treatment of disease with high levels of synthetic glucocorticoids; it takes months to recover from this inhibition when the high levels of steroid are removed.

Conditional Feedback in the Hypothalamic-Pituitary-Adrenal Axis

Up to this point, glucocorticoid feedback properties have been discussed with respect to the normal unstressed organism. Under conditions of persistent or chronic stress, the axis appears to change, and sensitivity to the feedback action of corticosteroids is slightly to markedly reduced. Thus, under chronic stress, mean daily plasma corticosteroid concentrations increase, frequently only because circadian trough levels are elevated but occasionally because there are major stressor-induced elevations throughout the circadian cycle. With chronic stress, the degree of the inhibition of stimulated ACTH secretion by exogenous (or endogenously secreted) glucocorticoids is decreased. In rats, chronic stress often stimulates increased expression of AVP in CRH-synthesizing neurons, thus providing a means for amplifying the corticotroph response to the CRH and AVP secreted. However, it also appears that neural sites upstream from the final hypothalamic CRH and AVP motor neurons of the HPA axis are less sensitive to corticosteroid feedback.

A decreased number of GRs has been reported, primarily in hippocampus, after many chronic stressors and after treatment with exogenous glucocorticoids, suggesting that one mechanism of reduced feedback sensitivity may reside in GR downregulation. This is not the only explanation for reduced feedback sensitivity during chronic stress, however, because there are several examples in which both MR and GR numbers are normal throughout brain but glucocorticoid feedback insensitivity is found.

Because the strength of inputs to the CRH and AVP cells stimulates dose-related output, it is likely that, although corticosteroid dose-related functions are occurring normally under chronic stress conditions, the level of input to the CRH and AVP cells increases. Thus, normal responsivity in the HPA axis is maintained, whereas the apparent feedback efficacy of glucocorticoids is reduced. It does appear that new stimuli presented to chronically stressed animals causes facilitated responses in the central neural pathways to the CRH and AVP neurons.

The result of the apparent decrease in glucocorticoid feedback under conditions of chronic stimulation of the HPA axis is that there is dampening of the response to the ongoing stimulus but full or even exaggerated responsiveness to a new and different stimulus. Both effects are useful – the degree of hyperglucocorticoidism is limited by ongoing glucocorticoid feedback, but the organism is still capable of responding to a new stimulus that may demand a momentary shot of the hormones for optimal response.

Site(s) of Negative Feedback in the Hypothalamic-Pituitary-Adrenocortical Axis

Feedback is primarily exerted in the brain under normal conditions, with only moderate increases in mean corticosteroid levels or low-magnitude acute stressors. Although the CRH and AVP neurons in the PVN are plentifully supplied with GRs, this site does not appear to be inhibited directly by the naturally occurring corticosteroids. Instead, the corticosteroids appear to inhibit the activity of neuronal pathways that eventually impinge on CRH and AVP neurons. At high sustained corticosteroid levels, there is also clearly negative feedback on anterior pituitary corticotrophs.

Feedback in the Brain

Microinfusions of low amounts of MR and GR antagonists into the cerebral ventricles or into specific brain sites augment the magnitude of ACTH responses to a variety of stressors, strongly suggesting that stress-induced glucocorticoid secretion decreases the stimulatory input to the PVN during both the fast- and intermediate-feedback time domains. Small crystalline implants of corticosterone placed chronically into prefrontal cortex, the preoptic area, and the dorsal hippocampus have been shown to reduce stress or adrenalectomy-induced ACTH secretion. However, it appears that steroids implanted into brain must bathe those neurons that are activated by the specific stressor used to excite the HPA axis. That is, there appear to be distributed sites at which steroids may inhibit HPA responses to stressors, not a single feedback site that globally inhibits PVN neuronal responses to stressors. Corticosteroids, acting through both MRs and GRs, have been shown to alter neuronal properties and activity in the hippocampus, and antagonists infused into both the amygdala and hippocampus have been shown to alter conditioned behaviors. However, it has not yet been directly demonstrated that implants in these sites alter the amount of ACTH secreted in response to a stressor. It may well be that corticosteroid receptors in these sites have little to do with modulating CRH and AVP secretion directly. In the brain, it appears that for feedback effects of steroid implants to be observed on ACTH secretion the steroid must act on sites that are also activated by stress; the feedback action is selective and specific.

Feedback at the Pituitary

Corticotrophs contain GRs but not MRs, and the direct inhibitory effects of corticosteroids are evident at the anterior pituitary. The concentrations of the naturally occurring steroids required to effect the inhibition of ACTH secretion are relatively high. This is probably because corticotrophs contain the high-affinity CBG corticosteroid binder apparently taken up from the circulation. The CBG in the corticotrophs sequesters the natural corticosteroids and high concentrations (10^{-8} M) are required to observe inhibition, although dexamethasone, which does not bind to CBG, is a more effective inhibitory agent. Moreover, corticotrophs tend to maintain sensitivity to AVP, although sensitivity to CRH decreases when corticosteroid levels are elevated. The relative insensitivity of the corticotroph to corticosteroid inhibition is useful because it allows the corticotroph to be the site of last resort, requiring the highest levels of signal, for the global inhibitory control of the HPA axis.

See Also the Following Articles

Feedback Systems; Glucocorticoids, Effects of Stress on.

Further Reading

Antoni, F. A. (1993). Vasopressinergic control of pituitary adrenocorticotropin comes of age. *Frontiers in Neuroendocrinology* **14**, 76–122.

Bamberger, C. M., Schulte, H. M. and Chrousos, G. P. Molecular determinants of glucocorticoid receptor function and tissue sensitivity to glucocorticoids. *Endocrine Review* **17**, 245–261.

Dallman, M. F., Akana, S. F., Cascio, C. S., Darlington, D. N., Jacobson, L. and Levin, N. (1987). Regulation of ACTH secretion: variations on a theme of B. In: Clark, J. H. (ed.) *Recent progress in hormone research*, pp. 113–173. Orlando, FL: Academic Press.

Dallman, M. F., Akana, S. F., Scribner, K. A., et al. (1992). Stress, feedback and facilitation in the hypothalamo-pituitary-adrenal axis. *Journal of Neuroendocrinology* **4**, 517–526.

Dallman, M. F. and Bhatnagar, S. (1999). *Chronic stress and energy balance: role of the hypothalamo-pituitary-adrenal axis*. Washington, DC: American Physiological Society.

De Kloet, E. R. (1991). Brain corticosteroid receptor balance and homeostatic control. *Frontiers in Neuroendocrinology* **12**, 95–164.

Joels, M. (1997). Steroid hormones and excitability in the mammalian brain. *Frontiers in Neuroendocrinology* **18**, 2–48.

Keller-Wood, M. E. and Dallman, M. F. (1984). Corticosteroid inhibition of ACTH secretion. *Endocrine Review* **5**, 1–24.

B. Corticotropin Regulatory Factors and Receptors - Proopiomelanocortin - ACTH

Corticotropin-Releasing Hormone and Urocortins: Binding Proteins and Receptors

M O Huising
The Salk Institute for Biological Studies, La Jolla, CA, USA and Department of Animal Physiology, Radboud University Nijmegen, Nijmegen, The Netherlands
W W Vale
The Salk Institute for Biological Studies, La Jolla, CA, USA

Discovery of CRF and Its Role in the Stress Response

Corticotropin-releasing factor (CRF) was identified in 1981 as the key hypothalamic factor to induce the release of adrenocorticotropic hormone (ACTH) from the anterior pituitary gland. This feat was accomplished by the purification of the peptide from sheep hypothalami. CRF is the most potent known stimulator of ACTH release, although other hypothalamic factors, most notably arginine vasopressin (AVP) and oxytocin, can synergize with CRF to augment the release of ACTH. Nevertheless, the observation that the release of ACTH from the anterior pituitary gland is almost completely blocked by administration of CRF antisera established that CRF is the predominant regulator of pituitary ACTH release. Mature bioactive CRF is a 41-amino-acid neuropeptide that is cleaved from a larger precursor protein lacking intrinsic biological activity (**Figure 1**). CRF is produced in the parvocellular neurons of the paraventricular nucleus (PVN) of the hypothalamus. These neurons project to the median eminence and release their neuropeptide content into the capillary bed of the hypophysial portal system. This portal system carries CRF to the anterior pituitary corticotropes, which respond by releasing ACTH into the general circulation to induce the release of glucocorticoids from the adrenal cortex. This endocrine axis, referred to as the hypothalamic–pituitary–adrenal (HPA) axis, controls reactions to stress. The stress response is an adaptive response aimed at maintaining or restoring homeostasis in the face of a plethora of potentially adverse stimuli from diverse origins. The glucocorticoids – cortisol in humans and corticosterone in rodents – that are released as a result of HPA axis

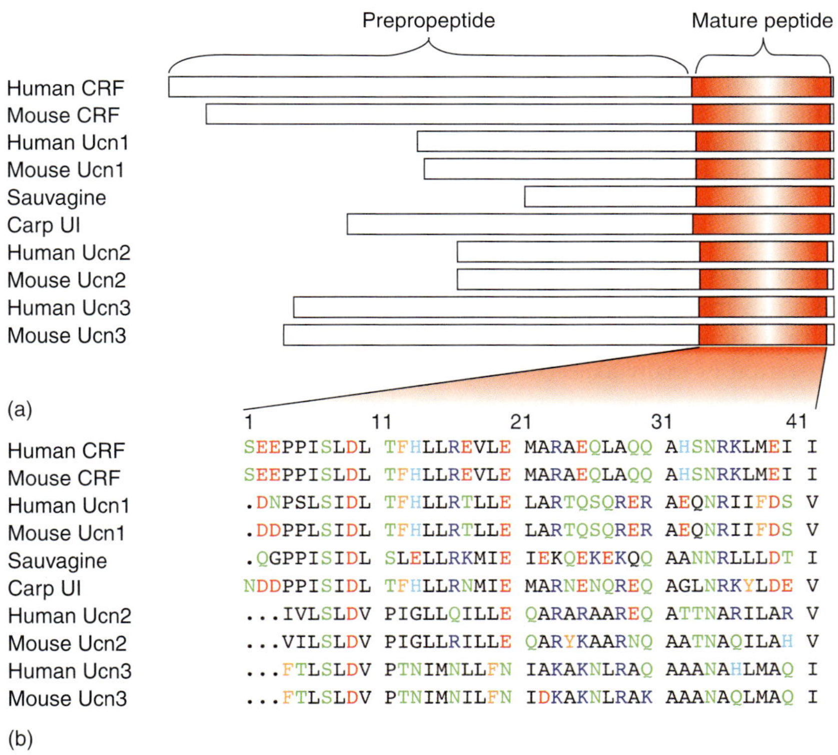

Figure 1 Corticotropin-releasing factor (CRF) family ligands (Ucn1, Ucn2, and Ucn3; urocortins) are encoded as preprohormones. (a) The C-terminal mature neuropeptides are liberated from the prepropeptide sequence by cleavage at mono- or dibasic cleavage sites. At the amino acid level CRF and urocortins share moderate amino acid similarity. (b) Amino acids with similar biochemical properties are color-coded for clarity.

activation are responsible for many of the hallmarks of the stress response, such as increased energy mobilization via enhanced liver glycogenolysis and the general inhibition of vegetative functions, including digestion, growth, reproduction, and immunity. Importantly, glucocorticoids engage in negative feedback at the level of both the pituitary gland and the hypothalamus to inhibit the synthesis and release of ACTH and CRF, aimed at a timely termination of the stress response. Many of the behavioral effects that are associated with stress, such as increased anxiety, improved cognition, increased depression, and reduced feeding behavior, are often the direct effect of the activation of central CRF circuits.

CRF: Founding Member of a Small Family of Neuropeptides

Shortly after the discovery of CRF in sheep, the CRF genes of humans, mice, rats, and other mammals were identified. Urotensin-I (UI), a peptide resembling CRF, was isolated from a fish species (*Catastomus commersonii*) following the discovery of CRF in mammals. This peptide was initially regarded as the fish ortholog (i.e., the same gene in a different species) of mammalian CRF, until a second peptide also resembling CRF was identified from the same fish species. As this second CRF-like peptide shared much higher similarity with mammalian CRF, it was clear that it represented the actual ortholog of mammalian CRF. The mammalian ortholog of fish UI was identified in 1995 with the isolation and characterization of urocortin 1 (Ucn1). Another peptide with resemblance to the Ucn1 of mammals and the UI of fishes was isolated from the skin of the waxy monkey tree frog (*Phylomedusa sauvagei*), a species from the Amazonian rain forest. This peptide was named sauvagine and although it is only known from the skin of a single amphibian species, sauvagine has been frequently used in the characterization of many aspects of CRF signaling. In recent years, two additional members of the CRF family of neuropeptides were independently discovered by two groups employing a bioinformatics approach. The current nomenclature for these peptides is urocortin 2 (Ucn2) and urocortin 3 (Ucn3), although one of the identifying groups initially named them stresscopin-related peptide and stresscopin, respectively. All members of the vertebrate CRF family have several characteristics in common with CRF. All are preprohormones that contain at their C-termini mature neuropeptides that are presumed to be liberated by cleavage at a mono- or dibasic cleavage site (**Figure 1**). In keeping with their discovery via bioinformatics, the existence of mature neuropeptides for Ucn2 and Ucn3 has been predicted, and their bioactivity following *de novo* synthesis has been established, but neither mature peptide has been directly isolated from an endogenous source.

CRF Family Neuropeptides Signal via One of Two CRF Receptors

Two receptors for CRF have been identified and are termed CRFR1 and CRFR2. Both are class B (secretin-like) seven-helix transmembrane G-protein-coupled receptors and consist of 395 to 440 amino acids. CRFR1 and CRFR2 share approximately 70% amino acid identity, with most of their amino acid differences concentrated in the N-terminal region. As the N-terminal domain (together with the extracellular loops) is responsible for ligand binding, this accounts for the substantial differences in the pharmacology of the receptors. CRFR1 is the principal receptor activating pituitary corticotropes during the stress response and has nanomolar affinity for CRF. CRFR1 binds Ucn1 with a similarly high affinity, but has no appreciable affinity for physiological doses of Ucn2 and Ucn3. The CRFR2 receptor has highest affinity for Ucn1 and also binds Ucn2 and Ucn3 with high affinity. The affinity of CRFR2 for CRF is about 10- to 30-fold lower than its affinity for the urocortins, but is still below 100 nM. This illustrates the redundancy of the CRF system, wherein multiple ligands share, and under certain circumstances may even compete for, two different receptors (**Figure 2**).

A further layer of complexity is added to CRF signaling by the observation that multiple transcripts can be generated from both CRFR genes. The CRFR1 gene (*CRHR1*, humans; *Crhr1*, rodents) consists of 14 exons in humans and 13 exons in rodents. More than one dozen alternative transcripts have been found that result from the skipping of one or several exons during gene transcription. The predicted proteins from some of these splice variants partially or completely lack the extracellular domain (ECD), or lack one or several transmembrane domains. Nevertheless, the mechanism responsible for these CRFR1 splice isoforms is unknown and the physiological roles played by CRFR1 splice variants remain presently unclear; direct evidence for the presence of corresponding CRFR1 proteins is lacking for most of these splice isoforms.

A clear example of how alternative splicing can generate functionally different receptor proteins is found in the mammalian gene encoding CRFR2. Two different receptor isoforms, CRFR2α and CRFR2β, are transcribed from the *CRFR2* gene by splicing alternative start exons onto a common set of downstream exons. A third isoform, CRFR2γ, is produced in a similar fashion in primates only. The resulting

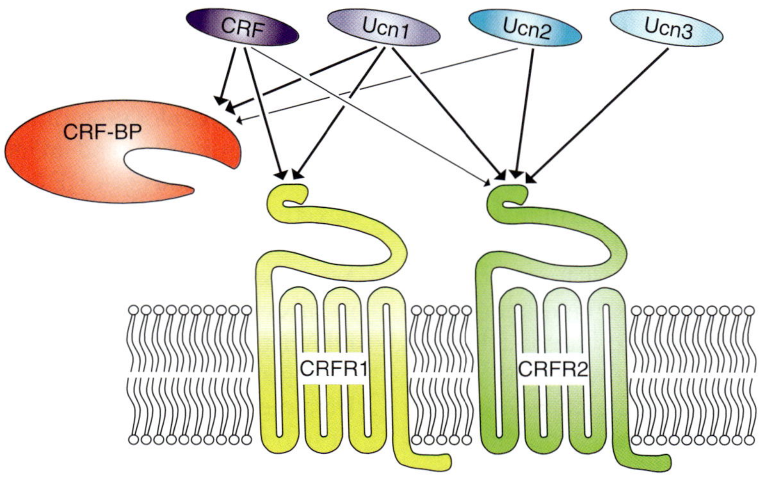

Figure 2 Corticotropin-releasing factor (CRF) and the urocortins (Ucn1, Ucn2, and Ucn3) signal through one of two CRF receptors (CRFR1 and CRFR2). Both CRF receptors differ in the repertoire of ligands that they bind. Furthermore, CRF and Ucn1, and to a lesser extent Ucn2, bind to CRF-binding protein (CRF-BP). The arrows pointing away from each ligand indicate the ligand potential targets. The thickness of the arrows indicates the approximate affinity for each of the ligands.

receptor proteins differ only at the extreme N-terminus of their ECD. As the majority of the ECD is encoded by exons four, five, and six, which are shared by all CRFR2 isoforms, their pharmacological properties do not differ substantially. Nevertheless, the different CRFR2 isoforms vary markedly in their central and peripheral tissue distribution, as the transcription of each isoform is driven by its own unique promoter sequence. In rodents, the expression of CRFR2α is largely restricted to the central nervous system (CNS), with expression in the olfactory bulb, ventromedial hypothalamus (VMH), the lateral septum (LS), and the bed nucleus of the stria terminalis (BNST). In contrast, the expression of CRFR2β within the CNS is restricted to the choroid plexus. In the periphery of rodents, the situation is completely reversed. Expression of CRFR2β is widespread, with highest expression levels in skeletal muscle, heart, and skin. Interestingly, CRFR2α is the predominantly expressed isoform in the human periphery. By comparison, CRFR1 is expressed in brain and pituitary as well as in peripheral sites, including adrenal gland, spleen, testis, and skin.

Recently, several other splice variants were discovered that are generated from the CRFR2 gene. One particularly interesting splice variant stems from the deletion of exon six, resulting in a premature stop codon caused by a shift in the amino acid reading frame. The resulting 143-amino-acid protein consists of the complete ECD of CRFR2α followed by a unique hydrophilic 38-amino-acid C-terminal tail. The resulting soluble CRFR2α can abrogate the response to CRF and Ucn1 *in vitro* and may serve as a natural modulator of the actions of CRF and urocortins.

A two-step model has been proposed for hormone binding and receptor activation of CRF receptors. First, the C-terminus of the ligand binds the extracellular domain of the receptor, followed by the partial insertion of its N-terminus into the transmembrane region. This results in a conformational change that leads to exchange of guanosine diphosphate (GDP) for guanosine triphosphate (GTP) on the Gα subunit of the G-protein that is coupled to the third intracellular loop of the receptor. The activated Gα subunit dissociates from the G$\beta\gamma$ dimer, and both species can activate various downstream signaling pathways. In many cells, activation of the G-protein activates the adenylyl cyclase–cyclic adenosine monophosphate (cAMP)/protein kinase A (PKA) pathway. This pathway results in downstream modulation of target proteins by PKA as well as transcriptional regulation via cAMP response element-binding protein (CREB). Depending on the cell type that expresses CRF receptors, other signaling pathways can be activated downstream of CRF receptors via different G-proteins. These pathways include extracellular signal-regulated kinase/mitogen-activated protein kinase (ERK/MAPK), protein kinase C (PKC), nuclear factor-kappa B (NF-κB), and several others.

CRF-Binding Protein

A unique player in the network of CRF signaling exists in the form of a soluble 37 kDa protein that binds CRF with high affinity. This CRF-binding protein (CRF-BP) was initially discovered in late gestational maternal plasma, where it prevents activation of the stress response via the substantial amounts of CRF from placental origin that circulate prior to parturition. The CRF-BP gene consists of seven exons that encode a protein of 322-amino-acids, unrelated to the CRF receptors. In fact, its primary amino acid sequence bears no resemblance to that of any other known protein. CRF-BP is characterized by ten conserved cysteine residues that form five consecutive disulfide bridges, and a single N-linked glycosylation site. CRF-BP orthologs have been demonstrated for a number of vertebrate species and were recently discovered in species of insects. In mammals, CRF-BP binds CRF and Ucn1 with an affinity that is several fold higher than the affinity of CRF receptors for either peptide. Human CRF-BP also binds mouse, but not human, Ucn2 with nanomolar affinity and does not bind Ucn3 (**Figure 2**). Interestingly, several peptide fragments, such as CRF(6–33) and CRF(9–33), which consist only of the core of the mature peptide hormone, retain the capacity to bind to CRF-BP with high affinity, but have lost the ability to activate CRF receptors. This indicates that different areas of the peptide hormone are involved in binding to the receptor and to the binding protein.

The high affinity of CRF-BP for CRF and Ucn1 suggests an antagonistic role by preventing these hormones from activating their receptors. Indeed, CRF-BP is expressed in anterior pituitary corticotropes and is capable of abrogating the CRF-induced release of ACTH from pituitary cells *in vitro*. CRF-BP is widely expressed within the CNS, including the cerebral cortex, the amygdala, BNST, olfactory bulb, and various nuclei within the brain stem and hypothalamus. Peripherally, complexes of CRF-BP and CRF are rapidly cleared from the circulation, supporting an antagonistic role for CRF-BP.

Central CRF Pathways Are Involved in Anxiety and Depression

Although initially discovered as an activator of the HPA axis, CRF is produced at many other sites in the brain outside of the parvocellular section of the PVN. Within the hypothalamus CRF is produced in several other nuclei, including the preoptic, supraoptic, and suprachiasmatic nuclei. Prominent sites of CRF localization outside of the hypothalamus include the cortex, the central nucleus of the amygdala (CeA), the BNST, the locus coeruleus (LC), and the parabrachial nucleus (PB). These nuclei are generally associated with autonomic function. Consensus is that within the CNS, CRF acts as a neurotransmitter by activating downstream neurons.

Central CRF pathways are involved in behavioral patterns that are commonly associated with stress, such as changes in arousal and anxiety. Several rodent models have been developed for the measurement and quantification of the behavioral manifestations of arousal and anxiety. Transfer of a rodent from a familiar nonstressful environment, such as its home cage, to a completely new environment is considered an acutely stressful event for the animal. This transition is immediately reflected in a series of behavioral changes that can be measured as a reduction in locomotor activity and reduced exploration of the novel environment, a reduction in rearing, and an increase in grooming and freezing. Injections of CRF (intracerebroventricularly; directly into the ventricles of the brain) can reproduce this panel of behaviors associated with novelty stress. Mice that lack CRFR1 display a marked reduction in anxiety-related behaviors in addition to blunted HPA activation. This suggests that the majority of the anxiogenic effects of CRF are mediated via CRFR1. Data regarding the role of CRFR2 in anxiety are less clear. Both anxiogenic (anxiety-promoting) and anxiolytic (anxiety-reducing) effects have been attributed to CRFR2, and the direction and magnitude of the effects mediated via CRFR2 may be dependent on the precise anatomical location of CRFR2 expression as well as on confounding factors such as gender.

Dysregulation of CRF pathways is implicated in the etiology of depression. CRF concentrations are significantly elevated in the cerebrospinal fluid of depressed patients, and reduction of these levels by electroconvulsive therapy correlates with alleviation of depression symptoms. Several rodent models have been developed that display behavior reflecting some traits associated with depression in human patients. In one of these models a mouse is suspended by the tail and the severity of depression is quantified as the fraction of the time the animal is immobile. In another test mice are subjected to involuntary swimming and depression is measured as a reduction in swimming and climbing behavior and increased immobility. In these animal models for depression, selective CRFR1 antagonists reduce immobility, implicating central CRF pathways that employ CRFR1 in the pathophysiology of depression. Recently, mice were generated that are deficient for the selective CRFR2 agonist Ucn2. One of the major findings in these Ucn2-deficient mice is their antidepression-like phenotype, as measured by reduced immobility in the forced swim test and the tail suspension tests. These experiments demonstrate a prominent role for CRFR1 and CRFR2 in the development of depressive disorders.

Feeding, Digestion, and Metabolism

Several CRF pathways are involved in the regulation of feeding and digestion. Central circuits employing CRF regulate key aspects of appetite control and feeding behavior, while peripheral CRF receptors relay signals that affect gastrointestinal motor functions. Much of the integration of central metabolic cues with peripheral indicators of nutrient status, such as circulating levels of leptin and insulin, takes place in the hypothalamus. It has long been known that injection of CRF and Ucn1 directly into the brain ventricle produces anorexic effects. Activation of either CRF receptor produces anorexic effects, but with different kinetics. Intracerebroventricular injection of CRFR1-specific agonists results in a rapid inhibition of food intake, while the specific activation of CRFR2 results in prolonged anorexia that requires several hours to establish. These findings are supported by studies on CRF-deficient mice: mice lacking CRFR1 are insensitive to short-onset anorexia induced by a general CRF receptor agonist such as Ucn1, while CRFR2-deficient mice fail to mount prolonged hypophagia following Ucn1 administration. The arcuate nucleus has strong CRFR1 expression while the ventromedial hypothalamus features prominent CRFR2 expression. Both nuclei play key roles in the regulation of food intake and metabolism. The VMH receives abundant projections of Ucn3, and, to a lesser extent, Ucn1, while it is only sparsely innervated by CRF. Ucn2 and Ucn3 are also detected in the arcuate nucleus. These observations suggest that many of the anorectic effects of CRF family peptides are mediated via CRFR2 and that the urocortins constitute its endogenous ligands, modulating appetite control and feeding behavior. CRFR2 expression levels in the VMH drop during fasting and are correlated with circulating leptin levels, suggesting that plasma leptin levels directly or indirectly affect the level of CRFR2 expression in this nucleus. Direct stimulation of the VMH by CRFR2 agonist injection or electrical stimulation not only results in reduced food intake, but also activates the sympathetic nervous system. Via this route energy expenditure is increased through the stimulation of brown adipose tissue (BAT) thermogenesis. Thus, feeding behavior is enhanced and BAT thermogenesis is decreased during starvation, when plasma leptin and consequently VMH CRFR2 expression are low. During times of surplus body energy stores, increased leptin concentrations and CRFR2 levels drive increased BAT thermogenesis and inhibit food intake.

CRF signaling is involved in the regulation of gastrointestinal motor function. Although the inhibition of gastromotor function that is observed during stress is partially mediated via central CRFR2, CRF and urocortins have direct effects on the gastrointestinal tract. Peripheral administration of urocortins delays gastric emptying and inhibits gut motility. These inhibitory effects on gastromotor functions are blocked by selective CRFR2, but not CRFR1, antagonists. In contrast to the inhibition of gastric motility by central and peripheral CRFR2 activation, colonic motility can be stimulated during stress via CRFR1-mediated activation of the parasympathetic nervous system as well as via CRFR1 present in the colonic myenteric nervous system. The physiological relevance of the dichotomy in the activation of different stretches of the gastrointestinal tract is explained by adaptive value in times of stress. Inhibitions of gastric and gut activity and colon evacuation are different ways of inhibiting digestion, thus contributing to the maximal allocation of resources toward responding to stress.

Cardiovascular Effects of Urocortins via CRFR2

It has long been known that CRF influences cardiovascular function. During acute stress, heart rate, blood pressure, and cardiac output increase as the result of activation of the sympathetic nervous system. This overall stimulation of the cardiovascular system is an important adaptive response, assisting an animal to actively cope with a stressful event. Central injection of CRF mimics the cardiovascular effects that are normally observed following stress, provided that the sympathetic nervous system is intact. Since coadministration of a CRFR1-specific antagonist attenuates CRF-induced increases in heart rate, the CRF-induced activation of the sympathetic nervous system is, at least in part, mediated via CRFR1.

In contrast to the generally stimulatory effects of central CRF injections on the cardiovascular system, CRF delivered peripherally causes vasodilatation and a drop in mean arterial blood pressure. Systemic CRF and Ucn1 also increase cardiac contractility. These direct effects of systemically administered CRF and Ucn1 on the cardiovascular system suggest the presence of local CRF receptors. Indeed, CRFR2 is expressed in significant amounts in cardiac tissue, including myocardium, epicardium, arterioles of atrium and ventricle, and aorta. Its role in the cardiovascular system was elegantly demonstrated by comparing the hemodynamic properties of normal mice with mice lacking CRFR2. The latter mice have an elevated mean arterial blood pressure that is insensitive to systemic Ucn1 administration, whereas normal mice respond to Ucn1 with significant and prolonged (>1 h) hypotension. Ucn1 and Ucn2 are potential endogenous ligand (s) for CRFR2 in the cardiovascular system, as both urocortins are expressed in isolated cardiac myocytes. Alternatively, it is possible that CRF family peptides reach the heart via nerve terminals or through the general circulation to activate cardiac CRFR2.

In addition to the effects on blood pressure and cardiac contractility mediated via CRFR2 *in vivo*, urocortins display cardioprotective effects. The expression of Ucn1 and Ucn2 in cultured cardiomyocytes is increased after hypoxia followed by reoxygenation, a model for cardiac ischemia. The presence of urocortin peptides in media reduces the percentage of cultured cardiomyocytes that can enter apoptosis and necrosis following hypoxia. CRFR2 is required for these cardioprotective effects, since Ucn2 and Ucn3 fail to rescue cardiomyocytes isolated from CRFR2-deficient mice from apoptosis. Moreover, the administration of Ucn2 and Ucn3 immediately following experimentally induced ischemia of the intact rat heart results in a substantial reduction of the infarct zone. These cardioprotective effects of urocortins acting through CRFR2 are of particular interest in the context of cardiac ischemia. In particular, the fact that Ucn2 and Ucn3 lack the affinity for CRFR1 required for HPA activation or induction of anxiety makes them promising targets in the quest for therapeutical interventions aimed at alleviation of the adverse outcome of cardiac ischemia in humans.

CRF and Pregnancy

CRF and Ucn1 as well as their cognate receptors and CRF-BP are expressed in different tissues of the female reproductive system. CRF plays a remarkably versatile role affecting pregnancy, from blastocyst implantation to parturition. Mammalian reproduction, in which the fetus is carried inside the womb, is an awkward phenomenon from an immunological point of view. The developing fetus is only 50% 'self': the paternal contribution to the fetus qualifies it as a foreign body and would as such subject it to attack by the maternal immune system. For obvious reasons, this would be incompatible with successful reproduction. CRF protects the fetus from attack by the maternal immune system and simultaneously prevents the developing fetal immune system from attacking maternal tissues. Around the time of blastocyst implantation into the uterus, CRF is produced in the embryonic trophoblast and the maternal decidua, the contact interface of maternal and fetal tissues. Locally, CRF increases the expression of an important proapoptotic factor, Fas ligand (FasL), via CRFR1. FasL induces apoptosis in cells carrying its cognate binding partner, Fas, which is expressed by many immune cells. As Fas only appears at the cell surface following leukocyte activation, CRF-induced upregulation of FasL at the site of implantation allows the specific deletion of only those immune cells that are activated at the maternal–fetal interface.

CRF is expressed in the placenta of primates, but not rodents, and CRF from placental origin is detectable in the maternal circulation beginning approximately halfway through gestation. Circulating CRF levels rise sharply toward the end of pregnancy and, close to term, reach levels equivalent to peak CRF levels measured in the hypothalamic–pituitary capillary bed during acute HPA activation. Yet, these high levels of CRF do not activate the HPA axis, because they are bound to a surplus of CRF-BP, which is also produced by the placenta. In the fetal circulation, increasing levels of CRF will activate the fetal HPA axis. This results in glucocorticoid release from the fetal adrenal gland, a process that drives the maturation of a number of fetal organs, including the lungs in preparation for delivery.

Throughout much of gestation, CRF in the placenta evokes quiescence of uterine smooth muscle cells via the CRFR1-dependent activation of the PKA pathway. In a series of intricate molecular switches that involve the oxytocin-dependent phosphorylation of CRFR1, CRFR1 is coupled to a different G-protein toward parturition. This causes a shift in the intracellular cascade that is activated upon ligand binding to CRFR1 from PKA to PKC. Instead of inducing myometrial relaxation, CRF now can assist in the induction of myometrial contractility and labor.

Summary

CRF was initially noted for its potent capacity to activate the stress response. In the decades that followed its discovery, three additional ligands related to CRF, as well as two receptors and a soluble binding protein, have been discovered. While CRF still has strong ties to 'stress,' we now know that CRF signaling is involved in a multitude of other central and peripheral processes. These include the regulation of anxiety, arousal, and depression, the modulation of food intake and sympathetic nervous system activation, control of cardiovascular output as well as cardioprotection, and a combination of fascinating roles in the regulation of human reproduction. Many of these processes are at the heart of human well-being, which has sparked widespread interest in CRF. The challenge that lies ahead will be the development of strategies to intervene in isolated CRF pathways without causing widespread activation of CRF receptors throughout the body.

See Also the Following Articles

Corticotropin-Releasing Hormone: Integration of Adaptive Responses to Stress; Hypothalamic–Pituitary–Adrenal (HPA) Axis; Stress Response: Neural and Feedback Regulation of the HPA Axis.

Further Reading

Charmandari, E., Tsigos, C. and Chrousos, G. P. (2005). Endocrinology of the stress response. *Annual Review of Physiology* 67, 259–284.

Chen, A., Perrin, M., Brar, B., et al. (2005). Mouse corticotropin-releasing factor receptor type 2α gene: Isolation, distribution, pharmacological characterization and regulation by stress and glucocorticoids. *Molecular Endocrinology* **19**, 441–458.

Coste, S. C., Quintos, R. F. and Stenzel-Poore, M. P. (2002). Corticotropin-releasing hormone-related peptides and receptors: Emergent regulators of cardiovascular adaptations to stress. *Trends in Cardiovascular Medicine* **12**, 176–182.

Heinrichs, S. C. and Koob, G. F. (2004). Corticotropin-releasing factor in brain: A role in activation, arousal, and affect regulation. *The Journal of Pharmacology and Experimental Therapeutics* **311**, 427–440.

Hillhouse, E. W. and Grammatopoulos, D. K. (2002). Role of stress peptides during human pregnancy and labour. *Reproduction* **124**, 323–329.

Hillhouse, E. W. and Grammatopoulos, D. K. (2006). The molecular mechanisms underlying the regulation of the biological activity of corticotropin-releasing hormone receptors: Implications for physiology and pathophysiology. *Endocrine Reviews* **27**, 260–286.

King, B. M. (2006). The rise, fall, and resurrection of the ventromedial hypothalamus in the regulation of feeding behavior and body weight. *Physiology & Behavior* **87**, 221–244.

Lewis, K., Perrin, M. H., Blount, A., et al. (2001). Identification of urocortin III, an additional member of the corticotropin-releasing factor (CRF) family with high affinity for the CRF2 receptor. *Proceedings of the National Academy of Sciences of the United States of America* **98**, 7570–7575.

McLean, M. and Smith, R. (2001). Corticotrophin-releasing hormone and human parturition. *Reproduction* **121**, 493–501.

Owens, M. J. and Nemeroff, C. B. (1991). Physiology and pharmacology of corticotropin-releasing factor. *Pharmacological Reviews* **43**, 425–473.

Reyes, T. M., Lewis, K., Perrin, M. H., et al. (2001). Urocortin II: A member of the corticotropin-releasing factor (CRF) neuropeptide family that is selectively bound by type 2 CRF receptors. *Proceedings of the National Academy of Sciences of the United States of America* **98**, 2843–2848.

Westphal, N. J. and Seasholtz, A. F. (2006). CRH-BP: The regulation and function of a phylogenetically conserved binding protein. *Frontiers in Bioscience* **11**, 1878–1891.

Winsky-Sommerer, R., Boutrel, B. and de Lecea, L. (2005). Stress and arousal: The corticotrophin-releasing factor/hypocretin circuitry. *Molecular Neurobiology* **32**, 285–294.

Zorilla, E. P., Taché, Y. and Koob, G. F. (2003). Nibbling at CRF receptor control of feeding and gastrocolonic motility. *Trends in Pharmacological Sciences* **24**, 421–427.

Urocortins

É M Fekete and E P Zorrilla
The Scripps Research Institute, La Jolla, CA, USA

This is a revised version of the article by E P Zorrilla and G F Koob, Encyclopedia of Stress, First edition, volume 3, pp 637–642, © 2000, Elsevier Inc.

Glossary

Adrenocorticotropic hormone (ACTH) — A hormone released into systemic circulation by the anterior pituitary as part of the HPA-stress response. ACTH, or corticotropin, induces the release of glucocorticoids from the adrenal cortex.

Corticotropin-releasing factor (CRF) — Isolated by Vale and colleagues in 1981, the first hypothalamic ACTH secretagogue to be identified. In addition to its hypothalamic endocrine function, extrahypothalamic CRF is important in behavioral and autonomic stress responses.

Edinger-Westphal nucleus — An oculomotor nucleus of the midbrain that has parasympathetic projections to the ciliary ganglion and descending inputs to the brain stem and spinal cord.

Hypothalamic-pituitary-adrenocortical (HPA) axis — The neuroendocrine system which, during stress, amplifies a neural signal of physiological or psychological stress into a systemic, endocrine response. Hormones secreted as part of the HPA stress response cascade equip the organism to mobilize and utilize energy resources more effectively and, more generally, respond to the stressor.

Stresscopin — An N-terminally extended analog of urocortin 3 that binds exclusively and with high affinity to the CRF_2 receptor.

Stresscopin-related peptide — An N-terminally extended analog of urocortin 2 that binds selectively and with high affinity to the CRF_2 receptor.

Since the isolation of corticotropin-releasing factor (CRF) in 1981, three more endogenous CRF-like peptides have been identified in mammals. The first of these – urocortin 1 (Ucn 1) – was identified in 1995 for its similar primary structure and bioactivity to suckerfish urotensin I and CRF. Ucn 1 exhibited greater affinity for and activation of type 2 CRF receptors (CRF_2) than CRF and was hypothesized to be a natural CRF_2 receptor ligand. Urocortin 2 (Ucn 2) and urocortin 3 (Ucn 3), 38-amino-acid residue peptides, were then identified in 2001 for their structural relation to both CRF and Ucn 1 and were named urocortins due to their predominant affinity for the CRF_2 receptor. Although the urocortins share sequence identity with one another and with CRF, each is phylogenetically distinct, with the CRF peptide family resulting from multiple gene duplication events. Each peptide has a unique anatomical distribution under the control of different genes. Consequently, despite a structural family resemblance, the natural functions of urocortins and CRF in stress responses *in vivo* may differ significantly.

Structure of Urocortins, CRF, and Related Peptides

The rat Ucn 1 cDNA was cloned from a rat midbrain mRNA library in 1995. The gene codes for a 122-residue prohormone that contains Ucn 1 in the C-terminus. Ucn 1 genes also have been cloned in mouse, human, hamster, sheep (*Ovis aries*), frog (*Xenopus laevis*), and capuchin monkey (*Cebus apella*) and are similar across species. The human Ucn 1 gene lies on chromosome 2 (2p23-p21) and has two exons, with the second exon comprising the coding region, like the CRF gene. The Ucn 1 promoter is regulated by several transcription factor binding sites, including a TATA box, GATA-binding sites, a C/EBP-binding site, a Brn-2 binding site, and a cyclic AMP responsive element (CRE). Upstream of the CRE site (four base pairs), the Ucn 1 promoter contains a consensus half site for glucocorticoid response elements (GREs), consistent with the finding that glucocorticoids upregulate Ucn 1 mRNA synthesis.

The cDNAs for Ucn 2 and Ucn 3 were identified from sequence homology searches of the mouse and human genomes, with the putative Ucn 2 peptide (an N-terminally shortened sequence of stresscopin-related peptide) contained in the C-terminus of a 112-amino-acid residue proprotein, and the putative Ucn 3 peptide (an N-terminally shortened sequence of stresscopin) encoded in a 161-residue precursor. The identity of the endogenous peptides derived from the Ucn 2 and Ucn 3 preproteins remains predicted, as mature peptide sequences have not been definitively isolated and sequenced. Whether a mature Ucn 2 peptide sequence is processed in humans remains uncertain because of the lack of a consensus proteolytic processing site at the C-terminus of the putative sequence. Preproteins for rat Ucn 2 and for chimpanzee and frog Ucn 3 have also been identified. The human genes for Ucn 2 and Ucn 3 lie on chromosomes 3 (3p21.3) and 10 (10p15.1), respectively. The Ucn 2 promoter contains several GREs and is positively regulated by glucocorticoids.

Ucn 1 resembles CRF in primary structure (see **Figure 1**) more so than it resembles Ucn 2 and Ucn 3. In contrast, Ucn 2 and Ucn 3 resemble one another more than they do CRF, a distinction, coupled with their greater CRF_2 receptor selectivity, that has led to their characterization as type 2 urocortins. An ancient gene duplication event is believed to have given rise to separate Ucn 1/CRF vs. Ucn 2/Ucn 3 lineages, with subsequent gene duplications events differentiating paralogs within each evolutionary branch (see **Figure 1**).

Distribution of Urocortins

Central Nervous System

Ucn 1 has a restricted, subcortical, predominantly caudal distribution in brain. The major site of brain Ucn 1 synthesis is the Edinger-Westphal nucleus (E-W), a dorsal midbrain structure known for its role in oculomotor function. The prominent synthesis of Ucn 1 in the E-W is conserved across rats, sheep, humans, and frogs. Descending Ucn 1-like immunoreactive (LI) positive fibers of possible E-W origin are observed in (1) midbrain: substantia nigra, periaqueductal gray, interpenduncular nucleus, and red nucleus; (2) caudal midbrain/rostral pons: dorsal raphe nucleus, ventral tegmentum, basilar pontine nuclei, and parabrachial nucleus; (3) medulla, including the facial, lateral reticular, and spinal trigeminal nuclei, inferior olive, and the dorsal column nuclei, nucleus of the solitary tract (NTS), and area postrema; (4) cerebellum: in the flocculus and paraflocculus as well as deep cerebellar and vestibular nuclei; and (5) spinal cord: throughout the spinal gray and, less so, in the dorsal and ventral horns. Ascending Ucn 1-LI-positive projections, possibly from the E-W, target the septal/preoptic region and, less heavily, the hypothalamus and thalamus. Validated secondary sites of brain Ucn 1 synthesis include the lateral superior olive, the supraoptic nucleus of the hypothalamus (SON), the lateral hypothalamic area, and several brain stem and spinal cord motoneuron nuclei. Ucn 1-LI is scarce in many regions in which CRF is prominent, including the external layer of the median eminence, the hypophysiotropic, dorsal medial parvocellular subdivision of the paraventricular nucleus of the hypothalamus (PVN), basal ganglia, amygdala, hippocampus, locus coeruleus (LC), and cerebral cortex.

Ucn 2 also exhibits a restricted, subcortical expression in rodent brain. Like Ucn 1, Ucn 2 mRNA is present in the SON and magnocellular subdivision of

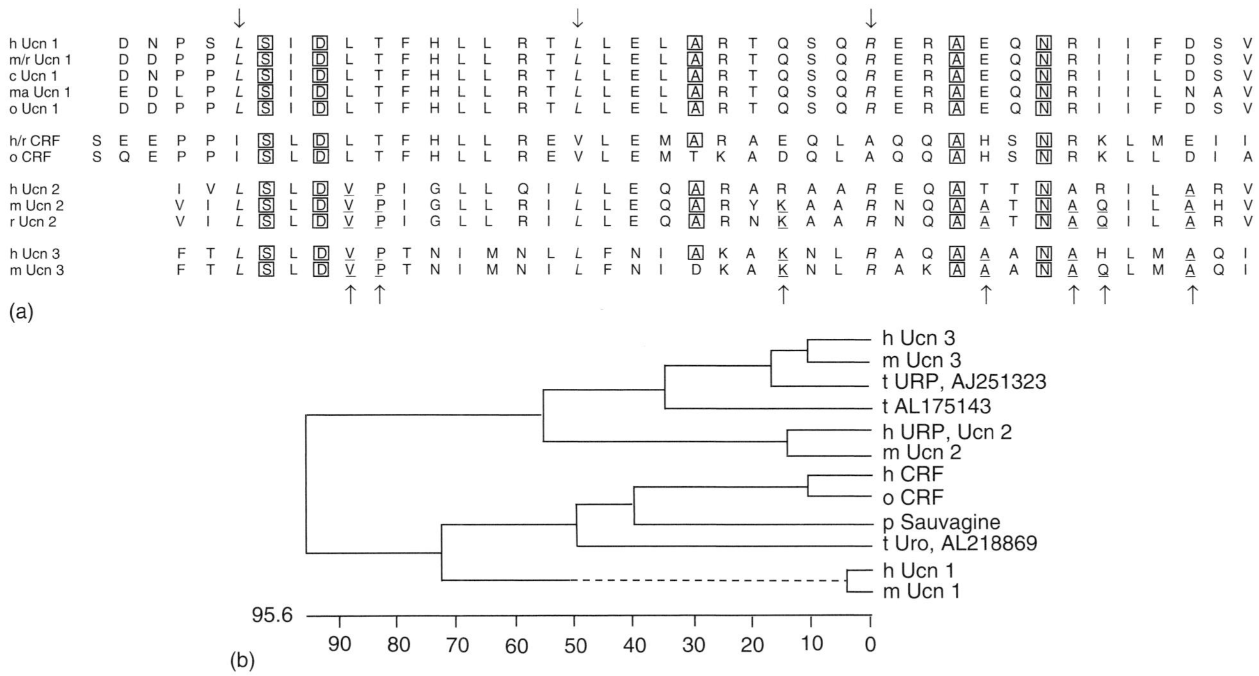

Figure 1 (a) Comparison of the primary structures of mammalian CRF family peptides. Selected putative amino acid sequences for CRF and urocortins 1, 2, and 3 across human (h), murine (*Mus musculus* [m]), rat (*Rattus norvegicus* [r]), monkey (*Cebus paella* [c]), hamster (*Mesocricetus auratus* [ma]), and sheep (*Ovis aries* [o]). Boxed regions indicate CRF superfamily homology; residues in italics and marked by down arrows are shared among all the urocortins; underlined residues marked by up arrows are shared among the type 2 urocortins (Ucn 2 and Ucn 3), but not by Ucn 1. (b) The phylogenetic tree associates human and mouse Ucn 3 and Ucn 2 with pufferfish (*Takifugu rubripes* [t]) urocortin-related peptide (URP). The more distantly related lineage is composed of ovine and human CRF, human and mouse Ucn 1, frog (*Phyllomedusa sauvagei* [p]) sauvagine, and pufferfish urotensin (tUro). The scale beneath the tree reflects sequence distances. Genbank accession sequences are provided for pufferfish-derived peptides. The phylogenetic tree was adapted from Lewis et al. (2001). *Proceedings of the National Academy of Sciences USA* **98,** 7570–7575.

the PVN, in brain stem motoneurons, and in the spinal cord. Unlike Ucn 1, Ucn 2 also is expressed in the arcuate nucleus of the hypothalamus and the LC. The projection targets of Ucn 2 neurons are unknown. Nonneuronal Ucn 2 expression also is present in meninges, but not glia.

Ucn 3 exhibits the most rostral, but again subcortical, distribution of the urocortins. The three main sites of forebrain Ucn 3 synthesis are (1) the median preoptic nucleus of the hypothalamus, (2) a perifornical hypothalamic region bordered laterally by the fornix and medially by the PVN, and (3) the dorsal medial amygdala. Less prominent forebrain sites of Ucn 3 synthesis include the dorsomedial hypothalamus, both magnocellular and parvocellular components of the PVN, a region dorsal to the SON, and the posterior cortical and amygdalohippocampal transition areas of the amygdala. Ucn 3-LI-positive fibers of uncertain origin project heavily to the ventromedial nucleus of the hypothamalus (VMH) and arcuate nucleus and less so to the ventral premammillary nucleus. Outside the hypothalamus, forebrain Ucn 3 fibers of uncertain origin are abundant in the lateral septum, posterior bed nucleus of stria terminals (BNST), and the medial amygdala. The topographical distribution of Ucn 3 in the LS differs from that of Ucn 1, with the latter innervating ventral and intermediate aspects of the structure, and the former innervating dorsal aspects. Caudally, Ucn 3 cell bodies are found in the auditory complex, and scattered Ucn 3 fibers are present in the periaqueductal gray, superior and inferior colliculi, and the ventral lateral lemniscus.

Periphery

Urocortins also are distributed in the periphery. Ucn 1 expression has been observed in adipose tissue, heart, and immune tissue, including thymus, spleen, and skin. Ucn 1 also is present in the enteric nervous system of the duodenum, small intestine, and colon, as well as in testis, kidney, adrenals, pancreas, and, possibly, anterior (but not posterior) pituitary. Ucn-1-LI also has consistently been observed in parietal and oxyntic cells of the stomach. Whether this Ucn 1 is actually synthesized by gastric tissue remains uncertain, however, as Ucn 1 is synthesized by lamina propria macrophages, components of the stomach's inflammatory mucosal immune system. Finally, Ucn 1-LI is abundant in human placenta and fetal membranes.

In humans, Ucn 2 gene expression was detected in most peripheral tissues analyzed by polymerase chain reaction analysis, with the highest levels observed in heart, lung, muscle, stomach, and adrenal and peripheral blood cells, but not skin. In the mouse, Ucn 2 gene expression was high in skeletal muscle and skin (unlike humans), moderate in lung, stomach, adrenal, ovary, brown fat, spleen, and thymus, and low in uterus, testes, kidney, white fat, and intestine. Unlike in humans, only low Ucn 2 mRNA expression is seen in murine heart. Skin, but not skeletal muscle, expression of Ucn 2 mRNA in the mouse appears to be inversely related to circulating glucocorticoid levels.

Ucn 3 gene expression is present in adipose tissue, heart, muscle, adrenal gland, and skin, albeit at levels considerably lower than those of Ucn 2. Ucn 3 also is present in thyroid, adrenals, β cells of the pancreas, spleen, and the muscularis mucosa of the gastrointestinal (GI) tract, especially in the stomach, small intestine, and colon, but not esophagus or rectum.

Pharmacology of Urocortins

Ucn 1 binds with high affinity to every mammalian CRF binding site identified to date, including the CRF_1 and CRF_2 receptor families and the CRF-binding protein (CRF-BP). This nonselectivity differs from that of the type 2 urocortins, which have selective CRF_2 affinity and less affinity for the CRF-BP. Three CRF receptor subtypes have been identified (CRF_1, CRF_2, CRF_3), two of which have been observed in mammals (CRF_1, CRF_2). CRF receptors are encoded by separate genes, share high sequency homology, and have unique tissue distributions and pharmacological affinity profiles, permitting a diversity of function. CRF receptors belong to the G-protein-coupled, seven transmembrane domain receptor (GPCR) family.

CRF_1 Receptors

The CRF_1 receptor is a class B (secretin-like) GPCR spanning 415 amino acids. Many alternatively spliced transcripts of CRF_1 have been identified in humans, rats, mice, and hamsters. However, only one of these splice variants is known to induce signal transduction in humans and rodents ($CRF_{1(a)}$), so the following pharmacological characterization pertains mainly to the $CRF_{1(a)}$ isoform. Ucn 1 exhibits reversible, saturable, high-affinity binding to CRF_1 receptors transfected in stable cell lines. Ucn 1 is two to six times more potent than CRF at binding to the CRF_1 receptor and two- to threefold more potent than CRF in stimulating the production of cAMP from CRF_1 expressing cells *in vitro*. Ucn 1's affinity for the CRF_1 receptor is determined by regions in the first three extracellular domains of the receptor. In contrast to Ucn 1, the type 2 urocortins have very low potencies to activate adenylate cyclase via CRF_1 ($EC_{50} > 100$ nM), and Ucn 3 shows negligible potency to stimulate ACTH release *in vitro* ($\gg 1$ μM), a CRF_1-mediated bioassay. The CRF_1 receptor can employ multiple signal transduction pathways when stimulated by Ucn 1. These include activation of adenylate cyclase and protein kinase A-dependent pathways, activation of phospholipase C and protein kinase C-dependent pathways, mitogen-activated protein (MAP) kinase-dependent pathways, nitric oxide production, and proximate interactions with calcium channels.

CRF_2 Receptors

CRF_2 receptors also are class B GPCRs. To date, four major CRF_2 splice variants have been identified, including membrane-bound and soluble isoforms of $CRF_{2(a)}$ and membrane-bound $CRF_{2(b)}$ and $CRF_{2(c)}$ receptors. The membrane-bound CRF_2 receptors are, respectively, 411, 431, and 397 residues in length, differing only in their extracellular N-terminus, with the $CRF_{2(c)}$ receptor observed thus far only in human limbic circuits. Unlike CRF, all urocortins bind with high affinity to membrane-bound CRF_2 receptors transfected in stable cell lines. Ucn 1 is slightly more potent than the type 2 urocortins, but is 10–40 times more potent than CRF at binding to membrane CRF_2 receptors. However, the type 2 urocortins are much more (>1000-fold) selective CRF_2 agonists than Ucn 1. The CRF_2 receptor also can activate the MAP kinase pathway, with some evidence suggesting that Ucn 3 may be less efficacious than Ucn 2 and, especially, Ucn 1 at engaging this signal transduction mechanism. The soluble $CRF_{2(a)}$ isoform was identified in mice and results from a frameshift deletion of exon 6. In contrast to membrane-bound CRF_2 receptors, the soluble $CRF_{2(a)}$ receptor unexpectedly shows high affinity for Ucn 1 and CRF (classically, CRF_1 ligands) and low affinity for Ucn 2 and Ucn 3. Similar to the CRF-BP (see below), the soluble $CRF_{2(a)}$ receptor may curb CRF_1 signaling by competitively sequestering ligand.

CRF-Binding Protein (CRF-BP)

The CRF-BP is a conserved 37-kDa secreted glycoprotein that binds CRF and Ucn 1 with high affinity, thereby potentially reducing their bioavailability. Ucn 1 and CRF are approximately equipotent at binding to the CRF-BP. Ucn 1 can displace CRF from the CRF-BP (and vice versa), thereby allowing the possibility that each ligand modulates levels of free CRF receptor agonist in the brain. The region of Ucn 1 that has affinity for the CRF-BP (residues 4–28) differs from that which underlies its affinity for CRF receptors. Ucn 1 is the main natural ligand for the CRF-BP in sheep brain and dissociates from the CRF-BP more slowly than CRF. In contrast to CRF and Ucn 1, mUcn 3 does not bind with high affinity to the human or rat CRF-BP, and mUcn 2 binds with an order lower affinity than CRF or Ucn 1 to the rat CRF-BP and with negligible affinity to the human CRF-BP.

Physiological and Behavioral Effects of Urocortins

Hypothalamic-Pituitary-Adrenocortical (HPA) Axis

Although exogenous administration of Ucn 1 can potently activate the HPA axis, it is doubtful that endogenous urocortin 1 is a physiological regulator of the HPA axis. Unlike CRF-deficient mice, Ucn 1-deficient mice exhibit normal basal and stress-induced HPA hormone levels. Similarly, unlike CRF antisera, peripheral administration of specific Ucn 1 antisera does not modify basal, stress-induced, or adrenalectomy-induced ACTH levels. Finally, unlike the distribution of CRF, Ucn 1-immunoreactive fibers are scarce in the PVN and the external layer of the median eminence under basal conditions. Unlike both CRF and Ucn 1, intravenous Ucn 2 and Ucn 3 do not increase ACTH or corticosterone secretion, consistent with the absence of CRF_2 on pituitary corticotroph cells. However, type 2 urocortins might locally modulate CRF synthesis at the hypothalamic level, because immobilization stress increases Ucn 2 and Ucn 3 mRNA in the parvocellular PVN.

Osmoregulation

Because Ucn 1 and Ucn 2 are synthesized by magnocellular neurons of the SON and because Ucn 1 fibers are present in the posterior pituitary, an osmoregulatory role for urocortins is hypothesized. Supporting this possibility, salt loading, dehydration, and hypophysectomy increase Ucn-LI in magnocellular SON and PVN neurons, and food deprivation decreases Ucn-LI in the SON. Salt loading also increases SON Ucn 1 mRNA expression. Finally, chronic osmotic stimulation increases CRF_2 mRNA levels in the SON and magnocellular PVN, potentially increasing sensitivity to local urocortin action. Collectively, the findings support a potential endogenous role for central urocortins in the regulation of salt/water balance. Peripheral urocortins also may control body fluid homeostasis as a result of their ability to stimulate atrial natriuretic peptide (ANP) release from cardiomyocytes, again through a putative CRF_2 mechanism. ANP, present in cardiac atrial tissue, has profound effects on salt and water homeostasis, as it acutely reduces blood volume by sequestering plasma and over the longer term by promoting renal salt and water excretion.

Energy Balance

Exogenous urocortin administration promotes negative energy balance, both by increasing energy expenditure and by decreasing food intake. The distribution of the urocortins supports the hypothesis that they may physiologically regulate energy balance via actions at CRF_2 receptors, exemplified by concordant hypothalamic expression in the VMH (Ucn 3), arcuate nucleus (Ucn 2, Ucn 3), and PVN (Ucn 1, Ucn 2) and in the NTS of the caudal hindbrain (Ucn 1). Furthermore, levels of VMH CRF_2 mRNA covary with circulating leptin levels, providing a homeostatic mechanism for modulating sensitivity to catabolic urocortin action. The presence of urocortins in the GI tract, glucose-regulating organs, and adipose tissue also is consistent with a possible peripheral role for urocortins in energy balance regulation.

With respect to energy expenditure, Ucn 1 (intracerebroventricular [ICV] administration) increases whole body oxygen consumption as measured by indirect calorimetry and increases sympathetic nervous system activity. The hypothalamus is a candidate site for metabolic action for urocortins, as intra-PVN Ucn 1 increases plasma leptin levels, induces intrascapular brown adipose tissue (BAT) uncoupling protein-1 (UCP1) mRNA synthesis, and increases the relative utilization of fat as an energy substrate. Whether energy expenditure-increasing effects of Ucn 1 are mediated in part by CRF_2 receptors and shared by the type 2 urocortins is unclear.

With respect to energy intake, peripheral Ucn 1 or stresscopin administration potently reduces food intake in rodents, possibly in part by slowing gastric emptying (see below). Central infusion of urocortins also potently suppresses feeding and reduces gastric emptying, effects that were shown to be at least partly CRF_2-mediated from studies that used selective agonists (type 2 urocortins), antagonists, antisense knockdown of receptor expression, and knockout mice. Unlike CRF_1 agonists, type 2 urocortins do not produce malaise, arousal, or anxiety-like effects at central anorectic doses in the rat. The degree to which endogenous brain urocortins produce these effects under physiological conditions remains unclear. In addition to the CRF_2-mediated urocortin anorexia, brain Ucn 1 may also reduce food intake via a separate CRF_1-dependent mechanism. Possible loci for Ucn 1-CRF_1-mediated anorexia include the dorsomedial nucleus of the hypothalamus, the parabrachial nucleus, and caudal hindbrain glucoregulatory sites.

Ucn 3 is present in pancreatic islet β cells, with pancreatic Ucn 3 levels responsive to changes in local glucose levels. Exogenous Ucn 3 administration increases glucagon and insulin levels *in vivo* and *in vitro*, resulting in a net increase in blood glucose levels. Glucoregulatory effects of Ucn 3 were abolished by pretreatment with a selective CRF_2 antagonist. Altogether, findings suggest an autocrine or paracrine regulation of glucose homeostasis by pancreatic Ucn 3.

Gastrocolonic Motility and Function

Stress also releases CRF-related peptides, possibly including urocortins, which slow gastric emptying through CRF_2 receptor systems. Through vagal efferents, central infusion of CRF receptor agonists reduce antral gastric motility, inhibit high-amplitude gastric contractions, and shift duodenal activity from fasted to fed motor patterns. Parallel to the central CRF_2 pathway for stress-induced gastric stasis, peripheral CRF_2 receptor activation delays gastric emptying, with peripheral (intravenous [IV] or intraperitoneal [IP]) administration of agonists with high (i.e., Ucn 1) or selective (i.e., Ucn 2 or Ucn 3) CRF_2 affinity delaying gastric emptying more potently than CRF. Like central infusion, peripheral Ucn 1 administration reduces antral gastric motility in fed rats and shifts gastric motor patterns from a fasted to fed state. Ucn 1 also hyperpolarizes stomach smooth muscle. Candidate regions that subserve CRF_2 receptor-mediated gastric stasis include, centrally, the PVN and dorsal vagal complex and, peripherally, myenteric fibers of the enteric nervous system. A physiological role for urocortins in stress-induced slowing of gastric emptying is supported by the presence of urocortins in the PVN, NTS of the caudal hindbrain, GI tract, and enteric nervous system.

Gastric Ucn 1 also may regulate gastric acid secretion, as peripheral administration of CRF_2 receptor agonists inhibits gastric acid secretion and increases gastric mucosal blood flow. Anatomical evidence supports such a relation. Ucn 1 colocalizes with tyrosine hydroxylase in parietal cells of the stomach, in proximity to CRF_2, but not CRF_1 receptors. CRF_2 receptors, in turn, colocalize with H^+/K^+-ATPase, the enzyme gastric proton pump, and somatostatin, which inhibits parietal cell activity and secretion of gastrin and histamine.

In contrast to their effects on gastric motor function, stressors stimulate colonic motility. Indicating a role for urocortin/CRF systems in these effects, central and peripheral administration of CRF_1, but not CRF_2, agonists likewise stimulates colonic motility, and selective CRF_1, but not CRF_2, antagonists attenuate stress-induced stimulation of colonic motility. Candidate substrates for CRF_1-mediated stimulation of colonic motor function include, centrally, the PVN and LC/Barrington nuclei that activate sacral parasympathetic nervous system activity and, peripherally, the colonic myenteric nervous system. Ucn 1 is expressed in these tissues, and, therefore, endogenous Ucn 1 may partly mediate the colonic-stimulating effects of stress.

Cardiovascular Function

Intravenous administration of urocortins more potently reduces blood pressure and has greater vasodilating effects than CRF. The relaxant effects of urocortin are mediated by arteriole and possibly cardiac CRF_2 receptors and appear to involve activation of protein kinase A and MAP kinase signaling pathways as well as inhibition of a PKC-dependent contractile mechanism. CRF_2-deficient mice have elevated mean arterial pressure, suggesting a physiological function of urocortin/CRF_2 interactions on vasculature *in vivo*. Independent of its effects on peripheral vascular resistance, systemic Ucn 1 infusion also had prolonged cardiac inotropic actions in sheep, increasing cardiac contractility, heart rate, and aortic blood flow.

Urocortins also are increasingly recognized to have cardioprotective and cardiovascular function-enhancing effects on compromised heart. Urocortins protect cardiac tissue from ischemia-reperfusion injury or hypoxia-reoxygenation injury via CRF_2 mechanisms. The cardioprotective effects of urocortins appear to involve activation of ERK1/2-p42, 44 signaling pathways, the phosphatidylinositol-3 (PI-3) kinase/Akt pathway, and protein kinase C epsilon isozyme activation. The cardioprotective effects also appear to involve reduced mitochondrial damage, achieved by increasing mitochondrial K_{ATP} channel opening. In addition to its cardioprotective effects, exogenous Ucn 1 also has cardiac hypertrophic effects, involving an Akt-dependent pathway.

Supporting a physiological cardioprotective role for urocortins, Ucn 1, 2, and 3 are present in the heart, with Ucn 2 and Ucn 3 abundant in myocardium. Plasma Ucn 1-IR increases in human systolic heart failure, and Ucn 1 expression increases more than ninefold in viable human myocytes after surgical cardioplegic arrest-reperfusion. Finally, cardiac myocytes isolated from CRF_2-deficient mice are more susceptible to ischemia-reperfusion injury.

Immune Function

As described previously, urocortins are expressed in immune tissue, including thymus, spleen, and/or skin, with Ucn 1 seen at the cellular level in lymphocytes, macrophages, fibroblasts, and mast cells. Exogenous Ucn 1 administration has palliative effects on experimental autoimmune encephalomyelitis and thermal injury-induced edema (although this may reflect glucocorticoid, vasodilatory, or direct cytoprotective mechanisms, as opposed to immunomodulating mechanisms). However, converging lines of evidence suggest that immune-derived urocortins locally modulate proinflammatory responses to perceived environmental insults.

For example, Ucn 1 mRNA is expressed in lamina propria macrophages, and Ucn 1-IR is detected throughout the entire lamina propria layer of the intestine. Intestinal Ucn 1 activity may be regulated by changes in the intestinal milieu, such as passage of dietary factors or food-associated bacterial antigens. Ucn 1-IR is elevated in the intestinal lamina propria macrophages of patients with ulcerative colitis, in which it is hypothesized to have a proinflammatory CRF_1-mediated effect. Intraperitoneal administration of CRF_1 agonists, such as Ucn 1, also increases intestinal mucosal permeability to macromolecules.

Other inflammatory conditions also are accompanied by increased Ucn 1 expression. In rheumatoid arthritis (but not osteoarthritis), Ucn 1-IR and Ucn 1 mRNA are elevated in synovium, and the number of Ucn 1-positive cells in synovia, including leukocytes and macrophages, is not only higher, but also correlates with the degree of inflammation. Supporting a proinflammatory property of secreted Ucn 1, Ucn 1 stimulates proinflammatory cytokine production by peripheral blood mononuclear cells *in vitro*, presumably, like CRF, via a CRF_1-mediated mechanism.

Some stress-related dermatological inflammatory conditions also have altered urocortin/CRF signaling. Mast cells, which play a role in allergy and inflammation, are widely distributed in the skin and synthesize and secrete both CRF and Ucn 1 in response to psychosocial stress or immunoglobulin E receptor cross-linking. Mast cells also express CRF receptors, activation of which leads to the release of proinflammatory mediators. Thus, atopic dermatitis, psoriasis, and alopecia areata have been hypothesized to involve a stress-related precipitation or exacerbation of mast cell activation via local CRF/ Ucn 1–CRF receptor signaling.

The reproductive tract also contains mast cells. Ucn 1-IR is increased more than 10-fold in spontaneous abortion products from women with a history of multiple nonelective abortions relative to products from elective or nonhabitual abortions. Supporting the hypothesis that the observed increase in Ucn 1-IR is related to mast cell activation, levels of tryptase, which constitutes one-fifth of all protein in mast cells, and IL-8, an abortogenic mast cell-derived cytokine, also are robustly elevated in habitual spontaneous abortion products. Endometriosis also is associated with an increased number of activated mast cells in association with strong Ucn 1 immunostaining. Normal endometrium, in contrast, shows low tryptase and Ucn 1 immunoreactivity. Thus, Ucn 1 expression and mast cell activation are both elevated in inflammatory conditions of the reproductive tract and may correlate with increased risk for spontaneous abortion.

Finally, Ucn 1-IR is increased in stomach biopsies from patients with active gastritis. Unlike the colon, the stomach is much richer in CRF_2 than in CRF_1 receptors. As a result, in contrast to the CRF_1-mediated proinflammatory effects of intestinal Ucn 1, stomach Ucn 1 has been hypothesized, via CRF_2 receptors, to reduce/repair injury to gastric mucosa following noxious stimuli. Consistent with this perspective, Ucn 1-IR increases in treatment-responsive, but not treatment-resistant, patients during recovery from gastritis.

Reproductive Function

In addition to mast cells within the reproductive system, the human reproductive system itself expresses Ucn 1, CRF receptors, and CRF-BP. Ucn 1-IR is produced by choriodecidual and placental tissue and is elevated in maternal plasma from midgestation through birth. Placental Ucn 1 appears to act as a vasoactive relaxant factor on uteroplacental vasculature via local action at CRF receptors. Supporting the physiological relevance of this mechanism, pregnant women who have impaired uterine artery blood flow have significantly reduced circulating Ucn 1 levels in proportion to the degree of increased arterial resistance. Urocortins also may stimulate uterine contractility, as myometrium expresses both CRF_1 and CRF_2 receptors. Whereas CRF inhibits contractility via CRF_1 receptors, urocortins increase myometrial contractility via local CRF_2-mediated actions. Thus, urocortins may regulate placental vessel resistance to blood flow and stimulate uterine contractility.

Anxiety-Related Behavior

Central administration of Ucn 1, like CRF, has anxiogenic-like properties in many rodent anxiety models that are mediated at least partly by CRF_1 receptors. Ucn 1's effects on acoustic startle responding appear to differ from those of CRF, however, as exogenous Ucn 1 dampens rather than potentiates the acoustic startle response. Contrary to the effects of CRF_1 receptor agonists, ICV type 2 urocortin administration does not consistently increase anxiogenic-like behavior. For example, Ucn 3 did not increase anxiety-like behavior in the open field, elevated plus maze, light/dark box, social interaction, or defensive burying tests. Ucn 2 (ICV) similarly lacked acute anxiogenic-like effects in the rat open field and elevated plus maze tests. In fact, ICV Ucn 3 acutely produced anxiolytic-like changes in the elevated plus maze and light/dark box tests, and Ucn 2 had delayed, anxiolytic-like effects in the plus maze and reversed the anxiogenic-like effects of CRF in the open field. Similarly, whereas CRF_1 agonists increased activity in familiar environments, type 2 urocortins had mild motor suppressing effects.

However, stress-like effects of CRF_2 receptor activation also have been reported following local micro-infusion into discrete brain regions, including the lateral septum and dorsal raphe, findings somewhat incongruous with the reviewed effects of ICV type 2 urocortin administration. Furthermore, unlike in rats, exogenous ICV administration of Ucn 2 to mice increased anxiety-like behavior in the plus maze as well as acoustic startle responses. Thus, although it is accepted that CRF_1 receptor activation has anxiogenic-like effects, general conclusions about the anxiety-related effects of central administration of the CRF_2-selective type 2 urocortins are not yet entirely possible and may involve brain region or species specificity. The endogenous roles of urocortins similarly remain unclear, as one Ucn 1-deficient mouse model exhibited normal anxiety-like behavior, whereas another showed increased anxiety-like responses.

Hearing

Ucn 1 may be required for normal hearing, as Ucn 1-deficient mutant mice have shorter hair cells in the inner spinal bundle of the organ of Corti and a higher response threshold in the auditory brain stem response examination than wild-type littermates. Perhaps reflecting this difference, a second murine model of Ucn 1 deficiency exhibited a reduced acoustic startle response. Anatomically supporting a relation of Ucn 1 to audition, Ucn 1-IR neurons are present in the lateral superior olive as well as in the inner spiral bundle of the organ of Corti. In the organ of Corti, Ucn 1 appears at 8 days of age, present only in the inner hair cell region, in proximity to CRF_1 and CRF_2 receptors.

Acknowledgments

This work was supported by NIH grants DK70118, DK64871 and DK26741 from the National Institute of Diabetes and Digestive and Kidney Diseases. This is publication number 17400-NP from the Scripps Research Institute.

See Also the Following Articles

Blood Pressure; Cardiovascular System and Stress; Central Stress Neurocircuits; Corticotropin Releasing Factor-Binding Protein; Corticotripin-Releasing Factor Receptors; Cytokines; Immune Response; Immunity; Macrophages.

Further Reading

Bale, T. L. and Vale, W. W. (2004). CRF and CRF receptors: role in stress responsivity and other behaviors. *Annual Review of Pharmacology and Toxicology* **44**, 525–557.

Hashimoto, K., Nishiyama, M., Tanaka, Y., et al. (2004). Urocortins and corticotropin releasing factor type 2 receptors in the hypothalamus and the cardiovascular system. *Peptides* **25**, 1711–1721.

Scarabelli, T. and Knight, R. (2004). Urocortins: take them to heart. *Current Medicinal Chemistry: Cardiovascular and Hematological Agents* **2**, 335–342.

Suda, T., Kageyama, K., Sakihara, S., et al. (2004). Physiological roles of urocortins, human homologues of fish urotensin I, and their receptors. *Peptides* **25**, 1689–1701.

Theoharides, T. C., Donelan, J. M., Papadopoulou, N., et al. (2004). Mast cells as targets of corticotropin-releasing factor and related peptides. *Trends in Pharmacological Sciences* **25**, 563–568.

Zorrilla, E. P., Taché, Y. and Koob, G. F. (2003). Nibbling at CRF receptor control of feeding and gastrocolonic motility. *Trends in Pharmacological Sciences* **24**, 421–427.

Corticotropin-Releasing Factor Receptors

D E Grigoriadis
Neurocrine Biosciences, Inc., San Diego, CA, USA

This is a revised version of the article by D E Grigoriadis, Encyclopedia of Stress, First edition, volume 1, pp 586–593, © 2000, Elsevier Inc.

Glossary

Adenylate cyclase — One of the signaling molecules for G-protein-coupled receptors. On activation by a specific G-protein, this transmembrane protein either increases or decreases the rate of conversion of ATP to cAMP.

Corticotropin releasing factor (CRF) — A 41-amino-acid peptide primarily secreted by the hypothalamus into the hypophysial portal vasculature to act on the pituitary and cause the release of adrenocorticotropic hormone.

G-protein — A heterotrimeric protein that has high affinity for GTP and interacts with the cytoplasmic domains of a receptor, transducing the signal from the activated (ligand-bound) receptor to the second-messenger signaling protein inside the cell.

G-protein-coupled receptor — A protein that typically spans a cell membrane seven times with extracellular and intracellular loops coordinating the binding of a ligand outside the membrane with a signal transduction mechanism inside the membrane.

Hypothalamic-pituitary-adrenal (HPA) axis — The hormonal pathway that is thought to mediate the primary stress response. CRF secreted from the hypothalamus acts on the anterior pituitary to release adrenocorticotropin (ACTH), which in turn acts on the adrenals to produce and release glucocorticoids. Glucocorticoids feed back to the pituitary to decrease ACTH release and also act on the hypothalamus to decrease CRF release in a negative feedback loop.

Introduction

More than half a century ago, Geoffrey Harris first proposed the concept that the hypothalamus plays a primary role in the regulation of the pituitary-adrenocortical axis and extended the notion put forth by Walter B. Cannon that an organism's ability to maintain homeostasis in the face of external stressors was coordinated by a specific portion of the central nervous system (CNS) operating in an automatic fashion. Subsequently, during the 1950s, Guillemin and Rosenberg and Saffran and Schally independently observed the presence of a factor in extracts of the hypothalamus that could stimulate the release of adrenocorticotropic hormone (ACTH, corticotropin) from anterior pituitary cells *in vitro*. This extract was termed corticotropin releasing factor (CRF). Although CRF was the first hypothalamic hypophysiotropic factor to be recognized, its chemical identity remained unknown largely due to the presence in hypothalamic extracts of other weaker secretagogues of ACTH secretion such as vasopressin, catecholamines, and angiotensin II. These agents, along with their synergistic effects with CRF on ACTH secretion and in combination with the relative lack of specificity of the *in vitro* bioassays, hindered the purification of this peptide. The development of radioimmunoassays for ACTH and quantitative *in vitro* methods for assaying hypophysiotropic substances along with the use of ion exchange and high-performance liquid chromatographic techniques led to the successful purification of CRF from sheep hypothalamic extracts in 1981 by Vale and his colleagues at the Salk Institute. They were the first to report the isolation, characterization, synthesis, and *in vitro* and *in vivo* biological activities of a 41-amino-acid hypothalamic peptide that fulfilled all the criteria for a corticotropin releasing factor. Thus, from the first basic understanding of homeostasis in the early 1940s, this neuropeptide has gained widespread acknowledgement of its role in mediating the HPA axis and regulating an organism's response to physical, emotional, and environmental stress.

Since the elucidation of the structure of CRF, there have been countless studies that have demonstrated the importance of this peptide and its role as a neurotransmitter and neuromodulator in the CNS apart from its role in the direct stimulation of ACTH from the pituitary through hypothalamic release. These reports have detailed the anatomical distribution of both CRF-containing cell bodies and fibers in the CNS and have identified the peptide in regions of the brain shown to clearly regulate autonomic function and mediate the behavioral responses to stress. For example, the neocortex contains high densities of CRF-containing neurons that are localized primarily to prefrontal, cingulate, and insular areas and that appear to regulate behavioral actions of the peptide. This extrahypothalamic distribution of CRF suggests that this peptide has numerous effects in the brain, and its widespread but discrete localization in various brain regions, both rat and human, place it in a position to regulate mood and stress-related behaviors. In fact, the exogenous administration of CRF into discrete brain regions has demonstrated direct interactions between the CRF and the norepinephrine systems (such as in the locus coeruleus) or the serotonergic systems (such as in the dorsal and median raphe nuclei) and corresponds to the effects seen under various stress paradigms in which these systems are activated. This further implicates this particular neuropeptide in mediating the central mechanisms through which various stressors can alter behavior.

The relatively recent cloning of multiple CRF receptor subtypes and the identification of a specific binding protein for the peptide (known as CRF-BP) has precipitated a new era in CRF research. In addition, the identification of a new related family of endogenous peptides, the urocortins, has expanded the notion that this system is under multiple regulatory factors and plays a much more complex role in the CNS than previously thought. This article focuses primarily on recent studies that elucidate the molecular biological, pharmacological, anatomical, and functional characteristics of mammalian CRF receptors.

Corticotropin Releasing Factor Receptor Family

Molecular Biology/Receptor Structure

The CRF receptors belong to the superfamily of G-protein-coupled receptors and, as such, have been shown to contain seven putative transmembrane domains and function through the coupling of a stimulatory guanine-nucleotide binding protein. These receptors also fall within the recently described, and still-growing, family of gut–brain neuropeptide receptors, which includes receptors for calcitonin, vasoactive intestinal peptide (VIP), parathyroid hormone, secretin, pituitary adenylate cyclase-activating peptide, glucagon and growth hormone-releasing factor. These receptors all share considerable sequence homology, and all stimulate adenylate cyclase in response to their respective agonist activation. Almost all of the initial characterization of the CRF receptors was performed using various native tissues from a variety of species. As such, there was only one form of the receptor that could be experimentally discerned. As will be described later in the chapter, this form was subsequently identified as the CRF_1 receptor. It has been very difficult to pharmacologically study the CRF_2 receptor in native tissues due to its discrete localization and relatively low abundance. Cloning of these receptor subtypes however, has enabled the pharmacological and biochemical characterization of these proteins and allowed the discovery of potential therapeutics through a variety of chemical-screening strategies.

CRF_1 Receptors

Vale and colleagues first cloned the CRF_1 receptor in 1993 from a human Cushing's anterior pituitary corticotropic adenoma using the technique of expression cloning. The protein was characterized as a 415-amino-acid protein with seven putative transmembrane domains and five potential extracellular N-linked glycosylation sites. In addition, the protein contained putative sites for protein kinase C phosphorylation in the first and second intracellular loops and in the C-terminal tail, as well as casein kinase II and protein kinase A phosphorylation sites in the third intracellular loop. The human gene was subsequently localized on chromosome 17 at position 17q12–22. Shortly after the elucidation of this human form, several groups identified the CRF_1 form of the receptor from a variety of other species. All species of CRF_1 mRNAs thus far identified encode proteins of 415 amino acids that are 98% identical to one another. The human CRF_1 gene contains at least two introns and is found in a number of alternative splice forms. none of which to date has been found to have any physiological significance. This is in contrast to the mouse, in which the gene has been identified as containing at least 12 introns. The various kinase and phosphorylation sites predicted on these proteins, although not fully characterized, may serve as regulatory elements in the control of receptor expression and/or function. The potential N-linked glycosylation sites on the N-terminal extracellular domain are characteristic of most G-protein-coupled receptors and confirm the glycosylation profiles determined by earlier chemical-affinity cross-linking studies. Indeed, the molecular weight predicted from the deglycosylated forms of the CRF_1 in the earlier biochemical studies was virtually identical to that obtained from the cloned amino acid sequence. Furthermore, mRNA distribution of the CRF_1 in the rat or human brain correlates extremely well with the previously identified biding sites for radiolabeled CRF using autoradiographic techniques in frozen brain sections. This correlation was expected (retrospectively) because the peptide CRF itself has a low affinity for the CRF_2 and does therefore not label this subtype in brain sections to any detectable level. There have been reports in the literature of splice variants of the CRF_1 mRNA; however, these have not yet been shown to produce physiologically functional proteins. This does not preclude the notion that splice variants of the CRF_1 may exist; however, their full characterization will have to await functional elucidation in a native tissue.

CRF_2 Receptors

Shortly after the cloning and characterization of the CRF_1, another subtype of this family for this hormone was identified through homology. This receptor constituted the CRF_2 subtype of the family and initially represented two splice forms termed $CRF_{2(a)}$ and $CRF_{2(b)}$. The $CRF_{2(a)}$, originally described by Lovenberg et al., is a 411-amino-acid protein with approximately 71% identity to the CRF_1. The $CRF_{2(b)}$, which has been cloned from rat, mouse, and human, contains 431 amino acids and differs from the $CRF_{2(b)}$ isoform in that the first 34 amino acids in the N-terminal extracellular domain are replaced by a unique sequence, 54 amino acids in length. The CRF_{2c} has most recently been identified and, thus far, is found only in the human brain. This splice variant uses yet a different 5′ alternative exon for its N-terminus and replaces the first 34-amino-acid sequence of the $CRF_{2(a)}$ with a unique 20-amino-acid sequence. Between the CRF_1 and CRF_{2s}, there exist very large regions of amino acid identity, particularly between transmembrane domain five and transmembrane domain six. This similarity strongly argues for conservation of biochemical function because it is this region that is thought to be the primary site of G-protein coupling and signal transduction. All three CRF_2 Receptors contain five potential N-glycosylation sites, which are analogous to those found on the CRF_1. The genomic structure of the human CRF_2 gene is similar to that of the mouse CRF_1, already described, and has 12 introns, the last 10 of which interrupt the coding region in identical positions. These gene sequences, however, diverge significantly at the 5′ end. The chromosomal mapping of the human CRF_2 gene has been localized to chromosome 7 p21–p15.

Endogenous Ligands

The peptide structure of CRF, once the amino acid sequence was determined, was found to bear strong similarities to two nonmammalian peptides, sauvagine from the frog and urotensin I from the fish. All of these peptides have the ability to potently release ACTH from cultured rat pituitary cells, which identifies them as high-affinity agonists for CRF Receptors. Although the mammalian CRF peptides from a variety of species all had high affinity for the CRF_1, they had lower affinity for the CRF_2, creating some doubt as to the likelihood that these peptides were the physiological activators for the CRF_2. It was interesting and quite unexpected, however, that, in addition to their high affinity for the CRF_1, the nonmammalian peptides sauvagine and urotensin I also had a high affinity for the CRF_2. In 1995, using antibodies for urotensin I, the first of a unique and novel family of mammalian peptides related to CRF was discovered in the rat and termed urocortin (UCN)1. UCN1 had a high affinity for both CRF Receptor subtypes, also bound with high affinity to the CRF-BP, and was localized in areas corresponding to the distribution of the CRF_2 itself. The human homolog of UCN was later identified and cloned from a human brain library and defined as the endogenous ligand for the CRF_2. Since then, two other mammalian peptides have been identified from the mouse and human, termed UCN2 (also referred to as stresscopin-related peptide) and UCN3 (also referred to as stresscopin). Unlike UCN1, UCN2 and UCN3 are much more selective for the CRF_2 subtype and have little or no affinity for the CRF-BP. These peptides have enabled a greater understanding of this increasingly complex system in the regulation of central stress responses.

To date, there are no known endogenous physiological antagonists for the CRF Receptor system; however, various truncations of the agonist peptides, with deletions of the first 8–11 N-terminal amino acids, have resulted in potent peptide antagonists. Of these, α-helical CRF(9–41), d-Phe CRF(12–41), and astressin are among the most potent and well characterized, having a high affinity for both the CRF_1 and CRF_2 receptors and being able to functionally block receptor activity both *in vitro* and *in vivo*. Recently, chemical modifications have resulted in two additional peptides that now have 400- to 500-fold selectivity for the CRF_2 over the CRF_1. Antisauvagine-30, an N-terminally truncated form of sauvagine, and the more recent cyclized astressin-2B have been used to dissect out specific roles of the CRF_2 subtype in a variety of *in vivo* studies. The pharmacological profiles of these peptide agonists and antagonists have elucidated some of the discrete biochemical requirements of the two receptor subtypes and have greatly enhanced the understanding of the physiology of the CRF system and the important role this neurohormone plays in mediating the stress response. Furthermore, there is now increasing evidence that this system is fully integrated in diseases such as anxiety and depression and may provide a target for novel therapeutics in the treatment of these disorders.

Pharmacological Characteristics

The rat and human forms of the CRF Receptor family have been transfected into a variety of mammalian cell lines that do not normally express these receptors, including COS-7 (monkey kidney), CHO (Chinese hamster ovary), and Ltk^- (mouse fibroblast) cells. Although rat tissue was commonly available for the study of the CRF_1, the expression in stable mammalian cell lines of the human forms of the CRF Receptor subtypes enabled, for the first time, direct biochemical and pharmacological study without the requirement for scarce human brain tissue.

The CRF Receptor subtypes exhibit a clear and distinct pharmacological profile with respect to the endogenous and related peptides known to activate this system. In addition, the $CRF_{2(a)}$ and $CRF_{2(b)}$ display very subtle differences in the pharmacological profiles with respect to one another, which suggests that some specific conformation of the protein can be attributed to the N-terminal extracellular domains and is critical for the high-affinity binding of peptides. As a direct result of the distinct pharmacological difference between the CRF_1 and CRF_2 subtypes, it became necessary to radiolabel a nonmammalian CRF-like ligand ($[^{125}I]$sauvagine) in order to completely characterize the CRF_2 subtype. Previous studies examining the detailed binding characteristics of the CRF peptides with respect to the peptide structure have revealed that all the CRF peptides – be they agonist or antagonist – must be amidated at their C-terminus for potent activity. The deamidation of any of these peptides results in a virtually complete loss of activity at either receptor subtype, suggesting that at least some similarity between the two subtypes must exist.

Ligand Binding Profile of CRF_1 Receptors

CRF_1 receptors expressed in the mammalian cell lines described demonstrate reversible, saturable, high-affinity binding to CRF and its related peptides with the pharmacological and functional characteristics comparable to those found in the variety of animal or human tissues previously described in the literature. Human and rat CRF_1 receptors in stably transfected Ltk^- cells demonstrate binding to a single homogeneous population of receptors with apparent affinities (K_D) of 130 and 168 pM and receptor densities (B_{max}) of 97 and 588 fmol/mg protein, respectively. The pharmacological rank orders of potency in the stably transfected cell lines with either the human or rat CRF_1 receptors were identical to the established profile for the CRF receptor in the rat frontal cortex, where UCN1, urotensin I, sauvagine > ovine CRF (oCRF), rat/human CRF (r/hCRF), bovine CRF > astressin > D-Phe r/hCRF(12–41) > α-helical oCRF (9–41) ≫ UCN2, UCN3, astressin-2B, r/hCRF(6–33), r/hCRF(9–33), r/hCRF(1–41)OH, VIP, arginine vasopressin (AVP). These data demonstrate that, although there are subtle differences between the rat and human forms of the receptor in terms of amino acid sequence, the differences are not significant enough to alter the ability of these peptides to bind or interact with this subtype.

Ligand Binding Profile of CRF_2 Receptors

The CRF_2 isoforms have also been expressed in stable mammalian cell lines and demonstrated to bind CRF-related peptides and function through the stimulation of cAMP production. In general, although some minor differences exist in the rank order profile of the CRF_2 splice variants to one another (mainly related to fragments of CRF peptides), as a subtype they are quite distinct from either the CRF_1 subtype or the CRF-BP. When expressed in stable cell lines, these receptors exhibit the following pharmacological rank order profile: UCN1, UCN2, sauvagine, urotensin I, astressin-2B > UCN3 > astressin > r/hCRF > D-Phe CRF(12–41), α-helical CRF(9–41) ≫ oCRF ≫ r/hCRF(6–33), oCRF(6–33), r/hCRF(1–41)OH, GHRH, AVP, and VIP. The data thus far on the $CRF_{2(a)}$ suggests a rank order of potencies similar to the other two splice variants with UCN, sauvagine > urotensin I > r/hCRF. Without exception, it is clear that the mammalian CRF peptides oCRF and r/hCRF have weaker affinity for the CRF_2 subtype, whereas UCN has equal affinity for both the CRF_1 and CRF_2 receptors and UCN2 has selectivity for the CRF_2 receptors. Interestingly, the relatively weaker affinity of UCN3 for the CRF_2 receptors may indeed suggest that this peptide is the endogenous ligand for a different and thus far undiscovered CRF receptor subtype.

Guanine Nucleotide Characteristics of Corticotropin Releasing Factor Receptors

Characteristic of receptor systems that are coupled to adenylate cyclase as a second-messenger system is the exclusive link to a guanine nucleotide-binding protein. These transducing proteins mediate the ligand-binding event at the receptor to an activation of an intracellular pathway, in this case beginning with the conversion of ATP to cAMP. *In vitro*, guanine nucleotides have been shown to decrease the specific binding of agonists for a great number of seven-transmembrane neurohormone or neurotransmitter receptors coupled to G-proteins, presumably by uncoupling the G-protein from the receptor and changing its conformation such that it now has low affinity for its agonist. Both CRF receptor subtypes transfected in stable mammalian cell lines were used to determine the guanine nucleotide sensitivity of the cloned receptors. Guanine nucleotides inhibited the binding of [^{125}I]oCRF (for CRF_1 receptors) or [^{125}I] sauvagine (for either CRF_1 receptors or CRF_2 receptors) by 50–70% (where 100% inhibition was defined by 1 μM unlabeled r/hCRF). The nonhydrolyzable forms of guanine nucleotides, Gpp(NH)p and GTP-γ-S, were more potent than GTP itself. The order of potencies were GTP-γ-S > Gpp(NH)p > GTP with median effective dose (ED_{50}) values of ~20–45, 200–800 and 2500–3000 nM, respectively. These effects on the binding in both human and rat CRF_1- or CRF_2-stable cell lines were specific for the guanine nucleotides because the adenosine nucleotide ATP was ineffective in altering the binding at equimolar concentrations ($ED_{50} > 10\,000$ nM). Recently, using a variety of peptide ligands in conjunction with the guanine nucleotide GTP-γ-S, three distinct receptor states have been elucidated for the CRF_1. These states represent RG, the G-protein-coupled form of the receptor sensitive to guanine nucleotides; R, the G-protein-uncoupled form of the receptor; and R0, a high-affinity uncoupled state of the CRF_1 that is GTP-γ-S insensitive. Although the nature of this state requires much further investigation for the CRF system, this conformation has been described for other GPCRs, including the β_2-adrenergic, M2 muscarinic, formyl peptide, and natural killer (NK)1 cell receptors where they have been identified to be in a complex with arrestin. Significantly, these three states for the CRF_1 have also been confirmed to exist in native rat tissues such as the cerebellum and may offer new approaches for the discovery of molecules targeting conformationally restricted binding sites.

Second-Messenger Characteristics of Corticotropin Releasing Factor Receptors

In addition to the adenylate cyclase system, other signal transduction mechanisms have been postulated to be involved in the actions of CRF. For example, CRF has been shown to increase protein carboxylmethylation and phospholipid methylation in AtT-20 cells. Preliminary evidence suggests that CRF may regulate cellular responses through products of arachidonic acid metabolism. Furthermore, although the evidence in anterior pituitary cells suggests that CRF does not directly regulate phosphotidylinositol turnover or protein kinase C activity, the stimulation of protein kinase C, either directly or by specific ligands (vasopressin or angiotensin II), enhances CRF-stimulated adenylate cyclase activity, ACTH release, and inhibits phosphodiesterase activity. Thus, the effects of CRF in native tissues such as the anterior pituitary cells, neurons, and other cell types expressing CRF receptors are likely to involve complex interactions among several intracellular second-messenger systems. All this evidence has thus far been gathered from native tissues that exhibit binding profiles consistent with the CRF receptor. These studies have most probably been examining second-messenger profiles of the CRF_1 in various tissues, primarily due to the ubiquitous nature of this subtype compared to the CRF_2 in the rat. Clearly, the most common and well-studied second-messenger system for the CRF receptor is the coupling to the adenylate cyclase system. In fact, there is no evidence to date that the heterologous expression of hCRF receptors transfected into mammalian cells function in any manner other than through the stimulation of the production of cAMP, unless forced to couple through overexpressed, genetically manipulated cell systems.

In the pituitary gland, CRF initiates a cascade of enzymatic reactions, beginning with the receptor-mediated stimulation of adenylate cyclase, which ultimately regulates proopiomelanocortin (POMC) peptide secretion and possibly synthesis. POMC-derived peptide secretion mediated by the activation of adenylate cyclase is dose-related and exhibits appropriate pharmacology consistent with the activation of the CRF_1. Similarly, in the brain and also in spleen, the pharmacological rank order profile of CRF-related peptides for stimulation of adenylate cyclase is analogous to the profile seen in the pituitary and in keeping with the affinities of these compounds for receptor binding. In addition, the putative CRF receptor antagonist α-helical oCRF(9–41) inhibits the CRF-stimulated adenylate cyclase observed in brain and spleen homogenates.

To further characterize the stable CRF receptor transfectants, the ability of CRF-related and unrelated peptides to stimulate CRF_1- or CRF_2-mediated cAMP production from the cells has been examined. The rank order of the peptides in stimulating cAMP production in these cells was in keeping with their rank order in inhibiting [^{125}I]oCRF and [^{125}I]sauvagine binding to the CRF_1 and CRF_2, respectively, and at least for the CRF_1, this rank order was virtually identical to the second-messenger pharmacological profile previously reported in the brain, pituitary, and spleen.

In addition to the stimulation studies, CRF-stimulated cAMP production could be competitively inhibited by the putative peptide antagonists D-Phe CRF(12–41) and α-helical CRF(9–41) in both CRF_1- and CRF_2-expressing cell lines, demonstrating that the expressed CRF receptors in these cell lines were indeed functional. Interestingly, both D-Phe CRF (12–41) and α-helical CRF(9–41) inhibited the stimulated cAMP response with the same median effective concentration (EC_{50}) in both receptor subtype preparations. This suggests that, although there is some fundamental difference in the pharmacological specificity of these two receptor subtypes when examining agonists, they must still possess some similarities in their structure of the binding site, at least as far as peptide antagonists are concerned. These results clearly suggest that not only subtype-specific and subtype-selective compounds can be identified for these two receptor subtypes but that mixed antagonists are possible and could bring to light possible subtle functions of the two receptor subtypes.

Distribution of Corticotropin Releasing Factor Receptor Subtypes

Receptor autoradiographic studies and more recent *in situ* hybridization and immunocytochemical studies have localized CRF binding sites and CRF Receptor mRNA, respectively, in slide-mounted sections of many tissues from a variety of species, identifying these proteins in anatomically and physiologically relevant areas. For example, in the pituitary gland, CRF_1 expression is detectable in both the anterior and intermediate lobes, with particularly high expression in clusters within the anterior lobe. In fact, there exists a good correlation between the actions of CRF on corticotropes of the anterior pituitary and the distribution of [^{125}I]oCRF or [^{125}I]sauvagine binding sites and CRF_1 mRNA. Within the anterior lobe, CRF_2 expression is detectable in only a few scattered cells. Thus, in terms of HPA axis activity, CRF_2 receptors may mediate CRF effects at the level of the hypothalamus, whereas CRF_1 receptors are responsible for CRF-induced changes in ACTH release in pituitary corticotropes.

Although there is a general correspondence of the distribution of [^{125}I]oCRF or [^{125}I]sauvagine binding sites and CRF_1 or CRF_2 mRNA in the brain with the functional actions of CRF, there are several brain areas with some apparent discrepancies. For example, CRF has potent electrophysiological and behavioral effects in the locus coeruleus, but the distribution of binding sites and CRF_1 or CRF_2 mRNA is not noteworthy in this brain-stem nucleus. Physiologically, it is tempting to speculate that other subtypes that are as yet unidentified may be responsible for the actions of the neurotransmitter in those regions where CRF seems to have profound actions but no appreciable labeling of the receptor is observed. The localization and distribution of CRF_2 Receptors in the mammalian brain, coupled with the discovery of the urocortins, has accounted for some of these discrepancies. However, species differences in the localization of receptor subtypes and peptides among rodent, nonhuman primate, and human tissues have made it somewhat difficult to extrapolate behavioral studies in rodent models to human effects. It is important to note that, because most of the autoradiographic studies in the literature thus far in rodents have used [^{125}I] oCRF or various forms of [^{125}I]rat/human CRF, the primary labeling, localization, and distribution are almost exclusively attributable to the CRF_1 subtype.

Within the rat brain, CRF_1 expression was very high in neocortical, cerebellar, and sensory relay structures, whereas CRF_2 expression was generally confined to subcortical structures, including the lateral septal region, the bed nucleus of the stria terminalis, the amygdaloid area, and the olfactory bulb. The contrast in expression patterns between CRF Receptor subtypes was particularly evident within the septal region; CRF_2 mRNA expression was very high in the lateral septal nuclei but very low in the medial septum, a region where CRF_1 mRNA abundance was most evident. The lateral septum, by virtue of widespread reciprocal connections throughout the brain, is implicated in a variety of physiological processes. These range from higher cognitive functions, such as learning and memory, to autonomic regulation, including food and water intake. In addition, the septum plays a central role in classic limbic circuitry and is thus important in a variety of emotional conditions, including fear and aggression. The lateral septum thus acts as both an integrator of limbic circuitry and an interface between the telencephalic and diencephalic areas. The high-level of CRF_2 expression in this area suggests a role for CRF_2 Receptors in modulating limbic circuitry at the level of the lateral septum.

The heterogeneous distribution of CRF_1 and CRF_2 mRNA suggests distinctive functional roles for each receptor in CRF-related systems. CRF_2 mRNA was evident throughout the rostrocaudal extent of the hypothalamus, particularly within the paraventricular nucleus (PVN), whereas CRF_1 expression was limited. The distribution of cells expressing CRF_2 mRNA within the PVN coincides with the cellular distribution of CRF mRNA, suggesting a possible autoreceptor role for CRF_2 Receptors in this nucleus. Because the CRF neurons of the PVN play a classical hypophysiotropic role in controlling ACTH release from the anterior pituitary, it is tempting to speculate that CRF_2 Receptors may act to selectively regulate hypophysiotropic-and/or autonomic-related CRF neurons. As such, this receptor subtype may be central to the control of the mammalian HPA stress system. Further, more detailed studies using double-labeling of the peptides and their receptors are required to determine the discrete role of this subtype. Whatever the case may be, the high level of CRF_2 expression within the hypothalamic structures is certainly suggestive of a role for CRF_2 Receptors in modulating autonomic CRF neurons. With regard to HPA axis activity, we may speculate that the PVN

CRF_2 Receptors could also act to modulate CRF neurosecretory neurons in response to stress, in essence providing a short-loop feedback role. Ono and colleagues have proposed such a role for CRF in a positive ultrashort-loop feedback effect on stress-induced ACTH release. In this regard, the comparatively lower affinity of CRF for the CRF_2 subtype may be of physiological design to allow activation of CRF_2 Receptors only under conditions of chronic stress or prolonged CRF release.

A more detailed examination of the precise localization of the CRF_2 splice variants, $CRF_{2(a)}$ and $CRF_{2(b)}$, indicates discrete anatomical distributions in the rat. The $CRF_{2(a)}$ form is primarily expressed within the brain, whereas the $CRF_{2(b)}$ variant is localized in both the CNS and periphery. Within the brain, it appears that the $CRF_{2(a)}$ form represents the predominant neuronal CRF_2 variant, whereas the $CRF_{2(b)}$ splice form is localized on nonneuronal elements, such as the choroid plexus of the ventricular system and cerebral arterioles. In the periphery, $CRF_{2(b)}$ mRNA is expressed at high levels in both the cardiac and skeletal muscle, with lower levels evident in both the lung and intestine. The $CRF_{2(c)}$ isoform has yet to be identified in the rodent; however, reverse transcription polymerase chain reaction (RT-PCR) analysis of human brain mRNA demonstrated expression in the septum, amygdala and hippocampus, and frontal cortex. The full characterization of the $CRF_{2(c)}$ subtype has not yet been elucidated in terms of native characteristics and function largely due to its nonexistence in rodent tissues. This type of species selectivity will make it difficult to completely examine the role of the CRF_2 subtype unless suitable animal models can be found.

Finally, in addition to the expression in the CNS, CRF receptors have been localized to a number of peripheral tissues. The gastrointestinal (GI) tract is an organ system that has a discrete localization pattern of CRF_1 and CRF_2 and is sensitive to a variety of stressors thought to act via the CRF system, both centrally and peripherally. GI responses are differentially affected by stress and these can be reproduced by the central administration of CRF. For example, stress decreases gastric emptying (upper GI tract) while increasing colonic motility and transit (lower GI tract). These effects seem to be independent of the HPA response and most likely reflect central autonomic function mediated by central CRF_2 and CRF_1, respectively. The fact that both these receptor subtypes are also found throughout the stomach and bowel, including the colon, suggests a much more complex interaction of this stress response system in the gut and that the precise mechanisms of regulation remain to be elucidated.

Summary and Conclusion

CRF is the primary regulator of the endocrine, autonomic, and behavioral response to stress via mechanisms in both the brain and the periphery. The endocrine stress response begins with the activation of the HPA axis, resulting in the release of CRF into the hypophysial portal vasculature. CRF then mediates its actions through cell surface receptors coupled to the activation of adenylyl cyclase. Centrally, CRF is found throughout the brain and plays a major role in mediating emotional, psychological, or behavioral stress. As described here, CRF receptors can be classified into two distinct subtypes: the CRF_1 (411 amino acids) and CRF_2, with the latter comprising three different isoforms, $CRF_{2(a)}$, $CRF_{2(b)}$, and $CRF_{2(c)}$ (encoded by 415, 431, and 397 amino acid proteins, respectively). These receptors differ with respect to their structures, tissue distributions, and pharmacological specificities for CRF-related ligands. UCN1, a mammalian CRF-related peptide with close sequence homology to fish urotensin, interacts with a high affinity with all CRF receptors, whereas UCN2 and UCN3 are more selective for the CRF_2 subtype. The areas of distribution of these CRF receptors in the brain are correlated well with the immunocytochemical distribution of the CRF and urocortin pathways as well as the pharmacological sites of action of CRF and the urocortins. The species differences that exist with respect to the distinct subtypes of the CRF_2 precludes our complete correlation of animal studies with humans; however, the identification of the multiple subtypes has led to an enhanced understanding of this complex system. It is becoming increasingly clear that the multiple receptor subtypes must mediate different functional and pathophysiological actions of this family of neuropeptides, and future studies aimed at identifying additional subtypes or peptides will serve to fully elucidate the role of this key neurohormone in the pathophysiology of stress and stress-related disorders.

Further Reading

Chen, R., Lewis, K. A., Perrin, M. H., et al. (1993). Expression cloning of a human corticotropin-releasing-factor receptor. *Proceedings of the National Academy of Sciences USA* **90**(19), 8967–8971.

De Souza, E. B. (1987). Corticotropin-releasing factor receptors in the rat central nervous system: characterization and regional distribution. *Journal of Neuroscience* 7(1), 88–100.

Grigoriadis, D. E. (2005). The corticotropin releasing factor receptor: a novel target for the treatment of depression and anxiety-related disorders. *Expert Opinion on Therapeutic Targets* **9**(4), 651–684.

Grigoriadis, D. E., Haddach, M., Ling, N., et al. (2001). The CRF receptor: structure, function and potential for therapeutic intervention. *Current Medicinal Chemistry: Central Nervous System Agents* **1**, 63–97.
Hauger, R. L., Grigoriadis, D. E., Dallman, M. F., et al. (2003). International Union of Pharmacology. 36: Current status of the nomenclature for receptors for corticotropin-releasing factor and their ligands. *Pharmacological Reviews* **55**(1), 21–26.
Heinrichs, S. C. and Tache, Y. (2001). Therapeutic potential of CRF receptor antagonists: a gut-brain perspective. *Expert Opinion on Investigational Drugs* **10**(4), 647–659.
Hoare, S. R. J. (2005). Mechanisms of peptide and nonpeptide ligand binding to class B G-protein coupled receptors. *Drug Discovery Today* **10**(6), 417–427.
Kehne, J. and De Lombaert, S. (2002). Non-peptidic CRF1 receptor antagonists for the treatment of anxiety, depression and stress disorders. *Current Drug Targets: CNS & Neurological Disorders* **1**(5), 467–493.
Keller, P. A., Elfick, L., Garner, J., et al. (2000). Corticotropin releasing hormone: therapeutic implications and medicinal chemistry developments. *Bioorganic & Medicinal Chemistry* **8**(6), 1213–1223.
Kostich, W. A., Chen, A., Sperle, K., et al. (1998). Molecular identification and analysis of a novel human corticotropin-releasing factor (CRF) receptor: the CRF2gamma receptor. *Molecular Endocrinology* **12**(8), 1077–1085.
Liaw, C. W., Lovenberg, T. W., Barry, G., et al. (1996). Cloning and characterization of the human corticotropin-releasing factor-2 receptor complementary deoxyribonucleic acid. *Endocrinology* **137**(1), 72–77.
Monnikes, H., Tebbe, J. J., Hildebrandt, M., et al. (2001). Role of stress in functional gastrointestinal disorders: evidence for stress-induced alterations in gastrointestinal motility and sensitivity. *Digestive Diseases* **19**(3), 201–211.
Perrin, M. H. and Vale, W. W. (1999). Corticotropin releasing factor receptors and their ligand family. *Annals of the New York Academy of Sciences* **885**, 312–328.
Sanchez, M. M., Young, L. J., Plotsky, P. M., et al. (1999). Autoradiographic and in situ hybridization localization of corticotropin-releasing factor 1 and 2 receptors in nonhuman primate brain. *Journal of Comparative Neurology* **408**(3), 365–377.
Skelton, K. H., Owens, M. J. and Nemeroff, C. B. (2000). The neurobiology of urocortin. *Regulatory Peptides* **93** (1–3), 85–92.
Tache, Y., Martinez, V., Wang, L., et al. (2004). CRF1 receptor signaling pathways are involved in stress-related alterations of colonic function and viscerosensitivity: implications for irritable bowel syndrome. *British Journal of Pharmacology* **141**(8), 1321–1330.
Vale, W., Spiess, J., Rivier, C., et al. (1981). Characterization of a 41-residue ovine hypothalamic peptide that stimulates secretion of corticotropin and beta-endorphin. *Science* **213**(4514), 1394–1397.

Corticotropin Releasing Factor Receptor Deficiency in Mice

N J Justice and K-F Lee
The Salk Institute, La Jolla, CA, USA

Glossary

Corticotropes — Endocrine cells in the anterior pituitary that release adrenocorticotropic hormone into the bloodstream.

Corticotropin releasing factor (CRF) family — A family of peptide ligands that bind CRF receptors; they were identified based on homology to CRF.

CRF receptor-deficient mice — The mice resulting from genetic manipulation of DNA to remove the genes encoding CRF receptors.

CRF receptors — Two seven-transmembrane G-protein-coupled receptors that are bound and activated by CRF family peptide ligands.

Hypothalamic-pituitary-adrenal (HPA) axis — The neuroendocrine circuit that coordinates the release of corticosteroids into the bloodstream in response to stress.

Paraventricular nucleus of the hypothalamus (PVN) — A nucleus in the hypothalamus containing neurons that release factors into portal circulation, which then stimulate the release of hormones from the anterior pituitary into the bloodstream.

Stress response — The cumulative physiological and behavioral response to real or perceived threats to homeostasis.

Corticotropin releasing factor (CRF) is released from the paraventricular nucleus of the hypothalamus (PVN) into the portal circulation in response to stress. In the anterior pituitary, CRF receptors on pituitary corticotropes respond to CRF by releasing adrenocorticotropic hormone (ACTH), which circulates in the bloodstream and, in turn, causes the release of glucocorticoids from the adrenal cortex. These corticosteroids are the primary effectors of the hypothalamic-pituitary-adrenal (HPA) axis stress response. CRF and its family of peptide ligands are also released at many other sites in the brain and in the periphery, where they effect cellular and physiological changes in addition to the activation of the HPA axis. The nature of these changes is determined by where CRF and related ligands bind and activate CRF receptors. Loss-of-function studies in mice deficient for CRF receptors have confirmed the importance of these receptors in bringing about corticosteroid release and have provided evidence for additional roles of CRF receptors in modulating the amplitude, duration, and behavioral outcome of the stress response. Here, we review what these receptor-deficient mice have taught us about how CRF receptors function to mediate and modulate stress.

Corticotropin Releasing Factor Receptors and Ligands

Two receptors for CRF have been identified. CRF type 1 receptor (CRFR1) is a high-affinity receptor for CRF that mediates the response of anterior pituitary corticotropes to CRF. CRF type 2 receptor (CRFR2), which shares 70% amino acid identity with CRFR1, has a lower affinity for CRF than the other CRF family peptide ligands. Urocortin (UCN1), a peptide ligand with homology to CRF, binds both CRFR1 and CRFR2 with high affinity, whereas urocortin 2 (UCN2) and urocortin 3 (UCN3) bind only CRFR2 with high affinity. Each peptide ligand has a unique distribution in the brain and peripheral tissues and overlaps in distinct areas with CRFR1 and CRFR2. For example, CRFR1 is expressed in the anterior pituitary, where it responds to CRF release from the PVN. In contrast, CRFR2 is expressed in the lateral septum, where it most likely responds to UCN1 from the Edinger–Westphal nucleus and UCN3 from the parafornical region of the hypothalamus. The discrete localization of each unique receptor–ligand pair suggests a distinct role for each receptor in the stress response. By selectively removing these genes from mice, we have begun to understand these roles.

CRFR1-Deficient Mice Have a Defective Hypothalamic-Pituitary-Adrenal Axis Response to Stress

CRFR1-deficient mice display abnormally low levels of circulating corticosteroids. This can be explained by a lack of responsiveness of anterior pituitary cells to CRF. The inability to stimulate ACTH release, which then activates corticosteroid release, not only blunts the stress response but also prevents the proper development of the adrenal cortex. The ACTH-responsive zona fasiculata of the adrenal gland fails to develop appropriately and undergoes atrophy in CRFR1-deficient animals. The supplementation of ACTH in postnatal animals (postnatal day 10 to postnatal day 21) can rescue adrenal gland development, indicating that an early postnatal CRFR1-dependent release of ACTH is necessary for proper adrenal gland development. The combination of adrenal gland atrophy and reduced ACTH release from the pituitary results in a profoundly reduced corticosteroid release in response to stress. Consistent with the notion that CRF and CRFR1 function as a ligand–receptor pair, this CRFR1-deficient phenotype mirrors the phenotype observed in CRF-deficient mice.

In addition to having a defective HPA axis, CRFR1-deficient animals display reduced anxiety-like behavior. In the elevated plus-maze and in the dark–light emergence task, two well-defined behavioral paradigms that measure anxiety-related behavior, CRFR1-deficient animals display decreased anxiety. This could be due to a blunted HPA response in mutant animals or a function of CRFR1 at other sites in the nervous system. To distinguish between these possibilities, investigators provided exogenous corticosteroids, which failed to rescue the anxiety-like behavioral phenotype. These data suggest that CRFR1 might modulate stress-induced behavior through actions in the brain, independent of HPA axis stimulation. Indeed, data from a forebrain-specific CRFR1-deficient animal support this interpretation. In the forebrain-specific loss of function, the pituitary retains expression of CRFR1. These animals have normal resting ACTH and corticosteroid levels as well as an intact HPA response. However, they display a reduction in anxiety-related behavior similar to full animal CRFR1-deficiency. Together, these findings strongly suggest that CRFR1 is involved in generating anxiety-like behavior through action in the forebrain, independent of its role in activating the HPA axis in the pituitary.

CRFR2-Deficient Mice Are Hypersensitive to Stress

In contrast to CRFR1-deficient mice, CRFR2-deficient mice display a hyperactive HPA axis and increased anxiety-like behavior. ACTH levels in CRFR2-deficient mice rise to approximately twice that of wild-type littermates following 2 min of restraint stress. Corticosteroid levels also remain elevated for a longer period of time following stress in the CRFR2 mutants. Consistent with overactive HPA axis dynamics, CRFR2-deficient animals appear more anxious than their wild-type littermates. In the elevated plus-maze and open field test, CRFR2-deficient mice display increased anxiety-like behavior. This might be due to a lack of modulation of the HPA axis, which is normally provided by CRFR2. Alternatively, it could be due to independent functions of CRFR2 apart from the regulation of the HPA axis.

CRFR2 is the most widely expressed CRF receptor in peripheral tissues. It was discovered based on its high levels of expression in the heart and skeletal muscle. Recently, additional functions for CRFR2 have been suggested by peripheral phenotypes observed in the CRFR2-deficient animal. For example, CRFR2-deficient animals have elevated blood pressure and fail to respond to UCN1 with an increase in heart contractility. In addition, an increase in temperature of the interscalpular brown adipose tissue of CRFR2-deficient animals has been reported, suggesting metabolic abnormalities. Consistently, these animals consume more food and gain less body fat when fed a high fat diet. These findings highlight the importance of CRF receptors in mediating peripheral changes in response to stress as well as central nervous system and neuroendocrine stress responses.

UCN1-Deficient Mice Have Increased Anxiety and Hearing Impairment

In order to gain more insight into the CRFR2-deficient mouse phenotype, a UCN1-deficient mouse has been generated. Interestingly, UCN1-deficient animals display increased anxiety-like behavior, similar to the CRFR2-deficient animal. Indeed, when the investigators examined CRFR2 expression in the lateral septum, where UCN1 projections meet CRFR2-expressing neurons, they saw greatly reduced levels of CRFR2 expression. This finding is consistent with a role for UCN1/CRFR2 in the lateral septum to control anxiety-related behavior. This control, however, must be independent of the modulation of the HPA by CRFR2 because the UCN1-deficient animal displays no changes in the dynamics of HPA function. This suggests that the role played by CRFR2 in regulating the HPA is either independent of UCN1 or that other ligands for CRFR2 function redundantly in the absence of UCN1.

An additional phenotype observed in the UCN1 knockout mouse is hearing impairment. UCN1-deficient mice showed an approximately twofold increase in the threshold for reaction to an auditory stimulus compared with wild-type mice. Although a role for UCN1 in development of the auditory system was not expected, it is consistent with CRFR1 and CRFR2 expression in the organ of Corti. Moreover, UCN1 is expressed on fibers of the lateral superior olive that project to the inner hair cells of the organ of Corti. Curiously, the change in auditory threshold indicates a problem with the outer hair cells. The investigators hypothesize that UCN1 from the inner hair cells is involved in a paracrine signal to the outer hair cells, which is required during development of the organ.

CRFR1/CRFR2-Double-Deficient Animals Have a Blunted Hypothalamic-Pituitary-Adrenal Axis Stress Response

The CRFR1-deficient mouse has an impaired HPA axis and displays decreased anxiety-like behavior, whereas the CRFR2-deficient mouse has a hypersensitive HPA axis and increased anxiety-like behavior. How do mice deficient for both CRFR1 and CRFR2 respond to stress? CRFR1-CRFR2-deficient mice have a decreased HPA response and decreased anxiety-related behavior, displaying a very similar phenotype to CRFR1-deficient animals. This suggests that the deletion of CRFR1 has a dominant impact on behavioral phenotypes associated with loss of CRF receptors, whereas CRFR2 most likely modulates behavior through central nervous system actions. The central functions of CRFR1and CRFR2 can affect the HPA axis by changing neural activity in the PVN. CRFR1 activates the PVN, whereas CRFR2 might decrease activity in the PVN to modulate HPA dynamics. The modulations made by central actions of CRFR1 and CRFR2, however, cannot override the changes in behavior that result from a defective HPA due to CRFR1 deficiency. Research is in progress to further understand how the complex actions of these receptor systems in the brain coordinate with the HPA axis to influence behavior.

Conclusion

CRFR1- and CRFR2-deficient mice have improved our understanding of the prominent roles these receptors play in the stress response. CRFR1 functions to activate the HPA axis and generate anxious behavior. Within the HPA axis, CRFR2 functions to control overactivity. In addition, CRFR1 and CRFR2 act within the central nervous system to influence behavior. CRFR2 also acts in the periphery to alter metabolism and cardiac function. UCN1 has an unexpected role in the development of the auditory system (**Table 1**). The diverse effects of CRF receptor deficiency on HPA axis, central nervous system, and

Table 1 CRF receptor- and ligand-deficient mouse phenotypes

Genotype	*HPA function*	*Anxiety-related behavior*	*Peripheral tissue development/function*	*Source*[a]
CRFR1-deficient	Inactive	Decreased anxiety	Abnormal adrenal cortex development	6, 7
CRFR2-deficient	Hyperactive	Increased anxiety	Altered cardiac function, altered metabolism	1, 2, 3, 4
CRF-deficient	Inactive	Not reported	Abnormal adrenal cortex development	5
UCN1-deficient	Normal	Increased anxiety	Hearing impairment	8

[a]Data from:
[1]Bale, T. L., Contarino, A., Smith, G. W., et al. (2000). Mice deficient for corticotropin-releasing hormone receptor-2 display anxiety-like behaviour and are hypersensitive to stress. *Nature Genetics* **24,** 410–414.
[2]Carlin, K. M., Vale, W. W. and Bale, T. L. (2006). Vital functions of corticotropin-releasing factor (CRF) pathways in maintenance and regulation of energy homeostasis. *Proceedings of the National Academy of Sciences USA,* **103,** 3462–3467.
[3]Coste, S. C., Kesterson, R. A., Heldwein, K. A., et al. (2000). Abnormal adaptations to stress and impaired cardiovascular function in mice lacking corticotropin-releasing hormone receptor-2. *Nature Genetics* **24,** 403–409.
[4]Kishimoto, T., Radulovic, J., Radulovic, M., et al. (2000). Deletion of crhr2 reveals an anxiolytic role for corticotropin-releasing hormone receptor-2. *Nature Genetics* **24,** 415–419.
[5]Muglia, L., Jacobson, L., Dikkes, P., et al. (1995). Corticotropin-releasing hormone deficiency reveals major fetal but not adult glucocorticoid need. *Nature* **373,** 427–432.
[6]Smith, G. W., Aubry, J. M., Dellu, F., et al. (1998). Corticotropin releasing factor receptor 1-deficient mice display decreased anxiety, impaired stress response, and aberrant neuroendocrine development. *Neuron* **20,** 1093–1102.
[7]Timpl, P., Spanagel, R., Sillaber, I., et al. (1998). Impaired stress response and reduced anxiety in mice lacking a functional corticotropin-releasing hormone receptor 1. *Nature Genetics* **19,** 162–166.
[8]Vetter, D. E., Li, C., Zhao, L., et al. (2002). Urocortin-deficient mice show hearing impairment and increased anxiety-like behavior. *Nature Genetics* **31,** 363–369.

peripheral tissue functions demonstrate the important contributions of CRF and its family of peptide ligands to adaptive responses to stress.

See Also the Following Articles

Corticotripin-Releasing Factor Receptors; Genetic Polymorphisms in Stress Response; Urocortins.

Further Reading

Bale, T. L., Contarino, A., Smith, G. W., et al. (2000). Mice deficient for corticotropin-releasing hormone receptor-2 display anxiety-like behaviour and are hypersensitive to stress. *Nature Genetics* **24,** 410–414.

Bale, T. L., Picetti, R., Contarino, A., et al. (2002). Mice deficient for both corticotropin-releasing factor receptor 1 (CRFR1) and CRFR2 have an impaired stress response and display sexually dichotomous anxiety-like behavior. *Journal of Neuroscience* **22,** 193–199.

Bale, T. L. and Vale, W. W. (2004). CRF and CRF receptors: role in stress responsivity and other behaviors. *Annual Review of Pharmacology and Toxicology* **44,** 525–557.

Carlin, K. M., Vale, W. W. and Bale, T. L. (2006). Vital functions of corticotropin-releasing factor (CRF) pathways in maintenance and regulation of energy homeostasis. *Proceedings of the National Academy of Sciences USA* **103,** 3462–3467.

Coste, S. C., Kesterson, R. A., Heldwein, K. A., et al. (2000). Abnormal adaptations to stress and impaired cardiovascular function in mice lacking corticotropin-releasing hormone receptor-2. *Nature Genetics* **24,** 403–409.

Kishimoto, T., Radulovic, J., Radulovic, M., et al. (2000). Deletion of *Crhr2* reveals an anxiolytic role for corticotropin-releasing hormone receptor-2. *Nature Genetics* **24,** 415–419.

Muglia, L., Jacobson, L., Dikkes, P., et al. (1995). Corticotropin-releasing hormone deficiency reveals major fetal but not adult glucocorticoid need. *Nature* **373,** 427–432.

Muller, M. B., Zimmermann, S., Sillaber, I., et al. (2003). Limbic corticotropin-releasing hormone receptor 1 mediates anxiety-related behavior and hormonal adaptation to stress. *Nature Neuroscience* **6,** 1100–1107.

Owens, M. J. and Nemeroff, C. B. (1991). Physiology and pharmacology of corticotropin-releasing factor. *Pharmacological Reviews* **43,** 425–473.

Rivier, C., Brownstein, M., Spiess, J., et al. (1982). In vivo corticotropin-releasing factor-induced secretion of adrenocorticotropin, beta-endorphin, and corticosterone. *Endocrinology* **110,** 272–278.

Smith, G. W., Aubry, J. M., Dellu, F., et al. (1998). Corticotropin releasing factor receptor 1-deficient mice display decreased anxiety, impaired stress response, and aberrant neuroendocrine development. *Neuron* **20,** 1093–1102.

Timpl, P., Spanagel, R., Sillaber, I., et al. (1998). Impaired stress response and reduced anxiety in mice lacking a functional corticotropin-releasing hormone receptor 1. *Nature Genetics* **19,** 162–166.

Vale, W., Spiess, J., Rivier, C., et al. (1981). Characterization of a 41-residue ovine hypothalamic peptide that stimulates secretion of corticotropin and beta-endorphin. *Science* **213,** 1394–1397.

Vetter, D. E., Li, C., Zhao, L., et al. (2002). Urocortin-deficient mice show hearing impairment and increased anxiety-like behavior. *Nature Genetics* **31,** 363–369.

Corticotropin Releasing Factor-Binding Protein

P J Lowry, C F Kemp and R J Woods
University of Reading, Reading, UK

This article is reproduced from Encyclopedia of Stress, First edition, volume 1, pp 582–585, © 2000, Elsevier Inc.

Glossary

Corticotropin releasing factor (CRF) — A hypothalamic peptide comprising 41 amino acid residues that is secreted in response to stressful stimuli into the hypothalamic-pituitary portal system causing release of adrenocorticotropic hormone (ACTH) from the anterior pituitary gland.

Corticotropin releasing factor-binding protein (CRF-BP) — A 37-kDa protein that binds CRF and is found in the circulation of higher primates as well as, in both membrane-bound and free forms, in the brain of all vertebrates hitherto examined.

Introduction

Under experimental conditions, the corticotropin releasing hormone-binding protein (CRF-BP) is able to bind CRF and render it biologically inactive. Because CRF-BP expression overlaps with CRF receptor expression in several areas of the brain, including the pituitary gland, it has been postulated that its function is to modulate the neuroendocrine and transmitter activities of CRF. The presence of CRF-BP in the periphery of higher primates as well indicates that this protein is involved in modulating the action of CRF in the periphery, where CRF has known proinflammatory effects (this is in contrast to the centrally derived anti-inflammatory action of CRF via the release of cortisol). Thus, the CRF-BP may play a pivotal role in the crossover of endocrine, immune, and higher functions in both acute and chronic stress responses.

Distribution

Central Corticotropin Releasing Factor-Binding Protein

From histochemistry and *in situ* hybridization, membrane-bound CRF-BP is observed to be expressed in the rat brain predominantly in the cerebral cortex, including archipaleo- and neocortical fields (see **Figure 1**). It is present also in subcortical limbic structures (amygdala and bed of the stria terminalis) and sensory relays of the auditory, olfactory, vestibular, and trigeminal systems; several raphe nuclei; and some cell groups of the brain stem reticular core. Hypothalamic expression occurs only in the ventral premammillary and dorsomedial nuclei. It is expressed in both neurons and glial astrocytes as well as in pituitary corticotrophs. Its wide distribution does not consistently match the more limited distribution of CRF, and the expression of the CRF 1 receptor (CRF-R1) and CRF 2a receptor (CRF-R2a) in the brain does not coincide completely with either CRF or CRF-BP mRNA.

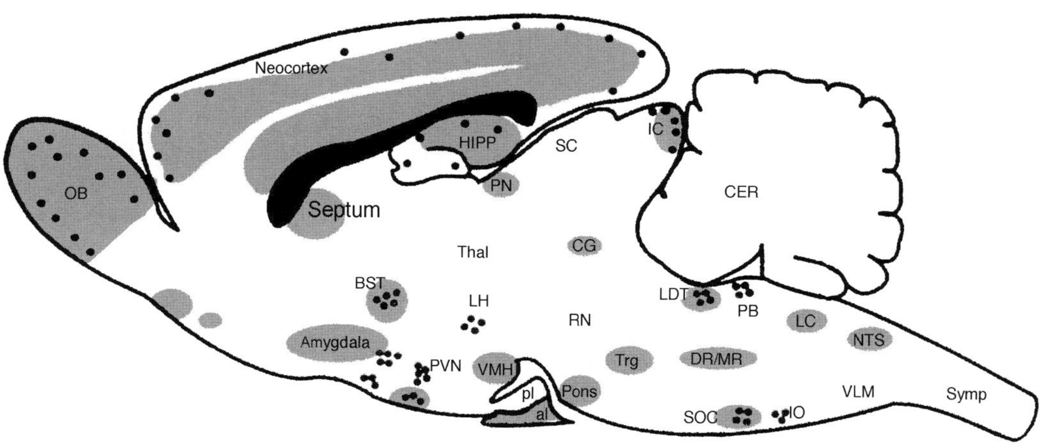

Figure 1 The distribution of the corticotropin releasing factor-binding protein in the rat brain. al, ; BST, bed nucleus of the stria terminalis; CER, cerebellum; CG, central grey; DR/MR, dorsal/medial raphe nucleus; HIPP, hippocampus; IC, inferior colliculus; IO, inferior olive; LC, locus cereolus; LH, lateral hypothalamus; LTD, lateral dorsal tegmental nucleus; NTS, nucleus of the solitary tract; OB, olfactory bulb; PB, parabrachial nucleus; pl, ; PN, perfect nucleus; Pons, pontine nuclei; PVN, paraventricular nucleus; RN, red nucleus; SC, superior colliculus; SOC, superior olivary complex; Symp, sympathetic related areas; Thal, thalamus; Trg, trigeminal; VLM, ventrolateral medulla; VMH, ventromedial hypothalamic nucleus.

Peripheral Corticotropin Releasing Factor-Binding Protein

It is suspected that, in addition to the brain form, only higher primates have circulating CRF-BP. Humans express CRF-BP in the liver, and it circulates in the plasma of both sexes at concentrations, measured by immunoradiometric assay, of between 50 and 100 μg liter^{-1}. The liver is the probable source of CRF-BP in plasma because concentrations are much reduced in patients with chronic liver disease. By contrast, kidney failure is associated with elevated plasma levels, indicating that CRF-BP (not bound to ligand) is normally cleared by the renal route. Plasma levels are remarkably constant from day to day. In molar terms, plasma CRF-BP vastly exceeds CRF and therefore never approaches saturation by ligand except in the last few weeks of pregnancy. The placenta of primates also expresses CRF, and it has been suggested that the binding protein serves in late pregnancy to help prevent the stimulation of the maternal pituitary by releasing large amounts of placental CRF into the circulation. Not only is hormonal activity abolished after binding to CRF-BP, but it is in the bound form that most CRF may be removed from the maternal circulation. The CRF-BP is also measurable in fetal blood and amniotic fluid and may have a further role in the modulation of CRF activity associated with the onset of labor. CRF stimulates the release of prostaglandins from fetal membranes and potentiates their induction of myometrial contractility. These activities are presumed to be modulated by CRF-BP in the fetal and maternal circulation.

In contrast to late pregnancy, when the plasma levels of CRF-BP are lower than normal, in both rheumatoid arthritis and septicemia the concentrations are significantly elevated (by up to 50%). Whereas the lowering of CRF-BP levels in pregnancy seems to be triggered by the secretion of placental CRF, the raised levels in these active immune states appear to be caused by increased secretion by the liver. Presumably this is due to the activation of the acute-phase response elements found in the 5′ flanking region of the CRF-BP gene. It is likely that the bioactivity of circulating CRF is always attended by some degree of modification imposed by the presence of its binding protein.

Properties

Ligand Binding

The affinity of human CRF-BP for human CRF is high ($K_d = 0.1$ nM). That for ovine CRF, which differs at 7 of the 41 amino acid residues, is 200-fold lower; however, CRFs from both species have equal affinities for the pituitary CRF-R1. Sheep CRF-BP has an 86% homology in its amino acid sequence with human and rat CRF-BP, yet it binds human CRF with a 10-fold higher affinity than ovine (CRF $K_d = 0.15$ nM, as opposed to 1.75 nM). Furthermore, a truncated version of human CRF, CRF(6–33), binds CRF-BP with reduced affinity but does not bind to CRF-R1, CRF-R2a, or CRF-R2b. These considerations indicate that the structural determinants required for ligand binding by the binding proteins and CRF-R1 are very different. The recent discovery of urocortin, a new member of the CRF family of peptides, has shown that CRF receptor–binding protein interactions may be further complicated by the participations of additional ligands. Discrepancies in the central distribution of the CRF receptors, CRF-BP, and CRF terminals is evidence that novel ligands for CRF-BP remain to be discovered. The relative affinities for CRF and CRF-like ligands are shown in **Table 1**.

Table 1 Order of ligand affinities for CRF-BP and the CRF receptors

CRF-BP	Urotensin > urocortin ≥ hCRF > sauvagine > oCRF
CRF-R1	Urocortin > hCRF = oCRF = urotensin = sauvagine
CRF-R2a	Urocortin > sauvagine > urotensin > hCRF > oCRF
CRF-R2b	Urocortin > sauvagine = urotensin > hCRF = oCRF

With the exception of the synthetic peptide antagonist α-helical CRF(9–41), CRF-like ligands interacting with CRF-BP *in vitro* induce dimerization. The formation of dimers has not been demonstrated to occur *in vivo*, but CRF administered to humans intravenously is cleared rapidly from the circulation. The possibility therefore exists that CRF-BP not only inactivates CRF but, by dimerizing, targets the ligand for elimination.

Physicochemical Properties

CRF-BP has a molecular mass of 37 kDa, and the mature polypeptide consists of 298 amino acid residues. Its structure is composed predominantly of a β-sheet with little evidence of α-helical folding.

CRF-BP is subject to two posttranslational modifications. These have been investigated using human recombinant CRF-BP. It has a consensus sequence for N-glycosylation of asparagine residue 204. Enzymic removal of the glycosyl moiety does not affect the binding of CRF. A potential phosphorylation site exists at serine residue 233, although phosphorylation has been found by experiment to occur instead at serine 206. On storage, affinity-purified recombinant CRF-BP also undergoes cleavage between amino acid residues 234 and 235, even in the presence of protease inhibitors, yielding fragments of 28 and 9.6 kDa molecular mass. Some degree of protein unfolding has been observed, by tryptophan excitation fluorescence, to occur prior to this *in vitro* cleavage. It is not known whether it is accompanied by dephosphorylation. Protein fragments of similar size have been observed in the synovial fluid of patients suffering from rheumatoid arthritis, although it is not clear whether this is a consequence of the inflammation or if it is involved in the pathogenesis of this condition. Under nonpathological conditions, insulinlike growth factor (IGF)-binding proteins also undergo dephosphorylation and cleavage, both of which are regulated by and affect ligand binding. In the case of IGF-binding protein-3, cleavage is regulated by IGF-1. The cleavage of IGF-binding proteins reduces their affinity for ligand, whereas, after cleavage of CRF-BP, the binding of human CRF to the 28-kDa N-terminal fragment is unimpaired.

Regulation of Gene Expression

The characterization of the upstream region of the CRF-BP gene has revealed acute-phase response elements, one of which (located at −305) is known to bind the transcription factor nuclear factor (NF)-κβ. This factor, which regulates immunoglobulin and interleukin expression, is thought to be important in activating liver-specific genes, such as angiotensin, in response to acute stress, inflammation, and injury. Another element (located at −676) binds interferon (INF)-1, which is known to regulate the interferon gene.

More recent evidence has revealed multiple potential transcription-factor binding sites in the 5′ flanking region of both the rat and human CRF-BP gene. These include a cAMP response element binding protein (CREB)/activating transcription factor (ATF) site, a liver factor (LF)-A1 site, an oxytocin (OTX) site, an activating enhancer binding protein (AP)-2 site, two stimulating protein (Sp)1 sites, and two AP-1 sites, as well as those mentioned previously. The CREB/ATF and AP-2 sites suggest that cAMP may be important for the regulation of the CRF-BP gene, and this is corroborated by the fact that primary rat neuronal or astrocyte cultures, stimulated with forskolin or isobutylmethylxanthine, have been shown to increase levels of CRF-BP mRNA. It has also been demonstrated using the G_s-protein-coupled CRF receptor in the AtT-20 pituitary cell line that CRF-BP gene expression is positively regulated by CRF, suggesting a mechanism for refining the action of CRF on the stress axis at the level of gene expression.

Role of Corticotropin Releasing Hormone-Binding Protein in the Stress Response

The stress axis and the immune system are interrelated, and stress influences the course and pathology of the immune response to infectious disease and to autoimmune stimuli. Intravenous administration of CRF, a key component of the stress axis, elicits visceral and neuroendocrine changes that mimic the body's reaction to stress. Peripheral CRF receptors have been identified on cells of the testes, ovaries, adrenal medulla, heart, uterus, skeletal muscle, lung, kidney, and vasculature. Furthermore, CRF receptors have been reported to exist on circulating lymphocytes and macrophages as well as on mast cells. There is evidence for the hypothesis that peripheral proinflammatory effects of CRF in humans may be modulated by circulating CRF-BP, whereas the central anti-inflammatory response to stress may be modulated by membrane-bound CRF-BP in the brain. It has been shown that CRF is displaced from CRF-BP when human brain tissue is treated with an analog of CRF that displaces bound CRF. *In vivo,* the displacement of CRF from CRF-BP by the central administration of a truncated form of CRF (CRF(6–33)) to rats had an anxiolytic effect. It improved learning and memory presumably by making more free CRF available to interact with CRF receptors. These observations demonstrate that CRF-BP is certainly capable of modulating the actions of CRF.

See Also the Following Articles

Corticotripin-Releasing Factor Receptors.

Further Reading

Behan, D. P., De Souza, E. B., Lowry, P. J., et al. (1995). corticotropin releasing factor (CRF) binding protein: a novel regulator of CRF and related peptides. *Frontiers in Neuroendocrinology* **16**, 362–382.

Behan, D. P., Maciejewski, D., Chalmers, D., et al. (1995). Corticotropin-releasing factor binding protein (CRF-BP) is expressed in neuronal and astrocytic cells. *Brain Research* **689**, 259–264.

Chalmers, D. T., Lovenberg, T. W., Grigoriadis, D. E., et al. (1996). Corticotropin-releasing factor receptors: from molecular biology to drug design. *TiPS* **17**, 166–172.

Kemp, C. F., Woods, R. J. and Lowry, P. J. (1998). The corticotropin releasing factor-binding protein: an act of several parts. *Peptides* **19**(6), 1119–1128.

Linton, E. A., Wolfe, C. D. A., Behan, D. P., et al. (1988). A specific carrier substance for human corticotropin releasing factor in late gestational maternal plasma that could mask its ACTH releasing activity. *Clinical Endocrinology* **28**, 315–324.

Turnbull, A. V. and Rivier, C. (1997). Corticotropin-releasing factor (CRF) and endocrine responses to stress: CRF receptors, binding protein and related peptides. *Proceedings of the Society for Experimental Biology and Medicine* **215**, 1–10.

Anti-CRF

E P Zorrilla, Y Zhao and G F Koob
The Scripps Research Institute, La Jolla, CA, USA

Glossary

Adrenocorticotropic hormone (ACTH, also known as adrenocorticotropin) — A hormone released into systemic circulation by the anterior pituitary as part of the hypothalamic-pituitary-adrenal (HPA)-stress response. ACTH induces the release of glucocorticoids from the adrenal cortex.

cLogP/cLogD — Calculated partition coefficients that express a compound's lipophilicity. A partition coefficient expresses the differential solubility of a compound in two solvents, with the log ratio of the concentrations of a neutral molecule partitioned between two solvents, classically octanol and water, called LogP. LogD expresses the partition coefficient at a specified pH, thereby accounting for charged forms of the molecule at a physiologically relevant pH (most typically that of blood, which has a pH of 7.4). Druglike substances have lipophilicities within a limited range, associated with favorable absorption, bioavailability, hydrophobic drug–receptor interactions, metabolism, and toxicity.

Corticotropin-releasing factor (CRF) — Isolated by Vale and colleagues in 1981, the first hypothalamic ACTH secretagogue to be identified. In addition to its hypothalamic endocrine function, extra-hypothalamic CRF is important in behavioral and autonomic stress responses.

Hypothalamic-pituitary-adrenal (HPA) axis — The neuroendocrine system which, during stress, amplifies a neural signal of physiological or psychological stress into a systemic, endocrine response. Hormones secreted as part of the HPA stress response cascade equip the organism to mobilize and utilize energy resources more effectively and, more generally, respond to the stressor.

Paralog — A gene (or gene product) related to a second gene (or gene product) by descent from an ancestral genetic duplication event. Although descended from common ancestral deoxyribonucleic acid (DNA) sequences, paralogs generally evolve new, distinct functions, though often related to that of the original sequence/gene product.

Pharmacophore — Term coined by Paul Ehrlich in 1909 as "a molecular framework that carries (*phoros*) the essential features responsible for a drug's (pharmacon's) biological activity." Updated by Peter Gund in 1977 to describe "a set of structural features in a molecule that is recognized at a receptor site and is responsible for that molecule's biological activity."

Urocortins — Structurally related mammalian paralogs of corticotropin-releasing factor (CRF). Though these three known peptides (urocortins (Ucn) 1, 2, and 3) share sequence identity with CRF, each CRF family peptide is coded by a different gene and has different pharmacological properties, tissue distributions, and regulatory pathways, leading to their diverse roles in stress responses to homeostatic threats. Urocortins, unlike CRF, exhibit high affinity for CRF_2 receptors.

Corticotropin-releasing factor (CRF) receptor antagonists have been sought since the isolation of the eponymous stress-related adrenocorticotropin-releasing peptide in 1981 by Vale and colleagues. Discovered for its hypophysiotropic function in the hypothalamic-pituitary-adrenal (HPA) axis, CRF and, later, urocortins (Ucn)-1, -2, and-3, paralogs of CRF, were subsequently found also to play roles in diverse homeostatic stress responses, via extra-hypothalamic brain sites and peripheral tissues. CRF receptor antagonists have potential therapeutic applications in cases where these responses are inappropriate in magnitude, timing, or context.

Pharmacology of Corticotropin-Releasing Factor/Urocortin Receptor Systems

CRF-related peptides interact with two known mammalian CRF receptor subtypes, CRF_1 and CRF_2, both belonging to the class B1 (secretinlike) subfamily of G-protein-coupled receptors for polypeptide hormones. The CRF_1 receptor has been cloned in humans, mice, rats, and tree shrews, among other species, and exists in multiple isoforms (e.g., CRF_{1a}–CRF_{1h}), with the best known and functional isoform being the $CRF_{1(a)}$ subtype. The CRF_2 receptor has three known functional membrane-associated subtypes in humans, $CRF_{2(a)}$, $CRF_{2(b)}$, and $CRF_{2(c)}$, as well as a ligand-sequestering, soluble $CRF_{2(a)}$ isoform discovered in mice. CRF_2 and CRF_1 receptors have ~70% sequence identity. Whereas CRF has high, preferential affinity for CRF_1 versus CRF_2 receptors, Ucn 1 is a high-affinity agonist at both receptors. The type 2 Ucns, Ucn 2 and Ucn 3 are more selective for membrane CRF_2 receptors. Because of this pharmacological profile, references to antiCRF treatments most often refer to functional or competitive antagonists of CRF_1 receptor-mediated effects, whereas antitype 2 Ucn treatments might target CRF_2 receptors. The biological actions of CRF, Ucn-1, and Ucn-2 in rodents also are modulated by a CRF-binding protein (CRF-BP), a 37-kD secreted glycoprotein that binds and putatively immunosequesters CRF and Ucn-1 with equal or greater affinity than do CRF receptors. However, structural requirements for binding to CRF receptors and the CRF-BP differ, so many (if not most) CRF receptor antagonists do not interact with the CRF-BP.

Nonneuroendocrine Distribution of CRF_1 Receptors

CRF_1 receptors mediate not only the HPA-axis neuroendocrine response to stress, but also other aspects of organism stress responses. In brain, the distribution of CRF_1 receptors is highly conserved in stress-responsive brain regions, including neocortex, the extended central amygdala, medial septum, hippocampus, hypothalamus, thalamus, cerebellum, and autonomic midbrain and hindbrain nuclei. This receptor distribution, concordant with that of its natural ligands (CRF, Ucn-1), is consistent with the proposed role for extrahypothalamic CRF_1 receptors in behavioral and autonomic stress responses. Accordingly, excessive CRF_1 signaling putatively has a pathophysiologic role in several stress-related disorders, including anxiety and depressive disorders, substance dependence, and irritable bowel syndrome. Hereafter, the identity and potential therapeutic indications for CRF_1 receptor antagonists are summarized.

Selected Corticotropin-Releasing Factor Receptor Antagonists

Nonselective Peptide Corticotropin-Releasing Factor Receptor Antagonists

N-terminally truncated and substituted analogs of CRF can act as competitive partial agonists or full receptor antagonists (**Table 1**). Examples of these, in chronological order of discovery, include the partial agonist [Met^{18},Lys^{23},$Glu^{27,29,40}$,$Ala^{32,41}$,$Leu^{33,36,38}$] r/h$CRF_{9\text{-}41}$ (also known as α-helical $CRF_{9\text{-}41}$); and the full receptor antagonists [D-Phe^{12},$Nle^{21,38}$ Cα$MeLeu^{37}$] r/h$CRF_{12\text{-}41}$ (also known as D-Phe-$CRF_{12\text{-}41}$); cyclo(30-33)[D-Phe^{12},$Nle^{21,38}$,Glu^{30},Lys^{33}] r/h$CRF_{12\text{-}41}$ (also known as astressin); and cyclo (30-33)[D-Phe^{12},Nle^{21},Cα$MeLeu^{27}$,Glu^{30},Lys^{33}, Nle^{38}, Cα$MeLeu^{40}$]Ac-r/h$CRF_{9\text{-}41}$ (also known as astressin-B). These peptide ligands have roughly the same order of binding and antagonist potency at CRF_1 versus CRF_2 receptors and do not cross the blood–brain barrier. Thus, they are subtype nonselective, peripherally acting CRF receptor antagonists.

Subtype-Selective Peptide Corticotropin-Releasing Factor Receptor Antagonists

Antisauvagine-30 was reported as the first preferential CRF_2 antagonist. Following its development, several subsequent series of CRF_2 receptor peptide antagonists have been identified, each of which is more potent, selective, and enzymatic degradation resistant than antisavuagine-30. These new antagonists included the antisauvagine-30 analogs K31440 and K41498; [Tyr^{11}, His^{12}, Nle^{17}]$SVG_{10\text{-}40}$, which has 2360-fold selectivity and subnanomolar affinity for the CRF_2 receptor; and astressin$_2$-B, a long-acting, potent, and selective CRF_2 antagonist (**Table 1**).

Table 1 Alphabetical selection of peptide CRF receptor antagonists

Familiar name	*CRF receptor binding affinity* (IC_{50} *or* K_i)		*Chemical structure*
	CRF_1 (nM)	*CRF_2 (nM)*	
α-helical $CRF_{9\text{-}41}$	19	1.1	[Met^{18},Lys^{23},$Glu^{27,29,40}$,$Ala^{32,41}$,$Leu^{33,36,38}$]-rat/human $CRF_{9\text{-}41}$
Antisauvagine-30	400	1.1	[D-Phe^{11},His^{12}]-sauvagine$_{11\text{-}40}$
Astressin	13.2	1.5	Cyclo(30-33)[D-Phe^{12},$Nle^{21,38}$,Glu^{30},Lys^{33}]-rat/human $CRF_{12\text{-}41}$
Astressin-B	High affinity	Moderate affinity	Cyclo(30-33)[D-Phe^{12},Nle^{21},Cα$MeLeu^{27}$,Glu^{30},Lys^{33},Nle^{38}, Cα$MeLeu^{40}$]acetyl-rat/human $CRF_{9\text{-}41}$
Astressin$_2$-B	>500	1.3	Cyclo(31-34)[D-Phe^{11},His^{12},Cα$MeLeu^{13,39}$,Nle^{17},Glu^{31}, Lys^{34}]acetyl-sauvagine$_{8\text{-}40}$
D-Phe-$CRF_{12\text{-}41}$	19.2	4.4	[D-Phe^{12},$Nle^{21,38}$,Cα$MeLeu^{37}$]-rat/human $CRF_{12\text{-}41}$
K31440	288	1.5	Acetyl-[D-Tyr^{11},His^{12},Nle^{17}]-sauvagine$_{11\text{-}40}$
K41498	425	0.7	[D-Phe^{11},His^{12},Nle^{17}]-sauvagine$_{11\text{-}40}$

CRF, corticotropin-releasing factor; IC_{50}, concentration required for 50% inhibition.
Data from Zorrilla et al., 2003 (with permission of Elsevier).

Although these antagonists do not oppose the classic stress-related effects of CRF reviewed above, they do reverse stress-induced CRF_2-mediated endpoints, some of which are recruited by Ucns and some by CRF. Such endpoints include, for example, stress-induced gastric stasis and, possibly a component of stress-induced anorexia.

Selective CRF_1 peptide antagonists also appear to have been identified recently in the course of seeking minimal peptide fragments with CRF receptor antagonist activity. For example, Yamada and colleagues followed upon a patent application (W01/29086) of the Solvay pharmaceutical group which described a peptide comprising the 12 *C*-terminal residues of astressin as a potent antagonist of CRF receptors. Through amino acid substitution, of Nle38 with the bulkier, lipophilic cyclohexylalanine residue and of Ala31 with an unnatural residue (D-Ala), they identified a metabolically stable, high-affinity ($K_i \sim 3$ nM) CRF_1 antagonist that potently (0.1 mg kg^{-1} intravenous; IV) reduced adrenocorticotropic hormone (ACTH) secretion in a rat model of sepsis. This peptide is likely a selective CRF_1 antagonist because the Solvay group concurrently published their findings on the patented 12-residue *N*-terminal truncated astressin derivative on which Yamada and colleagues began their investigation. The disclosed fragment not only retained CRF_1 affinity, but was inactive at the $CRF_{2(a)}$ receptor. Thus, it appears that lactam bridge-constrained *N*-terminally truncated astressin derivatives of 12–15 residue length may be selective CRF_1 receptor peptide antagonists. Such compounds could be useful for the treatment of pathologies that involve only peripheral CRF_1 hyperactivation.

Small-Molecule CRF_1 Receptor Antagonists

Pharmacophore and selectivity Small molecules that penetrate the blood–brain barrier with high and selective CRF_1 (versus CRF_2) affinity also have been identified (**Table 2**) and reviewed in considerable detail recently. With few exceptions, every known CRF_1 antagonist follows a common pharmacophore. Prototypical compounds (see **Figure 1**) share one or two lipophilic top/side units, a central mono-, bi- or tricyclic ring core, and a conformation-stabilizing di- or trisubstituted aromatic bottom group. Each ring core contains a putative proton-accepting ring nitrogen, and the hydrogen-bond accepting core is thought to interact with histidine-199 of the CRF_1 receptor, a polar amino acid in the third transmembrane domain that is not shared in the CRF_2 receptor or CRF-BP sequences. Therefore, CRF_1 antagonists with this pharmacophore are highly selective (CRF_1 versus CRF_2 and CRF-BP). Most known small-molecule CRF_1 receptor antagonists also show at least 1000-fold binding selectivity relative to other receptors, ion channels, and reuptake sites screened to date. However, this is not universal as one exception, R278995 (also known as CRA0450), actually exhibits 50-fold greater affinity for the σ_1 receptor than for the CRF_1 receptor.

The binding site of the classic pharmacophore also differs from the agonist binding site, whose confirmation is allosterically modified by CRF_1 antagonists, making these small molecules noncompetitive antagonists of peptide ligands. Exceptions to the pharmacophore include oxo-7*H*-benzo[*e*]perimidine-4-carboxylic acid derivatives, which are subtype nonselective CRF receptor antagonists discovered by Alanex; CC 2064460, a moderately potent arylamidrazone CRF_1 antagonist that lacks a central ring core with the customary hydrogen-bond accepting nitrogen; and stereospecific *N*-phenylphenylglycines, which also lack a ring core but were identified through computational screening based on a classic pharmacophore training set.

Lipophilicity An obstacle in the clinical use of CRF_1 antagonists is that most preclinical structures have been excessively lipophilic with poor water solubility, bioavailability, and pharmacokinetic properties. For example, the rank-ordered oral bioavailabilities of antalarmin (19%) < CP-154,526 (27%) < DMP904 (33%) < DMP696 (37–50%) follow the inverse rank of their cLogDs and cLogPs. Accordingly, the oral dose (30 mg kg^{-1}) of CP-154,526 needed to achieve the anxiolytic-like threshold of brain CRF_1 receptor occupancy in rats (~50–60% of receptors bound) is one order higher than that required by the similar affinity, but much less hydrophobic, compounds DMP696 (1–3 mg kg^{-1}), R121919 (2.5 mg kg^{-1}), and SSR125543A (6.5 mg kg^{-1}). Because of their high lipophilicity, many CRF_1 receptor antagonists have very high estimated bioconcentration factors at physiological pHs, a potential index of toxicity liability. Most early CRF_1 antagonists also failed Lipinski's "rule of 5" criteria for drug candidates, derived from a review of physiochemical properties of compounds within the United States Adopted Names database, due to excessive lipophilicity (cLogP > 5). Due to unfavorable pharmacokinetics, this degree of lipophilicity is rare for effective central nervous system (CNS)-acting agents. Of more than 100 drugs marketed as of 1992 for CNS indications, not one had a logD greater than 4; most (~85%) had a logD of 0–3. Much preclinical discovery since 2002 has therefore focused on identifying less hydrophobic CRF_1 antagonists, with recent success. Early studies indicate that CRF_1 antagonists as a class do not share some of the drawbacks of

Table 2 Alphabetical selection of small-molecule CRF_1 receptor antagonists

Familiar name	*CAS registry number*[c]	*CRF receptor binding affinity*		*Chemical structure*
		CRF_1 (nM)	*CRF_2 (nM)*	
Antalarmin	157284-96-3	1	>10 000	*N*-butyl-*N*-ethyl[2,5,6-trimethyl-7-(2,4,6-trimethylphenyl)-7*H*-pyrrolo[2,3-*d*]pyrimidin-4-yl]-amine
CC 2064460	438552-89-7	35	ND	Propanimidic acid, *N*-(3-ethynylphenyl)-2-oxo-, 2-(2-chlorophenyl)hydrazide (9Cl)
CP-154,526	157286-86-7	2.7	>10 000	*N*-butyl-*N*-[2,5-dimethyl-7-(2,4,6-trimethylphenyl)-7*H*-pyrrolo [2,3-*d*]pyrimidin-4-yl]-*N*-ethylamine
CRA0165	402751-10-4	10	>10 000	4-[5,6-dihydro-3-(2-methylphenyl)-1(2*H*)-pyridinyl]-*N*-ethyl-6-methyl-*N*-[4-(1-methylethyl)-2-(methylthio)phenyl]
CRA1000	226948-11-4	16-21	>10 000	*N*-ethyl-4-[4-(3-fluorophenyl)-1,2,3,6-tetrahydro-1-pyridinyl]-*N*-[4-isopropyl-2-(methylsulfanyl) phenyl]-6-methylpyrimidin-2-amine
CRA1001	229346-94-5	19-22	>10 000	2-[*N*-(2-bromo-4-isopropylphenyl)-*N*-ethylamino]-4-[4-(3-fluorophenyl)-1,2,3,6-tetrahydropyridin-1-yl]-6-methylpyrimidine
DMP695	354994-31-3	3.3	>10 000	*N*-(2-chloro-4,6-dimethylphenyl)-1-1-methoxymethyl-(2-methoxyethyl]-6-methyl-1*H*-1, 2,3-triazolo[4,5-*c*]pyridin-4-amine mesylate
DMP696	202578-52-7	1.7	>10 000	4-(1,3-dimethoxyprop-2-ylamine)-2,7-dimethyl-8-(2,4-dichlorophenyl)-pyrazolo[1,5-*a*]-1,3,5-triazine
DMP904	202579-74-6	1.0	>10 000	*N*-(1-ethylpropyl)-3-(4-methoxy-2-methylphenyl)-2,5-dimethyl-pyrazolo[1,5-*a*]pyrimidin-7-amine
LWH63	276890-57-4	0.7	>10 000	4-ethyl([2,5,6-trimethyl-7-(2,4,6-trimethylphenyl)-7*H*-pyrrolo[2,3-*d*] pyrimidin-4-yl]amino)-1-butanol
MJL-1-109-2	596107-16-3	1.9	ND	pyrazolo[1,5-*a*]-1,3,5-triazin-4-amine, 8-[4-(bromo)-2-chlorophenyl]-*N,N*-bis(2-methoxyethyl)-2,7-dimethyl-(9Cl)
NBI-27914	184241-44-9	2	>10 000	5-chloro-*N*-(cyclopropylmethyl)-2-methyl-*N*-propyl-*N'*-(2,4,6-trichlorophenyl)-4,6-pyrimidinediamine
NBI-30545	195054-99-0	2.8	ND	pyrazolo[1,5-*a*]pyrimidin-7-amine, 3-(2,4-dimethoxyphenyl)-*N*-(2-methoxyethyl)-2,5-dimethyl-*N*-propyl-(9Cl)
NBI-35965	354999-74-9	4	>10 000	ND
R121919[a]	195055-03-9	3.5	>10 000	pyrazolo[1,5-*a*]pyrimidin-7-amine, 3-[6-(dimethylamino)-4-methyl-3-pyridinyl]-2,5-dimethyl-*N,N*-dipropyl-(9Cl)
R121920	195055-01-7	4	ND	3-[6-(dimethylamino)-3-pyridinyl]-2,5-dimethyl-*N,N*-dipropyl-pyrazolo[1,5-*a*]pyrimidin-7-amine
R278995[b]	N/A	54	>10 000	1-[8-(2,4-dichlorophenyl)-2-methylquinolin-4-yl]-1,2,3,6-tetrahydropyridine-4-carboxamide benzenesulfonate
SC241	392336-72-0	5	>10 000	3-[(2-bromo-4-isopropylphenyl)-5-methyl-3*H*-[1,2,3]triazolo[4,5-*d*] pyrimidin-7-yl]-bis-(2-methoxy-ethyl)-amine
SN003	197801-88-0	6.8	ND	(+/−)-*N*-[2-methyl-4-methoxyphenyl]-1-(1-(methoxymethyl) propyl)-6-methyl-1*H*-1,2,3-triazolo[4,5-*c*]pyridin-4-amine
SSR125543A	321839-75-2	2	>10 000	4-(2-chloro-4-methoxy-5-methylphenyl)-*N*-[2-cyclopropyl-1(*S*)-(3-fluoro-4-methylphenyl)ethyl]-5-methyl-*N*-(2-propynyl)thiazol-2-amine hydrochloride

[a]Also known as NBI-30775;
[b]Also known as CRA0450;
[c]CAS, Chemical Abstract Service, a database of chemical substance information; ND, not determined.
Table modified from Zorrilla et al., 2003 (with permission from Elsevier) and Zorrilla & Koob, 2004 (with permission from *Expert opinion on Investigational Drugs*).

benzodiazepines, such as tolerance, sedative-hypnotic, or amnestic effects, or abuse liability. They also do not lead to HPA-axis insufficiency at preclinically therapeutic doses, but isolated reports of liver enzyme elevations led to the discontinued clinical development of R121919, which had shown dose-related efficacy in an open-label Phase IIa clinical trial of patients with major depression.

Therapeutic Potential of CRF_1 Antagonists

Endocrine Disorders

CRF released into the portal blood from the median eminence stimulates ACTH release from the anterior pituitary into systemic circulation, which elicits the synthesis and release of glucocorticoids from the

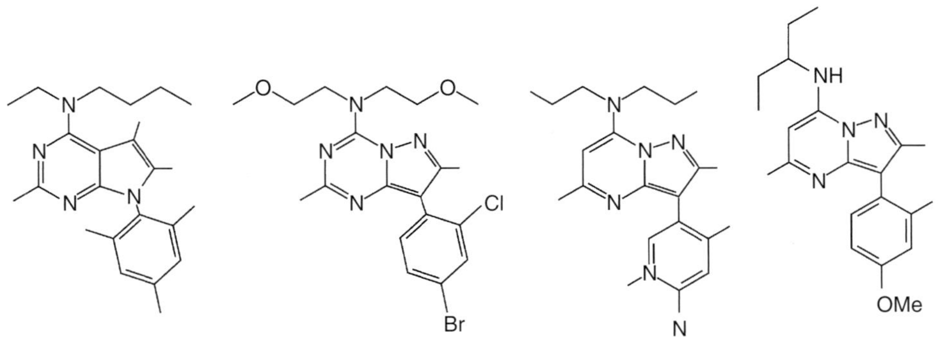

Figure 1 Representative selection of heterocyclic, small-molecule selective CRF_1 receptor antagonists that conform to the classic CRF_1 antagonist pharmacophore. See text for description of pharmacophore structural features and **Table 2** for chemical structure, CAS registry numbers, and binding properties of each compound.

adrenal cortex – the classic HPA-axis stress response. HPA-axis dysregulation can result in endocrine disorders of hypercortisolemia, including Cushing's syndrome. Most cases of Cushing's syndrome are iatrogenic (e.g., from synthetic glucocorticoids), or due to ACTH- or cortisol-hypersecreting tumors and hyperplasias. However, central hypersecretion of neuroendocrine CRF leads to a Cushingoid state, exemplified in CRF-overexpressing transgenic mice. Likewise, clinical syndromes with hypothalamic CRF-driven chronic hypercortisolemia, including severe alcohol dependence, visceral obesity, melancholic major depression, and anorexia nervosa, are marked by Cushingoid somatic and endocrine features that remit when cortisol levels normalize. Peripherally acting, long-acting peptide CRF receptor antagonists, such as astressin-B, have been especially effective in opposing CRF-evoked ACTH release and therefore may have a therapeutic role in managing Cushingoid consequences of these disorders, if not also the disorders themselves.

Sympathoadrenomedullary Response

Intracerebroventricular (ICV) CRF administration evokes the sympathoadrenomedullary stress response in animal models, as it elevates blood pressure and heart rate; increases circulating levels of catecholamines, glucagon, and glucose; increases body temperature; and raises energy expenditure. Conversely, in animal models, CRF receptor antagonists, in particular those for the CRF_1 subtype such as CP-154,526, attenuate both CRF- and stress-induced tachycardia, hypertension, and hyperthermia.

Central Nervous System-Related Disorders

Anxiety disorders Consistent with autonomic findings, clinical data suggest that brain CRF is hypersecreted in some pathological anxiety conditions. Cerebrospinal (CSF) CRF levels, which mostly reflect nonneuroendocrine brain CRF secretion, are high in some patients with posttraumatic stress disorder, underweight patients with anorexia nervosa, ethanol withdrawn alcoholics, and some adults with obsessive–compulsive disorder, all conditions marked by high anxiety levels. Conversely, effective treatment of juveniles with obsessive–compulsive disorder with the tricyclic antidepressant clomipramine decreased their CSF CRF levels.

The anxiolytic-like actions of nonselective peptide and small-molecule CRF_1 receptor antagonists, CRF_1 knockout, and CRF_1 antisense knockdown all collectively emphasize an endogenous role for extrahypothalamic, limbic CRF_1 neurotransmission in hyperarousal and anxiety. For example, ICV α-helical CRF_{9-41}, a nonselective CRF receptor partial agonist, reversed the ability of restraint, foot shock, or social isolation to wake rodents prematurely from pentobarbital-induced sleep, and small-molecule CRF_1 antagonists like CRA1000 and R121919 also mitigate insomnia-like effects of stress on sleep. Stress or CRF administration also increase locomotor activity in familiar environments, a sign of behavioral hyperarousal that is blocked by pretreatment with CRF_1 receptor antagonists and absent in CRF_1-deficient mice.

Nonselective or CRF_1 receptor antagonists also reduce the avoidance of unfamiliar, exposed areas in the open field, elevated plus maze, defensive withdrawal, or light/dark box tests by rodents that were stressed by restraint, swim stress, social defeat, conspecific stress, ethanol withdrawal, conditioned effects of psychostimulants, or novelty (but these actions are not observed in unstressed rodents). Knockout of CRF_1, but not CRF_2, receptors in mice or antisense knockdown of CRF_1, but not CRF_2, receptors in rats likewise produces anxiolytic-like effects in exploration-based models of anxiety. Anxiolytic-like actions of nonselective or CRF_1 receptor antagonists are not limited to exploration-based models as they also were seen in rodent models of foot shock or conditioned freezing, fear- or light-potentiated acoustic startle, shock-induced defensive burying, social interaction, neonatal isolation-induced pup ultrasonic vocalization, and in unconditioned conflict models, such as punished drinking and punished crossing. Peptide nonselective or nonpeptide CRF_1 antagonists also reduced stress-induced anorexia in rats and unconditioned submissive/defensive behaviors in social defeat models. In nonhuman primates, CRF_1 exhibited oral anxiolytic-like action as well. For example, in rhesus monkeys, DMP904 (effective dose inducing 50% reduction (ED_{50}) 21 mg kg^{-1}) reduced stereotypical mouthing of rhesus monkeys in a human intruder test, and antalarmin (20 mg kg^{-1}) attenuated behavioral signs of anxiety, normalized exploratory, and sexual activity, and decreased HPA-axis and sympathoadrenomedullary hormone responses. Finally, depressed patients who participated in the open-label clinical trial with R121919 reported a reduction of anxious symptoms (and improved sleep quality) in relation to escalating doses of the small-molecule CRF_1 antagonist.

Anxiolytic-like efficacy of antagonists is evident once they occupy 50–60% of brain CRF_1 receptors in rats, with further efficacy seen with incremental brain receptor occupancy. Acute anxiolytic-like efficacy of CRF_1 antagonists does not depend on actions at the HPA axis, as at least six compounds (antalarmin, CP-154,526, CRA1000, CRA1001, DMP904, and R121919) reduced anxiety-like behavior at doses that did not reduce ACTH or corticosterone responses to stress. The importance of central as opposed to pituitary CRF_1 receptors in anxiety-like behavior is highlighted by the finding that limbic-selective deletion of CRF_1 receptors in mice is sufficient to produce anxiolytic-like effects. Anxiogenic-like CRF signaling may be mediated by mitogen-activated protein (MAP) kinase extracellular signal-related kinase 1/2 (ERK1/2) pathways in the forebrain. Consistent with these findings and sites of anxiogenic-like action by exogenous CRF, the locus coeruleus, bed nucleus of the stria terminalis, and amygdala are sensitive to site-specific anxiolytic-like CRF_1 antagonist administration.

Depression Evidence for increased extrahypothalamic CRF activity, perhaps due to tonic, stimulatory glucocorticoid action on CRF synthesis, has also been observed in affective disorders and may contribute to depressive symptomatology. Patients with major depression exhibit signs of chronic hypothalamically driven HPA-axis hyperactivation, including hypercortisolemia, blunted ACTH responses to CRF infusion, nonsuppression in the dexamethasone suppression test, and increased numbers of paraventricular nucleus (PUN) CRF neurons postmortem. The resulting excess glucocorticoid levels exert positive feedback on extrahypothalamic CRF systems in the amygdala and bed nucleus of the stria terminalis, and thereby may lead to behavioral symptoms of depression. Accordingly, abnormally high CSF CRF levels are seen in severely depressed patients, who frequently exhibit comorbid pathological anxiety. Although CSF CRF concentrations are not elevated in patients with bipolar disorder, chronic administration of effective pharmacotherapies for bipolar disorder decreases amygdala CRF_1 receptor synthesis or expression in rats. Finally, very high CSF CRF levels and downregulated cortical CRF receptor binding and mRNA expression also were seen postmortem in patients who committed suicide.

Consistent with the therapeutic potential of CRF_1 antagonists for major depression, subchronic dosing with DMP696 or R121919 reduced mouse forced-swim immobility, and acute antalarmin reduced forced-swim immobility in CRF_2 knockout mice, a genetic model of high-stress responsiveness. Also, antalarmin, SSR125543A, or CRA1000 reduced forced-swim immobility in outbred rats, and chronic SSR125543A treatment increased swimming in Flinders Sensitive Line rats, a putative genetic model of depression. Findings are somewhat equivocal, however, as antalarmin, CP-154,526, DMP904, R121919, and DMP696 had no reliable effect on forced-swim immobility in normal mice, with negative findings seen after acute, subchronic, and even chronic (16 days) dosing, unlike positive antidepressant controls. Each of these antagonists, as well as R278995, also lacked activity in the tail suspension test with acute dosing.

CP-154,526, CRA1000, and R2789995 also can reduce the acquisition of learned helplessness. However, despite an initial report with CP-154,526 that showed reversal of shuttlebox escape deficits, subsequent studies with CP-154,526, DMP904, DMP696, or CRA1000 have not found that CRF_1 antagonists could acutely reverse learned helplessness in rats, once established.

R278995 reduced hyperemotionality of olfactory bulbectomized rats, regarded by some as a depression model, though it lacked antidepressant-like activity in the rat differential-reinforcement-of-low-rate 72-sec model. Chronic antalarmin or SSR125543A treatment also improved physical coat appearance in a mouse model of chronic mild stress, a fluoxetine-like effect that correlated with reversal of stress-induced suppression of hippocampal neurogenesis. The chronicity of treatment may be relevant for antidepressant CRF_1 action as repeated administration of CRF_1 antagonists has somewhat more often resulted in antidepressant-like activity. Consistent with this perspective, depressed patients treated with escalating doses of R121919 in an open-label study reported reduced depressive symptoms and showed normalization of sleep electroencephalography. Clinically, CRF_1 gene haplotypes also predict differential treatment response to fluoxetine in anxious, depressed Mexican-American people.

As was observed for anxiolytic-like activity, antidepressant-like activity appears to be dissociable from acute actions on HPA-axis activity, supporting the role of extrahypothalamic CRF in proximately mediating depressive-like symptoms. For example, acute R121919, CP-154,526, and R278995 failed to reduce rat forced-swim immobility, despite the fact that R121919 could reduce concurrent swim-induced ACTH secretion. Conversely, LWH234 (a different CRF_1 antagonist) did reduce forced-swim immobility, but at a dose which had no effect on swim-induced ACTH secretion.

Gastrointestinal Disorders

CRF_1-receptor antagonists also might be promising tools for the treatment of functional gastrointestinal disorders, including irritable bowel syndrome. In animal models, diverse stressors delay gastric emptying and stimulate colonic motor function, and endogenous CRF, through both brain and peripheral receptors, mediates these stress-induced changes in gastrocolonic motility. The colonic-stimulating effects of stress are observed as colonic hypermotility, decreased transit time, defecation, and watery diarrhea and are mimicked by ICV administration of CRF or Ucn-1 in rats, mice, and Mongolian gerbils. Central or peripheral administration of selective CRF_1, but not CRF_2, agonists stimulates colonic motility, and selective CRF_1, but not CRF_2, antagonists attenuate stress- or CRF/Ucn-1-induced stimulation of colonic motor function. For example, selective CRF_1 receptor antagonists such as CP154,526, CRA1000, NBI-35965, NBI-27914, and antalarmin, injected peripherally or ICV, blunted the acceleration of colonic transit induced by restraint; the defecation induced by water avoidance stress, restraint, or social stress; and the diarrhea induced by morphine withdrawal. Likely substrates for CRF_1-mediated stimulation of colonic motor function include, centrally, the PVN and locus coeruleus/Barrington nuclei that activate sacral parasympathetic nervous system activity, and, peripherally, the colonic myenteric nervous system.

CRF_1 receptor signaling is also involved in visceral hyperalgesia. For example, both stress and ICV CRF induce visceral hyperalgesia to colorectal distention in rats, and these actions of stress can be blocked by ICV α-helical $CRF_{9\text{-}41}$. More recently, systemic administration of NBI-35965, a nonpeptide CRF_1 antagonist, was found to block water avoidance stress-induced hyperalgesia to colorectal distention in adult offspring of maternal separation. Antalarmin (by intraperitoneal (IP) route) likewise reduced ICV CRF-induced hypersensitivity to colorectal distention and also blunted the visceral hyperalgesia of high-anxiety strain rats. Finally, α-helical $CRF_{9\text{-}41}$ attenuated electrical stimulation-induced visceral symptoms in patients with diarrhea-predominant irritable bowel syndrome.

CRF_1 receptors are involved in the early phase of postoperative gastric ileus. Peripheral CP-154,526 administration prevented abdominal surgery-induced slowing of gastric emptying. Similarly, CRF_1 knockout mice did not show postoperative gastric ileus, whereas abdominal surgery inhibited postoperative gastric emptying by 75% in wild-type mice.

CRF_2 receptor antagonists might be effective treatments to relieve stress-induced gastric stasis and perhaps other adverse gastroparesis. Stress or central infusion of CRF receptor agonists, through vagal effectors, delay gastric emptying, reduce antral gastric motility, inhibit high-amplitude gastric contractions, and shift duodenal activity from fasted to fed motor patterns, actions reversed by central $astressin_2$-B (CRF_2), but not NBI-27914 treatment. Complementing the central CRF_2 pathway for slowing gastric emptying, peripheral (by IV or IP route) injection of high-affinity and/or selective CRF_2 agonists (Ucn-1, Ucn-2, or Ucn-3) also delays gastric emptying more potently than CRF. Conversely, systemic pretreatment with CRF_2 (e.g., antisauvagine-30 or $astressin_2$-B), but not CRF_1 (e.g., CP-154,526, DMP904, and NBI-27914) antagonists blocks the gastromotor inhibiting effects of Ucns as well as restraint stress-induced gastric stasis. Thus, stress releases CRF like peptides that inhibit gastric motility through the brain–gastrointestinal tract CRF_2 receptor systems. Likely substrates include the PVN and dorsal vagal complex in the brain, and myenteric fibers of the enteric nervous system in the periphery.

Urologic Disorders

Epidemiologic and clinical findings indicate comorbidity of anxiety with several urologic problems, including overactive bladder, interstitial cystitis, and incontinence. In feline models of interstitial cystitis, CSF CRF levels are increased and subjects show exaggerated acoustic startle reactivity. This is somewhat expected because of the overlap in neuroanatomical substrates of CRF-related emotional responding and of micturition and pelvic viscerosensation. Shared neural substrates include Barrington's nucleus, amygdala, hippocampus, and prefrontal cortex. CRF also appears to play a role in the control of micturition and bladder sensation via the spinal cord. In particular, CRF immunoreactivity is present in intermediolateral cell column, suggesting a role in urinary motor function, and in sensory processing areas, including the dorsal horn, medial and lateral collateral pathways, dorsal intermediate gray, and laminas VII and X. Early studies indicate that CRF dose-dependently promotes micturition in awake animals, whereas CRF receptor antagonists have an inhibitory effect. Furthermore, CRF receptor antagonists have reversed bladder overactivity in animal models.

Pregnancy and Parturition

Changes in circulating CRF, Ucn-1, and CRF-BP levels help coordinate the events of pregnancy and parturition. CRF is produced in the hypothalamus and placenta during pregnancy, and placental CRF accesses both maternal and fetal circulations. During pregnancy, placental CRF secretion increases exponentially, peaking at birth. Accordingly, maternal plasma CRF levels increase from the second trimester exponentially towards term, rise dramatically during labor, and fall quickly after birth. Unbound (free) CRF levels are regulated by CRF-BP levels, which normally decrease near term (36 weeks' gestation), resulting in a dramatic increase in bioavailable maternal plasma CRF. Women with preterm labor show high CRF and low CRF-BP levels, suggesting an involvement of high bioavailability of maternal CRF in the onset of parturition. Consistent with this perspective, maternal free CRF measurement predicts outcome of certain at-risk pregnancies, and the regulation of the length of gestation by CRF has been termed a placental clock. For example, the highest levels of maternal CRF at 20 weeks' gestation are observed in high-risk populations that ultimately deliver before 34 weeks. A prospective study of 232 pregnancies likewise observed that elevated maternal plasma CRF levels at 33 weeks' gestation carried a 3.3-fold greater risk of preterm birth, whereas women who delivered postterm had lower circulating CRF levels at that time than mothers who delivered at term. Similarly, a prospective study of 282 pregnancies found that maternal plasma CRF levels at 18–20 weeks and 28–30 weeks' gestation were higher in women who ultimately delivered preterm. Thus, CRF_1 antagonists might delay premature birth. Supporting this hypothesis, CRF_1 receptor antagonists delayed the onset of labor in sheep model studies.

Inflammatory States

CRF is a proinflammatory peptide via direct autocrine/paracrine actions in immune and immune lineage cells. In brain, CRF and/or its receptors are localized in microglia, astrocytes, and infiltrating monocytes/macrophages. In the periphery, CRF receptors are found in macrophages, lymphocytes, and mast cells. Immune CRF and Ucn-1 are expressed by human cord blood-derived cultured mast cells by the 10th gestational week and also are produced by human leukemic mast cell lines. In addition to mast cells, Ucn-1 also is seen in lymphocytes, macrophages, and fibroblasts, a cellular distribution that underlies moderate overall expression in thymus, spleen, and skin.

Supporting proinflammatory properties for CRF and Ucn-1, both peptides provoke resting monocytes to secrete interleukin (IL)-1β and IL-6 *in vitro* via a CRF_1-mediated mechanism, and CRF triggers lymphocyte proliferation. CRF activates microglia, stimulates astrocytosis and monocyte migration, and augments macrophage production of free radicals and arachidonic acid. CRF receptor ligands also activate mast cells *in vitro*, an action that can be blocked by the CRF_1 antagonist antalarmin, but not the CRF_2 antagonist astressin$_2$-B and which leads to release of vascular endothelial growth factor, which is elevated in arthritis, psoriasis, and other chronic inflammatory conditions. The findings suggest a potential anti-inflammatory role for CRF_1 antagonists.

Inflammatory disorders Correspondingly, CRF immunoreactivity is elevated in local immune accessory cells in experimental models of arthritis and uveitis, and increased CRF or Ucn-1 immunoreactivity also are evident in human inflamed tissue, including joints of patients with rheumatoid arthritis, lamina propria macrophages of patients with ulcerative colitis, reproductive tissue of patients with endometriosis, and thyroid glands of patients with Hashimoto's thyroiditis. The number of Ucn-1-positive cells in synovia of arthritic patients correlates strongly with inflammation severity. Conversely, chronic systemic antalarmin treatment reduced joint inflammation in an adjuvant-induced arthritis model in LEW/N rats. Also, CRF_1 agonists (IP) increase intestinal mucosal permeability to macromolecules, and chronic psychosocial stress reduces intestinal host defense and initiates intestinal inflammation through a mast cell CRF_1 receptor-dependent mechanism.

Neurological insults Excitotoxic, ischemic, and hypoxic brain insults upregulate CRF production in topographic and temporal relation to neuronal injury, and CRF potentiates ischemia-induced neuronal apoptosis in the presence of microglia *in vitro*. Conversely, CRF receptor antagonists reduced neuronal death induced by diverse brain injuries independent of the adrenocortical axis. R121920, a small-molecule

CRF_1 antagonist, reduced infarct volume at 24 h in subtemporal and intraluminal suture middle cerebral artery occlusion models even when treatment was delayed up to 1 h postocclusion. Astressin, a nonselective peptide CRF antagonist also ameliorated the effects of 15-min ischemia in a Schaffer collateral-CA1 field potential hippocampal slice model. Central astressin treatment, prior to, or following, infantile seizures also decreased damage in hippocampal cell fields by 84%, perhaps also reflecting the antiexcitotoxic and not only anti-inflammatory properties of CRF_1 receptor antagonists.

Atopic/allergic disorders Stress worsens cutaneous diseases, such as psoriasis and atopic dermatitis. Recent evidence suggests that CRF/Ucn-1 crosstalk between mast cells, neurons, and keratinocytes underlie such exacerbation. Skin mast cells, which play a role in allergy and inflammation by releasing histamine, proteases, proteoglycans, prostaglandin D2, and leukotriene C4, secrete CRF and Ucn-1 in response to psychosocial stress. Accordingly, acute psychosocial stress increases skin CRF levels and triggers mast cell-dependent vascular permeability, which also results from intradermal CRF application. CRA1000, a CRF_1 antagonist, blocks the actions of repeated stress to thicken the epidermis and increases mast cell numbers in dermis, suggesting a role for CRF_1 receptors in chronic contact dermatitis. Mast cells also release CRF and Ucn-1 in response to immunoglobulin E receptor cross-linking, suggesting a general role for CRF1 activity in atopic disorders.

Acknowledgments

Supported by NIH grants DK64871 and DK26741 from the National Institute of Diabetes and Digestive and Kidney Diseases. The authors thank Mike Arends for editorial assistance. This is publication number 18309 from The Scripps Research Institute.

See Also the Following Articles

Blood Pressure; Cardiovascular System and Stress; Central Stress Neurocircuits; Corticotropin Releasing Factor-Binding Protein; Corticotripin-Releasing Factor Receptors; Cytokines; Immune Response; Immunity; Macrophages; Urocortins.

Further Reading

Chen, C. (2006). Recent advances in small molecule antagonists of the corticotropin-releasing factor type-1 receptor – focus on pharmacology and pharmacokinetics. *Current Medicinal Chemistry* **13**, 1261–1282.

Gravanis, A. and Margioris, A. N. (2005). The corticotropin-releasing factor (CRF) family of neuropeptides in inflammation: potential therapeutic applications. *Current Medicinal Chemistry* **12**, 1503–1512.

Kalantaridou, S. N., Makrigiannakis, A., Zoumakis, E., et al. (2004). Reproductive functions of corticotropin-releasing factor. Research and potential clinical utility of antalarmins (CRF receptor type 1 antagonists). *American Journal of Reproductive Immunology* **51**, 269–274.

Nemeroff, C. B. and Vale, W. W. (2005). The neurobiology of depression: inroads to treatment and new drug discovery. *Journal of Clinical Psychiatry* **66**, 5–13.

O'Kane, M., Murphy, E. P. and Kirby, B. (2006). The role of corticotropin-releasing factor in immune-mediated cutaneous inflammatory disease. *Experimental Dermatology* **15**, 143–153.

Taché, Y., Million, M., Nelson, A. G., et al. (2005). Role of corticotropin-releasing factor pathways in stress-related alterations of colonic motor function and viscerosensibility in female rodents. *Gender Medicine* **2**, 146–154.

Zorrilla, E. P. and Koob, G. F. (2004). The therapeutic potential of CRF1 antagonists for anxiety. *Expert Opinion in Investigational Drugs* **13**, 799–828.

Zorrilla, E. P., Taché, Y., and Koob, G. F. (2003). Nibbling at CRF receptor control of feeding and gastrocolonic motility. *Trends in Pharmacological Science* **24**, 421–427.

Pro-opiomelanocortin (POMC)

A B Bicknell
University of Reading, Reading, UK

This is a revised version of the article by A B Bicknell and P J Lowry, Encyclopedia of Stress, First edition, volume 3, pp 257–265, © 2000, Elsevier Inc.

Glossary

Adrenocorticotropin (ACTH) A 39-amino-acid peptide released from the pituitary in response to stress that acts on the adrenal cortex promoting the synthesis and release of corticosteroids.

α-Melanocyte-stimulating hormone (α-MSH) A peptide consisting of the first 13 residues of ACTH, produced mainly in the intermediate lobe of the pituitary. This peptide plays a role in the control of skin color in lower animals and in the control of feeding in mammals.

Immunoprecipitation A purification process in which a specific antibody is used to capture a protein or peptide from a complex mixture (e.g., cell extract).

Prohormone convertases A family of serine proteases that cleave proteins in the Golgi apparatus/secretory granule before they are secreted into the circulation.

Pro-opiomelanocortin (POMC) A 30 kDa protein synthesized predominantly in the pituitary that is the common precursor to ACTH and several other biologically active peptides.

SDS-PAGE (Sodium dodecyl sulfate polyacrylamide electrophoresis) A method to separate proteins by size using electrophoresis through a gel matrix.

Introduction

Adrenocorticotropin (ACTH), like the vast majority of peptide hormones, is synthesized as part of a large, biologically inactive precursor protein that is then proteolytically processed to release the active peptides. ACTH is derived from pro-opiomelanocortin (POMC), a 30-kDa protein that is the common precursor to a number of biologically distinct peptides, an N-terminal region (N-POMC 1–76), ACTH, and β-lipotropin (β-LPH). These peptides can be further cleaved to give β-endorphin, corticotropin-like intermediate peptide (CLIP), and N-POMC 1–49. POMC also contains three copies of the melanocyte-stimulating hormone (α-, β-, and γ-MSH) sequence. The name of the protein thus encompasses the names of the peptides it encodes.

Discovery of POMC

The concept of hormone precursors was developed in the 1960s when it was shown that insulin was synthesized as a larger molecule, pro-insulin, and was released by limited proteolysis. During the 1970s evidence accumulated that implied a very close link between ACTH and β-LPH. The two peptides were released in approximately equimolar amounts from the pituitary, while immunocytochemistry showed the two peptides colocalized in the same cells. This evidence suggested that the peptides were derived from the same precursor, and in 1977 this hypothesis was proved to be correct when two groups showed, in two entirely different ways, that indeed ACTH and β-LPH were derived from the same molecule. Mains and Eipper used a pulse chase approach with the mouse pituitary tumor cell line AtT-20, which secretes large amounts of ACTH. They incubated the cells with radiolabeled amino acids (the pulse) and then washed the radioactivity away after a short period (the chase), thus labeling all proteins synthesized during the period of the pulse. By taking the cells at different times after the chase and immunoprecipitating the cellular protein using either an ACTH or β-endorphin antisera followed by SDS-PAGE analysis, they identified a common 31-kDa protein that became progressively smaller with time after the pulse until it became fully processed.

The second group, headed by Ed Herbert, also used the AtT-20 cell line together with a cell free translation system. Messenger RNA was purified from the cells and expressed in the cell free system. In this way a 28-kDa protein was identified that was recognized by both ACTH and β-endorphin antisera. The apparent difference in size was accounted for by the absence of glycosylation.

Although these experiments gave conclusive evidence that indeed ACTH and β-LPH were derived from the same protein, it was not until 1979, when the cDNA encoding POMC was cloned from both the bovine intermediate lobe and the mouse pituitary cell line AtT-20, that the true structural relationship between ACTH and β-LPH was revealed. Since then the POMC gene has been cloned and sequenced from a variety of organisms. In every species examined, it has been found that there is a single functional copy of the gene, and the overall gene structure, with the exception of the loss of γ-MSH in the salmon, has remained conserved throughout evolution. In the human it consists of three exons and two introns. Exons 2 and 3 are translated, with exon 2 coding for

44 amino acids; the remaining 223 residues are coded for by exon 3. The precursor molecule (pre-POMC) has a 26-amino-acid signal sequence followed by a 76-residue peptide (N-POMC or pro-γ-MSH) that contains one copy of the MSH sequence. This is followed by a joining peptide, ACTH, whose sequence encompasses the second MSH sequence (α-MSH), and finally β-LPH at the C-terminus, the sequence of which includes that for β-endorphin and the third MSH sequence. All the bioactive peptides within POMC are flanked by dibasic amino acid residues, e.g., Arg-Lys, Arg-Arg, Lys-Arg, and Lys-Lys. The structure of POMC and the major peptides released as a result of proteolytic cleavage are shown in **Figure 1**.

Sites and Tissue-Specific Processing of POMC

The main site of POMC expression is the anterior and intermediate lobes of the pituitary. In the anterior lobe, POMC represents approximately 1% of total protein, while it represents up to 10% in the intermediate lobe. Although these two tissues make up the principle sources of circulating POMC, it is also expressed and processed in several other tissues throughout the body, including the adrenal, gut, reproductive tract, placenta, leukocytes, spleen, lung, liver, thyroid, heart, skin, and brain.

One advantage of producing peptides from a larger precursor is that the precursor can be cleaved in a tissue-specific manner to give a different set of products depending on tissue that the precursor is synthesized in. POMC is the classical example of this so-called tissue-specific processing, with the major sites of synthesis being the anterior and intermediate lobes of the pituitary. Classically, the pituitary can be divided into three distinct tissues:

1. The anterior pituitary or pars anterior contains a mixed population of cells, some of which, named corticotrophs, secrete POMC peptides that are involved mainly in the control of adrenal function.
2. The intermediate lobe or pars intermedia consists solely of melanotrophs that secrete POMC-derived peptides that are involved mainly with skin and hair pigmentation.
3. The posterior pituitary or pars nervosa stores and releases vasopressin and oxytocin produced in the hypothalamus.

In the rat these three tissues can be clearly defined, but in adult humans there is no distinct pars intermedia. It is present in fetal life but disappears soon after birth, leaving just a few scattered cells throughout the anterior lobe, giving the adult anterior lobe the collective name of pars distalis. The region between the anterior and posterior lobes is sometimes called the zona intermedia.

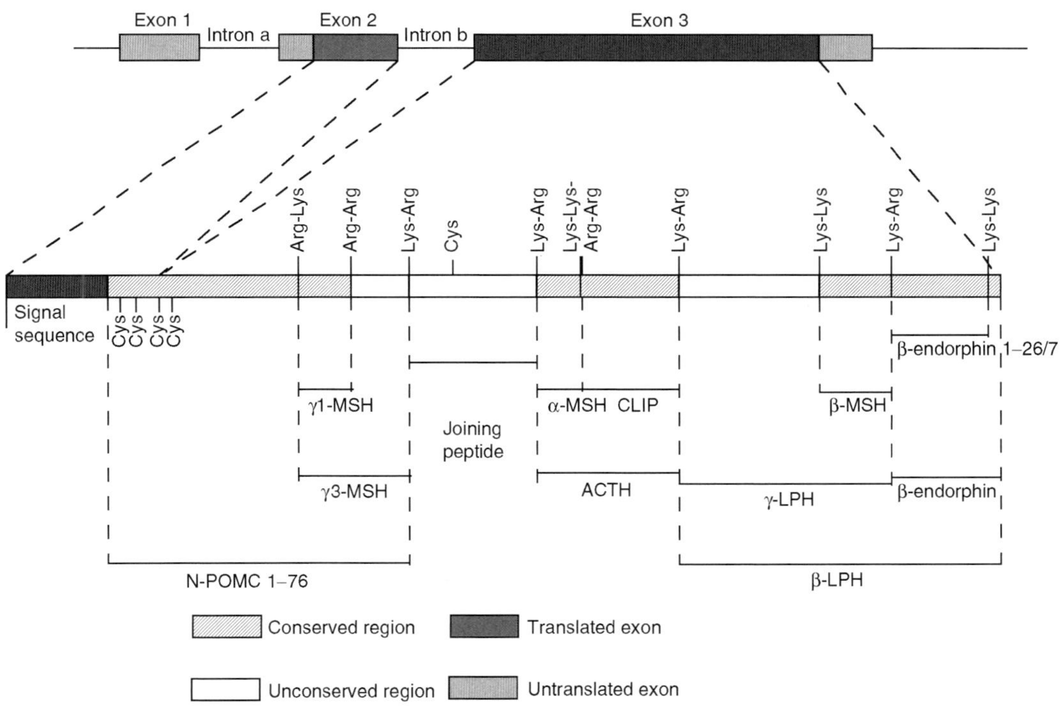

Figure 1 Structure of the POMC gene and the protein it encodes. Positions of the dibasic residues and the Cys residues are shown. Regions of the precursor conserved between species are also shown.

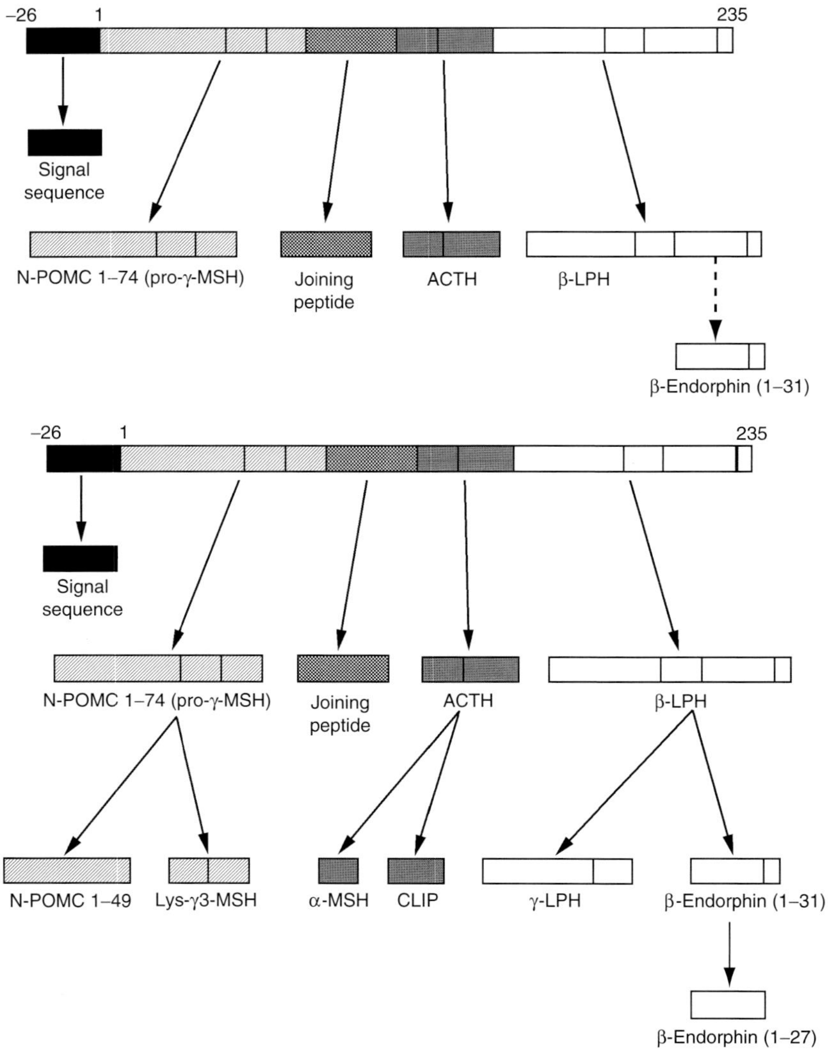

Figure 2 Processing of POMC in anterior and intermediate lobes of the pituitary. Dibasic cleavage sites are shown as vertical lines. Dashed arrow indicates incomplete processing.

Processing of POMC in the Anterior Pituitary

Processing of the POMC in the anterior pituitary is summarized in **Figure 2**. The mouse anterior pituitary cell line AtT-20 has been used extensively as an *in vitro* model for processing in the anterior lobe. Using pulse chase experiments it was determined that the major products were a 16-kDa N-terminal fragment, ACTH, and β-LPH. β-endorphin can also be formed from sequential cleavage from β-LPH (not from direct cleavage of POMC) but is only a minor product.

Processing of POMC in the Pars Intermedia

Within the pars intermedia, processing is more extensive, with the sequential cleavage of peptides produced in the anterior lobe. ACTH is cleaved to α-MSH and CLIP, while β-LPH is virtually completely processed to β-endorphin, and γ-LPH β-endorphin (1–31) is cleaved at the C-terminus to give β-endorphin(1–27), β-endorphin(1–26), and a dipeptide glycylglutamine. The majority of the β-endorphin is N-acetylated. The N-terminal fragment N-POMC 1–76 is partially cleaved at an Arg-Lys site to give N-POMC 1–49 and Lys-γ3-MSH. This latter peptide contains an additional dibasic site (although not in all species) but does not appear to be cleaved to any significant extent.

Molecular Basis of Tissue-Specific Processing

POMC is itself biologically inactive and must be processed correctly to its biologically active peptides. During and after sorting and packaging of the POMC precursor into the regulated secretory vesicles, and prior to the release of the nascent secretory vesicles from the trans Golgi network, it is endoproteolytically cleaved. Cleavage is normally elicited at dibasic amino acid residues and follows a common route involving three different enzymes:

1. An endoprotease that cleaves on the C-terminal side of the basic amino acid pair.
2. A carboxypeptidase-B-like activity that removes the basic amino acid left after cleavage. Carboxypeptidase E (CPE) (also called CPH) specifically removes the basic residues from the C-terminus of a peptide.
3. A C-terminal amidating enzyme that catalyses the amidation of peptides terminating in glycine. The enzyme pepitidylglycine alpha-amidating monooxygenase (PAM) catalyses this reaction and utilizes a glycine situated on the N-terminal side of the dibasic cleavage site as the nitrogen donor for the amide group.

These processing events are carried out in an acidic environment within the trans Golgi network or within the immature secretory vesicles and are necessary for the optimum activity of the processing enzymes as well as to induce conformational changes in the protein to expose the basic amino acid residues for cleavage.

In most cases, specific processing of prohormones occurs on the carboxyl side of pairs of basic amino acids, usually Lys-Arg or Arg-Arg sites. Processing can also occur at the tetrabasic sequence Arg-X-Lys/Arg-Arg and less frequently at monobasic sites. The enzymes that have implicated in the specific processing of POMC are known as prohormone convertases 1 and 2 (PC1 and PC2). These two enzymes are members of the subtilisin family of Ca^{2+}-dependent serine proteinases.

Identification of the Enzymes Involved in POMC Processing

During the early 1990s the identification of the prohormone converting enzymes was a major aim of researchers in the field. The breakthrough came with the cloning of a yeast gene called KEX2. The product of the KEX2 gene, known as kexin, is a protease that cleaves the yeast alpha factor mating pheromone. Cellular expression of the gene demonstrated that the enzyme belongs to the subtilisin family of Ca^{2+}-dependent serine proteinases. KEX2 has the ability to selectively cleave a number of mammalian prohormones, and this led to the hypothesis that similar mammalian counterparts existed.

The first mammalian gene to be identified as a potential processing enzyme came as a consequence of computer alignment of the amino acid sequences surrounding the serine and catalytically important asparagine of kexin against known protein sequences. By this method, a human gene of unknown function was identified, named *fur*, which lies upstream from the tyrosine kinase *fps/fes* proto-oncogene. The product of this gene, to become known as furin, was to become the first mammalian processing enzyme identified.

Using the sequence of the two eukaryotic proteases and several other subtilisin sequences, Smeekens and Steiner designed degenerate oligonucleotides corresponding to the conserved active site. By utilizing these in the polymerase chain reaction (PCR) with cDNA isolated from a human insulinoma library as template, they generated a fragment that was then used to probe that library. A full-length cDNA was identified that encoded for a protease that became known as PC2. Concurrently, Seidah and colleagues, using a similar procedure with the sequence of furin and a mouse pituitary library, identified two cDNA clones that were to become known as PC2 and PC1.

Elegant studies performed *in vitro* using cell-based assays and recombinant enzymes, together with studies looking at PC1 and PC2 knockout animals, have revealed the molecular basis of the tissue-specific processing observed in the anterior and intermediate lobes. In the anterior lobe, PC1 is the predominant enzyme present, and due to its more limited proteolytic activity, results in the generation of ACTH. However, in the intermediate lobe, both PC1 and PC2 are present, and their coordinate actions result in the generation of the smaller POMC peptides.

Cleavage of POMC occurs in a specific order and is summarized in **Figure 3**.

Regulation of the Expression of the POMC Peptides

As the processing of POMC occurs in a tissue-specific manner, it follows that the control of POMC expression and secretion of the derived products are also tissue specific.

Anterior Pituitary

With POMC produced in the pituitary, it followed logically that its secretion was under the control of factors released from the hypothalamus. In 1981 Vale identified the first of these as a 41-amino-acid peptide called corticotropin-releasing hormone (CRH). However, CRH does not stimulate ACTH release to the same extent as hypothalamic extracts, and it became clear that at least one other substance stimulated the release of ACTH. This second substance

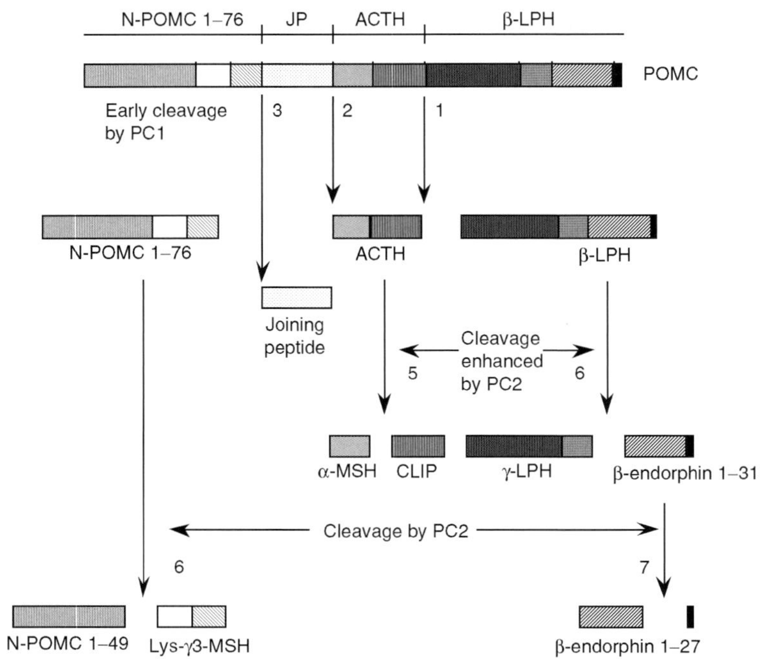

Figure 3 Processing of POMC by PC1 and PC2. The order of cleavage is dictated by the numbers showing that PC2 acts on the products of PC1 cleavage.

was identified by Lowry, McCann, Antoni and other investigators as arginine vasopressin, which potentiates the ACTH-releasing activity of CRH. Stimulation by CRH results in an increase in POMC mRNA levels as well as an increase in secretion of peptides. The two main factors are also potentiated by the action of several other weak secretagogues, namely, epinephrine, norepinephrine, oxytocin, and angiotensin II.

Observations after treatment with exogenous glucocorticoids or adrenalectomy have long implicated a role for glucocorticoids in the control of POMC peptide secretion. They exert their effects both at the hypothalamus, by decreasing CRH secretion, and at the corticotroph, by decreasing POMC synthesis.

Pars Intermedia

As would be expected, the regulation of POMC expression and secretion in the pars intermedia is quite distinct from that in the pars anterior. Glucocorticoids have no influence on POMC expression; although receptors are present, they do not seem to elicit any control over POMC gene expression.

POMC gene expression is enhanced by stress CRH and β-adrenergic agonists All exert their actions via cAMP.

Dopamine decreases POMC expression by binding to D2 receptors, which are thought to block the activation of adenylate cyclase, although there may be more direct effects.

Posttranslational Modifications of POMC

POMC and its peptides undergo a number of different modifications following POMC's synthesis and removal of the signal peptide.

Disulfide Bridge Formation

Human POMC contains five Cys residues, one more than every other species. Four occur close to the N-terminal at positions 2, 8, 20, and 24, while the fifth occurs in the joining peptide. The four N-terminal Cys residues form intramolecular disulfide bridges between 4 and 24 and 8 and 20. The fifth Cys, contained within the joining peptide and unique to humans, leads to its secretion as a homodimer, which may indicate that human POMC is produced as a dimer.

Glycosylation

In all species Asn 65 is N-linked glycosylated in the consensus sequence Asn-X-Ser. O-linked glycosylation also occurs at Thr 45 in the human and porcine pituitary.

Phosphorylation

Serine 31 of ACTH is phosphorylated in the rat, human, and mouse, although its presence has no effect on biological activity.

Acetylation

α-MSH and β-endorphin are found as des-, mono- and diacetylated forms, although the precise form varies between tissue and species. The N-terminal Ser of α-MSH may be acetylated through either the hydroxyl or amide group, acetylation increasing both its biological activity and half life, in contrast to β-endorphin, which reduces its biological opiate activity.

Biological Activity of the POMC Peptides

The peptides contained with the POMC precursor have a wide spectrum of biological activity that is briefly described in the following sections.

Adrenocorticotropin (ACTH)

The main role of ACTH is to promote steroidogenesis within the adrenal cortex. It exerts its actions by binding to the melanocortin 2 receptor (MC2R), leading to a rise in the levels of cAMP and activation of protein kinase A, resulting in secretion of glucocorticoids, androgenic steroids, and, to a lesser extent, mineralocorticoids. The acute effect of ACTH is to increase the rate of conversion of cholesterol to pregnenolone, the first and rate-limiting step in the steroidogenic pathway. The chronic effects of ACTH result in an upregulation of the expression of most of the enzymes involved in the steroidogenic pathway.

ACTH has also been implicated in the maintenance of adrenal weight. The evidence for this is based heavily on the observation that long-term glucocorticoid therapy results in adrenal atrophy. However, since all POMC peptides are downregulated during such treatment and administration of ACTH alone does not totally reverse the atrophy, it is clear that other POMC peptides play a role in the control of adrenal weight.

N-Terminal Peptides and Adrenal Growth

The role of the N-terminus of POMC in adrenal growth was originally proposed in the early 1980s, when a series of elegant studies demonstrated that N-terminal peptides could stimulate mitogenesis in adrenal cell cultures. It was also shown that immunoneutralization of N-POMC peptides resulted in the inhibition of the compensatory growth response observed following unilateral adrenalectomy.

However, N-POMC 1–76 is itself inactive, but peptides derived from its N-terminus, not containing γ-MSH, are potent adrenal mitogens. Since these shorter peptides are not generated during normal pituitary processing, it was proposed that N-POMC 1–76 is cleaved after secretion. Considerable weight has recently been added to this argument with the identification of an adrenal protease that appears to cleave N-POMC to the shorter forms.

Melanocyte-Stimulating Hormone

There are three copies of the MSH sequence in the POMC precursor: α-MSH in ACTH, β-MSH in β-LPH, and γ-MSH in N-POMC 1–76. The biological role of the MSH peptides in lower vertebrates such as frogs was known before the discovery of POMC. α-MSH produced by the pars intermedia causes the darkening of skin to match a darker background. Both α-MSH and β-MSH share the common core sequence Met-Glu-His-Phe-Arg-Trp-Gly, which is essential for biological activity. γ-MSH contains the sequence Met-Gly-His-Phe-Arg-Trp-Asp and was named due to its similarity to the other MSH sequences. However, it has no melanotropic activity.

The role of the MSH peptides in skin pigmentation in humans is not clear. Injection of the peptides into humans does result in skin darkening. Also, in Nelson's syndrome, a condition in which there are high levels of POMC peptides, skin darkening is observed. However, in the normal human this role is debatable. Humans do not have any pars intermedia tissue, and certainly there are no detectable amounts of α-MSH in the periphery, although mRNA encoding POMC can be detected in human skin.

Role of MSH Peptides in the Regulation of Feeding

Mammals regulate their energy stores relatively constantly despite a large variation in both food availability and physical activity. The control of energy expenditure has been shown to be the result of a complicated endocrine loop involving a number of neuropeptides, including the melanocortins.

POMC is synthesized in the hypothalamic arcuate nucleus, where it is processed in a manner similar to that observed in the intermediate lobe. It has been generally assumed that α-MSH is the most important peptide since it is the ligand with highest affinity for the two melanocortin receptors – the MC3R and MC4R expressed in the hypothalamus. Genetic and pharmacological disruption of this loop causes obesity in both humans and rodents. The POMC knockout mouse is hyperphagic and obese, whereas infusion of α-MSH (or synthetic agonists) results in anorexia and weight loss.

The complete subtle architecture of this system is still far from clear, but the system's potential as a therapeutic target for the treatment of obesity has made it the focus of intense research over the past few years.

γ-MSH and Steroidogenesis

γ-MSH is generated from N-POMC in the intermediate lobe of the pituitary. It contains a slightly modified core sequence, Met-Gly-His-Phe-Arg-Trp-Asp, and has a biological role distinct from that of α-MSH.

Studies performed by Alastair Brownie in the early 1980s identified γ-MSH as a regulator of hormone sensitive lipase (HSL). This enzyme is found in steroidogenic tissues and breaks down cholesterol esters to free cholesterol, which then feeds into the steroidogenic pathway. Several groups demonstrated that although not directly steroidogenic, this peptide can synergize with ACTH and result in an increase in steroid output. The receptor through which this peptide acts is unclear, since although the MC3R has been shown to be the only melanocortin receptor with significant affinity for γ-MSH, its expression profile and pharmacology suggest that it does not play a role in this system.

Joining Peptide

The joining peptide has no known biological function. Its role, like the C-peptide of insulin, is probably only to provide a spacer between the different peptides. One interesting feature of human joining peptide is that it uniquely contains a cysteine that has been implicated in dimer formation.

β-Endorphin

β-endorphin is one of several endogenous opioids that exert their actions by binding to receptors within the central and peripheral nervous systems. It is part of a larger family whose members include dynorphin and the enkephalins. The opioids bind to three receptors known as the μ, κ, and δ opioid receptors. The receptors derive their names from the opiate agonists that bind to them: morphine and ketocyclazocine for the μ and κ receptors, and the vas deferens for the δ receptor, where it is located. The receptors differ in their affinity for the different opioids, although not one is specific for a single ligand. β-endorphin and Met-enkephalin bind to the μ and δ receptors, while dynorphin binds to the κ receptor. All the receptors are G-coupled and recognize a common motif consisting of a protonated amine adjacent to an aromatic amine, for example, the tyrosine residue at the N-terminus of the enkephalins. The opioid actions of β-endorphin are dependent on its C-terminal residues. Removal leads to a decrease in both its analgesic properties and binding affinity for the receptors. Thus, the shorter endorphins lack opioid activity, as does N-acetylation of the peptide. The N-terminal portion of β-endorphin is required for binding to the opiate receptors, whereas the C-terminal residues are thought to enhance the binding affinity.

Conclusions

Most peptide hormones are produced as inactive precursor molecules that are subsequently cleaved at dibasic residues to release the active peptides. As the first such multihormone to be discovered, over a quarter of a century ago, POMC has been extensively studied and characterized. Its role in the control of adrenal function by the actions of ACTH on steroidogenesis, as well as N-POMC on the control of adrenal tonic state, are central to the stress axis as a whole.

See Also the Following Articles

Obesity, Stress and.

Further Reading

Bertagna, X. (1994). Proopiomelanocortin-derived peptides. *Endocrinology and Metabolism Clinics of North America* **23**, 467–485.

MacNeil, D. J., Howard, A. D., Guan, X., et al. (2002). The role of melanocortins in body weight regulation: opportunities for the treatment of obesity. *European Journal of Pharmacology* **450**, 93–109.

Raffin-Sanson, M. L., de Keyzer, Y. and Bertagna, X. (2003). Pro-opiomelanocortin, a polypeptide precursor with multiple functions: from physiology to pathological conditions. *European Journal of Endocrinology* **149**, 79–90.

Smith, A. I. and Funder, J. W. (1988). Proopiomelanocortin processing in the pituitary, central nervous system and peripheral tissues. *Endocrine Reviews* **9**, 159–179.

Steiner, D. F. (1998). The proprotein convertases. *Current Opinion in Chemical Biology* **2**, 31–39.

Beta-Endorphin

M Lee and S L Wardlaw
Columbia University College of Physicians and Surgeons, New York, NY, USA

This is a revised version of the article by J J Puder and S L Wardlaw, Encyclopedia of Stress, First edition, volume 1, pp 321–324, © 2000, Elsevier Inc.

Glossary

Adrenocorticotropin (ACTH) — The pituitary hormone that regulates adrenal corticosteroid synthesis and release. ACTH, like β-endorphin, is derived from proopiomelanocortin.

Endogenous opioid peptides — Peptides with morphine-like actions that are synthesized in the brain and in peripheral tissues.

Endorphins — A general term that refers to all of the endogenous opioid peptides. β-endorphin refers to a specific peptide.

Naloxone — A compound that binds to opiate receptors and blocks the effects of morphine and the endogenous opioid peptides.

Proopiomelanocortin — The larger precursor protein from which β-endorphin is derived.

β-endorphin is an endogenous opioid peptide that is synthesized primarily in the pituitary gland and in the brain. Stress stimulates the release of β-endorphin in both the pituitary and the brain. β-endorphin and the other endogenous opioid peptides have been implicated in analgesia and in neuroendocrine regulation during times of stress, including the suppression of reproductive function. These peptides also play a role in autonomic regulation, modulation of cardiovascular responses and cerebral blood flow, and the regulation of behavior and immune function.

Structure, Synthesis, and Localization

β-Endorphin is a 31-amino-acid peptide that is derived from the larger molecular weight precursor protein proopiomelanocortin (POMC). β-Endorphin is one of the three major classes of endogenous opioid peptides. The other two classes are composed of the enkephalins and the dynorphins, which are derived from separate precursor proteins. POMC is synthesized independently in the anterior and intermediate lobes of the pituitary gland, in the brain, and in several peripheral tissues, including the gastrointestinal tract, reproductive tract, placenta, and cells of the immune system. The posttranslational processing of POMC is tissue specific and results in the production of peptides with very different biological activities. In the anterior pituitary, POMC is processed predominantly to adrenocorticotropin (ACTH) and β-lipotropin (β-LPH), but some β-endorphin is also produced. ACTH is secreted from the pituitary into the peripheral circulation and is critical for the maintenance of adrenocortical function and cortisol secretion. β-endorphin is also secreted in parallel with ACTH. In the brain, ACTH and β-LPH are further processed to yield α-melanocyte-stimulating hormone (α-MSH) and β-endorphin. The regulation of POMC processing is potentially important, as α-MSH has been shown to antagonize some of the effects of β-endorphin. The regulation of POMC gene expression and peptide release is also tissue specific, but under conditions of stress, β-endorphin is released from both the pituitary and the brain. The hypothalamic releasing factor corticotropin-releasing hormone (CRH), which plays a key role in coordinating the organism's response to stress, has been shown to stimulate pituitary and brain β-endorphin. β-endorphin exerts its effects by binding to specific opioid receptors, particularly the mu and delta receptors, which have been recently cloned and localized throughout the brain.

β-Endorphin is released from the anterior pituitary into the peripheral circulation in parallel with ACTH in response to a variety of stresses. Numerous studies have documented parallel increases in peripheral blood levels of ACTH and β-endorphin in response to exercise. This appears to be related to the intensity and duration of the exercise. A number of correlations between β-endorphin levels in blood and central nervous system or cardiovascular responses during stress have been reported. One must be cautious, however, in attributing a causal relationship for circulating β-endorphin, because in many instances, brain β-endorphin may also be stimulated at the same time. In addition, peripherally released β-endorphin does not readily cross the blood–brain barrier. In the brain, β-endorphin is synthesized in only two regions, the arcuate nucleus of the hypothalamus and the nucleus of the solitary tract in the brain stem, but β-endorphin fibers project widely to many regions throughout the brain.

β-Endorphin and Neuroendocrine Responses

Endogenous opioid peptides have multiple effects on pituitary function. Effects on gonadotropin (luteinizing hormone [LH] and follicle-stimulating hormone

[FSH]), prolactin, ACTH, vasopressin, and oxytocin release have all been demonstrated. There is evidence for a specific role for β-endorphin during stress with respect to the regulation of LH and the hypothalamic-pituitary-gonadal (HPG) axis, of ACTH and the hypothalamic-pituitary-adrenocortical (HPA) axis, and of prolactin release. Stress is known to impair reproductive function in many species. Stress has been shown to suppress the release of LH from the pituitary with subsequent suppression of ovarian and testicular function. Such suppression has been seen with many types of stress ranging from exercise and weight loss to inflammatory and psychological stress. CRH, which is released from the hypothalamus during stress, has been shown to cause a similar suppression of the HPG axis. There is convincing evidence that the suppressive effects of stress and CRH on the HPG axis are mediated by β-endorphin. Thus, both CRH and β-endorphin are important in suppressing reproductive function during times of stress. Exogenous and endogenous opioids also have well-documented effects on the HPA axis. There are some differences, however, depending on the dose and duration of treatment and the species studied. In the human, morphine and β-endorphin have been shown to suppress ACTH and cortisol release in normal subjects and to blunt the HPA response to surgical stress. β-Endorphin has been shown to suppress CRH release from the hypothalamus *in vitro* and to suppress CRH release into hypophysial portal blood *in vivo*. Conversely, opioid antagonism has been reported to stimulate the HPA axis and to enhance the HPA response to stress. Thus, β-endorphin may be important in limiting the HPA response under conditions of stress.

β-Endorphin and Stress-Induced Analgesia

It has long been known that pain perception is affected by stress. Electrical stimulation of specific brain regions has been shown to induce analgesia that was blocked by treatment with naloxone and other opioid antagonists, implying that this analgesia was mediated by the release of endogenous opioids. Certain forms of stress-induced analgesia are also blocked by naloxone. It is now clear that stress-induced analgesia is mediated by both opioid and nonopioid pathways. There is considerable pharmacological and neuroanatomic evidence to implicate β-endorphin as a mediator of stress-induced analgesia. Recently, a genetic approach has been used to generate mice that are unable to synthesize β-endorphin. These transgenic mice do not exhibit the naloxone-reversible analgesia normally seen after a mild swim stress, supporting a role for β-endorphin in this process. β-Endorphin is also synthesized by immune cells and is known to play a role in mediating analgesia at sites of inflammation. Studies in rats have demonstrated that β-endorphin is released by immune cells at sites of inflammation and can induce analgesia by interaction with receptors on peripheral terminals of sensory nerves. These studies provide convincing evidence that β-endorphin plays an important role within the brain in mediating stress-induced analgesia and can also act locally to affect pain perception at sites of inflammation.

β-Endorphin and the Immune System

Both stress and opioids have suppressive effects on immune function. Naloxone has also been shown to block stress-induced immune suppression, indicating a role for endogenous opioids in this process. β-Endorphin-deficient mice possess enhanced immune responses as measured by increased splenocyte proliferation and inflammatory cytokine production, consistent with an inhibitory effect of endogenous β-endorphin on immune function. β-Endorphin is produced by cells of the immune system and may have local paracrine effects on immune function. Circulating, pituitary-derived β-endorphin, which increases with stress and with inflammation, may also affect immune function. In addition, β-endorphin may affect immune function indirectly by modulating neuroendocrine and autonomic function.

β-Endorphin and Cardiovascular Responses

The endogenous opioid peptides are localized to regions within the brain that are important in controlling the autonomic nervous system and cardiovascular responses. β-Endorphin is synthesized in the nucleus of the solitary tract in the medulla, an area important in cardiovascular regulation. The effects of opioids on cardiovascular function are complex and depend on the type of opioid injected, the site of injection, and whether the animal is anesthetized or stressed. Although discrepancies exist, it appears that in general, opioids diminish stress-induced cardiovascular effects. Opioid mechanisms appear to facilitate parasympathetic and inhibit sympathetic nervous system reactivity during stress. High-dose infusion of β-endorphin in human subjects reduces blood pressure and circulating norepinephrine levels. Several studies have demonstrated activation of the endogenous opioid system in hemorrhagic shock, sepsis, and trauma and shown that this system plays a complex role both centrally and peripherally in modulating autonomic and cardiovascular responses. Endogenous opioid peptides are also important in regulating cerebral blood flow, especially during periods of hypoxia. β-Endorphin, in particular, has been shown to regulate hypothalamic blood flow.

β-Endorphin and Stress-Induced Feeding and Other Behaviors

Pharmacological studies have shown that opioids generally stimulate food intake. Rats subjected to mild stress exhibit stress-induced eating that can be attenuated by treatment with naloxone, thus implicating a role of endogenous opioids in this process. β-Endorphin administration in rodents has also been shown to stimulate food intake. However, more recently, studies with transgenic mice deficient in β-endorphin indicate that the role of endogenous opioids in modulating feeding and energy homeostasis is quite complex and that β-endorphin may be important in primarily increasing the motivational and reward components of feeding. Finally, there is evidence that endogenous opioids may affect other behavioral and psychological responses to stress, but a specific role for β-endorphin remains to be defined.

Further Reading

Akil, H., Watson, S. J., Young, E., et al. (1984). Endogenous opioids: biology and function. *Annual Reviews of Neuroscience* 7, 223–255.

Benyó, Z. and Wahl, M. (1996). Opiate receptor-mediated mechanism in the regulation of cerebral blood flow. *Cerebrovascular Brain Metabolism Reviews* **8**, 326–357.

Bodnar, R. J. (2004). Endogenous opioids and feeding behavior: a 30-year historical perspective. *Peptides* **25**, 697–725.

Castro, M. G. and Morrison, E. (1997). Post-translational processing of proopiomelanocortin in the pituitary and in the brain. *Critical Reviews in Neurobiology* **11**, 35–57.

Cozzolino, D., Sasso, F. C., Cataldo, D., et al. (2005). Acute pressor and hormonal effects of β-endorphin at high doses in healthy and hypertensive subjects: role of opioid receptor agonism. *Journal of Clinical Endocrinology and Metabolism* **90**, 5167–5174.

Ferin, M. (1999). Stress and the reproductive cycle. *Journal of Clinical Endocrinology and Metabolism* **84**, 1768–1774.

Ferin, M., Van Vugt, D. and Wardlaw, S. L. (1984). The hypothalamic control of the menstrual cycle and the role of endogenous opioid peptides. *Recent Progress in Hormone Research* **40**, 441–485.

Goldfarb, A. H. and Jamurtas, A. Z. (1997). β-endorphin response to exercise. *Sports Medicine* **24**, 8–16.

Low, M. J., Hayward, M., Appleyard, S. M. and Rubinstein, M. (2003). State-dependent modulation of feeding behavior by proopiomelanocortin-derived β-endorphin. *Annals of the New York Academy of Sciences* **994**, 192–201.

Mansour, A., Fox, C. A., Akil, H. and Watson, S. J. (1995). Opioid-receptor mRNA expression in the rat CNS: anatomical and functional implications. *Trends in Neuroscience* **18**, 22–29.

McCubbin, J. A. (1993). Stress and endogenous opioids: behavioral and circulatory interactions. *Biological Psychology* **35**, 91–122.

Molina, P. E. (2002). Stress-specific opioid modulation of haemodynamic counter-regulation. *Clinical and Experimental Pharmacology and Physiology* **29**, 248–253.

Morely, J. E. and Levine, A. S. (1980). Stress-induced eating is mediated through endogenous opiates. *Science* **209**, 1259–1261.

Pechnik, R. N. (1993). Effects of opioids on the hypothalamo-pituitary-adrenal axis. *Annual Reviews in Pharmacology and Toxicology* **32**, 353–382.

Refojo, D., Kovalovsky, D., Young, J. I., et al. (2002). Increased splenocyte proliferative response and cytokine production in β-endorphin deficient mice. *Journal of Neuroimmunology* **131**, 126–134.

Rubinstein, M., Mogil, J. S., Japón, M., et al. (1996). Absence of opioid stress-induced analgesia in mice lacking β-endorphin by site-directed mutagenesis. *Proceedings of the National Academy of Sciences USA* **93**, 3995–4000.

Stein, C. R., Hassan, A. H. S., Przewlocki, R., et al. (1990). Opioids from immunocytes interact with receptors on sensory nerves to inhibit nociception in inflammation. *Proceedings of the National Academy of Sciences USA* **87**, 5935–5939.

III. ADRENAL GLANDS

A. Cortex - Corticosteroids

Adrenal Cortex

G P Vinson
Queen Mary, University of London, London, UK
B J Whitehouse
King's College London, London, UK
J P Hinson
Queen Mary, University of London, London, UK

This is a revised version of the article by G P Vinson, B J Whitehouse, and J P Hinson, Encyclopedia of Stress, First edition, volume 1, pp 42–51, © 2000, Elsevier Inc.

Glossary

Aldosterone	The principal mineralocorticoid secreted by the adrenal cortex.
Angiotensin II	An octapeptide that provides the major hormonal support of the growth and function of the zona glomerulosa of the adrenal cortex and of aldosterone secretion.
Cortex	The outer, steroid-forming part of the adrenal gland.
Corticosteroids	The collective name for the steroid hormones (glucocorticoid and mineralocorticoid) that are secreted by the adrenal cortex.
Corticosteroid-binding globulin (CBG)	The carrier protein to which cortisol binds in the circulation.
Corticotropin (corticotropin, adrenocorticotropic hormone, ACTH)	The pituitary hormone that largely controls growth and activity of the adrenal cortex, particularly the zona fasciculata and cortisol secretion.
Cortisol	The principal glucocorticoid secreted by the adrenal cortex.
Cytochrome-P450	A family of enzymes associated with the synthesis of steroid hormones that utilize molecular oxygen to form hydroxyl groups on the steroid molecule.
Dehydroepiandrosterone (DHEA, or DHA)	By amount the major androgen-like hormone secreted by the adrenal cortex.
Glucocorticoids	Steroid hormones (especially cortisol) from the zona fasciculata of the adrenal cortex that affect carbohydrate metabolism.
Medulla	The inner, catecholamine (adrenaline)-secreting core of the adrenal gland.
Mineralocorticoids	Steroid hormones (especially aldosterone) from the zona glomerulosa of the adrenal cortex that affect mineral (especially sodium/potassium) homeostasis.
Renin-angiotensin system (RAS)	The blood-borne complement of enzymes and substrates that gives rise to angiotensin II.
Zona fasciculata	The middle part of the adrenal cortex, secreting glucocorticoids, especially cortisol.
Zona glomerulosa	The outer, mineralocorticoid (especially aldosterone)-secreting part of the adrenal cortex.
Zona reticularis	The inner part of the adrenal cortex, secreting both glucocorticoids and androgens, but also containing apoptotic (dying) cells.

Structure of the Adrenal Cortex

The adrenals are paired glands lying close to the anterior part of the kidney. Their combined wet weight is about 0.01–0.02% of the total body weight, and thus they weigh about 8 g in the adult human in both males and females.

Morphology

The gland has two main parts, the medulla at the center and the cortex surrounding it. These two parts have different developmental origins; the medulla forms part of the sympathetic nervous system, whereas the cortex, like the gonads, has a distinct embryological origin in the germinal ridge. The medulla and cortex also have different functions, though both are associated with the response to stress. Their functional differences lie both in the nature of the hormones they produce – catecholamines such as adrenaline and noradrenaline from the medulla and steroids from the cortex – and the ways in which these secretions are controlled – by neural stimulation in the case of the medulla, but by other hormones circulating in the blood in the case of the cortex.

Histologically, the cells of the adrenal cortex are arranged as three major layers, or zones, organized as concentric shells. The cells of the different zones are generally distinguished by their shape and size and by their ultrastructure as well as by their arrangement and position within the gland. The three zones are called the *zona glomerulosa*, the *zona fasciculata*, and the *zona reticularis*. Broadly, the zona glomerulosa lies just below the connective tissue capsule and consists of whorl-like arrangements of cells. Cells of the zona fasciculata are arranged as a series of cords running centripetally, which extend to the less clearly organized network of cells of the zona reticularis (see **Figures 1** and **2**).

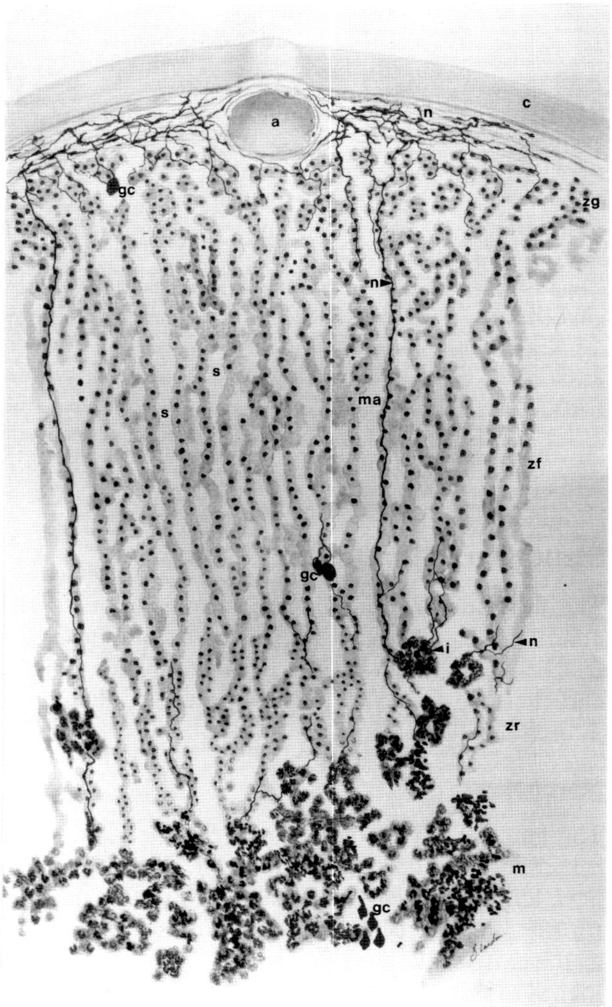

Figure 1 General structure of the mammalian adrenal cortex showing the positions of the zona glomerulosa (zg), zona fasciculata (zf), and zona reticularis (zr) and their relationship to the capsule (c), nerve cells (n), arteriolar supply (a), medullary arteries (ma), sinuses (s), medulla (m), and isolated islets (i) of chromaffin (medullary) cells lying in the inner cortex. Drawing by Bridget Landon. Figure reproduced with permission from G. P. Vinson, J. P. Hinson, and I. E. Toth. (1994). The neuroendocrinology of the adrenal cortex. *J. Neuroendocr.* **6**, 235–246, Blackwell, Oxford.

Other zones are recognized in different species, although these are usually smaller and may be transient. In humans, the most prominent of these is the fetal cortex (see below). The cells of the cortex are renewed from a region just below the glomerulosa; this may be the role of the cells of the zona intermedia, which has been described as a small band of cells in some species. The cells migrate centripetally over a period of time, and as they do so, they acquire the functional and morphological characteristics of the cells of the zones that they pass through.

In humans, the zona glomerulosa seldom occupies more than 5% of the total cortical volume and its cells are gathered into more or less isolated islets. The cells are relatively small and round, with a high nuclear-to-cytoplasmic ratio. Ultrastructurally, the mitochondria of zona glomerulosa cells are characterized by their lamelliform or shelflike cristae. The smooth endoplasmic reticulum is sparse: ribosomes and polysomes are visible throughout the cytoplasm.

The zona fasciculata cells are larger, with abundant cytoplasm, and the mitochondria contain tubulovesicular cristae, although these may vary between the outer and inner parts of the zone. In conventional stains, these cells are lighter in appearance than zona reticularis cells and hence have been termed *clear cells* as opposed to the *compact cells* of the zona reticularis, which stain more deeply.

The zona reticularis occupies one-third of the cortex, and its cells are intermediate in size between those of the zona glomerulosa and zona fasciculata. The mitochondria of zona reticularis cells are elongated with tubulovesicular cristae; microbodies (lipofuchsin granules) and lipid droplets also occur.

In humans the adrenal is prominent in fetal life, when it reaches a maximum of about 0.3% of body weight. This declines slightly in the third trimester and precipitously in the neonate. The large size of the gland is attributable to the presence of an additional zone – the fetal zone – which lies between the definitive cortex and the medulla. The cells of the fetal zone are larger than those of other zones and stain only palely in conventional histology. In the fetus, the cells of the definitive cortex contain lamelliform cristae (like the zona glomerulosa of the adult gland), whereas the mitochondria of the fetal zone cells are tubulovesicular. Studies on the origin and ultimate fate of the cells of the fetal zone are inconclusive. Some have held that the fetal zone cells arise from a second discrete proliferation, although this has been contested, and they may arise, like the reticularis, from the outer zones. Similarly, there are two explanations for its disappearance after birth; one that the zone involutes, the other that it is transformed into elements of the definitive cortex.

Circulation and Innervation

The intraglandular circulatory system deserves some attention, particularly because of its responses during stimulation. The adrenal is one of the most highly vascularized organs within the body, and detailed studies have shown that virtually every cell borders the thin and attenuated endothelial cells which line the vascular space (see **Figure 1**). The general pattern in mammals is as follows: a variable number of arteries supply the gland which divide in the capsular or subcapsular region to form an arteriolar plexus. Two types of vessels arise from this plexus: first, there

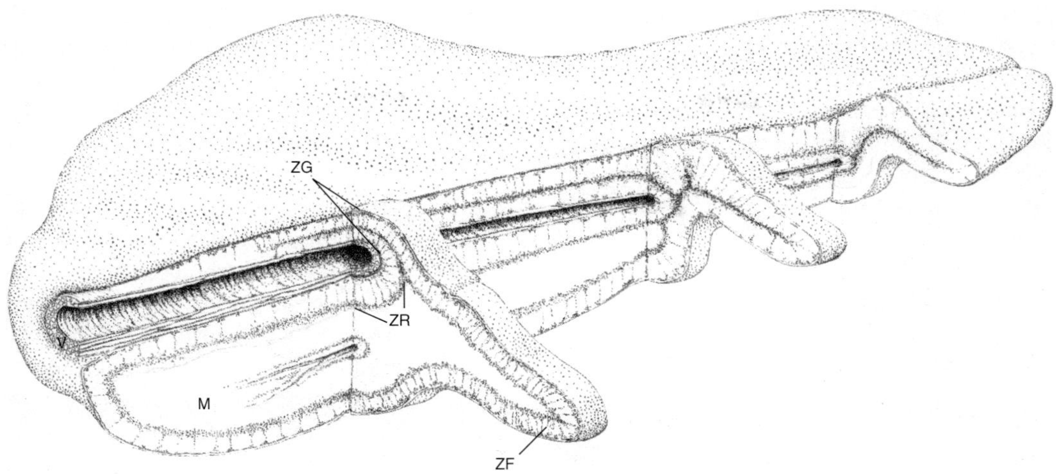

Figure 2 General structure of the human adrenal gland. Arrangement of adrenal cortex in the region of the cortical cuff. Notice the folding results in a doubling of the cortical thickness and the juxtaposition here of the inner zona glomerulosa and the central vein in cortical cuff region. M = medulla; ZG = zona glomerulosa; ZF = zona fasciculata; ZR = zona reticularis; V = central vein. Drawing by B. Landon. Figure reproduced with permission from G. P. Vinson and J. P. Hinson, *The Adrenal Gland* (V. H. T. James ed.), pp. 71–85, Raven Press. ©1992 Lippincott Williams & Wilkins.

are the thinly walled capillaries, frequently called sinuses, which run centripetally through the cortex. These are the most abundant of the cortical vessels and may be assumed to supply all of the cortical cells. Second, there are the much more sparsely distributed medullary arteries, with thicker walls, which run through the cortex to supply the medulla directly. It is likely that blood from the cortical sinuses and the medullary arteries mixes in the medulla, and, on the basis of the relative abundance of the vessels, it is reasonable to assume that the medulla receives most of its supply from the sinuses. Accordingly the cortex exerts an endocrine control over the medulla, and, in particular, glucocorticoids (see below) are required for the development in the medulla of a key enzyme required for the synthesis of adrenaline. It is in the medulla that the sinuses are drained into the single common vein for the whole gland (see **Figure 1**). In the human gland there are also arteriovenous loops in which blood is apparently carried from the subcapsular arterioles in vessels which sweep down through the zona glomerulosa and the zona fasciculata, then loop back to the exterior of the gland to sites close to their origins. Also, as the vein leaves the gland, a portion of the cortex is introverted from the exterior to surround the vessel as the cortical cuff (**Figure 2**).

Most early studies reported that nerve fibers which entered the gland passed straight to the medulla without branching and with no evidence of nerve endings. In fact much evidence now shows that nerve fibers reach the cortex, arising partly from the medulla, but also partly through direct innervation. In general, neural arborization is most dense in the capsular and subcapsular regions and nerves may contact both adrenocortical cells and blood vessels. Both catecholaminergic and peptidergic fibers have been identified.

Hormones of the Adrenal Cortex

The hormones of the adrenal cortex are steroids: compounds that contain the *perhydrocyclopentanophenanthrene* structure consisting of four linked rings, three of six carbon atoms and one of five. There are four major groups of these compounds, classified according to the number of carbon atoms they contain.

1. C_{27} compounds. These are the sterols, including cholesterol.
2. C_{21} steroids. These include progesterone, the hormone of pregnancy and of female cyclic reproductive function, as well as the compounds produced more or less exclusively by the adrenal cortex. The adrenal C_{21} steroids, collectively termed corticosteroids, are of two major types according to their activities, the mineralocorticoids and the glucocorticoids. The activity of the mineralocorticoids is primarily concerned with the regulation of sodium and potassium homeostasis. The most potent mineralocorticoid in all mammals is aldosterone, although other corticosteroids possess some mineralocorticoid activity. The glucocorticoids were originally defined on the basis of their actions on carbohydrate metabolism but are known to have a wide variety of functions (see below). In humans and many other species

(including canine, ovine, bovine) cortisol (hydrocortisone) is the most prominent secreted glucocorticoid, and smaller amounts of cortisone and corticosterone are also produced. In the rat and some other rodents (and in many nonmammalian vertebrates), adrenal 17α-hydroxylase activity (see below) is weak, and corticosterone is the major secreted adrenocortical product.

3. C_{19} steroids. These include the androgens, which support male structure and reproductive function. Of these, testosterone is the most potent but is normally produced in only small amounts by the adrenal. However, androstenedione, dehydroepiandrosterone (DHEA), and its sulfate (DHEAS) are prominent adrenal secretory products which may be converted to testosterone peripherally.

4. C_{18} steroids. These include the estrogens, female sex hormones, which are not usually secreted by the adrenal. However, androstenedione and DHEA(S) from the adrenal may be converted to estrogens elsewhere and this is the major source of circulating estrogen in postmenopausal women. In the fetus, DHEAS from the fetal adrenal is converted first to 16α-hydroxy-DHEAS and then to estriol sulfate by placental enzymes.

The circulating concentrations of the major adrenal steroids are shown in **Table 1**.

Biosynthesis of the Corticosteroids

Although their biological activities may be very different (see below), the close structural similarities of the corticosteroids reflect their biosynthetic relationship. Several groups of enzymes are involved in their synthesis within the adrenal cortex, and these are summarized in **Figure 3** and in **Table 2**.

Table 1 Examples of plasma concentrations of adrenal hormones in normal subjects[a]

Steroid	*Concentration*
Aldosterone (pmol per L)	100–400
Androstenedione (nmol per L)	
Adults	2–13
Children	<2
Cortisol (nmol per L)	
07.00–09.00 h	280–720
21.00–24.00 h	60–340
Dehydroepiandrosterone sulfate (μmol per L)	
Adults	2–11
Children	<2

[a]Values may show considerable variations as all adrenal steroids show a diurnal rhythm, and steroid secretion may also be affected by age, nutritional status, and stage of the menstrual cycle.

Steroid hormones are formed from cholesterol. Cholesterol may be formed *de novo* from acetate in the adrenal or it may be imported into the gland from circulating low-density lipoprotein (LDL) through a process of receptor-mediated endocytosis. Cholesterol is stored as esters in the lipid droplets within the adrenocortical cell.

The rate-limiting step in these sequences is thought to be (1) the delivery of cholesterol to the inner mitochondrial membrane and CYP11A. Current evidence suggests that this is primarily facilitated by a specific protein, designated the steroidogenic acute regulatory, or StAR, protein. (2) Much evidence suggests that a second "late pathway" rate-limiting step lies between 18-hydroxydeoxycorticosterone or corticosterone and aldosterone.

However, since CYP11B2 (aldosterone synthase) can catalyze all of the steps between deoxycorticosterone and aldosterone, this could only be achieved by the regulation of the supply of the alternative precursors.

Inborn errors of steroid metabolism exist which may result from congenital defects in the enzymes involved in steroid biosynthesis. A feature of all of these is that the end-product of biosynthesis (for example, cortisol) is produced in inappropriately low amounts. Accompanying this may be the excessive production of the steroid intermediate that immediately precedes the enzyme block. For example, 21-hydroxylase deficiency, the most common form, results in excessive secretion of 17α-hydroxyprogesterone (cf. **Figure 3**). This has little intrinsic biological activity, though it can be converted to androgens, resulting in virilization and hirsutism. Another defect, of 11 β-hydroxylase, may result in the secretion of large amounts of 11-deoxycorticosterone, which can have profound mineralocorticoid effects, with excessive sodium retention resulting in hypertension. The lack of cortisol in these patients results in enhanced secretion of ACTH, leading both to the excessive secretion of steroid intermediates and also to the growth (hyperplasia) of the gland – hence the general term *congenital adrenal hyperplasia* or CAH. These fortunately rare conditions can usually be treated by administration of cortisol.

Knowledge of the mechanisms for corticosteroid biosynthesis have led to the development of numerous and more or less specific inhibitors of adrenal steroidogenesis. These are listed in **Table 3**.

Transport and Metabolism of Corticosteroids

Under normal conditions around 90% of the circulating cortisol is bound to a specific plasma binding protein, called corticosteroid binding globulin (CBG). There is no comparable plasma binding

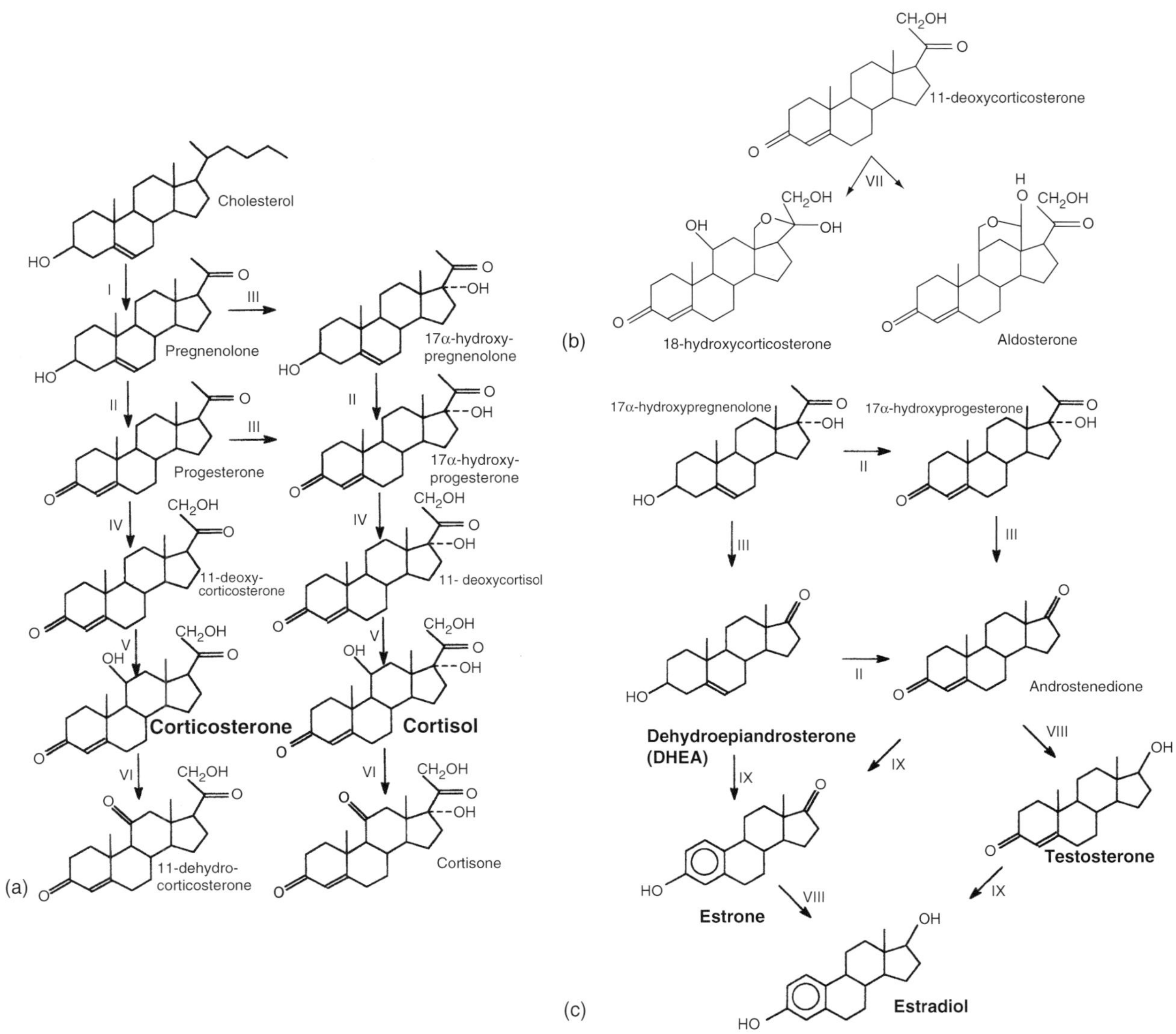

Figure 3 Pathways for biosynthesis of (a) glucocorticoids, (b) aldosterone, and (c) androgens and estrogens. The formation of aldosterone from 11-deoxycorticosterone is catalyzed by a single enzyme, CYP11B2 (aldosterone synthase). This may include the formation of other intermediates, corticosterone and/or 18-hydroxydeoxycorticosterone, that are not shown. Cortisol and, to a lesser extent, corticosterone are the major end-products of the glucocorticoid pathway, though cortisone and 11-dehydrocorticosterone (which are biologically inactive) may also be secreted. All of the dehydrogenase-catalyzed reactions may be reversible, however, i.e., cortisol may be formed from cortisone and androstenedione from testosterone.

protein for aldosterone, which may be loosely bound to plasma albumin. It is generally thought that only the unbound steroid fraction is biologically active. This view has, however, been questioned, but the conditions required for bioactivity of the bound fraction remain unclear.

The liver is the major site for corticosteroid metabolism, and in humans metabolites are generally excreted in the urine rather than by the biliary/fecal route, which predominates in some other species. The main reactions involved are reduction of ring A, hydroxylation, and conjugation as sulfates or glucuronides.

Control of Adrenocortical Secretion

Control of Cortisol Secretion

Cortisol (together with cortisone and corticosterone) is produced exclusively by the zona fasciculata and the zona reticularis of the adrenal cortex. Its secretion is almost entirely related to the degree of stimulation by circulating adrenocorticotropic hormone (ACTH), which is secreted by the anterior pituitary gland. In the absence of ACTH (e.g., after removal of the pituitary, or hypophysectomy), glucocorticoid levels in the blood fall to about 5% of normal values within 2 h, and this fall may be reversed by administration of

Table 2 Enzymes involved in steroid biosynthesis

Number[a]	*Type*	*Systematic designation*	*Other names*	*Activity*
I	Cytochrome-P450	CYP11A	P-450$_{SCC}$	Cholesterol side-chain cleavage
II	Dehydrogenase	3β-Hydroxysteroid-dehydrogenase, isomerase		Conversion pregnenolone to progesterone
III	Cytochrome-P450	CYP17	P450$_{17\alpha}$, 17-hydroxylase, 17-lyase	Hydroxylation at C-17, 20 lyase (side-chain cleavage)
IV	Cytochrome-P450	CYP21	P450$_{21}$, 21-hydroxylase	Hydroxylation at C-21
V	Cytochrome-P450	CYP11B1	P450$_{11\beta/18}$, 11β-hydroxylase type II	Hydroxylation at C-11 (and C-18)
VI	Dehydrogenase	11β-Hydroxysteroid-dehydrogenase		Conversion cortisol to cortisone
VII	Cytochrome-P450	CYP11B2	Aldosterone synthase	Conversion 11-deoxycorticosterone to aldosterone (and 18-hydroxycorticosterone)
VIII	Dehydrogenase	17-Hydroxysteroid dehydrogenase		Conversion androstenedione to testosterone, estrone to estradiol and reverse
IX	Cytochrome-P450	CYP18	Aromatase	Conversion c-19 steroids (e.g., testosterone, DHEA) to estrogens

[a]See **Figure 3**.

Table 3 Inhibitors of steroidogenesis in the adrenal cortex

Drug	*Principle enzymic site of action*[a]
Aminoglutethimide	CYP11A, cholesterol side-chain cleavage
Metyrapone	CYP11B1, 11 β-hydroxylase
Etomidate	CYP11B1, 11 β-hydroxylase
Trilostane	3 β-hydroxysteroid-dehydrogenase/ isomerase
Ketoconazole	CYP17, 17 α-hydroxylase

[a]Cf. **Table 2**.

ACTH. Under normal conditions, cortisol secretion has a clear diurnal rhythm, paralleling the pattern of ACTH secretion, with an early morning peak and an evening nadir. However, the secretion of ACTH is itself stimulated by all forms of stress, whatever the time of day.

Physiologically, the acute actions of ACTH are as follows: (1) to increase secretion of corticosteroids and (2) to increase blood flow through the gland. Chronically, as well as maintaining elevated glucocorticoid levels, ACTH brings about increased gland weight, which is attributable both to an increase in adrenocortical cell size and to increased blood content. Though also having some effect on cell number *in vivo*, other related pituitary peptides may stimulate adrenal mitogenesis. ACTH is also required to maintain steroid synthetic enzymes, which decline after a few days in the hypophysectomized animal. Adrenocorticotropic hormone is also required to maintain steroid synthetic enzymes which decline after a few days in the hypophysectomized animal. Morphologically, the effects of hypophysectomy on adrenal weight are attributable to the degeneration of the zona fasciculata and zona reticularis, while the zona glomerulosa is comparatively unaffected. In the inner zones, cell numbers decline markedly (through *apoptosis*), and the remaining cells are shrunken because of major decreases in mitochondrial volume and smooth endoplasmic reticulum.

Control of Glomerulosa Function and Aldosterone Secretion

Physiologically, the most important stimuli for aldosterone secretion are altered electrolyte and fluid status (particularly sodium loss) or extracellular fluid volume reduction by hemorrhage, the use of diuretics, and postural changes: aldosterone levels are increased by upright posture. Restriction of dietary sodium intake causes hypertrophy of the zona glomerulosa and elevation of aldosterone secretion, with no concomitant effect on glucocorticoids.

The action of sodium depletion and other physiological stimulation of the zona glomerulosa is attributable to the actions of several stimulants which may act in concert. The renin–angiotensin system is especially important. This mechanism, which becomes more active when sodium intake is decreased (or sodium loss increased) or when blood volume decreases, has as its end-product the formation of a peptide hormone, called angiotensin II, which acts on zona glomerulosa cells to stimulate the secretion of aldosterone. Administered chronically, it can also reproduce the morphological changes in the zona glomerulosa which are associated with sodium depletion.

Other stimulants of aldosterone secretion include ACTH (though only transitorily) and potassium ions, whereas the atrial natriuretic peptides (ANP) cause a decrease in circulating aldosterone concentrations.

There are numerous other factors that stimulate aldosterone secretion and zona glomerulosa function under experimental conditions, although the physiological importance of their actions remains to be clarified. These include serotonin, catecholamines, acetylcholine, vasoactive intestinal peptide, vasopressin, oxytocin, other neuropeptides, and prostaglandin E. Other inhibitors include somatostatin and dopamine.

Control of Adrenal Androgen Secretion

Adrenal androgen secretion [androstenedione and DHEA(S)] rises throughout childhood, paralleling the increase in adrenal size, and peaks just before the onset of puberty in a period that has been termed adrenarche. Secretion of these hormones remains high until 40–50 years of age, when they begin to decline (the *adrenopause*). The mechanism for regulation of adrenal androgen secretion is not completely clear, and although ACTH is a potent stimulant, the secretion of cortisol and the adrenal androgens may be dissociated under some conditions, during adrenarche, for example, when adrenal androgen secretion rises while cortisol is unchanged.

Actions of Corticosteroids

Early in the study of adrenal physiology it was discovered that this gland is essential for life because of the actions of the adrenocortical hormonal products, not those of the medulla. Among the effects of loss of adrenocortical hormones are depletion of sodium ions from the body, decreased blood volume, hypotension, increased plasma potassium levels, muscular weakness, reduced cardiac contractility, and depletion of liver and muscle glycogen together with a generally impaired capacity to respond to physical stress. It was from these beginnings that it became clear that two types of corticosteroid activity were involved. **Table 4** shows the relative glucocorticoid and mineralocorticoid activity *in vivo* of some common steroids, and it can be seen that, in practice, few corticosteroids are completely specific in their effects. Thus cortisol, which normally shows about 1/1000th the mineralocorticoid activity of aldosterone *in vivo*, may have appreciable effects on electrolyte metabolism when plasma levels are elevated as in Cushing's syndrome.

Table 4 Relative glucocorticoid and mineralocorticoid activity of corticosteroids

Steroid	*Mineralocorticoid activity*	*Glucocorticoid activity*
Aldosterone	1	0.15
Cortisol	0.001	1
Deoxycorticosterone	0.03	0.02
Corticosterone	0.004	0.4

Although the hormones were first classified on the basis of their physiological actions, they may also be differentiated on the basis of their binding affinity for tissue receptors. There are two main types of receptor: type I, originally detected in the kidney, was considered to be the mineralocorticoid receptor, and the more widely distributed type II receptor was thought to be responsible for glucocorticoid actions. More recently, with the cloning and characterization of the receptors, an unexpected finding has been that the recombinant mineralocorticoid (type I) receptor does not show the expected steroid specificity *in vitro* since it binds aldosterone and cortisol with equal affinity. As the levels of glucocorticoids in plasma may be up to 1000 times higher than those of aldosterone (**Table 1**), this raises the problem of how a specific mineralocorticoid effect can be exerted in the intact animal. Currently, it is believed that the presence of 11β-hydroxysteroid dehydrogenase type II (cf. **Figure 3a** and **Table 2**) in mineralocorticoid target tissues explains this paradox. The enzyme converts glucocorticoids to their 11-keto derivatives (cortisone and 11-dehydrocorticosterone), which do not bind effectively to the receptor. In this way, the receptor is protected, and cortisol and corticosterone do not cause sodium retention at normal physiological levels. Conversely, the type I enzyme, which catalyses the reverse reaction, thus converting cortisone to cortisol, may enhance local availability of cortisol.

Mineralocorticoid Actions

The main actions of hormones which bind to type I (mineralocorticoid) receptors are to increase the reabsorption of sodium in the kidney and at other secretory epithelial sites, thus reducing the sodium content of urine, sweat, saliva, and so on. Effectively, sodium ions are exchanged for hydrogen and potassium ions, leading to decreased sodium and increased potassium excretion and increased urine acidity. With prolonged mineralocorticoid treatment, extracellular fluid volume expansion occurs, but after a few days the kidney escapes from the mineralocorticoid effect on sodium but not potassium excretion, and thus a major effect of prolonged mineralocorticoid exposure is that body potassium levels are reduced. Hypertension (high blood pressure) is a well-known consequence of excess corticosteroid secretion and is seen in conditions with elevated aldosterone secretion such as Conn's syndrome as well as in conditions of elevated cortisol secretion such as Cushing's syndrome. The mechanisms by which steroids increase blood pressure is not fully understood. In both old age and chronic illness, there is also a dissociation between circulating cortisol and DHEA, with cortisol remaining unchanged, or decreasing, while DHEA secretion declines.

Glucocorticoid Actions

The effects of glucocorticoid receptor activation are varied and complex. Almost all tissues of the body have been found to contain type II receptors and a very large number of systems and processes are affected by these steroids. They are essential for the maintenance of cardiovascular and metabolic homeostasis, particularly during physically stressful conditions. In addition, they play a role in modulating inflammatory and immune responses and affect central nervous system function. In the perinatal period, glucocorticoids are particularly important in controlling lung development and maturation, which may present particular problems in premature infants who have not been sufficiently exposed to glucocorticoid.

The major metabolic effects of glucocorticoids are the stimulation of protein catabolism and hepatic glycogen synthesis. The actions essentially oppose those of insulin and are most evident in the unfed state. General inhibition of protein synthesis may be partly responsible for the inhibition of growth caused by corticosteroid administration to young subjects.

In general, glucorticoids exert powerful suppressive effects on the immune and inflammatory systems, and synthetic glucocorticoids are widely used to control the symptoms of many inflammatory and autoimmune diseases. These effects seem to be produced through the ability of the hormones and drugs to inhibit the production and actions of the cytokines that mediate the responses. Paradoxically, however, it has recently been recognized that endogenous corticosteroids may also augment some aspects of the immune response.

Corticosteroids can freely cross the blood–brain barrier and exert complex effects on behavior. Approximately 70% of patients with Cushing's syndrome are reported to be depressed; in contrast, treatment with exogenous glucocorticoid is commonly associated with improved mental state.

Stress

The relationship between increased adrenocortical activity and stresses of many different types has been known since the 1930s, and levels of cortisol in plasma are frequently measured as an index of stress. However, the mechanisms through which glucocorticoids confer resistance to stress is still debated. There is general agreement that the actions of glucocorticoids in the cardiovascular system which increase vascular reactivity and improve cardiac performance are beneficial under acutely stressful conditions. However, in the past it was often considered that the suppressive effects of glucocorticoids on the inflammatory and immune systems could not be rationalized in the context of protection against stress. More recently it has been suggested that glucocorticoids, by virtue of their ability to suppress the response to infection and injury, may protect against the overreaction of these systems and the risk of excessive vasodilatation, edema, and other damaging effects. The corollary of this is that an inadequate adrenocortical response to stress may be harmful in that defence reactions will proceed unchecked. This may be true of some patients; for example, in active rheumatoid arthritis or, possibly, in chronic fatigue syndrome. In some senses, glucocorticoids appear to regulate defence mechanisms in two opposing ways. In their permissive mode (at levels found in the normal diurnal cycle) the hormones act to prime the body for normal activity, whereas the suppressive effects (at levels found during severe stress) prevent overreaction.

Chronic excess of glucocorticoids also has deleterious effects on the organism. This is most obvious in Cushings syndrome, the symptoms of which include depression, hypertension and cardiovascular disease, osteoporosis, immunosuppression, visceral obesity, insulin resistance, and metabolic abnormalities. It has also been argued that more subtle forms of exposure to increased levels of corticosteroids such as might be experienced in chronic psychosocial stress could increase susceptibility to infection and tumors and be associated with severe depression and aging-related memory impairment.

See Also the Following Articles

Adrenal Medulla; Angiotensin; Corticosteroids and Stress; Cushing's Syndrome, Medical Aspects.

Further Reading

Barnes, P. J. and Adcock, I. (1993). Anti-inflammatory actions of steroid: molecular mechanisms. *Trends in Physiological Science* **14**, 438–441.

Belloni, A. S., Mazzochi, G., Mantero, F. and Nussdorfer, G. (1987). The human adrenal cortex: ultrastructure and base-line morphometric data. *Journal of Submicroscopic Cytology* **19**, 657–658.

Bravo, E. L. (1986). Aldosterone and other adrenal steroids. In: Zanchetti, A. & Tarzi, R. C. (eds.) *Handbook of hypertension: pathophysiology of hypertension-regulatory mechanisms,* (Vol. 8), pp. 603–625. Amsterdam: Elsevier.
Chrousos, G. P. (1995). The hypothalmic-pituitary-adrenal axis and immune-mediated inflammation. *New England Journal of Medicine* **332**(20), 1351–1362.
Chrousos, G. P. and Gold, P. W. (1998). A healthy body in a healthy mind and vice versa: the damaging power of uncontrollable stress. *Journal of Clinical Endocrinology and Metabolism* **83**, 1842–1845.
Flower, R. J. and Rothwell, N. J. (1994). Lipocortin-1: cellular mechanisms and clinical relevance. *Trends in Physiological Science* **15**, 71–76.
Gaillard, R. C. and Al-Damluji, S. (1987). Stress and the pituitary–adrenal axis. *Baillière's Clinical Endocrinology and Metabolism* **1**(2), 319–354.
Holmes, M. C., Yau, J. L., Kotelevtsev, Y., Mullins, J. J. and Seckl, J. R. (2003). 11 Beta-hydroxysteroid dehydrogenases in the brain: two enzymes two roles. *Annals of the New York Academy of Sciences* **1007**, 357–366.
Kino, T. and Chrousos, G. P. (2004). Glucocorticoid and mineralocorticoid receptors and associated diseases. *Essays in Biochemistry* **40**, 137–155.
McEwen, B. S. (1998). Protective and damaging effects of stress mediators. *New England Journal of Medicine* **338**(3), 171–179.
Miller, W. L. and Tyrell, J. B. (1999). The adrenal cortex. In: Felig, P., Baxter, J. D. & Frohman, L. A. (eds.) *Endocrinology and metabolism* (3rd edn., pp. 555–711). New York: McGraw Hill.
Payne, A. H. and Hales, D. B. (2004). Overview of steroidogenic enzymes in the pathway from cholesterol to active steroid hormones. *Endocrine Review* **25**, 947–970.
Seckl, J. R. (2004). Prenatal glucocorticoids and long-term programming. *European Journal of Endocrinology* **3**(Supplement), U49–U62.
Stocco, D. M. (2001). Tracking the role of a star in the sky of the new millennium. *Molecular Endocrinology* **15**, 1245–1254.

Adrenocortical Function, Factors Controlling Development Thereof

T Else and G D Hammer
University of Michigan, Ann Arbor, MI, USA

Glossary

Adrenal steroidogenesis — Process by which steroid hormones are synthesized from the cholesterol precursor. This multistep process involves several enzymes that together form the adrenal steroidogenic pathways of mineralocorticoid (aldosterone), glucocorticoid (cortisol) and androgen (dehydroepiandrosterone [DHEA]) synthesis.

Adrenocortical primordium — Structure within the craniomedial part of the urogenital ridge that harbors the precursor cells for the adrenal cortices. Arises from the adrenogonadal primordium.

Genetically engineered animals — Knockout animals are engineered for loss of a gene. Transgenic animals harbor genetically engineered multiple copies of one gene in their genome. Tissue-specific knockout/transgenic animals are engineered animals that display loss or transgenic gain of a gene in a tissue-specific manner.

Hypothalamus-pituitary-adrenal (HPA) axis — Endocrine stress axis. Higher brain centers control hypothalamic CRH (corticotropin-releasing hormone) release, which in turn leads to the release of ACTH (adrenocorticotropin) from the pituitary corticotroph cells. ACTH stimulates cortisol synthesis and release in the adrenal gland.

Nuclear hormone receptor (NHR) — Family of transcription factors, usually activated by hormone/ligand binding (e.g., estrogen receptor, glucocorticoid receptor). Further members of the NHR family referred to as orphan NHRs, for which a ligand is unknown to date, have been discovered through homology screening.

POMC, ACTH — ACTH is the main tropic pituitary hormone for stimulating adrenal glucocorticoid release. It is derived from a peptide precursor, proopiomelanocortin (POMC), which also gives rise to several other peptides with diverse function, e.g., N-POMC (N-terminal POMC fragment) stimulating adrenocortical cell growth and MSH (melanocyte-stimulating hormone) stimulating skin pigmentation and regulating satiety circuits.

Renin-angiotensin-aldosterone (RAA) system System to regulate body sodium homeostasis and blood pressure. Aldosterone release from the zona glomerulosa cells is regulated by angiotensin II and potassium. Angiotensin II is generated by conversion of angiotensinogen to angiotensin I by renin and subsequent conversion of angiotensin I to angiotensin II by angiotensin-converting enzyme.

Transcription factor Protein factor that influences ([trans] represses or [trans]activates) gene expression through binding to certain response elements within the DNA of a gene promoter or enhancer. Transcription factors can interact with each other and mutually modify their ability to activate or repress gene transcription.

Urogenital ridge Embryonic precursor that is visible as a ridgelike structure on both sides of the dorsal developing body cavity (coelom). The urogenital ridge gives rise to the adrenal cortex, the gonad (testis or ovary), and the kidney.

To serve as the functional end organ of the hypothalamus-pituitary-adrenal (HPA) axis and the renin-angiotensin-aldosterone (RAA) system, the adrenal gland needs to develop into an organ that is capable of responding to specific extrinsic stimuli with the release of different steroid hormones. While the ortholog of the adrenal cortex in lower species, the interrenal organ, consists of intermingled steroidogenic cells within the renal organ, the mammalian adrenal gland is organized into a distinct organ, which is morphologically and functionally zonated. The definitive adult human adrenal cortex comprises three functional zones: the outermost mineralocorticoid-producing zona glomerulosa, the glucocorticoid-secreting zona fasciculata, and the inner zona reticularis, which mainly secretes adrenal androgens.

The regulation of the embryonic development of the adrenal cortex can be divided into three consecutive steps. The first of these is a spatially and temporally regulated program of expression of developmental factors, mainly transcription factors, which induce differentiation and morphological shaping of the adrenogonadal primordium and the later adrenocortical primordium within the urogenital ridge. Second, during late pregnancy functional differentiation becomes increasingly controlled by endocrine factors, secreted by the pituitary (adrenocorticotropin [ACTH] and other proopiomelanocortin [POMC] peptides). The importance of this step is evident in autopsy findings from anencephalic fetuses, in which the adrenal cortex is usually hypoplastic and lacks a sufficient functional zonation. Last, in adult life the adrenal cortex is a dynamic organ, undergoing a constant cell renewal. Steroid output and tissue growth are regulated dynamically to fit the homeostatic needs of the organism.

Development of the Adrenal Cortex: From the Urogenital Ridge to the Definitive Adrenal Gland

The adrenal gland is of mesodermal origin and is a derivative of the urogenital ridge. The ridgelike impression of this precursor organ becomes evident on both sides of the coelomic cavity in the second month of human embryonic development and is mainly formed by the developing mesonephros. Though the actual origin of the earliest adrenal precursor cells is still enigmatic, with recent observations suggesting a contribution of the intermediate mesoderm, classical studies describe a proliferation and condensation of coelomic epithelial cells lining the mesonephros as the earliest event of adrenocorticogenesis. The adrenogonadal primordium can be visualized within the urogenital ridge by positive staining for the common marker steroidogenic factor-1 (SF1). This common structure further gives rise to the adrenocortical and gonadal primordium. At approximately 8 weeks, two different zones can be distinguished in the adrenocortical primordium, the outer definitive and the inner fetal zone. It is not yet established whether this morphological change is caused by a differentiation event of preexisting cells or a distinct migratory event of precursor cells. By the end of the ninth week, the developing adrenal gland becomes encapsulated, and migrating cells of neural crest origin form the precursor cells of the adrenal medulla. The clear demarcation of the two organ structures, cortex and medulla, becomes evident around term, when most of the fetal zone cells undergo apoptosis. Therefore, at birth the human adrenal cortex consists of the derivatives of the definitive zone (zona glomerulosa and zona fasciculata) and a regressing fetal zone. Later in life, at the time of adrenarche, a third zone appears between the zona fasciculata and adrenal medulla, the androgen producing zona reticularis. This zone is unique to primate species.

Notably, defects occurring at particular stages of adrenocortical development can additionally manifest in defective development of other urogenital ridge derived organs, namely, the gonad or kidney.

Transcription Factors Involved in Adrenocortical Development

There is emerging evidence of a myriad of signaling pathways and transcription factors involved in adrenocortical development. As a result of the elucidation of the molecular basis of the genetic disorder cytomegalic adrenal hypoplasia congenita (AHC) and the investigation of several mouse models of disturbed adrenal development, it has become clear that the two orphan nuclear hormone receptors (NHRs), DAX1 (dosage-sensitive sex reversal-adrenal hypoplasia region on the X chromosome) and SF1, can be considered to comprise a central signaling network of adrenal development and differentiation. On the molecular level, there are several functional interactions between these factors that mutually influence their potential for transcriptional regulation as well as their own expression levels.

Steroidogenic Factor-1

SF1 belongs to the NHR superfamily and shares an overall domain homology with other members of this transcription factor family. SF1 harbors a classical zinc finger domain, which enables it to bind to its cognate response element in the promoter of SF1-regulated genes. The two activation function domains (AF-1, AF-2) of SF1 direct interaction with other transcription factors (e.g., WT1, SRY-related HMG box gene 9 [SOX9], GATA-binding protein 4 [GATA-4]), coactivators (e.g., CREB-binding protein [CBP/p300], steroid receptor coactivator 1), and corepressors (e.g., nuclear receptor corepressor [NCoR]). These interactions are dependent on posttranslational modifications such as phosphorylation, through the mitogen-activated protein kinase (MAP kinase) signaling pathway, and sumoylation. In the case of steroidogenic genes, SF1 has been shown to enhance transcription via the cAMP/PKA (cyclic adenosine monophosphate/protein kinase A) and the MAP kinase pathway. The molecular bases of these mechanisms are not well understood.

The recent description of the crystal structure of Sf1 revealed phospholipids in the pocket of the ligand-binding domain. Future experiments need to determine whether binding of these lipid moieties serves as a regulatory mechanism or as a constitutional part of the SF1 complex.

SF1 is a critical determinant of adrenocortical growth and differentiation. SF1 is the earliest marker of the adrenogonadal primordium in the urogenital ridge and is an essential factor for expression of several steroidogenic genes. Mice deficient in Sf1 die perinatally due to adrenal insufficiency and exhibit complete absence of adrenal glands and gonads, loss of pituitary gonadotropes, and absence of the ventromedial hypothalamus. Increased apoptosis can be detected within the adrenal primordium and the genital ridge of *Sf1*$^{-/-}$ mice, outlining the role of SF1 and SF1-induced genes as crucial survival factors for the adrenogonadal primordium.

The importance of Sf1 in murine adrenocortical growth and development has been further underscored by the finding that *Sf1* haploinsufficient mice have a decreased cell number in the adrenal primordium and adult adrenal gland, while the degree of steroidogenic potential per cell is elevated.

Recently, several human patients with mutations in *SF1* have been described. Partially resembling the *Sf1* knockout model, and in accordance with a crucial role of *SF1* in adrenogonadal primordium differentiation, these patients display varying degrees of XY sex reversal and adrenal insufficiency, confirming the essential role of SF1 in growth regulation of the adrenal cortex.

DAX1

DAX1 was initially cloned as the gene responsible for the most common variant of congenital AHC, cytomegalic AHC. Male XY patients with *DAX1* mutations present with hypogonadotropic hypogonadism and adrenal insufficiency. AHC is defined as a hypofunctional adrenal gland composed of a retained cytomegalic (non-regressed) fetal zone and dysfunctional definitive zone. In the adrenogonadal primordium, Dax1 is detectable shortly after Sf1, which induces *DAX1* expression through binding to the *DAX* promoter.

Like SF1, DAX1 belongs to the family of NHR, but represents a rather atypical member of this family, as it contains the conserved ligand-binding domain but lacks the typical zinc finger DNA-binding motif. DAX1 contains three copies of a novel 67- to 69-amino-acid repeat that alternately has been reported to bind DNA or polyadenylated RNA and can therefore regulate gene expression on the transcriptional as well as translational level. DAX1 negatively regulates SF1-mediated gene expression via two main mechanisms. First, DAX1 can directly bind SF1 through one of its N-terminal LXXLL motifs; second, it binds to particular DNA structures in the promoter regions of certain genes, e.g., steroid acute regulatory protein gene (*StAR*). Interaction with the corepressor Alien and NCoR may be partly responsible for DAX1-mediated gene repression.

DAX1 function provides a feedback mechanism for SF1-mediated transcription, because SF1 induces its own repressor (DAX1) and successively inhibits SF1 function. Though there is a significant overlap of *DAX1* and *SF1* expression, not all *DAX1*-expressing cells stain positive for SF1, giving evidence for functions independent of repression of SF1-mediated transactivation. Indeed, DAX1 has been shown to repress the function of several other ligand-activated NHR.

Additional complexity arises from the description of a novel *DAX1* splice variant in human tissue. As a result of splicing to two alternative exons, the *DAX1* gene gives rise to two isoforms: DAX1 and DAX1A. Though DAX1A does not show a high degree of phylogenetic conservancy and its physiological significance has yet to be proven, the occurrence of a C-terminal truncated DAX1 is of special interest, because this isoform has been shown to transcriptionally synergize with SF1 in contrast to the mutual inhibitory effect of the classical DAX1 and SF1.

Other Factors

Several other signaling pathways and transcription factors have been implicated in adrenocortical development. Most of our knowledge about these factors is derived from genetically engineered mouse models and rare human disorders. Depending on the temporal expression of a given transcription factor during adrenocorticogenesis from the urogenital ridge, the formation of additional organs can be compromised. For example, disruption of *Wt1* (Wilms tumor 1) results in a renal and gonadal phenotype, and, on certain mouse strain backgrounds, the absence of the adrenal gland is evident.

Other common developmental pathways, such as the Wnt- or hedgehog-signaling networks, are involved in adrenocortical development as well. Disturbed hedgehog signaling, as in Pallister–Hall syndrome, causes not only skeletal deformation but also a varying degree of adrenal hypoplasia or complete absence of the organ, demonstrating the pleiotropy of these signaling pathways. The Wnt-signaling pathway is of special interest, as its downstream activated transcription factor β-catenin and SF1 can act synergistically to activate gene transcription.

Recent descriptions of knockout mouse models for the transcription factor *Pbx* and the transcriptional cofactor *Cited2* added two animal models displaying absence of the adrenal gland.

Future tissue-specific (adrenal-specific, e.g., *Sf1-Cre*-driven) knockouts of developmental factors will help clarify the complex transcriptional control of adrenocortical development.

Transcriptional Establishment of Adult Adrenocortical Function

The establishment of a fully functional adult organ requires the regulated expression of the various steroidogenic enzymes that generate steroid hormones from the precursor, cholesterol. This is achieved by the activation of tissue-specific transcription factors, e.g., SF1, that orchestrate the activation of steroidogenesis in response to the stress-induced release of tropic hormones, e.g., ACTH or angiotensin. While acute ACTH-mediated steroid output is not dependent on acute transcriptional activation (transcriptional effects occur within hours, while cortisol release occurs within minutes), ACTH signaling induces steroidogenic gene transcription to ensure sufficient steroidogenic potential and ultimate steroid secretion. Expression levels of critical steroidogenic enzymes match the functional needs of the endocrine response. The main ACTH-signaling pathway is the cAMP/PKA pathway, but others have also been shown to be important (e.g., mitogen-activated protein kinase pathways). The transcriptional regulation of steroidogenic genes is outlined with two examples: *StAR*, which encodes a non-zonal-specific mitochondrial cholesterol transporter, and the zone-specific genes encoding CYP11B1, which converts deoxycortisol to cortisol and is predominantly expressed in the zona fasciculata, and CYP11B2, which is specifically expressed in the zona glomerulosa and catalyzes the last step in aldosterone synthesis.

StAR

StAR-mediated cholesterol transport is a rate-limiting event in steroidogenesis and is in great part regulated posttranslationally, e.g., direct protein phosphorylation by PKA. In addition, the transcriptional regulation of *StAR* is an example of tissue-specific as well as dynamically regulated (stress-induced and endocrine-mediated, e.g., ACTH stimulation) gene expression. Tissue specificity is achieved by transcriptional regulation through SF1 and DAX1. In the human promoter, two binding sites for SF1 regulate basal expression of StAR. Through the mutual antagonism of DAX1 and SF1, StAR expression can be downregulated directly by DAX1 interference of SF1-mediated transactivation of the StAR promoter. Furthermore, DAX1 has been shown to directly bind to a hairpin loop and repress transcription independent of SF1. Other basal transcription factors, which in part may play a role in tissue specificity as well as regulating basal transcription, are SP1 and GATA4. Most of the acute induction of human StAR promoter activity is provided by SF1, underlining the importance of SF1 not only for tissue specificity, but also for regulated transactivation upon stimulation with tropic hormones/cAMP. For the mouse StAR promoter, interaction of phosphorylated CREB (cAMP-responsive element binding protein), the classical downstream transcription factor of the cAMP/PKA pathway, with a DNA element in the StAR promoter has also been recently reported.

CYP11B1 and *CYP11B2*

These two enzymes differ considerably in their intra-adrenal expression patterns, in accordance with their functions. *CYP11B1*, an enzyme mainly of the cortisol synthesis pathway, is expressed in the glucocorticoid-secreting zona fasciculata and is, like the *StAR* gene, regulated by SF1. *CYP11B2*, however, as the final enzyme in aldosterone synthesis, is expressed in the mineralocorticoid-secreting zona glomerulosa. Therefore, transcription of this gene needs to be regulated in a zone-specific pattern and needs to respond to angiotensin II and potassium as the main stimuli for mineralocorticoid production. Recently, nerve growth factor-induced clone B (NGFIB) and Nur-related factor 1 (NURR1) have been shown to selectively induce *CYP11B2* transcription. *NURR1* has further been shown to be expressed upon angiotensin and potassium stimulation. Moreover, the expression level of *NURR1* is highest in the zona glomerulosa and decreases in a centripedal pattern. Therefore, NURR1 is an illustrative example of a distinct spatial- and stimuli-dependent transcription factor specific for zona glomerulosa function and mineralocorticoid synthesis within the adrenal gland.

See Also the Following Articles

Adrenal Cortex; Adrenal Insufficiency; Anatomy of the HPA; Angiotensin; Cholesterol and Lipoproteins; Comparative Anatomy and Physiology; Corticosteroids and Stress; Glucocortoids, Overview; Pro-opiomelanocortin (POMC); Steroid Hydroxylases.

Further Reading

Achermann, J. C., Ito, M., et al. (1999). A mutation in the gene encoding steroidogenic factor-1 causes XY sex reversal and adrenal failure in humans. *Nature and Genetics* 22(2), 125–126.

Bardoni, B., Zanaria, E., Guioli, S., et al. (1994). A dosage sensitive locus at chromosome Xp21 is involved in male to female sex reversal. *Nature and Genetics* 7(4), 497–501.

Clipsham, R. and McCabe, E. R. (2003). DAX1 and its network partners: exploring complexity in development. *Molecular Genetics and Metabolism* 80(1–2), 81–120.

Else, T. and Hammer, G. D. (2005). Genetic analysis of adrenal absence: agenesis and aplasia. *Trends in Endocrinology and Metabolism* 16(10), 458–468.

Gallo-Payet, N. and Payet, M. D. (2003). Mechanism of action of ACTH: beyond cAMP. *Microscopy Research and Technique* 61(3), 275–287.

Hammer, G. D. and Ingraham, H. A. (1999). Steroidogenic factor-1: its role in endocrine organ development and differentiation. *Frontiers in Neuroendocrinology* 20(3), 199–223.

Hammer, G. D., Parker, K. L. and Schimmer, B. P. (2005). Minireview: transcriptional regulation of adrenocortical development. *Endocrinology* **146**(3), 1018–1024.

Keegan, C. E. and Hammer, G. D. (2002). Recent insights into organogenesis of the adrenal cortex. *Trends in Endocrinology and Metabolism* 13(5), 200–208.

Lalli, E. and Sassone-Corsi, P. (2003). DAX-1, an unusual orphan receptor at the crossroads of steroidogenic function and sexual differentiation. *Molecular Endocrinology* 17(8), 1445–1453.

Ludbrook, L. M. and Harley, V. R. (2004). Sex determination: a 'window' of DAX1 activity. *Trends in Endocrinology and Metabolism* 15(3), 116–121.

Luo, X., Ikeda, Y. and Parker, K. L. (1994). A cell-specific nuclear receptor is essential for adrenal and gonadal development and sexual differentiation. *Cell* 77(4), 481–490.

McCabe, E. R. (2001). Adrenal hypoplasias and aplasias. In: Scriver, C. R., Beaudet, A. L., Sly, W. S., et al. (eds.) *The metabolic and molecular bases of inherited disease* (Vol. III), pp. 4263–4274. New York: McGraw-Hill.

Mesiano, S. and Jaffe, R. B. (1997). Developmental and functional biology of the primate fetal adrenal cortex. *Endocrinology Reviews* 18(3), 378–403.

Wrobel, K. H. and Suss, F. (1999). On the origin and prenatal development of the bovine adrenal gland. *Anatomy and Embryology (Berlin)* 199(4), 301–318.

Zazopoulos, E., Lalli, E., Stocco, D. M. and Sassone-Corsi, P. (1997). DNA binding and transcriptional repression by DAX-1 blocks steroidogenesis. *Nature* 390(6657), 311–315.

Glucocorticoids, Overview

B E Pearson Murphy
McGill University Health Center, Montreal, PQ, Canada

This is a revised version of the article by B E P Murphy, Encyclopedia of Stress, First edition, volume 2, pp 244–260, © 2000, Elsevier Inc.

Glossary

Glucocorticoids (From Greek γλυκος meaning sweet and Latin *cortex* meaning bark.) Steroids produced by the adrenal cortex which regulate carbohydrate metabolism; however their actions are by no means confined to carbohydrate metabolism.

Steroids Chemicals containing the cyclopentanoperhydrophenanthrene nucleus (**Figure 1**).

Introduction

Chemistry

Structurally glucocorticoids (GCs) are all modifications of corticosterone (**Table 1**). Modifications which enhance activity include the addition of a 17α-hydroxy group (cortisol, **Figure 2**), a Δ1-double bond (prednisolone), a 9α-fluoro (fludrocortisol), a 16α- or 16β-methyl or a 16α-hydroxy group. The 11-keto analogs of these compounds are often included because, although they themselves are biologically inactive, they are readily converted to the active 11-hydroxylated forms. Cortisone, the 11-keto derivative of cortisol, was identified before cortisol, so that for many years cortisol was known as hydrocortisone (i.e., cortisone), with two additional hydrogens giving the 11-hydroxyl group. Oral cortisone and prednisone, the 11-keto analog of prednisolone, are widely used therapeutically since they are about 80% converted to the active forms as they pass through the liver after absorption in the gastrointestinal tract.

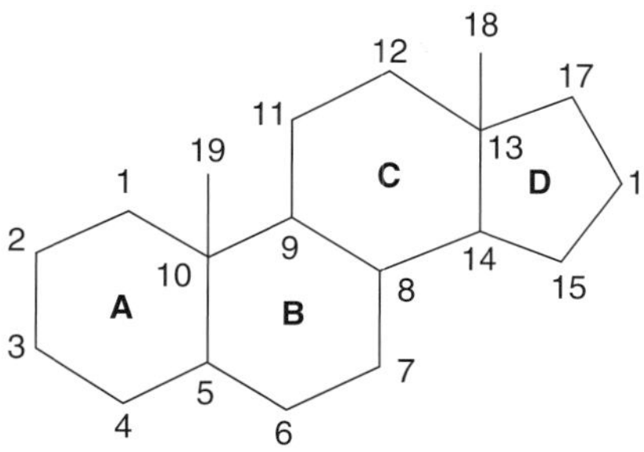

Figure 1 Cyclopentanoperhydrophenanthrene nucleus.

History

In the late 1930s and early 1940s many steroids were isolated from the adrenal cortex of animals and man. Glands from 20 000 cattle were collected to give 1000 kg of tissue from which 25 g of material was further processed to determine more than 30 different steroids, including the GCs and mineralocorticoids.

Evolution

Steroids are present throughout the whole of the biosphere of the Earth, and are thought to be ancient bioregulators, present throughout the plant and animal kingdoms, which evolved prior to the appearance of eukaryotes. They seem to be primordial biomolecules which are among the earliest chemical information transmitters and have had a crucial role in the evolution of life. Even bacteria, viruses, and blue–green algas contain steroids.

Table 1 Modifications of corticosterone to give other glucocorticoids, and their relative potencies in humans

Steroid	*Modification of corticosterone*	*Anti-inflammatory potency*	*Salt-retaining potency*	*LHPA-axis suppression*
Corticosterone	–	0.35	15	
Cortisol	17α-OH	1	1	1
Prednisolone	Δ^1-, 17α-OH	4	0.75	4
Methylprednisolone	6α-methyl-, Δ^1-, 17α-OH	6	0.5	4
Fludrocortisol	9α-fluoro-, 17α-OH	15	280	
Dexamethasone	16α-methyl-, Δ^1-, 9α-fluoro-, 17α-OH	26	<1	17
Betamethasone	16β-methyl-, Δ^1-, 9α-fluoro-, 17α-OH	25	<1	
Triamcinolone	16α-hydroxyl-, Δ^1-, 9α-fluoro-, 17α-OH	5	<1	4

LHPA, limbic-hypothalamic-pituitary-adrenal.

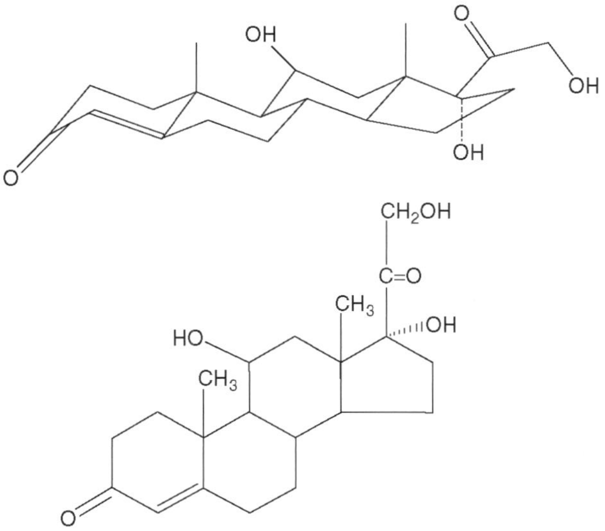

Figure 2 Structure of cortisol. Top: The three-dimensional structure. A dotted line denotes that the C17 OH is below the plane of the molecule, while a straight line, as for the C18- or C19-hydroxyl denotes that the CH_3 is above the plane. Asterisks indicate asymmetric carbon atoms. Bottom: Depicted in the customary fashion and showing numbering of the carbon atoms.

GCs are secreted in all vertebrates, but not in other life forms. In mammals and bony fish, the main GC is cortisol, except in some rodents where it is corticosterone. In birds, reptiles, amphibians, and cartilaginous fish, the main GC is corticosterone.

Binding Proteins

There are two types of binding proteins for steroids: one type which inactivates them, and the other which activates them.

Transport Proteins

Corticosteroid-binding globulin (CBG), present in blood, binds GCs noncovalently in such a way that their biological activity is suppressed; thus it is the unbound or free hormone which is active. These proteins are found in virtually all vertebrates and their specificities for GCs vary; in some cases the binding is very highly specific and can be used to measure the steroid that is bound. They are saturable so that at high levels of GCs, proportionally less is bound. Such proteins are important in the transport of GCs since they prevent undue transfer of the steroid into tissues where it would be subject to enzymatic action and/or degradation. They thus provide a reservoir to damp down rapid changes. In conditions of severe stress, they are reduced. GCs are also bound reversibly and noncovalently to albumin, but this is a nonspecific and loose type of binding.

Glucocorticoid Receptors

Another kind of protein that binds GCs is the GC receptor (GR), which mediates the action of the steroid and is found in or on the target cells for the hormones. This binding is of high affinity and specificity and is saturable. In the nucleus, the hormone-receptor complex is activated and binds to deoxyribonucleic acid (DNA), leading to transcription.

The actions of GCs are mediated by two types of receptors: GRs and mineralocorticoid receptors (MRs). GRs bind GCs but not aldosterone, while MRs bind both GCs and aldosterone, the selectivity of the MRs being dependent upon the presence of 11β-dehydrogenase (particularly in the kidney) to inactivate the GCs. In the hippocampus where MRs are present in high concentrations, GCs serve to activate both.

Biosynthesis

The synthetic pathway appears to be much the same throughout the vertebrates: acetate → cholesterol → pregnenolone → corticosterone and/or cortisol (**Figure 3**). Each step is catalyzed by an enzyme. Some of these enzymes are known to occur also in plants and bacteria.

Steroidogenic tissues can take up low-density lipoprotein cholesterol from the plasma (about 80%), mobilize intracellular cholesteryl ester pools, or synthesize cholesterol *de novo* from acetate. GCs are synthesized from cholesterol by the P450 group of enzymes (oxidative enzymes that have a characteristic 450-nm absorbance maximum when reduced with carbon monoxide). The first step is achieved by $P450_{scc}$, the side-chain cleavage (SCC) enzyme, which cleaves the side chain from the C20 to give pregnenolone. This occurs in the inner mitochondrial membrane. 21-Hydroxylation occurs in the smooth endoplasmic reticulum while 11-hydroxylation occurs in the mitochondrion. In humans, the route to corticosterone and aldosterone production takes place in the adrenal zona glomerulosa while that to cortisol occurs in the zona fasciculata and the reticularis; the 11-hydroxylating enzymes involved differ slightly in the two regions, while the $P450_{C17}$-hydroxylase is lacking in the zona glomerulosa. The $P450_{C17}$ enzyme also cleaves the C20–C21 from C17, giving rise to dehydroepiandrosterone (DHEA) and the adrenal androgen pathway. If the GC pathway is blocked, as in congenital adrenal hyperplasia, this route becomes prominent. DHEA is sulfated in the reticularis to give DHEA sulfate (DHAS), which is quantitatively, though not physiologically, the most important product of the adult adrenal cortex.

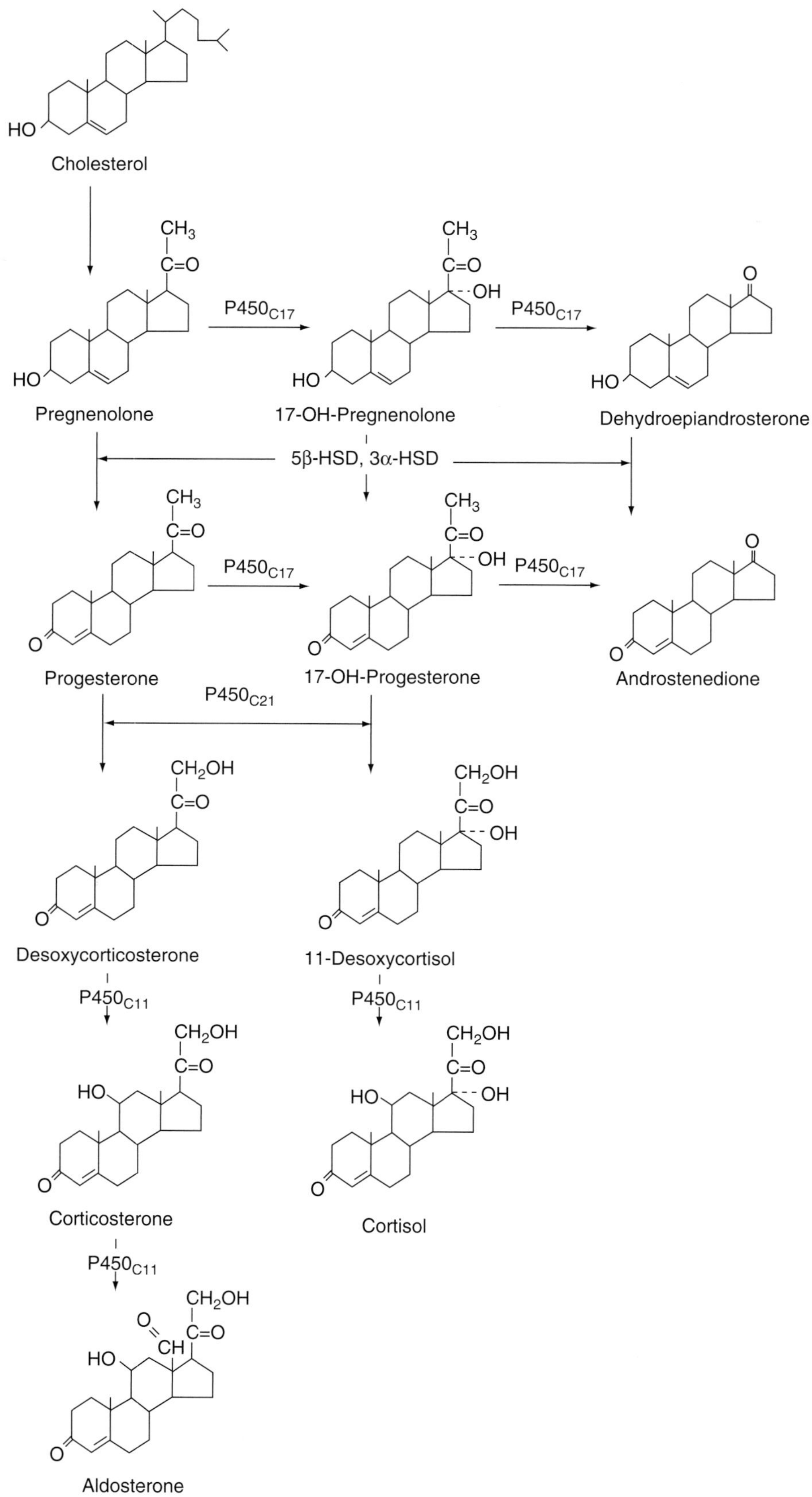

Figure 3 Biosynthesis of adrenal corticosteroids. 3α-HSD, 3α-hydroxysteroid dehydrogenase; 5β-HSD, 5β-hydroxysteroid dehydrogenase.

In fetal primates, the adrenal is relatively much larger than in the adult, and is made up mainly of a fetal zone which is lost at about the time of birth. This zone lacks 3β-hydroxysteroid dehydrogenase isomerase so that the major steroid produced by this zone is DHEA, mainly in the sulfated form. The function of this zone remains speculative.

Actions

GCs are necessary for life and affect every cell of the body. They are thought to enter the cell mainly by passive diffusion, and then bind to the GR. They also act nongenomically at membrane receptors.

Carbohydrate Metabolism

Adrenalectomized animals become hypoglycemic because they cannot maintain their hepatic glycogen stores. GCs activate glycogen synthase and inactivate the phosphorylase which mobilizes glycogen. Although glucagon and epinephrine are also gluconeogenic, they are ineffective in the absence of GCs which act permissively.

GCs enhance gluconeogenesis from protein, thereby raising blood glucose and repleting liver glycogen. This is accomplished by increasing release of glucogenic amino acids from peripheral tissues such as skeletal muscle. GCs also activate gluconeogenic enzymes, including glucose-6-phosphatase and phosphoenolpyruvate carboxykinase. Large amounts result in negative nitrogen balance, and if prolonged, depletion of body protein, observed clinically as thinning of the skin, muscle wasting, myopathy, osteoporosis, and in children, retarded growth.

Fat Metabolism

GCs, administered acutely, activate lipolysis in adipose tissue, so that plasma free fatty acid levels are reduced. However, when given chronically, increased availability of carbohydrate produces an antiketogenic effect, and clinically a redistribution of fat from the extremities to the face and trunk, especially in the supraclavicular and dorsocervical areas, the latter producing the characteristic buffalo hump seen in Cushing's syndrome.

Electrolyte and Water Metabolism

Although much less potent than the mineralocorticoids, GCs in high doses may produce sodium and water retention, hypokalemia, and hypertension. Conversely, in their absence, there is renal sodium wasting, with a concomitant loss of water, hemoconcentration, hyponatremia, and hypovolemia. Hypotension may occur, although this is usually avoided if sufficient mineralocorticoid is present. Vasopressin (VP) is increased and free water clearance is decreased in GC insufficiency, which may help to maintain normal blood pressure. GCs stimulate plasma atrial natriuretic peptide (ANP) production, and potentiate ANP action on the kidney.

Immunologic Function and Inflammation

GCs alter immune responses and inhibit inflammatory reactions. These actions can have both beneficial and deleterious results. While GCs are essential to maintain life in the face of stressors, excessive GCs may cause reactivation of latent infections such as tuberculosis. In contrast, they may benefit autoimmune diseases. A local inflammatory response involves the movement of cells and fluid to the site of inflammation. Histamine, a potent vasodilator, is released at the site, and prostaglandins are involved. Within 4 h after a rise in GCs in response to stress, peripheral lymphocyte and monocyte numbers fall, but granulocytes enter the circulation from lymphatic tissues and sites of inflammation. GCs inhibit synthesis of cytokines, proliferation of monocytes and their differentiation into macrophages; they also inhibit the phagocytic and cytotoxic functions of macrophages.

Effects on Bone and Connective Tissue

If GC excess is prolonged, osteopenia occurs because GCs inhibit osteoblast function – including downregulation of insulin-like growth factor I (IGF-I) which promotes osteoblast proliferation – thereby decreasing new bone formation. Osteoclast numbers and activity are increased. Intestinal calcium absorption is decreased and parathyroid hormone levels are secondarily increased; these effects can be reversed by giving vitamin D and calcium. Renal calcium reabsorption is decreased resulting in an increase in calcium excretion, and which may cause the formation of renal stones.

Since GCs also suppress synthesis of the extracellular matrix components collagen and hyaluronidate, clinically excessive GCs can impair wound healing and make connective tissue more friable, resulting in easy bruisability.

Oral administration of GCs may be associated with symptoms of gastric or duodenal ulcer; possibly this is only apparent, as ulcers caused by other factors, and which would heal if left alone, may become clinically troublesome if wound healing is impaired.

Neuropsychiatric Effects

GCs are released during learning and are necessary for establishment of an enduring memory. However excessive amounts impair spatial learning. Such processes involve the hippocampus.

Cortisol increases brain excitability, and emotional disturbances and even psychoses may occur in states either of deficiency or excess. In states of GC excess – either endogenous as in Cushing's syndrome or exogenous from therapeutic administration – altered behavior has been frequently noted.

Interestingly, in adrenal insufficiency, depression is also common, usually in association with apathy and lethargy; it improves with GC replacement.

The actions of GCs in the brain are mediated both genomically, whereby they enhance transcription, and nongenomically by direct effects on the excitability of neuronal networks, especially in the hippocampus, where GRs are present in the highest density. They can affect many neurotransmitter systems, including noradrenergic, serotonergic, cholinergic, dopamine, and GABAergic activity.

Development

Excessive concentrations of GCs, either endogenous or exogenous, inhibit skeletal growth in children. In the human fetus, the concentrations of circulating and tissue cortisol are kept low by the action of 11β-hydroxysteroid dehydrogenase type 2, which converts cortisol to inactive cortisone in almost all tissues until close to birth.

However GCs are important in stimulating differentiation of many cell types. In lung, they induce surfactant production, which is necessary for infant mammals to adapt to air-breathing at birth. GCs cause differentiation of the neural crest precursor cells of the adrenal medulla to differentiate into chromaffin cells which produce catecholamines.

Metabolism

Steps Involved

The GCs are metabolized primarily in the liver, and are excreted mainly through the kidneys in a series of steps catalyzed by enzymes (**Figure 4** and **Table 2**). These include:

1. Oxidation of the C11-hydroxyl to a ketone – the only reaction which is readily reversible
2. Reduction of the double bond at C4–5 to give 5α- and, mainly 5β-dihydro derivatives – these are almost entirely further reduced at the 3-ketone
3. Reduction of the 3-ketone to give 3α (mainly) and 3β-tetrahydro derivatives, which are in part further reduced at the C20-ketone
4. Reduction of the C20-ketone to give 20α- and (mainly) 20β-derivatives of any of the above compounds, but mainly of the tetrahydro derivatives to give the cortols (retaining the 11β-hydroxyl group) and cortolones (with the 11-ketone group)
5. Cleavage of the side chain of tetrahydrocortisol to give etiocholanolone
6. Oxidation of the 21-OH of the cortols to give the cortolic acids, and of the cortolones to give the cortolonic acids
7. Conjugation of the various metabolites with glucuronic acid (mainly at the 3β-hydroxyl) or sulfate (mainly 3α-hydroxyl), rendering the steroids more water-soluble
8. 6β-Hydroxylation of cortisol to give 6β-hydroxycortisol, also a much more water-soluble steroid

Factors Affecting Hepatic Metabolism

The following factors affect hepatic metabolism.

1. Thyroid hormones influence the rates of metabolism. In hyperthyroidism, metabolism of GCs is accelerated, while the opposite occurs in hypothyroidism. While these changes affect urinary excretion of metabolites, plasma corticoid levels are maintained, owing to the feedback mechanism which remains unaltered
2. In states of GC excess, hydroxylation to 6β-hydroxycortisol increases
3. In old age, corticoid metabolism decreases to some extent, while clearance of glucuronides is decreased; plasma levels usually rise slightly
4. In cirrhosis of the liver, 5-reduction is decreased
5. In obesity, greater amounts of metabolites are excreted, but the plasma levels remain essentially unchanged
6. Various drugs affect metabolism, e.g., rifampin accelerates metabolism, particularly to 6β-hydroxycortisol. Phenytoin, phenobarbital, and mitotane all divert metabolism toward 6β-hydroxycortisol

Extrahepatic Metabolism of Glucocorticoids

The kidney is another important site of metabolism, since its 11β-hydroxysteroid dehydrogenase (type 2) converts cortisol to cortisone, thereby limiting access of cortisol to the MR which binds both aldosterone and cortisol equally. Since aldosterone is present in much smaller amounts than cortisol, this permits aldosterone to exert its physiological action on the receptor. Genetic or pharmacologic alterations in the enzyme may cause mineralocorticoid problems.

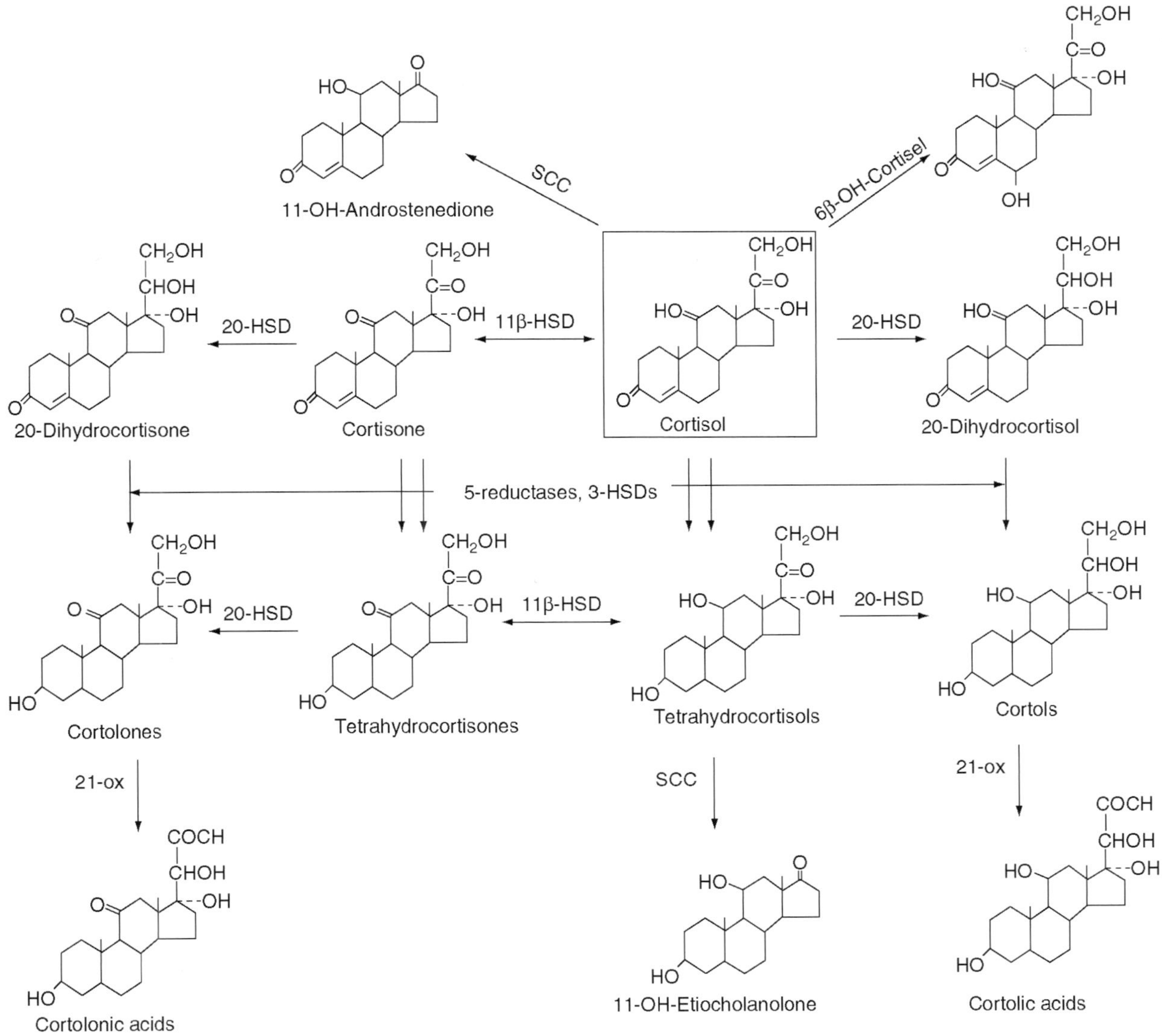

Figure 4 Metabolism of cortisol. HSD, hydroxysteroid dehydrogenase; ox, oxidase; SCC, side-chain cleavage.

Table 2 Cortisol and its metabolites in human urine[a]

Steroid	*Approximate % of total*
Tetrahydrocortisols (5β > 5α; 3α > 3β)	20
Tetrahydrocortisones (5β > 5α; 3α > 3β)	20
Cortolones	20
Cortols	10
Cortolic and cortolonic acids	10
11-OH-etiocholanolone	5
6β-OH-cortisol	1
11-OH-androstenedione	1
Cortisone, conjugated	1
Cortisol, conjugated	1
Cortisone, unconjugated	0.3
Cortisol, unconjugated	0.1

[a]With the possible exception of 6β-hydroxycortisol, all the metabolites occur mainly as conjugates, glucuronides exceeding sulfates.

Absorption

While steroids are generally administered via the oral route, they can be given effectively in many other ways including percutaneous, vaginal, rectal, nasal, and pulmonary, as well as intravenously, subcutaneously, and intramuscularly.

Intravenously administered steroids are diluted throughout the whole blood volume within a few minutes; subcutaneously injected steroids are absorbed within minutes to a few hours; intramuscularly injected steroids are more slowly absorbed, particularly if diluted in a medium which slows absorption, in which case absorption may be delayed for days to weeks. Absorption through skin (especially damaged skin) is rapid – usually detectable 30–100 min after application, and maximal by 16–24 h.

Regulation of Levels of Glucocorticoids

The Limbic-Hypothalamic-Pituitary-Adrenal Axis

Stimuli reaching the brain from extracerebral sites impact on the limbic system, where they are relayed to the hypothalamus, causing stimulation of corticotropin-releasing hormone (CRH) and VP. CRH and VP pass via the portal blood to the pituitary, causing pro-opio-melanocortin to be processed into adrenocorticotropic hormone (ACTH), endorphin, and other peptides, which enter the systemic circulation. ACTH stimulates the adrenal to produce cortisol and/or corticosterone which in turn feed back on GRs in the limbic system (principally the hippocampus and amygdala), hypothalamus, and pituitary to quench the stimulation, thus maintaining an ever-changing but essentially constant equilibrium (**Figure 5**).

Adrenocorticotropin ACTH acts by increasing synthesis of GCs, since adrenal storage of corticoids is minimal. ACTH stimulates the processing of cholesterol to Δ5-pregnenolone, the rate-limiting step in synthesis. It does this by binding to specific cell-surface receptors present on the adrenal cells, which activates adenylate cyclase thereby increasing cyclic adenosine monophosphate (cAMP), in turn activating cAMP-dependent protein kinase and phosphorylation of a number of proteins. If stimulation continues for more than a few minutes, increased synthesis of the various enzymes of the steroidogenic pathway are stimulated, as well as cell growth; if prolonged, the adrenal hypertrophies. Conversely, if ACTH levels fall for a prolonged period of weeks or months, the adrenal atrophies.

Other possible stimulators include direct effects of cytokines on the adrenal cortex and stimulation through neural connections.

Dexamethasone suppression test The dexamethasone-suppression test is often used to assess the suppressibility of the limbic-hypothalamic-pituitary-adrenal (LHPA) axis in humans; most commonly a 1 mg dose is given at bedtime, and blood samples are drawn once or more during the next day. The test is considered normal if the levels fall below 140 nmol l^{-1} (5 μg dl^{-1}, or preferably below 60 nmol l^{-1} (2.2 μg dl^{-1})).

Insulin tolerance test The insulin tolerance test is commonly used to evaluate the integrity of the LHPA axis. It measures the response to hypoglycemia induced by giving an injection of insulin, usually 1 μg, and following glucose and GC levels at 30, 60, and 90 min after injection. With normal CBG levels, the cortisol level should reach at least 500 nmol l^{-1} (18 μg dl^{-1}).

Plasma Levels of Glucocorticoids under Various Conditions

Plasma levels of GCs are generally in the range of 10–1000 nM. They vary diurnally, being highest shortly after awakening, and gradually falling during

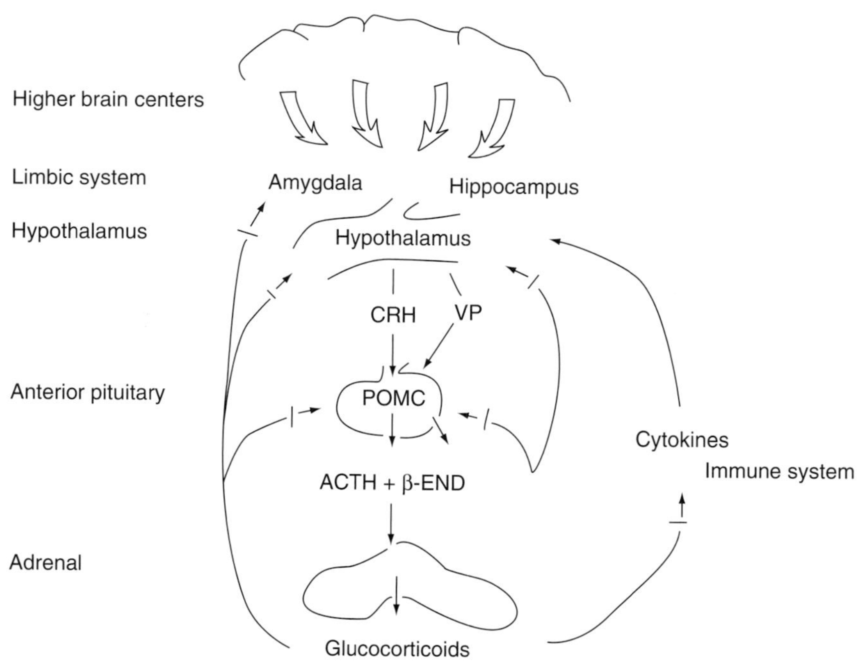

Figure 5 The limbic-hypothalamic-pituitary-adrenal (LHPA) axis. CRH, corticotropin-releasing hormone; VP, vasopressin; POMC, pro-opiomelanocortin; ACTH, adrenocorticotropic hormone; β-END, β-endorphin.

the period of activity (e.g., during the night in rodents, during the day in humans and monkeys). Plasma levels among species vary depending on the affinity and level of their CBG in plasma and of the GRs in the hippocampus, hypothalamus, and pituitary. GCs are also present in red blood cells in appreciable amounts.

In humans in the unstressed state, the plasma level of cortisol is 50–600 nmol l^{-1} during the day, being highest at 6–7 a.m. and lowest at midnight; corticosterone levels are about 10% of these and cortisone levels about 20%. Levels of cortisol in squirrel monkeys are higher at about 3000 nmol l^{-1} although their CBG levels are virtually undetectable. In rats, cortisol is absent, and corticosterone ranges at 50–200 nmol l^{-1}. Levels of corticosterone in fish (e.g., 15–200 nmol l^{-1} in trout) and reptiles are somewhat lower. In salmonids, and many animals, cortisol levels change seasonally, often in conjunction with CBG levels. In stressed animals, the levels of GCs rise within minutes to levels up to 10 or more times the resting levels.

Levels of Glucocorticoids in Other Tissues

GC levels in brain are as high or higher than those of plasma because brain is a fatty tissue and GCs are very fat soluble. GCs are found in all tissues but levels are usually lower than those in plasma and lymph. Levels are low in cerebrospinal fluid because the CBG level is low. They are very high in the adrenal cortex, the site of synthesis.

Cortisol–Cortisone Interconversion

Although in adult humans the level of cortisol greatly exceeds that of cortisone, the reverse is true in fetuses where oxidation by 11β-hydroxydehydrogenase (11β-HSD) greatly exceeds reduction. 11β-HSD consists of two enzymes: type 1 which predominates in adult liver and converts cortisone to cortisol; and type 2 which predominates in adult kidneys, allowing aldosterone to act in the presence of a 100-fold molar excess of circulating cortisol by converting cortisol to cortisone. This type is also high in skin, salivary glands, and nonpregnant uterus.

In the fetus, type 2 predominates in all tissues except liver and intestine. It is particularly high in the placenta, converting maternal cortisol to cortisone, and corticosterone to 11-dehydrocorticosterone. This conversion, which inactivates cortisol and corticosterone, protects the fetus from excessive GCs which would interfere with growth. Type 2 11β-HSD is inhibited by licorice. The same enzyme converts prednisolone to prednisone but does not act on dexamethasone.

The human uterus, though oxidative in the nonpregnant state, becomes strongly reductive in late pregnancy, increasing the cortisol level eightfold so that the membranes are in contact with an environment high in cortisol. This increased cortisol concentration may play an anti-immune role in the uterine wall, the single maternal tissue, apart from maternal blood, in direct contact with fetal tissue.

A similar relationship between corticosterone and its 11-keto analog has also been demonstrated in rodents.

Conditions of Glucocorticoid Excess

Cushing's syndrome In human Cushing's syndrome due to pituitary ACTH-secreting tumors (Cushing's disease), the morning cortisol levels are usually only minimally elevated, but the normal diurnal rhythm is lost so that the 24-h urinary cortisol, which reflects the integrated unbound cortisol level, is elevated. However the suppression of ACTH production by dexamethasone, although attenuated, is usually maintained.

In cases of ectopic ACTH-producing tumors, generally occurring in lung, cortisol levels are usually higher, and are frequently unsuppressed by dexamethasone.

Adrenal tumors cause varying levels of GCs, which are usually unresponsive to dexamethasone suppression, and are often associated with increases of adrenal androgens and/or mineralocorticoids.

Depression is common in Cushing's syndrome, and other behavioral disturbances may occur. In some cases the psychiatric features dominate over the physical features, leading to misdiagnosis. If the condition is successfully treated, either surgically or medically, the psychiatric manifestations usually subside.

Acute stress When an acute stress (threat to homeostasis) is perceived by the brain, impulses to the hypothalamus stimulate the production of CRH and VP, which, through ACTH, stimulate the production of GCs. If the stimulus is prolonged, the axis usually adapts to it over several days, so that ACTH and GCs return to normal.

In rats, it has been shown that the response of GCs to stress in later life can be modified by neonatal handling, which appears to increase the efficiency of the stress response, and to protect the animal from potentially damaging effects of GCs.

Chronic stress Should severe stress be continued for long periods, neurodegeneration or suppressed neurogenesis in the hippocampus occurs. Similar changes also occur after 3 weeks of treatment with a high dose of GCs.

Major depression Increased levels of GCs in major depression (seen in 60–70%) are the best-documented biochemical abnormality in psychiatric disease. There is also a decrease in the diurnal variation and, in about 50%, a resistance to suppression of cortisol by dexamethasone. Major depression is twice as common in women as in men. Although CRH levels are increased, ACTH levels are not increased, so that there appears to be an alteration in adrenal responsiveness which is not understood. These changes are reversed on remission.

Conditions of Glucocorticoid Deficiency

Adrenal insufficiency (Addison's disease) In adrenal insufficiency, first described by Addison in 1855, levels of GCs are low normal or low, and respond poorly or not at all to ACTH. Insufficiency may occur due to destruction of the adrenal cortex (primary), to deficient ACTH secretion (secondary), or to deficient hypothalamic secretion of ACTH secretagogues (tertiary).

Congenital adrenal hyperplasia (genetic defects in cortisol synthesis) Inherited enzymatic defects of GCs synthesis may become manifest in fetal life, the most common being due to lack of the various enzymes involved. In order to maintain adequate GCs levels, ACTH levels are increased to overcome the block, and hypertrophy and hyperplasia of the adrenal cortex occur. Also, due to increased ACTH, synthetic steps which are not blocked produce increased quantities of their products, particularly of precursors of GCs and of adrenal androgens. While males are usually asymptomatic, the excess androgens usually cause ambiguous genitalia in female fetuses. When initially recognized, this syndrome of masculinization of female fetuses associated with enlarged adrenal glands was called the adrenogenital syndrome.

21-Hydroxylase deficiency is the most common defect accounting for 95% of all cases of congenital adrenal hyperplasia and is particularly prevalent among the Yupik Eskimos, where the incidence is 1 in 500 births and the heterozygote frequency is 1 in 11. Milder cases of 21-hydroxylase deficiency are masculinized while more severely affected infants have the salt-losing form, causing hyponatremia, hyperkalemia, acidosis, and dehydration, sometimes leading to vascular collapse. Very mild cases may not become manifest until puberty, when hirsutism becomes prominent. If suspected, this defect can be diagnosed prenatally and treated with small doses of dexamethasone, which crosses the placental barrier (unlike cortisol, which is converted to cortisone in the placenta).

Deficiency of the following enzymes may also occur but is rare: cholesterol desmolase, 3β-hydroxysteroid dehydrogenase/isomerase, 17-hydroxylase, and 11β-hydroxylase.

Measurement

Competitive Protein-Binding Assays

GCs are currently usually measured by competitive protein-binding (CPB, displacement analysis). In this type of assay, the steroid is measured according to its ability to displace a tracer form of itself from a protein which binds it with high affinity and specificity. Such proteins include endogenous plasma proteins (CBGs), endogenous GR proteins, enzymes, or most commonly, antibodies raised to GCs modified to make them antigenic. The sensitivity of such methods is very great (usually a few picograms) and depends on the affinity of the steroid for the protein (usually of the order of $10^9\ M^{-1}$ or greater); thus for plasma only a few microliters of sample is required for the determination of cortisol or corticosterone concentrations. The specificity varies with the binding protein used, with the method of separating bound and free moieties, and with the steroid milieu in which the GCs are being measured. Since no protein is absolutely specific for any single ligand, each method must be carefully validated for the circumstances under which it is being used. The sample to be measured must be freed of any binding proteins that may interfere.

Assays Using Corticosteroid-Binding Globulin

Assays employing CBG were the first such assays to be used for GCs, and were introduced in 1963. Human CBG was the first to be used, but is less specific for cortisol than are dog or horse CBG. Each CBG has its own spectrum of specificity and can be chosen according to the milieu in which the GC is to be measured. These assays have the advantages that the binding properties of the CBG are essentially invariant, so that it is not necessary to determine the specificity or affinity of each batch of protein; also, no preparation beyond dilution is required.

Radioreceptorassays and Radioenzymaticassays

Receptor proteins can be used to measure their ligands, and enzymes can be used to measure their substrates in similar fashion, but are not usually used for GCs.

Radioimmunoassays

Immunoassays have the important advantage that a suitable protein can be raised to virtually any steroid, and since each antibody is slightly different, the most suitable one for the milieu in which the GC is to be measured can be chosen. A disadvantage is that each batch, even from the same animal, may vary with respect to affinity and specificity and must be characterized separately to ensure consistent results. Initially it was thought that the use of monoclonal antibodies might be advantageous but the sensitivity attained is usually less than with polyclonal antibodies.

Although radioactive isotopes have been the most common labels used (hence the term radioimmunoassay), other labels are now available (see below).

Fluorescence Immunoassays

Fluorescence immunoassays employ either a fluorophore label, or utilize enzyme-immunoassays in which substrates are converted to fluorescent endproducts.

Chemiluminescence Immunoassays

Chemiluminescence immunoassays use luminescent compounds which emit light during the course of a chemical reaction, usually enzymatic. Such assays have achieved the highest levels of sensitivity to date.

Determinations in Various Body Fluids

Plasma It is important to suit the method to the purpose. For example, a method which may be adequate for the measurement of cortisol in adult human blood may be, and usually is, entirely unsuitable for its measurement in neonatal or cord blood, which contain many steroids in high concentrations (e.g., progesterone and 17-hydroxyprogesterone) that are not present or are present in only minimal amounts in nonpregnant adult blood.

Urine Similarly, such a method is rarely, if ever, adequate to measure cortisol in urine, where there are very large amounts of competing steroids, so that extra steps such as extraction and chromatography must be performed first. Although the true mean value in human urine was established in 1980 to be about 60 nmol day^{-1}, published values continue to exceed these by a factor of 2–10 throughout the literature, so must be carefully scrutinized.

Saliva In saliva, which is convenient for the taking of samples, and more closely approximates free GCs, it must be taken into consideration that the level of cortisone (at least in humans) may exceed that of cortisol, so may interfere even with an antibody that ostensibly binds cortisone poorly. While saliva does not contain CBG, the salivary glands do contain 11β-hydroxysteroid hydroxylase type 2, which converts about half the cortisol reaching them to cortisone, so that salivary cortisol levels are about 50% of those of unbound plasma cortisol.

Indirect Methods

Prior to the development of CPB assays, GCs were measured by indirect methods. All of these are much less specific and less sensitive than CPB methods. They include fluorescence methods (steroids with an 11-hydroxyl group fluoresce under ultraviolet light in alkali or acid), the measurement of 17-hydroxycorticoids (Porter-Silber chromogens) as an approximation of GCs, the use of tetrazolium salts to measure compounds containing an α-ketol group, 17-ketogenic steroids minus 17-ketosteroids as an approximation of GCs, ultraviolet absorption after chromatography, and double isotope dilution derivative assay.

Antiglucocorticoids

Inhibitors of steroidogenesis

A selection of inhibitors of steroidogenesis is given in Figure 6.

Metyrapone mainly inhibits $P450_{C11}$, preventing 11-desoxycortisol from being hydroxylated at C11 to give cortisol, and 11-desoxycorticosterone from being converted to corticosterone, thereby lowering cortisol, corticosterone, and aldosterone and resulting in excessive amounts of the precursors due to stimulation of ACTH secretion.

Mitotane, which is related to the insecticide DDT (4,4′-(2,2,2-trichloroethane-1,1-diyl)bis(chlorobenzene)), is toxic to adrenal tissue, causing necrosis and hemorrhage. It also affects peripheral metabolism of cortisol, greatly increasing its conversion to 6β-hydroxycortisol

Aminoglutethimide affects GC synthesis in several ways: it inhibits $P450_{scc}$, thus decreasing the conversion of cholesterol to pregnenolone and the production of all the adrenal steroids. Although it may be useful in decreasing hypercortisolism, the blockade is often overridden by increased secretion of ACTH in response to the lowered cortisol levels.

Cyanoketone inhibits 3β-hydroxysteroid dehydrogenase but it is not currently used clinically.

Ketoconazole is an antifungal agent which inhibits $P450_{scc}$ and $P450_{C11}$.

Etomidate is an anesthetic agent and its main effect is on $P450_{C11}$, although it also affects $P450_{scc}$.

Inhibitor of Glucocorticoid Receptor

Mifepristone (RU 486) inhibits GCs production by binding to the GR, and has been used successfully in

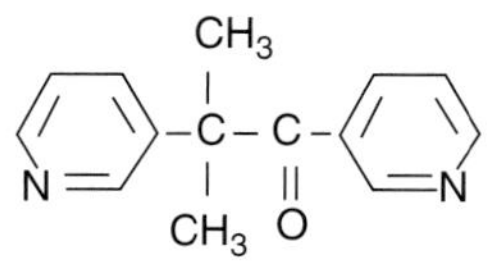

Metyrapone

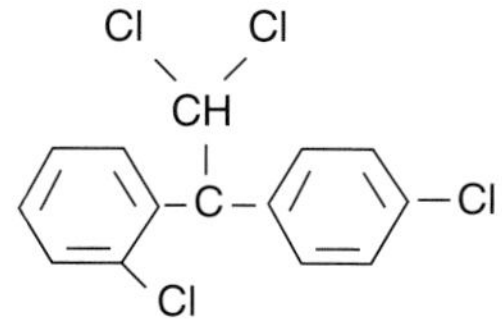

Mitotane (o,p′-DDD)

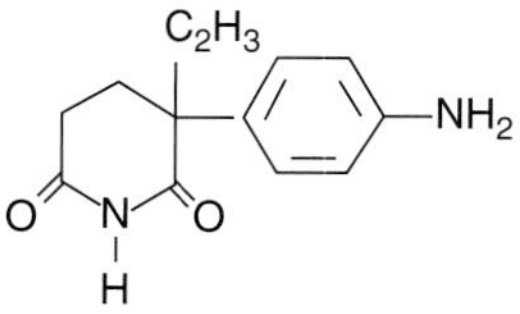

Aminoglutethimide

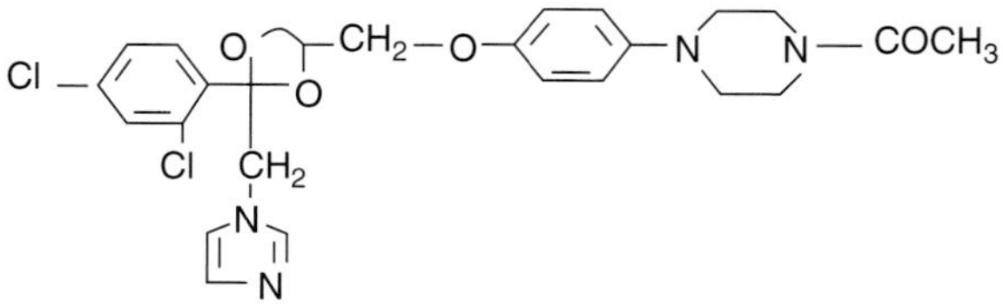

Ketoconazole

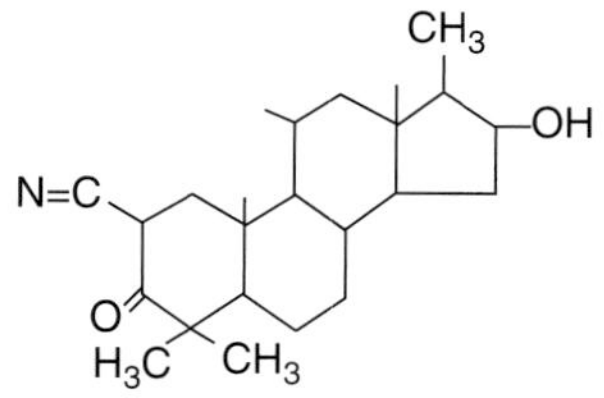

Cyanoketone

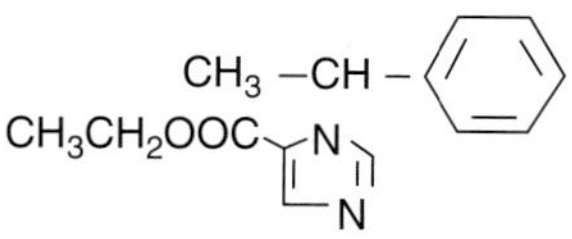

Etomidate

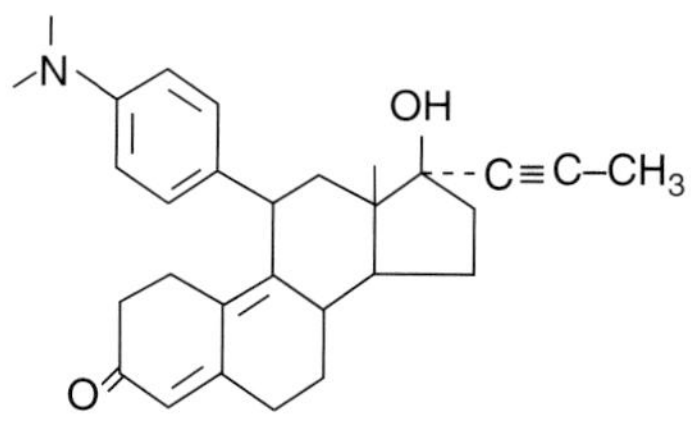

Mifepristone (RU 486)

Figure 6 Structures of selected antiglucocorticoids.

some cases of Cushing's syndrome. As with agents that directly interfere with synthesis, the blockade caused by this receptor inhibitor tends to be overcome by increased production of CRH and ACTH.

Uses of Glucocorticoids and their Inhibitors as Therapeutic Agents

Therapeutic Uses of Glucocorticoids

The first therapeutic use of GCs was that of cortisone by PS Hench and his coworkers in 1949 to treat rheumatoid arthritis. Since then, a great many disorders have been treated using a variety of GCs, including allergic diseases such as asthma and dermatitis, autoimmune diseases such as systemic lupus erythematosis and Graves' ophthalmopathy, and inflammatory disorders such as ulcerative colitis. They have also been used to decrease cerebral edema associated with intracerebral masses, to treat septic shock, and to suppress graft rejection after transplantation of organs.

When GCs are given therapeutically, a feeling of euphoria is commonly experienced, although prolonged use often results in depression, and less often mania, especially if higher doses are used. There is no typical presentation as a variety of mental symptoms is observed, including often irritability, insomnia, obsessive–compulsive behavior, and anxiety. Altered perception, sensory flooding, delusions and hallucinations, delirium, and even frank dementia may occur in about 5% of cases. The time required for mental symptoms to occur on treatment varies from almost immediate to several months, with a median onset of 11 days. These effects are usually largely reversible after reduction of dose or discontinuation of the steroid.

Cortisone itself is inactive but it is rapidly converted to cortisol in the liver. Although the natural GCs are very effective for many purposes, if given in large amounts they have many undesirable side effects, including bloating, hypertension, peptic ulcer, trunkal obesity, osteoporosis, and depression or mania.

Since GCs have so many different biological actions, much effort has been made to develop synthetic GCs that have a particular spectrum of effects deemed desirable but lack other effects deemed undesirable (**Table 1**). Examples are steroids which have strong anti-inflammatory effects but lack the mineralocorticoid effects. The modification of a double bond at C1–2 as in prednisolone (or its cortisone-like 11-keto analog prednisone) increases the GC activity while reducing the mineralocorticoid activity. Addition of a fluorine atom at C9 increases both GC (about 12-fold) and mineralocorticoid (about 25-fold) activity. Including both these modifications and adding a 16α-methyl group gives dexamethasone which has about 30-fold greater GC activity but relatively little mineralocorticoid activity. Since the steroids themselves are relatively insoluble in water, they are often formulated as organic esters such as acetates, which are somewhat more soluble, or as salts such as sodium succinates which are freely soluble.

Although extremely useful, GCs must be used with considerable caution, and preferably for only limited periods, because of their important side effects that can occur with all forms, and include bloating, osteoporosis, trunkal obesity, and other signs and symptoms of GC excess.

One of the most dangerous effects of large doses of GCs, whether natural or synthetic, is suppression of the LHPA axis. This can occur after only a few weeks of high-dose GC therapy and may require several months for recovery to occur. For this reason, therapy is never stopped abruptly but only very slowly so that the organism has time to adjust.

Uses of Antiglucocorticoids as Therapeutic Agents

Inhibitors of steroidogenesis are used to treat conditions of GC excess, including the various forms of Cushing's syndrome, and more recently, major depression. These agents may be effective for short periods, but their effects are often overcome after a few weeks or months by the normal feedback mechanism. In depressed patients, this may be long enough to induce a remission, in which case the levels remain normal after stopping the medication.

See Also the Following Articles

11ß-Hydroxysteroid Dehydrogenases; Corticosteroid Receptors; Corticosteroid-Binding Blobulin (Transcortin); Corticosteroids and Stress; Cushing's Syndrome, Medical Aspects; Gleucocorticoid Negative Feedback; Glucocorticoids, Effects of Stress on; Glucocorticoids – Adverse Effects on the Nervous System; Steroid Hydroxylases.

Further Reading

DeKloet, R. E., Vreugdenhil, E., Oitzl, M. S., et al. (1998). Brain corticosteroid receptor balance in health and disease. *Endocrine Reviews* **19**, 269–301.

Dixon, P. F., Booth, M. and Butler, J. (1967). The corticosteroids. In: Gray, C. H. & Bacharach, A. L. (eds.) *Hormones in blood,* 2nd ed., vol. 2, London: Academic Press.

Ehrhart-Bornstein, M., Hinson, J. P., Bornstein, S. R., et al. (1998). Intraadrenal interactions in the regulation of adrenocortical steroidogenesis. *Endocrine Reviews* **19**, 101–143.

Falkenstein, E., Tillmann, H.-C., Christ, M., et al. (2000). Multiple actions of steroid hormones – a focus on rapid nongenomic effects. *Pharmacological Reviews* **52**, 513–555.

Fieser, L. F. and Fieser, M. (1959). *Steroids.* New York: Reinhold Publishing Corporation.

Meaney, M. J., Mitchell, J. B., Aitken, D. H., et al. (1991). The effects of neonatal handling on the development of the adrenocortical response to stress: implications for neuropathology and cognitive deficits in later life. *Psychoneuroendocrinology* **16**, 85–103.

Murphy, B. E. P. (1967). Some studies of the protein-binding of steroids and their application to the routine micro and ultramicro measurement of various steroids in body fluids by competitive protein-binding radioassay. *Journal of Clinical Endocrinology and Metabolism* **27**, 973–990.

Murphy, B. E. P. and Branchaud, C. L. (1994). The fetal adrenal. In: Tulchinsky, D. & Little, B. (eds.) *Maternal-fetal endocrinology,* 2nd edn., pp. 275–295. Philadelphia: W. B. Saunders.

Murphy, B. E. P., Ghadirian, A. M. and Dhar, V. (1998). Neuroendocrine responses to inhibitors of steroid biosynthesis in patients with major depression resistant to antidepressant therapy. *Canadian Journal of Psychiatry* **43**, 279–286.

Sandor, T. and Mehdi, A. Z. (1979). Steroids and evolution. In: Barrington, E. J. W. (ed.) *Hormones and evolution,* vol. 1, pp. 1–72. New York: Academic Press.

Stewart, P. M. (2003). The adrenal cortex. In: Larsen, P. R., Kronenberg, H. M., Melmed, S., et al. (eds.) *Williams textbook of endocrinology* (10th edn., pp. 491–551). New York: W. B. Saunders.
Westphal, U. (1986). *Steroid-protein interactions II*. New York: Springer-Verlag.
Wild, D. (ed.) (2001). *The immunoassay handbook*, 2nd edn.). New York: Nature Publishing Group.
Wolkowitz, O. M. and Reus, V. I. (1999). Treatment of depression with antiglucocorticoid drugs. *Psychosomatic Medicine* **61**, 698–711.

Corticosteroids and Stress

A Munck
Dartmouth Medical School, Lebanon, NH, USA

This is a revised version of the article by A Munck, Encyclopedia of Stress, First edition, volume 1, pp 570–577, © 2000, Elsevier Inc.

Glossary

11β-Hydroxysteroid dehydrogenase type 2 (11β–HSD2) — An enzyme in mineralocorticoid target cells (e.g., the kidney and some brain cells) that inactivates glucocorticoids, thus allowing aldosterone access to the mineralocorticoid receptors; may also regulate glucocorticoid concentrations in some glucocorticoid target cells.

Adrenocorticotropic hormone (ACTH) — A peptide that controls the synthesis and secretion of glucocorticoids from the adrenal cortex.

Cytokines — Peptide hormones, produced particularly by activated cells of the immune system, that transmit signals between cells and organs via specific cell membrane receptors.

Glucocorticoid receptors (GRs) — Protein molecules with a relatively low-affinity ($K_d \sim 40$ nM) specific binding site for glucocorticoids that are present in the cytoplasm and nucleus of almost all nucleated cells; bind to chromatin and regulate gene expression when activated by ligand binding.

Glucocorticoids (GCs) — Cortisol and corticosterone, the steroidal stress hormones produced by the adrenal cortex under the control of ACTH; they act on almost all nucleated cells, influencing innumerable metabolic and physiological functions. The term also refers to synthetic analogs such as dexamethasone.

Hypothalamic-pituitary-adrenal (HPA) axis — The physiological link between the central nervous system and adrenocortical production of GCs. In response to signals including stress, decreased feedback from GCs, and certain cytokines, the hypothalamus produces the peptides corticotropin releasing hormone and vasopressin, which regulate the pituitary output of ACTH.

Mineralocorticoid receptors (MRs) — Protein molecules with high-affinity ($K_d \sim 2$ nM) specific binding site for aldosterone, cortisol, and corticosterone; present in the cytoplasm and nucleus of the kidney, brain, and some other cells. It binds to chromatin and regulates gene expression when activated by ligand binding.

Mineralocorticoids — Aldosterone, the steroid hormone produced in the adrenal cortex under control of angiotensin II, which stimulates mainly kidney cells to reabsorb sodium and water; also used for the much weaker natural steroid deoxycorticosterone and for synthetic analogs.

Glucocorticoids, Mineralocorticoids, and Stress

Although Thomas Addison's discovery of the essential role of the adrenal gland for survival dates back to the mid-nineteenth century, it was not until the 1930s that Hans Selye promulgated the physiological concept of stress and implicated the hormones of the adrenal cortex in protecting the organism against stress. By then Walter Cannon had established the role of the adrenal medulla and the sympathetic system in fight-or-flight responses, but the adrenal medulla, in contrast to the cortex, is not essential for life. An intimate relation between the adrenal cortex and stress became evident from observations that stress from all kinds of challenges to homeostasis – cold, infection, inflammation, trauma, hypoglycemia, psychological shock, emotional distress, pain, heavy exercise, hemorrhage, and others – stimulates the secretion of adrenocortical hormones and causes hyperplasia of the adrenal cortex. Furthermore, Addisonian patients, adrenalectomized animals, and other adrenally insufficient organisms were the least capable of resisting the sometimes fatal onslaught of stress, but were protected by the administration of adrenocortical extracts.

At first the adrenal cortex was thought to regulate a multitude of effects on metabolism and salt and water balance, along with stress, through a single hormone. Eventually, two principal types of steroid hormones were identified, the GCs and the mineralocorticoids. Each was found to be essential for survival, the mineralocorticoids by controlling electrolyte and water balance, mainly via actions on the kidney, and the GCs by protecting against stress through mechanisms that were to remain obscure for decades. This article discusses the mechanisms by which GCs protect against stress from a modern perspective.

Basal and Stress-Induced Glucocorticoid Levels: Functions in Stress?

As shown schematically in **Figure 1**, basal levels of cortisol in humans and primates (and of corticosterone in rats and mice) vary in a characteristic circadian pattern, rising during sleep to a maximum at the start of the waking period and then subsiding during the active period. Superimposed on this periodicity are erratic spikes in cortisol levels caused by brief episodes of secretion. Stress at any time causes a rapid increase in GC secretion to peak GC levels that may be several times higher than those attained under basal conditions.

Here, we discuss the questions: What role do basal GC levels play in protecting the organism against stress? Is there some significance to the pattern of circadian variation? What role do stress-induced GC levels play? Tentative answers to these questions are already intimated in **Figure 1**. Basal levels of GCs exert mainly permissive actions that prepare or prime some of the organism's homeostatic defense mechanisms for action, reaching a peak of preparedness as the diurnal activities begin. Stress-induced levels probably function mainly to suppress such defense mechanisms in order to prevent them from overshooting and damaging the organism. To answer the questions posed more completely, it is necessary first to survey some of the basic mechanisms and physiological consequences of GC actions.

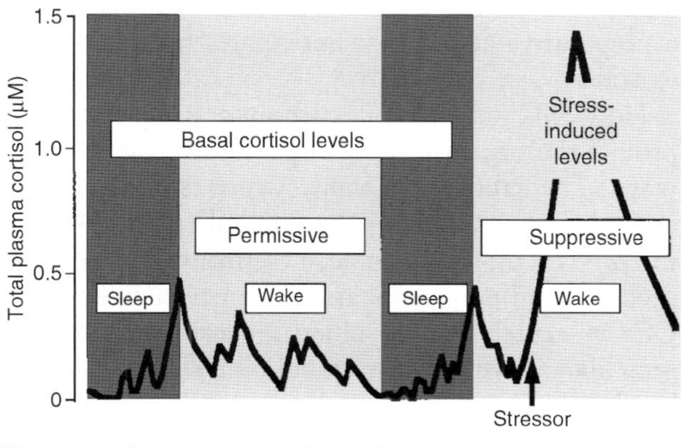

Figure 1 Schematic depiction of diurnal variation of basal cortisol levels in humans and a stress-induced surge. Permissive and suppressive refer to the roles proposed for each of these glucocorticoid regimens in protecting against stress.

Corticosteroid Receptors

The intracellular receptors for the GCs and mineralocorticoids, the GRs and MRs, respectively, were identified during the 1960s and cloned in the 1980s. GRs were characterized by their presence in GC target cells and their ability to specifically bind radioactively labeled cortisol and related GCs. MRs were characterized in mineralocorticoid target tissues by their ability to bind labeled aldosterone. Cortisol and corticosterone, the natural GCs, bind to GRs with dissociation constants in the range of normal GC concentrations in the blood. Similarly, aldosterone binds to MRs with a dissociation constant in the range of normal aldosterone concentrations in the blood, which are 100–1000 times lower than GC concentrations.

In the late 1980s, cortisol and corticosterone were found to bind to MRs with almost the same dissociation constant as aldosterone, that is, with a much higher affinity than to GRs. That posed a major quandary – because GCs would normally be expected to flood mineralocorticoid target cells and saturate MR binding sites, how does aldosterone bind to MRs? The quandary was resolved with the identification in mineralocorticoid target cells of the enzyme 11β–HSD2, which protects the MRs by rapidly inactivating GCs to their 11-keto forms, allowing aldosterone access to MRs. MRs in certain cells are unprotected by 11β–HSD2 and respond to GCs at concentrations far lower than those required to activate the GRs. Some cells in male and female reproductive tracts have 11β–HSD2 that may protect them from excessive levels of GCs.

The role of MRs as mediators of GC actions has been studied most extensively in the central nervous system. Both GRs and MRs are found in the brain and spinal cord, MRs being particularly abundant in the dentate gyrus and pyramidal cells of the hippocampus as well as other regions of the limbic system. There appears to be no 11β–HSD2 in the hippocampus, so hippocampal MRs are bound and activated mainly by GCs. Only the MRs in the anterior hypothalamus and circumventricular organs are protected by 11β–HSD2 and are therefore controlled by aldosterone. GRs are more widely dispersed in the central nervous system than MRs and are present in both neurons and glial cells.

GRs and MRs, when activated by hormone binding, initiate hormone actions by translocating to the nucleus and activating or repressing particular genes. Most GC and mineralocorticoid actions are thought to be produced through such genomic mechanisms, which are relatively slow, usually taking hours to become manifest. There is mounting evidence, however, that certain rapid effects of these and other steroid hormones, particularly in the nervous system, may be mediated by nongenomic effects transmitted through membrane receptors.

Permissive and Suppressive Glucocorticoid Actions

In the 1950s, Dwight Ingle found that adrenalectomized animals can respond normally to moderate stress if administered GCs at basal levels and concluded that, although stress-induced levels are required to protect against severe stress, they may not be necessary for moderate stress. He proposed that basal GC levels have permissive effects that are necessary for some homeostatic functions to respond to stress, distinguishing those effects from the regulatory effects of high GC levels espoused by Selye. Selye had introduced a unified theory of stress and proposed the controversial hypothesis that, by increasing levels of adrenocortical hormones, stress causes such diseases of adaptation as rheumatoid arthritis and allergy.

Permissive actions of the GCs on many defense mechanisms have since been found. They are generally produced by basal levels of GCs and often enhance the actions of such mediators of stress-induced responses as catecholamines and other stress hormones. Permissive actions thus occur during the unstressed periods indicated in **Figure 1** and can be regarded as preparing for a stressful episode. They can account for the substantially improved resistance to moderate stress of organisms lacking adrenocortical function, including Addisonian patients, when given maintenance levels of GCs. Among several mechanisms for permissive actions is the induction by the GCs of receptors for mediators of stress responses. Some other ways GCs are known to increase the sensitivity of signaling pathways are by strengthening coupling of a receptor to G-proteins and by increasing cAMP synthesis.

The suppressive actions of GCs are better known than the permissive actions. They have been extensively investigated because of their close link to the widespread clinical applications of GCs as immunosuppressants, as anti-inflammatory agents, and for treatment of lymphoproliferative diseases. For many years after they were described in 1949, the anti-inflammatory and immunosuppressive actions were regarded as the pharmacological effects of great therapeutic value but no physiological significance. Usually they are manifested at relatively high, stress-induced GC levels. They are exerted through many mechanisms; one mechanism that is fairly general is the suppression of cytokines and other mediators of stress responses.

Metabolic Actions

Early observations that GCs raise and maintain blood glucose levels gave the hormones their name. They also stimulate hepatic glycogen deposition. Long, Katzin, and Fry, in a classic 1940 paper, showed that GCs stimulate gluconeogenesis from amino acids derived from protein catabolism and decrease glucose oxidation. Ingle later found that GCs decrease glucose use and cause insulin resistance. Much work since then has elucidated some of the molecular mechanisms of these and other actions. In the case of gluconeogenesis, there is increased activity of phosphoenolpyruvate carboxykinase and other rate-limiting enzymes. The inhibition of glucose transport and insulin resistance are due to decreased translocation of glucose transporters to the cell membrane and decreased synthesis of insulin receptor substrate-1 (IRS-1). Liver glycogen is increased partly in response to the activation of glycogen synthase. Selye suggested that GCs protect against stress by providing an increased need for glucose. This idea did not survive experimental tests, which showed that glucose alone cannot substitute for GCs.

GCs are permissive for gluconeogenesis and glycogenolysis stimulated by catecholamines and glucagon, reactions that respond to stress in a fight-or-flight situation as well as to insulin-induced hypoglycemia. GC induction of glycogen synthesis can be regarded as a preparative action that anticipates future stressful episodes.

How GC actions on carbohydrate metabolism protect the organism may be viewed in two distinct ways. The ethological view, which considers how evolutionary pressures have molded GC actions for the survival of, for example, a confrontation between predator and prey, emphasizes the permissive role of GCs in acutely raising blood glucose levels to fuel muscular activity. The metabolic view, on the other hand, sees GCs, through their anti-insulin and permissive actions, as protecting the organism from insulin-induced hypoglycemia, as can occur after a meal. GCs share this role with other counterregulatory hormones, catecholamines and glucagon.

Cardiovascular Actions

It has long been known that Addisonian patients, adrenalectomized animals, and other organisms deficient in GCs or GC activity are relatively insensitive to the actions of vasoactive agents such as norepinephrine, vasopressin, and angiotensin II. GCs at basal levels permissively enhance that sensitivity in both vascular and cardiac tissues. These actions may be due partly to the enhancement of α1B and β2 catecholamine receptors and angiotensin II type 1 receptors in smooth muscle cells, as well as increased sensitivity of the G-protein-coupling receptor and adenylyl cyclase. GCs also increase cardiac output, which may be related to induction in cardiocytes of Na,K-ATPase. Despite evidence that GCs suppress catecholamine release, which counters the permissive actions, permissive enhancement clearly predominates in the cardiovascular stress response.

Actions on Electrolyte and Fluid Volume Balance

GC deficiency is associated with decreased ability to excrete water, which at one time was used as a test for GC insufficiency. It appears to be due to a decreased rate in glomerular filtration and an increased synthesis of vasopressin (VP), both of which are reversed by administered GCs. The underlying mechanisms are not known, but they may be related to the glucocorticoid-induced synthesis and secretion of atrial natriuretic peptide (ANP) and increased levels of ANP receptors on endothelial cells. The inhibition of VP synthesis is part of the negative feedback mechanism by which GCs regulate their own concentration and appears to be due to the decreased synthesis of VP.

Some of these actions are central to the role of GCs in stress. In rats, the stress of hemorrhage has been found to elicit a powerful vasoconstrictor response from VP, catecholamines, and renin. Without GCs, the VP response can overshoot, leading to ischemia and death in adrenalectomized animals. Stress-induced GCs protect the organism by limiting the increase in VP levels and hence the ischemia.

Anti-inflammatory and Immunosuppressive Actions

High levels of GCs suppress many functions. The inflammatory and immune systems are among those in which suppressive actions are most pronounced. Thymus enlargement in the absence of the adrenal cortex was recognized before 1900. Selye showed that stress causes thymus atrophy, a GC action now known to be due to the induction of lymphocyte apoptosis.

The anti-inflammatory actions of GCs, which account for most clinical applications of these hormones, were reported in 1949 by Hench, Kendall, Slocumb, and Polley, who found that treatment with GCs dramatically improved the symptoms of patients with rheumatoid arthritis. These observations had two unexpected consequences: (1) they contradicted Selye's hypothesis of diseases of adaptation, which rapidly lost support, and (2) GC physiologists were unable to reconcile the finding that GCs suppressed a defense mechanism, in this case inflammation, with their longstanding belief that stress-induced GC levels helped resist stress by enhancing activity of defense mechanisms. Despite an alternative view proposed by Marius Tausk (in a 1951 review that unfortunately had very limited circulation), physiologists categorized the anti-inflammatory actions as the pharmacological consequences of high unphysiological levels of GCs. The closely related immunosuppressive actions suffered the same fate. As a result, the spectacular development of new applications and synthetic analogs for GCs, the miracle drugs of the 1950s, proceeded with little or no involvement by GC physiologists.

The view advanced in germinal form by Marius Tausk in the context of GC therapy was revived independently in 1984 in the context of GC physiology. It held that the anti-inflammatory and immunosuppressive actions of GCs, far from being pharmacological, are prototypes for the physiological role of stress-induced GCs in stress – that role is to prevent stress-induced defense reactions from overshooting and harming the organism.

A great deal of evidence now supports the view that anti-inflammatory and immunosuppressive actions are physiological and are exerted by endogenous GCs. In rats, for example, adrenalectomy or administration of the glucocorticoid antagonist RU486 increases inflammatory responses, showing that endogenous GCs can control inflammation. Autoimmune reactions are also under the control of endogenous GCs. Striking experiments have shown that Lewis rats, which are extremely sensitive to arthritis after injection with streptococcal cell wall polysaccharide (SCW) and to experimental allergic encephalomyelitis (EAE) after injection with myelin basic protein, have a defect in biosynthesis of corticotropin releasing hormone (CRH), the hypothalamic hormone that, along with VP stimulates ACTH, is released by the pituitary. That defect reduces the ACTH, and hence the GC, response to an antigenic challenge. As expected, treatment with GCs protects Lewis rats from SCW.

GCs may also influence immune responses through permissive actions. For example, mitogenic responses of rat peripheral or splenic T cells in culture are reduced if the rats have been adrenalectomized. The responses can be restored by treating the rats with low physiological doses of corticosterone, as well as by brief exposure of the cells to low concentrations of corticosterone or aldosterone. These observations led to the suggestion that the permissive effects in this case were mediated by MRs, and possibly involve induction of interleukin (IL)-2 receptors. The acute phase response is a case in which GCs both potentiate the induction of acute phase proteins by cytokines such as IL-1 and IL-6 and suppress the production of the cytokines.

The permissive actions of GCs at stress-induced levels were revealed by experiments in which normal humans were given an endotoxin to stimulate increases in plasma tumor necrosis factor (TNF)-α and IL-6. At various times before or after the endotoxin, cortisol was infused at rates that gave stress-induced levels. When given within 6 h of the endotoxin, cortisol suppressed the cytokine response, but, when given 12, 32, 72, or 144 h before endotoxin, cortisol markedly enhanced the response.

Actions on the Central Nervous System

Electrophysiological experiments have been conducted with hippocampal tissue isolated from adrenalectomized rats and treated with GCs at various concentrations. Low concentrations of corticosterone, which mainly activate the MRs, were found to decrease after hyperpolarization of the neuronal membranes and enhance neuronal excitability, whereas high concentrations of corticosterone, or specific glucocorticoid agonists that activate the GRs but not MRs, suppressed excitability. Thus, GCs at low concentrations, corresponding to basal levels, permissively maintain neuronal excitability via the MRs, whereas GCs at high concentrations, corresponding to stress-induced levels, suppress stimulated neuronal activity via the GRs.

Effects via Cytokines and Other Mediators

As already indicated, suppressive actions of GCs are often due to the inhibition of production or activity of cytokines, the hormones of the immune system, and of other mediators. Such mediators constitute a communications network between cells of defense systems that respond to stress-induced challenges. Stress-induced mediators known to be suppressed by GCs are listed in **Table 1**. Neurotransmitters, such as the catecholamines, respond to sudden fight-or-flight challenges; inflammatory agents respond to tissue damage; cytokines and chemokines respond to infection and inflammation; and so on. Mediators are essential for propagating stress responses. By blocking them, GCs can dampen the stress responses, preventing them from overshooting and damaging the organism. At the same time, GCs also protect the organism from toxicity of most of these mediators when they are present in excess.

Many well-known GC effects on cell traffic may be initiated through the inhibition of chemokines (also known as chemotactic cytokines), which regulate the traffic and homing of leukocytes by binding to cell-surface receptors and which are actively secreted during inflammation. Some mediators are suppressed by GCs under some conditions and stimulated under

Table 1 Effects of glucocorticoids on mediators and mediator receptors[a]

	Mediators suppressed	*Mediators suppressed/ stimulated*[b]	*Mediator receptors induced*
Cytokines	IL-1, IL-2, IL-3, IL-5, IL-6, IL-11, IL-12, IL-16, IFN-γ, TNF-α, GM-CSF	IL-4, IL-10, TGF-β	IL-1, IL-2, IL-4, IL-6, IFN-γ, GM-CSF
Chemokines	IL-8, MCP-1, RANTES, MIP-1α, CINC/gro, LIX, SCF		
Inflammatory agents	5-HT, bradykinin, histamine, eicosanoids, Cox-2, collagenase, elastase, MMP-9, plasminogen activator		5-HT
Hormones and neurotransmitters	ACTH, CRH, VP, oxytocin, β-endorphin, LH, insulin, norepinephrine, nitric oxide, substance P	Epinephrine	CRH, VP, insulin, norepinephrine
Cell adhesion molecules	ICAM-1, LFA-1, e-selectin ELAM-1		

[a]5-HT, serotinin; ACTH, adrenocorticotropic hormone; CINC/gro, cytokine-induced neutrophil chromoattractant/growth-induced gene product; Cox, cyclo-oxygenase; CRH, corticotropin releasing hormone; ELAM, enothelial-leukocyte adhesion molecule; GM-CSF, granulocyte macrophage colony stimulating factor; ICAM, intercellular adhesion molecule; IFN, interferon; IL, interleukin; LFA, lymphocyte function-associated antigen; LIX, lipopolysaccharide-induced CXC chemokine; MCP, monocyte chemoattractant protein; MIP, macrophage inflammatory protein; MMP, matrix metalloproteinase; RANTES, regulated on activation, normal T-cell-expressed and secreted; SCF, stem-cell factor; TGF, tumor growth factor; TNF, tumor necrosis factor; VP, vasopressin.
[b]Mediators suppressed by GCs under some conditions and stimulated under others.

others. There are also mediators, such macrophage colony stimulating factor (M-CSF), that appear not to be affected by GCs at all.

Table 1 lists several mediators that have receptors that are induced by GCs. The possibility that the induction of mediator receptors accounts for some permissive actions has already been noted. Some cytokines, such as IL-1 and IL-6, not only communicate between cells of the immune and inflammatory systems, but also, as first proposed be Besedovsky and Sorkin, may signal the HPA system that the immune system is activated, thereby constituting a negative feedback loop through which GCs are summoned to control activated immune reactions.

Unified View of the Protective Roles of Glucocorticoids in Stress

As described so far, GCs exert actions that are predominantly permissive on the cardiovascular system; that are mainly suppressive on other systems, such as inflammation; and that are both permissive and suppressive on still other systems, such as the neural and immune systems. How are these opposing influences reconciled when both are present, with one enhancing and the other suppressing the defense response? This question can be analyzed with a simple but fairly realistic model in which suppressive actions are assumed to be due to the reduction in the concentration of a mediator and permissive actions are due to the induction of the mediator's receptors, as illustrated in **Figure 2**.

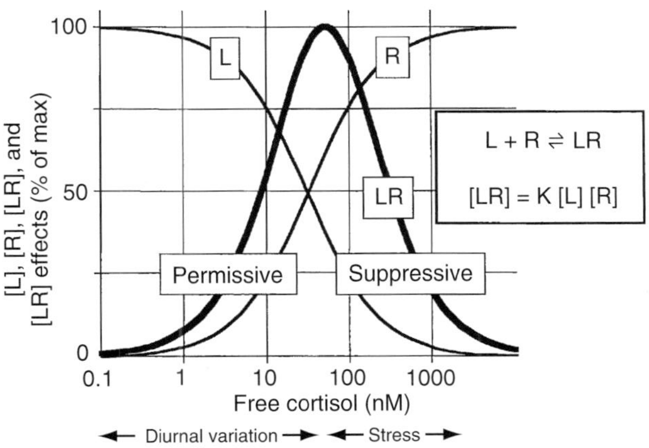

Figure 2 Model of a cortisol-regulated lymphokine system. Cortisol is assumed to permissively increase the concentration of lymphokine receptors (R) and to suppress the concentration of the lymphokine (L), according to dose–response curves that correspond to binding of cortisol to GRs with a dissociation constant of 30 nM. The concentration and activity of the lymphokine–receptor complex (LR) is determined by the equations in the inset, yielding the bell-shaped curve with a rising permissive branch at basal cortisol concentrations and a falling suppressive branch at stress-induced concentrations. Brackets denote concentration. Below the cortisol concentration scale the ranges covered during basal diurnal variation and stress are indicated roughly.

In **Figure 2**, a lymphokine receptor (R) is permissively induced by cortisol over a concentration range corresponding roughly to that in **Figure 1** (keeping in mind that at low cortisol concentrations less than 10% of total cortisol is free), following a dose–response curve chosen to parallel the binding of cortisol to GRs. Lymphokine (L) is suppressed according to an identical dose–response curve of opposite sign. Through these actions, cortisol regulates the concentration of the lymphokine–receptor complex (LR), as determined by the equations in the inset. The bell-shaped curve for LR and LR activity is, then, a composite dose–response curve that represents schematically the outcome of permissive and suppressive GC actions on the hypothetical defense mechanism that the lymphokine regulates (the simple curves for R and L represent the outcome for defense mechanisms subject to pure permissive and suppressive actions, respectively).

This model assumes that both permissive and suppressive actions are mediated by GRs. If permissive actions were mediated by MRs, the dose–response curve for induction of R and the ascending limb of the bell-shaped curve would be shifted to the left, as would the peak of the bell-shaped curve; similar qualitative conclusions would apply, however.

It should be evident that any permissive and suppressive actions with roughly comparable dose–response curves, whether transmitted via a lymphokine or other mechanism, will yield similar bell-shaped curves. Such curves correspond well with the physiological roles of GCs we have sketched earlier. Basal GC concentrations fluctuate during normal diurnal variation from the left end of the cortisol scale in **Figure 2** to approximately where the bell-shaped curve peaks and can be viewed as permissively priming some of the organism's defense mechanisms in preparation for a period of activity. Suppressive actions are present at all cortisol concentrations, but they predominate only at high stress-induced levels toward the right end of the cortisol scale, where they are required to prevent defense mechanisms from overshooting. In the absence of GCs, an organism may succumb to stress either because its defense mechanisms are not adequately primed (perhaps what happens in Addisonian crisis if the cardiovascular system cannot respond) or because the defense mechanisms overshoot (as occurred in the examples cited earlier after hemorrhage or an inflammatory challenge), depending on the nature of the stressor.

Thus, in summary, GCs can be thought of as protecting the organism from stress through two separate but related mechanisms. First, they are essential before a stressful episode to permissively prime certain defense mechanisms, a task generally accomplished by basal GC levels. Second, they are essential after a stressor to prevent some defense mechanisms from overshooting, a task generally requiring stress-induced GC levels.

Further Reading

Besedovsky, H. O. and del Rey, A. (1996). Immuno-neuro-endocrine interactions: facts and hypotheses. *Endocrine Review* **17**, 64–102.

de Kloet, R. E. (2003). Hormones, brain and stress. *Endocrine Regulation* **37**, 51–68.

Ingle, D. J. (1954). Permissibility of hormone action: a review. *Acta Endocrinologica* **17**, 172–186.

Makara, G. B. and Haller, J. (2001). Non-genomic effects of glucocorticoids in the neural system: evidence, mechanisms and implications. *Progress in Neurobiology* **65**, 367–390.

Munck, A., Guyre, P. M. and Holbrook, N. J. (1984). Physiological functions of glucocorticoids in stress and their relation to pharmacological actions. *Endocrine Review* **5**, 25–44.

Reichardt, H. M., Umland, T., Bauer, A., et al. (2000). Mice with an increased glucocorticoid receptor gene dosage show enhanced resistance to stress and endotoxic shock. *Molecular and Cellular Biology* **20**, 9009–9017.

Sapolsky, R. M., Romero, L. M. and Munck, A. (2000). How do glucocorticoids influence stress responses? integrating permissive, suppressive, stimulatory, and preparative actions. *Endocrine Review* **21**, 55–89.

Selye, H. (1946). The general adaptation syndrome and the diseases of adaptation. *Journal of Clinical Endocrinology and Metabolism* **6**, 117–230.

Sternberg, E. M., Young, S. W., III, Bernardini, R., et al. (1989). A central nervous system defect in biosynthesis of corticotropin-releasing hormone is associated with susceptibility to streptococcal cell wall-induced arthritis in Lewis rats. *Proceedings of the National Academy of Sciences USA* **86**, 4771–4775.

Tausk, M. (1951). Hat die Nebenniere tatsächlich eine Verteidigungsfunktion? *Das Hormon* (Organon, Holland) **3**, 1–24.

Webster, J. I., Tonelli, L. and Sternberg, E. M. (2002). Neuroendocrine regulation of immunity. *Annual Review of Immunology* **20**, 125–163.

Wiegers, G. J., Labeur, M. S., Stec, I. E. M., et al. (1995). Glucocorticoids accelerate anti-T cell receptor-induced T cell growth. *Journal of Immunology* **155**, 1893–1902.

Glucocorticoids, Effects of Stress on

J C Buckingham
Imperial College School of Medicine, London, UK

This article is reproduced from Encyclopedia of Stress, First edition, volume 2, pp 229–237, © 2000, Elsevier Inc.

Glossary

Hypothalamo–hypophysial portal vessels — A specialized portal blood system responsible for the transportation of neurohormones (termed releasing hormones) from the median eminence area of the hypothalamus to the anterior pituitary gland.

Paraventricular nuclei (PVNs) — Specialized areas of the hypothalamus lying on either side of the third ventricle; these nuclei include the cell bodies of neurons that project to the median eminence area of the hypothalamus, and they play a key role in initiating the pituitary-adrenal response to stress.

The glucocorticoids (cortisol and/or corticosterone, depending on the species) are steroid hormones produced by cells in the zona fasciculata of the adrenal cortex under the influence of the hypothalamic-pituitary complex (**Figure 1**). They exert diverse actions in the body and thereby play a key role in the regulation of crucial homeostatic mechanisms, such as those concerned with metabolic control and immune/inflammatory responses. The actions of the steroids are effected intracellularly, mainly via glucocorticoid receptors (GRs) but also via mineralocorticoid receptors (MRs). In normal circumstances, the rate of glucocorticoid secretion is maintained within narrow limits, varying according to a circadian rhythm that is coupled to the sleep–wake cycle; serum levels of the steroids are thus normally maximal at the end of the sleep phase and fall to a nadir some hours after waking. However, glucocorticoid secretion is increased markedly in conditions of physical and emotional stress; hence, the glucocorticoids are frequently termed stress hormones. The stress-induced changes in circulating glucocorticoids are superimposed on the existing circadian tone and vary in their rate of onset, magnitude, and duration according to the nature, duration, and intensity of the insult. Significant

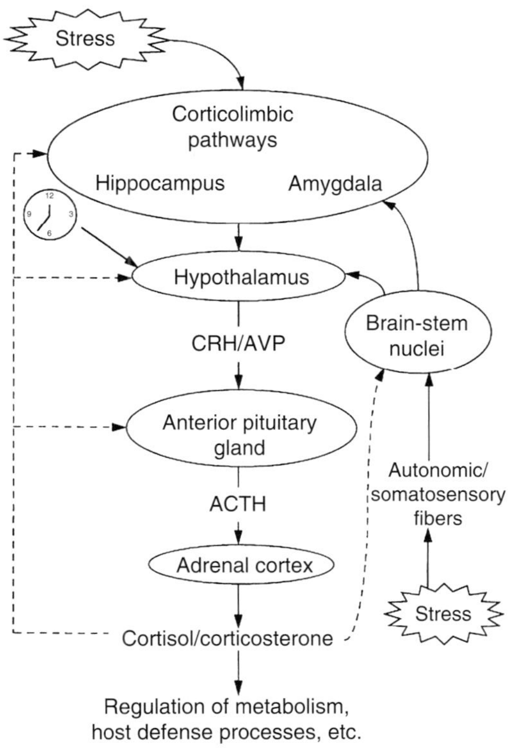

Figure 1 The hypothalamic-pituitary-adrenal axis. Dotted lines indicate inhibitory influences; intact lines indicate stimulatory influences; the clock indicates circadian influences. ACTH, adrenocorticotropic hormone; AVP, arginine vasopressin; CRH, corticotropin releasing hormone.

interspecies variations also occur; for example, humans are particularly sensitive to emotional trauma, whereas rats respond very readily to physical stimuli such as cold and pigs are relatively unresponsive to many stimuli (e.g., histamine and cold) but show a marked elevation in serum cortisol when deprived of food.

Mechanisms Controlling Glucocorticoid Secretion in Stress

The Hypothalamic-Pituitary-Adrenocortical Axis

The release of the glucocorticoids in stress is orchestrated mainly by the hypothalamus, which receives and integrates neural and humoral information from many sources and initiates the release of two neurohormones, termed corticotropin releasing hormone (CRH) and arginine vasopressin (AVP), into the hypothalamo-hypophysial portal vessels. These peptides are transported to the anterior pituitary gland via the portal vessels, where they act synergistically to cause the release of adrenocorticotropic hormone (ACTH), which, in turn, stimulates cortisol/corticosterone secretion. The hypothalamus thus provides a vital link between the perception of physical and emotional stress and the regulation of key homeostatic mechanisms. The responsivity of the hypothalamic-pituitary-adrenocortical (HPA) axis to incoming stimuli is modulated by a servo system through which the sequential release of CRH/AVP and ACTH from the hypothalamus and anterior pituitary gland, respectively, is regulated negatively by the glucocorticoids themselves (**Figure 1**); the magnitude of the HPA response to stress thus depends on the preexisting glucocorticoid tone.

Adrenocorticotropic Hormone and Steroidogenesis

Cortisol and corticosterone are not stored to any great degree in the adrenal cortex but are synthesized on demand and promptly pass by diffusion across the cell membrane into the systemic circulation. The primary trigger for the synthesis of the steroids is ACTH, a polypeptide hormone produced by a specialized subgroup of cells in the anterior pituitary gland, the corticotrophs. ACTH acts via specific membrane-bound receptors, termed type 2 melanocortin (MC2) receptors, to activate the rate-limiting enzyme in the steroidogenic pathway; it thus causes the conversion of cholesterol to pregnenolone, from which cortisol and corticosterone are formed rapidly. In addition, ACTH acts on the vasculature to increase adrenal blood flow and thereby aid the passage of the newly synthesized steroids out of the cells and into the general systemic circulation. Increases in circulating glucocorticoids may be apparent within 10 min of the onset of the stress, although, in some instances (e.g., following an immune insult) the response may be delayed. Approximately 95% of cortisol/corticosterone in blood is protein bound, mainly to a specific high-affinity corticosteroid-binding globulin (CBG) but also to albumin, which has a lower affinity for the steroids. In principle, only the free steroid has ready access to the corticosteroid receptors (GRs and MRs), which are located intracellularly in the target cells. However, local mechanisms that release the steroid from its carrier protein(s) appear to exist in at least some target tissues; these include (1) interactions of the carrier protein with cell surface CBG receptors and (2) enzymatic cleavage of CBG (e.g., by serine proteases in inflamed tissues), a process that lowers the affinity of the binding protein for the steroids. The access of the steroids to their receptors is further regulated within the target cells by 11β-hydroxysteroid dehydrogenase (11β-HSD) enzymes, which control the interconversion of cortisol and corticosterone to their inactive counterparts, cortisone and 11-dehydrocorticosterone. The biochemical half-life of the steroids is approximately 90 min, but the biological effects may be sustained for very much longer. Metabolism is hepatic and the resulting metabolites are conjugated and excreted in the bile and the urine.

Synthesis and Secretion of Adrenocorticotropic Hormone

ACTH is synthesized in the corticotrophs by the posttranslational cleavage of a large precursor molecule, proopiomelanocortin (POMC). POMC also gives rise to a number of other peptides that are coreleased with ACTH and are termed collectively ACTH-related or POMC peptides. These include an N-terminal peptide, N-POMC(1–76), of unknown function and β-lipotropin (β-LPH), which, in turn, may be partially degraded to β-endorphin (which is sometimes used as a marker of ACTH secretion) and γ-LPH. In some circumstances (e.g., adrenal insufficiency), more extensive N-terminal processing may occur, either within the pituitary gland or at the adrenal level, generating peptides that appear to augment the steroidogenic capacity of the adrenal cortex by potentiating the steroidogenic response to ACTH (γ-melanocyte-stimulating hormone) or enhancing adrenocortical mitogenesis (N-POMC(1–46)).

ACTH is released from the anterior pituitary gland into the bloodstream in an episodic manner under the direction of hypothalamic CRHs. The frequency of pulses is normally fairly constant over the 24-h period, and it is changes in the amplitude that give rise to the circadian profile of ACTH and, hence, glucocorticoid secretion. Increases in pulse amplitude also underpin the stress-induced excursions in pituitary-adrenocortical activity although, in some instances, changes in pulse frequency may also occur.

Hypothalamic Control of Adrenocorticotropic Hormone Secretion

The concept that the secretion of ACTH is driven by a neurohormone, termed corticotropin-releasing factor (CRF), that is released from the hypothalamus and transported to the pituitary gland via the hypothalamic-hypophysial portal vessels was first recognized in the late 1940s by Harris. However, some 35 years elapsed between Harris's pioneering work and the identification of the active principles. By the late 1970s it was becoming apparent that CRF activity of the hypothalamus could not be ascribed to a single factor, and the concept of a multifactorial CRF rapidly gained credence. Subsequent work identified a 41-amino-acid residue neuropeptide, termed CRH, as the principal component and also pointed to a key role for AVP.

Corticotropin releasing hormone The 41-amino-acid neuropeptide, CRH, was first identified in ovine hypothalami by Vale and colleagues; the human peptide was identified subsequently and shown to differ from the ovine peptide by seven amino acids but to be identical to the rat peptide. The CRH gene is well characterized in the rat, mouse, and human and is expressed at multiple sites within the central nervous system (e.g., the hypothalamus, amygdala, and brain stem) and also in the periphery. CRH destined for the anterior pituitary gland is synthesized in the cell bodies of parvocellular neurons, which originate in the paraventricular nucleus (PVN) of the hypothalamus and project to the external lamina of the median eminence. These neurons terminate in close apposition with the capillaries of the hypothalamo-hypophysial portal complex into which they release their secretory products for transportation to the anterior pituitary gland. The concentration of CRH in hypophysial portal blood is high (vs. peripheral blood) and alters in parallel with perturbations of pituitary-adrenal function (e.g., stress), as also does the expression of the peptide and its mRNA in the PVN–median eminence tract. The actions of CRH on the corticotrophs are effected by specific type 1 CRH receptors (CRH-R1s), and the blockade of these receptors with selective antagonists attenuates corticotropic responses to specific stressors and to exogenous CRH. The stress response is also impaired in mice in which genes encoding either CRH or CRH-R1 are ablated, although resting ACTH levels appear to be normal in mutant mice. CRH-R1s are coupled positively to adenylyl cyclase via a G_s-protein. The stimulation of the receptor therefore causes a rise in intracellular cAMP with subsequent activation of protein kinase A, which phosphorylates Ca^{2+} channels, thereby permitting Ca^{2+} influx and the release of ACTH by exocytosis. The activation of CRH-R1s in the pituitary gland also augments POMC gene expression and hence ACTH synthesis and, in the longer term, causes the proliferation of the corticotrophs.

Arginine vasopressin The ACTH-releasing activity of AVP was first recognized in the 1950s, and evidence that AVP may be an important component of a multifactorial corticotropin releasing complex emerged originally from studies performed in rats congenitally lacking AVP (Brattleboro strain) and was subsequently supported by work using specific antisera and antagonists to the peptide. AVP *per se* shows only weak ACTH-releasing activity, acting via the V1b subclass of AVP receptors, which use the phosphatidylinositol signal transduction system.

However, it also potentiates the corticotropic responses to CRH markedly and thus plays a key role in determining the magnitude of the stress response. Surprisingly, the biochemical basis of this important synergistic response is poorly defined, although it is apparent that the activation of the V1b receptor potentiates the accumulation of 3′5′ cAMP induced by CRH, probably by a mechanism involving protein kinase C-dependent protein phosphorylation. AVP destined for the corticotrophs is derived primarily from a population of CRH-containing parvocellular neurons projecting from the PVN to the median eminence; thus, as for CRH, the concentration of AVP in the portal system is relatively high (vs. peripheral blood) and is increased further by stress. In addition, some AVP may be directed to the corticotrophs from magnocellular neurons of the neurohypophysial system (the primary source of AVP in peripheral blood) via the interconnecting short portal vessels. Within the parvocellular system, CRH and AVP are colocalized in the same secretory granules and may therefore be cosecreted. However, histological studies suggest that not all CRH-positive neurons express AVP in normal circumstances, thus permitting the ratio of AVP : CRH released to vary in a stimulus-specific manner; equally, not all corticotrophs express receptors for AVP, thereby permitting another level of control. Although AVP is generally considered to be the second CRH, this is not always the case. For example, in the sheep, AVP has precedence over CRH; similarly, in rodents and possibly in humans, AVP appears to be the dominant factor driving ACTH release in conditions of repeated or sustained stress.

Other hypothalamic factors Other hypothalamic factors may also contribute to the regulation of ACTH, including the pituitary adenylyl cyclase-activating peptide (PACAP), which exerts a stimulatory influence, and atrial natriuretic peptide (ANP) and substance P, both of which exert inhibitory influences.

Stress-Induced Activation of Corticotropin Releasing Hormone/Arginine vasopressin Neurons

The parvocellular CRH/AVP neurons in the hypothalamus are well positioned to monitor, integrate, and respond to emotional insults and physical changes in the internal or external environment that threaten homeostasis (i.e., stress). Significantly, they receive inputs from many ascending and descending nervous pathways; in addition, they are sensitive to a variety of substances that may be relayed by the bloodstream or the cerebrospinal fluid (e.g., glucose and steroids) and to local factors released from interneurons or glial cells (e.g., eicosanoids and cytokines). Major roles have been identified for (1) inputs from the brain-stem nuclei, particularly the nucleus tractus solitarius (NTS), that relay sensory information directly to the PVN and also to other parts of the brain and (2) pathways projecting to the PVN from the prefrontal cortex and the limbic system (hippocampus; amygdala; lateral septum; and the bed nucleus of the stria terminalis, BNST), but other pathways, such as those arising from raphe nuclei, are also likely to contribute. Although the precise complement of neural pathways, humoral substances, and local mediators that orchestrates the release of CRH/AVP in stress almost certainly depends on the nature of the stimulus and the status of the individual at the time of the stress, some classification according to the type of stress is now possible. For example, HPA responses to visceral homeostatic stressors that lack a cognitive component (e.g., acute hypotension) are initiated by afferent fibers that signal via the brain-stem nuclei and the noradrenergic pathways that project from the brain stem to the PVN; some homeostatic stressors also signal via humoral mechanisms; for example, the responses to hypoglycemia and hypertonicity involve intrahypothalamic glucose- and osmotic-sensitive neurons, respectively. Visceral stressors with a significant cognitive component (e.g., restraint, foot shock, or cold) use somatosensory afferents and central pathways involving both the brain-stem nuclei and the corticolimbic system to activate the PVN. The corticolimbic system also plays a fundamental role in effecting the HPA responses to emotional stressors; the importance of the hippocampus, which is critical to cognitive function, particularly learning and memory function, is well documented in this regard, as is the role of the amygdala, a key area in coordinating the behavioral, autonomic, and neuroendocrine responses to fear or anxiety.

Challenges to the host defense system, such as those provoked by infection, injury, or inflammation, pose a major threat to homeostasis and thus constitute a severe stress. Not surprisingly, in experimental animals and in humans the HPA axis responds to such insults with a marked increase in its activity. This response is driven by the army of mediators (e.g., interleukins, eicosanoids, histamine, and phospholipase A2) released from the activated immune/inflammatory cells. Some of these agents may target the HPA axis directly, acting mainly at the hypothalamic level to trigger CRH/AVP release but also on the anterior pituitary gland and adrenal cortex to augment or sustain the final adrenocortical response. Others may act locally at the site of the infection or inflammatory lesion to stimulate sensory fibers and thereby activate the central pathways that precipitate CRH/AVP release. In addition, many of the mediators provoke widespread pathological effects in the body (e.g., hypotension or hypoglycemia), which themselves stimulate the axis by the mechanisms outlined earlier. The HPA response to immune insults is thus a complex event potentially requiring the integration of a broad spectrum of stimuli, the complement of which reflects the nature and intensity of the insult. Much research has focused on the influence of the cytokines, interleukin (IL)-1β and IL-6, which are particularly important in initiating the HPA response to bacterial and viral infections. Three main mechanisms have been proposed to explain their actions.

1. The cytokines act directly on the PVN to trigger CRH release via a mechanism dependent on prostanoid generation. This mechanism has been refuted on the basis that the cytokines, which are large polypeptides (17–26 kDa), are unlikely to penetrate the blood–brain barrier and thereby gain access to their targets. However, the possibility that cytokines enter the brain via fenestrated regions of the barrier (e.g., organum vasculosum lamina terminalis, OVLT), areas in which the permeability is increased by local inflammation, or the recently described transporter system cannot be discounted.
2. The cytokines act at the level of the blood–brain barrier itself, exerting prostanoid-dependent actions on the endothelium that trigger CRH/AVP release by mechanisms that may include the activation of neural pathways and/or induction of *de novo* synthesis of cytokines in the hypothalamus and elsewhere in the brain that are required to drive the neuroendocrine response. This concept is supported by the presence of IL-1 receptors in the endothelial cells and by increased IL-1 mRNA expression in the hypothalamus and other brain areas of rodents subjected to endotoxin challenge.
3. Hypothalamic responses to peripheral cytokines involve the sequential activation of sensory fibers, brain-stem nuclei (notably the NTS), and the ventral noradrenergic pathways (and possibly others) to the PVN. This view concurs with claims that the expression of IL-1β mRNA in the hypothalamus and the hypersecretion of ACTH release induced by endotoxin are both dependent on the integrity of the vagus and that HPA responses to local inflammatory lesions induced by turpentine require C fibers. However, it is at odds with reports that cytokines activate the NTS, and hence connections between the NTS and the PVN, by mechanisms that are independent of the vagus but which may involve local prostanoid-dependent interactions with the blood–brain barrier.

Negative Feedback Control of the Hypothalamic-Pituitary-Adrenal Axis

Role of glucocorticoids Adrenocortical responses to incoming stimuli are effectively contained within appropriate limits by the glucocorticoids themselves, which exert powerful inhibitory influences on the secretion of ACTH and its hypothalamic-releasing hormones. Thus, elevations in circulating glucocorticoid levels brought about, for example, by the administration of exogenous steroids effectively suppress the HPA responses to stress and also the circadian rise in pituitary-adrenocortical activity. Conversely, the ACTH response to stress is exaggerated in subjects with adrenocortical insufficiency (e.g., Addison's disease) but corrected by glucocorticoid replacement therapy. The feedback actions of the steroids are highly complex because they are exerted at multiple sites within the axis, effected by multiple molecular mechanisms, and operate over three time domains: rapid or fast feedback, early delayed feedback, and late delayed feedback.

Phases of steroid feedback Rapid feedback develops within 2–3 min of an increase in glucocorticoid levels. It is of short duration (<10 min) and is followed by a silent period during which the stress response is intact, even though the circulating steroid levels may remain elevated. Rapid feedback is sensitive to the rate of change rather than the absolute concentration of steroid in the blood and may therefore provide an important means whereby the HPA response to stress is terminated; alternatively, it may serve to blunt the responses to a second stress incurred at a time when the steroid levels are still rising in response to the first stress. The early delayed phase of feedback develops approximately 0.5–2 h after an acute elevation in plasma steroid levels. It is normally maximal within 2–4 h and, depending on the intensity of the stimulus, may persist for up to 24 h. Both the circadian and the stress-induced excursions in ACTH secretion are suppressed with an intensity that is directly proportional to the concentration of steroid previously reached in the blood. Late delayed feedback, which has a latency of approximately 24 h, develops only after a very substantial rise in steroid levels and is frequently the consequence of repeated or continuous administration of high doses of corticosteroids. It may persist for days or weeks after the steroid treatment is withdrawn and is thus largely responsible for the potentially life-threatening suppression of the HPA axis associated with abrupt cessation of long-term treatment with high doses of steroids in, for example, rheumatoid arthritis.

Mechanisms of glucocorticoid feedback The rapid feedback actions of the glucocorticoids are exerted primarily at the hypothalamic level; weaker actions also occur at the pituitary level, but the contribution, if any, of extrahypothalamic sites in the central nervous system is ill defined. The underlying molecular mechanisms are poorly understood. Although there are some reports to the contrary, the majority of data suggests that these effects are nongenomic (and hence do not involve MRs or GRs) and that they may be mediated by receptors that are located close to or within cell membranes and which, when activated, inhibit exocytosis, possibly by blocking Ca^{2+}. In contrast, the early and late delayed phases of feedback inhibition are mediated by classic intracellular corticosteroid receptors located primarily in the anterior pituitary gland, the hypothalamus, and the hippocampus, but also elsewhere in the brain. Both the high-affinity MRs and the lower-affinity GRs are involved. Current evidence suggests that MRs (located predominantly in the hippocampus) may maintain the tonic inhibitory influence of steroids on HPA function in nonstress conditions because these receptors, which are not protected by 11β-HSD, are normally almost fully occupied by glucocorticoids, even at the nadir of the circadian rhythm. GRs, however (found in particular abundance in the anterior pituitary gland and hypothalamus) are occupied extensively only when the glucocorticoid level is raised by stress, disease, or the administration of exogenous steroids; thus, unlike MRs, these receptors serve to detect phasic changes in steroid levels and to adjust the activity of the HPA axis accordingly. Early delayed feedback requires the *de novo* generation of protein second messengers that serve to inhibit the release of ACTH and its hypothalamic-releasing factors; several proteins are likely to be involved, including lipocortin 1 (LC1, annexin 1), a Ca^{2+}- and phospholipids-binding protein strongly implicated in the anti-inflammatory and antiproliferative actions of the steroids. The genes encoding POMC in the pituitary gland and CRH/AVP in the parvocellular PVN neurons may also be repressed during the early delayed phase of feedback; however, the consequent downregulation of ACTH, CRH, and AVP synthesis emerges relatively slowly and, with existing techniques, is not normally discernible until some hours after the onset of inhibition of peptide release. Late delayed feedback is characterized by the inhibition of the synthesis and the release of CRH/AVP and ACTH in the hypothalamus and anterior pituitary gland, respectively. The inhibition of synthesis again reflects the inhibitory influence of the steroids on the genes encoding each of the three peptides, but the concomitant inhibition of peptide release cannot be explained fully in this way because peptide stores are rarely fully depleted.

Short loop and ultrashort loop feedback mechanisms In addition to the corticosteroids, other hormones of the HPA axis participate in the feedback regulation of ACTH secretion. Of particular importance are the POMC-derived peptides, ACTH and β-endorphin, both of which have been shown to exert powerful inhibitory actions on the secretion of CRH/AVP by the hypothalamus. Because neither peptide penetrates the blood–brain barrier readily, their short loop feedback actions are probably exerted at the level of the median eminence, which lies outside the blood–brain barrier. Ultrashort loop feedback actions have been attributed to both CRH and AVP, but the physiological significance of such responses is unclear.

Glucocorticoid Secretion in Repeated or Sustained Stress

The bulk of studies on stress and HPA function have focused on acute stresses, and relatively little is known of either the characteristics or the mechanisms controlling the HPA responses to repeated or sustained stress. Such conditions are, of course, inherent to our lifestyle and environment, and a deeper understanding of their influence on neuroendocrine function is thus highly desirable. However, for both ethical and practical reasons, it is difficult to develop appropriate animal models and, as described later, the available data suggest that the profile of the HPA responses observed may vary considerably according to the nature of the stress.

In some cases, HPA responses to repeated (successive or intermittent) or sustained (chronic) stressful stimuli are attenuated. For example, tolerance develops to stresses such as cold, handling, saline injection, or water deprivation (induced by the replacement of drinking water with physiological saline). Some degree of cross-tolerance may occur between stresses that invoke similar pathways/mechanisms to increase CRH/AVP release. Thus, for example, repeated handling reduces the subsequent adrenocortical response to a saline injection; however, rats tolerant to the C fiber-dependent stress of exposure to a cold environment respond to the novel stress immobilization with a normal or even exaggerated rise in serum corticosterone. In other situations, however, tolerance does not develop; thus, HPA responses to intermittent stresses of electric foot shock, insulin hypoglycemia, or IL-1β are maintained or even enhanced, as are those to the chronic stress of septicemia.

The sustained release of ACTH in repeated/chronic stress appears to be driven mainly by AVP. Thus, in rats subjected to repetitive foot shock, brain surgery, or injection of IL-1β or lipopolysaccharide (LPS), AVP is synthesized in and released from parvocellular neurons in the PVN in preference to CRH; in addition, the sensitivity of the pituitary gland to AVP is well maintained, whereas that to CRH is reduced. Similarly, the expression of AVP, but not CRH, in the parvocellular PVN is increased in rats with experimentally induced arthritis; moreover, although the arthritic rats respond to LPS with a rise ACTH secretion, they are relatively unresponsive to a novel neurogenic stress normally driven mainly by CRH. The switch to AVP as the principal driving force to the corticotrophs in repetitive/chronic stress may reflect the disruption of the negative feedback mechanism for the expression of MRs in the hippocampus, and GRs in the PVN are reduced in conditions of chronic stress; moreover, the capacity of dexamethasone to block the HPA response to IL-1β is impaired in rats pretreated 3 weeks with the cytokine. In the same vein, AVP and disrupted feedback have both been implicated in the etiology of the hypercortisolemia evident in depression, although others have advocated a role for CRH.

Age- and Gender-Related Changes in the Stress Response

Development

The functional development of the HPA axis begins in fetal life, and in the later stages of gestation the fetus secretes substantial quantities of cortisol/corticosterone. It also responds to stress with increases in adrenocortical activity, which are driven by the hypothalamic-pituitary axis and which are sensitive to the negative feedback actions of the glucocorticoids. Paradoxically, in the rat and several other species, HPA function regresses postnatally and a period ensues during which the ability of the axis to respond to stress is compromised. In the rat, this stress hyporesponsive phase (SHRP) normally persists from postnatal day 5 (P5) to P14, although depending on the stimulus a mature stress response may not emerge for up to 5–6 weeks. The refractoriness of the HPA axis to stress in the SHRP is not absolute and may be at least partially overridden in certain cases. For example, IL-1β, hypoglycemia, glutamate, and histamine all elicit modest rises in serum ACTH and corticosterone throughout this period. Exceptionally, the hypersecretion of ACTH provoked by LPS in the SHRP matches that observed in the adult, although the associated rise in serum corticosterone does not; moreover, paradoxically, both the ACTH and the corticosterone responses to kainic acid are more robust at P12 than P18. These and many other data suggest that the processes involved in the maturation of the stress response are complex and stimulus-dependent. They are therefore likely to involve a variety of factors that act in concert at different levels of the axis during the developmental period. These include immaturity of the neural and humoral mechanisms effecting the release of CRH/AVP in stress, enhanced sensitivity of the axis to the regulatory actions of the glucocorticoids, and impairment of the synergy between CRH and AVP.

Perinatal Programming of the Stress Response

Glucocorticoids play a key role in developmental programming, and a growing body of evidence suggests that inappropriate exposure of the developing fetus/neonate to the steroids or to factors that influence the expression/function of their receptors may trigger a plethora of pathologies (e.g., growth retardation or impairment of central nervous system development) and predispose the individual in later life to conditions as diverse as hypertension, insulin resistance, cognitive and other behavioral disorders, and allergic/inflammatory disease. Because the SHRP coincides with an important phase of development, it seems likely that it may serve to protect the organism from the potentially harmful effects of overexposure to glucocorticoids.

Despite its tight control, the developing HPA axis exhibits a high degree of plasticity, and disturbances in its activity at critical stages of development precipitate abnormalities in glucocorticoid secretion that persist into adult life and may increase the susceptibility of the individual to disease. Perinatal manipulations that alter the expression of GRs (but not MRs) in the brain are particularly hazardous in this regard because, by disrupting the negative feedback mechanisms, they alter the responsivity of the HPA axis to stress throughout the lifetime of the individual. For example, exposure of neonatal rats to dexamethasone or LPS results in the adult in downregulation of GRs in the hippocampus and hypothalamus, decreased sensitivity of the HPA axis to the negative feedback actions of the glucocorticoids, and exaggerated HPA responses to stress. Similar long-term changes in GR expression occur in rats subjected to prolonged periods of maternal separation; the consequent impairment of the negative feedback system and changes in HPA function are associated with alterations in T-cell antibody responses and in the incidence of age-related neuropathies. In contrast, neonatal handling, which increases hippocampal GR expression by mechanisms involving serotonin, reduces the magnitude and duration of the stress response in the adult; maternal care may therefore help program events that regulate responses to stress in the adult and thus reduce vulnerability to disease.

Sexual Dimorphism in Hypothalamic-Pituitary-Adrenal Function

In adults, distinct sexually dimorphic patterns of glucocorticoid secretion emerge. Serum glucocorticoid concentrations are consistently higher in the female than in the male, with further increases occurring toward the middle of the menstrual/estrous cycle just prior to ovulation and in the late stages of pregnancy. These changes are due partly to the positive effects of estrogen on the expression of CBG. In addition, estrogen exerts significant effects at the hypothalamic level, increasing the synthesis and release of CRH, a phenomenon that may be implicated in the etiology of the relatively high incidence of emotional disorders (e.g., depression and anxiety) in the female that are characterized by enhanced CRH secretion. Further modulation may be brought about by progesterone, which, when present in large amounts (e.g., in the premenstrual phase or pregnancy), binds readily to but is only weakly active at MRs in the hippocampus.

Stress Responses in the Aging

In both sexes, serum glucocorticoid concentrations tend to increase in aging individuals, particularly in disease states; in addition, although sometimes delayed, the HPA responses to stress are frequently exaggerated and prolonged. This aging process has been attributed in part to the downregulation of the corticosteroid receptors (GRs and MRs) in the hippocampus and hypothalamus and to the consequent emergence of a resistance of the HPA axis to the negative feedback actions of the glucocorticoids. The consequences are potentially important because hyperglucocorticoidemia is considered to be an important contributory factor in a number of age-related diseases, including neurodegenerative conditions, cognitive dysfunction, osteoporosis, noninsulin-dependent diabetes mellitus, and the decline in immunocompetence.

See Also the Following Articles

Adrenal Cortex; Feedback Systems; Gleucocorticoid Negative Feedback; Glucocorticoids, Role in Stress.

Further Reading

Buckingham, J. C. (1996). Stress and the neuroendocrine immune axis: the pivotal role of glucocorticoids and lipocortin 1. *British Journal of Pharmacology* **118**, 1–19.

Buckingham, J. C., Gillies, G. E. and Cowell, A.-M. (1997). *Stress, stress hormones and the immune system.* Chichester, UK: John Wiley.

de Kloet, E. R., Vreugdenhil, E., Citzl, M. S., et al. (1988). Brain corticosteroid receptor balance in health and disease. *Endocrine Review* **19**, 269–301.

Ericsson, A., Arias, C. and Sawchenko, P. E. (1997). Evidence for an intramedullary prostaglandin-dependent mechanism in the activation of stress-related neuroendocrine circuitry by intravenous interleukin-1. *Journal of Neuroscience* **17**, 7166–7179.

Gillies, G. E., Linton, E. A. and Lowry, P. J. (1982). Corticotropin releasing activity of the new CRH is potentiated several times by vasopressin. *Nature* **299**, 355–357.

Harris, G. W. (1955). *Neural control of the pituitary.* London: Edward Arnold.

Kellerwood, M. E. and Dallman, M. F. (1984). Corticosteroid inhibition of ACTH secretion. *Endocrine Review* **5**, 1–25.

Li, H. Y. and Sawchenko, P. E. (1998). Hypothalamic effector neurons and extended circuitries activated in "neurogenic" stress: a comparison of footshock effects exerted accutely, chronically and in animals with controlled glucose levels. *Journal of Comparative Neurobiology* **393**, 244–266.

Lowry, P. J. (1984). Pro-opiocortin: the multiple hormone precursor. *Bioscience Reports* **4**, 467–482.

Muglia, L., Jacobson, L. and Majzoub, J. A. (1996). Production of corticotropin-releasing hormone deficient mice by targeted mutation of embryonic stem cells. *Annals of the New York Academy of Sciences* **780**, 49–59.

Rosenfeld, P., Surchecki, A. J. and Levins, S. (1992). *Neuroscience and Biobehavioral Reviews* **16**, 553–568.

Seckl, J. R. (1997). 11β-hydroxysteroid dehydrogenase in the brain: a novel regulator of glucocorticoid action? *Frontiers in Neuroendocrinology* **18**, 49–99.

Smith, G. W., Aubry, J. M., Dellu, F., et al. (1992). Corticotropin releasing factor receptor 1-deficient mice display increased anxiety, impaired stress response and observant neuroendocrine development. *Neuron* **20**, 1098–1102.

Tilders, F. J. and Solimidt, E. D. (1998). Interleukin 1β-induced plasticity of hypothalamic CRH neurons and long-term hyperresponsivity. *Annals of the New York Academy of Sciences* **840**, 65–73.

Vale, W., Spiess, J., Rivier, L., et al. (1981). Characterisation of a 41-residue ovine hypothalamic peptide that stimulates secretion of corticotropin and β-endorphin. *Science* **213**, 1394–1397.

Vamvakopoulos, N. C. and Chrousos, G. P. (1994). Hormonal regulation of human corticotropin releasing hormone gene expression: implications for the sexual dimorphism of the stress response and immune inflammatory reaction. *Endocrine Review* **15**, 409–420.

Steroid Hydroxylases

F H de Jong
Erasmus University Medical Centre, Rotterdam, The Netherlands

This is a revised version of the article by F H de Jong, Encyclopedia of Stress, First edition, volume 3, pp 505–507, © 2000, Elsevier Inc.

Glossary

Cytochromes P450 — Enzymes involved in the hydroxylation of endogenous or exogenous substrates.

Hydroxylation of steroids — Replacement of hydrogen (H) atoms in steroids by hydroxyl (OH) groups.

Localization of steroidogenic enzymes — Specific organs, cell types, or intracellular organelles in which the enzymes, responsible for the biosynthesis of steroids, can be found.

Regulation of steroidogenesis — Processes that play a role in increasing or decreasing the amounts of steroids formed.

Steroid biosynthesis — The process by which hormonally active steroids are formed from cholesterol.

Introduction

The cytochrome P450 (CYP) genes form a family, encoding a class of heme-thiolate enzymes active in the hydroxylation of endogenous and exogenous substances. They are involved in detoxification and catabolism of pharmacological substances and in biosynthesis of steroids. Homology between the various members is relatively high: CYPs in the same subfamily usually are about 70% similar. These enzymes are instrumental in conveying molecular oxygen to designated positions in the steroid skeleton, in this way introducing hydroxyl groups and determining which final hormonal steroids will be produced in the process of steroid biosynthesis. The specific roles of these enzymes in the pathway of steroidogenesis are indicated in **Figure 1.** The electrons necessary to drive this process are supplied by NADPH or NADH and are passed to mitochondrial CYPs by way of the flavoprotein adrenodoxin reductase to the iron-sulfur protein adrenodoxin. For the CYPs in the microsomal cell fraction, the role of adrenodoxin is taken over by P450 oxidoreductase; cytochrome b5 may play an additional role to support 17,20-lyase activity.

Cholesterol Side-Chain Cleavage Enzyme: CYP11A1

The enzyme CYP11A1 performs the conversion of cholesterol to pregnenolone, by first hydroxylating cholesterol at the 20α and 22 carbon atoms and then lysing the bond between these carbon atoms. The

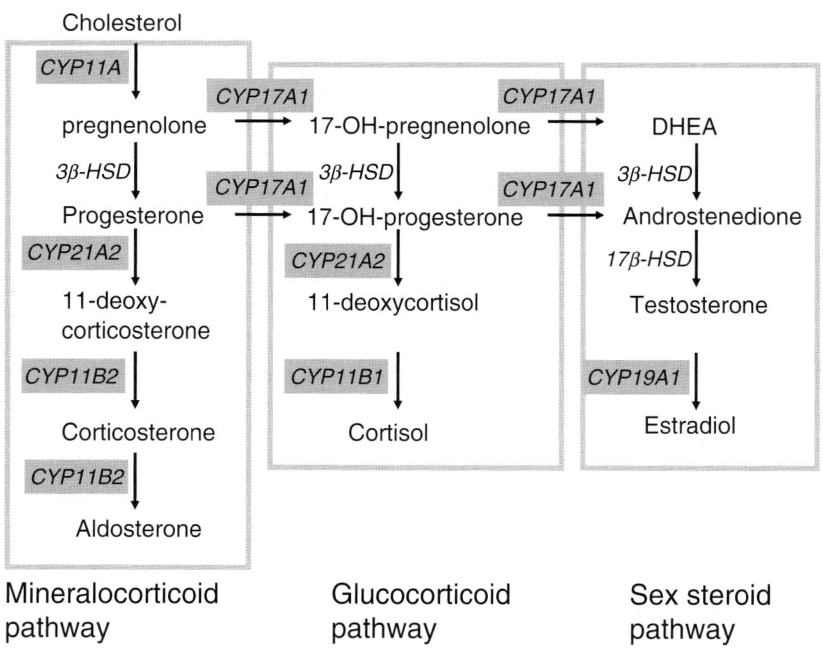

Figure 1 Localization of steroidogenic enzymes along the pathways leading to the biosynthesis of mineralocorticoids, glucocortoids, and sex steroids. Shaded boxes indicate the various cytochromes P450 (CYPs). DHEA, dehydroepiandrosterone.

enzyme, of which only one form is known, is localized in the adrenal glands, the gonads, the placenta, and the brain. Intracellularly, the location is in the inner mitochondrial membrane. Apparently, this localization is extremely important for the activity of the enzyme: transfection studies with constructs that direct the protein into the endoplasmic reticulum failed to show activity.

Regulation of the expression of CYP11A1 differs in different tissues. In organs where an acute stimulation of CYP11A1 transcription can take place under the influence of adrenocorticotropic hormone (ACTH) or gonadotropins, the adrenals, and the gonads, the responsible cyclic AMP-responsive elements differ from those in the placenta. Furthermore, a number of transcription factors, such as SF-1 and Sp-1, play a role in the stimulation of the transcription of CYP11A1. This transcriptional regulation of the amount of enzymes in the glands takes a relatively long time (2–4 h), whereas the stimulation of steroidogenesis may be much faster. These fast effects of increased cAMP levels are mediated through effects on the transport of cholesterol into the mitochondria by the steroidogenic acute regulatory protein (StAR), which enables cholesterol transport to the mitochondrial inner membrane. StAR is not expressed in brain or placenta. It has become apparent that the inability to lyse the C20–C22 bond of cholesterol, as present in congenital lipoid adrenal hyperplasia, may be due to inactivating mutations in CYP11A1, but can also be caused by inactivating mutations of StAR, indicating the crucial importance of this protein in steroidogenesis.

17-Hydroxylase: CYP17A1

After the conversion of cholesterol to pregnenolone in the mitochondria, further conversion of pregnenolone takes place in the endoplasmic reticulum by the conversion to 17-OH pregnenolone by CYP17A1 or to progesterone by 3β-HSD. Progesterone, in turn, can be converted to 17-OH progesterone by the same CYP17A1, which also contains 17,20-lyase activity to convert 17-OH pregnenolone to dehydroepiandrosterone (DHEA) and 17-OH progesterone to androstenedione. For this reason, CYP17A1 is at the bifurcation of the steroidogenic pathways to glucocorticosteroids and the sex steroids. CYP17 is expressed in the adrenal glands and in the gonads. The production of DHEA, which might be important as a neurosteroid through its interactions with γ-aminobutyric acid (GABA) and N-methyl-D-aspartate (NMDA) receptors, in the brain is an enigma so far because CYP17A1 has not been detected in the brain, which has led to alternative hypotheses for the mechanisms responsible for the production of this steroid involving reactive oxygen species. The expression of the CYP17A1 gene is mainly regulated by cAMP. Addition of cAMP derivatives can stimulate the transcription of the gene; this activity can be inhibited by the addition of phorbol esters, which act via protein kinase C and growth factors such as epidermal growth factor (EGF) and fibroblast growth factor (FGF).

The separate regulation of 17-hydroxylase and 17,20-lyase activity of the enzyme has been resolved on the basis of the finding of mutated genes, causing the production of 17-hydroxylated steroids, without removal of the C20,C21 side chain. These mutations are localized in the region of the protein, which interacts with the additional electron donor cytochrome b5; lyase activity appears to be more vulnerable to the disruption of interaction with this redox partner than the 17-hydroxylase reaction. Similarly, the changing ratios between the production of glucocorticoids and adrenal androgens, mainly DHEA sulfate, during human development is likely to be due to a changed expression of cytochrome b5.

The pivotal role of CYP17A1 in steroidogenesis is emphasized by the effects of inactivating mutations in this enzyme: a complete block of 17-hydroxylation leads to the inability to synthesize cortisol, whereas aldosterone will be produced in abundance, giving rise to hypertension. Furthermore, sex steroids cannot be produced, causing undervirilization in boys and absence of puberty in both sexes.

21-Hydroxylase: CYP21A2

CYP21A2 catalyzes the conversion of progesterone to 21-hydroxyprogesterone (deoxycorticosterone, DOC) and of 17-OH progesterone to 17,21-dihydroxyprogesterone (deoxycortisol, compound S). These reactions are a prerequisite to synthesize mineralocorticoids and glucocorticoids; the enzyme is expressed in the cortex of the adrenal gland and is not present in the gonads. Using reverse transcription polymerase chain reaction (RT-PCR), expression of CYP21A2 has also been detected in the brain stem, but not in other regions of the brain.

The expression of CYP21A2 is stimulated by cAMP- and protein kinase C-dependent pathways. In this way, the production of deoxycorticosterone in the zona glomerulosa of the adrenal cortex may be stimulated by angiotensin II, whereas the production of deoxycortisol in the zonae fasciculata and reticularis is ACTH dependent.

Due to the fact that an inactive pseudogene, CYP21A1P, exists in the neighborhood of the CYP21A2 gene on chromosome 6, frequent exchanges between these genes have taken place, leading to impairment of the functioning of the resulting protein, the inability to produce aldosterone, corticosterone, and cortisol, and overproduction of adrenal androgens (in humans). These enzyme deficiencies can lead to salt loss in newborn babies and severe masculinization in girls. In female patients with milder forms of the defect, late onset virilization or hirsutism may be found.

11β-Hydroxylases: CYP11B1 and CYP11B2

The further conversion of 21-hydroxylated steroids to the main mineralocorticoids and glucocorticoids (aldosterone and cortisol [humans] or corticosterone [rat and mouse]) is affected by CYP11B2 and CYP11B1, respectively. The genes encoding these members of the CYP family are found in close vicinity on chromosome 8q and probably arise from ancient gene duplication. The localization of these enzymes in the adrenal cortex is different: CYP11B1 is localized in mitochondria of the zona fasciculata, whereas CYP11B2 is found in mitochondria of the zona glomerulosa. Furthermore, using RT-PCR, mRNAs encoding these enzymes have been detected in various regions of the brain and in the heart.

The regulation of the expression of the two genes is also different. The expression of CYP11B1 is regulated by the ACTH-driven production of cAMP, followed by activation of a cAMP-responsive element, whereas CYP11B2 is stimulated mainly by angiotensin II, which stimulates the production of inositol triphosphate and diacylglycerol by phospholipase C. This leads to increased levels of intracellular calcium and increased activity of phosphokinase C. In this way, the expression of the two 11-hydroxylases can be regulated separately in the zona glomerulosa and zona fasciculata, respectively, of the adrenal cortex.

The clinical results of deficiencies of either of these enzymes can be predicted on the basis of the steroids, the biosynthesis of which will be blocked. Defective CYP11B1 gives rise to low levels of cortisol that can only be increased by supply of exogenous glucocorticoids. An insufficient production of aldosterone, caused by a mutation in CYP11B2, can be partially compensated by overproduction of deoxycorticosterone, which has mineralocorticoid activity.

Aromatase: CYP19A1

The final steroid-hydroxylating enzyme, which plays a role in the biosynthesis of steroids, is CYP19A1. It is responsible for the hydroxylation of carbon atom C19 of testosterone and androstenedione, the subsequent cleavage of the bond between C19 and C10, and subsequent redistribution of the electrons over the A ring to form the aromatic steroids estradiol and estrone, respectively. Only one copy of the gene has been found. It has a complex structure at the 5′ end, allowing start of transcription at a number of sites, under the control of various promoter sequences. This means that in various tissues, different mechanisms can be used for the stimulation of the transcription of the gene: in the gonads and adrenals, a cAMP-mediated mechanism is responsible for the stimulation of CYP19A1 by gonadotropins and ACTH, respectively, whereas in fat cells, cortisol can stimulate the production of estrogens. CYP19A1 is also expressed in a large number of other tissues, such as muscle, bone, and brain. In the latter, estrogens formed by this enzyme may play a role in sexual differentiation.

Defects of CYP19A1 are very rare. However, the clinical picture in patients with mutations in this gene shows profound changes of parameters of gonadal function, bone metabolism, and aspects of the metabolic syndrome, indicating the role of estrogens in the regulation of numerous aspects of homeostasis.

Steroid Catabolism by CYPs

Apart from their role in the biosynthesis of steroid hormones, enzymes of the CYP family also play important roles in the breakdown of steroids. The most important enzymes in this respect are those of the CYP1 and CYP4 subfamilies. Members of the CYP1 subfamily are important in the hydroxylation of mainly estrogens, where both C2 and C4 may be attacked. CYP4 family members hydroxylate corticosteroids and androgens at the 6 position and can also attach a hydroxyl group at C16. It is important to be aware of the fact that expression of all of these enzymes can be induced by xenobiotics, leading to aberrant metabolism of the steroid hormones and, for example, changes in the ratios between the serum levels of steroids produced in the adrenal gland, which might lead to erroneous conclusions of disturbed steroidogenesis.

See Also the Following Articles

11ß-Hydroxysteroid Dehydrogenases; Steroid Hormone Receptors.

Further Reading

de Ronde, W., Pols, H. A. P., van Leeuwen, J. P. T. M., et al. (2003). The importance of oestrogens in men. *Clinical Endocrinology* 58, 529–542.

Fujieda, K., Okuhara, K., Abe, S., et al. (2003). Molecular pathogenesis of lipoid adrenal hyperplasia and adrenal

hypoplasia congenita. *Journal of Steroid Biochemistry and Molecular Biolology* **85**, 483–489.
Grinberg, A. V., Hannemann, F., Schiffler, B., et al. (2000). Adrenodoxin: structure, stability, and electron transfer properties. *Proteins* **40**, 590–612.
Lewis, D. F. (2004). 57 varieties: the human cytochromes P450. *Pharmacogenomics* **5**, 305–318.
Lisurek, M. and Bernhardt, R. (2004). Modulation of aldosterone and cortisol synthesis on the molecular level. *Molecular and Cellular Endocrinology* **215**, 149–159.
Manna, P. R., Wang, X. J. and Stocco, D. M. (2003). Involvement of multiple transcription factors in the regulation of steroidogenic acute regulatory protein gene expression. *Steroids* **68**, 1125–1134.
Nebert, D. W. and Russell, D. W. (2002). Clinical importance of the cytochromes P450. *Lancet* **360**, 1155–1162.
New, M. I. (2003). Inborn errors of adrenal steroidogenesis. *Molecular and Cellular Endocrinology* **211**, 75–83.
Shimada, T. and Fujii-Kuriyama, Y. (2004). Metabolic activation of polycyclic aromatic hydrocarbons to carcinogens by cytochromes P450 1A1 and 1B1. *Cancer Science* **95**, 1–6.
Simpson, E. R., Misso, M., Hewitt, K. N., et al. (2005). Estrogen—the good, the bad, and the unexpected. *Endocrine Reviews* **26**, 322–330.
Stratakis, C. A. and Bossis, I. (2004). Genetics of the adrenal gland. *Reviews in Endocrine and Metabolic Disorders* **5**, 53–68.
You, L. (2004). Steroid hormone biotransformation and xenobiotic induction of hepatic steroid metabolizing enzymes. *Chemico-Biological Interactions* **147**, 233–246.

11β-Hydroxysteroid Dehydrogenases

J R Seckl
Edinburgh University, Edinburgh, UK

This is a revised version of the article by J R Seckl, Encyclopedia of Stress, First edition, volume 2, pp 413–420, © 2000, Elsevier Inc.

Glossary

11β-Hydroxysteroid dehydrogenase (11β-HSD) — An enzyme that catalyzes the interconversion of active cortisol (corticosterone in rats and mice) and inert cortisone (11-dehydrocorticosterone).

11β-HSD type 1 (11β-HSD1) — An isozyme that predominantly catalyzes the reduction of inert cortisone to active cortisol in intact cells and organs.

11β-HSD type 2 (11β-HSD2) — An isozyme that catalyzes the rapid dehydrogenation of active cortisol to inert cortisone.

Aromatase — The enzyme that catalyzes the conversion of androgens to estrogens.

Carbenoxolone — A nonselective 11β-HSD inhibitor.

Cushing's syndrome — The generic description of the phenotype observed with circulating glucocorticoid excess, due either to endogenous overproduction of cortisol or adrenocorticotrophic hormone (ACTH) or to exogenous pharmacotherapy.

Glucocorticoid receptor (GR) — Intracellular receptor for active cortisol.

Intracrine — The process whereby intracellular enzymic transformations of steroids alter their access to nuclear receptors.

Metabolic syndrome — The co-association of risk factors for atheromatous disease (insulin resistance, type 2 diabetes, dyslipidemia, and hypertension) and abdominal (visceral) obesity.

Mineralocorticoid receptor (MR) — Intracellular receptor for active cortisol, selectivity for aldosterone *in vivo* generated by 11β-HSD2.

Syndrome of apparent mineralocorticoid excess — A congenital syndrome of hypertension, hypernatremia, and hypokalemia due to inappropriate MR activation by glucocorticoids because of deleterious mutations of the 11β-HSD type 2 gene and hence lack of the enzyme in the kidney.

Definition: 11β-Hydroxysteroid Dehydrogenase

Elevated plasma cortisol or glucocorticoid pharmacotherapy has myriad adverse effects ranging from obesity, diabetes, and hypertension to depression and memory impairments. Glucocorticoid action is classically believed to be determined by the product of circulating glucocorticoid levels and the tissue density of corticosteroid receptors (GR and MR). However, recent discoveries suggest a key role for local enzymic tissue metabolism of glucocorticoids in determining receptor activation. The main enzymes involved are the 11β-hydroxysteroid dehydrogenases (11β-HSDs). These catalyze the interconversion of active cortisol (in humans and most mammals) and corticosterone

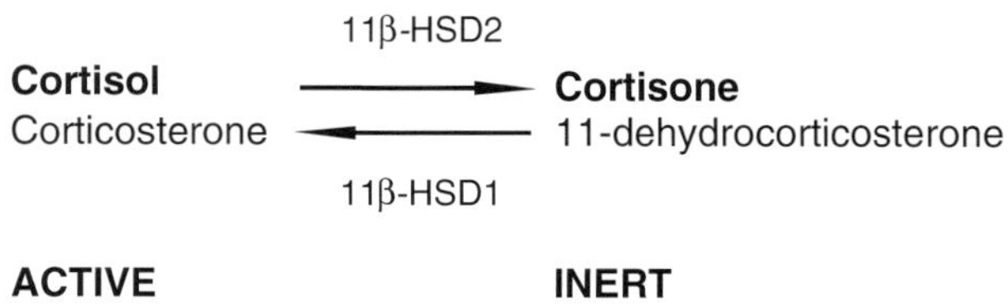

Figure 1 11β-Hydroxysteroid dehydrogenases. Type 1 acts as a ketoreductase, regenerating active cortisol (corticosterone), whereas type 2 acts as a dehydrogenase, rapidly inactivating these physiological glucocorticoids.

(in rats and mice) and inert 11-keto forms (cortisone, 11-dehydrocorticosterone) (**Figure 1**). The roles of these enzymes in determining glucocorticoid actions in the central nervous system (CNS) and periphery are now becoming apparent.

The Mineralocorticoid Receptor Paradox

Purified MR binds aldosterone, cortisol, and corticosterone with equal and high affinity *in vitro*, but *in vivo* only aldosterone binds to MR in the kidney, although there is much more glucocorticoid in the circulation. In resolution of this paradox, in 1988 groups in Edinburgh and Melbourne reported that 11β-HSD was a prereceptor enzymic mechanism that bestowed aldosterone selectivity on the intrinsically nonselective MR *in vivo*. The 11β-HSD activity associated with MR in the distal nephron acted as a dehydrogenase, rapidly inactivating physiological glucocorticoids (cortisol, corticosterone) to their inert 11-keto forms. Such 11β-HSD activity forms an intracellular barrier to glucocorticoids, preventing the occupation of MR. When the enzyme is congenitally deficient in the syndrome of apparent mineralocorticoid excess or is inhibited by liquorice, glucocorticoids inappropriately access MR, causing sodium retention, hypertension, and hypokalemia. Although an NADP(H)-associated 11β-HSD activity (now called 11β-HSD1) and its encoding cDNA were isolated from rat liver by Monder and colleagues in the mid-1980s, this was shown not to be responsible for renal MR selectivity: its encoding gene HSD11B1 was intact in patients with the syndrome. Subsequently a second 11β-HSD isozyme (11β-HSD2) was cloned from the kidney and placenta in a variety of species. This isozyme is a high-affinity 11β-dehydrogenase, which uses NAD as cofactor and is highly expressed in the distal nephron and placenta. Patients with the syndrome of apparent mineralocorticoid excess were homozygous or compound heterozygous for deleterious mutations in the HSD11B2 gene, and 11β-HSD2 knockout mice faithfully recapitulated the syndrome. This work underlined the fundamental principle that steroid access to nuclear receptors *in vivo* is regulated by prereceptor metabolism. Other examples include 5- and 5′-monodeiodinases (thyroid hormone receptors), 5α-reductase (androgen receptor), and aromatase (estrogen receptors).

11β-Hydroxysteroid Dehydrogenase Type 2 in the Adult Central Nervous System

Although the vast majority of MR in the CNS are nonselective and bind glucocorticoids (cortisol, corticosterone) *in vivo*, it is anticipated that any selective effects of aldosterone in the CNS will require MR gated by local 11β-HSD2. In this regard, aldosterone mediates the central regulation of blood pressure and salt appetite. Thus, aldosterone infused intracerebroventricularly (ICV) elevates blood pressure in the rat, whereas the same dose given peripherally is ineffective, demonstrating a specific central action. Corticosterone ICV does not reproduce this action, and indeed antagonizes aldosterone hypertension. Similarly, aldosterone exerts central actions on salt appetite that cannot be reproduced by corticosterone. 11β-HSD2 action in the CNS is therefore inferred. This is supported by ICV infusion of the 11β-HSD inhibitor carbenoxolone, which increases blood pressure in the rat, an effect reversed by an MR antagonist, suggesting central 11β-HSD2 prevents access of glucocorticoids to central MR. Although 11β-HSD2 mRNA is only found in a few discrete sites in the adult rat brain, these loci also express MR and are believed to underlie the selective central effects of aldosterone to increase blood pressure (nucleus tractus solitarius, NTS), and modulate salt appetite (ventromedial hypothalamus, subcommissural organ, and central nucleus of the amygdala). In the mouse there is an even more limited distribution of 11β-HSD2, with expression confined to the NTS. 11β-HSD2 was not found in the human forebrain, although the brain stem has not been investigated. Thus, there is very little 11β-HSD2 in the adult brain, located appropriately for the few CNS actions specifically ascribed to this hormone.

11β-Hydroxysteroid Dehydrogenase Type 2 in the Developing Central Nervous System

Prenatal glucocorticoid administration reduces brain weight at birth; delays the maturation of neurons, glia, and cerebral vasculature; and retards CNS myelination. Given such widespread effects, it is unsurprising that GR and MR are highly expressed in the developing brain. However, whether these receptors are occupied by endogenous glucocorticoids until late gestation is uncertain because there is also plentiful 11β-HSD2 in the CNS at midgestation in rodents and humans. This presumably functions to protect vulnerable developing cells from premature glucocorticoid action. Strikingly, 11β-HSD2 expression is dramatically switched off in a CNS at the end of midgestation, coinciding with the terminal stage of brain nucleus development. This appears to be an exquisitely timed system of cellular protection from circulating glucocorticoids.

11β-Hydroxysteroid Dehydrogenase Type 2 and Fetal Programming

Human epidemiological studies show that low birth weight at term is associated with an increased later occurrence of cardiovascular (hypertension and ischemic heart disease) and metabolic disorders (type 2 diabetes) in adult life. In rodents, sheep, and humans, excessive exposure to glucocorticoids during gestation, either bypassing of fetoplacental 11β-HSD2 with nonsubstrate glucocorticoid such as dexamethasone or using 11β-HSD inhibitors such as carbenoxolone, reduces birth weight. Although in such models, the weight deficit is regained soon after birth, the adult offspring show increased blood pressure and serum insulin and glucose levels. These effects are underpinned by an increased tissue sensitivity to glucocorticoids via increased GR density in key metabolic loci such as the liver and visceral adipose tissue depots.

Programming the Hypothalamic-Pituitary-Adrenal Axis and Behavior

Prenatal 11β-HSD2 inhibition or bypass with the nonsubstrate dexamethasone permanently increases basal plasma corticosterone levels in the offspring in rats. The density of GR and MR in the hippocampus are reduced in this model, which is anticipated to reduce hypothalamic-pituitary-adrenal (HPA) axis feedback sensitivity. Moreover the glucocorticoid excess may drive, at least in part, the hypertension and hyperglycemia observed in such prenatal programming models. Maternal undernutrition also lowers placental 11β-HSD2 and alters adult offspring metabolic, cardiovascular, and HPA axis function, suggesting that HPA programming may be a common outcome of prenatal environmental challenge. Overexposure to glucocorticoids *in utero* also leads to alterations in adult behavior to produce a phenotype reminiscent of anxiety. Prenatal glucocorticoid exposure also affects the developing dopaminergic system with clear implications for proposed developmental contributions to schizo-affective, attention-deficit hyperactivity and extrapyramidal disorders. Mechanistically, prenatal dexamethasone or 11β-HSD inhibition increases corticotropin-releasing hormone (CRH) mRNA levels specifically in the central nucleus of the amygdala, a key locus for the effects of the neuropeptide on the expression of fear and anxiety. Intriguingly, fetoplacental 11β-HSD inhibition also permanently increases GR and MR in the offspring amygdala. A direct relationship between brain GR levels and anxiety behaviors is supported by transgenic mice with selective loss of GR in the forebrain, which exhibit reduced fearfulness. Intriguingly, low-birth-weight humans also exhibit HPA hyperactivity in adult life.

11β-Hydroxysteroid Dehydrogenase Type 1 in the Brain

So what was the role of Monder's original 11β-HSD (type 1), highly expressed in liver, adipose tissue and the brain? Studies in intact cells from liver, fat, lung, and other sites have shown that 11β-HSD1, although bidirectional in tissue homogenates, is a predominant 11β-ketoreductase in intact cells. This reaction regenerates active glucocorticoids from inert 11-keto forms. A similar directional predominance is seen in the intact liver *ex vivo* and in rodents and humans *in vivo*. In the brain, 11β-HSD1-like immunoreactivity and mRNA are widespread. Fetal rat hippocampal cells in culture express 11β-HSD1 but no 11β-HSD2. Intact hippocampal cells show only 11β-reductase activity. This reaction direction increases intracellular glucocorticoid levels. In searching for functions, it was noted that licorice-derived 11β-HSD inhibitors given to rats alter hypothalamic secretagogs in pituitary portal blood *in vivo* and activate a series of regions of the CNS, including the hippocampus, a key glucocorticoid target with high GR and MR density where glucocorticoids act to suppress HPA activity and to modulate cognitive functions.

11β-Hydroxysteroid Dehydrogenase Type 1 and the Hypothalamic-Pituitary-Adrenal Axis

11β-HSD1 is expressed in the hippocampus, paraventricular nucleus of the hypothalamus (PVN) and pituitary, key sites of glucocorticoid negative feedback. 11β-HSD1 knockout (11β-HSD1$^{-/-}$) mice have hypertrophied adrenals and elevated basal adrenocorticotropic hormone (ACTH) and corticosterone levels at the nadir of the rhythm. These effects are compatible with the requirement for increased glucocorticoid production from the adrenal cortex in this mouse secondary to increased metabolic clearance of corticosterone because of the lack of glucocorticoid regeneration, notably in the liver. Unexpectedly, basal plasma corticosterone levels are also elevated in 11β-HSD1$^{-/-}$ mice, suggesting reduced glucocorticoid feedback on the HPA axis and increased forward drive on the HPA system. Altered central drive is rather unlikely because CRH mRNA levels in the PVN are unaltered. In contrast, some findings suggest that 11β-HSD1$^{-/-}$ mice have attenuated negative feedback because they show less suppression of corticosterone to exogenous cortisol 2 h prior to restraint stress. Interestingly, recent data show that obese Zucker rats have reduced 11β-HSD1 in the hippocampus, which may explain why this strain has reduced HPA feedback sensitivity and hence has increased corticosterone levels. Altered brain 11β-HSD1 has been reported in pregnancy, when the HPA axis becomes refractory to stressful stimulation. Interestingly, 11β-HSD1 activity is selectively increased in the PVN in pregnancy, so locally increased 11β-HSD1 may further amplify glucocorticoid feedback and hence attenuate HPA activity.

11β-Hydroxysteroid Dehydrogenase Type 1 and Brain Aging

A subgroup of aged rodents and humans shows the association of cognitive decline with a chronic elevation of plasma corticosterone levels. If glucocorticoids are maintained at low levels in rats, by adrenalectomy and low-dose corticosterone replacement, age-related impairments are reduced. The hippocampus requires glucocorticoids for neuronal function and survival but is especially vulnerable to the adverse effects of chronic glucocorticoid excess, which causes atrophy of dendrites and cognitive dysfunction. Therefore, chronic glucocorticoid overexposure has been implicated in the pathogenesis of age-related decline in hippocampus-associated cognitive functions.

In primary cultures of hippocampal cells, 11β-HSD1 potentiates kainic acid-induced neurotoxicity, not only by corticosterone but equally by intrinsically inert 11-dehydrocorticosterone, an effect prevented by carbenoxolone. 11-Dehydrocorticosterone increases kainic acid hippocampal toxicity *in vivo*, an effect also blocked by carbenoxolone. Crucially, old 11β-HSD1$^{-/-}$ mice learn as well as young mice in hippocampus tasks and avoid the cognitive decline seen in the majority of aged wild-type mice. This cognitive protection in aged 11β-HSD1$^{-/-}$ mice is associated with reduced intrahippocampal corticosterone levels, indicating the potency of intracellular metabolism by 11β-HSDs in determining effective glucocorticoid action on target receptors. *In situ* hybridization studies in postmortem human brain material show high expression of 11β-HSD1 mRNA in the hippocampus, prefrontal cortex, and cerebellum, mirroring rodent findings. In two small randomized double-blind placebo-controlled cross-over studies, the administration of the 11β-HSD inhibitor carbenoxolone improved verbal fluency after 4 weeks in ten healthy elderly men and improved verbal memory after 6 weeks in 12 elderly patients with type 2 diabetes. Plasma cortisol was unaltered, suggesting that 11β-HSD1 does not modulate HPA axis feedback in humans, at least at the morning peak. Intriguingly, 11β-HSD1 may play a role in pathogenesis because rare haplotypes of the HSD11B1 gene are associated with a risk of Alzheimer's disease.

Conclusion

11β-HSDs interconvert active glucocorticoids and inert 11-keto forms. This seemingly obscure reaction is important in peripheral tissues and the CNS, determining glucocorticoid access to nuclear receptors and hence biological effects in health and disease. 11β-HSD1 is an 11β-ketoreductase that amplifies intracellular glucocorticoid levels. Studies in 11β-HSD1$^{-/-}$ mice show a role in HPA feedback. Deficiency of 11β-HSD1 reduces intracerebral glucocorticoid levels and prevents the emergence of cognitive deficits with aging. 11β-HSD2 is a potent 11β-dehydrogenase, which is little expressed in the adult CNS but which plays an emerging role in preventing premature glucocorticoid actions on the developing nervous system. The maintenance of fetoplacental 11β-HSD2 and the inhibition of 11β-HSD1 have therapeutic potential.

Further Reading

De Kloet, E. R. (2004). Hormones and the stressed brain. Stress: current neuroendocrine and genetic approaches. *Annals of the New York Academy of Sciences* **1018**, 1–15.

Diaz, R., Brown, R. W. and Seckl, J. R. (1998). Ontogeny of mRNAs encoding glucocorticoid and mineralocorticoid receptors and 11β-hydroxysteroid dehydrogenases in prenatal rat brain development reveal complex control of glucocorticoid action. *Journal of Neuroscience* **18**, 2570–2580.

Edwards, C. R. W., Benediktsson, R., and Lindsay, R. (1993). Dysfunction of the placental glucocorticoid barrier: a link between the foetal environment and adult hypertension? *Lancet* **341**, 355–357.

Harris, H. J., Kotelevtsev, Y. and Mullins, J. J. 2001. 11β-hydroxysteroid dehydrogenase type 1 null mice have altered hypothalamic-pituitary-adrenal axis activity: a novel control of glucocorticoid feedback. *Endocrinology* **142**, 114–120.

Kotelevtsev, Y., Holmes, M. C. and Burchell, A. (1997). 11β-hydroxysteroid dehydrogenase type 1 knockout mice show attenuated glucocorticoid inducible responses and resist hyperglycaemia on obesity or stress. *Proceedings of the National Academy of Sciences USA* **94**, 14924–14929.

Kotelevtsev, Y., Brown, R. W. and Fleming, S. (1999). Hypertension in mice lacking 11β-hydroxysteroid dehydrogenase type 2. *Journal of Clinical Investigations* **103**, 683–689.

Liu, D., Dioria, J. and Tannenbaum, B. (1997). Maternal care, hippocampal glucocorticoid receptors, and hypothalamic-pituitary-adrenal responses to stress. *Science* **277**, 1659–1662.

Matthews, S. G. (2002). Early programming of the hypothalamo-pituitary-adrenal axis. *Trends in Endocrinology and Metabolism* **130**, 373–380.

McEwen, B. S. (1999). Stress and hippocampal plasticity. *Annual Review of Neuroscience* **22**, 105–122.

Moisan, M.-P., Seckl, J. R. and Edwards, C. R. W. (1990). 11β-hydroxysteroid dehydrogenase bioactivity and messenger RNA expression in rat forebrain: localization in hypothalamus, hippocampus and cortex. *Endocrinology* **127**, 1450–1455.

Mune, T., Rogerson, F. M. and Nikkilä, H. (1995). Human hypertension caused by mutations in the kidney isozyme of 11β-hydroxysteroid dehydrogenase. *Nature Genetics* **10**, 394–399.

Phillips, D. I. W., Walker, B. R. and Reynolds, R. M. (2000). Low birth weight predicts elevated plasma cortisol concentrations in adults from 3 populations. *Hypertension* **35**(6), 1301–1306.

Rajan, V., Edwards, C. R. W. and Seckl, J. R. (1996). 11β-hydroxysteroid dehydrogenase in cultured hippocampal cells reactivates inert 11-dehydrocorticosterone, potentiating neurotoxicity. *Journal of Neuroscience* **16**, 65–70.

Roland, B. L., Li, K. X. Z. and Funder, J. W. (1995). Hybridization histochemical localization of 11β-hydroxysteroid dehydrogenase type 2 in rat brain. *Endocrinology* **136**, 4697–4700.

Sandeep, T., Yau, J., MacCullich, A., et al. (2004). Effects of 11beta-hydroxysteroid dehydrogenase inhibition on cognitive function in healthy elderly men and patients with type 2 diabetes. *Proceedings of the National Academy of Sciences USA* **101**, 6734–6739.

Seckl, J. R. (2004). 11β-hydroxysteroid dehydrogenases: changing glucocorticoid action. *Current Opinions in Pharmacology* **4**, 597–602.

Seckl, J. R. (2004). Prenatal glucocorticoids and long-term programming. *European Journal of Endocrinology* **151**, U49–U62.

Seckl, J. R. and Walker, B. R. (2004). 11beta-hydroxysteroid dehydrogenase type 1 as a modulator of glucocorticoid action: from metabolism to memory. *Trends in Endocrinology and Metabolism* **15**, 418–424.

Stewart, P. M. and Krozowski, Z. S. (1999). 11 beta-hydroxysteroid dehydrogenase. *Vitamins and Hormones* **57**, 249–324.

Weaver, I., Cervoni, N., Champagne, F., et al. (2004). Epigenetic programming by maternal behavior. *Nature Neuroscience* **7**, 847–854.

Welberg, L. A. M., Seckl, J. R. and Holmes, M. C. (2000). Inhibition of 11β-hydroxysteroid dehydrogenase, the feto-placental barrier to maternal glucocorticoids, permanently programs amygdala glucocorticoid receptor mRNA expression and anxiety-like behavior in the offspring. *European Journal of Neuroscience* **12**, 1047–1054.

Yau, J. L. W., Noble, J., Kenyon, C. J., et al. (2001). Lack of tissue glucocorticoid reactivation in 11β-hydroxysteroid dehydrogenase type 1 knockout mice ameliorates age-related learning impairments. *Proceedings of the National Academy of Sciences USA* **98**, 4716–4721.

Congenital Adrenal Hyperplasia (CAH)

A Solomon and P-M G Bouloux
Royal Free Hospital and Medical School, London, UK

Glossary

Allele One of two or more copies of a particular gene located on a chromosome.

Androgens Sex steroids that stimulate the development of male sex organs and male secondary sexual characteristics.

Azoospermia The complete absence of sperm in seminal fluid.

Compound heterozygote A pair of alleles that are both mutated with abnormalities distinct from one another.

Homozygote A pair of genes that are identical.

Hyperplasia The increase in the size and number of normal cells in an organ or tissue.

Hypogonadism A condition that results from the failure of sex steroid production.

Phenotype The expression of the characteristics of a person as determined by his or her genes and influenced by environmental factors.

Virilization The clinical consequences of excessive androgen production in females; characterized by temporal balding, a male body form, muscle bulk, deepening of the voice, enlargement of the clitoris, and hirsutism.

Congenital adrenal hyperplasia (CAH; previously known as adrenogenital syndrome) represents a diverse range of inherited disorders resulting from altered activity in the enzymatic steps required in steroid hormone synthesis. In each, cortisol production is reduced, leading to an increase of pituitary adrenocorticotropic hormone (ACTH; corticotropin) secretion by negative feedback, which causes adrenal hyperplasia and the overproduction of either cortisol precursors or androgens. The incidence of the classic disorder is 1 in 5000–20 000 live births in most populations. This rate increases in certain specific geographic locations, including the Yupic population of Alaska, the island of La Réunion, Brazil, and the Philippines. There is wide racial variation and phenotypic heterogeneity. Among Caucasians a 1/60 carrier frequency is found; in the Ashkenazi Jewish population, the carrier rate for nonclassic CAH is up to 19%.

Classification

CAH can be classified according to the specific type of enzyme deficiency involved. Classic CAH refers to the more severe form of enzyme deficiency with a prenatal, neonatal, or early childhood presentation. Nonclassic CAH represents a milder variant of the disorder, associated with less severe enzyme deficiency, a later presentation, and usually mild hyperandrogenism, often mimicking polycystic ovarian syndrome (PCOS). When presenting in adulthood, symptoms may be unmasked by various factors including cytochrome p450-inducing drugs such as anticonvulsants. CAH can also be classified as salt-wasting, non-salt-wasting, virilizing, or feminizing (see **Table 1**).

Molecular Genetics

The gene encoding the 21-OH enzyme is found on chromosome 6 (6p.21.3), and within this locus are both active and inactive (pseudo-)genes known as CYP21A2 and CYP21A, respectively. Most mutations involve the recombination of active and inactive genes, creating compound heterozygotes (i.e., different mutations on the two alleles) – with phenotype correlating with the less severely mutant allele – explaining the phenotypic variability of the disorder. Alongside common mutations, novel, highly variable mutated alleles of CYP21A2 are increasingly being recognized, especially in the nonclassic phenotype. An unusual mechanism involving inactivating mutations of the P450 oxidoreductase enzyme causing simultaneous combined P450P17 and P450C21 deficiency has now been described in several families and provides significant insight into the pathophysiology of the disorder. Interestingly, *in vivo* this mechanism appears to confer a combination of androgen excess prenatally and androgen deficiency postnatally.

Biochemical Abnormalities

The family of disorders causing CAH are due to deficient activity (either the reduction in the amount of enzyme or impaired enzymatic function) in one of the five steps involved in cortisol biosynthesis (**Figure 1**). 21-Hydroxylase (21-OH) deficiency is the most frequent form. This enzyme converts progesterone to deoxycorticosterone and 17-hydroxyprogesterone (17-OHP) to 11-deoxycortisol in the endoplasmic reticulum (ER). Less commonly, deficient activity of 11β-hydroxylase (11β-OH) in the mitochondria or 3β-hydroxysteroid dehydrogenase (3β-HSD) and 17α-hydroxylase (17α-OH) in the ER can result in the syndrome. Last, the steroidogenic acute regulatory protein (StAR) is essential for transporting cholesterol to

Table 1 Classification and presentation of congenital adrenal hyperplasia at diagnosis[a]

Deficiency	*Salt-wasting*	*Virilization*	*Feminization (undervirilization)*	*Precocious puberty*	*Delayed puberty*	*Hypertension*	*Infertility, menstrual disturbance, hirsutism, and acne*
21-OH (>90%)	Yes (not in late onset nonclassic cases)	Yes (severity varies)	No	Yes (possible presenting complaint)	No	No	Yes
11β-OH (~5%)	No (almost all cases)	Yes (severity varies)	No	Yes	No	Yes (most cases)	Yes
3β-HSD	Yes	No (mild or none at birth)	Yes (in males with classic cases)	Yes	No	No	Yes
17α-OH	No	No	Yes	No	Yes	Yes	No
StAR	Yes	No	Yes	No	Yes	No	No

[a]3β-HSD, 3β-hydroxysteroid dehydrogenase; 11β-OH, 11β-hydroxylase; 17α-OH, 17α-hydroxylase; 21-OH, 21-hydroxylase; StAR, steroidogenic acute regulatory protein.

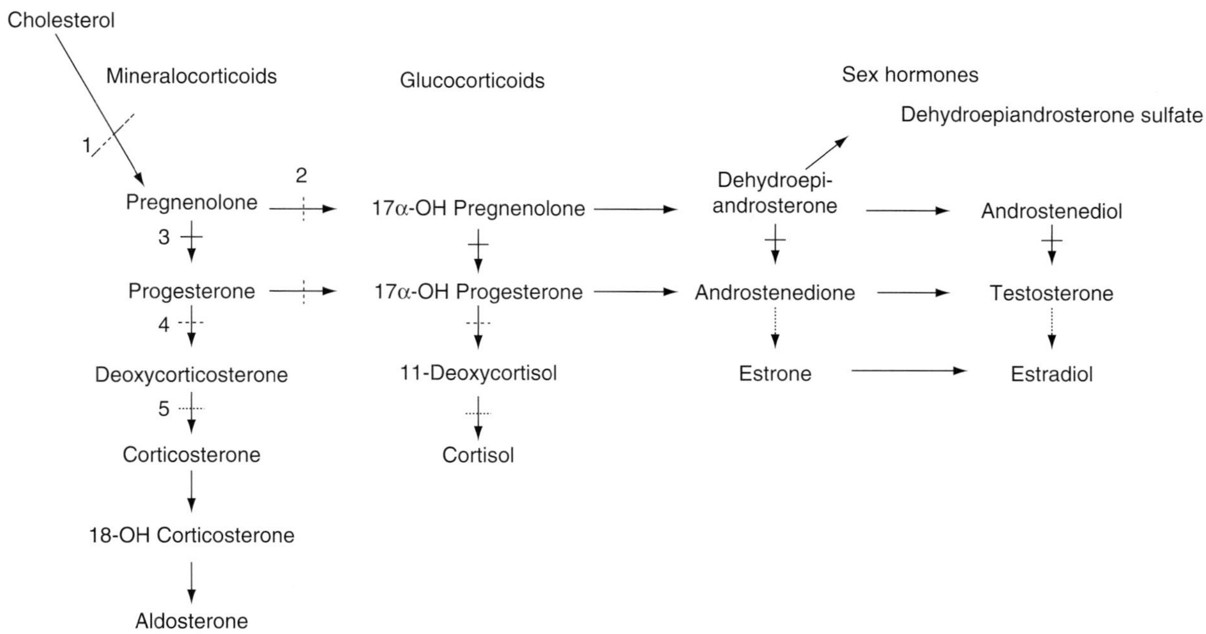

Figure 1 Adrenal steroidogenesis: (1) StAR; (2) 17α-OH; (3) 3β-HSD; (4) 21-OH; (5) 11β-OH.

the mitochondria for steroid biosynthesis in the adrenal and gonad, and an abnormality in the gene encoding this protein leads to the very rare but devastating congenital lipoid adrenal hyperplasia.

Figure 2 illustrates the mechanism whereby deficient 21-OH enzyme activity leads to a decrease in cortisol production and an increase in adrenal androgen production by the shunting of precursors through alternative steroidogenic pathways. The biochemical abnormalities resulting from enzyme blockade can be deduced by examining the site of the block (**Figure 1**).

Clinical Features

The clinical spectrum of mild to severe forms of CAH reflects the degree of deficiency in cortisol and aldosterone (or both) and also the excess or deficient production of androgens. This, in turn, is determined by the particular genetic abnormality (see **Table 1**).

Classic Congenital Adrenal Hyperplasia

Abnormal genitalia Abnormalities in all five steps of cortisol synthesis can present with abnormal genitalia. In the female, virilization of the external genitalia by adrenal androgens *in utero* leads to clitoromegaly, labial fusion, and formation of a urogenital sinus (called female pseudohermaphroditism). Severe cases can be mistakenly diagnosed as hypospadias with undescended testes and incorrect gender assignment at birth can result. Affected males may have normal sexual development. A further important clinical phenomenon is the occasional finding of testicular adrenal rest tumors; these masses occur under stimulation of high ACTH due to embryological similarity between the adrenal gland and genital ridge.

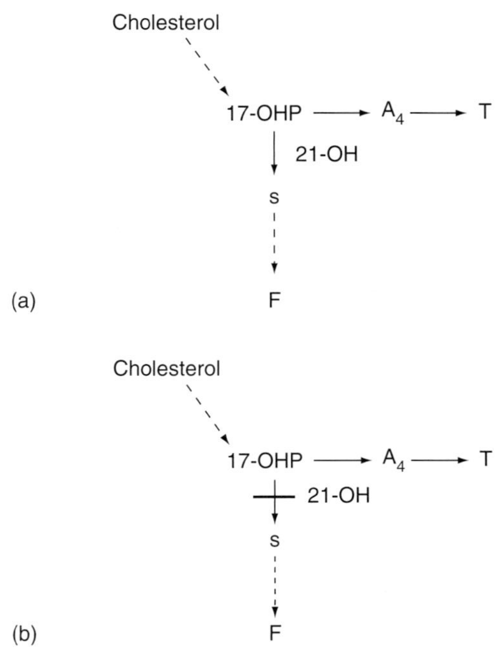

Figure 2 Biochemical consequences of enzyme blockade. a, Normal reaction pathway; b, pathway with 21-hydroxylase deficiency, leading to the shunting of cortisol precursors to increase adrenal androgen production. 17-OHP, 17-hydroxyprogesterone; A_4, androstenedione; F, cortisol; S, 11-deoxycortisol; T, testosterone.

They are detectable by ultrasonography and improve with compliance with glucocorticoid therapy.

Salt-wasting crisis Salt-wasting crisis may occur in all types of CAH except 11β-OH and 17α-OH deficiency. Most commonly an affected male infant 2–3 weeks old presents with failure to thrive followed by an acute illness consisting of diarrhea, vomiting, dehydration, and circulatory collapse. Plasma electrolytes typically show hyperkalemia, hyponatremia, and metabolic acidosis. Sodium conservation improves with age in some patients, although it is unclear why this should occur.

Virilization and precocious puberty In females, clitoral enlargement in early childhood may occur due to overproduction of adrenal androgens. In males, the penis may enlarge but the testes remain small. In both, pubic hair growth may occur early and excess linear growth with concomitant epiphyseal closure is common. Circulating androgens may prematurely activate the hypothalamic-pituitary-gonadal axis, and the child may have true precocious puberty. Short stature due to premature epiphyseal closure invariably occurs unless the condition is treated early.

Delayed puberty Delayed puberty is a rare manifestation of CAH and can occur in poorly controlled 21-OH deficiency with the suppression of gonadotropins by excess adrenal androgens.

Primary amenorrhea Primary amenorrhea is an uncommon presentation that may occur in less severe variants of 17α-OH deficiency or 3β-HSD deficiency when phenotypic females with poorly developed secondary sexual characteristics (breast development and pubic hair) fail to menstruate due to deficient production of ovarian estrogen.

Impaired fertility A degree of impaired fertility found in some patients is multifactorial. Live birth rates resulting from patients with classic CAH continue to improve – ovulation may be spontaneous or assisted by clomiphene and/or gonadotropins.

Nonclassic Congenital Adrenal Hyperplasia

Nonclassic forms of CAH have their onset of symptoms in late childhood or in adulthood.

Precocious puberty Less severe forms of CAH with no evidence of salt-wasting can present for the first time in later childhood. Accelerated linear growth and bone age can result in reduced ultimate adult height unless the correct diagnosis is made and treatment given.

Hypertension In those types of CAH in which excess mineralocorticoids are produced, hypertension may result, which may become apparent only in later life.

Acne and hirsutism in the female Nonclassic types of CAH with excess androgen production can be indistinguishable from those women with polycystic ovaries, which are frequently present on ultrasound. Approximately 1–3% of hyperandrogenism in adult females is due to late-onset CAH.

Impaired fertility and menstrual disorders Fertility can be impaired in both males and females with CAH. In females, this is due to excess progesterone and androgens suppressing the normal cyclicity of the hypothalamic-pituitary-gonadal axis plus various factors affecting fertilization and implantation. In males, azoospermia may be reversed with glucocorticoid replacement and various forms of assisted conception.

17α-Hydroxylase Deficiency

The specific condition of 17α-OH deficiency deserves highlighting due to the resultant deficiency of sex steroid production. It exhibits marked phenotypic heterogeneity, with a disproportionately higher prevalence found in Brazil. There may be a severely impaired development of external genitalia in both sexes; genotypic males are usually raised as females due to a lack of *in utero* and postnatal male phenotypic development. In addition, the mechanism of this metabolic defect generates excess mineralocorticoid with its associated clinical features.

Diagnostic Investigations

Once the clinical suspicion is raised, the diagnosis of CAH can be made by measuring the level of steroid precursors in the basal state (see **Table 2**) or after ACTH stimulation (see **Figure 3**). 17-OHP can also be measured in saliva; examining the urinary steroid profile for abnormal concentrations or ratios of metabolic products of the various steroids can be diagnostic (see **Table 2**). The adrenal glands can be imaged by ultrasound, computed tomography (CT) scan, or magnetic resonance imaging (MRI) and may show evidence of bilateral hyperplasia in contrast to the focal lesion, which may be seen with an adrenal tumor. Prenatal diagnosis can be made by the measurement of 17-OHP or androstenedione in amniotic fluid. Human leukocyte antigen (HLA) typing and linkage analysis of cultured fetal cells from chorionic villus sampling in the first trimester or amniocentesis later in gestation can reliably predict genotype for 21-OH deficiency. Automated sequencing and polymerase chain reaction using DNA extracted

Table 2 Basal biochemical profile in congenital adrenal hyperplasia[a]

Deficiency	*Serum*							*Urine*		
	17-OHP	*A_4*	*DHEAS*	*T*	*S*	*P*	*PRA*	*17KS*	*Pregnantriol*	*THS*
21-OH	↑↑	↓	–,↑	↑	–, ↓	–	–,↑↑	↑↑	↑↑	↓
11β-OH	–,↑	↓	↑	↑	↑↑	–	–, ↓↓	↑↑	↑	↑↑
3β-HSD	–,↑	2, ↑	↑	↓	–,↓	↓	↑	↑↑	2, ↓	2, ↓
17α-OH	↓	↓	↓	↓	↓	↑	↓	↓	↓	↓
StAR	↓	↓	↓	↓	↓	↓	↑	↓	↓	↓

[a]–, ; ↓, ;↑, ; 3β-HSD, 3β-hydroxysteroid dehydrogenase; 11β-OH, 11β-hydroxylase; 17α-OH, 17α-hydroxylase; 17KS, 17-ketosteroid; 17-OHP, 17-hydroxyprogesterone; 21-OH, 21-hydroxylase; A_4, androstenedione; DHEAS, dehydroepiandrosterone sulfate; P, PRA, S, 11-deoxycortisol; StAR, steroidogenic acute regulatory protein; T, testosterone; THS.

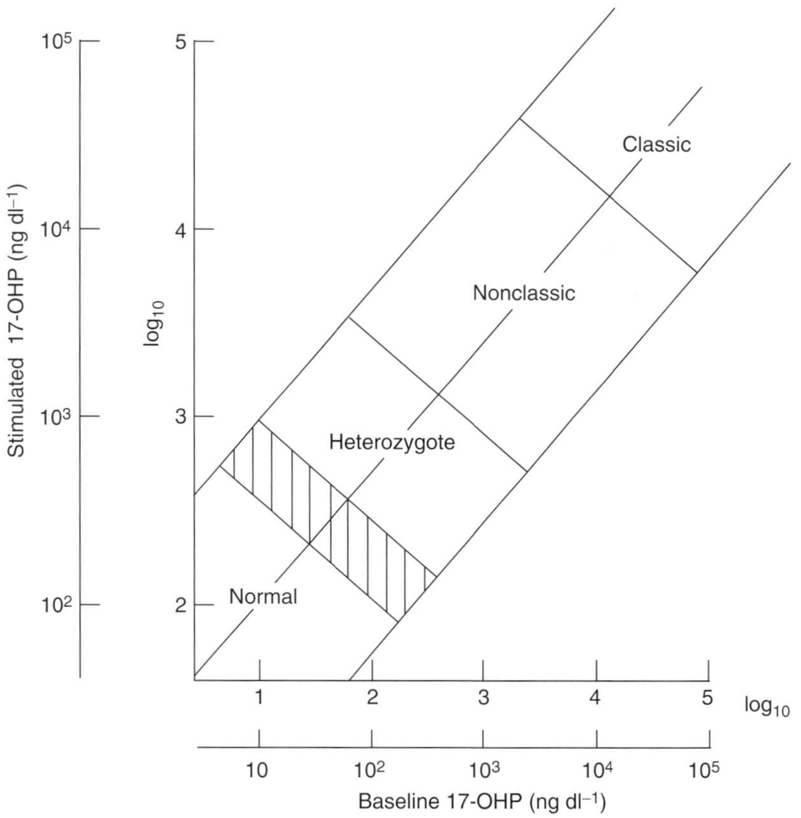

Figure 3 Nomogram for genotyping 21-OH deficiency based on baseline plasma 17-OHP and values obtained 60 min following stimulation with 250 μg ACTH (Synacthen). Note there is considerable overlap between the normal unaffected individual and the heterozygote. 17-OHP, 17-hydroxyprogesterone. From M. C. Young and I. A. Hughes, used with permission.

from uncultured or cultured fetal cells can be employed to screen for specific mutations in the genes responsible for CAH.

Treatment of Congenital Adrenal Hyperplasia

The aims of treatment are usually to correct cortisol and mineralocorticoid deficiency and to suppress adrenal androgen production, thereby preventing virilization. If successful, this should allow normal maturation, growth, development, and fertility in adult life. The patient should be monitored for the potential adverse effects of overtreatment with glucocorticoids.

The daily dose of glucocorticoid therapy should correspond to the normal adrenal production rate of approximately 7 mg/m^2/day usually given in split dosage. The decision on dosage schedule and preparation of replacement glucocorticoid is still controversial.

Larger dosing at night with longer-acting, more potent glucocorticoids such as dexamethasone decreases the exaggerated morning ACTH (and also adrenal androgen) peak of the circadian rhythm but theoretically can suppress nocturnal growth hormone release. The dosage of glucocorticoid should be increased two- to threefold in the event of a febrile illness, and for more severe stresses higher doses or even parenteral therapy may be required. The theoretical concern in relation to the bone density effects of glucocorticoids does not appear to be borne out by the evidence available from carefully treated patients. Glucocorticoids are not used for replacement in the treatment of nonclassic CAH but are used to suppress adrenal hyperandrogenism by inhibiting the morning ACTH peak by delivery of small doses of dexamethasone (e.g., 0.5 mg) or prednisone (e.g., 5 mg) at night. In the nonclassic and classic variants, an antiandrogen can be used in combination with glucocorticoids to treat symptoms of hyperandrogenism.

The adjustment of the dose of glucocorticoid depends on clinical assessment combined with the results of monitoring in the cases of 21-OH deficiency, 17-OHP, adrenal androgens, and/or urinary 17-ketosteroid production. These are, however, not ideal biomarkers, and efforts continue to find more specific ways of monitoring the disease.

Mineralocorticoid replacement therapy with 9α-fludrocortisone should be used in all those patients with salt-wasting forms of CAH. The use of mineralocorticoid therapy in nonclassic late-onset variants of the disorder with raised plasma renin activity, which reflects salt loss, often allows a reduction in the dosage of glucocorticoid and subsequently less risk of iatrogenic side effects. Renin levels can be used in the monitoring of fludrocortisone dosage. In refractory cases, especially when subfertility, obesity, and hirsutism may be prominent features, adrenalectomy is sometimes performed, followed by adrenal steroid replacement.

Prenatal treatment of affected females *in utero* with dexamethasone to prevent virilization of the fetus has been used with varying success. To be effective, treatment must be started at less than 10 weeks (preferably 5–7 weeks) gestation and continued until delivery in affected females but discontinued in males and unaffected females. Mendelian inheritance dictates that without diagnostic confirmation, treatment will only be appropriate in one out of eight fetuses. Maternal side effects such as weight gain, hypertension, diabetes, and edema are common but fortunately more severe side effects are rare. This field lacks consensus, and registries have been created in certain locations, such as Sweden, where the gold standard is that treatment is provided only within the framework of a prospective trial.

The timing of corrective surgery and correct gender assignment is the subject of much debate, with earlier single-procedure operations becoming more popular. There is still controversy over the ideal mechanisms for assigning gender, and multidisciplinary teams have been found to be the optimal strategy for handling the delicate issues involved. In severe forms of 21-OH and 11β-OH deficiency, virilization may be so severe that genotypic females may need to be raised as males and ovarectomy will be required with prostheses inserted into the scrotum at puberty. There is evidence that exposure to androgens *in utero* can alter gender and sexual identity in affected females, in whom there is an above-average increase in tomboyish behavior and lesbianism. These sequelae demonstrate the need for early and adequate treatment of the condition and long-term follow-up to ensure well-balanced individuals, progress through puberty, and the formation of stable relationships. Sexual function in adulthood is an area of increasing discussion, and the psychosocial impact of this condition has only recently been fully explored.

Conclusion

CAH is a heterogeneous condition that causes multiple imbalances in metabolic pathways of steroid hormone synthesis. Knowledge of the genetic basis for the condition has allowed increasingly specific methods of screening and treatment to be developed.

Further Reading

Arlt, W. and Stewart, P. M. (2005). Adrenal corticosteroid biosynthesis, metabolism, and action. *Endocrinology & Metabolism Clinics of North America* **34**(2), viii, 293–313.

Arlt, W., Walker, E. A., Draper, N., et al. (2004). Congenital adrenal hyperplasia caused by mutant P450 oxidoreductase and human androgen synthesis: analytical study. *Lancet* **363**(9427), 2128–2135.

Friaes, A., Rego, A. T., Aragues, J. M., et al. (2006). CYP21A2 mutations in Portuguese patients with congenital adrenal hyperplasia: identification of two novel mutations and characterization of four different partial gene conversions. *Molecular Genetics and Metabolism.*

Gonzalez, A. A., Reyes, M. L., Carvajal, C. A., et al. (2004). Congenital lipoid adrenal hyperplasia caused by a novel splicing mutation in the gene for the steroidogenic acute regulatory protein. *Journal of Clinical Endocrinology and Metabolism* **89**(2), 946–951.

King, J. A., Wisniewski, A. B., Bankowski, B. J., et al. (2006). Long-term corticosteroid replacement and bone mineral density in adult women with classical congenital

adrenal hyperplasia. *Journal of Clinical Endocrinology and Metabolism* **91**(3), 865–869.
Lajic, S., Nordenstrom, A., Ritzen, E. M., et al. (2004). Prenatal treatment of congenital adrenal hyperplasia. *European Journal of Endocrinology* **151**(supplement 3), U63–U69.
Loidi, L., Quinteiro, C., Parajes, S., et al. (2006). High variability in CYP21A2 mutated alleles in Spanish 21-hydroxylase deficiency patients, six novel mutations and a founder effect. *Clinical Endocrinology* (Oxford) **64**(3), 330–336.
Merke, D. P. and Bornstein, S. R. (2005). Congenital adrenal hyperplasia. *Lancet* **365**(9477), 2125–2136.
Ogilvie, C. M., Crouch, N. S., Rumsby, G., et al. (2006). Congenital adrenal hyperplasia in adults: a review of medical, surgical and psychological issues. *Clinical Endocrinology* (Oxford) **64**(1), 2–11.
Rumsby, G., Avey, C. J., Conway, G. S., et al. (1998). Genotype-phenotype analysis in late onset 21-hydroxylase deficiency in comparison to the classical forms. *Clinical Endocrinology* (Oxford) **48**(6), 707–711.
Seckl, J. R. and Miller, W. L. (1997). How safe is long-term prenatal glucocorticoid treatment? *Journal of the American Medical Association* **277**, 1077–1079.
Speiser, P. W. and White, P. C. (2003). Congenital adrenal hyperplasia. *New England Journal of Medicine* **349**(8), 776–788.
Wudy, S. A., Hartmann, M. F., Draper, N., et al. (2004). A male twin infant with skull deformity and elevated neonatal 17-hydroxyprogesterone: a prismatic case of P450 oxidoreductase deficiency. *Endocrine Research* **30**(4), 957–964.

Cushing's Syndrome, Medical Aspects

S R Bornstein and M Gruber
Technical University of Dresden, Dresden, Germany
H S Willenberg
University Hospital Duesseldorf, Duesseldorf, Germany
C A Stratakis and G P Chrousos
National Institute of Child and Health and Human Development, National Institutes of Health, Bethesda, MD, USA

This is a revised version of the article by S R Bornstein, C A Stratakis, and G P Chrousos, Encyclopedia of Stress, First edition, volume 1, pp 615–620, © 2000, Elsevier Inc.

Glossary

Adrenocorticotropic hormone (ACTH)	Pituitary hormone stimulating release of adrenal glucocorticoids.
Corticotropin-releasing hormone (CRH)	The main regulator of the endocrine stress access. Stimulates pituitary ACTH.
Cushing's syndrome	Caused by the state of hypercortisolemia.
Transsphenoidal surgery (TSS)	Surgical procedure of choice to remove pituitary tumors. This procedure utilizes the nasal approach, avoiding the necessity of opening the skull.

Epidemiology

The overall incidence of spontaneous Cushing's syndrome (CS) is approximately two to four new cases per million of population per year, with a female to male preponderance. Approximately 10% of these cases occur in children and adolescents. Adrenocorticotropic hormone (ACTH)-dependent CS accounts for about 85% of endogenous cases in adults, adolescents, and children older than 7 years of age (**Table 1**). Cushing's disease is responsible for 80% of these cases; the remaining 20% is caused by ectopic ACTH or, very rarely, ectopic corticotropin-releasing hormone (CRH) secretion. Benign cortisol-secreting adenomas or adrenocortical carcinomas are rare and account for 10–15% of endogenous cases in children older than 5. In children younger than 5, adrenocortical carcinomas and primary pigmented nodular adrenal disease (PPNAD) are the more frequent causes of endogenous CS. Primary pigmented nodular adrenal disease is a form of adrenal tumors that occurs frequently in association with Carney complex, a multiple endocrine neoplasia and lentiginosis syndrome. With the increasing utilization of glucocorticoids for a wide range of nonendocrine diseases, the exogenous, iatrogenic CS has become more frequent and is more prevalent than the endogenous forms.

Etiology

Endogenous CS results from increased secretion of cortisol by the adrenal cortex and is due to ACTH hypersecretion (ACTH-dependent CS) or the autonomous hyperfunction of the adrenocortical cells (ACTH-independent CS). Some forms of ACTH-independent

Table 1 Classification of Endogenous Cushing's Syndrome and Rate of Occurrence in Children Older than 7 Years[a]

Classification	*Percentage*
ACTH-dependent	**85**
Pituitary (Cushing's disease) (includes MEN-I)	80
Ectopic ACTH (includes MEN-I)	20
Ectopic CRH	Rare
ACTH-independent	**15**
Adrenal adenoma (includes MEN-I)	30
Adrenal carcinoma	70
Primary pigmented adrenocortical disease (PPNAD)	0.5–1
McCune-Albright's syndrome	Rare
"Transitional states"	Rare

[a]Modified from Magiakou and Chrousos (1994).

CS have recently been discovered to be due to aberrant expression of neuroendocrine or cytokine receptors (such as GIP, vasopressin, β-receptor, or interleukin-1), putting the adrenal tissue under a tropic stimulus, which is not under the control of the regular negative feedback. Cushing's disease, the ACTH-dependent form of endogenous CS, is due to an ACTH-secreting, benign corticotroph tumor of the anterior pituitary gland. Ectopic ACTH-secreting tumors occur mostly in patients with bronchial carcinoma. In addition, other tumors may present with ectopic ACTH production (thymus, liver, renal carcinoma, etc.). Exogenous CS results from chronic administration of glucocorticoids (for treatment of neoplastic, autoimmune, and other diseases) or ACTH (for the treatment of certain seizure disorders).

Pathophysiology

The main stimulus for the release of cortisol from the adrenal cortex is ACTH, which is produced by the corticotrophs of the anterior pituitary, which, in turn, are under the regulatory influence of hypothalamic CRH and vasopressin (**Figure 1**). The ambient plasma free cortisol levels regulate ACTH secretion in a negative feedback fashion. Normally, less than 10% of plasma cortisol is in the free form, with the majority being bound to cortisol-binding globulin (or transcortin).

In the physiological state, ACTH and cortisol have a circadian pattern of secretion, established early in infancy and in accordance with other human circadian biological activities. The peak of ACTH and cortisol secretion occurs in the morning (between 7:00 and 8:00 a.m.) and is lowest is in the late evening hours (around midnight). This physiological circadian rhythm is blunted in CS.

The adrenals have an amazing ability to adapt to states of hyper- or hypofunction. They use more than 10 times the cardiac output and blood volume that would correspond to their organ weight. Therefore, they are unique in demonstrating signs of hormonal excess and stress. Chronic stimulation of adrenal tissue with ACTH in Cushing's disease or ectopic ACTH-secreting tumors will cause hypertrophy of the adrenals, leading in particular to an increase in size of the zona fasciculata. The adrenal cortex undergoes hypervascularization and the cells increase in mitochondria, smooth endoplasmic reticulum, and filopodia, indicating increased activation of steroidosynthesis.

Glucocorticoids are vital for survival because they participate greatly in the stress response of humans. Glucocorticoids affect all tissues and organ systems, and the glucocorticoid receptor is ubiquitously present. Glucocorticoids have profound catabolic activities: they inhibit growth and reproduction, promote proteinolysis, and suppress the immune and inflammatory reaction. These effects are behind some of the cardinal clinical manifestations of CS: delayed growth and bone maturation, hypogonadism, dermopathy, loss of muscular tissue, and frequent fungal or saprophytic infections.

Clinical Picture

Table 2 summarizes the clinical features of CS in children and adolescents. An early and common sign in almost all patients is obesity, which is generalized or truncal and is characterized by moon facies (facial rounding) and plethora. Growth retardation or complete arrest is present in 90% of the children. Other clinical manifestations include sleep disturbances, muscle weakness and fatigue, hirsutism, and typical purple skin striae. Hypertension, carbohydrate intolerance or diabetes, amenorrhea, advancement or arrest of pubertal development, and easy bruising or spontaneous fractures of ribs and vertebrae may also be encountered. Although all patients may exhibit some of these features at the time of diagnosis, few, if any, will have all of them. Photographs of the patient, taken over a period of years, are helpful in the clinical evaluation.

The clinical presentation can identify the cause of CS in children and adolescents. Thus, severe and rapidly progressing CS points toward an adrenal neoplasm or, although rare in children, ectopic ACTH syndrome. Patients with adrenocortical carcinomas may be asymptomatic or may have abdominal pain or fullness, symptoms and signs of CS (30%), virilization (20%), combined symptoms of CS and virilization (30%), feminization (10%), or hyperaldosteronism (5–10%). CS is periodic or intermittent in a significant percentage (~10%) of children and adolescents.

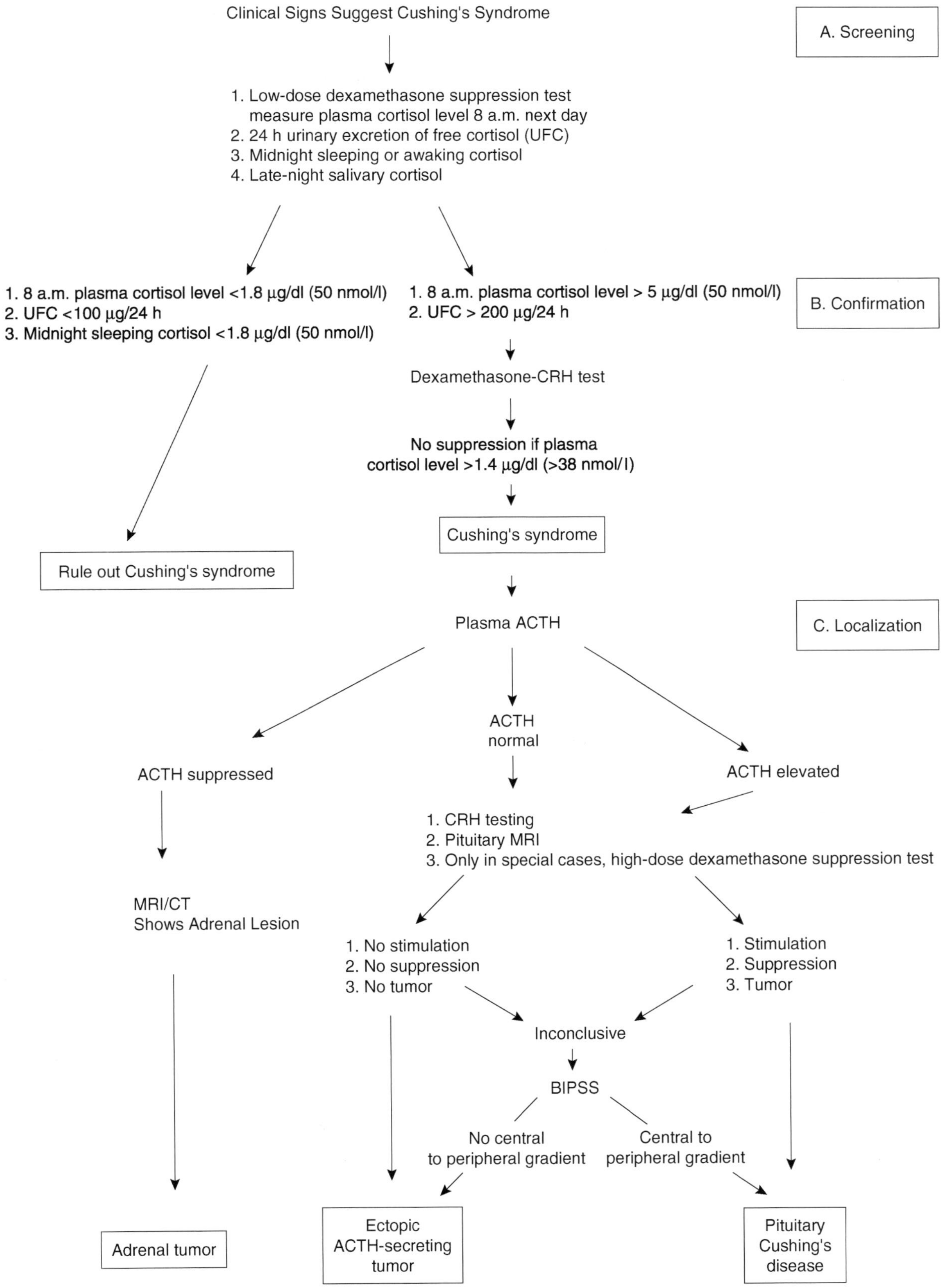

Figure 1 Diagnostic algorithm for Cushing's syndrome. Modified from Bornstein, S. R., Stratakis, C. A., and Chrousos, G. P. (1999). Adrenocortical tumors: recent advances in basic concepts and clinical management. *Annals of Internal Medicine* **130**, 711–759.

Table 2 Clinical presentation of CS in pediatric patients[a]

Symptoms/signs	*Frequency (percentage)*
Weight gain	90
Growth retardation	83
Menstrual irregularities	81
Hirsutism	81
Obesity (Body Mass Index .85 percentile)	73
Violaceous skin striae	63
Acne	52
Hypertension	51
Fatigue-weakness	45
Precocious puberty	41
Bruising	27
Mental changes	18
"Delayed" bone age	14
Hyperpigmentation	13
Muscle weakness	13
Acanthosis nigricans	10
Accelerated bone age	10
Sleep disturbances	7
Pubertal delay	7
Hypercalcemia	6
Alkalosis	6
Hypokalemia	2
Slipped femoral capital epiphysis	2

[a]Modified from Magiakou *et al.* (1994).

Laboratory Findings

The first step in diagnosing noniatrogenic CS is the biochemical documentation of endogenous hypercortisolism, which can usually be accomplished by outpatient tests. The first test is measurement of 24-h urinary free cortisol (UFC) excretion corrected for body surface area and/or the determination of 24-h urinary 17-hydroxycorticosteroid (17OHCS) excretion (corrected per gram of excreted creatinine). UFC excretion is a good first-line test for documentation of CS, with, assuming correct collection, very few false negative results. The second test is the single-dose dexamethasone suppression test. The overnight 1-mg (in young children, 15 μg/kg body weight) dexamethasone suppression test is a useful screening procedure for hypercortisolism. It is simple, with a low incidence of false normal suppression (less than 3%). The same test, however, has a high incidence of false positive results (approximately 20–30%). A plasma cortisol level >1.8 μg/dl (50 nmol/l) suggests endogenous hypercortisolism and needs to be followed by a 24-h urine collection for determination of UFC or 17OHCS levels.

CS is generally excluded if the aforementioned tests are normal, although one should remember that periodic and intermittent cortisol hypersecretion, which may occur in patients with CS of any etiology, may confuse the picture.

In the past few years, a simple test reached importance in the first-line diagnosis of CS, especially for outpatient assessment. The measurement of late-night salivary cortisol is easy, and the cortisol in this test is stable under room conditions. Because of the variety of the diagnostic ranges in this test, the cut-off point of the local laboratory has to be known. The sensitivity and the specificity of this test are between 95 and 98%.

Another important and highly sensitive test is the measurement of the midnight sleeping or awaking cortisol levels, because of the circadian rhythm of cortisol secretion in healthy persons. A sleeping midnight cortisol level of less than 1.8 μg/dl (50 nmol/l) excludes CS. Once CS has been diagnosed, the differential diagnosis is investigated via dynamic testing of the function of the hypothalamic-pituitary-adrenal (HPA) axis as well as imaging studies. It is essential that dynamic endocrine testing is performed while the patient is hypercortisolemic, and, in order to avoid mistakes, this state should always be documented at the time of testing. All adrenal blocking agents should be discontinued for at least 6 weeks prior to testing.

The major tests in the differential diagnosis of CS and their interpretations include the following (see also **Figure 1**):

1. Low-dose dexamethasone suppression test and dexamethasone-CRH test*:* The low-dose dexamethasone suppression test (0.5 mg every 6 h over 2 days) and the dexamethasone-CRH test are reliable procedures for differentiating Cushing's disease from subclinical CS. In the combined dexamethasone-CRH test, after application of 0.5 mg dexamethasone every 6 h over 2 days (start on first day at 12.00 a.m.; the finish dose is given at 6.00 a.m.), a CRH-stimulating test will follow at 8.00 a.m. If the plasma cortisol is lower than 1.4 μg/dl (38 nmol/l) after 15 min, the CS is excluded. In subclinical CS, the cortisol is depressed at this time.
2. CRH stimulation test. The ovine (o) CRH test is of greater value than the dexamethasone suppression test in differentiating Cushing's disease and ectopic ACTH syndrome.
3. Overnight 8-mg dexamethasone suppression test. This test is currently not recommended for routine use. Because of its sensitivity of about 80% of cortisol suppression in CS, it yields no further information than the low-dose test.
4. Petrosal-sinus sampling with CRH test. This procedure can help to differentiate between a pituitary and a non-pituitary source of corticotropin secretion: if there is a ratio of two between basal central and basal peripheral sampling of

corticotropin, or after stimulation with CRH a ratio of three, the diagnosis of Cushing's disease is clear.

Radiographic Findings

Imaging techniques can help clarify the etiology of hypercortisolism. These include computed tomographic (CT) scanning and magnetic resonance imaging (MRI) of the pituitary gland and CT scan, MRI, and ultrasound imaging of the adrenal glands. CT and MRI scans of the chest and abdomen are also used when tumors secreting ectopic ACTH are suspected.

Treatment

The preferred treatment for CS depends upon the specific cause of the hypercortisolism, which must be firmly and unequivocally established. The optimal treatment is correction of hypercortisolism without permanent dependence on hormone replacement.

Cushing's Disease

Transsphenoidal surgery (TSS) Transsphenoidal surgery is the treatment of choice for most cases of CS caused by pituitary microadenomas. It is indicated if the presence of a pituitary microadenoma can be demonstrated preoperatively by imaging techniques or bilateral inferior petrosalsinus blood sampling (BIPSS). In most specialized centers, the success rate of first TSS exceeds 90%. If BIPSS has lateralized the microadenoma and the surgeon cannot identify it at surgery, 75–80% of patients can be cured by ipsilateral hemihypophysectomy. Usually, successful TSS leads to the cure of hypercortisolism without using permanent glucocorticoid replacement. Approximately 5% of patients suffer recurrences; this is most common in patients with pituitary macroadenomas. The success rate of repeat TSS is considerably lower (approximately 50–60%). Complications include transient or permanent, partial or complete anterior pituitary insufficiency, including, in order of frequency, hypothyroidism, growth hormone deficiency, hypogonadism, and adrenal insufficiency. Transient diabetes insipidus and inappropriate antidiuretic secretion syndrome are also common. Success after TSS is defined as a decrease in serum cortisol or UFC to an undetectable level in the immediate postoperative period. After a successful TSS, a period of adrenal insufficiency occurs in most patients cured, during which glucocorticoids must be replaced at a dose of 12–15 mg/m^2/day. This abnormality of the HPA axis can last as long as a year or longer. It is rare, though possible, that it is permanent. The replacement dose of hydrocortisone is maintained for 3 months, and adrenocortical function is evaluated at that time with a rapid Cortrosyn test (250 mg ACTH 1–24 iv bolus, with plasma cortisol measured at 0, 30, and 60 min). If the test is normal (cortisol >18 and >20 μg/dl (500 nmol/l and 550 nmol/l) at 30 and 60 min, respectively), glucocorticoid replacement is discontinued. If the response is subnormal, the patient is reevaluated at 3-month intervals. About 70–80% of the patients will have a normal test at 6 months postoperation. Patients should be given extra glucocorticoids during stress (two times replacement dose for minor stress such as febrile illness or dental surgery, and 8–10 times replacement dose for major stress, such as major trauma or surgery).

Pituitary X-radiation with or without mitotane This is an alternative treatment that may be used after failure of TSS, when there is presence of cavernous sinus wall invasion by the tumor, or in patients judged unsuitable for surgery. The total recommended dosage of pituitary irradiation is 4500 to 5000 rad. High-voltage, conventional X-radiation is administered in 180- to 200-rad fractions over a period of 6 weeks. Success rate is ~40–50%, without mitotane and ~80% with mitotane (see later).

Pharmacotherapy Drug therapy alone is rarely used to treat Cushing's disease, except temporarily, prior to definitive treatment. Mitotane (Lysodren) is the only available pharmacological agent that both inhibits biosynthesis of corticosteroids and destroys adrenocortical cells secreting cortisol, thus producing a long-lasting effect. Therapy with mitotane (up to 3 g/day) is usually combined with radiotherapy. Aminoglutethimide, up to 1 g/day orally in four divided doses, or metyrapone, up to 1 g/day in four divided doses, may also be used alone or in combination with mitotane. During treatment, UFC excretion should be monitored and the regimen should be titrated to maintain this parameter in the normal range. If adrenal insufficiency is suspected, oral hydrocortisone should be added.

Ketoconazole (up to 1400 mg/day or 20 mg/kg/day) or trilostane have also been used alone or in combination with mitotane to control some of the symptoms and metabolic abnormalities associated with Cushing's disease. Combinations are recommended because they usually prevent breakthroughs that occur when the drugs are used alone. In addition, one can use moderate doses with less side effects from each agent.

There are also new compounds such as fluconazole and glitazones, and for ectopic CS there are somatostatin analogs such as octreotide, lanreotide, and cabergolin.

Bilateral adrenalectomy The indications for this procedure have been dramatically changed by the success and low morbidity of TSS. Bilateral adrenalectomy is a possible treatment for patients who have failed selective pituitary adenomectomy or hemihypophysectomy. The major disadvantages of this surgery are that the individual is committed to lifelong daily gluco- and mineralocorticoid replacements, it does not eliminate the cause underlying the hypersecretion of ACTH, and relapses, though rare, may occur as a result of growth of adrenal rest tissue or an adrenal remnant. Furthermore, perioperative mortality is approximately three times higher than that of TSS, although it can be minimized by careful perioperative preparation. Also, Nelson syndrome (i.e., large pituitary macroadenomas secreting great amounts of ACTH and lipotropin resulting in skin hyperpigmentation) may occur in approximately 10–15% of patients with Cushing's disease treated with bilateral adrenalectomy. These tumors can impair vision and should be treated surgically and by radiotherapy.

Ectopic ACTH-Dependent CS

The preferred treatment for ectopic ACTH secretion is surgery aimed at completely excising the tumor, if resectable and of known location. If there is evidence of adjacent lymph node invasion, local radiation can be recommended after surgery for some tumors, such as carcinoids. If surgical resection is impossible or if the tumor is hidden, blockade of steroidogenesis is indicated; if necessary, bilateral adrenalectomy is considered.

See Also the Following Articles

Adrenal Cortex.

Further Reading

Arnaldi, G., et al. (2003). Diagnosis and complications of Cushing's syndrome: a consensus statement. *Journal of Clinical Endocrinology and Metabolism* **88**(12), 555593–555602.

Aron, D. C., et al. (1997). Effectiveness versus efficacy. The limited value in clinical practise of high dose dexamethasone suppression testing in the differential diagnosis of ACTH-dependent Cushing's syndrome. *Journal of Clinical Endocrinology and Metabolism* **82**(6), 1780–1785.

Findling, J. W., et al. (2005). Screening and diagnosis of Cushing's syndrome. *Endocrinology and Metabolism Clinics of North America* **34**(2), 384–502.

Ilias, I., et al. (2005). Cushing's syndrome due to ectopic corticotropin secretion: twenty years' experience at the National Institutes of Health. *Journal of Clinical Endocrinology and Metabolism* **90**(8), 4955–4962.

Katabami, T., et al. (2005). Discrepancies in results of low- and high-dose dexamethasone suppression tests for diagnosing preclinical Cushing's syndrome. *Endocrinology Journal* **52**(4), 463–469.

Monson, J. P., et al. (2000). The epidemiology of endocrine tumours. *Endocrine-Related Cancer* **7**(1), 29–365.

Newell-Price, J., et al. (1995). A single sleeping midnight cortisol has 100% sensitivity for the diagnosis of Cushing's syndrome. *Clinical Endocrinology (Oxford)* **43**(5), 545–550.

Newell-Price, J., et al. (1998). The diagnosis and differential diagnosis of Cushing's syndrome and pseudo Cushing's states. *Endocrine Reviews* **19**(5), 647–672.

Newell-Price, J., et al. (2006). Cushing's syndrome. *The Lancet* **367**, 1605–1617.

Niemann, L. K., et al. (2002). Medical therapy of Cushing's disease. *Pituitary* **5**(2), 77–82.

Reimondo, G., et al. (2005). Evaluation of the effectiveness of midnight serum cortisol in the diagnostic procedures for Cushing's syndrome. *European Journal of Endocrinology* **153**(6), 803–809.

Riedl, M., et al. (2006). Long term control of hypercortisolism with fluconazole: case report and in vitro studies. *European Journal of Endocrinology* **154**(4), 519–524.

Terzolo, M., et al. (2004). Subclinical Cushing's syndrome. *Pituitary* **7**(4), 217–223.

Viardot, A., et al. (2005). Reproducibility of nighttime salivary cortisol and its use in the diagnosis of hypercortisolism compared with urinary free cortisol and overnight dexamethasone suppression test. *Journal of Clinical Endocrinology and Metabolism* **90**(10), 5730–5736.

Yaneva, M., et al. (2004). Midnight salivary cortisol for the initial diagnosis of Cushing's syndrome of various causes. *Journal of Clinical Endocrinology and Metabolism* **89**(7), 3345–3351.

Adrenal Insufficiency

H S Willenberg
University Hospital Duesseldorf, Duesseldorf, Germany
S R Bornstein
Technical University of Dresden, Dresden, Germany
G P Chrousos
Athens University Medical School, Greece

This is a revised version of the article by H S Willenberg, S R Bornstein, and G P Chrousos, Encyclopedia of Stress, First edition, volume 1, pp 58–62, © 2000, Elsevier Inc.

Glossary

Adrenal crisis	Acute manifestation of adrenal insufficiency with symptoms including hypotension, hypovolemic shock, fever, and/or hypoglycemia. This condition is a medical emergency.
Adrenal insufficiency	Characterized by hypocortisolism and/or hypoaldosteronism. See also Primary adrenal insufficiency, Secondary adrenal insufficiency, and Tertiary adrenal insufficiency.
AIDS	Aquired immunodeficiency syndrome.
Cushing's disease	State of chronic hypercortisolism due to increased secretion of corticotropin from pituitary adenomas. See also Cushing's syndrome.
Cushing's syndrome	State of chronic hypercortisolism in general with typical clinical features. See also Cushing's disease.
Primary adrenal insufficiency	State of hypocortisolism and/or hypoaldosteronism due to a pathologic process that involves the adrenal glands in the first place. See also Secondary adrenal insufficiency and Tertiary adrenal insufficiency.
Secondary adrenal insufficiency	State of hypocortisolism and/or hypoaldosteronism due to a diminished capacity of the pituitary gland to secrete corticotropin. See also Primary adrenal insufficiency and Tertiary adrenal insufficiency.
Sheehan's syndrome	Pathologic condition of a newborn characterized by intrapituitary postpartum hemorrhage.
Tertiary adrenal insufficiency	State of hypocortisolism and/or hypoaldosteronism due to a pathologic process that involves the hypothalamus in the first place. See also Primary adrenal insufficiency and Secondary adrenal insufficiency.

Definition and Etiology of Adrenal Insufficiency

Adrenal insufficiency (AI) is a heterogenous group of diseases leading to a functional impairment of the hypothalamic-pituitary-adrenal (HPA) axis (**Table 1**). Adrenal insufficiency is caused by a disease process located in the adrenal glands (primary), the pituitary (secondary), or the hypothalamus (tertiary) and describes a state of glucocorticoid deficiency, mineralocorticoid deficiency, or deficiency in adrenal androgen production. Depending on the lesion that causes the adrenal hypofunction, isolated or combined impairment of adrenal hormone secretion may ensue.

Primary adrenal insufficiency was first described by Thomas Addison one and half a centuries ago; therefore, all primary forms of this condition are also termed Addison's disease. Because clinical symptoms usually do not occur until more than 90% of the adrenal cortex is destroyed or nonfunctional, both organs have to be affected.

The autoimmune destruction of the adrenal glands is the most common cause of primary adrenal insufficiency in the industrialized world, accounting for the majority of cases. Autoimmune adrenalitis can occur isolated or in combination with other autoimmune diseases (**Table 2**). Combinations are termed autoimmune polyendocrinopathy syndrome (APS). The monogenetic form of this syndrome, autoimmune polyendocrinopathy–candidiasis–ectodermal dystrophy (APECED, APS type I), is due to mutations in the autoimmune regulatory (AIRE) gene located on chromosome 21q22.3 and usually develops early in life. APS type II, which is also called Schmidt's syndrome when Addison's disease and hypothyroidism are present, is a complex genetic disorder and often occurs spontaneously. Susceptibility to developing this disease is conferred by genes in the human leukocyte antigen (HLA) region on the short arm of chromosome 6, and different susceptibility and resistance alleles of the major histocompatibility complex (MHA) class II have been identified so far. Other candidate genes include the cytotoxic T-lymphocyte antigen 4 (CTLA4) coding region of chromosome 2 on q33.

Hereditary or congenital adrenal dysfunction is particularly important in the pediatric patient population and is in the majority of cases due to deficiencies of enzymes involved in adrenal steroidogenesis, of which defects in the CYP21 enzyme gene are the most frequent. Depending on the site and number of hits to the alleles that encode for the steroidogenic

Table 1 Etiology of adrenal insufficiency[a]

Primary adrenal insufficiency	Autoimmune (idiopathic) disease	
	Expansive disease	Infection (tuberculosis, fungi) Hemorrhage (sepsis, anticoagulants, trauma) Secondary tumor (metastasis)
	Congenital-hereditary diseases	Congenital adrenal hyperplasia Congenital adrenal hypoplasia Congenital unresponsiveness to ACTH X-linked adrenoleukodystrophy / adrenomyeloneuropathy
	Drugs	Inhibitors of steroidogenesis Adrenolytic agents Glucocorticoid antagonists
Secondary and tertiary adrenal insufficiency	Glucocorticoid withdrawal syndrome	Following glucocorticoid therapy Following neurosurgery
	Expansive disease	Primary or secondary tumor, infection (tuberculosis) Inflammation (autoimmune, sarcoidosis)
	Iatrogenic hypopituitarism	following surgery, following radiation
	Other	Postpartum hemorrhage (Sheehan's syndrome) Trauma Apoplexy
Isolated hypoaldosteronism		Hyporeninism Surgery Congenital-inherited biosynthetic defect Central diseases Protracted heparin treatment
Isolated adrenomedullary insufficiency		Tuberculosis Infiltration by tumors Surgery Congenital-inherited dysautonomia

[a]ACTH, adrenocorticotropic hormone.

Table 2 Clinical manifestations of autoimmune polyendocrinopathy syndromes

Autoimmune endocrine diseases	Autoimmune adrenalitis, Autoimmune thyroid disease Autoimmune hypergonadotropic hypogonadism Type 1 diabetes mellitus Chronic hypoparathyroidism Autoimmune hypophysitis
Autoimmune diseases of other tissues	Skin/ectodermal manifestations: chronic mucocutaneous candidiasis, vitiligo, alopecia, nail dystrophy, keratoconjunctivitis, enamel dysplasia Chronic atrophic gastritis with: pernicious anemia, hypergastrinemia with benign carcinoids Celiac disease with malabsorption Autoimmune hepatitis

cytochromes, different enzyme activities with different phenotypes result. Of these, the salt-wasting forms are the most severe and life-threatening conditions of congenital adrenal hyperplasia (CAH). In puberty and adults, hirsutism, irregularities in the menstrual cycle, acne, or hair loss may point to a heterozygous form of this condition.

Adrenal hypoplasia congenita (AHC) can occur in an X-linked trait due to a mutation of the DAX-1 gene. Hypogonadotropic hypogonadism or premature puberty can be combined with this disorder or represent the only clinical presentation. Isolated glucocorticoid deficiency, triple A syndrome, and the demyelinating X-linked lipid metabolism disorders adrenoleukodystrophy and adrenomyeloneuropathy are also forms to be considered in the workup of Addison's disease.

The destruction of the adrenal cortex can also be the consequence of chronic infectious diseases. Tests of adrenocortical reserve are frequently impaired in chronic systemic diseases, including tuberculosis, acquired immunodeficiency syndrome (AIDS), toxoplasmosis, histoplasmosis, sarcoidosis, and amyloidosis. Bilateral metastatic infiltration or intraadrenal hemorrhage due to sepsis (*Meningococcus*) or anticoagulation are rare. However, postprimary tuberculosis still accounts for approximately 10% of the cases in the industrialized world and the majority of cases with a low standard of living. This condition is usually complicated by the involvement of other organ systems. Nonetheless, autoimmune adrenalitis may occur in cases with tuberculosis too. Of the fungal infections that are also known to cause adrenocortical dysfunction, histoplasmosis is common. Other causes of primary adrenal insufficiency have a rather low prevalence.

Iatrogenic forms of primary adrenal insufficiency include bilateral adrenalectomy and treatment with glucocorticoid receptor antagonists, such as RU486 (mifepristone); adrenolytic agents, such as mitotane and suramin; and drugs that inhibit steroidogenesis, such as ethomidate, aminoglutethemide, metyrapone, ketoconazole, and trilostane.

Secondary adrenal insufficiency due to a diminished secretion of corticotropin is frequent. Iatrogenic suppression of the HPA axis or adrenal suppression in the course of glucocorticoid treatment and subsequent discontinuation is the most common cause. Also, adrenal suppression is observed in patients with endogenous Cushing's syndrome after correction of the hypercortisolism by curative surgery. Other iatrogenic causes of secondary adrenal insufficiency include hypopituitarism following surgical intervention for pituitary and hypothalamic tumors and radiation. Space-occupying lesions in the hypothalamic-pituitary area (e.g., pituitary adenomas, craniopharyngiomas, meningiomas, or even metastatic infiltration and vascular lesions) may result in hypopituitarism. In addition, trauma, Sheehan's syndrome (intrapituitary postpartum hemorrhage) and apoplexy are also possible causes of impaired pituitary-adrenocortical function. Rare conditions include hypophysitis and granulomatous disorders affecting the pituitary gland.

Usually, secondary forms of adrenal insufficiency are limited to glucocorticoid deficiency in both sexes and androgen deficiency in women.

Tertiary adrenal insufficiency is a rare form of adrenal insufficiency. Main causes include hemorrhage due to trauma, tumorous formations, and ischemia in the hypothalamus. In addition, the hypothalamus is also a site for the endocrine feedback regulation by glucocorticoids and, therefore, is involved in iatrogenic adrenal insufficiency, as already described.

Some disease states of unknown pathophysiology, such as posttraumatic stress disorder, chronic fatigue syndrome, and fibromyalgia, may also be associated with dysfunction of the HPA axis resulting in hypo- or hypercortisolism. Guidelines for the diagnosis and therapy of these controversially discussed conditions are under development. Psychological care, introduction into self-help groups, and symptomatic treatment are current therapeutic approaches.

In addition, there are disorders that cannot be classified within this scheme and are named relative adrenal insufficiency. In critical illness (e.g., sepsis and shock), it has been found that patients demonstrated high levels of corticotropin and cortisol. However, it has been shown that glucocorticoid therapy is beneficial in the survival for this subgroup of patients. Therefore, it has been suggested that the elevation of corticotropin in critical illness reflects a state of relative hypocortisolism. The elevation of inflammatory cytokines and presence of bacterial toxins cause a profound activation of the HPA axis and are believed to contribute to the development of relative adrenal insufficiency.

Clinical Presentation and Diagnosis

The main clinical manifestations of adrenal insufficiency are caused by hypocortisolism and hypoaldosteronism. All forms of adrenal insufficiency may present as an acute adrenal crisis or as chronic state with exacerbations. Acute symptoms include anorexia and/or vomiting, somnolence, orthostatic or persistent hypotension with dizziness, hypovolemic shock, fever, and hypoglycemia. Adrenal crisis is a medical emergency.

Patients with chronic adrenal insufficiency may present with weakness, failure to thrive (children), weight loss, anorexia, fatigue, nausea and vomiting, orthostatic hypotension, and abdominal pain. In primary adrenal insufficiency, lack of negative pituitary and hypothalamic feedback by glucocorticoids causes increased secretion of adrenocorticotropic hormone (ACTH), which has melanocyte-stimulating activity causing hyperpigmentation (creases of palms, buccal mucosa, breast areolas and nipples, and scars). In most forms of congenital adrenal hyperplasia, hyperandrogenism (virilization of girls and premature puberty of boys and girls) is observed. In combined glucocorticoid and mineralocorticoid deficiency, relative hypovolemia leads to compensatory secretion of antidiuretic hormone with resulting hyponatremia, whereas the lack of aldosterone leads to salt loss and retention of potassium and protons. The rare forms of defective 17α-hydroxylation lead to glucocorticoid and androgen deficiency in combination with mineralocorticoid excess.

An adrenal crisis can be diagnosed on the basis of a single cortisol measurement at the time of crisis. Low serum sodium concentrations in combination with hyperkalemia and elevated plasma renin and ACTH concentrations strongly suggest primary adrenal insufficiency, whereas elevated serum potassium levels are not typical for secondary forms of hypocortisolism. Hypoglycemia may occur in children, women, and very thin men. Lymphocytosis with eosinophilia, azotemia, and metabolic acidosis may be present, and the first results in the diagnostic workup. Routine laboratory parameters may demonstrate no abnormalities in early adrenal hypofunction. Specific study methods to ensure and further differentiate the diagnosis of adrenal insufficiency should not delay therapeutic intervention during an adrenal crisis.

Adrenal stimulation tests provide evidence of a dysfunction of the HPA axis. Among them the rapid (60-min) corticotropin test is useful for the diagnosis of adrenal insufficiency, whereas the corticotropin releasing hormone (CRH) test and the long 48-h ACTH stimulation tests are useful for the differentiation of primary and secondary adrenal insufficiency (**Table 3**). Although basal cortisol production may be normal, an impaired increase in steroid output may be present and difficult to diagnose. Therefore, these tests, particularly the fast one, are valuable tools in establishing the diagnosis of adrenal hypofunction in cases of decreased adrenal reserve and in monitoring the recovery of the HPA axis after the discontinuation of glucocorticoid therapy or correction of hypercortisolism.

In several countries, screening for congenital adrenal hyperplasia and genetic workup of heterozygous patients have been shown to decrease the risk of early death and to be cost-effective in health programs.

Autoantibodies can develop and are detectable in most cases of autoimmune adrenalitis. They are directed against CYP21, CYPscc, CYP17, or steroidogenic cells and more frequent in APS type I or II than in isolated autoimmune adrenalitis. In autoimmune polyendocrinopathy syndroms without adrenal insufficiency, they allow the prediction of a possible manifestation of this complication in 85% of patients.

Treatment

The therapeutic goal is an optimal replacement of glucocorticoids and, if necessary, mineralocorticoids. In addition, there is need of an additional glucocorticoid substitution therapy in certain stress-related circumstances. Therefore, all patients with this condition and their close relatives and friends need careful education about the management of their disease and should be handed out an Emergency Health Card, containing information on disease, regimen of hormone substitution and instructions how to avoid or deal with an adrenal crisis.

Usually, patients do very well with oral glucocorticoids. The treatment of choice is hydrocortisone. Doses of 10–20 mg in the early morning may be sufficient, especially in cases with mild secondary adrenal insufficiency. However, in primary forms or complete secondary hypocortisolism, 10–15 mg/m^2/day may be necessary. To simulate the circadian rhythm of glucocorticoid secretion split, doses are given: two-thirds in the morning and one-third in the afternoon (**Table 4**). Before surgery or dental extraction or during periods of intercurrent illness, steroid dosage has to be doubled or even tripled. During severe stress (such as car accidents, sepsis, or major surgery), an individual's intact adrenal gland will increase its cortisol secretion approximately fivefold. Therefore, during such situations, replacement doses higher than 200 mg day^{-1} are not required in patients with adrenal insufficiency. Following an operation, provided that there are no complications, the hydrocortisone doses should be returned to the normal replacement regimen within a few days. Parenteral administration may be required. Although cortisol and cortisone have mineralocorticoid effects, a dose of 30 mg day^{-1} covers only approximately 50% of the daily requirement. Therefore, 0.05–0.1 mg fludrocortisone, a synthetic mineralocorticoid, is given to Addisonian patients. Furthermore, these patients should be put on a sodium-enriched diet because they are frequently not able to conserve this electrolyte in spite of replacement therapy.

Table 3 Differentiation among primary, secondary, and tertiary adrenal insufficiency[a]

	Adrenal insufficiency		
	Primary	*Secondary*	*Tertiary*
Plasma ACTH, baseline	↑	↓	↓
Plasma ACTH after CRH	↑	↓ (response)	↑ (delayed)
Plasma cortisol, baseline during crisis	↓	↓	↓
Plasma cortisol after ACTH (60 min)	↓ (<20 μg dl^{-1})	↑ (<20 μg dl^{-1})	↑ (<20 μg dl^{-1})
Plasma cortisol after CRH	↓ (no elevation)	↓ (no elevation)	↑ or ↔
Urinary free cortisol or 17-hydroxysteroid excretion after 48-h ACTH infusion	↓ (no elevation)	↑ (two- to threefold elevation)	↑ (two- to threefold elevation)
Aldosterone	↓	↔	↔
Renin	↑	↔	↔

[a]ACTH, adrenocorticotropic hormone; CRH, corticotropin releasing hormone.

Table 4 Examples of glucocorticoid replacement therapy

Glucocorticoid	*Morning*	*Noon*	*Late afternoon*
Hydrocortisone[a]	15 mg	10 mg	5 mg
Cortisone actetate	25 mg	–	12.5 mg
Prednisone	5 mg	–	–

[a]Hydrocortisone is recommended.

Adrenal insufficiency may lead to a deficit in androgen secretion in women. The substitution of dehydroepiandrostendione in women with this disorder has been proven beneficial and is being considered for inclusion in the treatment regimen. Women with secondary or tertiary forms of adrenal insufficiency may be put on hormone replacement therapy with estrogens and a gestagen, which has a partial androgenic action.

In some cases of secondary and tertiary adrenal insufficiency, such as in dermatomyositis and multiple sclerosis, treatment with corticotropin may be more effective than glucocorticoid therapy. In fact, the administration of corticotropin leads to the secretion of adrenal androgens, glucocorticoids, and mineralocorticoids and generally prevents the adrenal glands from hypotrophy but not the hypothalamic-pituitary unit from suppression. Oral glucocorticoid replacement is generally sufficient and easier to adjust to the individual's requirements in the great majority of the patients.

In acute adrenocortical insufficiency, therapy should be initiated immediately after taking blood for the determination of cortisol and corticotropin levels. Hypovolemic shock requires the rapid replacement of sodium and water deficits. This is accomplished by the intravenous infusion of 5% glucose in normal saline solutions lacking potassium. Cortisol should be administered, starting with a bolus of 100 mg. An adrenal crisis is often precipitated by acute stress. Therefore, an appropriate increase in glucocorticoid replacement serves to restore glucocorticoid function. After successful treatment and improvement of the patient's condition, glucocorticoids can be administered orally and the doses can be lowered to maintenance levels. (The treatment of the different forms of congenital adrenal hyperplasia are not discussed in this article.)

Additional Aspects and Implications for Stress

Glucocorticoids do not participate only in endocrine feedback loops with corticotropin and CRH at the levels of the pituitary gland and the hypothalamus, respectively, but also in feedback loops with other peptides derived from the immune system. Of those mediators, interleukin-6 is a key interface between the immune system and the HPA axis. This cytokine is found to be elevated in patients with hypocortisolism and believed to play a role in the steroid withdrawal syndrome.

Glucocorticoids are associated with a switch in production from T helper cell (Th)1 to Th2 cytokines. The absence of glucocorticoids leads to an enhanced Th1 profile, promoting autoimmune and allergic phenomena, including autoimmune thyroid disease, rheumatoid arthritis, and asthma.

Adrenal insufficiency is a state of hypocortisolism and, thus, is a decreased effectiveness of the adaptive response. The profound dysregulation of the HPA axis with loss of drive (secondary and tertiary forms) or loss of feedback (primary forms) makes a balanced homeostasis impossible. Therefore, frequently, manifestations of adrenal insufficiency are observed under stressful conditions, such as inapparent infection, physical challenge, and surgery. Once the diagnosis of adrenal insufficiency has been established, careful diagnosis and causal therapy of a possible underlying disease are also pivotal.

When Brown-Sequard and Thomas Addison recognized that the adrenal glands were organs necessary for life, they did not have knowledge of Hans Selye's concept of stress. Adrenal dysfunction practically means the disintegration of the powerful stress system, which is necessary for maintenance of homeostasis. Cases of adrenal insufficiency document the importance of such a system. Its dysfunction may result in severe life-threatening disorders.

Further Reading

Bornstein, S. R. (1996). *The adrenal functional unit.* Stuttgart: Georg Thieme Verlag.

Chrousos, G. P. (1998). Stressors, stress, and neuroendocrine integration of the adaptive response: 1997 Hans Selye memorial lecture. *Annals of the New York Academy of Sciences* **851**, 311–335.

Eisenbarth, G. S. and Gottlieb, P. A. (2004). Autoimmune polyendocrine syndromes. *New England Journal of Medicine* **350**, 2068–2079.

Papanicolaou, D. A. (1997). Cytokines and adrenal insufficiency. *Current Opinion in Endocrinology and Diabetes* 4, 194–198.

Stratakis, C. A. and Chrousos, G. P. (1998). Adrenal diseases. In: Jameson, J. L. (ed.) *Principles of molecular medicine*, pp. 495–503. Totowa, NJ: Humana Press.

B. Corticosteroid Receptors

Steroid Hormone Receptors

M Beato
Centre de Regulació de Genòmica, UPF, Barcelona, Spain
J Klug
University of Giessen, Giessen, Germany

This is a revised version of the article by M Beato and J Klug, Encyclopedia of Stress, First edition, volume 3, pp 495–504, © 2000, Elsevier Inc.

Glossary

Chromatin A complex of nuclear DNA and basic proteins called histones. Every 146 bp of nuclear DNA is wrapped around a histone octamer into a nucleosome. A 30-bp DNA linker connects one nucleosome to the next, forming a nucleosome necklace.

Steroid hormone receptors (SHRs) Intracellular transcription factors that are induced by the specific and high-affinity binding of ligands to exert positive or negative effects on the expression of target genes by different mechanisms.

Steroid hormones Lipophilic hormones derived from cholesterol and synthesized in the adrenal cortex (glucocorticoids, mineralocorticoids, and adrenal androgens), the testes (testicular androgens and estrogen), and the ovary and placenta (estrogens and progestagens).

Transcription factors (TFs) Nuclear proteins interacting with the regulatory regions of genes, promoters, and enhancers. They can be divided into general transcription factors, forming the transcription initiation complex required for the transcription of all genes, and sequence-specific transcription factors, which bind to specific DNA sequences present in only a subset of genes and carry activation or repression domains that serve to activate or repress transcription.

Steroid hormone receptors (SHRs) are ligand-activated transcription factors and the key mediators of steroid hormone action. Lipophilic steroid hormones pass the cell membrane of target cells by simple diffusion and bind to soluble intracellular SHRs that are complexed to chaperones, such as Hsp90, or to a small fraction of membrane-tethered SHRs. Chaperones are proteins that help other proteins fold and prevent aggregation. The binding of agonistic or antagonistic ligands leads to different allosteric changes of receptors, making them competent to exert positive or negative effects on the expression of target genes by three mechanisms. First, ligand-bound SHR complexes can bind to short, specific DNA sequences in the vicinity of target genes, termed hormone response elements (HREs). The HRE-recruited hormone–receptor complexes are then able to relay activating or repressing signals to the target-gene transcription machinery (**Figure 1a**). Second, the SHR response can be integrated into intracellular signal transduction pathways that transmit an extracellular growth factor signal via mitogen-activated protein kinases (MAPKs) to a nuclear transcription factor that activates a target gene (**Figure 1b**). Third, through protein–protein interactions, SHRs can repress the activity of many genes that are switched on during the stress response (transrepression) (**Figure 1c**).

Historical Development

The gonads and adrenal gland produce five major groups of steroid hormones: estrogens, progestagens, androgens, glucocorticoids, and mineralocorticoids. The effects and clinical symptoms associated with a reduced level of these hormones were known long before the hormone concept was developed. Aristotle, for instance, identified the consequences of castration in humans and birds, and in 1855 Addison described the symptoms of chronic adrenal insufficiency. Moreover, since the nineteenth century it has been known that female sex steroid hormones play a pivotal role in promoting mammary tumor growth, similar to androgens promoting the growth of prostatic neoplasms. Between the tenth and sixteenth centuries, Chinese alchemists developed empirical methods to purify steroids to near homogeneity. In the first half of the twentieth century, it became possible to isolate individual steroids from extracts derived from source tissues by employing biological complementation assays. When tritium and ^{14}C-labeled hormone compounds of high specific activity became available in the late 1950s, it became possible to follow the fate of the steroid hormones up to their target tissues. Thus, it could be shown that the hormone itself, not a metabolite, produced the response via the activation of gene expression mechanisms. The concept that steroid hormones are involved in transcriptional control was also triggered by the observation of ecdysone-induced giant chromosome puffs by Clever and Karlson in 1960. Some 10 years later the groups of Jensen and Gorski had established a two-step model that involved the binding of the hormone to specific high-affinity SHRs within the target cells, followed by

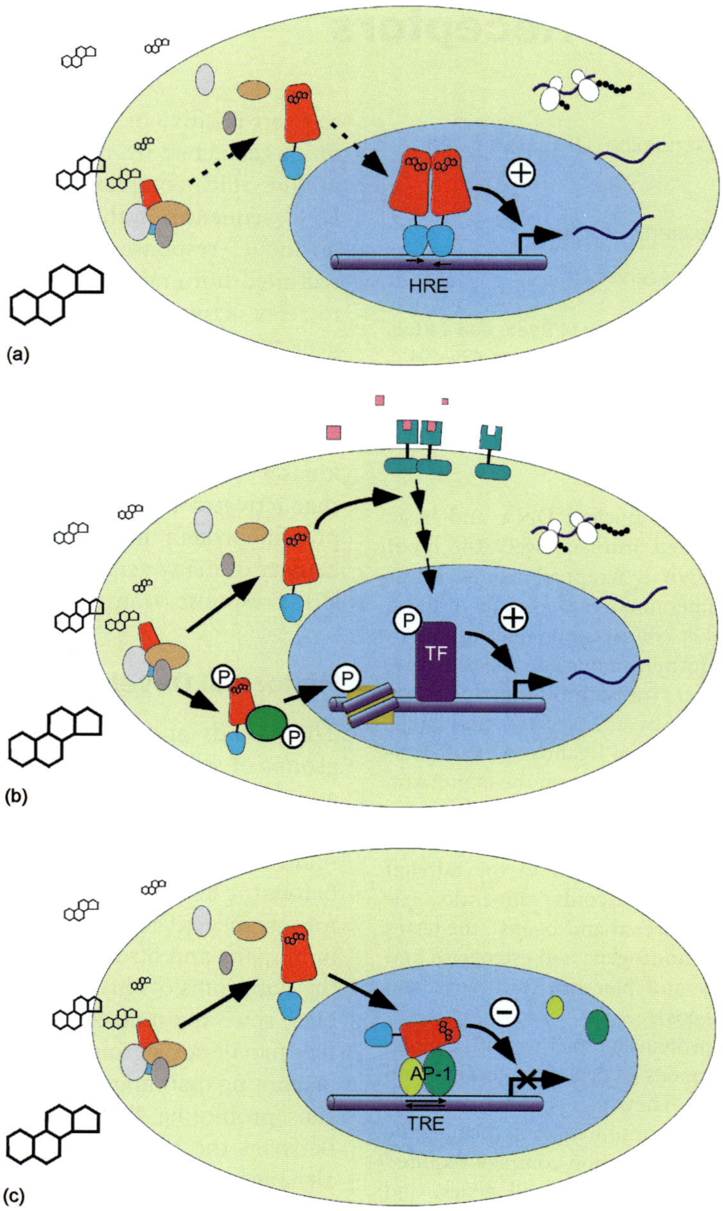

Figure 1 Three implementations of the SHR signal transduction pathway. a, Ligand-bound SHR complexes binding to short, specific DNA sequences in the vicinity of target genes; b, SHR response being integrated into intracellular signal transduction pathways; c, SHRs repressing the activity of genes that are switched on during the stress response. In a, the lipophilic steroid hormones (depicted by the chemical formula showing the central sterane building block of all steroid hormones) pass the cell membrane of target cells by simple diffusion and bind to soluble intracellular SHRs that are complexed to chaperones such as Hsp90 (shown as ellipses with various colors). Binding of the hormone leads to an allosteric change of the receptor, resulting in the dissociation of chaperones (dashed arrow). The liganded SHR-complexes dimerize, bind to hormone response elements (HREs, dashed arrow) in the vicinity of target genes, and transmit activating (or repressing) signals to the target genes' transcription machinery. In b, an extracellular polypeptide growth factor signal (pink squares) is received by the target cell via membrane receptors with kinase activity that dimerize on ligand binding. The dimerized growth factor receptors relay the signal through a cascade of mitogen-activated protein kinases (MAPKs; arrows) to sequence specific transcription factors (TFs) that are induced (or repressed) by phosphorylation (P) to activate the target gene. Hormone-activated SHRs can bypass a growth factor receptor-mediated signal by activating MAPKs and vice versa. In addition, hormone receptors form complexes with cytoplasmic kinases (green ellipsoid) such as ERK and MSK1 that are activated (phosphorylated) on hormone binding and activate (phosphorylate) the receptor. The complex of activated receptor and kinase(s) is recruited to the target promoter where it phosphorylates histones (brown rectangle) as a prerequisite for chromatin remodeling and transcriptional activation. In c, many immunoregulatory genes as well as genes involved in inflammation are positively regulated by the heterodimeric sequence-specific transcription factor activator protein 1 (AP-1) recognizing a TPA response element (TRE) within the promoter of a target gene. Through protein–protein interactions, ligand-activated SHRs are able to repress in trans the AP-1 activity (transrepression).

the activation of the hormone–receptor complex in order to induce the expression of hormone responsive genes (**Figure 1a**). After another 10 years, the hormone receptors for glucocorticoids and estrogens were cloned and thus became the first molecularly defined transcription factors for RNA polymerase II. At around the same time, the cloning of some SHR targets, such as the human metallothionein gene and the mouse mammary tumor virus genome, led to the identification of the first HREs. Within the last 15 years, many details of the SHR signal transduction pathway, including new mechanisms, have been discovered (**Figures 1b–c**).

Steroid Hormone Receptors Form a Subgroup within the Nuclear Receptor Family

In addition to the hormone receptors for glucocorticoids and estrogens, which were cloned first, receptors for the remaining three major steroid hormone classes have been identified and characterized extensively, as well as a second estrogen receptor and three estrogen-related receptors. All SHRs are characterized by a central DNA-binding domain (DBD) that targets the receptor to the HREs and by a ligand-binding domain (LBD) that is required for switching the receptor's functions. When the v-*erbA* oncogene was cloned, it turned out to also contain a DBD and a LBD that were homologous to the cognate regions of the known SHRs. Later on, the c-*erbA* locus was identified as the receptor for the thyroid hormone T_3, which is also a hormone found in the nucleus like steroid hormones. The identification of another structurally related receptor for the vitamin A metabolite retinoic acid solidified the concept of a nuclear receptor superfamily. Today, more than 520 different nuclear receptors have been described from more than 120 metazoan species, among them receptors for the known nuclear hormones and a vast number of so-called orphan receptors with no, or unknown and possibly novel, ligands. In order to avoid the coining of several trivial names for the same gene, an official nomenclature system has been in use since 1999 (NUREBASE). The SHRs and steroid hormone-like receptors form the nuclear receptor subfamily 3 (NR3), consisting of three groups: A, B, and C (**Figure 2a**). NR3 includes two receptors for estrogens (ERα and ERβ, or NR3A1 and NR3A2), three estrogen-related orphan receptors (ERRα, ERRβ, and ERRγ, or NR3B1, NR3B2, and NR3B3), and one receptor each for the other major steroid hormone classes: glucocorticoids (GR, or NR3C1), mineralocorticoids (MR, or NR3C2), progestagens (PR, or NR3C3), and androgens (AR, or NR3C4).

Domain Structure of Steroid Hormone Receptors

All SHRs are modular proteins composed of distinct regions, as shown in **Figure 2b** (top line). When the chicken estrogen receptor cDNA became available, comparison with the human estrogen and glucocorticoid receptor sequences led to the region A–F nomenclature, which is used for all members of the whole nuclear receptor superfamily today. From numerous functional and structural analyses, it became clear that these distinct regions correspond to functional and structural units called domains. Region C (the DBD) and region E (the LBD) display a high degree of sequence conservation, whereas no significant conservation is detected between paralogous SHRs for the regions A/B, D, and F.

Region D is considered a flexible hinge region between the DBD and LBD. Its very N-terminus is an integral part of the DBD and is involved in DBD dimerization. The F region is essential for hormone binding in the PR, GR, and AR but not in the ERα. This domain is also important for the discrimination between agonistic and antagonistic hormone ligands. The A region is highly conserved between chicken and human estrogen receptors, but this distinction is much less clear in the other steroid receptors. Therefore, regions A and B are combined into an A/B region in most cases.

Regions C and E are not only responsible for DNA and ligand binding, respectively, but they do encode other functions as well (**Figure 2b**, bottom). The intracellular distribution of steroid receptors is the result of nuclear-cytoplasmic diffusion and cytoplasmic-nuclear shuttling. At equilibrium, the majority of steroid receptors are in the nucleus due to the presence of nuclear localization signals (NLS), which are believed to be required for nuclear pore recognition. A constitutive NLS is located at the border of regions C and D, whereas a second NLS in the LBD is ligand-dependent. Intracellular localization is different for GR and MR because hormone-induced nuclear translocation has been reported in these cases.

Most SHRs bind as homodimers to their cognate response elements within the promoters of target genes, which is a specific characteristic of this subfamily within the nuclear receptor superfamily. It is also well known that the predominant form of the GR is monomeric in solution and that dimerization occurs only after binding to an HRE, accounting for the cooperativity observed during DNA binding. Responsible for dimerization are a weak dimerization domain encoded within the DBD and a strong dimerization interface provided by the LBD.

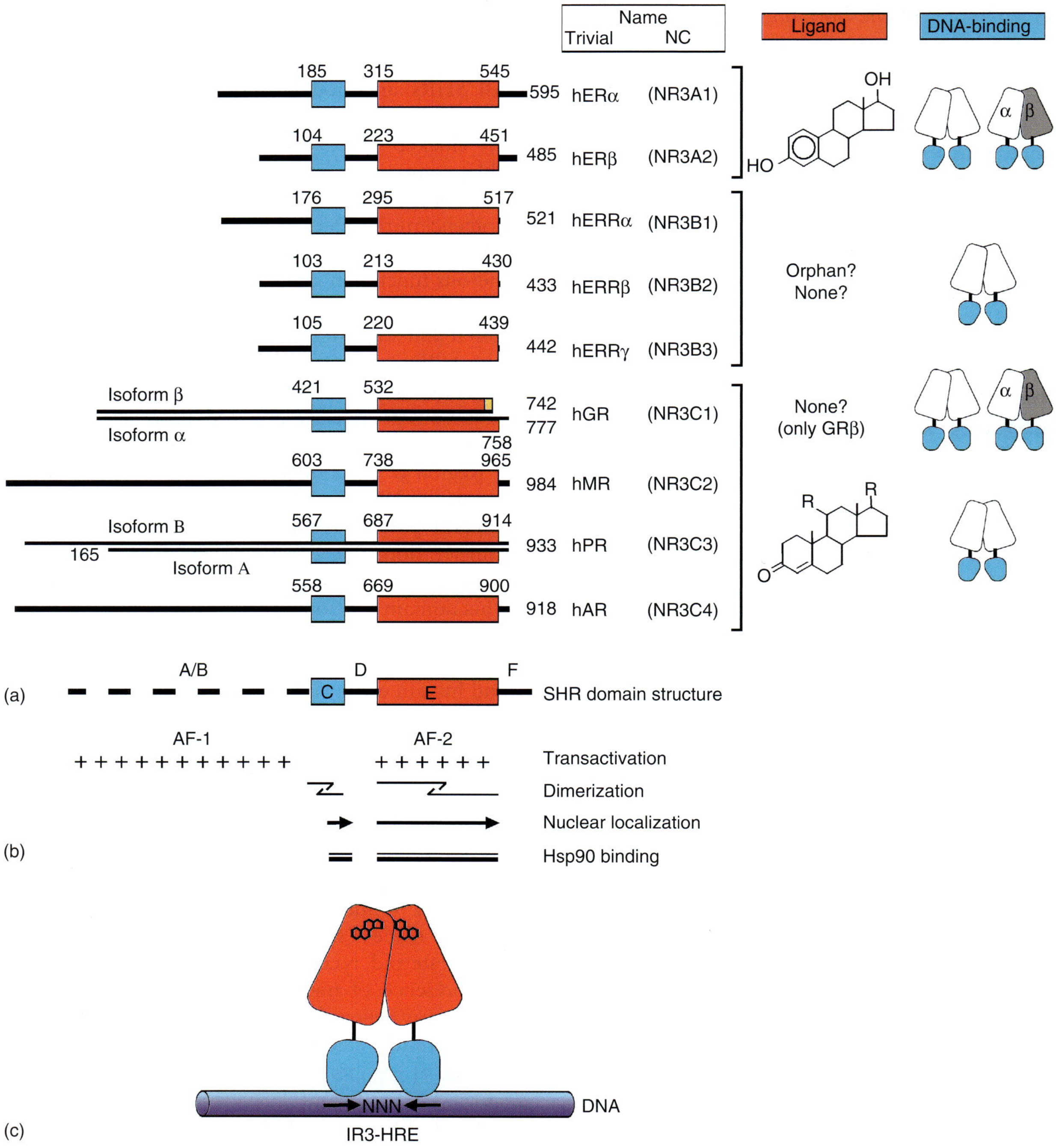

Figure 2 The human steroid hormone receptor family. a, Structure of all family members, cognate ligand, and DNA-binding mode; b, SHR domain structure and structure–function relationships; c, an SHR homodimer bound to its cognate hormone response element (HRE). In a, the numbers refer to amino acid positions. Highlighted are the DNA-binding domain (DBD; shown in blue) and the ligand-binding domain (LBD; shown in red). The A/B and F domains are drawn to scale, and the name of each receptor is indicated (trivial and name according to nomenclature scheme). In c, the HRE is of an inverted repeat (IR) type (palindrome), and half-sites (arrows) are separated by three unspecified (N) nucleotides (IR3-HRE); the hormone ligand is indicated by a sterane formula. AF-1 and-2, transcription activation functions 1 and 2; AR, androgen receptor; ER, estrogen receptor; ERR, estrogen-related receptor; GR, glucocorticoid receptor; h, human; MR, mineralocorticoid receptor; PR, progesterone receptor.

Ligand binding confers transcriptional competence on to SHRs that is exerted in most receptors by two independent transactivation functions: a constitutively active one in the A/B region located close to the DBD, referred to as activation function 1 (AF-1; also called τ-1 or enh-1), and a ligand-inducible activation function in the LBD, called AF-2. AFs connect the receptor to the transcription apparatus via direct interactions with basal transcription factors, sequence-specific transcription factors, and/or coregulators.

Individual Family Members

The human estrogen receptor (now called hERα, **Figure 2a**) was cloned from a cDNA expression library produced from the breast cancer cell line MCF-7. A second estrogen receptor, ERβ, has been characterized that is very similar to ERα in terms of structure and function but also shows subtle and important functional differences. Both receptors bind the ligands estradiol, diethylstilbestrol, estriol, and estrone with high affinity. cDNA clones for hERRα and hERRβ were isolated from a human testis cDNA library using the hERα DBD as a probe. Mouse ERRγ was identified by yeast two-hybrid screening, using the transcriptional coactivator GR interacting protein 1 as bait. It is still unclear whether the ERRs are true orphan receptors in search of a ligand or are ligand-independent.

For the GR, two different classes of cDNAs have been described in humans, termed hGRα and hGRβ, which are the result of alternative splicing from a single gene transcript. Both isoforms are identical up to amino acid 727 and then diverge, with hGRα being slighly larger (777 amino acids) than hGRβ (742 amino acids). In contrast to hGRα, which is commonly referred to as the bona fide hGR, hGRβ was long dismissed as a cloning artifact but has now been shown to be expressed at modest but varying levels in a range of tissues. Each variant mRNA is translated from at least eight initiation sites into multiple GRα and possibly GRβ isoforms, amounting to a multitude of GR monomers and probably a plethora of homo- or heterodimers of unknown function. hGRβ does not bind hormones, is transcriptionally inactive, and therefore acts as a ligand-independent negative regulator of glucocorticoid action in transfection experiments. However, the β isoform is not conserved across species, and functional evidence that implicates hGRβ in glucocortioid insensitivity is still missing. hGRα shows a high affinity for the artificial glucocorticoid dexamethasone, moderate affinity for the physiological steroids cortisol and corticosterone, and low affinity for mineralocorticoids and progesterone. In contrast to all other SHRs, GRα dimerizes only weekly.

The progesterone receptor was the first SHR shown to exist in two common isoforms generated by differential promoter use. One promoter initiates transcription at positions +1 and +15 of the gene, which gives rise to the longer isoform B (**Figure 2a**). The second promoter initiates hPR transcripts between +737 and +842, encoding the 164-amino-acid residues shorter hPR form A. Only PR-B harbors a third activation function (AF-3) at its specific N-terminus, which functions promoter- and cell-specificly. Both isoforms, therefore, display differential target gene specificity. First regarded as an exception in the family, differential promoter use and alternative splicing are now considered the rule for all members. Both PR isoforms show a high affinity for the natural ligand progesterone and the synthetic agonist R5020. Alternative splicing can also generate truncated forms of PR that are found in breast cancer.

The human mineralocorticoid receptor (hMR) and androgen receptor (hAR) were cloned 2–3 years after the GR was described. The hAR exists in two isoforms, hAR-A and hAR-B, which are structurally analogous to the two hPR isoforms. In contrast to hPR-A/B, hAR-A is expressed at substantially lower levels than the B form and its contribution to androgen action is not known. The hAR binds the two naturally occurring ligands dihydrotestosterone and testosterone with high affinity, whereas the hMR shows high and equivalent affinity for aldosterone, physiological corticosteroids, and progesterone.

Heterooligomeric Complex and Ligand and DNA Binding

Heterooligomeric Complex

In 1965, the groups of Jensen and Gorski showed that specific and high-affinity binding sites for estrogen existed in large heterooligomeric complexes migrating with 9S on low-salt sucrose gradients. This non-DNA-binding complex can be transformed into a more compact and protease-resistant 4S DNA-binding form by high salt and temperature or hormone. The 9S heterooligomeric receptor complexes were later shown to be composed of the two chaperones – heat shock protein (Hsp)90, recently identified as a member of the GHKL family of ATPases, and Hsp70 – plus a number of co-chaperones.

Hsps form an evolutionarily very conserved group of stress-inducible proteins. Contrary to their name, Hsps are strongly induced not only by heat shock, but are also expressed constitutively at physiological temperatures at significant levels. Hsps belong to a larger family of chaperones that are known to stabilize the native structure of other polypeptides by controlled binding to them.

Most investigations have been performed with the heterooligomeric GR complex that contains a dimer of Hsp90 and a substoichiometric amount of Hsp70 and one or two molecules of p23. The last two are required for the assembly of the final heterooligomeric complex. The crystal structure of full-length yeast Hsp90 in complex with an ATP analog and the yeast p23 homolog has been solved recently. For PR and AR, the LBD is sufficient for an interaction with Hsp90 that also requires ATP. In case of the GR, a seven-amino-acid segment overlapping the N-terminus of the LBD, which is located on the surface of the LBD at the opening of the ligand-binding pocket, is sufficient and required for Hsp90 binding. In case of the ER, in addition to the LBD, part of the hinge region D stabilizes the Hsp90–ER complex. From the known crystal structures of a number of LBDs of nuclear receptors and several biochemical studies, it becomes clear that Hsp90 recognizes two hydrophobic surfaces at opposite sides of the LBD located in the vicinity of the ligand-binding pocket. The large distance between the two hydrophobic surfaces probably accounts for the fact that two Hsp90 molecules are bound to SHRs. The LBD of the receptor must be in a complex with Hsp90 in order to have high ligand-binding activity. Hsp90 binding seems to be a characteristic of SHRs because other nuclear receptors, such as the retinoid, thyroid hormone, and vitamin D_3 receptors, do not associate efficiently with these Hsps.

The complexes also contain one of a number of tetratricopeptide (TPR) domain immunophilins that bind to a TPR acceptor site at the C-terminus of Hsp90. Immunophilins are characterized by their peptidylprolyl isomerase (PPIase or rotamase) domains and can function as chaperones like Hsps. SHR complexes contain one of three immunophilins (FKBP51, FKBP52 or CyP-40) or PP5, a protein phosphatase that contains both a TPR domain and a PPIase homology domain. The PPIase domain of immunophilins is a binding site for immunosuppressant drugs such as FK506 or cyclosporine A that inhibit PPIase activity on binding.

In hormone-free cells, steroid receptors shuttle between the cytoplasm and nucleus. The distribution may be predominantly cytoplasmic (GR) or nuclear (ERα). Steroid-dependent transformation of the GR triggers its rapid translocation to the nucleus, possibly involving movement along microtubules driven by the motor protein dynein. In wheat germ extracts, it was shown *in vitro* that wheat immunophilins can link the GR–Hsp90 heterocomplex to cytoplasmic dynein via conserved TPR and PPIase domain interactions. Immunoadsorption of GR from cell lysates of L cells coimmunoadsorbs Hsp90, the dynein intermediate chain, FKBP52, PP5, and dynamitin (a subunit of the dynein-associated dynactin complex). If the microtubules are stabilized by taxol, α-tubulin is coimmunoadsorbed as well.

All these data are derived from *in vitro* experiments with cell extracts in which the cellular microenvironments are destroyed, so that the observed complexes may be artificial. But a number of *in vivo* observations indicate that the heterooligomeric receptor complex is also of functional importance. Increased levels of FKBP51 have been reported to be the common cause of glucocorticoid resistance in three New World primates, due to delayed translocation of the GR to the nucleus. Likewise the overexpression of FKBP51 in COS cells reduces the hormone binding activity of GR and hence its transcriptional activity. In yeast cells, the overexpression of FKBP51 has no effect, whereas FKBP52 enhances GR-dependent transcription that is dependent on interaction with Hsp90 and PPIase activity. It could be shown that the binding of FKBP52 to Hsp90 potentiates glucocorticoid-dependent reporter gene activity in yeast and mammalian cells that is dependent on PPIase activity and increases the hormone binding affinity of the receptor. Moreover, differential binding of FKBP51 and-52 to dynein corresponds to a differential effect on nuclear translocation. The co-expression of dynamitin and the PPIase domain, as well as PPIase domain-swapping experiments, demonstrated the relevance of the dynactin complex for receptor function. Hsp90 and the co-chaperone p23 have been shown to colocalize *in vivo* at genomic HREs in a hormone-dependent manner. p23 seems to be involved in disrupting receptor-mediated transcriptional activation *in vivo* and *in vitro* and, thus, it could be involved in terminating the hormone response.

Therefore receptor-associated chaperones and co-chaperones can no longer be viewed as simple repressors that have to be removed by hormone in order to transform the non-DNA-binding heterooligomeric complex into a DNA-binding entity; they are, instead, viewed as chaperone complexes that accompany all steps in the life of these client proteins: folding, assembly of quaternary structures, intracellular transport, and targeting for proteolytic degradation.

Ligand Binding

Although not proven formally, it is believed that the lipophilic steroid hormones, as well as synthetic compounds with agonistic or antagonistic effects, enter the target cell by simple diffusion and bind to SHRs within the heterooligomeric complex. For hERα and hPR, the three-dimensional structure of their ligand-binding domains complexed with 17β-estradiol and the antihormone raloxifene or progesterone, respectively, have been determined. Like other known LBDs of nuclear receptors, the LBDs of SHRs are folded into a three-layer antiparallel α-helical sandwich that creates a wedge-shaped molecular scaffold with the ligand-binding cavity at the narrower end of the domain (**Figure 3**). This cavity is completely partitioned from the external environment and is closed by helix

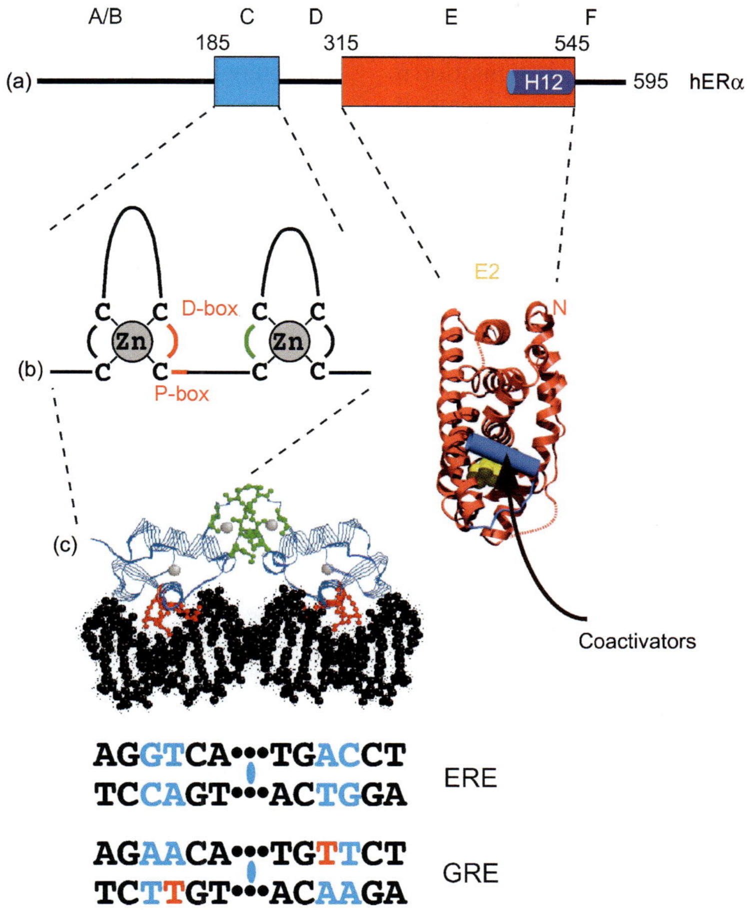

Figure 3 Structure of the human estrogen receptor α. a, Functional domains (A/B to F) of hERα at the primary structure level, with the DNA-binding domain (DBD) and the ligand-binding domain (LBD) highlighted; b, an exploded view of the secondary structure of the hERα DBD; c, crystal structure of the hERα DBD bound to DNA, followed by the sequences of the consensus estrogen response element (ERE) and a consensus glucocorticoid response element (GRE); d, crystal structure of the hERα LBD complexed with 17β-estradiol (E2). In a, The numbers refer to amino acid positions. DBD is highlighted in blue and the LBD in red. The A/B and F domains are drawn to scale. In b, the secondary structure of the DBD is characterized by two steroid hormone receptor-specific zinc fingers. Four cysteines each tetrahedrally coordinate one zinc ion (grey). The Proximal box (P-box) responsible for specific DNA recognition is shown in red; the Distal box (D-box) mediating DBD dimerization is shown in green. In the crystal structure in c, the four amino acid side chains of the P-box (red) are shown interacting with DNA bases (black). These residues are part of an α-helix responsible for specific DNA-sequence recognition that is positioned within the DNA's major groove (perpendicular to the paper plane). A second amphipathic α-helix can be seen to cross the recognition helix with the red P-box residues at a right angle. Between the two helices, the green D-box residues promoting DBD dimerization are located. Underneath the DNA, the sequences of the consensus ERE and a consensus GRE are shown. Both half-sites are organized as an inverted repeat with 3-bp spacing (IR-3). The symmetry axis is indicated by a blue ellipse. The bases that differ between ERE and GRE are highlighted in blue, and the thymine important for the discrimination between both response elements is highlighted in red. In the crystal structure in d, E2, a natural ligand, is shown in yellow. Decisive for a productive interaction with coactivators is the proper positioning of helix 12 (H 12) over the ligand-binding pocket. (We thank R. Hubbard and A. Pike, University of York, UK, for providing this part of the figure.)

12 of the LBD, operating as a lid after the hormone has entered the binding pocket. The relocation of this amphipathic helix 12 over the hormone-binding site generates a new surface that allows coactivators to bind to the LBD, thereby mediating the activity of AF-2, which forms the core of helix 12. The LBD dimerization interfaces are formed by α-helices that line up and/or intertwine and differ slightly between ERα and PR.

DNA Binding

The receptors for progestagens, glucocorticoids, mineralocorticoids, and androgens bind to the same HRE that is composed of two half-sites (AGAACA), which are arranged as inverted (palindromic) repeats (IR) with the half-sites being separated by three nucleotides (IR-3). The HRE half-site recognized by both ERs (AGGTCA) deviates in two nucleotides from this DNA sequence (**Figure 3c**). One HRE half-site is recognized by one receptor monomer, and the homodimer binds in a head-to-head orientation to an IR-3 element. The non-ERs recognize their half-site mainly by a hydrophobic interaction with the methyl group of the thymine in position 4 of the complementary strand (AGAACA) that is not present in the DNA sequence recognized by the ER. The half-site spacing of 3 bp is such that an SHR homodimer binds both half-sites on the same face of the DNA. In addition to IR-3 elements, only the AR is able to selectively recognize direct repeats of the two half-sites separated by three nucleotides (ADR-3 elements). In contrast to other nuclear receptors binding to DR elements, the AR homodimer also binds in a head-to-head orientation to an ADR-3 element.

The DBD of SHRs comprises approximately 80 amino acids encoded by region C plus some 14 N-terminal amino acids of region D. Domain C contains two patterns that are reminiscent of, but clearly distinguishable from, the zinc-finger motifs first observed in the *Xenopus laevis* transcription factor IIIA. The SHR zinc fingers are also able to tetrahedrally coordinate a zinc atom, but are of the type (Cys2-Cys2). Only very few amino acids, termed the proximal (P-)box, within the first SHR zinc finger are responsible for specific recognition of the cognate HRE. Another set of amino acids, called the distal (D-)box within the second SHR zinc finger, forms the weak dimerization interface of the DNA-binding domain (**Figure 3b**).

Activation of Transcription

To regulate transcription, agonist-liganded SHRs must talk to the general transcription machinery. This can be achieved either by a direct contact between SHRs and the general transcription factors (GTFs), which are building up the transcription preinitiation complex at the transcription start point, or by means of other cellular factors that do not bind to DNA directly but are recruited to the promoters by the SHRs via protein–protein interactions. Depending on the effect of these coregulators on gene expression, they can be divided into coactivators, which promote transcription mediated by SHRs, and corepressors, which suppress SHR-dependent gene transcription. Coregulators, other sequence-specific transcription factors, and chromatin factors all function as interpreters between SHRs and the general transcription machinery.

Coactivators

Coactivators were originally called transcriptional intermediary factors because they are supposed to bridge between DNA-bound sequence-specific transcription factors and GTFs. The suspicion that SHRs may require coactivators for activation was derived from the squelching phenomenon – the observation that an excess receptor can inhibit its own transactivation as well as transcription by other transactivators. One possible explanation for this behavior is that additional factors, which are present in limited amounts and required for transactivation, are trapped by excess SHRs in unproductive complexes. Conversely, by overexpressing coactivators, it is possible to reactivate a target promoter that has been squelched by excess SHR.

Today, more than 20 of these coactivators are known that were quickly identified within a decade. An important and well-characterized class of coactivators is the steroid receptor coactivator (SRC, or p160) family of coactivators, consisting of its three members SRC-1, SRC-2 (also known as transcription intermediary factor 2 or glucocorticoid receptor-interacting protein 1), and SRC-3. The three related proteins have partial overlapping specificity for hormone receptors and cell type. SRCs enhance hormone-dependent transcriptional activities of SHRs without altering the basal activity of a target promoter. The biological functions of SRCs have been revealed by gene-disruption experiments in mice. Whereas SRC-1-deficient mice display normal growth and fertility but partial resistance to a number of steroid hormones, SRC-2 knockout mice have reduced fertility due to gonadal failure and are leaner because the ratio of white and brown adipose tissue is decreased. The inactivation of SRC-3 has more dramatic effects and results in growth retardation and smaller body size as well as resistance to growth hormones (GHs) and estrogen. Like SHRs, coactivators are modular proteins with common functional domains such as one that possesses acetyltransferase activity. For the binding to agonist-liganded SHRs, one or several copies of an α-helical LXXLL signature motif, also called a nuclear receptor (NR) box, are required. After the binding of an agonistic ligand to the SHR, helix 12, containing the AF-2 core of the receptor, is relocated, exposing a hydrophobic cleft and an adjacent ionic clamp as the principal determinants for the interaction with an NR box.

In vivo coactivators are organized into complexes that are poised for interaction with SHRs in response to appropriate stimuli. Many of the characterized complexes share subunits, suggesting that a directed or cyclical assembly of coactivator complexes takes place. Current data support a model in which the initial binding of ligand results in the dissociation of corepressors and recruitment of chromatin remodeling machines such as SWI/SNF. The binding of SRCs and other coactivators such as CBP/p300 then results in local acetyltransferase activity and the opening of chromatin in the vicinity of the target promoter. C-terminal SRC-domains can recruit other coactivators, such as the coactivator-associated arginine methyltransferase-1 (CARM1) and cAMP responsive element binding protein (CREB)-binding protein (CBP), and the related protein p300 for complementing and potentiating histone acetyltransferase activity, respectively.

Coactivators are subject to a number of posttranslational modifications for modulating coactivator function. Acetylation and ubiquitination appear to alter the half-life of molecules, whereas phosphorylation is essential for the optimal activity of coactivators within the cell. Phosporylation of SRCs occurs in response to a plethora of stimuli, including epidermal growth factor, steroid hormones, cytokines, and increased intracellular cAMP. In turn, multiple kinases, such as MAPKs and IκB kinases, that are involved in a number of cellular signaling pathways are responsible for a distinct phosphorylation pattern on SRC-3, regulating its activity and, more important, its specificity. In contrast to SHRs, SRCs have a broad tissue distribution and coactivate an ever-expanding number of transcription factors. Therefore, coactivators, like SRCs, might serve as integrators of multiple afferent stimuli in order to produce an appropriate cellular response.

Cyclin D1, the regulatory subunit of a holoenzyme that phosphorylates and inactivates the retinoblastoma protein tumor suppressor and promotes progression through the G1-S phase of the cell cycle, has been identified as a coactivator for ERα recently. The *cyclin D1* gene is frequently overexpressed in human breast cancer and is capable of inducing mammary tumorigenesis when overexpressed in transgenic mice. Cyclin D1 binds to the N-terminal half of the ligand binding domain of ERα and enhances ligand-induced recruitment of ERα to an estrogen responsive element (ERE). More important, cyclin D1 antagonizes the repression of ERα activity mediated by the tumor suppressor gene product BRCA1, which is functioning as a corepressor of ERα in this context. Thus cyclin D1 and BRCA1 constitute an antagonizing pair of coregulators for ERα.

Corepressors

For some members of the nuclear receptor family, such as the thyroid hormone receptor (TR) and the retinoid acid receptors (RARs), that form heterodimers with the retinoid X receptor (RXR), it is well known that they repress basal transcription in the unliganded state. It has been shown that this silencing effect is mediated by corepressors that were called nuclear receptor corepressor (N-CoR) and silencing mediator for retinoid and thyroid hormone receptors (SMRT). N-CoR and SMRT associate with DNA-bound TR–RXR or RAR–RXR heterodimers in the absence of hormone but not in its presence. SMRT and N-CoR are multiprotein complexes that exhibit histone deacetylase activity. Both corepressors are also involved in steroid hormone action because it was demonstrated that the overexpression of N-CoR and SMRT represses the partial agonistic activity of both ERα bound to the antihormone tamoxifen and of PR bound to the antagonist RU486. Recognition by transcriptionally incompetent SHRs of corepressors is mediated by short amphipathic helical signature motifs, called CoRNR boxes, which are similar to the NR boxes of coactivators. Corepressor activity is mediated by histone deacetylation. Because corepressors lack intrinsic deacetylation domains, they recruit histone deacetylases for this task. Apparently, corepressors and coactivators are functionally similar proteins, so it is not surprising that a corepressor can also turn into a coactivator, as shown for N-CoR and RAR.

Recently, the tumor suppressor gene product BRCA1 has been shown to be a corepressor of ERα. BRCA1 is implicated in DNA repair mechanisms, and germ-line mutations in the BRCA1 gene predispose women to ovarian and breast cancer. BRCA1 inhibited estradiol-induced endogenous gene expression at levels of BRCA1 that are within the physiological range. Moreover, BRCA1 was shown to bind to ERα directly *in vitro* and the binding of BRCA1 to an estrogen responsive gene was reduced by estradiol *in vivo*. BRCA1 appears not to act on specific estrogen responsive genes or gene subsets but blocks the ability of estradiol to alter the expression of the vast majority of all estradiol responsive genes in MCF7 cells. BRCA1 downregulates the coactivator p300, and excess p300 rescues BRCA1 repression of ERα like cyclin D1 can. The physical association of cyclin D1 with ERα may exclude the direct association of BRCA1 with the receptor or alter the conformation of BRCA1 and/or the binding of other BRCA1-associated proteins and thereby contributes to activation at an ERE.

Altogether, SHRs can exist in a multitude of conformations, depending on the nature of bound ligand. The various interaction surfaces are mainly determined by helix 12 and most likely by the C-terminus beyond helix 12, the F region. The transactivation by SHRs appears to be not only a simple net activation but the sum of relief from repression by corepressors and activation by coactivators. The switch from the repressed to the activated state is initiated by the hormone ligand through an allosteric change in SHR structure followed by an intricate interplay of coregulators.

Interactions with Sequence-Specific Transcription Factors

SHRs control the activity of natural promoters through positive and negative interactions with sequence-specific transcription factors. Particularly interesting is an interaction that represses the activity of both partners, as exemplified in the case of hGR and the heterodimeric transcription factor AP-1. Similar interactions have been described between GR and the p65 subunit of the transcription factor nuclear factor (NF-)κB and the transcription factor GATA-1. From experiments with numerous SHR mutants, it can be concluded that repression is most likely mediated by a protein–protein interaction with an SHR monomer that requires the N-terminal portion of the receptor. Because most immunoregulatory genes as well as genes involved in inflammation are positively regulated by the transcription factors AP-1 and NF-κ B, it is conceivable that the immunosuppressive and anti-inflammatory activities of glucocorticoids are mediated through the inhibition of AP-1- and NF-κ B-mediated transactivation by GR (**Figure 1c**).

A novel biological action of GR was revealed by constructing mice with the hepatocyte-specific loss of GR that have a severe reduction in body weight due to decreased bone length and size of internal organs, very reminiscent of mice lacking the signal transducer and activator of transcription (STAT)5. In both mice strains, growth hormone (GH) signaling via the JAK–STAT pathway is impaired. GR directly interacts with both phosphorylated and unphosphorylated forms of STAT5, and both proteins are detectable at promoters of GH-regulated genes *in vivo*, which is essential for GH signaling. As shown by dimerization defective GR mutant (GR^{dim}) mice, GH signaling is independent of GR DNA binding and most likely mediated by protein–protein interaction with STAT5 transcription factors.

Interaction with Chromatin Factors

The interaction of SHRs with DNA, the general transcription machinery, coregulators, and sequence-specific transcription factors takes place in the nucleus with its DNA compacted into chromatin. Genetic analyses have demonstrated a widespread involvement of chromatin structure in gene regulation in general. For the GR, it was shown that components of the so-called SWI–SNF complex, a set of pleiotropic transactivators that counteract the repressive functions of chromatin, are required for transactivation in yeast. In human cells lacking brahma (hBrm), the homolog of the SWI–SNF complex subunit SWI2, transactivation by GR is weak and can be enhanced selectively by the ectopic expression of hBrm. Like SWI2 in yeast, hBrm is part of a large multiprotein complex that mediates the ATP-dependent disruption of a nucleosome. A direct interaction between nuclear receptors and components of hBrg1, a brahma-related ATPase complex, has been demonstrated, and chromatin immunoprecipitation experiments indicate that the hormone receptors recruit these ATP-dependent chromatin remodeling complexes to their target genes. In the case of the MMTV promoter, activation by glucocorticoids and progestins depends on the correct organization of the promoter sequences in nucleosomes so that some HREs of a larger cluster get exposed. The binding of the receptor to the exposed HREs leads to the recruitment of ATP-dependent chromatin remodeling activities that displace H2A–H2B dimers from the promoter and allow the binding of the ubiquitous transcription factor NF1 and the recruitment of more receptor molecules, followed by coactivators and the transcription preinitiation complex. Optimal activation requires the inclusion of linker histones that help to position nucleosomes and generate a more suitable platform for receptor binding.

Apart from the SWI/SNF complex and related ATP-dependent chromatin remodeling machines, increasing evidence has implicated the modification of histones in the regulation of gene transcription. Histones are composed of a histone fold domain, involved in wrapping the DNA in nucleosomes, and an N-terminal tail rich in lysine that protrudes out of the nucleosome. The acetylation of tail lysines reduces the affinity of histone tails for DNA greatly and is believed to render DNA more accessible to transcription factors while still maintaining a nucleosomal architecture. Moreover, some of the identified coactivators for SHRs, such as CBP/p300 and SRC1, as well as the largest subunit of the pivotal GTF TFIID, $TAF_{II}230/250$, turned out to be histone acetyl transferases (HATs). All of these observations led to the current two-step model for transcriptional activation by SHRs that is built on the hormone-mediated recruitment of coactivators and other transcription factors with HAT activity, resulting in the local destabilization of repressive histone–DNA interactions, followed by direct or indirect interactions with the basal transcription machinery. Histone arginine methyl transferases, such as CARM1, are also implicated in gene activation by steroid hormones. and recent evidence suggests a participation of kinases that phosphorylate core and linker histones. Altogether, these new findings emphasize the importance of chromatin remodeling in gene regulation by steroid hormones.

Recently, a detailed kinetic analysis by chromatin immunoprecipitation (ChiP) analyses of the assembly of transcription initiation complexes on the estrogen responsive promoter of the pS2 gene has revealed a sequence of cycles of formation of multiprotein complexes involving protein-modifying enzymes and ATP-dependent chromatin remodeling complexes, followed by ubiquitin/proteasome-mediated degradation of the receptor with a cycling amplitude on a time scale of minutes. The dynamic nature of transcriptional activation has also been assessed by single live-cell imaging of transcription factors tagged with fluorescent proteins. Contrary to the ChiP results, fluorescence recovery after photobleaching analyses have shown that SHRs and interacting coregulators rapidly exchange on large artificial HRE arrays on a time scale of seconds. In attempting to reconcile these contradictory results, we have to consider that ChIP is a composite freeze-frame of promoter occupancy in millions of cells, whereas live-imaging focuses on the chronology of events in a single cell.

Involvement of the Glucocorticoid Receptor in the Stress Response

Studies of human patients and adrenalectomized animals have shown that glucocorticoids have a plethora of functions, the most important being the stimulation of gluconeogenesis; decrease of glucose uptake by peripheral tissues; increase of glycogen deposition; increase of lipolysis; stimulation of protein and nucleic acid synthesis, predominantly in the liver; suppression of immune and inflammatory responses; inhibition of fibroblast proliferation and extracellular matrix deposition; maintenance of normal cardiovascular function and blood pressure; and regulation of calcium absorption. Many of these functions should prevent an overreaction of defense mechanisms to stress and be conducive to coping with the stress response. In line with this hypothesis, the synthesis and release of glucocorticoids are elevated during stress, and people with chronic adrenal insufficiency show "general languor and debility, remarkable feebleness of the heart's action, irritability of the stomach and a peculiar change in the color of the skin," as Addison described it in 1855. Although none of these symptoms is life-threatening, patients with Addison disease cannot withstand stress and are prone to suffering an acute adrenal crisis that can lead to shock or coma.

Until recently, it was believed that all these glucocorticoid effects were of a genomic nature, mediated by its receptor binding to glucocorticoid response elements (GREs) in the target genes. Given the multiple important functions of glucocorticoids, it was therefore not surprising to learn that GR-deficient mice, which were generated using gene knockout techniques, are not viable and die shortly after birth.

However, the cause of death – respiratory failure due to lack of lung maturation – does not seem to depend on genomic effects mediated by GREs. Contrary to GR-deficient mice, homozygous mice that express a mutated GR that is not able to dimerize appear almost normal and healthy under standard laboratory conditions. This dimerization-defective GR (GR^{dim}) can no longer bind efficiently to palindromic GREs, and these mutant mice do not respond to the administration of glucocorticoids by the induction of well-characterized hormone responsive genes. Clearly, GRE-mediated gene activation is not required for development and survival. On the other hand, GR^{dim} mice show a selective impairment of spatial memory in the water maze. It is known that the stress that is associated with a learning task – here orientation in a maze – leads to the activation of GRs in the brain, which is required for facilitated storage of the acquired information. Therefore, the facilitating effects of corticosterone on spatial memory seem to depend on DNA binding of the GR.

There is also increasing evidence that altered GR signaling is an important cause of the pathogenesis of major depression. The most consistent biological finding in patients with depression is hyperactivity of the hypothalamic-pituitary-adrenal (HPA) axis. Mutant mice with a 50% GR gene dose reduction have a disinhibited HPA axis like human patients and show increased helplessness after stress exposure, a behavioral correlate of depression in mice. In contrast, mice that overexpress GR demonstrate a reduced helplessness response after stress challenge. Also, human carriers of two polymorphisms in the GR gene had an increased risk of developing a major depressive mode.

Cross-Talk with Other Signal Transduction Pathways

Steroid hormones can either act via their cognate receptors that alter gene expression after binding to HREs in target genes (termed genomic or nuclear action) or act via membrane-bound or -localized SHRs or non-SHRs (termed nongenomic or cytoplasmic action). Whereas genomic action is slow and takes 30–60 min, nongenomic action is rapid and takes a couple of seconds or minutes. We now briefly summarize the important findings on nongenomic actions that involve the classical steroid receptors.

The existence of such nongenomic actions became apparent in experiments with GR knockout mice that die postnatally and with mice that express a dimerization-defective mutant GR and are viable. The dimerization-defective GR shows impaired GRE-dependent transactivation while functions that require cross-talk with other transcription factors remain intact. Moreover, many studies employing different techniques and assays have shown that a small pool of estrogen (some 2%) and ARs are associated with the plasma membrane. More specifically, both receptors have been identified in the caveolae, together with a number of signaling molecules. One of the actions of steroid receptors thought to take place in the caveolae is the estrogen-mediated rapid increase in endothelial nitric oxide synthase (eNOS) activity. The 110-kDa caveolin-binding protein striatin has been identified as a molecular interaction hub that organizes an ERα–eNOS membrane signaling complex engaging also the G-protein $G_{\alpha i}$. The disruption of the ERα–striatin interaction abolishes the rapid activation of MAPK, Akt kinase (also called protein kinase B), and eNOS by estrogen, whereas genomic signaling is not affected. But other proteins such as caveolin-1, modulator of nongenomic action of estrogen receptor (MNAR), Shc, or insulin-like growth factor-1 receptor are also implicated in tethering ERα to the inner face of the plasma membrane bilayer. Moreover, the steroid-independent palmitoylation of a cystine residue within the E domain has been observed. Palmitoylation facilitates caveolin-1 binding as well as membrane localization. Interestingly, A/B and C domain-deleted ERα still localizes to the membrane and signals to extracellular receptor kinase (ERK) like the wild-type receptor. Current evidence suggests that ERα membrane localization is required for kinase activation.

A well-known rapid response of steroid receptors is the activation of the c-Src–p21ras–ERK2 pathway by ligand-bound AR, ERα (but not ERβ), GR, MR, and PR-B. For all five SHRs MAPK activation is abrogated in the presence of antihormones, but this is less clear for MR. Although various mechanisms have been proposed, the interaction of SHRs with the kinase c-Src is an important aspect of cross-talk. Whereas AR interacts with the SH3 domain of c-Src, ERα interacts with the SH2 domain. AR activation of the ERK pathway is more effective if, in addition to AR binding to the SH2 domain, ERα simultaneously binds to the SH3 domain. In cells expressing both receptors, stimulation with androgen or estrogen induces a productive ERα–AR–c-Src complex that can be prevented by treating with either antiandrogens or antiestrogens. PR-B does not bind to c-Src directly, but requires the presence of ERα. In the absence of progestins, PR-B (but not PR-A) binds to ERα. Progestins release ERα from this complex and thus trigger the interaction of ERα with c-Src. In case of ERα, cross-talk is exemplified by epidermal growth factor (EGF) treatment of ovariectomized mice. This results in nuclear translocation and an altered phosphorylation state of ERα. Transient transfection studies showed that EGF, thus, can activate ERα.

The activation of the GR elicits apoptosis in T cells, but can paradoxically also promote thymocyte survival. This dual effect is reminiscent of the actions of the T-cell antigen receptor, which is essential for thymocyte survival but can also cause apoptosis. Interestingly, the activation of the T-cell antigen receptor blocks glucocortiocid-induced apoptosis, thus implying functional cross-talk between these two distinct signaling systems. The regulation of programmed cell death by glucocorticoids also involves the regulated expression and alternative splicing of the *bcl-X* gene and crosstalk with the STAT5 family of transcription factors. In lymphocytes, the apoptotic effect is mediated by a selective interaction of GR with activated STAT5a, whereas in mammary cells, equipped with STAT5b, glucocorticoids act as antiapoptotic factors.

The downstream targets of the rapid action of steroids remain to be fully uncovered, but in many cases the SHRs themselves – and their coactivators – are targeted. Therefore, one function of these rapid actions seems to be the potentiation of genomic action. All SHRs have been known to be phosphoproteins for many years. Most of the identified phosphorylation sites are serine and threonine residues, but some of the family members are also phosphorylated on tyrosine. In case of the chicken PR, for instance, four phosphorylated serines have been identified common to both isoforms, PR-A and PR-B. The two N-terminal sites are only moderately phosphorylated in the absence of hormone, whereas, after hormone treatment, an increase in the phosphorylation of these sites and the appearance of two new phosphorylation sites are observed. The mutation of these serine residues results in a cell- and promoter-specific variation of receptor activity when tested in transfection experiments. In case of ERα ERK, phosphatidylinositol 3-kinase, $p90^{RSK}$, a kinase downstream of Akt2, and Akt2 itself phosporylate discrete residues of the receptor, upregulating its transcriptional activity or stability.

See Also the Following Articles

Adrenal Insufficiency; Corticosteroids and Stress; Glucocortoids, Overview; Membrane Glucocorticoid Receptors.

Further Reading

Addison, T. (1855). *On the constitutional and local effects of disease of the suprarenal capsules.* London: D. Highley.

Baulieu, E. -E. and Kelly, P. A. (1990). *Hormones: from molecules to disease.* New York: Chapman and Hall.

Beato, M., Herrlich, P. and Schütz, G. (1995). Steroid hormone receptors: many actors in search of a plot. *Cell* **83**, 851–857.
Cato, A. C. B., Nestl, A. and Mink, S. (2002). Rapid actions of steroid receptors in cellular signaling pathways. *Science's Signal Transduction Knowledge Environment* **138**[Online].
Gronemeyer, H. and Laudet, V. (1995). Transcription factors 3: nuclear receptors. *Protein Profile* **2**, 1173–1308.
Nuclear Receptors Nomenclature Committee. (1999). Nuclear receptors nomenclature committee: a unified nomenclature system for the nuclear receptor superfamily. *Cell* **97**, 161.
Levin, E. R. (2005). Integration of the extranuclear and nuclear actions of estrogen. *Molecular Endocrinology* **19**, 1951–1959.
Lu, N. Z. and Cidlowski, J. A. (2006). Glucocorticoid receptor isoforms generate transcription specificity. *Trends in Cell Biology* **16**, 301–307.
Mangelsdorf, D. J., Thummel, C., Beato, M., et al. (1995). The nuclear receptor superfamily: the second decade. *Cell* **83**, 835–839.
McKenna, N. J. and O'Malley, B. W. (2002). Combinatorial control of gene expression by nuclear receptors and coregulators. *Cell* **108**, 465–474.
Metivier, R., Reid, G. and Gannon, F. (2006). Transcription in four dimensions: nuclear receptor-directed initiation of gene expression. *EMBO Reports* **7**, 161–167.
Parker, M. G. (1991). *Nuclear hormone receptors: molecular mechanisms, cellular functions, clinical abnormalities*. London: Academic Press.
Pratt, W. B., Morishima, Y., Murphy, M., et al. (2005). Chaperoning of glucocorticoid receptors. In: Gaestel, M. (ed.) *Handbook of experimental pharmacology. Vol. 172: Molecular chaperones in health and disease*, pp. 111–138. Berlin: Springer.
Wu, R. C., Smith, C. L. and O'Malley, B. W. (2005). Transcriptional regulation by steroid receptor coactivator phosphorylation. *Endocrine Reviews* **26**, 393–399.
Wintermantel, T. M., Berger, S., Greiner, E. F., et al. (2005). Evaluation of steroid receptor function by gene targeting in mice. *Journal of Steroid Biochemistry and Molecular Biology* **93**, 107–112.

Relevant Website

NUREBASE, http://www.ens-lyon.fr/LBMC/laudet/nurebase

Corticosteroid Receptor Genes: Functional Dissection in Mice

F Tronche
CNRS, Collège de France, Paris, France

Glossary

Additional transgenesis — Adding an extra gene to the mouse genome; often used for the random insertion of a synthetic gene into the mouse genome by injection into a monocellular zygote followed by the selection of a mouse colony carrying the desired gene.

Corticosteroid receptor genes — Genes encoding the glucocorticoid and mineralocorticoid receptors. These receptors are the intracellular receptors for corticosteroid hormones and function as transcription factors in the cell nucleus, controlling the expression of target genes. These genes are similar to those of the receptors for other steroid hormones: androgens, progesterone, and estrogens. All these genes are derived from a common ancestor, and they form the steroid receptor gene subfamily of the nuclear receptor gene family.

Gene targeting — A technique for the modification of a given chromosomal DNA sequence by homologous recombination in cultured mouse embryonic stem cells. Live animals carrying the mutation can be derived from this modified cell line.

Molecular genetics — The field of biology concerned with studies of the structure and function of genes at the molecular level. The development of reverse genetic tools, facilitating the introduction of the desired modification into the mouse genome has made it possible to investigate the consequences of targeted mutations at the level of a mammal organism.

Null allele — Often used to define a gene allele that cannot lead to the synthesis of gene product, synonym of (−) or knock-out. A major difficulty of gene targeting in mice is to ensure that the gene is indeed invalidated and that no wild-type or modified protein is produced.

Tissue-specific gene inactivation The deletion of a given gene from the mouse chromosome only in certain cell types, the gene remaining intact throughout the rest of the body. Such deletions are achieved by introducing two 34-bp DNA sequences – the *loxP* sites – on either side of the DNA segment to be deleted. These sites render the modified allele sensitive to Cre recombinase, which, if present in the desired cell type, binds to *loxP* sites and excises the intervening DNA segment from the chromosome. The *loxP* site and Cre recombinase are derived from the P1 bacteriophage.

The adaptation of organisms is based on their ability to respond to environmental variation by adapting their gene transcription profile to meet actual physiological needs. This is well illustrated by the adrenal release of glucocorticoids (GCs) in response to stress. These compounds may act on various tissues, coordinating immune, metabolic, endocrine, and behavioral responses by activating receptors, which, in turn, directly modulate gene transcription. This system is beneficial in healthy organisms, but dysfunctions in this system constitute a severe threat to the health and well-being of the organism. In humans, the dysregulation of the stress response is associated with the development of physiological and behavioral disorders, such as depression, anxiety, memory deficits, and drug dependence.

GCs bind to two related transcription factors, the ubiquitously expressed low-affinity glucocorticoid receptor (GR) and the high-affinity mineralocorticoid receptor (MR), which acts as a bona fide glucocorticoid receptor in a few cell types, such as hippocampal neurons, but is mostly expressed in cells involved in salt-balance control, in which it serves as a mineralocorticoid (aldosterone) receptor. In these cells, the MR is indeed protected from GCs by 11β-hydroxysteroid dehydrogenase (11β-HSD2), an enzyme that converts GCs into inactive forms.

The GR and MR genes belong to the nuclear receptor gene family, the members of which have several characteristics in common. The GR and MR proteins contain two highly structured domains: the DNA-binding domain (DBD) and the ligand-binding domain (LBD). In addition, two domains involved in controlling transcription (the activation function, AF, domains) are located in the N-terminal part of the protein and within the LBD. In the absence of ligand, the receptor exists in an inactive state as part of a large cytoplasmic complex. On hormone binding, the activated GR monomer translocates into the nucleus, where it modulates the transcription of target genes by remodeling chromatin and interacting with the basal transcriptional machinery, coactivators, and other transcription factors. The GR may activate or repress gene expression, by binding directly to its cognate response element in the promoter region of target genes and via DNA-binding-independent mechanisms involving other transcription factors (**Figure 1**). However, due to the wide-ranging effects of GCs, the precise mechanisms underlying the molecular actions of GR and MR and the nature of their cellular targets throughout the body remain largely to be defined with precision.

To address these issues, various animal models have been developed, based on the use of molecular genetic tools established for the precise modification of the mouse genome. These tools include classic gene inactivation or mutation by homologous recombination in embryonic stem (ES) cells and tissue-specific gene inactivation based on the Cre–*loxP* system, both of which affect the endogenous gene. Other approaches modify gene dosage by adding a transgene to the genome for the constitutive or inducible (tetracycline system) expression of GR or MR. Critical analysis of the phenotypes resulting from these modifications has both confirmed the expected roles of GR and MR and uncovered entirely unexpected functions.

Classic Inactivation of Glucocorticoid Receptor and Mineralocorticoid Receptor Genes

Glucocorticoid Receptor Is Absolutely Required for Survival

Homologous recombination in ES cells has been used to generate various mutations inactivating the GR gene in mice. The resulting phenotypes were somewhat different. The first attempt involved insertion of a DNA cassette within the second exon to prevent the processing of GR mRNA. This approach generated a hypomorphic allele because alternative splicing of the GR gene can lead to the formation of a truncated mRNA encoding an N-terminally truncated GR protein that contains the DBDs and LBDs (allele GR^{-} or GR^{hypo}; **Figure 2**). A second mutation was then designed to ensure complete gene inactivation. This mutation consisted of a deletion of the third exon (GR^{null} allele), which encodes an essential part of the DBD, and it introduced a frameshift in the open reading frame following the fusion of the second and the fourth exon. This mutation thus ensures that no GR protein isoform containing the DBDs and LBDs can be formed.

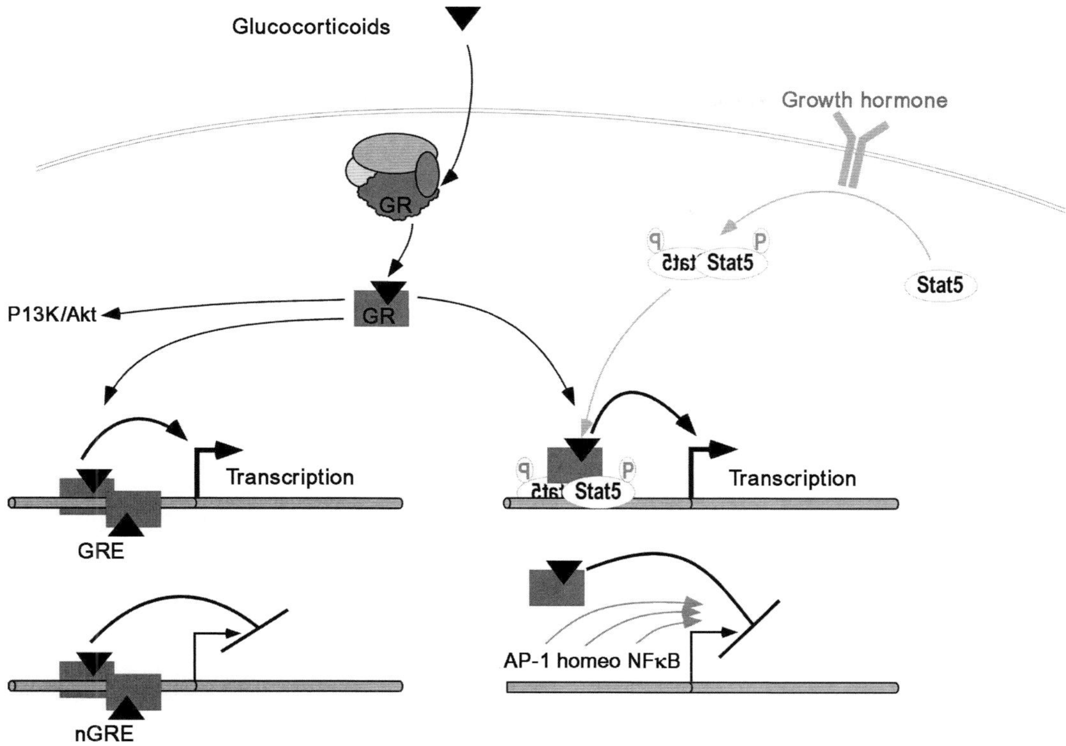

Figure 1 The glucocorticoid receptor acts by various molecular mechanisms. Due to their lipophilic nature, glucocorticoids can easily cross the cell membrane. Hormone binding to GR induces a change in the conformation of the receptor, leading to its release from an inactivating multiprotein complex and its translocation into the nucleus. The receptor then binds to glucocorticoid response elements (GRE) in DNA, as a dimer, or to negative GRE (nGRE), thereby activating or repressing the transcription of target genes. It can also modulate the activation of gene transcription by other factors, acting as a coactivator of Stat5 – a transcription factor induced by phosphorylation on GH binding to its receptor – or repressing transcription factors such as AP-1, NF-κB, or some homeoproteins. GR may also act by other modes, interfering with intracellular signaling cascades by stimulating Akt phosphorylation, for example.

$GR^{null/null}$ animals develop to term, but die at birth because they are unable to breathe due to collapsing of the lungs. They present defects in the maturation of several tissues, including a very thin stratum corneum (the outermost layer of the epidermis) and a defect in pancreas organization. GC levels are tightly controlled by an endocrine cascade (see), which is in turn regulated by a negative feedback loop. The absence of GR leads to a profound imbalance in the hypothalamic-pituitary-adrenal (HPA) axis. Corticotropin releasing hormone (CRH), adrenocorticotropic hormone (ACTH), and GC levels increase. Consistent with the increase in GC levels, the region responsible for GC synthesis – the adrenal cortex – is markedly enlarged and displays tissue disorganization. Surprisingly, adrenal chromaffin cell development is not impaired. Differentiated chromaffin cells are scattered throughout the gland, but are no fewer in number in mutant neonates than in wild-type neonates. This unexpected result demonstrates that GR is not essential for the development of this cell type *in vivo*, whereas the contrary is suggested by results obtained in cell culture. However, $GR^{null/null}$ chromaffin cells do not synthesize epinephrine due to a lack of expression of the gene-encoding phenylethanolamine *N*-methyltransferase (PNMT), the enzyme responsible for converting norepinephrine into epinephrine.

Hematopoietic stem cells from $GR^{null/null}$ animals have been used to demonstrate the role of GR activation in stress erythropoiesis. In the absence of GR, cultured erythroblasts proliferate poorly and rapidly differentiate into erythrocytes. *In vivo*, this has important consequences for survival and adaptation. Chimeric adult animals subjected to irradiation and grafted with mutant stem cells such that they carry only $GR^{null/null}$ erythroblasts cannot rapidly reconstitute a normal number of red blood cells after erythrolysis or bleeding. In hypoxic conditions, similar to conditions at an altitude of 5000 m, they are unable to adapt rapidly by increasing their number of red blood cells.

$GR^{hypo/hypo}$ animals (originally named $GR^{-/-}$) display a milder phenotype. Unlike $GR^{null/null}$ animals, all of which die at birth, 20% of $GR^{hypo/hypo}$ mice pass this stage, grow normally, and reach adulthood. Several of the phenotypes of $GR^{null/null}$ animals, such as the almost total absence of the stratum corneum

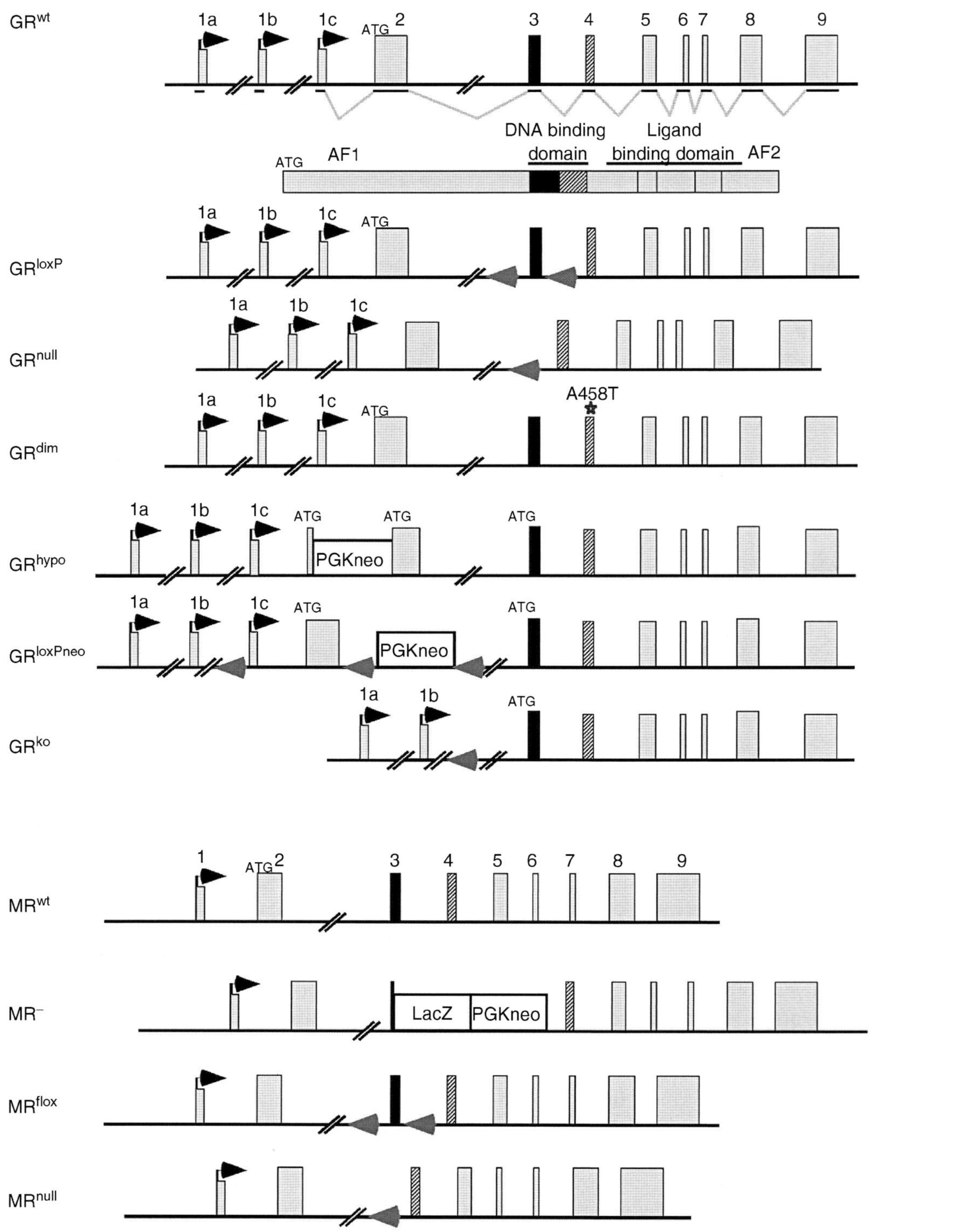

Figure 2 Schematic representation of the various GR and MR alleles generated in mice by gene targeting. Promoters are represented by black arrows, exons by boxes and *loxP* sites by gray arrows. The position of the *dim* point mutation is indicated by a star.

and the pancreatic defect, are not observed in $GR^{hypo/hypo}$ mice. The differences between the two mutations presumably result from the presence of residual GR protein isoforms in $GR^{hypo/hypo}$ animals. A third mutation involving the deletion of the alternative exon 1c and exon 2 has been generated (GR^{ko}). No skin or pancreas phenotypes have been reported for $GR^{ko/ko}$ animals. The inactivation strategy, consisting of the deletion of the second exon, is similar to that of the GR^{hypo} allele and may potentially allow the formation of proteins with a DBD. Further investigations are required to understand the differences between $GR^{ko/ko}$ and $GR^{null/null}$ animals.

Inactivation of the Mineralocorticoid Receptor Gene Leads to Type I Pseudohypoaldosteronism

Mineralocorticoid hormone (aldosterone) is a key element in homeostatic sodium balance control, activating MR in the polarized cells of sodium-transporting epithelia (distal part of the nephron, colon, salivary, and sweat glands). MR is also expressed in neurons, cardiomyocytes, and adipocytes, in which it may be activated by both mineralocorticoids and GCs. The MR gene has been inactivated by replacing the third exon with the *lacZ* gene in embryonic stem cells. This exon encodes the first zinc finger of the DBD. $MR^{-/-}$ animals develop normally but die approximately 10 days after birth due to a massive loss of renal sodium and water. Mutant animals present major dehydration, with a high hematocrit and hyperkalemia. The renin–angiotensin–aldosterone system (RAAS), which controls salt balance, is strongly induced. These symptoms correspond to exacerbated human type I pseudohypoaldosteronism, due to mutations in the MR (heterozygous) or ENaC genes. In $MR^{-/-}$ animals, the molecular mechanism underlying the major loss of renal sodium remains unclear. Amiloride-sensitive sodium reabsorption rates have been shown to be low, but the levels of ENaC mRNA encoding the amiloride-sensitive epithelial sodium channels remain unchanged, as do the sodium/potassium ATPase mRNA levels.

$MR^{-/-}$mice may be kept alive by salt supplementation. Animals may survive if they are given daily subcutaneous injections of NaCl solution until weaning and are supplied with oral NaCl thereafter. Adult animals display high levels of renal sodium excretion, hyperkalemia, and persistent activation of the RAAS. These survivors have been used to study other MR functions. MR is strongly expressed in brain structures, such as the hippocampus. In rescued adult $MR^{-/-}$ animals, the dentate gyrus region of the hippocampus is thinner than in control littermates due to lower levels of neurogenesis, resulting in a lower density of granule cells. The absence of MR may be the primary cause of this defect, but higher levels of GR signaling due to higher circulating GC levels may also be involved.

Tissue-Specific Corticosteroid Receptor Genes Inactivation

The early death of mice lacking the GR or the MR gene precludes the study of the functions of these genes in adult physiology or behavior. In addition, the disruption throughout the animal of genes expressed in many different cell types and encoding proteins with highly diverse functions, results in a phenotype reflecting the combined absence of these functions. This phenotype may therefore be difficult to interpret. The ability to inactivate a gene in a single cell type is therefore a major breakthrough and has clear advantages over the disruption of the gene throughout the body. The Cre–*loxP* system has been used to inactivate the GR and MR genes in a tissue-specific manner. This system is based on the use of CRE recombinase, which binds to a 34-bp DNA sequence (*loxP*) and excises any DNA segment flanked by two such sites. Therefore, if a *loxP* site is present on either side of a mouse gene, that gene will be selectively deleted in cell types expressing the Cre recombinase but will remain intact in the rest of the body (**Figure 3**). Conditional alleles have been generated by flanking the third exons of the GR and MR genes with two *loxP* sites, through homologous recombination in ES cells. This DNA modification is very small given the overall size of the GR and MR genes (34 bp versus >100 kb), particularly because the neomycin resistance gene, used for ES cell selection, is removed from these targeted alleles. The insertion of *loxP* sites has no effect on the endogenous expression of the genes, but it makes them sensitive to the presence of Cre recombinase. Mice carrying the GR^{loxP} or MR^{flox} alleles were crossed with transgenic animals expressing Cre recombinase in various tissues, leading to the conversion, in these tissues, of the GR^{loxP} or MR^{flox} alleles into null alleles. Analyses of mutant mice lacking GR or MR in particular tissues confirmed some known or suspected functions of the receptor and revealed a number of previously unsuspected functions. Using this approach, we were able to dissect *in vivo* some of the roles of GR because we were able to isolate its function in a given cell type from its effects in the rest of the body.

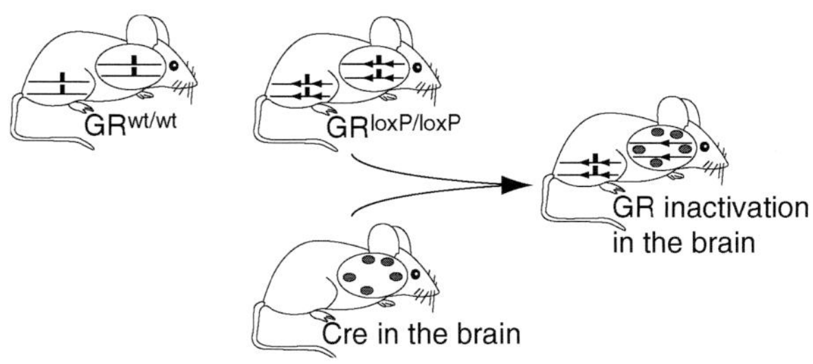

Figure 3 Principle of tissue-specific gene inactivation using the Cre–*loxP* system. When crossed with transgenic mice expressing the Cre recombinase in the brain (gray circle), the DNA fragment flanked with *loxP* sites in the same orientation (gray arrow) is deleted in this organ. It remains intact in all other cells of the organism.

Tissue-Specific Glucocorticoid Receptor Gene Inactivation

Liver-Specific Glucocorticoid Receptor Inactivation Results in Body-Growth Deficiency The GR gene was inactivated in hepatocytes, by expressing the Cre recombinase under the control of transcriptional regulatory elements from both albumin and α-fetoprotein genes, leading to early and robust recombination (AlfpCre transgene). These animals were crossed with mice carrying the GR^{loxP} allele. The resulting mutant mice ($GR^{loxP/loxP}$; Tg:AlfpCre) are referred to as $GR^{AlfpCre}$ mice. Surprisingly, mice lacking GR in their hepatocytes are much smaller than control mice. This difference is first observed at 3–4 weeks of age and is more pronounced in males, suggesting a dysfunction in growth hormone (GH)-dependent postnatal body growth. The defect is not systemic. GC and GH levels are normal, but the GH signaling pathway is not functional in hepatocytes. The binding of GH to its receptor activates the phosphorylation of signal transducer and activator of transcription 5 (Stat5), which in turn stimulates the transcription of GH-regulated genes. Some of these genes encode secreted factors mediating peripheral body growth. In the absence of GR, the expression of GH-regulated target genes controlled by Stat5, such as insulin-like growth factor (IGF-)I, Spi2.1, acid labile subunit (ALS), and major urinary protein (MUP), is strongly reduced. This may be accounted for by physical interaction between GR and Stat5, as shown by coimmunoprecipitation and chromatin immunoprecipitation (ChIP) experiments and by GR acting as a coactivator for Stat5-dependent transcription on GH stimulation. This hypothesis is supported by the similar growth phenotype observed in animals lacking Stat5 throughout the body ($Stat5^{-/-}$ animals) and by analyses of gene expression at the genomic scale, which have identified a subset of coregulated genes, including all known GH-regulated genes in the liver. Significantly, in addition to the role for hepatic GR in the control of body growth, this result demonstrates the essential role of the liver for body growth.

GCs were named based on the function of these molecules in the hormonal control of glycemia. They globally promote glycemia by acting on the fat tissue, muscles, pancreas, and liver, where they stimulate glucose synthesis. Glucose homeostasis was studied in $GR^{AlfpCre}$ animals to isolate the effects of GCs on hepatocytes from those on other cell types. Basal glycemia was normal in $GR^{AlfpCre}$ mice. However, in challenging situations, such as prolonged fasting, the induction of gluconeogenesis is impaired due to deficiencies in the induction of enzymes participating in this pathway, such as phosphoenol pyruvate carboxykinase (PEPCK), TAT, and glucose-6-phosphate (G6P). This leads to hypoglycemia in mutant animals, whereas control littermates maintain normal glucose levels. $GR^{AlfpCre}$ mice have also been studied in pathological situations. The contribution of hepatic GR to the hyperglycemia observed in diabetes was assessed by inducing type I diabetes mellitus, by streptozotocin injection, in $GR^{AlfpCre}$ and control animals. Hyperglycemia was less severe in the absence of hepatocytic GR, probably due to the observed defective induction of PEPCK, reducing gluconeogenesis.

$GR^{AlfpCre}$ mice were used by U. Schibler and colleagues to confirm *in vivo* an unexpected role for GCs – their contribution to resetting the circadian clocks in peripheral tissues. In mammals, the circadian system consists of a master pacemaker in the suprachiasmatic nucleus of the hypothalamus and slave clocks in most peripheral cell types. The mechanisms underlying the resetting of these peripheral clocks remain unclear, but GCs seem to play a role. The injection of dexamethasone, a synthetic GC, induces the expression of circadian genes and shifts the circadian phase of peripheral organs. This effect involves GR in peripheral cells, as shown in $GR^{AlfpCre}$ animals, in which a shift is observed after dexamethasone injection in all organs except the liver.

GR gene inactivation in the liver has also been reported in animals carrying a GR allele in which exon 1c and exon 2 are flanked by *loxP* sites and a neomycin resistance selection cassette. On recombination, this allele generates the GR^{ko} allele. Liver-specific mutants were obtained using a different Cre-expressing transgenic mouse line (AlbCre). Defective cell proliferation was observed after partial hepatectomy, but the body growth rate remained normal. This difference may be due to the use of the AlbCre transgene, which gives later recombination that AlfpCre for other *loxP* targets. It may also be due to differences in the GR mutation because removal of exons 1c and 2 is still potentially compatible with the formation of GR proteins with a DBD, as for the GR^{hypo} allele (as already discussed).

The Glucocorticoid Receptor Gene and Pancreas Programming There is considerable evidence to suggest that elevated maternal GC levels may influence embryonic development, with long-term consequences for the metabolism or behavior of the child into adulthood. Maternal food restriction results in a low birth weight and impaired glucose homeostasis in adulthood. This phenomenon may be related to the association between low birth weight and the appearance of cardiovascular diseases, obesity, insulin resistance, and diabetes at adulthood in humans. It has been suggested that maternal GCs may affect embryonic pancreas development because the consequences of maternal food restriction, including a reduction of the β-cell mass in the pancreas, can be blocked by adrenalectomy. In addition, the absence of GR in developing pancreatic cells leads to an increase in β-cell mass that persists into adulthood. This model was developed using a recombinase transgene expressed under the control of the pdx promoter (GR^{PdxCre} animals). Further studies on these animals should make it possible to analyze the role of pancreatic GR in adult animal metabolism.

The Glucocorticoid Receptor Gene and Mammary Glands GCs are known to influence mammary gland function *in vivo* and to stimulate milk-protein gene expression in cell culture. Mice deprived of GR in their mammary epithelial cells were obtained using a Cre recombinase transgene expressed under the control of the whey acidic protein (WAP) gene promoter ($GR^{WAPiCre}$). They produce and secrete milk and nurse their litters until weaning, suggesting that GCs do not act on the mammary gland via GR or that they act on other cells than those secreting WAP. The absence of GR reduces cell proliferation, retarding lobulo-alveolar development.

The Glucocorticoid Receptor Gene and T Cells GCs act as potent anti-inflammatory and immunosuppressive therapeutic agents. The endogenous production of these hormones is involved in the optimization of the immune repertoire during thymocyte maturation and in downregulating the immune response in mature T cells. The role of GR in T cells from animals carrying the GR^{ko} allele was studied by grafting hematopoietic stem cells from fetal $GR^{ko/ko}$ mouse liver into irradiated animals and using the lckCre transgenic line to invalidate the $GR^{loxPneo}$ allele in thymocytes (TGRKO). Analyses of these animal models demonstrated that GR is not required for T-cell development.

In vivo, $GR^{ko/ko}$ thymocytes are resistant to apoptosis induced by stimulation of the T-cell receptor (TCR). This is not a cell-autonomous property of $GR^{ko/ko}$ thymocytes because these cells display normal sensitivity *in vitro*, demonstrating that the evoked GC release on TCR stimulation is involved in this response. TCR stimulation in TGRKO animals is associated with a high mortality rate, probably due to the uncontrolled induction of cyclooxygenase-2 (COX-2) because the selective inhibition of this enzyme prevents the death of mutant mice.

Inactivation of the Glucocorticoid Receptor Gene in the Brain GCs affect many aspects of brain physiology, in addition to repressing the HPA axis by controlling the CRH and vasopressin expression in the neurons of the hypothalamic paraventricular nuclei. In response to stress, these hormones modulate the activity of several neurotransmitter systems and affect behavior. In healthy animals, this response helps the organism to adapt to its environment, but dysfunctions in this mechanism may be associated with the development of behavioral disorders.

GCs can affect neuronal activity and neurotransmitter release, modify cellular shape by remodeling dendritic formations, compromise neuronal survival, and reduce the rate of renewal of granule cells in the dentate gyrus by downregulating neurogenesis.

The GR gene was inactivated in the brain by crossing mice carrying the GR^{loxP} allele with transgenic animals expressing Cre recombinase in neuronal precursor cells under the control of the rat nestin promoter and a neuron-specific enhancer (the NesCre transgenic line). GR^{NesCre} mice, which have no GR in their neurons and glial cells, survive to adulthood. Because the GR-mediated negative feedback on the HPA axis is disrupted at the hypothalamic level in mutant mice, GC levels are 15 times higher than in control animals. The negative feedback loop continues to function in the pituitary gland (in which the GR gene is not inactivated), but this is clearly not sufficient to control hormone levels. The level of CRH production is very high in the hypothalamus of mutant animals, whereas vasopressin levels are unaffected. The increase in CRH levels induces ACTH production in the pituitary gland, and both mRNA and intracellular protein levels are high. Surprisingly, circulating ACTH levels are significantly reduced. This demonstrates that high GC levels are not sufficient to repress ACTH expression completely but are sufficient to repress ACTH secretion. The mechanisms responsible for higher levels of GC secretion in the presence of lower circulating ACTH circulating levels remain to be elucidated. A similar divergence between ACTH and GC levels is observed in other animal models and in some pathological situations, such as major depression. The high GC levels in GR^{NesCre} mice may have an effect on peripheral organs expressing GR, leading to symptoms reminiscent to those observed in patients with Cushing's syndrome (due to high GC levels), such as a reduced size, low bone density, and changes in fat distribution. GR^{NesCre} animals present a decreased food intake and a reduced metabolic efficiency. In GR^{NesCre} animals, GC levels cycle with a circadian rhythm and are further increased in response to stress.

In the brain of mutant mice, stress-released GCs are not perceived by GR that is absent. We therefore studied behaviors influenced by stress responses in GR^{NesCre} mice to distinguish between those involving GR activation in the brain and those involving other mechanisms. Mutant mice display lower levels of anxiety in the elevated zero maze and the dark-light box, two tasks based on a behavioral conflict between exploring and avoiding an aversive compartment. Despair or depression-like behavior, measured in the forced swim test, was also reduced in the absence of GR. CRH is often considered to be the anxiogenic mediator of the HPA axis. Interestingly, the fact that CRH expression is strongly induced in the hypothalamus of mutant animals, but unaffected in the amygdala, suggests that changes in CRH are not responsible for changes in the level of anxiety of GR^{NesCre} mice. This indicates that central GR may be directly involved in anxiety modulation. A more restricted deletion of the $GR^{loxPneo}$ allele, using a recombinase expressed in most forebrain neurons (FBGRKO mice), also affects emotional behavior. Despair behavior is more marked, but anxiety levels are reduced, in these mutants in the dark/light box and elevated plus-maze behavioral tasks. This difference between GR^{NesCre} and FBGRKO mice may reflect the restriction of the GR mutation to a neuronal subpopulation in FBGRKO mice. This mutation leads to an increase in GC levels that, in turn, may act on GR-positive neurons. More work is required to define the nature of the neuronal cells in which GR activation modulates particular types of behavior.

The absence of brain GR in GR^{NesCre} mice also has a weak effect on learning and memory retention in a water-maze task designed to test spatial memory. Learning is similar between mutant and control littermates, but retention is slightly affected in mutant mice. Further training sessions, however, overcame this memory impairment, indicating that GR is not essential for the formation of explicit memory.

Addiction is favored by stress responses. Physical and psychological stressors facilitate drug addiction in rodents. The acquisition of drug self-administration, its intensity, and the reinstatement of drug taking even after prolonged periods of withdrawal are facilitated or increased by stress. Even in the absence of stress, GR gene inactivation in GR^{NesCre} mice profoundly reduces the motivation for cocaine-induced self-administration, a test considered to be the best experimental model of drug abuse. In addition, cocaine-induced behavioral sensitization, a process implicated in the development of addiction and defining the increase in the behavioral effects of cocaine observed over repeated drug injections, is abolished in these mice. The molecular mechanisms underlying these effects are unknown, but the absence of GR leads to strong downregulation of the mitogen-activated protein kinase (MAPK) pathway responsible for impaired expression of the immediate early gene *Zif268* (also named *Egr-1*, *NGFI-A*, or *Krox24*). This is particularly evident in hippocampus GR^{NesCre} animals. The MAPK pathway and *Zif268* expression in the hippocampus of control animals are induced by immobilization – an acute stress for mice – but this induction is defective in GR^{NesCre} animals.

Tissue-Specific Mineralocorticoid Receptor Gene Inactivation

In the brain, MR is abundantly expressed in the hippocampus, where it serves as a high-affinity GR. Conditional MR gene inactivation was recently achieved by flanking the third exon with two *loxP* sites (MR^{flox} allele) and using a transgenic line expressing Cre recombinase throughout the forebrain, under the control of the CamKIIα gene on a bacterial artificial chromosome. The absence of MR does not affect the circadian rhythm or stress response of the HPA axis. $MR^{CamKCre}$ mice have a learning deficit in spatial navigation, as shown in a water-maze task, but display normal retention once the task is learned. $MR^{CamKCre}$ mice also display working memory impairment, as assessed in a radial maze. In contrast to what has been observed in GR mutant animals, anxiety is not affected by the mutation. Significantly, studies on $MR^{CamKCre}$ mice recently demonstrated that MR is responsible for certain rapid effects of GCs on hippocampal signaling that do not involve gene expression.

Function-Selective Glucocorticoid Receptor Mutation

GR acts via different molecular mechanisms involving specific protein–protein interactions, with itself or with other factors, to control gene expression (**Figure 1**). If these different interactions engage different protein interfaces, it should be possible to define mutations that selectively abolish a given mechanism without affecting the others. This is the case for a mutation in the D-loop region of the DBD that results in the replacement of alanine 458 by a threonine residue (GR^{dim}). This mutation affects the cooperative binding of GR homodimers to glucocorticoid-response elements (GREs), resulting in reduced occupancy of these binding sites. Interactions with other known proteins are not affected. Following its introduction into the mouse genome by homologous recombination in embryonic stem cells, this mutation was indeed shown to reduce the expression of genes known to be controlled via binding to GREs, such as the TAT gene in the liver. In contrast, the GR^{dim} protein is still able to repress the activating enhancer binding protein (AP-)1-dependent expression of the collagenase-3 (MMP-13) and stromelysin-1 (MMP-3) genes and pro-inflammatory NFκB activity and to activate the expression of Stat5-dependent genes in the liver. Surprisingly, all homozygous mutant mice survived to adulthood. The fact that $GR^{null/null}$ mice die shortly after birth, whereas $GR^{dim/dim}$ mice do not, indicates that the interaction of GR with other proteins is more important for survival than its ability to bind DNA cooperatively on GRE target sites. In adult mice, various phenotypes have implicated defects in GR binding to GREs. CRH synthesis and ACTH release are not impaired in these mice. In contrast, transcription of the *POMC* gene (encoding ACTH) is upregulated in corticotropic cells and therefore requires the binding of GR dimers to DNA. In the hippocampus, dimerization and cooperative DNA binding seem to be involved in neuronal activity. GR activation in $GR^{dim/dim}$ mice does not lead to increases in calcium currents or in the response to serotonin as in wild-type mice, indicating that dimerization is required for these responses.

Modifying Glucocorticoid Receptor and Mineralocorticoid Receptor Gene Dosage in an Organism or Cell Type

We have so far discussed studies aiming to define the function so the GR and MR genes by means of gene mutation abolishing expression or generating modified protein. The function of corticosteroid receptors has also been studied using approaches that increase or decrease the levels of the corresponding gene products. GR gene dosage has been increased by introducing two additional copies of the receptor gene into the mouse genome using yeast artificial chromosomes. As the entire GR gene, including all the regulatory elements responsible for gene transcription, is present in the 290-kb yeast artificial chromosomes (YAC) used, the expression of the GR transgene should mimic the endogenous expression profile. These animals have a downregulated HPA axis under basal conditions and after acute stress, and they display increased resistance to lipopolysaccharide-induced endotoxic shock. A behavioral analysis of this animal model showed lower levels of despair behavior, with a decrease in GR dosage ($GR^{null/wt}$ animals) giving the opposite response.

Mice over- or underexpressing GR in a given tissue have also been established by additional transgenesis. The first mice with impaired GR function were generated by overexpressing an antisense RNA directed against the 3′ prime untranslated region of the GR mRNA. This mouse model has been of great value for studying GR function, but it is problematic for several reasons. The main problem is that it is difficult to determine the actual levels of GR protein in a given cell because transgene expression varies as a function of cell type. In addition, the antisense RNA is expressed ectopically in organs outside the nervous system, probably due to positional effects relating to the use of the human neurofilament promoter. On average, GR levels were 50% lower than normal in the brain, resulting in changes to HPA axis regulation and stress-related behavior and in changes in energy balance and lipid metabolism. GR has been overexpressed in various tissues, including the pancreas, brain, and T cells, using tissue-specific promoters or the tetracycline inducible system.

MR function has also been investigated by means of conditional downregulation and overexpression strategies based on the tetracycline system. This approach revealed unexpected roles for MR in cardiac tissue. The heart-specific expression of an antisense mRNA directed against MR causes severe heart failure and cardiac fibrosis in the absence of hypertension or hyperaldosteronism, leading to massive water retention. In adult mice, this phenotype was fully reversed within a few days following the abolition of mRNA expression. Mice with conditional heart-specific MR overexpression in the heart also present a cardiac phenotype with marked arrhythmia and high early mortality rates, as observed in arrhythmia-related sudden death in humans.

The different animal models presented here are invaluable tools for the study of corticosteroid receptor gene function. They allowed us to define more precisely the known or expected corticosteroid receptor function, such as, the GR's roles in the HPA axis negative feedback loop and in glucose homeostasis and its functions in immunosuppression and anti-inflammation and the MR's role in the control of the body salt balance. These animal models also clarified the role of GR in the modulation of stress-related behaviors and revealed unexpected roles such as the requirement of GR for GH signaling in hepatocytes. The results are still fragmented, but further analysis of the existing models and of new models targeting other tissues should allow a more integrated understanding of corticosteroid receptor gene functions at the level of the organism. They should also allow us to distinguish in these functions the ones relevant for hormonal control and stress response from the ones that are not associated with the binding of corticosteroids. It is indeed now clear that, in some situations, steroid receptors may be activated by other means than ligand binding, such as phosphorylation. The generation of precisely modified animal models is fastidious and will undoubtedly benefit from complementary approaches, such the use of short interfering RNA (siRNA) or small molecules that will facilitate combinatorial studies targeting several genes simultaneously.

Acknowledgments

I thank Monique Lazar and Christoph Kellendonk for their critical reading of this review and all the members of the Molecular Genetics, Neurophysiology and Behavior laboratory for our stimulating discussions. I also thank Günther Schütz for his support and for having introduced me to this research field. The work in the CNRS UMR7148 unit is supported by the CNRS, the NRJ foundation, the MILDT, the FRM, the French Ministry of Research (ACI and ANR programs), and the European Union (EARNEST consortium).

See Also the Following Articles

Corticosteroid Receptors; Corticosteroids and Stress.

Further Reading

Balsalobre, A., Brown, S. A., Marcacci, L., et al. (2000). Resetting of circadian time in peripheral tissues by glucocorticoid signaling. *Science* **289**, 2344–2347.

Bauer, A., Tronche, F., Wessely, O., et al. (1999). The glucocorticoid receptor is required for stress erythropoiesis. *Genes & Development* **13**, 2996–3002.

Beggah, A. T., Escoubet, B., Puttini, S., et al. (2002). Reversible cardiac fibrosis and heart failure induced by conditional expression of an antisense mRNA of the mineralocorticoid receptor in cardiomyocytes. *Proceedings of the National Academy of Sciences USA* **99**, 7160–7165.

Berger, S., Bleich, M., Schmid, W., et al. (1998). Mineralocorticoid receptor knockout mice: pathophysiology of Na^{+} metabolism. *Proceedings of the National Academy of Sciences USA* **95**, 9424–9429.

Berger, S., Wolfer, D. P., Selbach, O., et al. (2006). Loss of the limbic mineralocorticoid receptor impairs behavioral plasticity. *Proceedings of the National Academy of Sciences USA* **103**, 195–200.

Boyle, M. P., Brewer, J. A., Funatsu, M., et al. (2005). Acquired deficit of forebrain glucocorticoid receptor produces depression-like changes in adrenal axis regulation and behavior. *Proceedings of the National Academy of Sciences USA* **102**, 473–478.

Boyle, M. P., Kolber, B. J., Vogt, S. K., et al. (2006). Forebrain glucocorticoid receptors modulate anxiety-associated locomotor activation and adrenal responsiveness. *Journal of Neuroscience* **26**, 1971–1978.

Brewer, J. A., Kanagawa, O., Sleckman, B. P., et al. (2002). Thymocyte apoptosis induced by T cell activation is mediated by glucocorticoids in vivo. *Journal of Immunology* **169**, 1837–1843.

Brewer, J. A., Khor, B., Vogt, S. K., et al. (2003). T-cell glucocorticoid receptor is required to suppress COX-2-mediated lethal immune activation. *Nature Medicine* **9**, 1318–1322.

Cole, T. J., Blendy, J. A., Monaghan, A. P., et al. (1995). Targeted disruption of the glucocorticoid receptor gene blocks adrenergic chromaffin cell development and severely retards lung maturation. *Genes & Development* **9**, 1608–1621.

Cole, T. J., Myles, K., Purton, J. F., et al. (2001). GRKO mice express an aberrant dexamethasone-binding glucocorticoid receptor, but are profoundly glucocorticoid resistant. *Molecular and Cellular Endocrinology* **173**, 193–202.

Delaunay, F., Khan, A., Cintra, A., et al. (1997). Pancreatic beta cells are important targets for the diabetogenic effects of glucocorticoids. *Journal of Clinical Investigations* **100**, 2094–2098.

Deroche-Gamonet, V., Sillaber, I., Aouizerate, B., et al. (2003). The glucocorticoid receptor as a potential target to reduce cocaine abuse. *Journal of Neuroscience* **23**, 4785–4790.

Finotto, S., Krieglstein, K., Schober, A., et al. (1999). Analysis of mice carrying targeted mutations of the glucocorticoid receptor gene argues against an essential role of glucocorticoid signalling for generating adrenal chromaffin cells. *Development* **126**(13), 2935–2944.

Froger, N., Palazzo, E., Boni, C., et al. (2004). Neurochemical and behavioral alterations in glucocorticoid receptor-impaired transgenic mice after chronic mild stress. *Journal of Neuroscience* **24**, 2787–2796.

Gass, P., Kretz, O., Wolfer, D. P., et al. (2000). Genetic disruption of mineralocorticoid receptor leads to impaired neurogenesis and granule cell degeneration in the hippocampus of adult mice. *EMBO Report* **1**, 447–451.

Gesina, E., Tronche, F., Herrera, P., et al. (2004). Dissecting the role of glucocorticoids on pancreas development. *Diabetes* **53**, 2322–2329.

Gold, P. W., Loriaux, D. L., Roy, A., et al. (1986). Responses to corticotropin-releasing hormone in the hypercortisolism of depression and Cushing's disease: pathophysiologic and diagnostic implications. *New England Journal of Medicine* **314**, 1329–1335.

Hubert, C., Gasc, J. M., Berger, S., et al. (1999). Effects of mineralocorticoid receptor gene disruption on the components of the renin-angiotensin system in 8-day-old mice. *Molecular Endocrinology* **13**, 297–306.

Karst, H., Berger, S., Turiault, M., et al. (2005). Mineralocorticoid receptors are indispensable for nongenomic modulation of hippocampal glutamate transmission by corticosterone. *Proceedings of the National Academy of Sciences USA* **102**, 19204–19207.

Karst, H., Karten, Y. J., Reichardt, H. M., et al. (2000). Corticosteroid actions in hippocampus require DNA binding of glucocorticoid receptor homodimers. *Nature Neuroscience* **3**, 977–978.

Kellendonk, C., Eiden, S., Kretz, O., et al. (2002). Inactivation of the GR in the nervous system affects energy accumulation. *Endocrinology* **143**, 2333–2340.

Kellendonk, C., Opherk, C., Anlag, K., et al. (2000). Hepatocyte-specific expression of Cre recombinase. *Genesis* **26**, 151–153.
Mittelstadt, P. R. and Ashwell, J. D. (2003). Disruption of glucocorticoid receptor exon 2 yields a ligand-responsive C-terminal fragment that regulates gene expression. *Molecular Endocrinology* **17**, 1534–1542.
Opherk, C., Tronche, F., Kellendonk, C., et al. (2004). Inactivation of the glucocorticoid receptor in hepatocytes leads to fasting hypoglycemia and ameliorates hyperglycemia in streptozotocin-induced diabetes mellitus. *Molecular Endocrinology* **18**, 1346–1353.
Ouvrard-Pascaud, A., Sainte-Marie, Y., Benitah, J. P., et al. (2005). Conditional mineralocorticoid receptor expression in the heart leads to life-threatening arrhythmias. *Circulation* **111**, 3025–3033.
Pazirandeh, A., Jondal, M. and Okret, S. (2005). Conditional expression of a glucocorticoid receptor transgene in thymocytes reveals a role for thymic-derived glucocorticoids in thymopoiesis in vivo. *Endocrinology* **146**, 2501–2507.
Pepin, M., Pothier, F. and Barden, N. (1992). Impaired type II glucocorticoid-receptor function in mice bearing antisense RNA transgene. *Nature* **355**, 725–728.
Reichardt, H. M., Kaestner, K. H., Tuckermann, J., et al. (1998). DNA binding of the glucocorticoid receptor is not essential for survival. *Cell* **93**, 531–541.
Reichardt, H. M., Tuckermann, J. P., Gottlicher, M., et al. (2001). Repression of inflammatory responses in the absence of DNA binding by the glucocorticoid receptor. *EMBO Journal* **20**, 7168–7173.
Reichardt, H. M., Umland, T., Bauer, A., et al. (2000). Mice with an increased glucocorticoid receptor gene dosage show enhanced resistance to stress and endotoxic shock. *Molecular and Cellular Biology* **20**, 9009–9017.
Revest, J. M., DiBlasi, F., Kitchener, P., et al. (2005). The MAPK pathway and Egr-1 mediate stress-related behavioral effects of glucocorticoids. *Nature Neuroscience* **8**, 664–672.
Ridder, S., Chourbaji, S., Hellweg, R., et al. (2005). Mice with genetically altered glucocorticoid receptor expression show altered sensitivity for stress-induced depressive reactions. *Journal of Neuroscience* **25**, 6243–6250.
Shteyer, E., Liao, Y., Muglia, L. J., et al. (2004). Disruption of hepatic adipogenesis is associated with impaired liver regeneration in mice. *Hepatology* **40**, 1322–1332.
Tronche, F., Casanova, E., Turiault, M., et al. (2002). When reverse genetics meets physiology: the use of site-specific recombinases in mice. *FEBS Letters* **529**, 116–121.
Tronche, F., Kellendonk, C., Kretz, O., et al. (1999). Disruption of the glucocorticoid receptor gene in the nervous system results in reduced anxiety. *Nature Genetics* **23**, 99–103.
Tronche, F., Kellendonk, C., Reichardt, H. M., et al. (1998). Genetic dissection of glucocorticoid receptor function in mice. *Current Opinion in Genetics and Development* **8**, 532–538.
Tronche, F., Opherk, C., Moriggl, R., et al. (2004). Glucocorticoid receptor function in hepatocytes is essential to promote postnatal body growth. *Genes & Development* **18**, 492–497.
Tuckermann, J. P., Reichardt, H. M., Arribas, R., et al. (1999). The DNA binding-independent function of the glucocorticoid receptor mediates repression of AP-1-dependent genes in skin. *Journal of Cell Biology* **147**, 1365–1370.
Wei, Q., Lu, X. Y., Liu, L., et al. (2004). Glucocorticoid receptor overexpression in forebrain: a mouse model of increased emotional lability. *Proceedings of the National Academy of Sciences USA* **101**, 11851–11856.
Wintermantel, T. M., Bock, D., Fleig, V., et al. (2005). The epithelial glucocorticoid receptor is required for the normal timing of cell proliferation during mammary lobuloalveolar development but is dispensable for milk production. *Molecular Endocrinology* **19**, 340–349.

Corticosteroid Receptors

O C Meijer and E R de Kloet
Leiden University, Leiden, Netherlands
B S McEwen
Rockefeller University, New York, USA

This is a revised version of the article by O C Meijer, E R de Kloet, and B S McEwen, Encyclopedia of Stress, First edition, volume 1, pp 557–569, © 2000, Elsevier Inc.

Glossary

Adrenalectomy — The surgical removal of the adrenal glands from the body.

Corticosteroid hormones — Hormones synthesized and secreted from the adrenal gland in response to stress and also during the diurnal rhythm. The main endogenous glucocorticoids are corticosterone (in rodents) and cortisol (in humans).

Corticosteroid receptors — Intracellular receptor molecules for corticosteroid hormones. On hormone binding, they function as transcription factors in the nucleus of the cell to change mRNA and protein synthesis of target genes. There are two types: mineralocorticoid receptors and glucocorticoid receptors.

Hypothalamic-pituitary-adrenal (HPA) axis	The brain-controlled activation pathway for the secretion of corticosteroid hormones after stress through a hormonal cascade, involving the release of corticotropin releasing hormone from the paraventricular nucleus of the hypothalamus in the brain and adrenocorticotropic hormone from the pituitary gland.
Hippocampus	A cortical brain structure involved in declarative and spatial memory and the cognitive aspects of emotions, with high expression of both types of corticosteroid receptors.
Stress	A state caused by a real or perceived challenge to homeostasis, which is accompanied by a hormonal stress response.

The effects of cortisol and corticosterone (CORT), the main glucocorticoid hormones in primates and rodents, respectively, are mediated by two types of intracellular receptor molecules: glucocorticoid receptors (GRs, or type II receptors) and mineralocorticoid receptors (MRs, or type I receptors). In peripheral tissues, CORT acts almost exclusively via GRs to affect energy stores, bone metabolism, and inflammatory and immune responses. MRs in epithelial cell types, as present in kidney and colon, are protected from endogenous CORT by the enzyme 11β-OH-steroid dehydrogenase (11β-HSD) so that aldosterone may bind to regulate the sodium balance in the body. In nonepithelial targets, such as the brain, both MRs and GRs function as receptors for CORT to act in either synergy or antagonism. GRs and MRs are members of the steroid hormone receptor superfamily and, accordingly, act as transcription factors to change the expression levels of target genes. These genomic effects have a relatively slow onset and long duration. However, CORT may also acutely affect the activity of neuronal cells via non-genomic mechanisms involving MR and possibly GR. However, no such receptors have been identified in mammals to date. MRs and GRs have different pharmacological properties and distributions in the brain. Corticosteroid receptors in the brain and pituitary play a crucial role in the regulation of the stress response and in mediating the effects of CORT on mood and cognition.

Corticosteroid Receptor Properties

Activation of Corticosteroid Receptors

The lipophilic CORT diffuses readily through the plasma membrane of cells to bind to its receptors. Corticosteroid receptors are part of a cytoplasmic multiprotein complex that consists of one receptor molecule and several heat shock proteins (HSPs). The binding of CORT leads to a rapid chain of events that consists of the dissociation of the HSP, multiple phosphorylation steps, and increased affinity of the ligand-activated receptor for nuclear domains: the Ligand–receptor complex translocates to the cell nucleus to exert its action on gene expression and protein synthesis (**Tables 1** and **2**).

An important determinant of corticosteroid receptor activation is access of the ligand to the receptor, which depends on several factors in addition to the total plasma concentration of CORT. First, the circulating hormone is bound to corticosteroid-binding protein (CBG)/transcortin and with a much lower affinity to serum albumin. Of the average CORT concentration circulating during a 24-h period in the rat, less than 5% is not bound to CBG, (i.e., is free and biologically available).

Second, the enzyme 11β–HSD type 2 converts cortisol and CORT to their inactive 11-dehydro metabolites in mineralocorticoid target tissues. Conversely, the 11β-HSD type 1 isoform, which is often colocalized with GRs, can catalyze the reverse reaction and generate cortisol from cortisone within a target cell. This reaction takes place in the liver and fat cells, and it may also be relevant for certain areas in the brain.

A third determinant of access, which particularly pertains to synthetic glucocorticoids, is the mdr1a P-glycoprotein. This protein is expressed in the apical membranes of endothelial cells of the blood–brain barrier. mdr1a P-glycoprotein functions as an energy-dependent pump that limits access to the brain

Table 1 Characteristics of the two corticosteroid receptor types

	Affinity	*Agonists*	*Antagonists*	*Distribution*
Mineralocorticoid receptor (type 1)	High affinity for cortisol and corticosterone ($K_d \approx 0.5$ nM)	Aldosterone (epithelial cell types as in kidney), cortisol (brain)	Spironolactone, RU 28328	Limited distribution in periphery (kidney, colon, lymphocytes) and brain (limbic brain)
Glucocorticoid receptor (type 2)	Lower affinity for cortisol and corticosterone ($K_d \approx 5.0$ nM)	Cortisol, dexamethasone, RU 28362	RU 38486	Ubiquitous expression in periphery and brain

Table 2 Milestones in brain corticosteroid receptor research

Year	*Milestone*
1968	First report on selective retention of [^{3}H]corticosterone in hippocampus
1975	Low retention of [^{3}H]dexamethasone in hippocampus; high in pituitary
1980	Selective MR agonists discriminate between MRs and GRs
1982	*In vitro* hippocampus and kidney cytosol contain MRs and GRs
1983	GR acts as transcription factor through DNA binding
1985	MR and not GR retains [^{3}H]corticosterone in hippocampus
1985	Cloning of GR
1985	First brain map of immunoreactive GR neurons
1987	Cloning of MR
1988	11β-HSD confers aldosteron specificity to MR
1990	Transrepression of AP-1-induced transcription via GR
1991	First brain map of immunoreactive MR neurons
1993	Differential effects of MR and GR on transrepression
1994	*In vitro* demonstration of MR/GR heterodimers
1994	Mechanistic differentiation between transactivation and transrepression GR
1995	mdr1a Pgp in blood–brain barrier hampers brain entry of dexamethasone
1995	GR knockout mice
1996	Colocalized immunoreactive MR/GR clusters in hippocampal neuronal nuclei
1998	Knock-in mice that express a dimerization-impaired mutant of GR
2005	Non-genomic effects in hippocampus via MR

of xenobiotic agents, including synthetic steroids. Accordingly, the brain (but not the pituitary) is resistant to the penetration of moderate amounts of dexamethasone.

Corticosteroid Receptor Diversity in Pituitary and Brain

Although the GRs and MRs act as high-affinity receptors for CORT in the brain, these receptor types differ significantly with respect to their pharmacology, distribution, and physiological effects.

Structure The human GR gene is localized on chromosome 5, whereas the MR gene is localized on chromosome 4, indicating an early duplication of their common ancestor during evolution. Despite this early divergence, their genomic organization is very similar, notwithstanding differences at the 5′ and 3′ ends. The overall structure of GR and MR proteins follows that of the other members of the steroid hormone receptor family. The molecules are generally viewed as consisting of three domains: a highly conserved DNA-binding domain (95% homology between the MR and the GR), flanked by the C-terminal ligand-binding domain (60%), and a large N-terminal domain that contains a transactivation function and is highly variable between the MR and the GR (15%) and among species.

Pharmacology Although GRs and MRs are high-affinity receptors for CORT, they differ in their affinities for several ligands. In the case of cortisol and CORT, an MR has an approximately 10-fold higher affinity than a GR. The important consequence of this is that GRs and MRs are occupied differentially during the day and during stress responses. MRs are already occupied extensively under basal trough conditions, whereas the saturation of GRs requires hormone levels that occur after stress or after the circadian peak. Because of the high, almost tonic, occupation of MRs, it has been hypothesized that the amount of bioactive receptor protein is an important level of regulation for MRs, whereas the GR signal depends primarily on ligand concentration. Synthetic glucocorticoids have higher affinity for GRs than for MRs, but their access to the brain GRs is hampered by the mdr1a gene-encoded P-glycoprotein.

Distribution GRs are expressed ubiquitously in many different tissues and cell types. In tissues such as the liver, lung, and adrenal medulla, GRs are crucial for appropriate development. MRs have a much more limited distribution, and as receptors for CORT (as opposed to mineralocorticoids), they have been characterized in the brain and some lymphoid tissues. The pituitary, outside the blood–brain barrier, contains GRs as well as MRs, although no specific function for MRs has been described for any of its cell types.

Throughout the brain, immunocytochemical and *in situ* hybridization procedures have shown a widespread distribution of GRs in neurons and glial cells. Particularly high GR concentrations are found in the limbic system (hippocampus, with relatively low concentrations in the CA3 region; septum; and amygdala), in the parvocellular neurons of the paraventricular nucleus (PVN) of the hypothalamus, and in the supraoptic nucleus. In the PVN, the biosynthesis and release of parvocellular vasopressine, corticotropin releasing hormone (CRH), and other neuropeptides are under glucocorticoid control. GRs are also present in relatively high concentrations in the ascending monoaminergic neurons of the brain stem. Moderate GR levels are also found in many thalamic nuclei and in patchlike distribution in the striatal areas, as well as throughout the cortical hemispheres (see **Figure 1**).

In the brain, MRs have a more restricted topography than GRs. High MR densities have been found in the neurons of the hippocampal formation, lateral

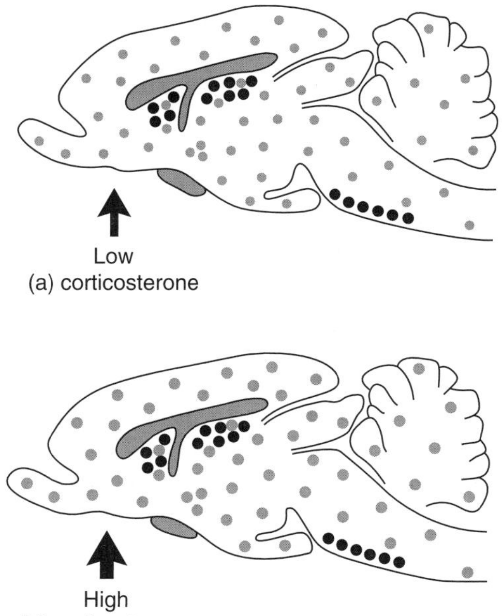

Figure 1 Distribution of MRs (black circles) and GRs (grey circles) in the rat brain. a, Basal corticosterone secretion; b, Peak corticosterone secretion. MR expression is more restricted and especially high in the hippocampus; the MRs are substantially occupied by corticosterone under basal conditions (i.e., at the circadian trough under nonstressed conditions). The GRs show a widespread distribution and are only partially occupied under basal conditions; they become more fully activated at the circadian peak of corticosterone secretion or after stress. Reprinted from M. Joëls and E. R. De Kloet (1992), Control of neuronal excitability by corticosteroid hormones. *Trends in Neuroscience* **15**, 25–30. Used with permission.

septum, medial and central amygdala, olfactory nucleus, layer II of the cortex, and in brain-stem sensory and motor neurons. This distribution of MRs is essentially the same as that discovered in 1968 by McEwen with the cell-nuclear retention of radioligand after the administration of tracer doses of [^{3}H]-corticosterone to adrenalectomized rats. Aldosterone-preferring MRs involved in salt homeostasis are localized in the anterior hypothalamus and circumventricular organs, such as the chorioid plexus.

The subcellular localization of MRs and GRs was studied in hippocampal neurons by dual labeling immunocytochemistry and confocal microscopy. It was observed that MRs and GRs are distributed nonhomogeneously over the nucleus. Both receptors are concentrated in approximately 1000 clusters scattered throughout the nucleoplasm. Many clusters contain exclusively either MRs or GRs, although a significant number of domains were found to contain both receptor types. The latter clusters are candidate sites where the two receptors could interact to establish a coordinated regulation of gene expression. This implies that GR and MR homodimers, as well as the possible MR–GR heterodimers, are associated with distinct nuclear domains.

Corticosteroid Receptor Variants Alternative splicing of the 3′ end of the human GR pre-mRNA creates an hGRβ variant in addition to the common hGRα variant. However, it should be noted that rodent GR pre-mRNA lacks this splice site and GRβ cannot be detected in rodent tissue. The translation of GRα and GRβ mRNA produces two proteins that are almost identical but that differ in their C-terminals, which implies that GRα binds cortisol, whereas GRβ does not. However, *in vitro* experiments suggest that GRβ is capable of binding to glucocorticoid-responsive elements (GREs) and can form homodimers as well as heterodimers with GRα. Accordingly, GRβ has been shown to block GR-mediated transactivation *in vitro*, whereas it does not seem to interfere with transrepression. In the human brain, GRβ mRNA is found in the hypothalamus and the hippocampus, but the relative abundance is subject to debate and may be only 1% relative to GRα. Thus, validation of the possible role of GRβ as a dominant-negative factor awaits further studies. Different forms of GR may also arise from the use of alternative translation start sites for its mRNA, adding yet another level of complexity to the receptor diversity.

The expression of the human MR gene may result in the formation of at least four transcripts, which are derived from two different promoters. The two main transcripts, MRα and MRβ, differ only in the 5′ untranslated exon 1 and thus are translated into the same 985-amino-acid MR protein. In rats, an MR transcript derived from exon 1 is detectable in very low amounts. Other intriguing splice variants have been described, including transcripts that code for truncated proteins. The use of an alternative splice site between exon 3 and 4 creates a 12-bp insertion, which, after translation, corresponds to four additional amino acids in the amino acid sequence bridging the two zinc finger domains of the DNA-binding domain. The functional analysis and relevance of these MR variants await further studies.

Variations in MRs and GRs in the form of single nucleotide polymorphism are quite frequent in the normal human populations. Although the biology of these variants is poorly understood, some of these variant receptors can be associated with the metabolic profile, stress responsiveness, and even life span.

Receptor variants may play an important role in disease states. Thus, individuals with familial glucocorticoid resistance may express a GR variant and, as a consequence, have deficient GR function and impaired glucocorticoid feedback resulting in hypercorticism. However, they lack the symptoms of

Cushing's syndrome because adrenocorticotropic hormone (ACTH) and cortisol levels are also at a higher set point and GRs are, in general, less sensitive to glucocorticoid activation. The symptomatology of familial glucocorticoid resistance is usually related to the overproduction of adrenal mineralocorticoids and androgens in response to ACTH. Although these severe inherited deficits in GRs, resulting in asymptomatic hypercorticoidism, are rare disorders in humans, there are also pronounced species differences in guinea pigs, prairie voles, and New World monkeys. These animals display a normal circadian rhythm in HPA axis activity, but ACTH and cortisol are circulating at a much higher level. Apparently, the elevated set point in HPA axis regulation is an adequate adaptation.

Regulation of Transcription through Corticosteroid Receptors

As members of the steroid hormone receptor superfamily, ligand-activated GRs and MRs exert their effects by acting as transcription factors to up- or downregulate protein and peptide levels in the cell. MRs and GRs may stimulate or repress transcription by several mechanisms (see **Figure 2**).

Transactivation via Glucocorticoid-Responsive Elements GRs and MRs contain a nearly identical DNA-binding domain that recognizes specific DNA elements in the regulatory regions of genes: glucocorticoid response elements (GREs; consensus sequence: GGTACAnnnTGTt/cCT). The steroid receptors bind as homodimers and perhaps also as heterodimers to GREs to stimulate transcription. In general, GRs are more potent activators of transcription than MRs, at least in *in vitro* conditions. Heterodimers of MRs and GRs have been shown in cell systems to have, at times, characteristics that are different from either type of homodimer. The strong synergizing effect of GR-activated transcription on multiple GREs is not observed with MR activation, probably due to the limited homology of the N-terminal sequences. Tyrosine amino transferase and phenylethanolamine-*N*-methyltransferase (PNMT) are examples of genes that are regulated via GREs.

Repression via Negative Glucocorticoid-Responsive Elements GRs (and possibly MRs) can also repress gene transcription by binding to DNA. DNA elements that are involved are known as negative GREs (nGREs). The sequence of nGREs can be highly variable and differs from the consensus sequence for positively acting GREs. The mechanism by which transcription is repressed also differs between cases. One mechanism involves the binding of GRs to the nGRE to occlude adjacent or overlapping binding sites on the DNA for positively acting transcription factors. An nGRE has been described for the human POMC gene.

Repression via Protein–Protein Interactions The mode of action generally referred to as transrepression involves the repression by GRs of gene transcription activated by other transcription factors,

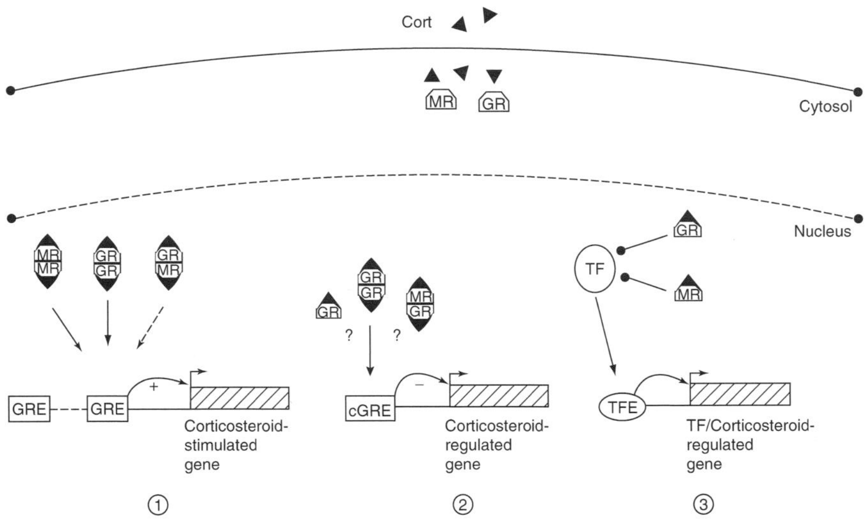

Figure 2 Three molecular mechanisms of regulation of gene expression. (1) GRs and MRs bind as homo- and heterodimers to GRE sequences to stimulate transcription. (2) GRs (and possibly MRs) bind to negative GRE sequences that diverge from consensus GRE. Through mechanisms such as occlusion of adjacent sites they repress transcription. (3) GRs and MRs interfere through protein–protein interactions with other transcription factors (TFs) at times independent of binding of the steroid receptors to the DNA. This results in antagonism of the effects of the TF (e.g., AP-1 or NF-κB).

such as activating protein (AP)-1, nuclear factor (NF)-κB, and cAMP response element binding protein (CREB). GRs interfere with these other factors via protein–protein interactions. This may happen independently of the binding of GRs to the DNA, and dimerization of GRs is not required. The target genes involved lacked GREs.

Corticosteroid receptors may also activate genes in synergy with other, nonreceptor transcription factors. On elements known as composite GREs (cGREs), GRs bind to the DNA in close proximity to another transcription factor and may either repress or enhance the effect of this other factor. In the case of the proliferin cGRE, the GR enhances the effect of the adjacently bound transcription factor AP-1 greatly if the latter consists of c-jun–c-jun homodimers. In contrast, GR binding leads to repression of the action of c-jun–c-fos heterodimers. Interactions with other transcription factors depend by definition on the presence of these factors, which can be regulated by extracellular signals other than steroid hormones. This demonstrates that the effects of CORT vary widely and are context-dependent.

Dissociation between MR- and GR-mediated events may arise through these cross-talk mechanisms because it has been shown that GRs suppresses AP-1 activity under conditions in which an MR is ineffective. It is probable that the unique N-terminal regions of the GR and the MR account for the different properties with respect to transrepression.

Cellular Effects of Corticosteroid Hormone Activation

The activation of intracellular corticosteroid receptors in many cell types may induce a variety of cellular responses, influencing diverse processes such as cellular structure, energy metabolism, or signal transduction. Changes in cellular structure usually develop over the course of several days, whereas effects on energy metabolism or signal transduction may already become apparent within an hour. In peripheral tissues, the activation of GRs leads to pronounced cellular effects, for example, apoptosis of thymocytes (via antagonism of NF-κB activity) and induction of gluconeogenesis in hepatocytes (through induction of critical enzymes). Here, focus lies on the effects of the MRs and GRs in the brain because these are important factors in the regulation of the HPA axis and of adaptation to stress in general. Although the delayed onset of the observed effects – as opposed to the rapidly induced effects by neurosteroids – favors gene-mediated effects via MRs and GRs, the molecular mechanism has, in many cases, not been resolved.

Differential Effects at the Level of a Single Structure: Mineralocorticoid and Glucocorticoid Receptors in the Hippocampus

The principal cell types in the hippocampus, a brain structure involved in declarative memory processes and (possibly) mood, express both MRs and GRs. The effects of differential occupation on firing characteristics have been particularly well studied for CA1 pyramidal cells. A conspicuous feature of CORT actions on cellular activity in the hippocampus is the apparent lack of effect when neurons are studied under basal conditions. Only when neurons are shifted from their basal condition (e.g., by the action of neurotransmitters) do CORT effects become visible. The general picture emerging is that conditions of predominant MR activation (i.e., at the circadian trough at rest) are associated with the maintenance of neuronal excitability, so excitatory inputs to the hippocampal CA1 area result in considerable excitatory hippocampal output. In contrast, additional GR activation (e.g., following acute stress) generally depresses the transiently activated CA1 hippocampal output. A similar effect is seen after adrenalectomy (ADX), indicating a U-shaped dose–response dependency of these cellular responses to corticosteroids. Most of the CORT effects on hippocampal physiology have been shown to depend on *de novo* protein synthesis and even on DNA binding of the GR, indicating that the effects on transcription of as yet unidentified target genes are responsible for the observed phenomena.

The U shape of CORT on neuronal excitability, which is determined by differential MR and GR activations, is reflected in a number of parameters. An intrinsic cellular property is the voltage-gated Ca current; this current is small under conditions of predominant MR occupation and is elevated when GRs become activated in addition. Basal and stimulus-induced intracellular Ca levels were also found to be increased by substantial GR activation, which may be explained by steroid effects on Ca-buffering or extrusion mechanisms. In accordance with these steroid effects, the Ca-dependent accommodation and afterhyperpolarization (AHP) amplitude were found to be small with predominant MR activation.

MR and GR activations also modulate the responses to several neurotransmitters. With respect to amino acid-mediated synaptic transmission in the hippocampus, responses to both excitatory (glutamatergic) and inhibitory (GABAergic) inputs are maintained at a stable level when MRs are predominantly activated (i.e., with low CORT levels). When GRs become occupied, in addition, as a consequence of rising CORT levels, excitatory transmission (and thus CA1 hippocampal output) is reduced. At very high steroid levels, inhibitory networks are also impaired. These GR-mediated effects may involve the impairment of energy metabolism. The high efficiency of amino acid transmission with predominant MR activation is also reflected in long-term plastic changes involving this hippocampal network. Plasticity-related phenomena are most pronounced with moderate CORT levels so that most of the MRs and only part of the GRs are activated; when CORT levels are either reduced or enhanced, synaptic potentiation/depression is far less effective. Thus, the varying concentrations of CORT as a consequence of stress will have consequences for the efficacy of synaptic potentiation in the hippocampus.

In addition to amino acid input, hippocampal neurons also receive considerable input mediated by biogenic amines such as acetylcholine, norepinephrine, and serotonin. Norepinephrine acts via a β-adrenergic receptor to increase excitability of the CA1 hippocampal area. High CORT levels, occupying GRs, reduce the norepinephrine effect, again leading to a reduction in responsiveness of the hippocampal neurons.

Serotonin (5-hydroxytryptamine, 5-HT) evokes many different effects in the CA1 hippocampal neurons, of which 5-HT-1A receptor-mediated hyperpolarization of the membrane is most prominent. This hyperpolarization is small in amplitude with predominant MR occupation; additional GR activation increases 5-HT responses. This is seen both when CORT is applied exogenously and after acute stress. Although CORT through MR activation also downregulates 5-HT-1A receptor mRNA expression and binding capacity, acute functional impairment is probably not brought about through reduced binding capacity.

Effects on Neurotransmitter Systems

CORT influences many cell types in the brain, and it is worthwhile to analyze its effects at the level of neurotransmitter systems, as opposed to a single cell type or nucleus. Major targets for coordinate regulation through corticosteroid receptors are the serotonin, dopamine, and norepinephrine systems. Modulation may take place at the level of both the presynaptic cell and the postsynaptic cell. As for most aspects of CORT action, the effects are permissive in nature – the genomic effects of steroid receptor activation are revealed in the context of activated systems.

Serotonin: Coordinate Regulation via Mineralocorticoid and Glucocorticoid Receptors A concept of coordinate regulation via MRs and GRs has emerged for the serotonin system, particularly in relation to its projection on the hippocampus. Under basal conditions, when corticosteroid levels are low, there is predominant activation of MRs. As described earlier, the response of hippocampal 5-HT-1A receptors under these conditions is low. In addition, MRs in certain hippocampal areas suppress the expression of the 5-HT-1A receptor. Thus, a situation of predominant MR occupation is associated with low responses to serotonin in the hippocampus. Serotonin release in the hippocampus is increased during and after stress conditions that are associated with increased levels of CORT, that is, increased activation of GRs in serotonergic and hippocampal neurons. When the stress-induced GR occupation is prevented, no increased release of serotonin is observed in animals. CORT acts via GRs, presumably on the activity of the rate-limiting enzyme for serotonin synthesis (tryptophan hydroxylase), and via the attenuation of negative feedback inhibition by serotonin in the serotonergic neurons in the midbrain. At the postsynaptic level in the hippocampus, acute GR activation leads to increased responses to 5-HT-1A receptor activation. Thus, whereas MR-mediated actions of CORT inhibit hippocampal responses, GR occupation is required for the stress-induced increased activity of serotonin cells and for the increased responsiveness of 5-HT-1A receptor-mediated responses.

When CORT is chronically elevated to levels in the GR-occupying range, hyporesponses to serotonin are observed in hippocampal neurons and endocrine challenge tests. It is unclear which molecular changes underlie the transition from stimulatory to inhibitory effects of high levels of CORT on serotonergic transmission.

Catecholamines Dopaminergic and catecholaminergic cells also depend on GR occupation for development and function. As in the case of stress-induced serotonin activity, increased activity of the mesolimbic dopamine system in the adult rat depends on GR activation. Dopamine (DA) release in the nucleus accumbens and neuronal and behavioral responses to dopamine agonists such as apomorphine are stimulated by CORT via GR. Sensitization to repeated treatment with drugs that increase dopaminergic transmission, such as cocaine, depend on GR activation. GR-mediated activation and sensitization of DA systems are important for understanding the relationship between stress and drug addiction in the context of individual response characteristics and have implications for psychopathology. Increased DA is involved in the symptoms of psychosis and depression, which are often associated with elevated basal levels of circulating CORT and escape from dexamethasone suppression.

In the periphery, there are clear effects of CORT on epinephrine – the expression of the PNMT gene in the adrenal medulla depends on GR activation. CORT also potentiates epinephrine responses at the target level. In the central nervous system, GRs are abundantly present in the majority of the neurons in midbrain norepinephrine cell groups. Although studies with ADX rats show a permissive function of corticosteroids for norepinephrine cells during ontogeny and stress (e.g., in relation to memory formation), the effect of GR activation in these cells and their postsynaptic targets are not as clear as for other transmitters.

Postsynaptically, CORT region-dependently regulates adrenergic receptor expression; that is, it induces the inhibitory α2 receptor in the hypothalamic PVN. In the hippocampus, the electrophysiological effects of norepinephrine are attenuated via a GR-dependent mechanism. Stress levels of CORT reduce the cyclic AMP generation induced by norepinephrine acting via β-adrenergic receptors in the hippocampus.

Neuropeptide Systems In addition to the classical neurotransmitter systems, many peptidergic systems are controlled via corticosteroid receptors, both at the level of peptide synthesis and at the level of postsynaptic receptors. These peptides are involved in many aspects of brain function, including hypothalamic control of the HPA axis and regulation of metabolism and feeding. The best-studied examples are POMC-derived peptides, CRH and arginine vasopressin (AVP) because of their critical role in the activation of the HPA axis. Both CRH and AVP mRNA levels are suppressed by CORT in the parvocellular division of the PVN, presumably via GR activation. However, this type of regulation is cell type-dependent because in the amygdala CRH mRNA is upregulated by corticosteroids. In the hippocampus, corticosteroid receptors mediate the regulation by CORT of neuropeptide Y and dynorphin mRNA levels; in the caudate-putamen and nucleus accumbens, corticosteroid receptors mediate regulation by CORT of preproenkephalin, neurokinin A, and preprodynorphin mRNA levels.

Cellular Viability

Structural changes of hippocampal neurons were observed both with chronic absence and chronic overexposure to CORT, indicating that the steroid-dependent expression of genes is of crucial importance for hippocampal integrity.

Chronic Absence of Corticosteroids The removal of the adrenal glands results within 3 days in apoptotic-like degeneration of mature granule cells in the rat dentatus gyrus but not in other hippocampal fields. The degeneration and associated loss of synaptic function can be prevented by treatment with MR ligands. In contrast to most brain regions, the dentate gyrus shows neurogenesis even during adulthood, which can be blocked by chronic stress and adrenal steroids. Lack of MR activation as a consequence of ADX results in increased cell birth and cell death. It has been argued that MR activation maintains the balance between cell birth and cell death in the dentate gyrus by enhancing the excitatory input to this region. However, newborn neurons in the dentate gyrus do not express corticosteroid receptors, suggesting that the steroid effects on neurogenesis are indirect and possibly involve the modulation of excitatory transmission and neurotrophins.

Chronic Exposure to High Corticosteroid Levels Ample evidence now shows that chronic elevation of CORT levels leads to atrophy in parts of the hippocampus, as well as to increased vulnerability to excitotoxic insults. CA3 pyramidal neurons seem to be particularly vulnerable, although effects in the CA1 and dentate subfield have also been reported. Three weeks of restraint stress in rats causes the regression of apical dendrites of hippocampal CA3 pyramidal neurons. This effect is mimicked by 3 weeks of treatment with a high dose of CORT and does not occur when CORT secretion is blocked by cyanoketone treatment. The regression occurring after 3 weeks of high levels of CORT is reversible, and available data support the view that an imbalance of excitatory over inhibitory signals, leading indirectly to an enhanced Ca influx in the CA3 pyramidal neurons, contributes to the observed degeneration. Lack of neurotrophic capacity may also contribute to enhanced neuronal vulnerability. Indeed, chronic stress or the administration of CORT affects brain-derived neurotrophic factor (BDNF), nerve growth factor (NGF), and basic fibroblast growth factor (bFGF), and tumor growth factor (TGF) expression in the hippocampus.

A critical duration of overexposure to steroids is essential for the atrophy of CA3 neurons to develop; temporary high levels of the hormone decrease responsiveness to excitatory amino acids and reduce excitability. It is only in conditions of chronically enhanced corticosteroid exposure that local depolarization is sustained and the breakdown of inhibitory networks occurs. Hippocampal neurons are subsequently subjected to a substantial GR-dependent rise in intracellular Ca levels. Following this line of reasoning, the beneficial effects exerted by phasic activation of GRs are turned into damaging actions when GRs are activated chronically.

Behavior and the Stress Response

The differential effects on neuronal functioning that CORT exerts via MRs and GRs, and the differential occupation of these receptors as a function of the behavioral state of the animal, suggest fundamentally different roles for CORT via MR- and GR-mediated processes. MRs are occupied by basal levels of CORT and thus mediate tonic hormonal influences. This might function to prepare the animal for upcoming challenges and determine the magnitude and/or nature of initial responses. This proactive mode of control includes the effects on the processing of sensory information, interpretation of environmental stimuli, and selection of the appropriate behavioral strategy. GRs, however, are occupied after plasma CORT levels have become elevated after challenges/stress. Their role may be to generally mediate reactive processes that serve to restore homeostasis, to facilitate behavioral adaptation of the animal, and to prepare the animal for a next exposure to a stressor.

Corticosteroid Receptors and Hypothalamic-Pituitary-Adrenal Axis Control

Both MRs and GRs are involved in the feedback control of HPA axis activity, but the temporal and neuroanatomical aspects of feedback differ substantially for each receptor type. Apart from primary feedback sites, the hippocampus has received a lot of attention, particularly because it contains the highest concentrations of both MRs and GRs in the brain.

Pituitary corticotrophs and PVN (being part of the HPA axis) contain the primary feedback sites for stress levels of CORT. The effects of CORT on pituitary, PVN, and brain-stem catecholaminergic nuclei involve the activation of GRs. Limbic inputs impinging on the PVN (via hypothalamic GABAergic neurons) express high levels of the MR in addition to the GR, suggesting the dual regulation of these inputs by CORT. Moreover, the effect of these inputs can be either inhibitory on HPA activity (from hippocampus) or excitatory (e.g., from amygdala).

Pharmacological experiments in rats have shown that MR occupation suppresses HPA axis activity under basal conditions around the circadian trough; in ADX animals, hormone levels can be normalized with a median inhibitory concentration (IC_{50}) of approximately 0.5 nM in terms of circulating free CORT, which is in the range of the MR K_d value. In intact animals, MR antagonists lead to an increase in CORT levels at the time of the circadian trough. Accordingly, MR activation serves to control HPA axis activity in a proactive manner.

At the circadian peak, much higher levels of exogenous corticosteroids are required to normalize ADX-induced increases in HPA axis activity, and half-maximal suppression is achieved by a free concentration of approximately 5 nM, close to the K_d of GRs. However, the exclusive activation of GRs is insufficient to suppress the circadian peak, and MR activation appears to be indispensable. One episodic rise in CORT levels by injection or ingestion via the normal evening drink is sufficient to occupy both receptor types and to maintain ACTH levels with small amplitude changes over the 24-h period. These GR-mediated effects observed after exogenous glucocorticoids thus are also involved in maintenance of HPA activity.

Elevated CORT facilitates the termination of the HPA response to stress, and various temporal (fast and slow feedback) domains have been distinguished. These GR-mediated effects triggered in response to stress represent the reactive mode of feedback operation.

Hippocampal Mineralocorticoid and Glucocorticoid Receptors Lesioning and electrical stimulation studies suggest an overall inhibitory influence of the hippocampus on HPA activity. The effects of intracerebroventricular MR antagonists in rats (see earlier discussion on the elevation of basal trough levels of CORT and enhanced adrenocortical responses to novelty) are likely mediated by hippocampal MRs. Consistent with the MR specificity of the response, a CORT implant in the dorsal hippocampus has been shown to suppress ADX-induced elevations in ACTH levels, whereas dexamethasone implants were ineffective. Finally, the systemic administration of spironolactone can increase basal HPA activity in humans, although this response has not been noted in all studies. Thus, hippocampal MRs appear to mediate the effect of CORT in maintaining the tone of basal HPA activity.

GR activation in the hippocampus, however, may not be involved in negative feedback but, rather, serves to suppress hippocampal output, leading to a disinhibition of the HPA axis. In fact, there is some experimental evidence that the intrahippocampal (in contrast to intracerebroventricular) administration of GR agonists does lead to an activation of the HPA axis. The nature of HPA regulation via hippocampal MRs and GRs is also consistent with the cellular actions they evoke in the hippocampus; predominant MR activation (comparable with local antiglucocorticoid application) maintains hippocampal excitability and, through transsynaptic inhibitory projections to the PVN, basal HPA activity. Conversely, with rising CORT concentration, GR activation suppresses the hippocampal output, resulting in a disinhibition of PVN neurons. The functions mediated by both receptor types are linked. A deficiency in an MR is predicted to allow a CORT response more readily, thus leading to more pronounced GR-mediated effects. This illustrates the importance of balance in MR- and GR-mediated effects involved in HPA regulation.

Indirect Effects Observations on HPA regulation have often been made without consideration of the steroid effects on higher brain functions involved in arousal and processing of information. Brain areas projecting to the PVN have profound and long-lasting consequences for feedback regulation. Many systems with inputs to the PVN generally express GRs and contain numerous colocalized neuropeptides, which also regulate PVN activity in their own right.

The activation of a particular afferent neuronal network innervating the PVN area is stressor-specific and depends on the nature of the stimulus. If it constitutes a direct threat to survival through physical stressors (e.g., respiratory distress, hemorrhage, inflammation, infection, and trauma), the ascending aminergic pathways promptly activate the autonomic and neuroendocrine centers in the hypothalamus. If sensory stimuli are subject to appraisal and interpretation, processing in higher brain regions is required, which may subsequently lead to the modulation of GABAergic tone and a change in synthesis of CRH, AVP, and other neuropeptides of the PVN secretagogue cocktail. The activation of brain stem and limbic circuitry is not separated but is, in fact, mutually interactive because stress-induced CORT enters the brain readily and feeds back on all components of the neural stress circuitry, but in a context-dependent manner.

Control over Learning and Memory via Mineralocorticoid and Glucocorticoid Receptors

The activation of central corticosteroid receptors does not necessarily cause a behavioral change but, rather, influences information processing, thereby affecting the likelihood that a particular stimulus elicits an appropriate behavioral response. For example, the GR-mediated effects on the dopaminergic reward system may render animals more susceptible to addiction but by themselves cause no such state. Through coordinate MR- and GR-mediated actions in higher brain areas (e.g., the neocortical regions and limbic areas such as the hippocampus, septum, and amygdala), CORT affects learning and memory processes. Therefore, when studying the modulation of behavioral responses by CORT, the time and duration of the hormone action, as well as its context, need to be considered.

The hippocampal formation plays a key role in animals' reactivity to novelty and provides an essential contribution to learning and memory. Stress hormones, including CORT, are secreted during learning and are necessary for the establishment of an enduring memory. In this context, the role of CORT on the acquisition, consolidation, and retrieval of information has been studied for more than 4 decades. Many different tests revealed that the administration of exogenous CORT in the appropriate temporal context (i.e., in close relation to training) potentiated memory in a dose-related fashion. From studies involving the use of specific corticosteroid receptor antagonists, antisense oligonucleotides, and transgenic animals, it is clear that these effects of corticosteroids require GR activation. These effects via GR in the context of stress-induced elevated hormone levels represent a reactive mode of action.

Studies with specific antagonists have shown that MRs modulate ongoing behavioral activity, as demonstrated by the effects of MR blockade during, but not after, the training session. These effects mediated by the MR regulate sensory integration underlying the evaluation of environmental information and response selection and thus have the capacity to subsequently affect memory storage for spatial and avoidance behavior. MR-mediated effects on behavioral response selection and reactivity may again be interpreted as a proactive mode of action, aimed to maintain homeostasis.

Thus, hippocampal MRs mediate the effects of CORT on the appraisal of information and response selection, whereas GR function does not so much modify these aspects of sensory integration as promote the processes underlying the consolidation of acquired information. However, exposure to high CORT levels in a different context (e.g., as a consequence of an additional stressor) may interfere with the consolidation processes because it may signal different, and more relevant, stimuli to the animal. The MR- and GR-mediated effects on information processing facilitate behavioral adaptation. This also promotes the inhibitory control exerted by higher brain circuits over HPA activity.

Corticosteroid Receptors in Pathology

The inappropriate activation of corticosteroid receptors through aberrant levels of hormone leads to well-known pathologies: Cushing's disease, immunosuppressed states (glucocorticoid excess), Addison's disease (glucocorticoid deficiency), and pseudomineralocorticoid excess states that are associated with high blood pressure. In the brain, the situation is much more complex. Depending on the region, both MRs and GRs can mediate the effects of CORT, and the balance in activation of these two receptor types may be critical in determining the effects of CORT on neuronal systems. For example, animal studies show that the balance of MR- and GR-mediated activities in hippocampal circuits determines excitability, stress responsiveness, and behavioral reactivity. Also, the effects of corticosteroid receptor activation often depend on the cellular context as a result of cross-talk with other signaling cascades. Genetically determined differences in any of the signaling pathways involved can lead to a predisposition to adverse effects of CORT.

Significant changes in CORT signaling in the brain can result from chronic stress exposure and the inefficient operation of the HPA axis, resulting in over- or underexposure to circulating CORT, and from genetically determined or acquired changes in relative abundance of MRs and GRs (and associated factors). All these changes may lead to disturbances in mood and affect and in neurodegenerative phenomena via direct actions on relevant brain structures, as well as via the modulation of the HPA axis activity. However, the specific contribution of brain MRs and GRs to these cognitive and affective deficits has not been established.

Disturbed CORT signaling in brain appears to be causally involved in enhancing vulnerability to depression. In this context, it is extremely interesting that the tricyclic antidepressants not only restore 5-HT and noradrenergic transmission in brain but also increase the expression of brain corticosteroid receptors, in parallel with the normalization of HPA tone. Recent data suggest that the blockade of central GRs can be used as an effective treatment against psychotic major depression. In contrast to depression, posttraumatic stress disorder, chronic fatigue syndrome, and fibromyalgia are associated with a hypoactivity of the HPA axis.

Evidence from animal experiments and in humans shows that a disregulated HPA axis, corticosteroid receptor deficits, and elevated CORT levels during stress are associated with age and may lead to an enhanced vulnerability to neurodegenerative disorders, particularly in the hippocampus. GR-mediated impairment in the energy metabolism of hippocampal pyramidal cells is thought to play a role here. The glucocorticoid cascade hypothesis has received much attention over the last years – hypercorticism leads, over time, to damage to the hippocampus, which in turn leads to the disinhibition of the HPA axis and further elevation of CORT levels. A central assumption of this hypothesis is that hippocampal GRs are thought to promote escape from negative feedback via downregulation. However, there is little evidence for a direct negative feedback function of hippocampal GRs; the role of the hippocampus appears to be indirect and involved more with the shutoff of the neural activity that drives HPA output, operating in concert with the output from the amygdala and pathways via the bed nucleus of the stria terminalis. Thus, the mechanisms that lead to the progressive hyperactivity and disregulation of the HPA axis in some individuals as they age are evidently more complex than envisioned in the glucocorticoid cascade hypothesis, and their elucidation will require a more extensive understanding of the role of other brain structures than the hippocampus and the hypothalamus in HPA regulation.

See Also the Following Articles

11β-Hydroxysteroid Dehydrogenases; Corticosteroids and Stress; Mineralocorticoid Receptor Polymorphisms.

Further Reading

Ahima, R., Krozowski, Z. and Harlan, R. (1991). Type 1 corticosteroid receptor-like immunoreactivity in the rat CNS: distribution and regulation by corticosteroids. *Journal of Comparative Neurology* **313**, 522–538.

Arriza, J. L., Weinberger, C., Cerelli, G., et al. (1987). Cloning of human mineralocorticoid receptor cDNA: structural and functional kinship with the glucocorticoid receptor. *Science* **237**, 268–275.

Belanoff, J., Rothschild, A., Cassidy, F., et al. (2002). An open label trial of C-1073 (mifepristone) for psychotic major depression. *Biological Psychiatry* **52**, 386–392.

Chandler, V. L., Maler, B. A. and Yamamoto, K. R. (1983). DNA sequences bound specifically by glucocorticoid receptor in vitro render a heterologous promoter hormone responsive in vivo. *Cell* **33**, 489–499.

Cole, T. J., Blendy, J. A., Monaghan, A. P., et al. (1995). Targeted disruption of the glucocorticoid receptor gene blocks adrenergic chromaffin cell development and severely retards lung maturation. *Genes & Development* **9**, 1608–1621.

De Kloet, E. R., Vreugdenhil, E., Oitzl, M. S., et al. (1998). Brain corticosteroid receptor balance in health and disease. *Endocrine Review* **19**, 269–301.

De Kloet, E. R., Wallach, G. and McEwen, B. S. (1975). Differences in corticosterone and dexamethasone binding to rat brain and pituitary. *Endocrinology* **96**, 598–609.

Edwards, C. R. W., Stewart, P. M., Burt, D., et al. (1988). Localization of 11β-hydroxysteroid dehydrogenase: tissue specific protector of the mineralocorticoid receptor. *Lancet* **2**, 986–989.

Funder, J. W., Pearce, P. T., Smith, R., et al. (1988). Mineralocorticoid action: target tissue specificity is enzyme, not receptor, mediated. *Science* **242**, 583–586.

Fuxe, K., Wikström, A. C., Okret, S., et al. (1985). Mapping of the glucocorticoid receptor immunoreactive neurons in the rat tel- and diencephalon using a monoclonal antibody against rat liver glucocorticoid receptors. *Endocrinology* **117**, 1803–1812.

Heck, S., Kullmann, M., Gast, A., et al. (1994). A distinct modulating domain in glucocorticoid receptor monomers in the repression of activity of the transcription factor AP-1. *EMBO Journal* **13**, 4087–4095.

Herman, J. P. and Cullinan, W. E. (1997). Neurocircuitry of stress: central control of the hypothalamo-pituitary-adrenocortical axis. *Trends in Neuroscience* **20**, 78–84.

Hollenberg, S. M., Weinberger, C., Ong, E. S., et al. (1985). Primary structure and expression of a functional glucocorticoid receptor cDNA. *Nature* **318**, 635–641.

Joëls, M. and De Kloet, E. R. (1992). Control of neuronal excitability by corticosteroid hormones. *Trends in Neuroscience* **15**, 25–30.

Jonat, C., Rahmsdorf, H. J., Park, K. K., et al. (1990). Antitumor promotion and antiinflammation: down-modulation of AP-1 (fos/jun) activity by glucocorticoid hormone. *Cell* **62**, 1189–1204.

Karst, H., Karten, Y. J., Reichart, H. M., et al. (2000). Corticosteroid actions in hippocampus require DNA binding of glucocorticoid receptor homodimers. *Nature Neuroscience* **3**, 977–978.

Karst, H., Berger, S., Turiault, M., et al. (2005). Mineralocorticoid receptors are indispensable for nongenomic modulation of hippocampal glutamate transmission by corticosterone. *Proceedings of the National Academy of Sciences of the USA* **102**, 19204–19207.

Krozowski, Z. S. and Funder, J. W. (1983). Renal mineralocorticoid receptors and hippocampal corticosterone-binding species have identical intrinsic steroid specificity. *Proceedings of the National Academy of Sciences USA* **80**, 6056–6060.

Liu, W., Wang, J., Sauter, N. K., et al. (1995). Steroid receptor heterodimerization demonstrated *in vitro* and *in vivo*. *Proceedings of the National Academy of Sciences USA* **92**, 12480–12484.

McEwen, B. S. (1999). Stress and hippocampal plasticity. *Annual Review of Neuroscience* **22**, 105–122.

McEwen, B. S., Weiss, J. M. and Schwartz, L. S. (1968). Selective retention of corticosterone by limbic structures in rat brain. *Nature* **220**, 911–912.

Moguilewsky, M. and Raynaud, J. P. (1980). Evidence for a specific mineralocorticoid receptor in rat pituitary and brain. *Journal of Steroid Biochemistry* **12**, 309–314.

Pearce, D. and Yamamoto, K. R. (1993). Mineralocorticoid and glucocorticoid receptor activities distinguished by non-receptor factors at a composite response element. *Science* **259**, 1161–1165.

Reichardt, H. M., Kaestner, K. H., Tuckermann, J., et al. (1998). DNA binding of the glucocorticoid receptor is not essential for survival. *Cell* **93**, 531–541.

Reul, J. M. H. M. and De Kloet, E. R. (1985). Two receptor systems for corticosterone in rat brain: microdistribution and differential occupation. *Endocrinology* **117**, 2505–2511.

Schinkel, A. H., Wagenaar, E., Van Deemter, L., et al. (1996). Absence of the mdr1a P-glycoprotein in mice affects tissue distribution and pharmacokinetics of dexamethasone, digoxin, and cyclosporin A. *Journal of Clinical Investigations* **96**, 1698–1705.

Trapp, T. and Holsboer, F. (1996). Heterodimerization between mineralocorticoid and glucocorticoid receptors increases the functional diversity of corticosteroid action. *Trends in Pharmacology* **17**, 145–149.

Van Steensel, B., Van Binnendijk, E. P., Hornsby, C. D., et al. (1996). Partial colocalization of glucocorticoid and mineralocorticoid receptors in compartments in nuclei of rat hippocampal neurons. *Journal of Cell Science* **109**, 787–792.

Veldhuis, H. D., Van Koppen, C., Van Ittersum, M., et al. (1982). Specificity of adrenal steroid receptor system in the rat hippocampus. *Endocrinology* **110**, 2044–2051.

Yudt, M. R. and Cidlowski, J. A. (2002). The glucocorticoid receptor: coding a diversity of proteins and responses through a single gene. *Molecular Endocrinology* **16**, 1719–1726.

Mineralocorticoid Receptor Polymorphisms

R H DeRijk and E R de Kloet
Leiden University Medical Center and Leiden University, Leiden, Netherlands

Glossary

Aldosterone — The classic salt-retaining steroid hormone secreted from the zona glomerulosa of the adrenal cortex; its release is stimulated by the renin–angiotensin system and rising plasma potassium concentrations.

Glucocorticoid hormones — Hormones synthesized and secreted from the zona fasciculata by the adrenal gland in response to stress and also during the diurnal rhythm. The main endogenous glucocorticoids are corticosterone in rodents and cortisol in humans.

Haplotypes — Combinations of several single-nucleotide polymorphism (SNP) alleles on the same chromosome. Here an allele is one variant of a sequence on the DNA, for example, a certain SNP. Often several haplotypes can be found in a gene due to unique combinations of SNPs.

Mineralocorticoid receptors (MRs) Intracellular receptors by which aldosterone acts in epithelial cells to promote sodium transport while mediating the glucocorticoid-like effects in nonepithelial cells. In the brain, MRs bind the glucocorticoid hormones (corticosterone and cortisol) and mediate the effect of these steroids on appraisal processes and the onset of the stress response.

Single-nucleotide polymorphism (SNP) A variation in DNA sequence that occurs with a frequency of at least 1%. SNPs can result in amino acid changes, if they are located in the coding region. If they are not in the coding region, they can influence gene regulation by effects on, for example, gene splicing or the promoter region or through the introduction of a stop codon.

Splice variant mRNA splicing occurs following transcription leading to alternative different mature mRNA molecules, so-called splice variants. Splicing can be tissue specific and context dependent with effects on mRNA expression levels and potentially leading to alternative different proteins.

Transactivational properties Effects different factors have on the control of gene expression.

Zinc fingers A highly conserved protein domain consisting of about 30 amino acid residues enabling corticosteroid receptors to bind DNA. Steroid receptors have typically two of these domains, encoded by exon 3 and 4. Each domain contains four cysteine residues interacting with one zinc ion, which is crucial for the stability of this domain.

Mineralocorticoid receptors (MRs) have similar affinity for the naturally occurring glucocorticoids (corticosterone and cortisol) and the mineralocorticoid aldosterone. In the epithelia, such as in the kidney, colon, sweat glands and circumventricular organ of the brain, these MRs selectively bind aldosterone, in spite of the approximately 100- to 1000-fold higher concentrations of glucocorticoid hormone in humans. MR selectivity for aldosterone is maintained through the activity of 11β-hydroxysteroid dehydrogenase (11βHSD) type 2, which converts cortisol and corticosterone to inactive metabolites. Through this mechanism, aldosterone can regulate the electrolyte balance, blood volume, and blood pressure. In nonepithelial cells residing in the heart, blood vessels and brain, the MRs are nonselective due to virtual absence of 11βHSD type 2. Accordingly, MRs are exposed to both aldosterone and excess glucocorticoid hormone.

In addition to the regulation of the electrolyte balance, aldosterone and MRs have been implicated in vascular inflammation and damage and in fibrosis in the heart. These actions seem to be relatively independent from the regulation of blood pressure and electrolyte balance. In the brain, the activation of MRs can induce drinking behavior, salt craving, and other effects aimed at reestablishing the electrolyte balance. However, MRs also play a crucial role in the maintenance of cellular stability, regulation of the hypothalamic-pituitary-adrenal (HPA) axis, behavioral adaptation, and cell homeostasis. The MRs involved in the latter functions are predominantly located in the hippocampus, where the receptors are activated by cortisol or corticosterone, due to the relative absence of 11βHSD type 2. Finally, recent data indicate the expression of the MRs in adipose tissue, regulating adipocytes differentiation and thermogenesis.

On the binding of the ligand, aldosterone or cortisol/corticosterone, MRs translocate from the cytosol to the nucleus and bind as a homodimer to hormone responsive elements (HREs). Transcriptional activation occurs through direct interactions with transcription factors and recruitment of co-regulator proteins. This recruitment is governed in part by the ligand and by the HRE. Co-regulator complexes are involved in chromatin remodeling and the recruitment of numerous other factors that are part of the transcriptional machinery.

Genetic variants of the MR gene (i.e. splice variants, deletions, insertions, or SNPs) probably have effects on these functions. These effects include not only an action on the electrolyte balance and cardiovascular control but also on vascular inflammation, behavior, HPA axis control, and homeostatic control mechanisms.

Mineralocorticoid Receptor Gene

The MR (NR3C2) is a member of the nuclear receptor family and resembles the glucocorticoid receptor (GR; NR3C1). In the DNA-binding domain, amino acid identity between MR and GR is approximately 94%, in the C-terminus 57%, and in the N-terminus less then 15%. Transcriptional regulation is mediated by the N-terminal part (exon 2, region AF-1a and AF-1b), plus a small part of the ligand-binding domain (C-terminus, AF-2). DNA binding involves residues in exons 3 and 4. Furthermore, exons 5–9 are involved in ligand binding, dimerization (with exons 3–4), heat shock protein (Hsp)90 binding, nuclear localization, and transcriptional regulation.

The MR gene is located on chromosome 4 (4q31.1) and has a size of approximately 350 kbp (this can be viewed on the Ensembl website). On a regular basis, new SNPs are being identified. The full protein contains 984 amino acids and has a size of approximately 107 kDa. Two (possibly three) exon 1s exist, which can join exon 2 (see **Figure 1**).

Genetic Variants in the Mineralocorticoid Receptor

Genetic Variability

Genetic variants can result from mutations causing deletions, insertions, or just changes of the nucleotide at a given position. Depending on the position in the genome, different effects on the phenotype can be observed. Genetic variants can affect protein structure or regulation through different mechanisms. Even single base pair substitutions can cause dramatic

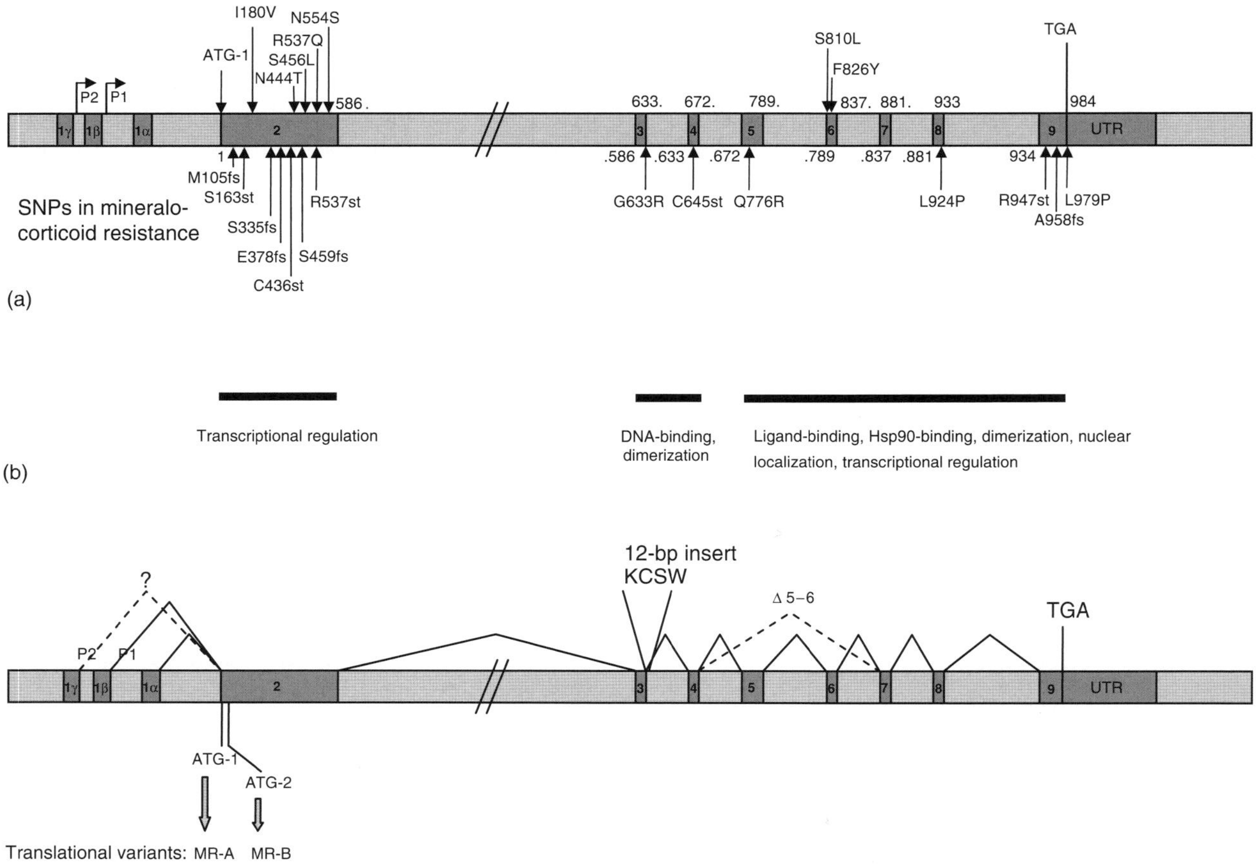

Figure 1 Human MR variants. a, Reported single-nucleotide polymorphisms (SNPs) leading to amino acid changes; b, the three functional domains; c, splice variants and translational variants. The number of the exon is in bold: **1α, 1β, 1γ, 2–9**. The exons are flanked by upper and lower numbers, which indicate the codon (or amino acid), ending with 984 in exon 9. If the number is followed by a dot, the codon spans both exons. Translation starts in the beginning of exon 2 and ends in exon 9 (TGA), followed by an untranslated region (UTR). In a (upper part), the indicated SNPs leading to amino acid changes are shown (from the Ensembl website), with the addition of S810L (associated with hypertension in pregnancy). In a (lower part), specific SNPs are shown that are found to be associated with mineralocorticoid resistance. These have a very low frequency and are only found in specific kindreds. The effects of these SNPs can involve a frameshift (fs) or the introduction of a premature stop codon (st). In b, the three functional domains are shown: the transcriptional active domain, the DNA-binding domain, and the ligand-binding domain (which has several other functions). In c, although both exon 1α and 1β can join exon 2, this is not clear for exon 1γ. In addition to most common annealing pattern (exons 2–9), exon skipping of exons 5 and 6 occurs, resulting in a frameshift with a new termination codon ending in exon 7 (position 2836). At the end of exon 3, 12 extra base pairs can be inserted due to alternative splicing (coding for Lys-Cys-Ser-Tyr), and joined with exon 4; this form is designated MR4+. KCSW, lysine-cysteine-serine-tryptophan.

changes to the phenotype; however, the vast majority of such changes which reach appreciable frequencies in the population (referred to as single nucleotide polymorphisms, SNPs) are benign.

The number of different SNPs in the human genome is probably in the range of 3–4 million out of a total of approximately 3 billion base pairs, counting only SNPs with a minor allele frequency of more then 1%. SNPs make up 90% of all human genetic variations, and two of every three SNPs substitute cytosine (C) with thymine (T), due to a high level of deamination of cytosine. These changes in nucleotide sequence give rise to alternative forms of a gene, named alleles. Combinations of several alleles on the same chromosomes are called haplotypes. However, not all possible combinations of the variants in a stretch of DNA are observed because of specific allele association or so-called linkage disequilibrium (LD). Often blocks of several SNPs are found, giving rise to several haplotypes in a gene.

SNPs are increasingly used to study the involvement of a certain gene and its protein product, in a complex phenotype, as is presented in psychiatric diseases. The association of an SNP in a given gene with a certain phenotype indicates the involvement of the gene. Alternatively, the carriers of a certain SNP/haplotype could represent a vulnerable (or protected) phenotype. Moreover, the determination of genetic variants could be used for more individual treatment of patients based on their specific needs, with respect to treatment efficacy and side effects.

However, several pitfalls are encountered when using variants in genetic research. Phenotyping is crucial because the effect of genetic variants are often moderate, which also calls for the use of large numbers of subjects in association studies. The elucidation of the molecular mechanism of a functional variant will strengthen the *a priori* hypothesis and will also help identify which genetic variant in a given haplotype causes the observed phenotype. Finally, the replication of an association in an independent cohort of subjects will overcome the often observed false-positive associations.

Variants of the Human Mineralocorticoid Receptor Gene

Splicing variants Several alternative splicing variants exist at the 5′ end of the gene: exon 1α, exon 1β, or exon1γ can join exon 2 (**Figure 1c**). The existence of exon 1γ is still not completely clear. Upstream of exon 1α and 1β, many regulatory sites have been identified, and this region (P2 and P1) is considered the proximal promotor. The effect of the alternative use of exon 1s is still unresolved. However, during development a differential regulation and response to adrenalectomy of 1α, 1β, or 1γ is observed in the rat hippocampal CA1, CA2, and CA3 pyramidal cell fields and the dentate gyrus (DG) neurons.

In the human MR, a 12-bp insert directly adjacent to the 3′ end of exon 3, as a result of alternative splicing, has been found. The result is four extra amino acids (lysine-cysteine-serine-tryptophan; KCSW) in between the two zinc (Zn)-fingers involved in DNA binding. No clear effect of this splice variant, especially on DNA binding, was found. It is, however, expressed in most human tissues, with relative levels varying from 5 to 50%, compared to the most common MR.

Another human MR isoform is derived from skipping exons 5 and 6 with a resultant premature stop, giving rise to a protein of 75 kDa, retaining DNA-binding capacity and ligand-independent transcriptional activity. The high level of expression of this splice variant makes it a potential important modulator of MR effects.

Translational variants also exist as a result of the alternative use of different translational start sites. Two different forms of the MR, designated MR-A and MR-B have recently been described, with different transcriptional activities.

Cardiovascular control Research into the molecular mechanism of mineralocorticoid resistance or pseudohypoaldosteronism (PHA1), characterized by urinary salt wasting and hypotension, has revealed several inactivating mutations in the MR gene. Two forms of PHA1 exist: an autosomal dominant form that is mild and a recessive form that is more severe due to defects in the epithelial sodium channel. In the autosomal dominant form, the target organ defect is confined to the kidney and clinical expression varies from asymptomatic to moderate. It may be severe at birth, with a failure to thrive, but symptoms often remit with age. The frequency of these mutations, including frameshifts, splice-site mutations, and premature stop codons, is quite low, which accords with the fact that PHA1 is a relatively rare disease. The usefulness of these mutations lies primarily in the understanding of MR protein activity with respect to DNA binding, translocation, and transactivational properties.

An activating mutation in the MR has been detected in patients with severe hypertension, which is exacerbated in pregnancy. The mutation, serine to leucine (S810L; **Figure 1a**), was found to alter the MR ligand specificity; progesterone and other steroids lacking the C-21-OH group became agonists.

Stress responsiveness Mutations of the MR may compromise the role of this receptor in the control of neuronal stability and stress responsiveness. Indeed

Brown Norway (BN) rats are, compared to Fisher rats, insensitive to adrenalectomy because there is no weight loss and resistance to saline intake. In the BN-rat MR gene, a tyrosine to cysteine (Y73C) substitution was detected. This mutation revealed a greater transactivational activity of aldosterone and, interestingly, also of progesterone, suggesting that the MR is constitutively more active in the BN rat. It is of interest to note that BN rats have a long life span and seem to have a relatively stable HPA axis, compared to other rat strains.

In humans, some SNPs have a high enough frequency to be potentially important for stress-related disorders, such as anxiety and depression. We found the MR 180V (MRI180V, isoleucine to valine; allele frequency 11%) to be associated with measures of depression in an elderly cohort. In human 180V carriers (i.e., the heterozygote I180V and the homozygote V180V genotypes), cortisol levels and heart rate were enhanced in response to psychological challenge evoked in the Trier Social Stress Test (), whereas the SNP was not associated with changes in blood pressure in response to salt loading as part of the Weinberger's test. Moreover, *in vitro* the response of the MR 180V allele to cortisol was attenuated, which was not observed with aldosterone. The finding suggests that such a subtle SNP can have profound effects on stress responsiveness with potentially important consequences for stress-related pathology.

See Also the Following Articles

Corticosteroid Receptors; Genetic Polymorphisms in Stress Response; Steroid Hormone Receptors.

Further Reading

Arriza, J., Weinberger, C., Cerelli, G., et al. (1987). Cloning of human mineralocorticoid receptor complementary DNA: structural and functional kinship with the glucocorticoid receptor. *Science* **237**, 268–275.

de Kloet, E. R., Joëls, M. and Holsboer, F. (2005). Stress and the brain: from adaptation to disease. *Nature Reviews Neuroscience* **6**(6), 463–475.

DeRijk, R. H., Wust, S., Meijer, O. C., et al. (2006). A common polymorphism in the mineralocorticoid receptor modulates stress responsiveness. *Journal of Clinical Endocrinology and Metabolism* Oct. 3 [Epub ahead of print].

Geller, D. S. (2005). Mineralocorticoid resistance. *Clinical Endocrinology* **62**, 513–520.

Vazquez, D. M., Lopez, J. F., Morano, M. I., et al. (1998). Alpha, beta, and gamma mineralocorticoid receptor messenger ribonucleic acid splice variants: differential expression and rapid regulation in the developing hippocampus. *Endocrinology* **139**, 3165–3175.

Zennaro, M. -C. and Lombes, M. (2004). Mineralocorticoid resistance. *Trends in Endocrinology and Metabolism* **15**(6), 264–270.

Relevant Website

Ensembl website.http://www.ensembl.org.

Membrane Glucocorticoid Receptors

P J Gasser and M Orchinik
Arizona State University, Tempe, AZ, USA

This article is reproduced from Encyclopedia of Stress, First edition, volume 2, pp 713–720, © 2000, Elsevier Inc.

Glossary

Corticosteroid-binding globulin (CBG or transcortin)	A plasma protein that specifically binds corticosteroids.
Corticotropin releasing factor (CRF)	A 41 amino acid residue hypothalamic peptide that mediates the neural control of pituitary adrenocorticotropin secretion.
Dexamethasone	A synthetic glucocorticoid.
EC_{50}	The dose of a hormone or drug necessary to produce 50% of the maximal response.
GABA	γ-Aminobutyric acid, an inhibitory neurotransmitter.
$GABA_A$ receptor	A membrane protein complex that forms an agonist-gated chloride ion channel and mediates fast inhibitory synaptic transmission.
K_D	Equilibrium dissociation constant. The concentration of ligand at which 50% of the receptors are occupied.
Nongenomic	A mechanism of steroid hormone action that does not initially involve modulation of gene transcription.
RU38486 (Mifepristone)	A synthetic progesterone receptor antagonist that binds with high affinity to the cytosolic glucocorticoid receptor.
TBPS (t-Butylbicyclophosphorothionate)	A competitor for binding of GABA to the $GABA_A$ receptor.
Triamcinolone acetonide	A synthetic glucocorticoid.

Glucocorticoid Receptors

Cellular and organismal responses to glucocorticoid hormones are complex and integrative, involving immediate, short-term, and long-term components. Target cell responses to glucocorticoids are initiated by two main mechanisms. In the classical, genomic mechanism, glucocorticoids interact with intracellular receptors, which act as ligand-gated transcription factors. The ligand–receptor complex then regulates the transcription of specific genes by interaction with hormone response elements and/or AP-1 transcriptional regulatory sites. This mechanism produces responses that are usually apparent in hours or days.

In the other, nongenomic, mechanism, glucocorticoids initiate immediate or very short latency responses in target cells. These short latencies preclude the genomic mechanism of transcriptional activation/inhibition and altered translation, although genomic responses may follow rapid responses. It is believed that these responses are mediated by glucocorticoid receptors that are integral to or associated with target cell plasma membranes. Membranal glucocorticoid receptors have not been cloned, but several membrane-associated glucocorticoid-binding proteins have been purified, and there are numerous reports of nongenomic physiological and behavioral responses to the hormones (**Table 1**). Receptor binding studies have characterized glucocorticoid binding to plasma membranes in various tissues from several species (**Table 2**), and some of the cellular signaling mechanisms activated by the hormones have been elucidated. Multiple classes of glucocorticoid-binding sites have been revealed in plasma membranes: (1) membranal glucocorticoid receptors distinct from intracellular glucocorticoid receptors, (2) membrane-associated forms of intracellular glucocorticoid receptors, (3) membrane receptors for corticosteroid-binding globulins (CBG), (4) membrane glucocorticoid-transporting proteins, and (5) other membrane proteins that also bind glucocorticoids. These proteins have been distinguished pharmacologically, based on binding specificity profiles for various natural and synthetic ligands, and immunologically, based on cross-reactivity with antibodies for intracellular glucocorticoid receptors. This article reviews the membrane glucocorticoid receptors and describes what is known of the mechanisms by which they initiate rapid cellular/organismal responses.

Glucocorticoid Receptors in Liver

The liver, a major target organ for glucocorticoid hormones during stress, shows both immediate and long latency physiological responses to glucocorticoid hormones and has both cytosolic and membrane glucocorticoid receptors. Radioligand binding and photoaffinity labeling reveal high-affinity (K_D = 7–12 nM) and low-affinity (K_D = 90–344 nM) membrane-binding sites for both dexamethasone and cortisol (see **Table 2**) in rat and chicken hepatocytes. The sites appear to be integral membrane proteins, as they can be extracted by detergent, but not by high salt. The sites for the two glucocorticoids also appear to be distinct from each other. Low-affinity dexamethasone binding is attributed to a 45-kDa protein, whereas two membrane proteins, 52 and 57 kDa, are responsible for cortisol binding. Glucocorticoid-binding sites have also been demonstrated visually in rat hepatocyte membranes. Gold-conjugated corticosterone–bovine serum albumin (BSA) specifically labels the apical, but not the lateral, membranes of hepatocytes (see **Table 2**).

During stress, glucose stores in the liver are mobilized rapidly by the activation of glycogen-degrading enzymes in the hepatocytes. This effect is largely due to the actions of catecholamines, but glucocorticoids also play a role. Corticosterone, dexamethasone, and cortisol increase the activity of glycogen phosphorylase, a glucose-liberating enzyme, in rat and chicken hepatocytes within 10 min of administration (see **Table 1**). Glucocorticoids act in this case via a Ca^{2+}-mediated signaling process, as the effect is diminished in Ca^{2+}-depleted medium. Other rapid effects of glucocorticoids in hepatocytes include increases in the phosphorylation of histone and nonhistone proteins and general activation of translational machinery, including increased synthesis of intracellular glucocorticoid receptors (see **Table 1**). These rapid effects may facilitate long-term, genomic responses to glucocorticoids.

Glucocorticoid Receptors in Lymphocytes

The immune system is another major target of glucocorticoid hormones. Membrane-mediated effects of glucocorticoids and membrane-associated forms of the intracellular glucocorticoid receptor have been demonstrated in various lymphocytes. In rat mast cells and basophils, cortisol inhibits the antigen-induced release of histamine and attenuates the antigen-induced release of Ca^{2+} from intracellular stores (see **Table 1**). This effect may be related to the potent antiallergic actions of glucocorticoids.

Studies with antibodies have demonstrated that a population of human lymphoma cells possesses a membrane-associated form of the intracellular glucocorticoid receptor (see **Table 2**). Cells that possess

Table 1 Selected membrane-mediated effects of glucocorticoids

Hormone	*Effect*	*Tissue*	*Dose (EC_{50})[a]*	*Organism*	*Reference*
Liver					
Corticosterone/ dexamethasone	↑ glycogen phosphorylase activity	Hepatocytes	1–10 μM B; 10–1000 nM Dex	Rat	Gomez-Munoz et al. (1989). *Biochem. J.* **262,** 417–423
Cortisol	↑ glycogen phosphorylase activity	Hepatocytes		Chicken	Sancho et al. (1986). *Biochim. Biophys. Acta* **88,** 249–255
Adrenal					
Corticosterone	↓ depolarization-induced calcium release	PC12 cells	100 nM–10 μM	Human	Lou and Chen (1998). *Biochem. Biophys. Res. Commun.* **244,** 403–407
Dexamethasone	↓ acetylcholine-induced current	Chromaffin cells	10 μM	Guinea pig	Inoue and Kuriyama (1989). *Am. J. Physiol.* **257,** C906–C912
Corticosterone	↓ steroid release	Interrenal tissue	10 μg/ml	Frog	Netchitailo et al. (1991). *J. Mol. Endocrinol.* **6,** 249–255
Intestine					
Cortisol	↑/↓ GABA-induced contractility	Ileum	1–10 pM (↑);10–1000 nM (↓)	Guinea pig	Ong et al. (1987). *Neurosci. Lett.* **82,** 101–106.
Endometrium					
Dexamethasone	↑ actin assembly	Endometrial cells	0.1 μM	Human	Koukouritaki et al. (1997). *J. Cell. Biochem.* **65,** 492–500
Immune system					
Cortisol	↓ histamine release	Mast cells	3 μM	Rat	Dukhanin et al. (1996). *Inflamm. Res.* **45,** S15–S16
Pituitary					
Corticosterone, cortisol, dexamethasone	↓ CRF-stimulated ACTH release	Pituitary	100 nM	Rat	Widmaier and Dallman (1984). *Endocrinology* **115,** 2368–2374
Dexamethasone	↓ AVP-stimulated ACTH release	Anterior pituitary	1 μM	Rat	Nicholson and Gillham (1989). *J. Endocrinol.* **122,** 545–551
Corticosterone	↓ CRF-stimulated ACTH release	Pituitary	45 μg/kg	Dog	Keller-Wood and Bell (1988). *Am. J. Physiol.* **255,** R344–R349
Cortisol/dexamethasone	↓ prolactin release	Rostral pars distalis	10 nM–1 μM	Tilapia	Borski et al. (1991). *Proc. Natl. Acad. Sci. USA* **88,** 2758–2762
Brain/neuronal tissue					
Corticosterone	↑ Ca^{2+} uptake	Synaptosomes	130 nM	Rat	Sze and Iqbal (1994). *Neuroendocrinology* **59,** 457–465
	↑ tryptophan uptake				Neckers and Sze (1975). *Brain Res.* **93,** 123–132
Cortisol/corticosterone	↓ calcium current	Hippocampal CA1 neurons	1 pM–100 nM (F) 10 pM–100 nM (B)	Guinea pig	ffrench-Mullen (1995). *J. Neurosci.* **15,** 903–911
Corticosterone	↓ vasopressin release	Hypothalamic slices	100 nM–100 μM	Rat	Liu and Chen (1995). *Brain Res.* **704,** 19–22
Corticosterone	↑/↓ somatostatin release	Hypothalamic neurons	100 nM–1 μM	Rat	Estupina et al. (1997). *Exp. Brain Res.* **113,** 337–342
Cortisol/corticosterone	↓ CRF release	Hypothalamic synaptosomes	750 nM (B) 6–60 nM (F)	Sheep	Edwardson and Bennett (1974). *Nature* **251,** 425–427
Cortisol	↑/↓ single-unit activity	Medial preoptic septal neurons	Iontophoresis	Rat	Kelly et al. (1977). *Exp. Brain Res.* **30,** 53–64

Corticosterone	↑/↓ firing rate	Pontine reticular neurons	2.5–3 mg/kg	Rat	Dubrovsky et al. (1985). *J. Neurosci. Res.* **14,** 117–128
Corticosterone	↑/↓ spontaneous and evoked activity	Hypothalamus, amygdala, midbrain	25–33 mg/kg	Rat	Feldman et al. (1983). *Exp. Neurol.* **80,** 427–438
Corticosterone	↓ population spike amplitude	Hippocampal pyramidal cells	100 nM–10 μM	Rat	Vidal et al. (1986). *Brain Res.* **383,** 54–59
Corticosterone	↓ population spike amplitude	Hippocampal pyramidal cells	0.05–5 nM	Rat	Talmi et al. (1992). *Neuroendocrinology* **55,** 257–263
Corticosterone	↑/↓ amplitude of sciatic-evoked responses	Pontine reticular neurons	2.5–3 mg/kg	Rat	Dubrovsky et al. (1985). *J. Neurosci. Res.* **14,** 117–128
Corticosterone/cortisol	↑/↓ activity	Hypothalamic neurons	Iontophoresis	Rat	Saphier and Feldman (1988). *Brain Res.* **453,** 183–190
Cortisol	↑/↓ sciatic-evoked responses	Hypothalamic neurons (MBH)	Iontophoresis	Rat	Mandelbrod et al. (1981). *Brain Res.* **218,** 115–130
Corticosterone/cortisol	↑/↓ TBPS binding	Synaptosomes	10–100 nM (↑); >100 nM (↓)	Rat	Majewska et al. (1985). *Brain Res.* **339,** 178–182 Majewska (1987). *Brain Res.* **418,** 377–382
Cortisol	↓ GABA-induced depolarization	Spinal ganglion neurons	5 μM–1 mM	Bullfrog	Ariyoshi and Akasu (1986). *Brain Res.* **367,** 332–336 Ariyoshi and Akasu (1987). *Brain Res.* **435,** 241–248
Corticosterone	↑/↓ activity	Medullary neurons	11–25 μg/animal	Newt	Rose et al. (1993). *Neuroendocrinology* **57,** 815–824 Rose et al. (1995). *Neuroendocrinology* **62,** 406–417
Behavioral effects					
Corticosterone	↓ courtship behavior		0.6 nM	Newt	Orchinik et al. (1991). *Science* **252,** 1848–1851 Moore and Miller (1984). *Horm. Behav.* **18,** 400–410
Corticosterone	↑ perch hopping		26 ng/ml	Sparrow	Breuner et al. (1998). *Gen. Comp. Endocrinol.* **111,** 386–394
Corticosterone	↑ locomotor response to novelty		2.5–5 mg/kg	Rat	Sandi et al. (1996). *Eur. J. Neurosci.* **8,** 794–800
Corticosterone	Stimulation of behavior during social challenge		2 mg/kg	Rat	Haller et al. (1997). *J. Neuroendocrinol.* **9,** 515–518
Corticosterone	↑ lordosis		200 μg/animal	Rat	Kubli-Garfias (1990). *Horm. Behav.* **24,** 443–449
Cortisol	↑/↓ aggression		1–10 μM	Hamster	Hayden-Hixson et al. (1991). *J. Neuroendocrinol.* **3,** 613–622

[a]B, corticosterone; F, cortisol; Dex, dexamethasone.

Table 2 Selected glucocorticoid-binding sites associated with plasma membranes

Hormone	K_D	*Organism*	*Reference*
Liver			
Cortisol	12 nM, 344 nM	Rat	Ibarrola et al. (1996). *Biochim. Biophys. Acta* **1284,** 41–46[a]
Dexamethasone	7 nM, 90 nM	Rat	Howell et al. (1989). *Biochem. J.* **260,** 435–441[a]
Cortisol	1.4 nM	Rat	Suyemitsu and Terayama (1975). *Endocrinology* **96,** 1499–1508
Corticosterone	None available	Rat	Spindler et al. (1991). *J. Steroid Biochem. Mol. Biol.* **39,** 315–322
Cortisol	4.5 nM	Chicken	Trueba et al. (1987). *Int. J. Biochem.* **19,** 957–962
Pituitary			
Corticosterone	3.2 nM	Rat	Koch et al. (1978). *J. Endocrinol.* **79,** 215–222
Corticosterone	None available	Mouse (AtT-20 cells)	Harrison et al. (1979). In: Leavitt and Clark (eds.) *Steroid hormone receptor systems*, pp. 423–443. New York: Plenum
Adrenal cortex			
Corticosterone	77 nM	Calf	Andres et al. (1997). *Cell. Mol. Life Sci.* **53,** 673–680
Brain			
Corticosterone	120 nM	Rat (synaptosomes)	Towle and Sze (1983). *J. Steroid Biochem.* **18,** 135–143
Corticosterone	6 nM (via CBG)	Vole (synaptosomes)	Orchinik et al. (1997). *J. Steroid Biochem. Mol. Biol.* **60,** 229–236
Corticosterone	0.5 nM	Newt (synaptosomes)	Orchinik et al. (1991). *Science* **252,** 1848–1851
Corticosterone	24.2 nM	Sparrow (synaptosomes)	Breuner et al. (1997). *Soc. Neurosci. Abst.* **23,** 1076
Lymphocytes			
Corticosterone	None available	Human (leukemic cells)	Gametchu et al. (1993). *FASEB J.* **7,** 1283–1292

[a]Indicates that the glucocorticoid-binding protein has been purified.

this form of the receptor are particularly sensitive to glucocorticoid-induced cytolysis.

Glucocorticoid Receptors in Adrenal Gland

Both the adrenal cortex and the adrenal medulla are targets of rapid glucocorticoid hormone action. Rapid effects in both areas appear to be related to the feedback regulation of adrenal hormone release. Corticosterone decreases the secretion of adrenal steroids from frog interrenal gland by 45–80%. This effect is not mimicked by dexamethasone and is not blocked by the specific glucocorticoid receptor antagonist RU43044 (see **Table 1**), indicating that this ultrashort feedback regulation of adrenal steroid secretion is mediated by another type of glucocorticoid receptor.

A membrane glucocorticoid-binding site in bovine adrenal cortex has high affinity ($K_D = 77$ nM) for corticosterone and very low affinity ($IC_{50} = 25$–50 μM) for dexamethasone, triamcinolone, and cortisol (see **Table 2**).

Chromaffin cells of the adrenal medulla secrete catecholamines in response to a variety of neurotransmitters, including acetylcholine. These cells are exposed to very high concentrations of glucocorticoids in venous blood from the adrenal cortex. At high concentrations (up to 10 μM), glucocorticoids modulate the responses of adrenal chromaffin cells to acetylcholine and to K^+-induced depolarization rapidly (see **Table 1**). Dexamethasone immediately diminishes the acetylcholine-induced current when applied extracellularly to dispersed guinea pig chromaffin cells, but has no effect when applied intracellularly. In PC12 cells from rat medullary tumors, corticosterone and corticosterone–BSA inhibit depolarization-induced intracellular Ca^{2+} release by a mechanism that involves G-protein-mediated calcium signaling.

Glucocorticoid Receptors in Pituitary

Several hypothalamic peptide hormones can cause cells of the anterior pituitary to release adrenocorticotropic hormone (ACTH), which in turn stimulates the release of glucocorticoid hormones from the adrenal cortex. Glucocorticoids regulate pituitary production/secretion of ACTH in a complex system of feedback inhibition. This inhibition occurs on rapid (seconds to minutes), delayed intermediate (10–15 min to hours), and delayed slow (hours to days) time courses. Rapid feedback inhibition of pituitary ACTH secretion by glucocorticoids is thought to be mediated by membrane receptors. The stimulation of ACTH release by CRF, oxytocin, vasopressin, and insulin is diminished rapidly by glucocorticoids, including corticosterone, cortisol, and dexamethasone (see **Table 1**). These effects are not completely understood, but appear to involve the attenuation of secretagogue-induced increases in second messenger accumulation. Some fast feedback effects, with latencies of 15–20 min, have been attributed to rapid protein synthesis.

Glucocorticoid-binding sites have been characterized in plasma membranes from rat and mouse pituitary cells (see **Table 2**). The rat membrane receptor has high affinity (K_D = 3.2 nM) for corticosterone and does not bind dexamethasone. Mouse pituitary tumor (AtT-20) cell membranes specifically bind corticosterone, but not dexamethasone or triamcinolone. This binding site appears to be a glycoprotein, as treatment of cells with proteases abolishes glucocorticoid binding and treatment with neuraminidase enhances binding.

The release of other pituitary hormones can also be modulated by glucocorticoids. In pituitaries of the teleost fish tilapia, cortisol inhibits the release of prolactin rapidly, apparently via the membrane-mediated modulation of Ca^{2+} and cAMP levels (see **Table 1**).

Glucocorticoid Receptors in Brain

Stress effects on neuronal activity and animal behavior are widely varied, stressor specific, and dependent on the endocrine/sensory history of the organism. Rapid glucocorticoid actions on neurophysiology and behavior show the same variability. In the brain, glucocorticoids can modulate both spontaneous and evoked neuronal activity rapidly. The direction of this modulation (increase or decrease) depends on the identity of the target neuron and is often context dependent. In the rat hypothalamus, for instance, corticosterone increases the activity of oxytocin-secreting neurons, but is mainly inhibitory to vasopressin neurons and neurons projecting to the median eminence (see **Table 1**). In the newt, corticosterone inhibits the responses of naive medullary reticular neurons to sensory stimuli, but it potentiates sensory responses of the same neurons when they have been previously exposed to vasotocin (see **Table 1**). Glucocorticoid-induced increases in sparrow perch-hopping behavior are dependent on photoperiod.

The best correlations between glucocorticoid-binding characteristics of membrane receptors and doses of glucocorticoids necessary for rapid physiological/behavioral effects have been demonstrated in the brains of rats and newts. In rat brain synaptosomes, corticosterone causes an increased uptake of Ca^{2+} and tryptophan (see **Table 1**). The EC_{50} for this effect (130 nM) is almost identical to the K_D (120 nM) determined for glucocorticoid binding to synaptic plasma membranes from the rat brain. In newts, corticosterone causes a rapid inhibition of male courtship behavior (see **Table 1**). This effect has an EC_{50} of 0.6 nM and is not mimicked by dexamethasone. The K_D for corticosterone binding to newt synaptic plasma membranes is 0.5 nM, and dexamethasone does not compete with corticosterone for this binding site.

Other effects of glucocorticoids in the brain include rapid modulation of neuropeptide release by hypothalamic neurons, modulation of spontaneous neuronal activity in various brain regions, and modulation of neuronal responses to sensory stimuli (see **Table 1**). It is likely that these rapid neuronal responses to glucocorticoids mediate rapid changes in behavior during stress.

Glucocorticoid Transport Proteins

There is still debate over the mechanisms by which glucocorticoid hormones cross plasma membranes. Certain membrane glucocorticoid-binding proteins also transport the steroids across the plasma membrane. One major membrane steroid transporter, P-glycoprotein, binds corticosterone, cortisol, and dexamethasone and transports them out of cells. This protein is expressed at high levels in epithelia of adrenal cortex, kidney proximal tubule, biliary hepatocytes, brain capillaries, small intestine, and colon.

Rat liver plasma membranes possess a bidirectional glucocorticoid transporter that is specific for corticosterone and cortisol. Immunochemical methods demonstrate that this binding site is distinct from P-glycoprotein. Specific transmembrane transport of glucocorticoids has also been demonstrated in membrane vesicles from pituitary and placenta.

Corticosteroid-Binding Globulins

Of the pool of glucocorticoid hormones circulating in the blood, a substantial fraction occurs bound to plasma proteins. Adrenal steroids (cortisol, corticosterone, and deoxycorticosterone) bind specifically and with high affinity to corticosteroid-binding globulin (or transcortin). While its functions are still unclear, CBG does interact specifically with a plasma membrane receptor. Specific, high-affinity CBG receptors have been purified from plasma membranes of rat and human liver and human endometrium and trophoblast cells. The interaction of the CBG–cortisol complex with trophoblast cell membranes causes activation of adenylate cyclase and accumulation of cAMP.

High affinity (K_D = 6 nM) binding of corticosterone to vole synaptic plasma membranes appears to involve one form of CBG. Specific binding to vole membranes was abolished by the saline perfusion of brains before binding studies, and vole plasma displayed a corticosterone-binding profile similar to that of synaptic plasma membranes (see **Table 2**).

Signal Transduction by Membrane Glucocorticoid Receptors

Pharmacological manipulations of nongenomic glucocorticoid effects (see **Table 1**) have revealed some aspects of the signal transduction mechanisms by which the hormones modulate cell physiology rapidly. These signaling mechanisms are nearly as diverse as the hormone effects. Existing data indicate that glucocorticoids can initiate rapid responses via (1) modulation of intracellular Ca^{2+}, often via G-protein-mediated pathways, and (2) activation/ inhibition of other signal transduction systems.

Modulation of Calcium Signaling

A large body of evidence indicates that glucocorticoids initiate rapid responses in many target cells by the modulation of intracellular calcium signaling. Cortisol inhibits N- and L-type Ca^{2+} currents in hippocampal neurons via a pertussis toxin-sensitive G-protein and protein kinase C (see **Table 1**). In rat brain synaptosomes, corticosterone enhances depolarization-induced Ca^{2+} influx rapidly and potentiates calmodulin-induced activation of voltage-sensitive calcium channels (see **Table 1**). Fish pituitary cells, rat lymphocytes, and PC12 cells respond to glucocorticoid treatment with rapid decreases in intracellular Ca^{2+} accumulation. In PC12 cells, this effect is diminished by pertussis toxin and by inhibitors of protein kinase C.

Many rapid effects of glucocorticoids are modulated by changes in extracellular calcium concentration. For example, the corticosterone-induced inhibition of vasopressin release from hypothalamic slices is potentiated in Ca^{2+}-rich medium and decreased in Ca^{2+}-depleted medium (see **Table 1**). The same manipulation of extracellular Ca^{2+} concentration attenuates/ enhances the corticosterone-induced decrease in population spike amplitude in hippocampal neurons (see **Table 1**). The corticosterone-induced increase in hepatocyte glycogen phosphorylase activity is diminished in Ca^{2+}-depleted medium.

Other Signaling Pathways

A variety of other signal transduction pathways have been implicated in the mediation of rapid glucocorticoid actions. The diversity of these pathways reflects the diversity of rapid glucocorticoid actions. Roles have been proposed for rapid glucocorticoid signaling via the $GABA_A$ receptor system, the cytoskeleton, the cAMP and cGMP pathways, and the nitric oxide system. Certain rapid effects of glucocorticoids result from the interaction of the hormones with other membrane proteins. One such protein is the $GABA_A$ receptor, a membrane protein complex that forms an agonist-gated chloride channel. Most studies indicate that metabolites of adrenal steroids, rather than the hormones themselves, modulate $GABA_A$ receptor function. However, there are reports of interactions between glucocorticoids and $GABA_A$ receptors. Glucocorticoids alter physiological responses to GABA and modulate agonist binding to the $GABA_A$ receptor (see **Table 1**). Other intracellular signaling pathways have been implicated in mediating the rapid effects of glucocorticoids. In human endometrial cells, dexamethasone induces rapid actin polymerization without concomitant changes in actin synthesis, implicating the cytoskeleton as another rapid glucocorticoid effector system (see **Table 1**). Cortisol inhibits cAMP phosphodiesterase in bovine testis and cardiac muscle homogenates and enhances guanylate cyclase activity in various tissues, indicating other possible mechanisms of rapid glucocorticoid signaling. Inhibitors of nitric oxide synthase prevent corticosterone-induced increases in the locomotor activity of rats in a novel environment (see **Table 1**).

See Also the Following Articles

Corticosteroid-Binding Blobulin (Transcortin); Glucocortoids, Overview.

Further Reading

Antoni, F. A., Hoyland, J., Woods, M. D. and Mason, W. T. (1992). Glucocorticoid inhibition of stimulus-evoked adrenocorticotropic release caused by suppression of intracellular calcium signals. *Journal of Endocrinology* **133**, R13–R16.

Fant, M. E., Harbison, R. D. and Harrison, R. W. (1979). Glucocorticoid uptake into human placental membrane vesicles. *Journal of Biological Chemistry* **254**, 6218–6221.

Gee, K. W., McCauley, L. D. and Lan, N. C. (1996). A putative receptor for neurosteroids on the $GABA_A$ receptor complex: the pharmacological properties and therapeutic potential of epalons. *Critical Review of Neurobiology* **9**, 207–227.

Grote, H., Ioannou, I., Voigt, J. and Sekeris, C. E. (1993). Localization of the glucocorticoid receptor in rat liver cells: evidence for plasma membrane bound receptor. *International Journal of Biochemistry* **25**, 1593–1599.

Harrison, R. W. and Yeakley, J. (1979). Evidence for glucocorticoid transport into AtT-20 cells. *Molecular and Cellular Endocrinology* **15**, 13–18.

Howie, J. G. R., Hopton, J. L., Heaney, D. J. and Porter, A. M. D. (1992). Attitudes to medical care. The organization of work and stress among general practitioners. *British Journal of General Practice* **42**, 181–185.

Lackner, C., Daufeldt, S., Wildt, L. and Allera, A. (1998). Glucocorticoid-recognizing and-effector sites in rat liver plasma membrane: kinetics of corticosterone uptake by isolated membrane vesicles. III. Specificity and

stereospecificity. *Journal of Steroid Biochemistry and Molecular Biology* **64**, 69–82.
Majewska, M. D. (1987). Antagonist-type interaction of glucocorticoids with the GABA receptor-coupled chloride channel. *Brain Research* **418**, 377–382.
Mechanic, D. (1972). General medical practice: some comparisons between the work of primary care physicians in the United States and England and Wales. In: *Public expectations and health care.* New York: Wiley.
Orchinik, M., Moore, F. L. and Rose, J. D. (1994). Mechanistic and functional studies of rapid corticosteroid actions. *Annals of the New York Academy of Sciences* **746**, 101–114.
Richardsen, A. M. and Burke, R. J. (1991). Occupational stress and job satisfaction among physicians: sex differences. *Social Science and Medicine* **33**, 1179–1187.
Riska, E. and Wegar, K. (1993). Women physicians: a new force in medicine? In: Riska, E. & Wegar, K. (eds.) *Gender, work and medicine.* London: Sage.
Rose, J. D., Kinnaird, J. R. and Moore, F. L. (1995). Neurophysiological effects of vasotocin and corticosterone on medullary neurons: implications for hormonal control of amphibian courtship behavior. *Neuroendocrinology* **62**, 406–417.
Schmidtke, J., Wienker, T., Flugel, M. and Engel, W. (1976). *In vitro* inhibition of cyclic AMP phosphodiesterase by cortisol. *Nature* **262**, 593–594.
Strel'chyonok, O. A. and Avvakumov, G. V. (1991). Interaction of human CBG with cell membranes. *Journal of Steroid Biochemistry and Molecular Biology* **40**, 795–803.
Sutherland, V. J. and Cooper, C. L. (1993). Identifying distress among general practitioners: predictors of psychological ill-health and job dissatisfaction. *Social Science and Medicine* **37**, 575–581.
Swanson, V., Power, K. G. and Simpson, R. J. (1998). Occupational stress and family life: a comparison of male and female doctors. *Journal of Occupational and Organizational Psychology* **71**, 237–260.
Winefield, H. R. and Anstey, T. J. (1991). Job stress in general practice: practitioner age, sex and attitudes as predictors. *Family Practice* **8**, 140–144.

Corticosteroid-Binding Globulin (Transcortin)

B E P Murphy
McGill University, Montreal, Canada

This is a revised version of the article by B E P Murphy, Encyclopedia of Stress, First edition, volume 1, pp 547–556, © 2000, Elsevier Inc.

Glossary

Affinity — The degree of association between two entities; expressed as the ratio of complexed to free reactants at equilibrium (the affinity constant), which is the reciprocal of the dissociation constant.

Binding capacity — An expression of the number of binding sites available for a ligand.

Corticosteroids — Steroids made by the adrenal cortex.

Ligand — An entity bound by noncovalent forces to another (usually larger, usually protein) entity.

Steroids — Molecules containing the perhydrocyclopentanophenanthrene nucleus, including sterols, bile acids, sex hormones, adrenocortical hormones, cardiac glycosides, and sapogenins.

Discovery and Definition of Corticosteroid-Binding Globulin

The presence of a human plasma protein binding corticosteroids with high affinity ($5–8 \times 10^7$ M^{-1}) and low capacity ($10^{-9}–10^{-8}$ M) was discovered in 1956 independently by I. E. Bush and by W. H. Daughaday. In 1958, A. A. Sandberg and W. R. Slaunwhite discovered a similar protein, which they called transcortin and which turned out to be identical with corticosteroid-binding globulin (CBG). Similar proteins have been found, many by U.S. Seal and R. P. Doe, in almost all species of vertebrates. A CBG-like protein has even been described in the eukaryotic fungus *Candida albicans*, with a K_a of 1.6×10^8 M^{-1} at 0°C, which might represent a primitive form of either the mammalian glucocorticoid receptor or of CBG.

CBGs differ from species to species in their relative affinities for various steroids. Most bind cortisol and corticosterone the most strongly; many bind progesterone very strongly; they bind aldosterone weakly. The guinea pig possesses a second corticosteroid-binding protein – progesterone-binding globulin (PBG) – in addition to CBG; PBG rises more than 100-fold during pregnancy. Although CBG binds testosterone and estradiol weakly, many species have, in addition to CBG, a sex hormone-binding globulin (SHBG), which binds these and related steroids more strongly. CBG is very low or undetectable in the plasma of the spiny anteater (an egg-laying mammal) and of the New World squirrel monkey.

Biological Role of Corticosteroid-Binding Globulin

Serum proteins such as albumin and CBG increase the solubility in biological fluids of steroids that are otherwise poorly soluble in aqueous solutions. However, the limited capacity and high affinity of CBG for glucocorticoids and progesterone has led to the accepted model of CBG action in which CBG provides a plasma store of tightly bound steroid that is less able to diffuse into cells, whereas free or unbound steroid passes freely across cell membranes to initiate hormone action. Because the binding to CBG is rapidly reversible, steroid may quickly be transferred from the bound to the free state. Thus CBG is a major determinant regulating the concentration of the hormones that it binds. On exposure to serine protease from inflammatory granulocytes, CBG is cleaved and releases all or most of its bound steroid; thus, it seems likely that this process may permit the enhanced delivery of cortisol to sites of inflammation. The binding of CBG to cell membranes and entry into cells may also be important in its action.

Changes of CBG in fetal life occur as a result of normal development, possibly promoting the delivery of glucocorticoids to sites of rapid growth and tissue remodeling.

In the human, the unbound fraction of cortisol is usually approximately 10% of total cortisol; in Cushing's syndrome, in which CBG levels are decreased and total cortisol levels increase, this fraction rises to approximately 25% of the total, whereas in adrenal insufficiency it falls to approximately 6% of total cortisol.

Physical Characteristics of Corticosteroid-Binding Globulin

Structure

The molecular weight of CBG is 50–60 kDa, and there is one cortisol-binding site per molecule. The degree of sequence similarity among species is 60–70%. CBG is a monomeric glycoprotein (with the possible exception of New World primate CBGs, which may circulate as dimers) consisting of approximately 380 amino acids with a molecular weight of approximately 42 000 (**Figure 1**). Relatively large differences in the apparent molecular size among species is probably due to variations in carbohydrate composition. The human CBG sequence is thought to contain six consensus sites for N-glycosylation. Only two of these sites have been retained throughout evolution, and these are located in highly conserved regions and may therefore be functionally important. The gene for CBG is localized to chromosome 14. The deduced primary structure of CBG suggests a greater than 30% homology with the SERPIN (serine protease inhibitor) superfamily of proteins. This family includes α_1-proteinase inhibitor (A1-P1), α_1-antichymotrypsin (ACT), and thyroxine-binding globulin. A1-P1 and ACT are located close to the region containing the human CBG gene. The PBG of guinea pig has a molecular weight of approximately 80 000 kDa and has one binding site per molecule. Its properties have been reviewed by Westphal.

Biosynthesis

The liver is the main site of CBG synthesis, and CBG is synthesized by hepatocytes in culture. CBG mRNA has been detected in the extrahepatic tissues (the spleen, ovary, testis, and lung) of various species but only in low amounts, and their significance is uncertain. CBG production is regulated independently in mother and fetus. Guinea pig PBG is made in only very small amounts by the liver, and the large rise in pregnancy is due mainly to synthesis by the placenta.

Degradation of Corticosteroid-Binding Globulin

The half-life of human CBG is approximately 5 days under usual circumstances but is decreased with severe stress. The serum clearance in early postnatal life in the rat is approximately twice as rapid (50% in ~7 h) as in the adult animal (~14 h).

Temperature Dependence

CBG binding in all species is temperature dependent, being maximal at approximately 4°C. At temperatures above 60°C, it is rapidly destroyed (in ~20 min). Stability is increased at higher cortisol concentrations. Between 37 and 40°C there is a rapidly increasing rate of dissociation, which may be important physiologically in febrile states, resulting in a more rapid release of cortisol to the tissues. Similarly, local elevation of temperature as a consequence of inflammation may contribute to more available cortisol at these sites. Binding activity is usually retained after a single freezing but is lost with repeated thawing and freezing. Many CBGs in serum are stable for long periods at 4°C; human CBG is stable for months or years provided bacterial contamination is prevented

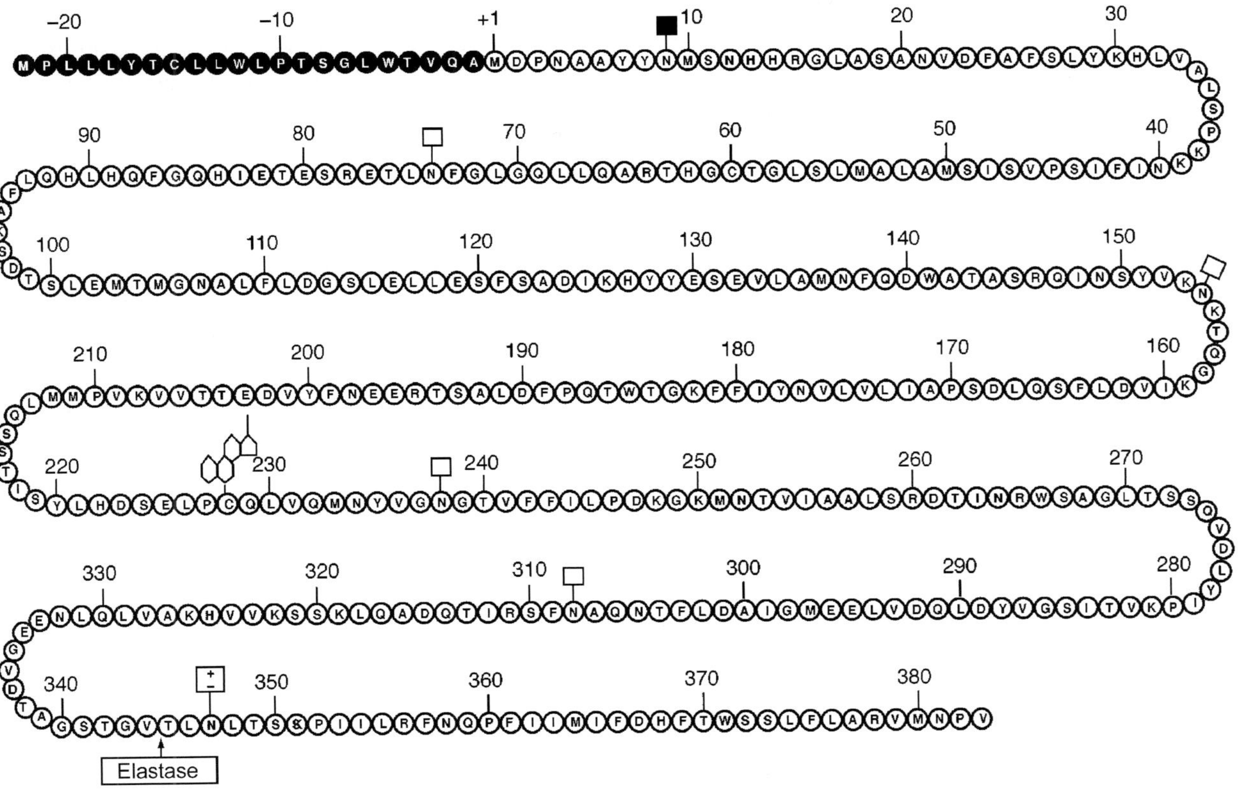

Figure 1 Primary structure of the human CBG precursor. The N-terminus of the mature polypeptide is inferred from published data, and the proposed signal peptide comprises 22 amino acids, shown in shaded circles. Potential sites for N-glycosylation are shown as squares, with a filled square indicating the site that is known to be used, and ± representing partial utilization. The elastase cleavage site is marked by an arrow, and the cysteine residue, which is conserved between species, is indicated. From Hammond, G. L. (1990), Molecular properties of corticosteroid binding globulin and the sex-steroid binding proteins, *Endocrine Reviews* **11**, 65–79. Copyright 1990, The Endocrine Society.

(e.g., by the addition of 0.1% sodium azide). Guinea pig PBG is more resistant to heating than most CBGs.

Affinity

The affinity constant for the binding of cortisol to human CBG is approximately 1×10^9 M^{-1} at 4°C and 5×10^7 M^{-1} at 37°C. The CBGs of most other species are in the range of 10^7–10^9 M^{-1} at 4°C and are also lower at 37°C. A relatively high association constant (0.9×10^8 M^{-1}) has been observed for ovine plasma at 37°C.

pH

Binding activity is also dependent on pH; for human CBG, it is maximal at approximately pH 8, but irreversible denaturation takes place below pH 5. In the guinea pig, PBG is more resistant to low pH than is CBG.

Electrophoresis

Electrophoretically, CBG behaves as an α_1-globulin.

Relationship to Albumin Binding

Steroids are also bound by albumin in all species. The free fraction is usually 6–14% of the total, with the CBG-bound fraction being 67–87% and the albumin-bound fraction 7–19%. In the squirrel monkey, approximately one-half is free and one-half is bound to albumin; this is the only vertebrate species in which CBG appears to be virtually absent.

Effect of Reducing Agents

The binding of cortisol and progesterone to purified human CBG is reversibly decreased by adding strong reducing agents such as dithiothreitol and β-mercaptoethanol but not by the milder sodium ascorbate. Only the affinity is decreased; the number of binding sites remains the same.

Binding Specificity

Mammals Although the specificity and affinity of the steroid-binding site vary among species, maximal binding usually coincides with the biologically more important glucocorticoid (either cortisol or corticosterone) in a given species. The ratio of cortisol to corticosterone varies widely among species, and the relative binding affinities for the two steroids also differ widely. In the green iguana there is high binding of cortisol (3056 nmol l^{-1}) but no detectable binding of corticosterone, whereas in the porcupine fish the binding to corticosterone (1250 nmol l^{-1}) is much higher than that of cortisol (67 nmol l^{-1}). For human plasma, Dunn et al. have calculated the binding distribution of endogenous steroids in normal men and in nonpregnant and pregnant women (**Table 1**).

In many species, progesterone, 11-desoxycortisol and desoxycortisol are also bound to CBG (**Table 2**). Alterations in ring A of strongly binding steroids cause a drastic drop in binding affinity; this is less marked in the CBG of avian species and in PBG.

Progesterone-binding globulin of guinea pig Whereas in human and many other species, CBG binds progesterone strongly, the guinea pig is the only species known to possess PBG, a separate CBG-like protein, which binds progesterone almost exclusively.

Marsupials The affinity of CBG in marsupials is similar to those of mammals, but the binding site concentrations are generally lower.

Synthetic steroids Some synthetic steroids, such as prednisolone, which is a glucocorticoid, and danazol (WII 131), which is not, also bind to CBG and compete with cortisol for binding sites. Dexamethasone, another synthetic glucocorticoid, is not bound to human CBG, but it does bind to chicken and dog CBG. Bovine serum is unusual in that, in addition to a CBG, which binds cortisol strongly, it contains a protein that binds triamcinolone acetonide, a synthetic glucocorticoid, approximately 50 times more strongly than cortisol.

Physiological Variation

In the human, the CBG binding capacity of men and women is similar (600–700 nM) and changes little from ages 1–60 years. Plasma levels of CBG vary from 10 to 500 nM in most vertebrate species. They are exceptionally high in the green iguana (3000 nM) and squirrel (2500 nM), and they are low in New World monkeys – only 1–10% of those in Old World primates and humans. The affinity is also lower, resulting in a much higher fraction of unbound plasma cortisol, possibly to compensate for the target organ resistance to glucocorticoids, which characterizes this group. In the squirrel monkey, the only mammal known that appears to lack CBG, half the cortisol is albumin-bound and half is free. In rat and guinea pig, female CBG levels are approximately twice those of males, a difference that is abolished by neonatal gonadectomy.

The concentration of CBG in the lymph is slightly lower than that in the blood, whereas concentrations in the synovial fluid and pleural effusion are higher and those in the spinal fluid and amniotic fluid are very low. CBG passes into milk – in human milk the concentration has been reported to be 1–15% that of plasma and in rat milk approximately 25% that of plasma. A CBG-like protein that binds progesterone

Table 1 CBG-bound endogenous steroids in human plasma[a]

Steroid	*Men*		*Women*					
	nmol/l[b]	*%*[c]	*Late pregnancy nmol/l*	*%*	*Follicular nmol/l*	*%*	*Luteal nmol/l*	*%*
Cortisol	400	90	740	95	400	90	400	90
Cortisone	72	38	110	5	54	39	54	38
Corticosterone	12	78	48	90	7.0	78	13	78
4-Androstene-3,17-dione	4.1	1.4	13	2.3	5.4	1.4	5.4	1.3
5-Pregnen-3β-ol-20-one	2.2	0.4	15	0.4	2.2	0.2	4.4	0.2
17-Hydroxyprogesterone	1.8	41	14	66	1.8	42	5.9	41
Androsterone	1.5	0.5	1.5	1.4	1.5	0.5	1.5	0.5
Testosterone	1.3	3.4	4.7	4.7	1.3	2.3	1.3	2.2
Etiocholanolone	1.2	0.4	1.2	1.3	1.2	0.5	1.2	0.4
Aldosterone	0.4	21	5.8	41	0.2	22	0.5	21

[a]Data from Dunn, J. F., Nisula, B. C. and Rodbard, D. (1981), Transport of steroid hormones: binding of 21 endogenous steroids to both testosterone-binding globulin and corticosteroid-binding globulin in human plasma, *Journal of Clinical Endocrinology and Metabolism* **53**, 58–68.

[b]Total concentration.

[c]Percentage bound to CBG.

Table 2 Steroid competition for sites on CBG in various species and on PBG of pregnant guinea pig[a]

Species	*Plasma concentration (%)*	*Steroid added*[b]							
		F	*B*	*S*	*P*	*H*	*E*	*T*	*A*
Human	2.5	100	82	89	20	73	16	4	3
Rhesus monkey	0.5	20	100	17	43	7	4	6	2
Dog	1.25	100	54	85	9	44	44	5	5
Cat	1.25	100	80	104	20	50	80	<1	<1
Beef	12.5	100	57	60	29	27	68	15	3
Rabbit	1.25	100	40	56	16	19	64	14	2
Rat	0.5	30	100	17	27	2	9	9	7
Mouse	0.5	12	100	15	6	15	0	0	0
Chicken	2.5	100	83	125	89	37	270	10	9
Horse	1.0	100	30	28	2	22	2	0.5	<1
Guinea pig[c]	0.025	<0.5	<0.5	0.9	100	0.6	<0.5	8	<0.5

[a]The tracer used was ^{3}H-corticosterone for all but pregnant guinea pig serum, in which ^{3}H-progesterone was used. The relative binding activity of the steroid added was determined at 50% displacement of the steroid indicated at 100%.
A, aldosterone; B, corticosterone; E, cortisone; F, cortisol; H, 17-hydroxyprogesterone; P, progesterone; S, 11-desoxycortisol; T, testosterone.
[b]Determined at 4–10°C, using Florisil as adsorbent (which gives slightly different values from equilibrium dialysis).
[c]PBG; serum from guinea pig in late pregnancy was used.

strongly has been reported in human breast cyst fluids. Because there is little or no CBG or albumin in saliva, salivary cortisol is often used as an index of free cortisol; however, the salivary gland contains 11-hydroxysteroid dehydrogenase type 2, which converts approximately half the cortisol to cortisone, so salivary values are approximately one-half those of free cortisol in plasma.

Pregnancy

In human pregnancy, CBG levels rise to levels more than twice those of nonpregnant women. The affinity is unchanged. The increase is due to the increased levels of estrogens in pregnancy. Progesterone binding, both free and total, increases steadily until the end of pregnancy; the free fraction rises from 6% of total at week 24 to 13% at week 40.

Elevated levels of CBG, up to 30-fold, have been observed by Seal and Doe to occur during pregnancy in mammals with a hemochorial type of placentation (rodents, cats, dogs, moles, shrews, manatees, and most primates) but not in those with other types such as endotheliochorial, choriovitelline, epitheliochorial, or syndesmochorial; the biological significance of this difference is not known. The increase in CBG is minimal in the rat (see **Figure 2**). In the guinea pig, CBG rises three- to fourfold, whereas PBG rises more than 100-fold. PBG differs from CBG in that it is not stimulated by estrogen.

Fetus and Neonate

Whereas fetal corticosteroid levels rise in many species during pregnancy, CBG levels vary considerably with species; in many, the levels fall rapidly postpartum. In most species, early postpartum fetal CBG levels are lower than adult values.

Compared to the adult (700 nmol l^{-1}), CBG levels are lower in the human fetus and neonate, approximately 250 nmol l^{-1} in late gestation and immediately postpartum; rise to approximately 500 nmol l^{-1} by 30 days postpartum; and rise to adult levels by several months of age.

The level of CBG in the fetal rat rises from approximately 1.3 mol l^{-1} at 16 days gestation to a maximum of approximately 2 $\mu\text{mol l}^{-1}$ at 28 days, after which it falls rapidly and subsequently rises slowly to adult values by 6 weeks (**Figure 2**). Thus CBG production is apparently independently regulated in mother and fetus. The decline in fetal rat CBG before birth may promote an increase in free corticosterone levels necessary for lung maturation. Despite the low neonatal values of CBG in rats, hippocampal glucocorticoid receptor occupancy/translocation (i.e., hormone-bound receptor) was noted by Viau et al. to be similar at all ages, both under basal conditions and following stress.

The sheep differs from this pattern; fetal CBG levels increase markedly over the last 2 weeks before term, from 50 nmol l^{-1} cortisol bound to 250 nmol l^{-1} at term, whereas unbound and albumin-bound cortisol increase from 3 to 58 nmol l^{-1} and the total cortisol rises 13- to 15-fold. During this time, no changes occur in the maternal plasma. After birth, the CBG binding capacity of the neonate falls rapidly to about 90 nmol l^{-1} by 4 days and to 17 nmol l^{-1} by 14 days; total and free corticoids also decrease, but more slowly. The increase of CBG in fetal sheep

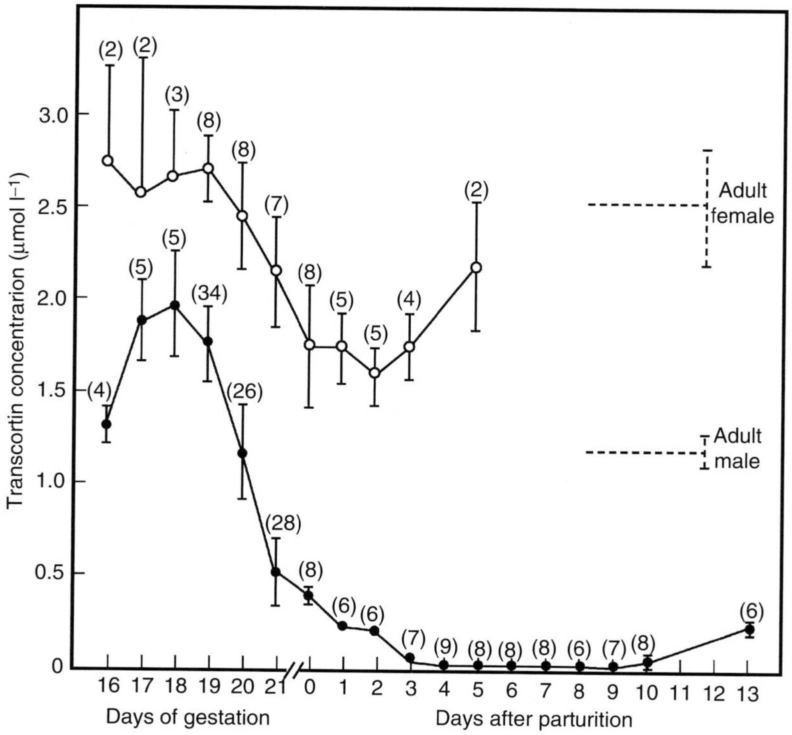

Figure 2 Serum CBG concentrations in fetal and neonatal rats (•) and in pregnant and lactating rats (o). The concentrations are expressed as means ±SD, and the number of animals or pools (days 16–18 for the fetuses) is given in parentheses. The normal serum concentration of four female and four male rats on day 154 of life is indicated on the right. From Van Baelen, H., Vandoren, G. and DeMoor, P. (1977), Concentration of transcortin in the pregnant rat and its foetuses, *Journal of Endocrinology* **75**, 427–431. Reproduced by permission of the Society for Endocrinology.

plasma before term has been shown to depend on an intact fetal pituitary. The affinity of fetal CBG is similar to that of adult CBG. Possibly the rise in CBG contributes to the onset of parturition because the administration of glucocorticoids induces parturition in this species.

In the baboon, fetal serum CBG capacity at 100–132 days gestation is similar to that of the mother and decreases at term by half. Fetal serum cortisol is low (~100 nmol l^{-1}) before 168 days gestation and reaches approximately 1400 nmol l^{-1} after term delivery. Affinity constants are the same throughout.

Hereditary Deficiency

Hereditary deficiency has been shown in a few human families, in which the concentration was reduced to approximately one-half the normal. However, familial low levels of CBG are rare and no convincing case of completely absent CBG in the human has been documented, suggesting that absence of CBG may be a lethal mutation, although cases with low CBG have no clinical apparent abnormalities. CBG appears to be identical in all human races. A variant of CBG, containing a slightly altered carbohydrate, occurs in pregnant women and accounts for 4–14% of total plasma CBG at term; its function is not yet clear.

Changes with Diet

Slight changes occur with diet; a high carbohydrate diet may result in a 20% fall in CBG.

Possible Fatal Drop in Corticosteroid-Binding Globulin

A remarkable change in CBG occurs in the male *Antechinus stuartii*, a shrewlike marsupial. In this species, all the males die within 3 weeks of the beginning of their first and only mating period in late winter. Over this period there is a precipitous fall in CBG levels, whereas the plasma corticosteroid concentrations remain high. No such changes occur in the females. Because these changes in the males result in a large increase in free cortisol, it is possible that the males die of hypercorticism.

Response of Corticosteroid-Binding Globulin to Stress

In humans, patients with septic shock or multitrauma have markedly low CBG levels in the early phase, with levels gradually increasing to normal by 7 days; in contrast, the free cortisol index shows high levels in the early phase, decreasing toward normal during the second phase. These observations suggest that CBG plays an active role by regulating availability to target tissues.

Acute severe stress in rats (e.g., immobilization for 1 h or tail shocks over 2 h) causes a fall in CBG, which is apparent by 6 h, maximal at 24 h, and persists for 24–48 h. Despite the low values of CBG in the neonatal rat, in response to stress (restraint for 1 h or separation from the mother) the adrenocorticotropic hormone (ACTH) and the free corticosterone levels increase, and this increase persists for 48 h. Such increases are associated with an increased glucocorticoid receptor occupancy/translocation similar to that of stressed adults.

In rats in which an inflammatory process was induced by a subcutaneous injection of turpentine, CBG levels had decreased by two-thirds, whereas the corticosteroid levels were very high. Although the high corticosteroid levels might be expected to decrease CBG levels, the effect was still present after adrenalectomy, suggesting that changes in glucocorticoid concentration are not necessary for this change. At the same time as the CBG levels were low, the levels of haptoglobin, an acute-phase serum protein rose 6- to 10-fold. CBG levels in pregnant rats treated similarly showed a threefold decrease of CBG, whereas their 19-day-old embryos were not affected.

Alexander and Irvine found that social stress in horses caused a decrease in CBG binding capacity (horses new to a herd were confined in a small yard with dominant resident horses for 3–4 h daily for 3–14 days). This decrease in CBG, seen after 3–4 days and increasing over the 2-week period, was accompanied by an increase in free cortisol, so that the total cortisol concentrations remained unaltered.

In comparing the homology of CBG cDNA, it was found that there is no sequence homology with any steroid hormone receptor. However, the homology with the SERPIN superfamily of proteins exceeds 30%. The proteins in the SERPIN superfamily share a typical tertiary structure responsible for the marked inhibition of serine proteases. In contact with neutrophil elastase, released by neutrophils in large amounts at sites of inflammation, CBG is cleaved, resulting in a 10-fold fall in its affinity for cortisol and thereby releasing its cortisol. Such a mechanism may permit the free cortisol to remain in high concentration at sites of inflammation while maintaining basal free cortisol concentrations at other sites.

Response of Corticosteroid-Binding Globulin to Other Pathological Factors in Humans

Increases in CBG also occur with the administration of oral contraceptive agents or other estrogen-containing preparations that increase synthesis. Tamoxifen and clomiphene also raise CBG levels. On the other hand, androgens such as testosterone decrease them; other anabolic steroids such as methandrostenolone and oxymetholone increase them slightly. CBG levels are reduced in patients with liver cirrhosis, nephrotic syndrome, and, in some cases, hypertension and hyperthyroidism, whereas elevated levels have been reported in some cases of acute leukemia, lymphoma, chronic active hepatitis, lung cancer, untreated adrenal insufficiency, adrenocortical hyperplasia, and disorders of male and female puberty. A slightly enhanced CBG capacity has been observed in juvenile-onset diabetics. A decreased CBG concentration, corrected by vitamin B_{12} administration, has been observed in some cases of pernicious anemia.

Glucocorticoids decrease CBG levels, so increased CBG levels are found after adrenalectomy, whereas decreased levels are found in Cushing's syndrome (whether endogenously or exogenously produced).

A rapid fall in CBG occurs in septic shock, reaching a nadir at approximately 24 h due to a marked increase in rate of removal because the half-life of CBG is approximately 5 days; this may occur by proteolysis at sites of inflammation. In cases of shock due to severe acute infection by *Candida albicans*, the CBG activity may be virtually absent.

Binding of Corticosteroid-Binding Globulin to Cell Membranes

A number of reports suggest that CBG binds to various cell membranes, including prostate, epididymis, testis, mammary carcinoma cells, uterus, pituitary, kidney, spleen, muscle, lung, and placenta. Although many of these await confirmation, it appears that CBG does bind to some cell membranes with a K_D of approximately 0.9 μM at physiological temperatures. This binding requires calcium and/or magnesium ions and is negligible at 4 or 23°C. The physiological significance of this binding is still unknown. In rat white adipose tissue, del Mar Grasa et al. found that CBG was seen in a thin layer surrounding the cells; they suggested that CBG in this location may act as a protective barrier limiting the access of glucocorticoids to adipocytes.

Measurement of Corticosteroid-Binding Globulin

CBG is measured either by its binding capacity for glucocorticoids (described by Westphal), by radioimmunoassay, or more recently by enzyme-linked immunosorbent assay.

Use of Corticosteroid-Binding Globulin to Measure Steroids by Competitive Protein Binding

Human CBG was the first protein used for the determination of glucocorticoids by B. E. P. Murphy in 1963 using the principle of competitive protein binding (displacement analysis and radiotransinassay), which is identical to that of radioimmunoassay. In this type of analysis, the specificity of the assay depends on the binding properties of the binding protein and the conditions under which the assay is carried out. The endogenous steroid or ligand is quantitated according to its competition with a tracer ligand, usually a radioisotopic form of the endogenous ligand, for binding sites on the protein, and the displacement of the tracer steroid is estimated against a series of standards of the ligand being measured. Thus, for example, the binding of radiolabeled cortisol will be gradually lowered by increasing amounts of endogenous cortisol, giving a standard curve.

Although no CBG is entirely specific for cortisol alone, the amounts of competing steroids in human plasma are usually small. In human pregnancy, progesterone is an important competitor, but it can be easily removed by extraction into hexane, which does not extract cortisol; the extracted progesterone can then itself be measured using CBG and a series of progesterone standards. Even better, progesterone may be measured using PBG of pregnant guinea pig serum, which has high specificity for progesterone and very little for cortisol or corticosterone. Because no protein is ever specific for a single ligand (and monoclonal antibodies are no exception), care must be taken to ensure that specificity is achieved under the conditions used. Because of the high affinity of CBG for cortisol, the sensitivity of such a method is very great, so that picogram amounts are readily measured. If chromatographic techniques are employed, other competing steroids can also be measured. Because different species of CBGs provide proteins with varying specificity and affinity, they can be used for the assay of many different steroids (**Table 1**). Maximum sensitivity is achieved by using a high dilution of the protein and a low volume for equilibration (usually 0.1 ml). Precision and accuracy are similar to those of radioimmunoassay.

See Also the Following Articles

Adrenal Cortex; Circadian Rhythms, Genetics of; Corticosteroids and Stress; Cushing's Syndrome, Medical Aspects; Gleucocorticoid Negative Feedback; Glucocortoids, Overview; Glucocorticoids, Role in Stress.

Further Reading

Alexander, S. L. and Irvine, C. H. G. (1998). The effect of social stress on adrenal axis activity in horses: the importance of monitoring corticosteroid-binding globulin capacity. *Journal of Endocrinology* **157**, 425–432.

Ballard, P. L., Kitterman, J. A. and Bland, R. D. (1982). Ontogeny and regulation of corticosteroid-binding globulin capacity in plasma of fetal and newborn lambs. *Endocrinology* **110**, 59–366.

Beishuizen, A., Thijs, L. G. and Vermes, I. (2001). Patterns of corticosteroid-binding globulin and the free cortisol index during septic shock and multitrauma. *Intensive Care Medicine* **27**, 1584–1591.

Breuner, C. W. and Orchinik, M. (2002). Beyond carrier proteins: plasma binding proteins as mediators of corticosteroid action in vertebrates. *Journal of Endocrinology* **175**, 99–112.

Dunn, J. F., Nisula, B. C. and Rodbard, D. (1981). Transport of steroid hormones: binding of 21 endogenous steroids to both testosterone-binding globulin and corticosteroid-binding globulin in human plasma. *Journal of Clinical Endocrinology and Metabolism* **53**, 58–68.

Hammond, G. L. (1990). Molecular properties of corticosteroid binding globulin and the sex-steroid binding proteins. *Endocrine Reviews* **11**, 65–79.

Murphy, B. E. P. (1967). Some studies of the protein-binding of steroids and their application to the routine micro and ultramicro measurement of various steroids in body fluids by competitive protein-binding radioassay. *Journal of Clinical Endocrinology and Metabolism* **27**, 973–990.

Rosner, W. (1991). Plasma steroid-binding proteins. *Endocrinology & Metabolism Clinics of North America* **20**, 697–720.

Seal, U. S. and Doe, R. P. (1967). The role of corticosteroid-binding globulin in mammalian pregnancy. In: Martin, L., (ed.) *Proceedings of Second International Congress on Hormonal Steroids,* pp. 697–706. Amsterdam, New York: Excerpta Medica Foundation.

Van Baelen, H., Vandoren, G. and DeMoor, P. (1977). Concentration of transcortin in the pregnant rat and its foetuses. *Journal of Endocrinology* **75**, 427–431.

Viau, V., Sharma, S. and Meaney, M. J. (1996). Changes in plasma adrenocorticotropin, corticosterone, corticosteroid-binding globulin, and hippocampal glucocorticoid receptor occupancy/translocation in rat pups in response to stress. *Journal of Neuroendocrinology* **8**, 1–8.

Westphal, U. (1971). *Steroid-protein interactions.* New York: Springer-Verlag.

Westphal, U. (1986). *Steroid-protein interactions II.* New York: Springer-Verlag.

Expression Profiling of Stress Responsive Gene Patterns

N A Datson and M C Morsink
Leiden University, Leiden, The Netherlands

Glossary

Corticosteroids Steroid hormones secreted at high levels during stress that regulate carbohydrate metabolism and influence the inflammatory response and cognition, mood, and behavior. Also known as glucocorticoids.

Glucocorticoid receptor (GR) An intracellular receptor that binds corticosteroids and then translocates to the nucleus, where it influences gene expression.

Hippocampus A complex neural structure (shaped like a sea horse) consisting of gray matter and located on the floor of each lateral ventricle; intimately involved in motivation and emotion as part of the limbic system; has a central role in the formation of memories.

Large-scale gene expression profiling A general name for molecular biological methods aimed at measuring expression levels of large numbers of genes (>100–30,000) simultaneously. Also known as transcriptomics or (pharmaco)genomics.

Limbic system A group of interconnected deep brain structures, common to all mammals, and involved in olfaction, emotion, motivation, behavior, and various autonomic functions.

Mineralocorticoid receptor (MR) An intracellular receptor that binds aldosterone and then translocates to the nucleus, where it influences gene expression. This receptor, which is colocalized with glucocorticoid receptor in several limbic brain structures, also has a high affinity for corticosteroids.

Introduction

The hypothalamic-pituitary-adrenal (HPA) axis is involved in regulation of stress responses in the organism. Under normal conditions, the adrenals secrete basal concentrations of corticosteroids into the bloodstream in a circadian manner. When the organism experiences a stressor, the activity of the HPA axis increases, which results in increased concentrations of corticosteroids. These corticosteroids (CORT) target many organs, exerting effects on blood glucose levels and immune function. Furthermore, corticosteroids are able to pass the blood–brain barrier, affecting brain functions such as cognition, behavior, and mood.

This article focuses on the effects of corticosteroids on gene expression in brain. These stress hormones have a profound effect on brain function. Moreover, exposure to chronic stress can precipitate the onset of central nervous system disorders such as depression.

Corticosteroids Modify Gene Expression

There are two endogenous receptors for CORT that are colocalized in several limbic brain structures such as the hippocampus and amygdala. The mineralocorticoid receptor (MR), which is expressed at high levels in the hippocampus, has a high affinity for its ligand and is already occupied under basal concentrations. The glucocorticoid receptor (GR) is ubiquitously expressed, has a tenfold lower affinity, and becomes occupied during rising concentrations of corticosteroids, for instance, during stress.

Both MR and GR belong to the superfamily of ligand-regulated nuclear receptors and are able to modify gene expression via two different mechanisms: (1) transactivation, in which the receptors bind to glucocorticoid-responsive elements (GREs) on the DNA and influence the transcription rate of the target genes, and (2) transrepression, in which the receptors interact with other transcription factors (such as activator protein-1 [AP-1] and nuclear factor-κβ [NF-κβ]), thereby inhibiting their transcriptional actions (**Figure 1**).

Effects of Stress on the Hippocampus

One of the major targets in the brain is the hippocampus, a structure that plays a crucial role in learning, memory, emotion, and regulation of the stress system. Several aspects of hippocampal cell function, such as neurotransmission and energy metabolism, are under the tight control of corticosteroids.

MR and GR, which are colocalized in hippocampal neurons, exert differential effects on hippocampal cell function. For instance, under low, basal concentrations in which only MR is occupied, neuroexcitability in hippocampal neurons is high, whereas under stress conditions, in which both MR and GR are occupied, neuroexcitability is low. Thus, MR is involved in maintenance of neuronal excitability and basal activity of the stress system, while GR activation results in reduced hippocampal output and is involved in negative feedback to restore homeostasis. Inadequate corticosteroid input as well as chronic occupation of GR results in degeneration of hippocampal neuronal circuits, accompanied by deficits in cognition and maladaptation to stress. A balanced activation of MR/GR is therefore an important determinant of neuronal excitability, stress responsiveness, and neuronal health.

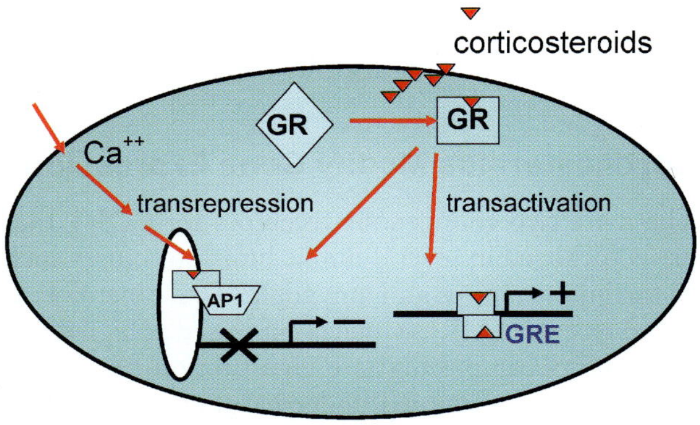

Figure 1 Molecular mechanisms of GR action on gene expression. Transactivation: after binding to corticosteroids, GRs translocate from the cytoplasm to the cell nucleus and bind to glucocorticoid-responsive elements (GREs) on the DNA, thereby influencing the transcription rates of target genes. Transrepression: corticosteroid-activated GRs bind to other transcription factors (such as AP-1), inhibiting their transcriptional actions.

Since (1) MR and GR are able to modify gene expression and (2) the majority of the effects of corticosteroids on hippocampal cell function develop in a delayed manner, it can be hypothesized that changes in gene expression underlie these CORT-induced effects. Therefore, by determining the CORT-induced changes in gene expression, the molecular mechanisms responsible for the actions of corticosteroids can be investigated. This entails measuring the expression levels of thousands of genes simultaneously, known as large-scale expression profiling, transcriptome analysis, or pharmacogenomics.

Large-Scale Gene Expression Profiling

In **Figure 2** the general outline for a large-scale gene expression profiling strategy is depicted. Instead of starting with a hypothesis, this strategy raises the question which genes are regulated by the hormone. Therefore, this type of research can be described as question-driven as opposed to hypothesis-driven research, and its primary goal is to generate gene expression profiles. When these profiles are established, candidate genes can be selected and hypotheses are generated as to how the selected candidate genes may play a role in the observed effects of corticosteroids on the hippocampal phenotype. Finally,

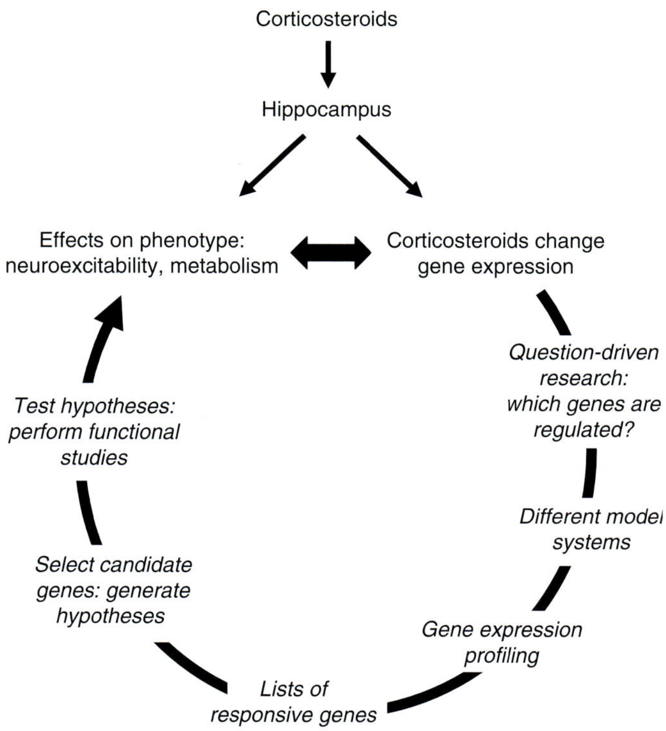

Figure 2 Outline for a large-scale gene expression profiling strategy. In order to elucidate the molecular mechanisms underlying the corticosteroid-mediated effects on the hippocampal phenotype, large-scale gene expression profiling techniques are used to assess corticosteroid-responsive genes. Candidate genes are selected and hypotheses are generated as to how these genes may play a role in the observed effects of corticosteroid on the hippocampus. These hypotheses are then tested in functional studies.

these hypotheses are tested in functional studies using *in vitro* systems such as cell lines or *in vivo* systems such as transgenic animals.

Large-scale gene expression profiling can be performed in a number of ways. Two of the more commonly used techniques are serial analysis of gene expression (SAGE) and DNA microarrays.

In SAGE, gene expression profiles are established by sequencing and counting 10-base-pair-long SAGE tags that are derived from a defined position within the 3′-untranslated region of each transcript. By sequencing and counting sufficient transcript-specific tags, a representative expression profile is obtained of a tissue under conditions of interest, for example, after hormone treatment (**Figure 3**).

DNA microarrays are glass microscope slides or silica chips on which a large number of DNA sequences representing a part of each transcript are deposited at a very high density. Depending on the type of microarray, the number of represented transcripts can range from 1000 to more than 20 000. Expression levels of each transcript are measured by hybridizing labeled RNA from a tissue of interest to the microarray, thus generating a hybridization signal (mostly fluorescent) that is a measure for the expression level of the corresponding transcript.

The use of DNA microarrays has been described as following a closed expression profiling strategy, since only the expression of a predefined set of genes (i.e., the sequences that are represented on the microarray) is profiled. In contrast, by using SAGE, no selection of transcripts is made beforehand; thus, this method can be considered an open expression profiling strategy.

Model Systems of Stress

The first step of an expression profiling strategy is the choice of the model system. Several model systems in which corticosteroid levels are pharmacologically manipulated can be used, although one must be aware that this only represents the hormonal part of the stress response and is not the same as stress. For instance, surgically removing the adrenals from rats results in complete absence of endogenous corticosteroids and lack of hippocampal MR and GR occupancy. Adrenalectomized rats can be further manipulated by (1) replacing them with low concentration corticosteroid-secreting pellets, resulting in occupancy of hippocampal MRs, and (2) administering high-concentration corticosteroid injections in order to additionally occupy hippocampal GRs.

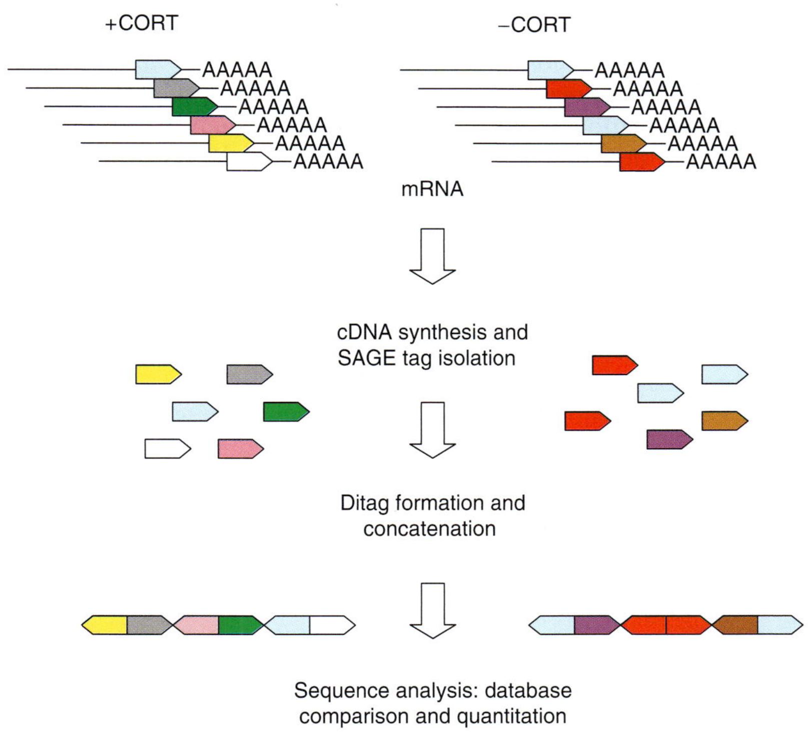

Figure 3 Serial analysis of gene expression (SAGE). In SAGE, 10-bp-long tags are generated from mRNA pools of different experimental treatment groups (for instance, corticosteroid-treated [+CORT] and control [−CORT)] groups). These mRNA-specific tags are ligated to produce concatemers, which are cloned and sequenced. By counting the tag abundancies, mRNA expression levels can be estimated and compared between the different experimental groups.

After isolating the hippocampi from these animals, gene expression profiles can be generated. Additionally, *ex vivo* hippocampal slices, which are derived from isolated hippocampi and are kept alive in carbogenated buffer, have also been used as a model to study the effects of corticosteroids on gene expression. In these slices, corticosteroid receptors can be directly activated by adding the hormone to the solution, thereby circumventing peripheral effects of injections into animals and removing the influence of projections from other brain areas to the hippocampus.

Another way of looking at the effects of stress on gene expression is to subject intact animals to a stressor, causing physiological activation of their HPA axis and a rise in plasma CORT levels. Several stress paradigms have been described in the literature, both for acute stress and for chronic stress. For example, placing a rat or mouse in a novel environment is sufficient to elicit a stress response, or placing a rat on top of the cage of a mouse will give rise to a stress response in the mouse. Purely physical stressors, such as cold stress or shaking stress, can be distinguished from psychological stressors such as psychosocial defeat and chronic unpredictable stress, in which experimental animals are subjected to a variety of different stressors in an unpredictable manner over several weeks.

A disadvantage of the physiological approach is that it can be difficult to control for interindividual differences in HPA response. Pharmacological manipulation of CORT levels in combination with a relevant psychological stressor may therefore be a good choice, depending on the focus of the study.

Stress-Responsive Gene Patterns in Brain

Different combinations of model systems and gene expression profiling techniques have been applied to analyze stress or corticosteroid-dependent changes in gene expression in brain. The vast majority of these studies focus on the hippocampus, because the activity of hippocampal neurons is modulated by elevated corticosteroid levels and it is the region with the highest expression of CORT receptors in the brain. Most of the studies have focused on GR-dependent gene expression. So far, not much is known about the genes regulated by MR as well as its molecular mode of action. It has been shown, using SAGE to analyze CORT-dependent gene expression in hippocampus of rats in which either MR or both MR and GR were occupied by pharmacological manipulation of CORT levels, that MR and GR activate or repress distinct yet partially overlapping sets of genes. This suggests that largely different signaling pathways are involved in maintenance of the basal activity of the stress system (MR dependent) and in the stress response (GR dependent).

In a study in tree shrews subjected to chronic psychosocial stress, reduced expression of four genes involved in cell differentiation in response to stress was found. This finding is in agreement with previous findings that this chronic psychosocial stress paradigm in tree shrews leads to structural alterations in hippocampal neurons such as dendritic retraction and impaired neurogenesis.

In a chronic psychosocial stress study performed in mice selected for attack latency (long attack latency [LAL]), hippocampal expression profiles were analyzed using DNA microarrays after 25 days of continuous sensory contact with an aggressive short attack latency (SAL) male. LAL mice but not SAL mice have been shown to display symptoms of chronic stress, such as increased CORT levels, decreased body weight, and lower hippocampal MR expression, using this paradigm. Interestingly, only downregulated genes were observed in response to this chronic psychosocial stress paradigm. The identified genes encoded a heterogeneous group of different proteins, the majority showing a subtle (less than twofold) downregulation. Several transcripts were identified to be involved in regulation of NF-κβ signaling, suggesting that NF-κβ may be involved in stress-induced functional changes in hippocampal neurons, thereby increasing their vulnerability.

Another study using *ex vivo* hippocampal slices investigated the gene expression response in time following GR activation. This revealed that corticosteroid effects are subtle and transient, with several subsequent waves of gene expression occurring after a single corticosteroid-pulse. Furthermore, within 5 h after activation of GR the gene expression response was comparable to the control group (non-activated GR).

Taking all these studies together, a general conclusion can be drawn that CORT-dependent gene expression encompasses a large variety of functional gene classes involved in energy metabolism, cell adhesion, synaptic transmission, oxidative stress, metabolism, neurogenesis, the cell cycle, and structural plasticity. In addition, the observed responses in hippocampus are subtle in magnitude. Therefore, it is very difficult to conclude which signaling pathways in the brain are most important and most profoundly affected by stress. It appears that corticosteroid stress hormones confer a pleiotropic signal to the neuron, affecting its excitability, connectivity to other neurons, metabolic rate, strength of its synaptic connections, differentiation from newborn neuron into mature neuron, and its vulnerability to metabolic damage. What exactly this means for neuronal function and vulnerability of the individual for stress-related brain disorders remains to be clarified.

The current expression profiling methodology has several limitations. It is still not possible today to perform genome-wide screening for genes regulated by stress due to the fact that annotation of the rat and mouse genome is not fully completed. Furthermore, so far low abundant genes such as neurotransmitter receptors and neurotrophic factors have been underrepresented due to sensitivity issues. Both these factors have also contributed to the currently incomplete picture of the effects of stress and corticosteroid stress hormones on hippocampal gene expression.

Future Perspectives

Since the hippocampus consists of many different cell types, it can be expected that by profiling whole hippocampus, CORT-dependent changes in expression that occur in a specific subpopulation of cells will be diluted to undetectable levels. Therefore, the feasibility of reducing the complexity of the tissue by using laser-microdissected hippocampal subregions has recently been evaluated. A high degree of differential expression between two different hippocampal subregions was identified, indicating that by isolating specific subregions of the hippocampus, detection efficiencies of transcripts with a subregion-specific expression or regulation may be improved. This type of approach combined with use of more genome-wide DNA microarrays and better bioinformatics tools to analyze this type of complex expression data should extend our knowledge on stress-dependent gene patterns in brain.

In conclusion, the application of large-scale expression profiling strategies has revealed a number of interesting candidate genes that may underlie some of the effects of corticosteroids on hippocampal cell function. Additionally, the use of laser-microdissected hippocampal subregions for expression profiling may increase the detection of low abundant genes, resulting in a more refined view on corticosteroid-responsive genes.

See Also the Following Articles

Corticosteroid Receptors; Corticosteroids and Stress; Hippocampus, Corticosteroid Effects on.

Further Reading

Alfonso, J., Pollevick, G. D., van der Hart, M., Flügge, G., Fuchs, E. and Frasch, A. C. C. (2004). Identification of genes regulated by chronic psychosocial stress and antidepressant treatment in the hippocampus. *European Journal of Neuroscience* **19**, 659–666.

Datson, N. A., van der Perk, J., de Kloet, E. R. and Vreugdenhil, E. (2001). Identification of corticosteroid-responsive genes in rat hippocampus using serial analysis of gene expression. *European Journal of Neuroscience* **14**, 675–689.

Datson, N. A., Meijer, L., Steenbergen, P. J., et al. (2004). Expression profiling in laser microdissected hippocampal subregions in rat brain reveals large subregion-specific differences in expression. *European Journal of Neuroscience* **20**, 2541–2554.

Feldker, D. M., Morsink, M. C., Veenema, A. H., et al. (2006). The effect of chronic exposure to highly aggressive mice on hippocampal gene expression of non-aggressive subordinates. *Brain Research* **1089**, 10–20.

Joëls, M. (2001). Corticosteroid actions in the hippocampus. *Journal of Neuroendocrinology* **13**, 657–669.

Karst, H., Karten, Y. J., Reichardt, H. M., de Kloet, E. R., Schutz, G. and Joëls, M. (2000). Corticosteroid actions in hippocampus require DNA binding of glucocorticoid receptor homodimers. *Nature Neuroscience* **3**, 977–978.

de Kloet, E. R., Joels, M. and Holsboer, F. (2005). Stress and the brain: from adaptation to disease. *Nature Reviews Neuroscience* **6**, 463–475.

McEwen, B. S. (1999). Stress and hippocampal plasticity. *Annual Reviews of Neuroscience* **22**, 105–122.

Morsink, M. C., Steenbergen, P. J., Vos, J. B., et al. (2006). Acute activation of hippocampal glucocorticoid receptors results in different waves of gene expression throughout time. *Journal of Neuroendocrinology* **18**, 239–252.

Oitzl, M. S. and de Kloet, E. R. (1992). Selective corticosteroid antagonists modulate specific aspects of spatial orientation learning. *Behavioral Neuroscience* **106**, 62–71.

Vreugdenhil, E., de Kloet, E. R., Schaaf, M. and Datson, N. A. (2001). Genetic dissection of corticosterone receptor function in the rat hippocampus. *European Neuropsychopharmacology* **11**, 423–430.

IV. AUTONOMIC NERVOUS SYSTEM - ADRENAL MEDULLA

Adrenal Medulla

R Kvetnansky
Slovak Academy of Sciences, Slovak Republic
R McCarty
Vanderbilt University, Nashville, TN, USA

This is a revised version of the article by R Kvetnansky and R McCarty, Encyclopedia of Stress, First edition, volume 1, pp 63–70, © 2000, Elsevier Inc.

Glossary

Adrenal medulla The inner portion of the adrenal gland that is part of the sympathetic-adrenal medullary system. The adrenal medulla receives neural input from sympathetic preganglionic fibers arising from the intermediolateral cell column of the thoracic and lumbar regions of the spinal cord. It is known primarily for its ability to synthesize and secrete the stress hormone epinephrine.

Chromaffin cell The cell type that makes up the bulk of the adrenal medulla, named for its capacity to take up and stain with chromium salts. In most mammalian species, there are two types of chromaffin cells: those that synthesize, store, and secrete norepinephrine and those that synthesize, store, and secrete epinephrine. These cells also synthesize, store, and secrete a range of biologically active peptides.

Dopamine-β-hydroxylase (DBH) An enzyme, contained within vesicles, that catalyzes the conversion of dopamine to norepinephrine.

Neuropeptide Y (NPY) A 36-amino-acid peptide found in cell bodies and nerve terminals of the central and peripheral nervous systems. This peptide is also localized within chromaffin cells of the adrenal medulla as well as other nonneuronal cells. It has important effects on the cardiovascular system and is also a smooth muscle cell mitogen.

Phenylethanolamine N-methyltransferase (PNMT) An enzyme localized within epinephrine-containing chromaffin cells of the adrenal medulla, adrenergic neurons of the central nervous system, and some other peripheral tissues (e.g., the heart). This enzyme catalyzes the conversion of norepinephrine to epinephrine.

Tyrosine hydroxylase (TH) An enzyme localized to catecholamine-synthesizing cells that catalyzes the conversion of tyrosine to dihydroxyphenylalanine. The hydroxylation of tyrosine is the rate-limiting step in catecholamine biosynthesis.

The adrenal medulla played a pivotal role in studies of the physiology of stress for most of the twentieth century. As the nineteenth century came to a close, the pharmacologist John Jacob Abel of Johns Hopkins University identified epinephrine (EPI) as the endogenous substance from the adrenal gland with pronounced effects on the cardiovascular system. Soon thereafter, Takamine identified the chemical structure and the synthesis of EPI was described. EPI was the first hormone with a known chemical structure. The physiologist Walter Branford Cannon of Harvard University conducted a series of seminal experiments on the importance of the adrenal medullary secretion of epinephrine during various types of stressful stimulation in animals and humans. Based on these studies, he introduced the terms homeostasis and fight-or-flight into the scientific literature, and these terms remain in use to the present. Another catecholamine, norepinephrine (NE), was identified in the middle of the twentieth century by Ulf S. von Euler of Karolinska University in Sweden as the neurotransmitter in sympathetic nerves.

The adrenal medulla of many mammalian species, including rats and humans, has both NE-containing and EPI-containing secretory cells. These two types of adrenal chromaffin cells are innervated by sympathetic preganglionic fibers of the splanchnic nerve. Each chromaffin cell contains approximately 10–30 thousand chromaffin granules in which catecholamines (CAs) are stored. Human adrenals contain approximately 6 mg of CAs (the ratio EPI : NE is approximately 4 : 1). The secretion of CAs from adrenal medullary chromaffin cells is controlled in part by the sympathetic preganglionic nerve fibers, and the CAs, secreted via exocytosis, are carried from the site of release by blood that drains from the adrenal medulla and into the adrenal vein. NE and EPI are then carried throughout the body (with the exception of those portions of the central nervous system where the blood–brain barrier is intact) and exert effects on most of the major organ systems of the body.

Biosynthesis and Release of Adrenal Medullary Catecholamines

The CA biosynthetic pathway is summarized in **Table 1**. CAs are synthesized from the amino acid precursor tyrosine. There are two primary sources of tyrosine: the diet and hydroxylation of the amino acid phenylalanine in the liver.

Table 1 Overview of the biosynthetic pathway of catecholamines in the adrenal medulla

Epinephrine
↑ Phenylethanolamine-*N*-methyltransferase
Norepinephrine
↑ Dopamine-β-hydroxylase
Dopamine
↑ Aromatic amino acid decarboxylase
Dihydroxyphenylalanine
↑ Tyrosine hydroxylase
Tyrosine

On entry into an adrenal chromaffin cell, tyrosine is converted to dihydroxyphenylalanine (DOPA) by the soluble cytoplasmic enzyme tyrosine hydroxylase (TH). TH activity is regulated in part by concentrations of Fe^{2+}, O_2, Mg^{2+}, adenosine triphosphate (ATP), and the cofactor tetrahydrobiopterin. Under most conditions, TH is the rate-limiting step in CA biosynthesis. DOPA is converted into dopamine (DA) by a nonspecific enzyme, aromatic amino acid decarboxylase (AADC). AADC activity depends on levels of its cofactor pyridoxal phosphate. DA is taken up into storage vesicles and converted to NE by dopamine-β-hydroxylase (DBH), an enzyme found in soluble and membrane-bound forms within storage vesicles. DBH activity is influenced by levels of copper, ascorbic acid, and O_2. NE is then converted to EPI by the soluble cytoplasmic enzyme phenylethanolamine *N*-methyltransferase (PNMT), which uses *S*-adenosyl-methionine as the cofactor.

Separate populations of adrenal chromaffin cells contain NE and EPI as the final products of CA biosynthesis. The latter are distinguished from the former by the presence of PNMT. Under resting conditions, low levels of EPI (but very little NE) are released into blood from the adrenal medulla. During some types of stressful stimulation, however, significant amounts of NE may be released from the adrenal medulla and may compose up to 35% of the total circulating NE. The remaining 65% of NE is released from sympathetic nerve terminals and enters blood from the site of release at the neuroeffector junction.

As already mentioned, NE and EPI are stored in chromaffin granules that are formed from the Golgi apparatus and enclosed by a single membrane. The chromaffin granules contain water, various proteins, ATP, and lipid, in addition to either NE or EPI. The most prominent proteins include the chromogranins. The release of CAs together with other compounds from adrenal chromaffin cells is via exocytosis.

Until the mid-1980s, the view of the adrenal medullary system was relatively simplistic. Acetylcholine was released from sympathetic preganglionic nerve terminals and bound to nicotinic cholinergic receptors on the adrenal chromaffin cells. The interaction of acetylcholine with its nicotinic receptor led to a depolarization of the chromaffin cell membrane, resulting in an increase in membrane permeability to sodium. Increased intracellular sodium initiated a series of events that led to an increase in the influx of calcium. Amine storage vesicles fused with the chromaffin cell membrane and released their contents of EPI or NE via exocytosis. Although it was known in the mid-1980s that chromogranins, ATP, and a fraction of the soluble DBH were released during exocytosis, the focus of attention was on EPI and its biological effects.

Since the mid-1980s, a wealth of new information has accumulated and the adrenal medulla can no longer be viewed as a tissue that is under the exclusive control of acetylcholine and concerned primarily with the synthesis, storage, and secretion of CAs (**Table 2**). Indeed, more than 30 biologically active substances have been localized to adrenal chromaffin cells, and a number of them have been shown to be released following depolarization of the chromaffin cell membrane. In addition, various biologically active neuropeptides are colocalized with acetylcholine within sympathetic preganglionic nerve terminals. Several of these neuropeptides, including substance P, NPY, vasoactive intestinal peptide (VIP), and pituitary adenylate cyclase-activating polypeptide (PACAP), appear to act as neuromodulators of cholinergic transmission. Finally, chromaffin cells have a range of membrane-bound receptors for various biologically active molecules that are released from preganglionic nerve terminals or are delivered to chromaffin cells via the circulation. These substances may also interact in complex ways to regulate secretory patterns of adrenal chromaffin cells. Each chromaffin cell may also have its own secretory phenotype based on the complement of peptide and classical neurotransmitter receptors contained on its outer cell membrane.

In some instances, peptides released from adrenal chromaffin cells may exert negative feedback effects on continued chromaffin cell secretory activity by stimulating chromaffin cell receptors. This type of intramedullary feedback loop introduces a new layer of complexity to the regulation of adrenal medullary secretion.

Stress Effects on the Biosynthetic Capacity of the Adrenal Medulla

Plasma Epinephrine and Stress

Many different approaches have been taken to assess the functional status of the adrenal medulla.

Table 2 Partial listing of neuropeptides in adrenal medullary chromaffin cells and in preganglionic nerve terminals and medullary ganglion cells and of neurotransmitter and neuropeptide receptors on adrenal medullary chromaffin cells[a]

Chromaffin cell peptides	*Nerve terminal peptides*	*Receptors*
Calcitonin gene-related peptide	Calcitonin gene-related peptide	Nicotinic
Enkephalins	Enkephalins	Muscarinic
Galanin	Galanin	Substance P
Substance P	Substance P	Bradykinin
Neuropeptide Y	Neuropeptide Y	Vasopressin
Vasoactive intestinal polypeptide	Vasoactive intestinal polypeptide	Neurotensin
Neurotensin	Neurotensin	Angiotensin II
Somatostatin	Somatostatin	Atrial natriuretic factor
Dynorphin	Dynorphin	Cholecystokinin
Adrenomedullin	Cholecystokinin	Neurokinins
Vasopressin	PACAP	Endothelins
Guanylin		
CRH		
ACTH		
Renin		
Chromogranins A, B, and C		
Chromostatins		
Secretogranins		
Secretoneurin		
Synaptophysin		
Interleukin-1		
Natriuretic peptides		
Endothelins		
Erythropoietin		
Endorphins		
Cerebellin		
Parathyroid hormone-related protein		

[a]ACTH, adrenocorticotropic hormone; CRH, corticotropin releasing hormone; PACAP, pituitary adenylate cyclase activating peptide.

Beginning in the 1950s, fluorometric assays of CAs were employed to study the effects of stress on whole gland content of EPI and NE. In addition, fluorometric assays allowed for quantification of urinary excretion rates of CAs in laboratory animals and in humans. The earliest studies of plasma levels of CAs also made use of fluorometric assays. However, studies of plasma CAs in laboratory animals and in humans were greatly facilitated by the introduction of highly sensitive radioenzymatic thin-layer chromatographic techniques in the 1970s and high-pressure liquid chromatography with electrochemical detection (HPLC-EC) beginning in the 1980s.

Studies of plasma levels of EPI revealed a number of facets of adrenal medullary regulation. The adrenal medulla is for all intents and purposes the sole source of circulating EPI in all mammalian species that have been studied, including humans. Gene expression of PNMT and levels of PNMT protein have also been detected in several other organs such as the heart, spleen, thymus, and some brain-stem nuclei. However, EPI synthesized in these tissues has mainly a local function and practically does not influence the EPI concentration in circulation. In all studies dealing with levels of circulating EPI and NE, the subjects must be surgically prepared with indwelling arterial or venous catheters to reduce to the greatest extent possible any stress associated with blood collection. Basal plasma levels of EPI in laboratory rats and in humans are often less than 50 pg ml^{-1}. Plasma EPI levels increase rapidly in response to even minor stressors, and there is a monotonic relationship between the intensity of a stressor and the increment above the baseline in plasma levels of EPI.

Prior stress history exerts a profound effect on the secretory response of the adrenal medulla to subsequent exposure to a stressor. For example, if a laboratory rat is exposed to the same stressor each day for several weeks, the adrenal medullary response to the next exposure to that same stressor is reduced significantly compared to first-time-stressed controls. In contrast, if these same chronically stressed animals are instead exposed to a novel stressor, the adrenal medullary response is significantly greater compared to a first-time-stressed control group. The former pattern has been referred to as habituation, and the latter response has been referred to as sensitization. The mechanisms explaining these effects are not fully understood even if changes in gene expression of CA-synthesizing enzymes are in a good correlation with changes in CA secretion. However, it has been assumed that splanchnic stimulation of the adrenal medulla is reduced during the development of habituation and is enhanced during a sensitizing experience.

An important research question since the late 1960s has been the processes by which the adrenal medulla responds to acute versus chronic intermittent exposure to stressful stimulation. This research question has been subject to ongoing refinement as new and more sensitive neurochemical and molecular biological techniques have become available. Most of the studies in this field of inquiry have focused on regulatory processes affecting CA biosynthesis and release. However, although the adrenal medulla secretes a complex array of biologically active peptides, many fewer studies have examined how the biosynthesis and release of these neuropeptides are affected by chronic intermittent stress and exposure to novel stressors.

Exposure to a single episode of immobilization stress for up to 2 h is attended by a significant decrease of 15–20% in the total adrenal medullary content of EPI. An animal or human experiencing this sustained exposure to an acute stressor does not know when the stressor will be terminated and, once terminated, if and when the stressor will begin again. In the face of this uncertainty, how does the adrenal medulla meet the immediate needs of replenishing supplies of EPI in adrenal chromaffin cells and what, if any, provisions are made for an uncertain future?

Given that the synthesis of EPI within the adrenal medulla involves a complex interplay of several different enzymes, studies have focused on three key enzymes: TH, DBH, and PNMT. Recently, these enzymes were intensively studied at the level of their gene transcription and translation to protein, as well as the regulation of these processes by transcription factors. The most extensive literature is available for TH because of its role as the rate-limiting step in CA biosynthesis; however, the other two enzymes have also received considerable attention. The discussion here focuses in large part on the effects of acute versus repeated immobilization stress in laboratory rats because there is an extensive literature relating to this stressor and the studies have been performed in a systematic fashion.

Effects of Acute Immobilization Stress on Adrenal Catecholamine Synthesizing Enzymes

Following a single 2-h period of immobilization stress, there are profound changes in mRNA levels of adrenal biosynthetic enzymes but very little change in enzyme activity and protein levels. Compared to values in unstressed controls, TH mRNA levels increase by approximately 600%, DBH mRNA levels increase by approximately 100%, and PNMT mRNA levels increase by approximately 200% (**Table 3**). In contrast, following a single 2-h period of immobilization stress TH, DBH, and PNMT enzyme activities and protein levels do not change significantly. Note here the dissociation between the levels of message for the CA biosynthetic enzymes versus the actual levels of enzyme activity. Note, too, that increases in DBH mRNA levels are just as likely to not be increased significantly following a single episode of immobilization stress.

These changes in mRNA levels for adrenal CA-synthesizing enzymes following a single period of immobilization stress are transient and reach the peak levels 3 h after the immobilization is completed. Twenty-four hours following a single 2-h period of immobilization stress, mRNA levels for TH, DBH, and PNMT return toward baseline levels and are no longer significantly different from unstressed control levels (**Table 3**).

Recently, methods for quantitative evaluation of gene expression of CA biosynthetic enzymes became available. Kvetnansky and coworkers for the first time quantified basal and stress-induced concentrations of TH, DBH, and PNMT mRNA in rat adrenal medulla, sympathetic ganglia, and various brain nuclei by the reverse transcription (RT)-competitive polymerase chain reaction (PCR) method using corresponding competitors of known concentration.

In the adrenal medulla, the basal concentration of TH mRNA was approximately 0.5 amol ng^{-1} of total RNA. DBH mRNA was approximately 12 times higher (6.0 amol ng^{-1} RNA) and PNMT mRNA was approximately 56 times higher (28.0 amol ng^{-1} RNA) than TH mRNA. In the stellate ganglia, the basal concentration of TH mRNA was approximately 30 times lower than in the adrenal medulla, but the concentration of DBH mRNA in the ganglia was similar to the adrenal medulla. Unexpectedly, the presence of a low level of PNMT mRNA has been

Table 3 Adrenal mRNA levels (in arbitrary units) of TH, DBH, and PNMT under basal conditions and immediately and 24 h following one 2-h period of immobilization stress

Enzyme	*Baseline*	*Post-IMMO*	*24 h post-IMMO*
TH	1.00 ± 0.21	7.50 ± 0.50**	1.60 ± 0.25
DBH	1.00 ± 0.10	1.88 ± 0.49*	1.42 ± 0.50
PNMT	1.00 ± 0.32	3.00 ± 0.33**	1.52 ± 0.20

Values are means ± SEM. * indicates $P < 0.05$ and ** indicates $P < 0.01$ compared to unstressed controls. DBH, dopamine-β-hydroxylase; IMMO, immobilization stress; PNMT, phenylethanolamine-N-methyltransferase; TH, tyrosine hydroxylase.

detected for the first time in the sympathetic ganglia of rats.

Immobilization stress produced approximately a sixfold increase of TH mRNA (3.0 amol ng^{-1} RNA), a 2.5-fold increase of DBH mRNA (15.0 amol ng^{-1} RNA), and approximately a fivefold increase in PNMT mRNA (140.0 amol ng^{-1} RNA), in spite of the fact that basal levels of PNMT mRNA were already very high. Twenty-four hours after the end of immobilization exposure, the mRNA concentrations of all three adrenomedullary enzymes returned to control values (in the sympathetic ganglia, in contrast, the highest concentrations were detected during this time interval). Thus, the lowest concentration of TH mRNA in the adrenal medulla and sympathetic ganglia supports the hypothesis that TH is the rate-limiting step in the biosynthesis of CAs.

Effects of Repeated Immobilization Stress on Adrenal Catecholamine-Synthesizing Enzymes

The adrenal response to repeated immobilization stress is summarized in **Table 4**. Compared to unstressed control rats, rats exposed to immobilization stress for 2 h per day for 6 consecutive days had significant elevations in adrenal medullary mRNA levels of TH, DBH, and PNMT even 24 h after the last stress exposure. In addition, TH, DBH, and PNMT enzyme activities and protein levels were already increased significantly, and each of these changes persisted for at least 24 h. A similar pattern of results was obtained following as few as two consecutive daily bouts of immobilization stress. However, repeated immobilization does not produce further increases in mRNA concentrations compared to the elevated values found in the adapted control group (measured 24 h after six daily immobilization periods). The levels of enzyme immunoproteins both in the adrenal medulla and sympathetic ganglia were significantly increased only after repeated immobilization.

These findings reveal that the adrenal medulla exhibits a transient increase in TH, DBH, and PNMT transcriptional activities following a single 2-h period of immobilization stress. However, these increases in transcriptional activities are not accompanied by increases in enzyme proteins and activities. If animals are exposed daily to immobilization stress for 2–6 days, increases in TH, DBH, and PNMT transcriptional activities, as well as levels of enzyme protein and activity, are enhanced and these increases are maintained for at least 24 h. Thus, the adrenal medulla of repeatedly stressed animals exhibits a significant and long-lasting enhancement of CA biosynthetic capacity already at the level of gene expression. However, as previously noted, these increases in CA biosynthetic capacity develop as the adrenal medulla habituates to repeated immobilization stress and actually releases significantly less EPI with each repeated daily exposure to stress. The importance of the increase in CA biosynthetic capacity is unmasked when a repeatedly stressed animal is exposed to a novel stressor and EPI release from the adrenal medulla is amplified over and above that of a first-time-stressed control.

The pattern of transcriptional activation and translational control of CA-synthesizing enzymes differs in other models of stress. For example, in animals continuously exposed to a cold environment, TH mRNA levels increased by approximately threefold above baseline within 3–6 h after the start of cold exposure and remained elevated throughout. Levels of TH protein peaked after 3 days of continuous cold exposure and TH activity peaked after 6–7 days of continuous cold exposure. Other stressors such as insulin-induced hypoglycemia, administration of 2-deoxyglucose, and hypoxia have also been shown to affect increases in mRNA, protein levels, and activity of these enzymes in the adrenal medulla. Even social hierarchy affects the gene expression of these enzymes in rats. Gene expression and protein levels were higher in subordinate than in dominant rats.

Finally, it is important to note that stress-induced increases in CA biosynthetic enzymes also occur in tissues other than the adrenal medulla. For example, such changes have been described in various sympathetic ganglia, the heart (PNMT only), several hypothalamic nuclei, and noradrenergic cell bodies of the nucleus locus ceruleus and other brain-stem nuclei.

Table 4 Adrenal mRNA levels and activities of TH, DBH, and PNMT under basal conditions and immediately following six daily 2-h periods of immobilization stress[a]

Enzyme	*Baseline*	*mRNA levels post-IMMO*[b]	*Enzyme activity post-IMMO*[b]
TH	100 ± 25	375 ± 20**	320 ± 25**
DBH	100 ± 15	385 ± 40**	255 ± 25**
PNMT	100 ± 10	330 ± 25**	160 ± 10*

[a]Values are means ± SEM. * indicates $P < 0.05$ and ** indicates $P < 0.01$ compared to unstressed controls. DBH, dopamine-β-hydroxylase; IMMO, immobilization stress; PNMT, phenylethanolamine-N-methyltransferase; TH, tyrosine hydroxylase.
[b]Expressed as percentage of unstressed controls.

Factors Influencing Gene Transcription in the Adrenal Medulla during Stress

The Splanchnic Nerve

The chromaffin cells of the adrenal medulla are innervated by terminals arising from the splanchnic nerve. It has been hypothesized that splanchnic input is critical for the enhanced transcription of genes for TH, DBH, PNMT, and various neuropeptides during stressful stimulation. Kvetnansky, Sabban, and their colleagues tested this hypothesis by examining the effects of adrenal denervation on the transcriptional activation of TH, PNMT, and NPY by various stressors.

In their first experiment, the right adrenal gland was intact and the left adrenal gland was denervated in a group of laboratory rats. These animals were then immobilized for 2 h and were sacrificed 3 h later. The results indicated that the immobilization-induced increases in mRNAs for PNMT and TH were not dependent on an intact splanchnic nerve. In contrast, splanchnectomy abolished the stress-induced increase in NPY mRNA (**Table 5**). In other experiments, it has been shown that an intact splanchnic nerve is required for the increase in enzyme activites for TH and PNMT following immobilization stress. Taken together, these results demonstrate that the splanchnic nerve does play a critical role in the immobilization-stress-induced increase in NPY mRNA and in the increase in TH and PNMT enzyme activities. However, other as yet unidentified factors are responsible for the immobilization-stress-induced increases in TH mRNA. It should be noted that glucocorticoids are an important regulator of PNMT gene expression.

In another set of experiments, Kvetnansky, Sabban, and their coworkers examined the role of splanchnic input on increases in TH mRNA following three different stressors: cold exposure, insulin-induced hypoglycemia, and immobilization (**Table 6**). With chronic cold exposure and with insulin-induced hypoglycemia, TH mRNA increased several-fold above basal levels in the intact adrenal, but this increase was completely abolished in the denervated adrenal. In contrast, with immobilization stress there was a significant increase in TH mRNA levels in both the intact and the denervated adrenals. Additional experiments demonstrated that the immobilization-induced increase in adrenal medullary TH mRNA levels is also not dependent on the pituitary gland. The administration of adrenocorticotropic hormone (ACTH) elicited the induction of TH and DBH gene expression in the rat sympathetic ganglia but not in the adrenal medulla. The ganglia (not the adrenal medulla) were found to express mRNA for melanocortin (MC-2) receptors, which increased after immobilization. Thus, ACTH via the MC-2 receptors may be directly involved in the stress-elicited regulation of NE biosynthesis in the sympathetic ganglia but not in the adrenal medulla. The factors that regulate the increase in TH mRNA in the adrenal medulla of immobilized animals are as yet unknown.

Modulation of Transcription

The expression of genes that encode CA biosynthetic enzymes in the adrenal medulla is mediated by transcriptional mechanisms. The persistence of

Table 5 Influence of the splanchnic nerve on transcriptional activation of TH, PNMT, and NPY under basal conditions and 3 h following one 2-h period of immobilization stress

Treatment	*TH mRNA*	*PNMT mRNA*	*NPY mRNA*
Sham	100 ± 33	100 ± 17	100 ± 29
Sham + IMMO	479 ± 76**	863 ± 82**	259 ± 35*
Denervated	100 ± 21	110 ± 21	88 ± 35
Denervated + IMMO	426 ± 72**	776 ± 132**	79 ± 14

Reproduced from Sabban, E. L., Nankova, B., Hiremagalur, B., et al. (1996), Molecular mechanisms in immobilization stress elicited rise in expression of genes for adrenal catecholamine biosynthetic enzymes, neuropeptide Y and proenkephalin. In: McCarty, R., Aguilera, G., Sabban, E. L. & Kvetnansky. R. (eds.) *Stress: molecular genetic and neurobiological advances,* pp. 611–628. New York: Gordon and Breach. Values are means ± SEM and are expressed as a percentage of the sham-operated right adrenal gland. * indicates $P < 0.05$ and ** indicates $P < 0.01$ compared to the appropriate sham or denervated control group. IMMO, immobilization stress; NPY, neuropeptide Y; PNMT, phenylethanolamine-N-methyltransferase; TH, tyrosine hydroxylase.

Table 6 Influence of the splanchnic nerve on transcriptional activation of TH under basal conditions and after exposure to three stressors[a]

Treatment	*Cold stress*[b]	*Insulin*[c]	*IMMO*[d]
Sham control	100 ± 5	100 ± 23	100 ± 30
Sham + stress	302 ± 36**	375 ± 68**	478 ± 77**
Denervated control	106 ± 12	101 ± 34	100 ± 19
Denervated + stress	104 ± 13	112 ± 37	425 ± 70**

[a]Adapted from Kvetnansky, R. and Sabban, E. L. (1998). Stress and molecular biology of neurotransmitter-related enzymes. In Csermely, P. (ed.) *Special issue on stress of life: from molecules to man. Annals of the New York Academy of Sciences* **851**, 342–356. Values are means ± SEM and are expressed in arbitrary units. ** indicates $P < 0.01$ compared to the appropriate sham or denervated control group. IMMO, immobilization stress; TH, tyrosine hydroxylase.

[b]Cold stress for 5 days at 5°C.

[c]Insulin-induced hypoglycemia (5 h after administration of 5.0 IU/kg).

[d]Single 2-h period of immobilization stress with sacrifice 3 h later.

transcription depends on the duration and repetition of stress stimuli. Recent work identified various transcription factors that are associated with brief or intermediate duration of a single or repeated stressors.

A detailed discussion of the transcription factors and promotors involved in stress-induced increases in mRNAs for TH, DBH, PNMT, and various neuropeptides is beyond the scope of this article. However, it has been shown that the genes coding for the CA biosynthetic enzymes contain several regulatory genomic elements in their promoters. These include the CRE, GRE, API, AP2, POU/Oct, and SP1 sites. The signaling molecules that may influence the transcription rates of the genes for TH, DBH, and PNMT include P-cAMP response element binding protein (-CREB), c-Jun N-terminal kinase (JNK), c-fos, Egr-l, Fra-1, Fra-2, and others. These and other promoters and signaling molecules interact in a complex fashion to regulate mRNA levels for the various adrenal medullary biosynthetic enzymes and neuropeptides under basal conditions and during exposure to stress. The involvement of transcription factors in regulation of gene expression of CA biosynthetic enzymes during stress is not clear yet. However, the present status in the adrenal medulla is as follows. A single episode of stress response-triggered the elevation of c-fos and Fras, activation of the mitogen-activated protein kinase (MAPK) JNK, and induction of AP-1 factors, Egr-1, and phosphorylation of CREB. With repeated daily stress exposure, Fra-2 was a major AP-1 factor induced in the adrenal medulla but Egr-1 levels were also markedly elevated. For PNMT gene expression, two transcription factors are especially important: glucocorticoid receptor and Egr-1. The crucial role of glucocorticoids in PNMT gene regulation has also been confirmed in corticotropin releasing hormone (CRH) knockout mice.

Thus, different transcription pathways are involved in the mediation of the elevated gene expression of CA biosynthetic enzymes during acute or chronic/repeated stress. Recently, the genetic determinants of the sympathoadrenal response to stress have been mapped.

Summary and Conclusion

The adrenal medulla and the concept of stress are inextricably intertwined. The adrenal medulla may function in concert with the sympathetic nervous system, or it may function somewhat independently in meeting the homeostatic demands presented by a variety of stressful stimuli. Although EPI secretion has been the primary focus of physiological studies of the adrenal medulla, it is now apparent that the adrenal medulla secretes a complex array of neuropeptides that exerts effects in the adrenal medulla and throughout the body. The adrenal medulla is innervated by preganglionic sympathetic nerve terminals that release acetylcholine and various colocalized peptides.

A major focus of studies beginning in the early 1970s concerned the ways in which the adrenal medulla responds to acute versus repeated exposure to stress. With the advent of sensitive and specific assay techniques, it has been shown that a complex cascade of biosynthetic changes occurs within the adrenal medulla as animals adapt to stressful stimuli.

Finally, an important lesson that has been learned relates to the stressor-specific pattern of molecular responses of the adrenal medulla. Although many stressors result in increases in mRNA levels for TH and other biosynthetic enzymes, these changes may be dependent on an intact splanchnic nerve or on an as yet unidentified mechanism that is independent of the splanchnic nerve.

In spite of thousands of experiments on the adrenal medulla and stress, there are many important questions that await answers. What mechanism explains the reduced secretion of EPI from the adrenal medulla of animals exposed to chronic intermittent stress and the enhanced secretion of EPI following the exposure of chronically stressed animals to a novel stressor? What factors regulate the increased levels of mRNAs for TH, DBH, and PNMT in the adrenal medulla versus other organs following exposure to various stressors? What are the roles played by the various neuropeptides that are released from splanchnic nerve terminals and from adrenal medullary chromaffin cells, and how do these substances interact with EPI? What is the exact mechanism of the transcription process and involvement of transcription factors during a single and chronic stress exposure? These and other questions are being addressed by many research groups throughout the world. As answers become available, our knowledge of the physiological and molecular aspects of stress will be enhanced.

See Also the Following Articles

Adrenal Cortex; Adrenaline.

Further Reading

Goldstein, D. S. (2001). *The autonomic nervous system in health and disease*. New York: Marcel Dekker.

Goldstein, D. S. (2003). Catecholamines and stress. *Endocrine Regulations* 37, 69–80.

Johnson, E. O., Kamilaris, T. C., Chrousos, G. P., et al. (1992). Mechanisms of stress: a dynamic overview of hormonal and behavioral homeostasis. *Neuroscience and Biobehavioral Reviews* **16**, 115–130.

Klimes, I., Weston, K., Gasperikova, D., et al. (2005). Mapping of genetic determinants of the sympathoneural response to stress. *Physiological Genomics* **20**, 183–187.

Kubovcakova, L., Tybitanclova, K., Sabban, E. L., et al. (2004). Catecholamine synthesizing enzymes and their modulation by immobilization stress in knockout mice. *Annals of the New York Academy of Sciences* **1018**, 458–465.

Kvetnansky, R. (2004). Stressor specificity and effect of prior experience on catecholamine biosynthetic enzyme phenylethanolamine N-methyltransferase. *Annals of the New York Academy of Sciences* **1032**, 117–129.

Kvetnansky, R., Jelokova, J., Rusnak, M., et al. (2002). Novel stressors exaggerate tyrosine hydroxylase gene expression in the adrenal medulla of rats exposed to long-term cold stress. In: McCarty, R., Aguilera, G., Sabban, E. L. & Kvetnansky, R. (eds.) *Stress: neural, endocrine and molecular studies*, pp. 121–128. London: Taylor and Francis.

Kvetnansky, R., Micutkova, L., Kubovcakova, L., et al. (2004). Localization and regulation of phenylethanolamine N-methyltransferase gene expression in the heart of rats and mice during stress. *Annals of the New York Academy of Sciences* **1018**, 405–417.

Kvetnansky, R., Micutkova, L., Rychkova, N., et al. (2004). Quantitative evaluation of catecholamine enzymes gene expression in adrenal medulla and sympathetic ganglia of stressed rats. *Annals of the New York Academy of Sciences* **1018**, 356–369.

Kvetnansky, R., Nankova, B. B., Rusnak, M., et al. (2002). Differential gene expression of tyrosine hydroxylase in rats exposed long-term to various stressors. In: Nagatsu, T., Nabeshima, T., McCarty, R. & Goldstein, D. S. (eds.) *Catecholamine research: from molecular insights to clinical medicine*, pp. 317–320. New York: Kluwer Academic/Plenum.

Kvetnansky, R. and Sabban, E. L. (1993). Stress-induced changes in tyrosine hydroxylase and other catecholamine biosynthetic enzymes. In: Naoi, M. & Parvez, S. H. (eds.) *Tyrosine hydroxylase: from discovery to cloning*, pp. 253–281. Utrecht: VSP Press.

Kvetnansky, R. and Sabban, E. L. (1998). Stress and molecular biology of neurotransmitter-related enzymes. In: Csermely, P. (ed.) *Special issue on stress of life: from molecules to man. Annals of the New York Academy of Sciences* **851**, 342–356.

McCarty, R. and Gold, P. E. (1996). Catecholamines, stress and disease: a psychobiological perspective. *Psychosomatic Medicine* **58**, 590–597.

Pohorecky, L. A., Blakley, G. G., Kubovcakova, L., et al. (2004). Social hierarchy affects gene expression for catecholamine biosynthetic enzymes in rat adrenal glands. *Neuroendocrinology* **80**, 42–51.

Sabban, E. L., Hebert, M. A., Liu, X., et al. (2004). Differential effects of stress on gene transcription factors in catecholaminergic systems. *Annals of the New York Academy of Sciences* **1032**, 130–140.

Sabban, E. L. and Kvetnansky, R. (2001). Stress-triggered activation of gene expression in catecholaminergic systems: dynamics of transcriptional events. *Trends in Neurosciences* **24**, 91–98.

Sabban, E. L., Nankova, B., Hiremagalur, B., et al. (1996). Molecular mechanisms in immobilization stress elicited rise in expression of genes for adrenal catecholamine biosynthetic enzymes, neuropeptide Y and proenkephalin. In: McCarty, R., Aguilera, G., Sabban, E. L. & Kvetnansky, R. (eds.) *Stress: molecular genetic and neurobiological advances*, pp. 611–628. New York: Gordon and Breach.

Sabban, E. L., Nankova, B. B., Serova, L. I., et al. (2004). Molecular regulation of gene expression of catecholamine biosynthetic enzymes by stress: sympathetic ganglia versus adrenal medulla. *Annals of the New York Academy of Sciences* **1018**, 370–377.

Sabban, E. L., Nankova, B. B., Serova, L. I., et al. (2002). Dynamics of transcriptional events in stress-triggered regulation of adrenal catecholamine biosynthetic enzymes. In: Nagatsu, T., Nabeshima, T., McCarty, R. & Goldstein, D. S. (eds.) *Catecholamine research: from molecular insights to clinical medicine*, pp. 321–324. New York: Kluwer Academic/Plenum.

Tank, A. W., Augonis, C. A., Best, J. A., et al. (1996). Regulation of tyrosine hydroxylase gene expression by multiple receptor-mediated pathways during stress or nicotine treatment. In: McCarty, R., Aguilera, G., Sabban, E. L. & Kvetnansky, R. (eds.) *Stress: molecular genetic and neurobiological advances*, pp. 647–662. New York: Gordon and Breach.

Wong, D. L., Ebert, S. N. and Morita, K. (1996). Glucocorticoid control of phenylethanolamine N-methyltransferase gene expression: implications for stress and disorders of the stress axis. In: McCarty, R., Aguilera, G., Sabban, E. L. & Kvetnansky, R. (eds.) *Stress: molecular genetic and neurobiological advances*, pp. 677–693. New York: Gordon and Breach.

Wong, D. L., Tai, T. C., Wong-Faull, D. C., et al. (2004). Genetic mechanisms for adrenergic control during stress. *Annals of the New York Academy of Sciences* **1018**, 387–397.

Autonomic Nervous System: General Overview

N R Keller and D Robertson
Vanderbilt University, Nashville, TN, USA

Introduction

The autonomic nervous system (ANS) is composed of the sympathetic, parasympathetic, and enteric neurons, and the adrenal medulla. It is one of two major divisions of peripheral nerves, the other being the sensorisomatic nervous system. Reciprocally integrated with central autonomic foci, the ANS maintains homeostasis and adaptive responses to physical and mental stress virtually beyond the awareness of the host. The sympathetic system controls fight-or-flight reactions by increasing sympathetic outflow to the heart and other viscera, while the parasympathetic system maintains basal regulation of bodily functions. The enteric nervous system, on the other hand, manages peristalsis and influences glandular secretions. Among the many different aspects of the ANS, this article focuses primarily on neurotransmission within the sympathetic branch (**Figure 1**).

Neurotransmitters were first proposed as chemical stimulants released by nerve terminals early in the twentieth century. Research in the past 10 to 20 years has generated substantial progress in identifying intra- and extracellular signaling molecules, developmental regulatory transcription factors, metabolic pathways, targeted pharmacologic agents, and the influence of genetic mutations in the pathogenesis of autonomic dysfunction. Along with these discoveries, our understanding of the mechanisms underlying various neurotransmitter disorders has also grown. A sampling of genetic, metabolic, and transport errors is highlighted herein.

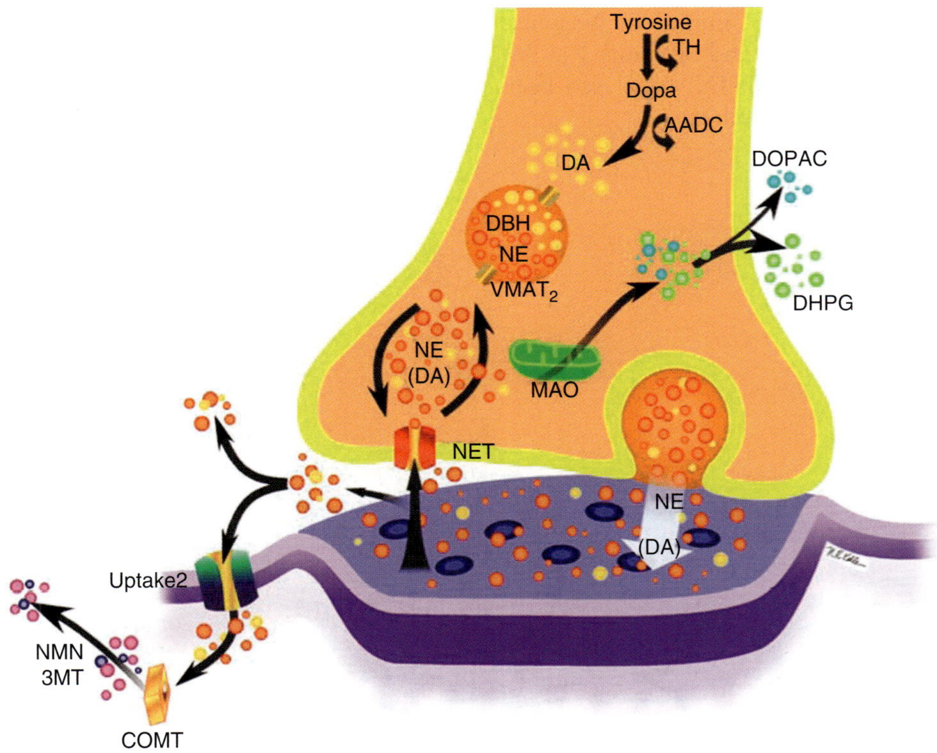

Figure 1 Normal sympathetic neurotransmission. Norepinephrine (NE) is the major neurotransmitter in postganglionic sympathetic and central noradrenergic neurons. Enzymatic conversion of tyrosine to dopamine (DA) takes place in the cytoplasm, whereas transformation of dopamine to NE occurs within the storage vesicles. After release into the synapse, residual catecholamines are pumped back into the presynaptic neuron by the norepinephrine transporter (NET), and returned to storage vesicles by the vesicular monoamine transporter 2 ($VMAT_2$). A smaller portion of the surplus transmitters diffuse into the extracellular space; these transmitters are cleared by the low-affinity, high-capacity 'Uptake 2' transporter, which has recently been renamed the 'extraneuronal monoamine transporter' in humans. Breakdown of cytosolic catecholamines is accomplished in part by monoamine oxidases (MAOs), while extracellular metabolism is conducted by catechol-*O*-methyltransferase (COMT). NMN, normetanephrine; 3MT, 3-methoxytyramine; DBH, dopamine β-hydroxylase; TH, tyrosine hydroxylase; Dopa, dihydroxyphenylalanine; DOPAC, 3,4-dihydroxyphenylacetic acid; AADC, L-aromatic amino acid decarboxylase; DHPG, 3,4-dihydroxyphenylglycol.

Synthesis

Dopamine β-Hydroxylase

Dopamine β-hydroxylase deficiency Dopamine β-hydroxylase (DBH) is an oxidoreductase of the copper type II, ascorbate-dependent monooxygenase family, and is responsible for conversion of dopamine (DA) to norepinephrine (NE). DBH deficiency is an autosomal recessive disorder of heterogeneous nature. The human DBH gene contains 12 exons and is situated at the 9q34 locus, immediately adjacent to the blood group locus ABO. All DBH-deficient patients characterized thus far carry one copy of an IVS1 + 2T → C mutation in intron 1 that prevents appropriate splicing. *In vitro* analysis, however, has shown that this mutation does not entirely explain undetectable levels of DBH protein in plasma, because some properly spliced DBH message can be detected. Instead, concomitant genetic changes such as −1021C → T, which is linked with very low plasma DBH activity, are suspected as inhibitory transcriptional modulators. Thus, NE deficiency may only occur in the context of a specific haplotype, not merely as the result of an individual mutation. Missense mutations of exon 2 (D100E) and of exons 1 and 6 residing *in cis* (V87M and D331N) have also been suggested as pathogenic accomplices.

Both norepinephrine and epinephrine (EPI) are completely absent in plasma, urine, and cerebrospinal fluid (CSF) of humans with DBH deficiency (**Figure 2**), since the enzyme is vital for conversion of DA to NE. Untreated individuals experience a lifetime of severe orthostatic hypotension and mild eyelid ptosis, with some skeletal muscle hypotonia and nasal stuffiness. Perinatal progress is understandably precarious; near-fatal events in the first few days of life include hypotension, hypoglycemia, hypothermia, and seizures. In survivors, delay in eye opening may occur. Because neonates with undetected enzyme insufficiency may succumb to such complications, it is possible that the incidence of DBH deficiency is greater than predicted based on the number of affected adults, although it is still quite rare.

The lack of sympathetic tone severely limits the hemodynamic response to upright posture, with systolic blood pressure (BP) routinely falling well below 100 mmHg with a relatively small increase in heart rate (HR). Presyncopal dizziness is often accompanied by dyspnea, nuchal discomfort, and occasional chest pain. Dizziness is exacerbated by warm environmental temperature. For these reasons, individuals with DBH deficiency are not able to tolerate physical exercise. Hypothermia is seen in infants. Male reproduction is complicated by retrograde ejaculation.

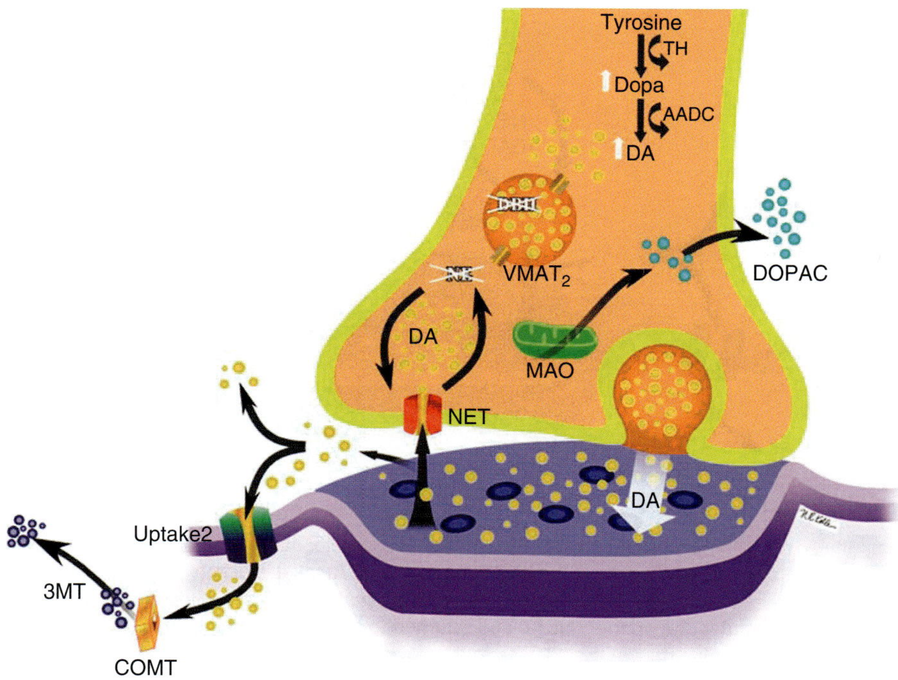

Figure 2 Dopamine β-hydroxylase (DBH) deficiency. Lack of DBH causes the total absence of norepinephrine (NE) in noradrenergic nerve terminals. Sympathetic neurotransmission, therefore, results in the release of dopamine (DA). Because there is no NE-mediated negative feedback on tyrosine hydroxylase (TH), DA production is increased. Reuptake of synaptic DA occurs through the norepinephrine transporter (NET). Enzymatic breakdown yields increased DA metabolites. (Other abbreviations as in **Figure 1**.)

Autonomic testing in DBH deficiency is abnormal for sympathetic function. No increase in BP is elicited in the cold pressor test, isometric handgrip, or phase IV of the Valsalva maneuver. Patients are normal, however, with respect to sweating, lacrimation, salivation, corneal and deep tendon reflexes, sensory function, and the senses of taste and smell. Gastrointestinal function is within normal limits, and bladder function is preserved. Nocturnal polyuria with increased dopamine-mediated natriuresis is a shared feature of the disease.

Sympathetic nerve endings in DBH deficiency appear normal and stain positive for cytosolic tyrosine hydroxylase, the rate-limiting enzyme in DA synthesis. Normally, DA is taken into the vesicles for conversion to NE by DBH. Without dopamine transformation, however, it is released from stimulated noradrenergic nerve terminals in place of NE. DBH is also present in the normal adrenal medulla, thus the effects of enzyme failure are undetectable tissue EPI and NE.

Without NE-mediated negative feedback on tyrosine hydroxylase, cytosolic DA production is amplified. Plasma levels of DA, therefore, are notably elevated; approximately five- to tenfold. Urine DA is more than doubled and CSF levels are also increased. The DA metabolites homovanillic acid (HVA) and 3-methoxytyramine (3MT) are roughly double normal values in urine. Plasma and CSF dihydroxyphenylalanine (DOPA) levels are double to triple normal values. As might be expected, prolactin is low. The NE metabolites 3-methoxy-4-hydroxyphenylglycol (MHPG) and normetanephrine (NM) are below detectable limits in urine.

Patients can be successfully treated with droxidopa (dihydroxyphenylserine, or L-DOPS), which is endogenously converted to NE by L-aromatic amino acid decarboxylase (AADC). Both intraneuronal and extraneuronal conversions take place, since AADC is present in most tissues. Adrenomedullary conversion of DA to NE does not occur, however, and EPI levels remain undetectable. With drug administration, BP increases dramatically and NE concentrations approach the normal range in plasma and urine. Consequently, standing time is greatly enhanced, as is quality of life – so improved, in fact, that in 2005 a 26-year-old patient treated with droxidopa for less than 2 years of her life was able to compete in and finish a 26-mile marathon.

Menkes Disease

Menkes disease is an X-linked fatal neurodegenerative disease caused by impaired copper transport in the gastrointestinal tract, placenta, and the blood–brain barrier, resulting in systemic deficiency of the element. Mutations in the *ATP7A* gene are responsible for the defective protein, MNK, a P-type ATPase that belongs to the CPx-type family of transmembrane enzymes necessary for ATP-dependent translocation of metal cations across cell membranes. MNK typically resides in the *trans*-Golgi network, where it delivers copper to local enzymes, including DBH. The ATPase can also be found in cytosolic vesicular compartments and the plasma membrane, where it mediates efflux of excess copper.

Copper is an essential cofactor for DBH. Consequently, plasma catecholamines are abnormally low, although NE levels in the CSF may be normal or elevated. Typically, however, because DBH activity is impaired, plasma and CSF DOPA, DA, and dihydroxyphenylacetic acid (DOPAC) are elevated. Ratios of plasma DOPA to dihydroxyphenylglycol (DHPG), the chief neuronal metabolite of NE, are increased approximately sevenfold, and DOPAC to DHPG ratios are about fivefold greater. CSF ratios follow a similar pattern. In addition, the proportion of HVA to vanillylmandelic acid (HVA:VMA) increases in the urine.

Early detection and treatment of the disease is crucial, since copper deficiency begins during gestation. Affected infants often appear normal until 2 to 3 months of age. Clinical symptoms vary somewhat depending on the exact mutation, but most neonates experience seizures, severe hypotonia, hypothermia, and extreme developmental delay. Connective tissue abnormalities due to impaired lysyl oxidase may appear as hyperelastic skin, hernias, and aortic aneurysms. Copper administration, however, does not correct these developmental defects. The most striking outward symptom may be the appearance of the hair, which is unusually short, sparse, coarse, and twisted, and is often lightly pigmented. It has been compared to steel wool, and the disease was formerly referred to as the 'kinky hair syndrome.' The first indicators of autonomic dysfunction are likely temperature instability and hypoglycemia. Without treatment using parenteral copper-histidine, death typically occurs by 3–4 years of age. Copper-histidine therapy for 3 months ordinarily normalizes serum copper, ceruloplasmin, DA, and NE levels.

Tetrahydrobiopterin

Hyperphenylalaninemia (HPA) and phenylketonuria (PKU) are the result of impaired enzymatic action of phenylalanine-4-hydroxylase (PAH). Underlying the PAH malfunction, however, is an array of direct and indirect mechanisms ultimately linked to tetrahydrobiopterin (BH4) deficiency. BH4 is a cofactor for

PAH, tyrosine-3-hydroxylase (TH), and tryptophan-5-hydroxylase (TPH). Impaired hydroxylation of tyrosine and tryptophan results in catecholamine and serotonin deficiencies. Determination of pterins and neurotransmitter metabolites in CSF is paramount in establishing an early treatment plan.

Clinical features, along with specific biochemical criteria, distinguish disease variants. The terms 'severe' (typical, general) and 'mild' (atypical, peripheral, partial) are used to describe symptoms, and indicate the need for treatment with neurotransmitter precursors. Symptoms may not be obvious within the first few weeks of life, but are usually apparent by the fourth month. Severe forms of BH4 deficiency manifest as mental retardation, tone and posture abnormalities, convulsions, somnolence, irritability, dyskinesias, hypersalivation and difficulty swallowing, and intermittent hyperthermia without underlying infection. Neurologic symptoms may follow a diurnal pattern, being worst in the evenings and less bothersome in the mornings after rest and neurotransmitter precursor replenishment.

Cofactor deficiency is attributable to genetic mutations in the enzymes responsible for BH4 biosynthesis or regeneration. Here, focus is limited to faulty metabolic pathways causing catecholamine deficiency. Catechol replacement usually consists of droxidopa, with carbidopa added to inhibit peripheral DA production. Levels of plasma phenylalanine warrant close attention when administering neurotransmitter therapy, since high concentrations of phenylalanine can hinder precursor membrane transport or compete with tyrosine.

The form of HPA encountered most is 6-pyruvoyl-tetrahydropterin synthase (PTPS) deficiency, which also exhibits the largest amount of genetic variability. Over 50% of BH4 deficiencies are PTPS and about 80% of affected individuals have the severe form of the disease. Phenotypic expression ordinarily reflects homozygous, compound heterozygous, and obligate heterozygous enzyme activities. Mutations in the PTS gene have been located in all six exons and generally result in a deficient or inactive enzyme product. An exception is the K129E mutant, which demonstrates heightened enzyme activity in a cell-specific manner *in vitro*, suggesting that posttranslational modification plays a role in inducing the upper limits of enzyme performance.

Analysis of urinary pterins discloses that severe PTPS produces the highest amount of neopterin of the BH4 deficiencies, while levels in the mild form are comparable to the pterin-4α-carbinolamine dehydratase (PCD) deficiency profile. Neurotransmitter metabolites are often normal in the CSF of persons with the mild version, as they are in the rarer intermediate form of PTPS deficiency, whereas urinary pterin concentrations are similar to the severe variety. Milder symptoms can worsen with age, and CSF neurotransmitter levels, although normal soon after birth, decrease in accordance with neurological decline.

Most patients with dihydropteridine reductase (DHPR) deficiency lack enzyme activity entirely, or nearly so. Thus, the majority of patients have the severe phenotype. About half are found in southern Europe. Again, mutations are distributed fairly evenly throughout the gene, and most are of the missense type. Urine biopterin levels are higher than in any other BH4 deficiency, and pterin synthesis in general is increased due to lack of feedback inhibition of GTP cyclohydrolase I (GTPCH). Neopterin is normal or slightly elevated. The CSF neurotransmitter metabolic profile is similar to severe PTPS deficiency, with HVA levels more than twice those of 5-hydroxyindoleacetic acid (5HIAA). An unrelated consequence of DHPR deficiency is central folate depletion, presumed to be due to accumulation of 7,8-dihydrobiopterin that competitively interferes with reduction of 7,8-dihydrofolic acid to the active tetrahydrofolic acid.

Both GTP cyclohydrolase I (GTPCH) deficiency and PCD are relatively rare compared to other BH4 disease varieties, with the former being somewhat variable clinically but in general, more severe. Pterins are virtually undetectable in urine from GTPCH patients since the enzyme participates in early pterin synthesis, while neopterin is elevated in PCD. In CSF, pterins follow a similar trend, although both neopterin and biopterin are increased in PCD. Neurotransmitter metabolites are below normal in both disorders as well.

Metabolism

Monoamine Oxidase

Monoamine oxidase (MAO) is located in the outer mitochondrial membrane where oxidative deamination of neuroactive, vasoactive, and xenobiotic amines occurs (**Figure 3**), producing hydrogen peroxide and aldehydes. MAO-A and MAO-B are encoded by two adjacent gene products on the X-chromosome, with different molecular weights and immunological properties. They share about 70% homology and neurons routinely contain both forms. Norepinephrine and serotonin (5-hydroxytryptamine; 5-HT) are preferential substrates for MAO-A, while dopamine, phenylethylamine, and benzylamine are metabolized by MAO-B. Dopamine, tyramine, and tryptamine are substrates of both isoenzymes.

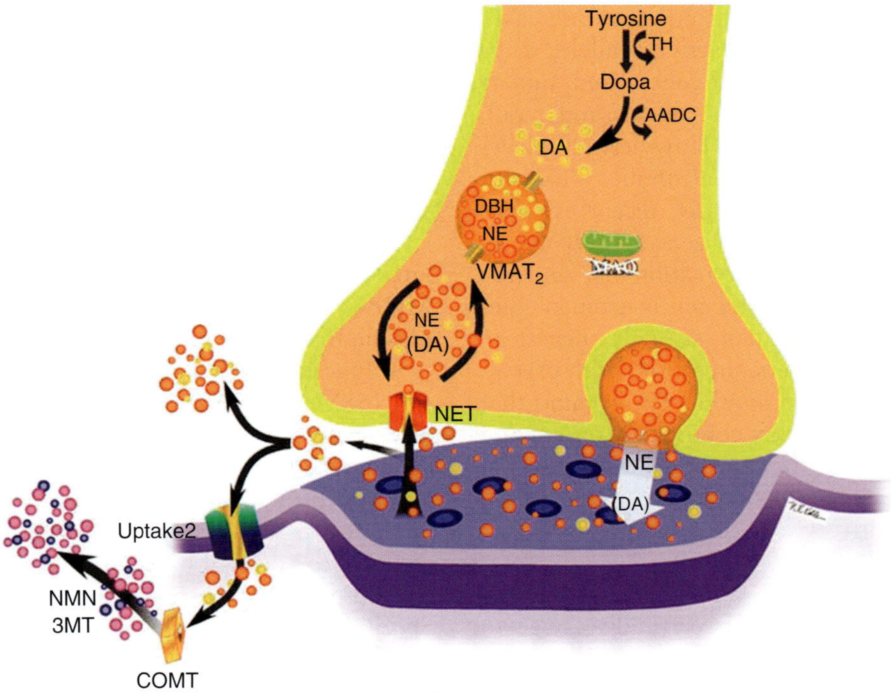

Figure 3 Monoamine oxidase (MAO) deficiency. Norepinephrine (NE) and 5-hydroxytryptamine are metabolized by MAO-A, while dopamine (DA), phenylethylamine, and benzylamine are broken down by MAO-B. Dopamine, tyramine, and tryptamine are substrates of both isoenzymes. Deficiency of only one gene product is reflected by the absence of its corresponding metabolites. Without oxidative deamination of NE by MAO-A in sympathetic nerves, for example, 3,4-dihydroxyphenylglycol will not be formed. Lack of both enzyme subtypes would result in the loss of both 3,4-dihydroxyphenylglycol and 3,4-dihydroxyphenylacetic acid. Metabolites of catechol-*O*-methyltransferase (COMT) will increase. (Other abbreviations as in **Figure 1**.)

MAO has been implicated in the pathogenesis of neurodegeneration, including that underlying Parkinson's disease. Active transport of catecholamines into neuronal vesicles is dynamically opposed by passive leakage into the cytoplasm. Historically, neurotoxicity has been explained by nonenzymatic autooxidation of cytoplasmic catecholamines and the formation of reactive quinones, free radical production, and formation of alkaloids via condensation reactions. The oxidative by-products of MAO, on the other hand, are deaminated catecholaldehyde metabolites. In fact, 3,4-dihydroxyphenylacetaldehyde (DOPAL) and 3,4-dihydroxyphenylglycolaldehyde (DOPEGAL) are formed in such a manner by deamination of DA and NE/EPI, respectively, by MAO and are highly reactive. Prompt aldehyde metabolism to deaminated acids by aldehyde dehydrogenase or to deaminated alcohols by aldose or aldehyde reductase normally neutralizes the deleterious effects. However, any cytoplasmic imbalance that interferes with vesicular uptake, increases vesicular leakage, or inhibits aldehyde metabolism theoretically favors accumulation of neurotoxins and impending cell damage. Centrally, this could be associated with neurodegenerative changes in dopaminergic neurons and parkinsonian-like movement disorders, whereas buildup of toxic NE metabolites in cardiac sympathetic nerves has been postulated to play a role in orthostatic hypotension due to sympathetic denervation of the heart. Unfortunately, we do not have experimental evidence which implicates all these mechanisms in human disease. If such mechanisms are found to be operative, then MAO inhibitors might reduce neurodegeneration caused by overproduction and/or reduced metabolism of cytoplasmic catecholaldehydes.

MAO inhibitors have long been used in the treatment of depression, and the significance of MAO polymorphisms in psychiatric illness has been widely investigated. Deficiency of either isoenzyme alone or the combination of both will yield characteristic neurochemical profiles. One MAO-A mutation found in a Dutch pedigree yields no active enzyme and is associated with mental retardation and impulsive–aggressive behavior in males. Follow-up animal models have also revealed an aggressive phenotype in male mice lacking MAO-A.

In other human studies, significant variations in upstream coding sequences of the MAO-A gene were found across ethnic groups, consisting of 30 bp repeats present in 2, 3, 3.5, 4, or 5 copies. The polymorphism proved to be functional in regulating the MAO-A promoter, and alleles with a higher number of repeat copies (3.5, 4, and 5) demonstrate increased transcriptional activity. High-activity alleles have been associated with panic and generalized anxiety disorders in females, neuroticism in males, and impulsivity and aggression in males. Low-activity alleles have been associated with male alcoholics with antisocial personality disorder. Finally, recent evidence suggests that increased MAO-A gene activity due to incomplete X chromosome inactivation may underlie the greater prevalence of depression in women compared to men. While these data strongly suggest an association of specific genetic mutations with psychiatric disorders, the reader should keep in mind that different groups often report contrasting results and resolution has proved difficult in some instances. Repeat studies and larger sample sizes are clearly necessary before a definitive association can be claimed for any given diagnosis.

MAO-A and-B deficiency (and Norrie disease gene) The MAO genes are situated next to the Norrie disease (ND) gene on the X chromosome. ND is a neurodevelopmental disorder characterized by congenital blindness caused by incomplete retinal vascularization. Approximately one-third of patients also suffer sensorineural deafness. Mental retardation is not uncommon, but the degree of severity is variable. Patients with atypical ND, by contrast, exhibit profound mental retardation, autistic-like behavior, hypogonadism, atonic seizures, altered peripheral autonomic function, and aberrant biogenic amine metabolism. Such severity is ascribed to large deletions encompassing the MAO and ND gene loci together. Combined MAO-AB deficiency results in >93% reductions in plasma DHPG, MHPG, and VMA, along with elevated plasma normetanephrine and metanephrine resulting from increased catechol-O-methyltransferase (COMT) metabolism. Individuals lacking the ND and MAO-B genes, on the other hand, show no signs of mental retardation or disruptive behavior. MAO-B deficiency is characterized by undetectable levels of platelet MAO-B activity and increased urinary phenylethylamine.

Catechol-*O*-Methyltransferase

Most extraneuronal catecholamine metabolism is accomplished by COMT in the liver and kidney. In addition to catecholamines, COMT also metabolizes L-DOPA, DHPG, DOPAC, and catechol estrogens. Conversion of catechols to their O-methylated metabolites requires *S*-adenosyl-L-methionine as a methyl donor. Two isoenzyme forms of COMT exist, one soluble and the other membrane bound. Soluble COMT is present in most tissues and has higher activity levels compared to the membrane-bound form. The main exception is the adrenal medulla, in which membrane-bound COMT is most prevalent. Pheochromocytomas, catecholamine-producing tumors at adrenomedullary and extraadrenal sites, contain vast amounts of membrane-bound COMT and generate high concentrations of O-methylated metabolites, primarily metanephrine and MHPG. Diagnosis is best accomplished by assaying plasma free metanephrines.

A functional polymorphism of the COMT gene (Val158Met) has been identified that causes amino acid substitution. The wild-type Val allele is associated with high enzyme activity, while the Met substitution produces three- to fourfold lower activity. Globally, there is wide allelic variation, with persons of European descent having the greatest heterozygosity compared to those of African or Asian heritage. Specifically, Europeans have nearly equal frequencies of the two alleles, whereas the majority of populations in other parts of the world express the high-activity allele. Furthermore, high-activity COMT is primarily found in nonhuman primates, implying it is the ancestral allele in humans.

A large genetically homogeneous population-based study conducted in Norway recently revealed an association of the Val/Val genotype with systolic BP $\geq$140 mm Hg compared to either Val/Met or Met/Met genotypes. Although the underlying mechanism was not accounted for, the authors postulate that altered dopamine catabolism may be involved. Dopamine-mediated natriuresis is believed to be important in long-term control of BP. Therefore, elevated COMT activity in the kidney would likely increase dopamine breakdown, thus increasing sodium levels and, ultimately, BP.

The COMT polymorphism has been extensively investigated in anxiety disorders. Despite early promising findings, later studies revealed conflicting results and failed to replicate a significant association of this polymorphism with various subtypes of anxiety, including obsessive–compulsive, general anxiety, and panic disorders, or phobias.

A secondary role for COMT is methylation of 2-OH and 4-OH catechol estrogens. Transformation to methoxy estrogens lowers the risk of breast cancer associated with estrogen-mediated DNA adduct formation or oxidative damage arising from catechol estrogen quinone–semiquinone redox cycling. Cancer risk examined by *in vitro* analysis of the COMT Val $\rightarrow$ Met polymorphism demonstrated that the low-activity Met variant produced two- to threefold lower levels of methoxy estrogens in breast cancer cells compared to the wild-type variant. Therefore, estrogenized women with lower COMT activity may be at increased risk for breast cancer due to elevated tissue concentrations of prooxidative 4-OH catechol estrogens, and lower levels of 2-methoxyestradiol, an antiproliferative metabolite.

Reuptake

Norepinephrine Transporter Dysfunction

Norepinephrine is rapidly recycled by the presynaptic neuron for rerelease. Most NE is removed from the synaptic cleft by active transport via the norepinephrine transporter (NET). The NET is a member of Na^+/Cl^--dependent transporters sharing similar amino acid sequences and pumping mechanisms. Transporters were historically considered to be static proteins intrinsic to the cell surface. Recent evidence, however, has revealed that NET is usually tethered to neuronal vesicles until transmitter release, and that phosphorylation is crucial to cell surface expression. NET is dynamically regulated by both intra- and extracellular signaling molecules, as well as targeted by a host of long-term therapeutic agents and drugs of abuse. Indeed, NET expression is recognized as a means of neuronal adaptation to changes in transmission. Endogenous regulators of NET expression include norepinephrine, acetylcholine, γ-aminobutyric acid (GABA), angiotensin, insulin, natriuretic peptide, nerve growth factor, estrogens, and nitric oxide.

A substitution mutation in the NET gene was discovered in a large family in which affected individuals had orthostatic tachycardia and postural tachycardia syndrome (POTS). The A457P mutation resulted in decreased plasma membrane concentrations of NET in heterozygous individuals. In fact, the altered protein was shown to bind native transporter and reduce its trafficking to the cell surface, making this a dominant-negative mutation. (General NET deficiency is shown in **Figure 4**.) Analysis of 254 additional POTS patients has not yielded similar functional NET mutations to account for diminished NE reuptake. Therefore, POTS remains a dysautonomia of heterogeneous etiology, with NET deficiency a very rare etiology.

POTS is an often debilitating autonomic disorder characterized by excessive tachycardia on standing, elevated plasma NE spillover, and presyncopal/syncopal

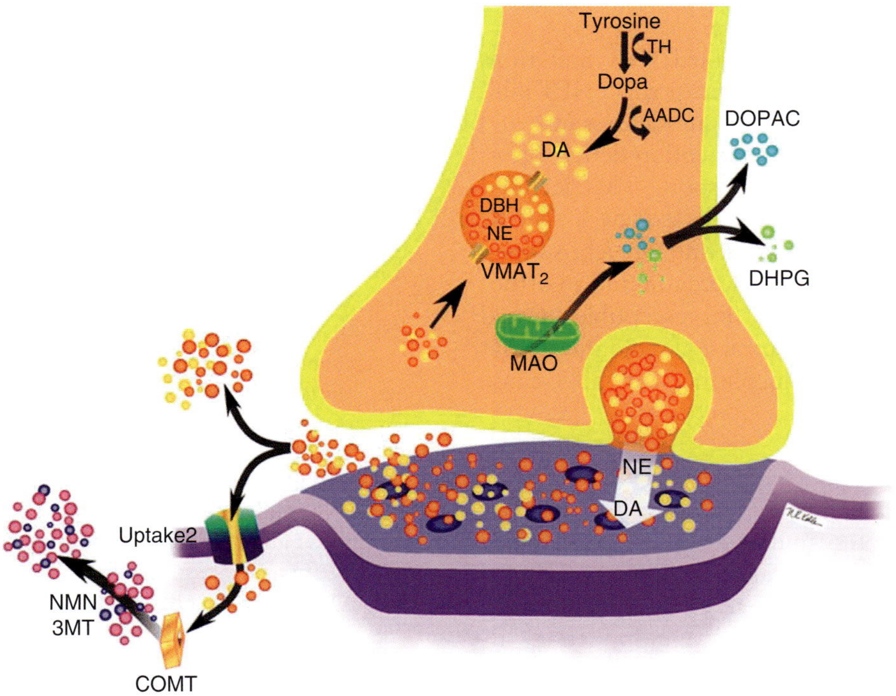

Figure 4 Norepinephrine (NE) transporter deficiency. Residual NE and dopamine (DA) are removed from the synaptic cleft by active transport through the NE transporter. The absence of NE transporter results in an increased concentration of catecholamines in the synapse, prolonging noradrenergic signaling and elevating levels of plasma NE and DA. Because monoamine recycling does not occur, conversion of DA to NE is increased. Continuous neurotransmission can deplete intraneuronal stores of NE, resulting in greater release of precursor and decreased production of 3,4-dihydroxyphenylglycol (DHPG). Metabolites of catechol-*O*-methyltransferase (COMT) are increased. (Other abbreviations as in **Figure 1**.)

episodes. Affected individuals are young and primarily women. In addition to syncopal symptoms, common complaints include dizziness, visual changes, head and neck discomfort, poor concentration while standing, fatigue, palpitations, tremor, and anxiety. In familial POTS, levels of plasma NE increase approximately twice as high as in normal individuals on standing. DHPG concentration is decreased supine and upright, thereby lowering the DHPG:NE ratio. This is in contrast to idiopathic POTS, in which NE spillover is similar to that in normal individuals, both supine and standing.

Numerous naturally occurring single-nucleotide polymorphisms (SNPs) have been identified in the NET gene; these SNPs alter protein synthesis or maturation, transport mechanics, antagonist interactions, and kinase-mediated regulation. Many were discovered in cardiovascular phenotypes, and the role of similar functional mutations has been examined in psychiatric profiles. One such case is an A $\rightarrow$ T polymorphism at −3081 upstream of the transcription initiation site. The T allele was shown to decrease NET promoter function by allowing the binding of transcriptional repressors. A significant association of the mutation was demonstrated with attention-deficit/hyperactivity disorder (ADHD) in a relatively small sample size, but more extensive investigation is needed to confirm these findings.

Although detection of functional NET mutations has thus far been limited, pharmacological NET inhibition is very common. Many antidepressants and medications used in treating attention-deficit disorders block or alter NET transport. This includes first-generation tricyclics as well as newer specific NET inhibitors (e.g., atomoxetine or reboxetine). Pharmacological NET blockade can mimic an orthostatic tachycardia phenotype in susceptible normal subjects. Yohimbine, a central α-2 antagonist that increases synaptic norepinephrine, can also cause orthostatic tachycardia.

Conclusion

In summary, neurotransmitter disorders occur when there is insufficient or exaggerated neurochemical transmission, and can be due to either direct or indirect causes. For example, genetic mutations may affect essential enzymes directly in the synthesis pathway, or indirectly by limiting cofactor function. Multiple mechanisms exist for the clearance and recycling of catecholamines, and gain-of-function or loss-of-function mutations that alter synaptic, cytosolic, or vesicular concentrations often underlie aberrant neurotransmission. Continued investigation of genotype–phenotype associations will provide a better understanding of the pathophysiology of neurotransmitter disorders, allowing new methods for diagnosis and adjustment of treatment options to meet individual needs.

Further Reading

Blakely, R. D., DeFelice, L. J. and Galli, A. (2005). Biogenic amine neurotransmitter transporters: Just when you thought you knew them. *Physiology* **20**, 225–231.

Blau, N., Thony, B., Cotton, R. R. H., et al. (2001). Disorders of tetrahydrobiopterin and related biogenic amines. In: Scriver, C. R., Beaudet, A. L., Sly, W. S., et al. (eds.) *The Metabolic and Molecular Bases of Inherited Disease*, pp. 1725–1776. New York: McGraw-Hill.

Carrel, L. and Willard, H. F. (2005). X-Inactivation profile reveals extensive variability in X-linked gene expression in females. *Nature* **434**, 400–404.

Cox, D. W. and Moore, S. D. P. (2002). Copper transporting P-type ATPases and human disease. *Journal of Bioenergetics and Biomembranes* **34**, 333–338.

Daniel, K. G., Harbach, R. H., Guida, W. C., et al. (2004). Copper storage diseases: Menkes, Wilson's, and cancer. *Frontiers in Bioscience* **9**, 2652–2662.

Eisenhofer, G., Kopin, I. J. and Goldstein, D. S. (2004). Catecholamine metabolism: A contemporary view with implications for physiology and medicine. *Pharmacological Reviews* **56**, 331–349.

Garland, E. M., Hahn, M. K., Ketch, T. P., et al. (2002). Genetic basis of clinical catecholamine disorders. *Annals of the New York Academy of Sciences* **971**, 506–514.

Goldstein, D. S., Eisenhofer, G. and Kopin, I. J. (2003). Sources and significance of plasma levels of catechols and their metabolites in humans. *Journal of Pharmacology and Experimental Therapeutics* **305**, 800–811.

Hagen, K., Pettersen, E., Stovner, L. J., et al. (2007). High systolic blood pressure is associated with Val/Val genotype in the catechol-O-methyltransferase gene. *American Journal of Hypertension* **20**, 21–26.

Hahn, M. K., Mazei-Robison, M. S. and Blakely, R. D. (2005). Single nucleotide polymorphisms in the human norepinephrine transporter gene affect expression, trafficking, antidepressant interaction, and protein kinase C regulation. *Molecular Pharmacology* **68**, 457–466.

Keller, N. R. and Robertson, D. (2006). Familial orthostatic tachycardia. *Current Opinion in Cardiology* **21**, 173–179.

Mandela, P. and Ordway, G. A. (2006). The norepinephrine transporter and its regulation. *Journal of Neurochemistry* **97**, 310–333.

Oeltmann, T., Carson, R., Shannon, J. R., et al. (2004). Assessment of O-methylated catecholamine levels in plasma and urine for diagnosis of autonomic disorders. *Autonomic Neuroscience* **116**, 1–10.

Palmatier, M. A., Kang, A. M. and Kidd, K. K. (1999). Global variation in the frequencies of functionally different catechol-O-methyltransferase alleles. *Biological Psychiatry* **46**, 557–567.

Robertson, D., Biaggioni, I., Burnstock, G., et al. (eds.) (2004). *Primer on the Autonomic Nervous System*, 2nd edn). San Diego: Elsevier Academic Press.

Robertson, D., Goldberg, M. R., Onrot, J., et al. (1986). Isolated failure of autonomic noradrenergic neurotransmission: Evidence for impaired beta-hydroxylation of dopamine. *New England Journal of Medicine* **314**, 1494–1497.

Sabol, S. Z., Hu, S. and Hamer, D. (1998). A functional polymorphism in the monoamine oxidase A gene promoter. *Human Genetics* **103**, 273–279.

Shannon, J. R., Flattem, N. L., Jordan, J., et al. (2000). Orthostatic intolerance and tachycardia associated with norepinephrine-transporter deficiency. *New England Journal of Medicine* **342**, 541–549.

Shih, J. C., Chen, K. and Ridd, M. J. (1999). Monoamine oxidase: From genes to behavior. *Annual Review of Neuroscience* **22**, 197–217.

Vincent, S., Bieck, P. R., Garland, E. M., et al. (2004). Clinical assessment of norepinephrine transporter blockade through biochemical and pharmacological profiles. *Circulation* **109**, 3202–3207.

Zahniser, N. R. and Doolen, S. (2001). Chronic and acute regulation of Na^+/Cl^--dependent neurotransmitter transporters: Drugs, substrates, presynaptic receptors, and signaling systems. *Pharmacology and Therapeutics* **92**, 21–55.

Zhu, B. T. (2002). Catechol-O-methyltransferase(COMT)-mediated methylation metabolism of endogenous bioactive catechols and modulation by endobiotics and xenobiotics: Importance in pathophysiologoy and pathogenesis. *Current Drug Metabolism* **3**, 321–349.

Relevant Websites

http://www.genetests.org – Medical genetics information resource (funded by the National Institutes of Health).

http://www.bh4.org – Tetrahydrobiopterin deficiencies research (Zürich Research Group).

Autonomic Nervous System

W R Lovallo
Veterans Affairs Medical Center and University of Oklahoma Health Sciences Center, Oklahoma City, OK, USA
J J Sollers III
Department of Psychology, Ohio State University, Columbus, OH, USA

This is a revised version of the article by W R Lovallo and J J Sollers III, Encyclopedia of Stress, First edition, volume 1, pp 275–283, © 2000, Elsevier Inc.

Glossary

Brain stem The portion of the brain connecting the cerebral hemispheres with the spinal cord, consisting of the midbrain, the pons, and the medulla.

Endocrine Pertaining to the secretory glands of the body, which release hormones that circulate in the blood to act on distant glands and target tissues to regulate their function.

Ganglion A specialized collection of interconnected nerve cell bodies.

Homeostasis A concept expressing the collective actions of the autonomic nervous system and endocrine system to maintain physiological systems within a range of optimal values consistent with the maintenance of life.

Hypothalamus The collection of brain nuclei located below the thalamus that act to regulate the endocrine system and the autonomic nervous system to maintain homeostatic processes.

Limbic system Brain structures of the cortex and basal ganglia that are involved with motivation and the emotions.

Neurotransmitter A chemical substance supporting communication across a synapse or neuroeffector junction.

Receptor A complex protein molecule that is embedded within a cell membrane having chemical affinities for one or more neurotransmitters and that initiates a response by the cell.

In the course of daily life, we must rest or be active, obtain food and digest it, and, occasionally, cope with an exceptional challenge. At all times, during normal activity and during extreme stress, our brain coordinates the actions of our vital organs and our muscles to ensure our survival. The brain uses two systems to do this, the nervous system and the endocrine system. This article describes one branch of the nervous system, called the autonomic nervous system, which plays a central role in the stress response and in normal regulation.

Background

The peripheral nervous system has two branches: the somatic motor system, which controls voluntary movement, and the autonomic nervous system (ANS), which regulates the internal organs and the eyes. There are five main points to consider regarding the ANS and its role in the stress response: (1) the ANS, along with the endocrine system, regulates the vital organs and coordinates their functions; (2) the ANS is part of a layered set of controls over organ function, starting at the local organ and ending with the brain; (3) the ANS is controlled directly by two brain areas, the brain stem and hypothalamus, and indirectly by higher brain centers, including the prefrontal cortex; (4) during normal activity, the vital organs regulate themselves with little outside help, but during stress the ANS is needed to coordinate their actions; and (5) during psychological stress, the bodily responses we experience originate in higher brain centers that act on the brain stem and hypothalamus to cause changes in the body via the ANS.

Two historic figures have shaped our understanding of the functions of the ANS during stress: Claude Bernard (1813–1878), the French physiologist, who showed that living things must respond to changes in their external environment and in the internal environment (the blood and bodily fluids) to maintain proper cellular and organ function, and Walter Cannon (1871–1945), an American physiologist, who coined the term "homeostasis" to describe these processes of self-regulation. He showed that homeostasis was served primarily by actions of the ANS along with the endocrine system. Cannon demonstrated that the ANS reacts to emergencies in a pattern of widespread activation that he called the fight-or-flight response.

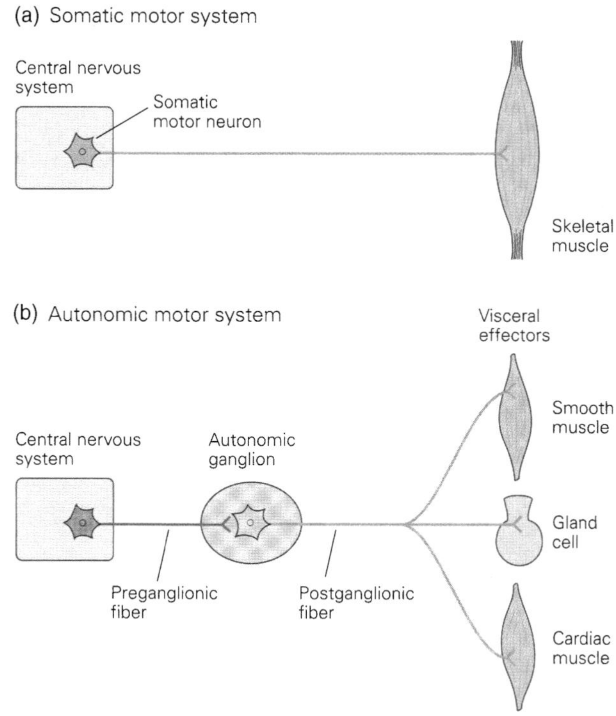

Figure 1 Neurons innervating the skeletal muscles (a) and the vital organs (b). (a) Skeletal motor nerves. Motor neurons that control the skeletal muscles travel from the motor portions of the cerebral cortex, down the spinal cord, and directly to individual muscle fiber bundles without synapsing with other neurons. (b) Autonomic nerves. The autonomic nervous system has two sets of neurons. Preganglionic neurons originate in the pons and medulla of the brain stem. They descend by way of the spinal cord and travel to autonomic ganglia, where they synapse with postganglionic neurons that travel to specific effector organs. There are three types of autonomic effectors: smooth muscle cells, secretory cells, and cardiac muscle. From Iversen, S., Iversen, L. and Saper, C. B. (2000). The autonomic nervous system and the hypothalamus. In: Kandel, E. R., Schwartz, J. J. & Jessel, J. H. (eds.) *Principles of neural science* (4th edn., pp. 960–981). New York: McGraw-Hill. Copyright The McGraw-Hill Companies, Inc. Used with permission.

Autonomic Nervous System Compared to the Somatic Motor System

There are four points of comparison between the somatic motor nervous system and the ANS: (1) both of them are motor systems that regulate the activity of muscle fibers or secretory cells; (2) the somatic nervous system allows voluntary control over muscles, while the ANS automatically regulates the vital organs and related tissues without voluntary control; (3) somatic nerves always activate contraction of the somatic muscles, while ANS fibers will either activate or inhibit the vital organs; and (4) there are two anatomical differences between the somatic nervous system and the ANS (**Figure 1**). In the somatic nervous system, a nerve fiber goes directly from the central nervous system to a skeletal muscle. The ANS is more complex, with two sets of nerve fibers: preganglionic fibers that travel from the central nervous system to a peripheral autonomic ganglion, where they synapse with postganglionic fibers that travel to a target organ.

Autonomic Nervous System Has Three Branches

The ANS has three branches: the sympathetic, parasympathetic, and enteric nervous systems. The two major branches, the sympathetic and parasympathetic, are diagrammed in **Figure 2**.

Sympathetic Branch

Sympathetic preganglionic fibers exit from the middle, thoracic, and lumbar segments of the spinal

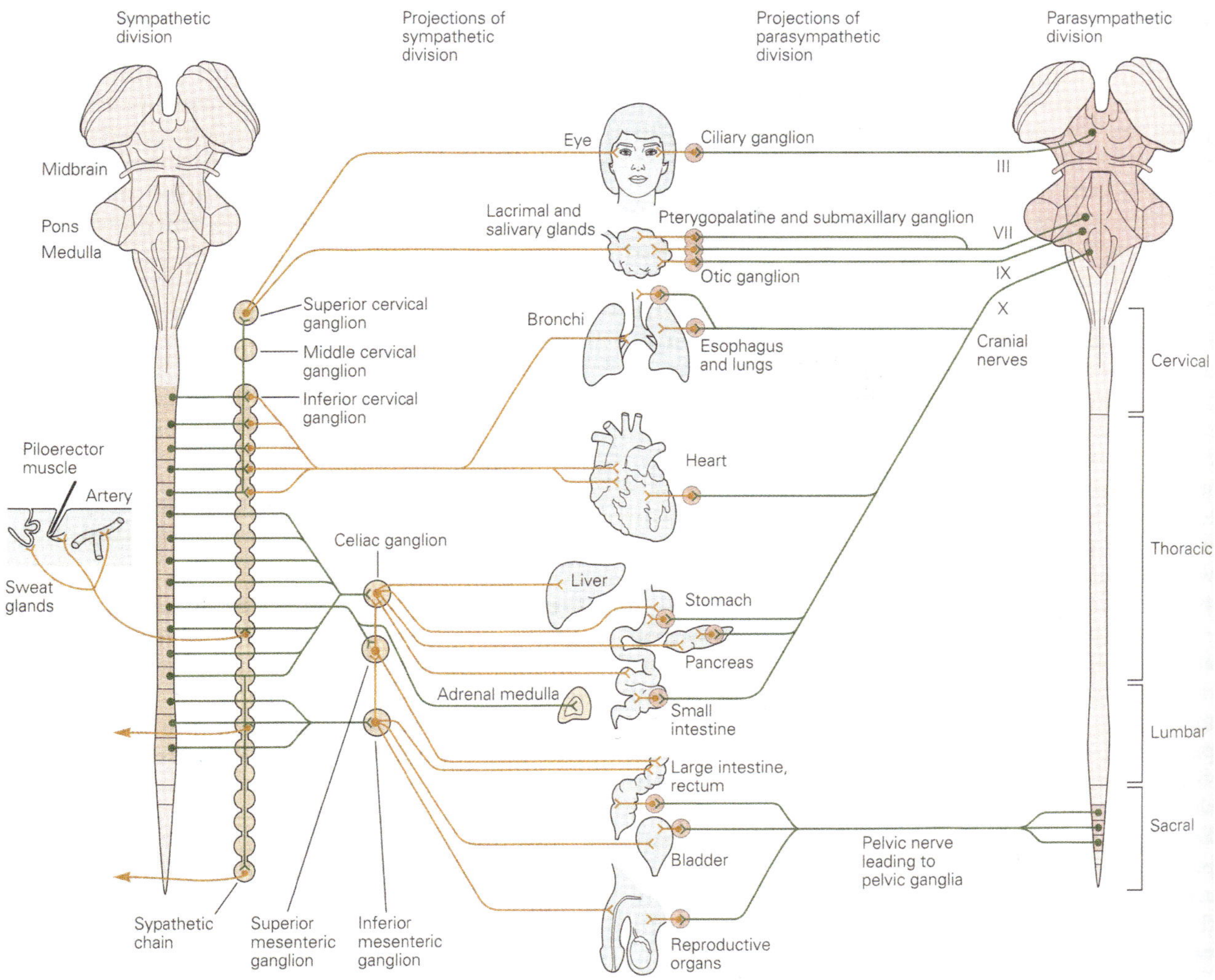

Figure 2 The sympathetic and parasympathetic branches of the autonomic nervous system. The sympathetic branch has preganglionic fibers that exit the spinal cord at the thoracic and lumbar vertebrae. These travel to the sympathetic chain ganglia, located near the spinal cord, or to the celiac or mesenteric ganglia of the gut. The sympathetic postganglionic fibers then exit their respective ganglia and travel to distant target organs. The parasympathetic preganglionic fibers exit the central nervous system either from the pons and medulla or from the sacral level of the spinal cord. The preganglionic fibers travel along several cranial nerves or the splanchnic nerve, and they travel some distance to their ganglia, located near or within the target organs. The postganglionic fibers then travel short distances to their target tissues. From Iversen, S., Iversen, L. and Saper, C. B. (2000). The autonomic nervous system and the hypothalamus. In: Kandel, E. R., Schwartz, J. J. & Jessel, J. H. (eds.) *Principles of neural science* (4th edn., pp. 960–981). New York: McGraw-Hill. Copyright The McGraw-Hill Companies, Inc. Used with permission.

cord. The sympathetic branch is so named because it operates in a coordinated fashion and in sympathy with the emotions. In general, the sympathetic branch regulates energy-using functions and is most active during states of fight or flight in order to maintain homeostasis in the face of external threats. It is also active during normal activities, but less so.

Parasympathetic Branch

In the parasympathetic branch, preganglionic fibers leave the central nervous system at points above and below the sympathetic fibers, hence the name parasympathetic. The upper group of neurons exits the medulla by way of the cranial nerves. These exit the central nervous system directly from the pons and medulla and serve the head, neck, cardiovascular system, and gut. The lower group exits the sacral segments of the spinal column. Parasympathetic activity generally serves energy-conserving functions that Cannon called rest-or-digest. It is active in energy intake, such as feeding and digestion, and during reproductive functions, and it is most active during routine activities.

Enteric Branch

As the name implies, the enteric system pertains exclusively to the organs of digestion, including the pancreas, the gall bladder, and the gastrointestinal tract. Some consider the enteric nervous system to be a branch of the ANS, while others view it as part of the digestive system. All three branches of the ANS are active during normal activities, and they coordinate their actions to maintain homeostasis. However, the sympathetic nervous system predominates, and the other branches are inhibited during states of acute stress, such as periods of fight or flight, when resources must be devoted to the task of immediate survival.

Neurons and Neurotransmitters

There are two points of communication in the ANS. At a ganglion, preganglionic neurons synapse with postganglionic neurons. At a target organ, the postganglionic neuron forms a neuroeffector junction with a muscle cell or a secretory cell.

At both places, neurons communicate using specialized chemicals called neurotransmitters. These are released onto specialized receptors that activate either a postganglionic neuron or an effector cell. There are two ANS neurotransmitters, acetylcholine and norepinephrine (also called noradrenalin).

Preganglionic neurons always use acetylcholine to communicate to their postganglionic neurons. Postganglionic neurons use two primary neurotransmitters to act on their target tissues. In the parasympathetic branch, postganglionic fibers secrete acetylcholine at neuroeffector junctions located at target tissues. In addition, there are parasympathetic postganglionic fibers to the digestive tract that use the purine adenosine triphosphate as their transmitter. These purinergic fibers are involved in relaxation of the esophagus, stomach, and intestines. In the sympathetic branch of the ANS, postganglionic fibers secrete norepinephrine at their neuroeffector junctions. There are two exceptions to this rule. The sympathetic nervous system uses acetylcholine as a transmitter in the neuroeffectors of two tissues: the specialized sweat glands of the skin and the medulla of the adrenal gland.

Autonomic ganglia have an important feature. They are not simply relay stations; instead, they have small neurons that communicate directly between the larger pre- and postganglionic neurons. These small neurons secrete the neurotransmitter dopamine, which inhibits the main ganglionic neurons. The autonomic ganglia use this local inhibition to produce the first level of integrative control over the vital organs.

Anatomy of the Autonomic Nervous System

The brainstem contains several autonomic control nuclei that regulate the actions of the sympathetic and parasympathetic branches. Preganglionic fibers descend from these control centers to their autonomic ganglia, and postganglionic fibers travel to the target organs.

Sympathetic Division

The sympathetic division serves the eye, salivary glands, lungs, heart, liver, spleen, stomach, gut, kidney, genitalia, and all blood vessels except those of the brain. The actions of these sympathetic inputs are summarized in **Table 1** for each effector organ.

Sympathetic fibers exit from the spinal cord at thoracic levels 1–12 and lumbar levels 1–3. As shown in **Figure 2**, there are two sets of sympathetic ganglia. The chain ganglia run parallel to the spinal column, and they are highly interconnected. A second, more distinct group includes the cervical and stellate ganglia, located in the neck, and the celiac, superior, and inferior mesenteric and renal ganglia found in the abdomen.

Sympathetic preganglionic fibers have four patterns of dispersal. Some preganglionic fibers enter the nearest ganglion and their postganglionic fibers exit at the same level of the ganglionic chain; other preganglionic fibers ascend the sympathetic chain ganglion to synapse in the cervical and stellate ganglia before they send postganglionic fibers to the eye, head, neck, mouth, and upper limbs and heart – the stellate ganglion serves the heart particularly. The blood vessels and skin of the lower body are served by postganglionic fibers that receive input from preganglionic fibers that descend from the lumbar and sacral ganglia; and, finally, certain preganglionic fibers pass directly through the chain ganglia without synapsing. They collect to form the three splanchnic nerves that pass through the diaphragm to enter the abdomen before arriving at the celiac, mesenteric, and renal ganglia.

A notable exception to this organization of sympathetic fibers is the innervation of the adrenal gland. In this case, sympathetic preganglionic fibers exit the spinal cord and travel directly to the adrenal medulla without synapsing at a ganglion.

The sympathetic nervous system is especially effective at promoting coordinated action of the bodily organs during states of stress. Its ganglia are close to the spinal cord and far from their target organs, and a single preganglionic fiber may send branches to several of the chain ganglia at different levels of

Table 1 Responses of Effector Organs to Autonomic Nerve Impulses[a]

Effector organs	*Sympathetic receptors*	*Sympathetic impulses and responses*	*Parasympathetic impulses and responses*
Eye			
Radial muscle, iris	α	Contraction (pupil enlargement) ++	—
Sphincter muscle, iris		—	Contraction (pupil constriction) +++
Cilary muscle	β_2	Relaxation for far vision +	Contraction or near vision +++
Heart			
SA node	β_1	Increase in heart rate ++	Decrease in heart rate; vagal arrest ++
Atria	β_1	Increase in contractility and conduction velocity ++	Decrease contractility, and (usually) Increase in conduction velocity ++
AV node	β_1	Increase in automaticity and conduction velocity ++	Decrease in conduction velocity; AV block +++
Ventricles	β_1	Increase in contractility, conduction Velocity, automaticity, and rate of idioventricular pacemakers +++	Slight decrease in contractility
Arterioles			
Coronary	α, β_2	Constriction +; dilation ++	Dilation +
Skin and mucosa	α	Constriction +++	Dilation
Skeletal muscle	α, β_2	Constriction ++	Dilation +
Cerebral	α	Constriction (slight)	Dilation
Pulmonary	α, β_2	Constriction +; dilation	Dilation
Abdominal viscera			
Kidney	α, β_2	Constriction +++; dilation +	—
Salivary gland	α	Constriction +++	Dilation ++
Veins (systemic)	α, β_2	Constriction ++; dilation ++	—
Lung			
Bronchial muscle	β_2	Relaxation +	Contraction ++
Bronchial glands	?	Inhibition (?)	Stimulation +++
Stomach			
Motility and tone	α, β_2	Decrease (usually) +	Increase +++
Sphincters	α	Contraction (usually) +	Relaxation (usually)
Secretion		Inhibition (?)	Stimulation +++
Intestine			
Motility and tone	α, β_2	Decrease +	Increase +++
Sphincters	α	Contraction (usually) +	Relaxation (usually) +
Secretion		Inhibition (?)	Stimulation ++
Gallbladder and ducts		Relaxation +	Contraction +
Kidney	β_2	Renin secretion ++	—
Urinary bladder			
Detrusor	β_2	Relaxation (usually) +	Contraction +++
Trigone and sphincter	α	Contraction ++	Relaxation ++
Ureter			
Motility and tone	α	Increase (usually)	Increase (?)
Uterus	α, β_2	Pregnant: contraction (a); nonpregnant: Relaxation (B)	Variable
Sex organs, male	α	Ejaculation +++	Erection +++
Skin			
Pilomotor muscles	α	Contraction ++	—
Sweat glands	α	Localized secretion +	Generalized secretion +++
Spleen capsule	α, β_2	Contraction +++, relaxation +	—
Adrenal medulla		—	Secretion of epinephrine and norepinephrine
Liver	α, β_2	Glycogenolysis, gluconeogenesis +++	Glycogen synthesis +
Pancreas			
Acini	α	Decreased secretion +	Secretion ++

Continued

Table 1 Continued

Effector organs	*Sympathetic receptors*	*Sympathetic impulses and responses*	*Parasympathetic impulses and responses*
Islets (B cells)	α	Decreased secretion +++	—
	β_2	Increased secretion +	—
Fat cells	α, β_1	Lipolysis +++	—
Salivary glands	α	Potassium and water secretion +	Potassium and water secretion +++
	β_2	Amylase secretion +	—
Lacrimal glands		—	Secretion +++
Nasopharyngeal glands		—	Secretion ++
Pineal gland	β_2	Melatonin synthesis	—

[a]Receptor types refer to receptors of the sympathetic nervous system. There are three types of sympathetic receptors: alpha (α), beta-1 (β_1), and beta-2 (β_2). α receptors are most sensitive to norepinephrine released from sympathetic nerve terminals. β_1 receptors are located only at the heart and in fat cells. These are sensitive to norepinephrine from sympathetic nerve terminals and to circulating epinephrine. β_2 receptors are mostly not innervated by sympathetic nerves. They are primarily sensitive to circulating epinephrine. The parasympathetic nervous system acts exclusively by secretion of acetylcholine on cholinergic receptors, regardless of the organ in question. The adrenal medulla is innervated by sympathetic preganglionic fibers that secrete acetylcholine. The sweat glands of the palms of the hands and soles of the feet are innervated by postganglionic sympathetic fibers that release acetylcholine. +, little action; ++, moderate effect; +++, large effect.

the spinal column. There is a ratio of 1 preganglionic fiber to 10 postganglionic fibers. This allows for coordinated activation of organs of the cardiovascular and pulmonary systems that are needed for coping with fight-or-flight situations. Epinephrine secreted by the adrenal medulla circulates throughout the body to act on noninnervated β receptors, further coordinating the organs sustaining fight or flight.

Parasympathetic Division

As shown in **Figure 2** and **Table 1**, parasympathetic ganglia are located close to or within the organs they innervate. Preganglionic fibers arise from the brain stem and sacral region of the spinal cord. The eye, face, and mouth are served by cranial verves III, VII, and IX. The cardiopulmonary and digestive systems are served by the vagus nerve (cranial nerve X), while the functions of excretion and control of reproductive organs are served by the splanchnic nerves.

The parasympathetic nervous system is designed to promote highly specific regulation of individual organs: (1) parasympathetic preganglionic fibers are long and travel to specific ganglia linked to specific organs; (2) postganglionic fibers are short and are sometimes found entirely within the innervated tissue; and (3) the ratio of pre- to postganglionic fibers is about 1:3, with one preganglionic fiber affecting only a single organ.

Autonomic Regulation of Specific Organs

Figure 2 and **Table 1** summarize how the ANS regulates specific organs. The activity of each organ involves interactions between the organ's intrinsic functioning and inputs from the ANS. In most cases, the sympathetic and parasympathetic branches of the ANS have opposite effects on the organs they innervate, and the balance of sympathetic to parasympathetic outflow determines the organ's final level of activity. This balance shifts constantly as the physiological and behavioral demands of the person change. During states of fight or flight, this balance is predominantly sympathetic in nature.

This regulatory interplay is illustrated in the activity of the heart. With no external controls, the heart beats automatically at a fixed rate of about 105–110 beats per minute. This rate is due to the heart's internal pacemakers, the atrioventricular and sinoatrial nodes. The pacemakers each have alternate phases of excitation and quiescence, and they interact to allow the heart to beat in a coordinated way. The heart's intrinsic force of contraction is determined by how well the ventricles fill with blood between beats and the resulting stretch on the walls of the ventricles. Greater wall tension results in a more effective contraction, with more blood being pumped on the next beat. These intrinsic mechanisms are entirely adequate to sustain life if conditions are constant and no threats to homeostasis are present.

The two branches of the ANS are active at all times, and they coordinate their actions to regulate the heart during all levels of demand on the circulation. During most normal behavioral states, the predominant ANS influence on the heart is through the parasympathetic branch. This branch acts on the heart by way of the vagus nerve, whose firing serves to lower the heart's rate and force of contraction. The heart's intrinsic rhythm is normally regulated by this parasympathetic input. Up to and including moderate demands on the circulation, the parasympathetic branch can allow the heart to pump more blood simply by firing less often and allowing the heart to increase its rate up to its intrinsic rate.

At times of increased demand, the ANS may cause the heart to change its rate and force of contraction, and it may have to coordinate these changes with changes in the state of the peripheral blood vessels. A rapid change in circulatory demand occurs, for example, when a person suddenly rises from a chair, at which time there is a danger of blood pooling in the legs, causing a loss of circulation to the brain. This danger is averted by a rapid increase in firing by the sympathetic nerves that increase the rate and force of the heart's contractions and also increase the constrictive force of the blood vessels of the lower extremities. During more severe and sustained demands, such as intense physical exercise, the parasympathetic outflow to the heart is almost absent, and the sympathetic influence increases toward a maximum. In addition, endocrine input to the heart by circulating epinephrine greatly augments the heart's contractions. These three influences can cause a sevenfold increase in the volume of blood the heart pumps each minute. In a trained athlete, such increases in circulation can be sustained for hours.

These examples illustrate that the heart can function without outside control if no response is called for. However, the ANS must provide external control to meet rapid or sustained demands on the circulation and to help the heart operate in concert with the blood vessels. Circulating hormones, such as epinephrine, compliment the actions of the ANS to achieve the necessary level and coordination of cardiovascular response during stress. Similar arguments apply to the ANS regulation of other organ systems.

Local Regulation of Autonomic Function

Since ANS controls, especially sympathetic activity, are more or less nonspecific for each organ, there has been considerable interest in local mechanisms that can fine-tune organ function. The previous section illustrated the interplay of intrinsic and extrinsic regulation of the heart. There is still another level of fine-tuning of ANS actions at a given tissue. In all organs, ANS input is regulated by locally released biochemicals classified as peptides, neuromodulators, or metabolites. These act by several mechanisms at either the smooth muscle or the autonomic-neuroeffector junction to modify ANS activity or its effectiveness.

An example of the action of such local modulators is seen in the regulation of blood flow. Blood flow into the tissues is regulated by sympathetic activity at local blood vessels in concert with local metabolic demands. To regulate the level of tonus at the blood vessel wall, sympathetic nerves release norepinephrine at the sympathetic neuroeffector junction, causing contraction of networks of smooth muscle cells, increasing constriction of the blood vessel. This constrictive force can reduce blood flow into a local volume of tissue. If this were the only influence, the cardiovascular system would not adequately regulate blood flow according to the specific needs of local tissues. However, this constrictive force is balanced by local chemical substances that act on the blood vessel wall in relation to the activity of the local tissues and their consequent need for increased blood flow. Metabolites produced by cellular activity can act locally on smooth muscle cells to regulate their activity. For example, carbon dioxide produced by tissue metabolism leads to local production of nitric oxide, and nitric oxide causes relaxation of vascular smooth muscle cells. This results in the relaxation of blood vessels, allowing improved blood flow to a local volume of tissue. In this process of local autoregulation, exercising muscles produce more carbon dioxide when they are working harder, causing greater relaxation in the local resistance vessels and increasing the local blood supply. Neuromodulators can act on the sympathetic nerves themselves to regulate their actions on smooth muscle cells. In the sympathetic nerves, adenosine diphosphate is released along with norepinephrine at the adrenergic nerve terminal. This adenosine diphosphate is rapidly metabolized to adenosine, which then acts on adenosine receptors located on local sympathetic nerve terminals to decrease the release of norepinephrine. The greater the level of sympathetic outflow, the greater the production of adenosine, and the greater the modulation of neurotransmitter release. In the case of the blood vessel wall, autoregulation and neuromodulation work together to balance the effects of sympathetic activation and constrictor tonus, allowing blood flow to be controlled according to local tissues needs. Similar processes occur in the heart muscle.

The balance of intrinsic regulation, ANS inputs, and local regulation occurs in all tissues. This interaction fine-tunes organ function to maintain homeostasis.

Physical and Psychological Stress

Physical and psychological stress result from very different causes, but they both influence the body by way of the ANS. The earlier example of a person arising from a seated position illustrates a physical challenge to homeostasis that results in a response by the ANS to maintain blood flow to the brain. This

ANS response is coordinated by reflex mechanisms in the large blood vessels and brain stem that sense an impending drop in blood pressure and orchestrate the shift toward a sympathetically dominated state until blood flow is normalized. Such ANS responses are referred to as bottom-up because their source is in the body, involving some physical threat to homeostasis.

Psychological stress has a different origin. Our bodies can undergo significant changes in activity when we are anxious, ruminating about past failures, or in an acute state of fear. However, these changes originate in the highest centers in the brain, including the prefrontal cortex and limbic system. These ruminations result in signals to the hypothalamus and brain stem that can cause changes in the state of the body through the ANS and endocrine systems. These brain mechanisms therefore exert a top-down effect on the state of the body. In this manner, psychological stimuli can act as stressors in themselves. These can alter the usual homeostatic balance of the body.

Summary

The ANS and the endocrine systems are the brain's two primary pathways for regulating the vital organs. The ANS innervates all tissues outside of the central nervous system. It regulates contraction of smooth muscle cells and cardiac muscle cells and output by secretory cells. Changes in the internal or external environment of the body are normally countered by the ANS, which serves to maintain homeostasis. The ANS itself is controlled by the brain stem and hypothalamus. The highest level of control is provided by the brain's limbic system and cerebral cortex. During times of emotional distress, influences descending from these higher centers alter the activity of the hypothalamus and brain stem. These psychologically induced influences can change the activity of the ANS to alter the state of the body and temporarily alter the homeostatic balance.

See Also the Following Articles

Adrenaline; Sympathetic Nervous System.

Further Reading

Burnstock, G. (1975). Comparative studies of purinergic nerves. *Journal of Experimental Zoology* **194**, 103–133.
Burnstock, G. and Hoyle, C. H. (eds.) (1992). *Autonomic neuroeffector mechanisms.* Reading, UK: Harwood.
Iversen, S., Iversen, L. and Saper, C. B. (2000). The autonomic nervous system and the hypothalamus. In: Kandel, E. R., Schwartz, J. J. & Jessel, J. H. (eds.) *Principles of neural science* (4th edn., pp. 960–981). New York: McGraw-Hill.
Karczmar, A. G., Koketsu, K. and Nishi, S. (eds.) (1986). *Autonomic and enteric ganglia: Transmission and its pharmacology.* New York: Plenum.
Lovallo, W. R. (2005). *Stress and health: Biological and psychological interactions* (2nd edn.). Thousand Oaks, CA: Sage.
Nilsson, S. and Holmgren, S. (eds.) (1914). *Comparative physiology and evolution of the autonomic nervous system.* Reading, UK: Harwood.
Smith, E. E., Guyton, A. C., Manning, R. D. and White, R. J. (1976). Integrated mechanisms of cardiovascular response and control during exercise in the normal human. *Progress in Cardiovascular Disease* **28**, 421–443.

Sympathoadrenal System: Neural Arm of the Stress Response

M Palkovits
Semmelweis University, Budapest, Hungary

The sympathetic nervous system, like the other major regulatory mechanisms of the central and peripheral nervous systems, can be divided into afferent and efferent arms. The somatosensory and viscerosensory projections carrying external and internal signals to the spinal and supraspinal compartments of the sympathetic nervous system represent its afferent arm. The efferent arm of the sympathetic nervous system (sympathetic outflow) appears to be organized into two major divisions: sympathoadrenal (SAS) and sympathoneural (SNS) systems. The term sympathoadrenal system is frequently used as a synonym for the sympathetic outflow or for the efferent arm of the sympathetic nervous system in general. It should be emphasized that according to their anatomical organization, neurotransmitter characteristics, and their functional role in the sympathetic outflow, the two systems are different: They may be independently activated, and they independently respond to stressful stimuli.

The activation of these two divisions of the efferent arm of the sympathetic nervous system is organized in a hierarchical manner (**Figure 1**). First, supraspinal (premotor sympathetic) neurons project to sympathetic preganglionic neurons in the thoracic spinal cord. Second, the sympathetic preganglionic neurons that represent the first compartment in both systems provide anatomical substrate through which selective regulation of sympathetic nervous system targets is accomplished. Fibers of the sympathetic preganglionic neurons innervate the adrenal medulla (SAS) and neurons in the sympathetic ganglia (SNS) (**Figure 2**). Third,

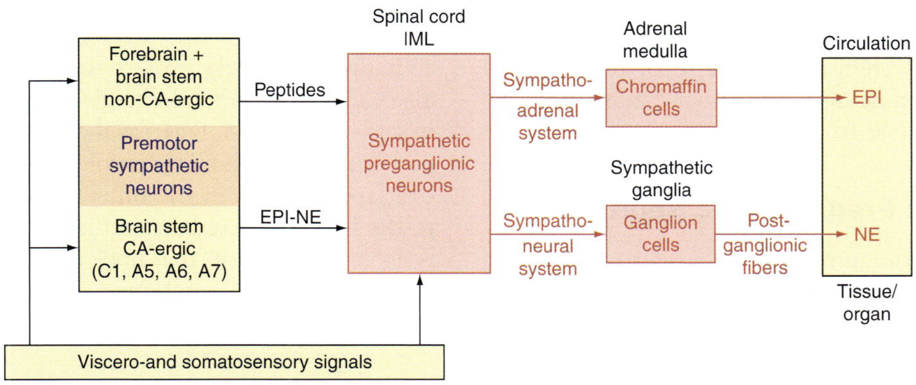

Figure 1 Neuroanatomical organization of the sympathetic nervous system. EPI, epinephrine; IML, intermediolateral cell column; NE, norepinephrine.

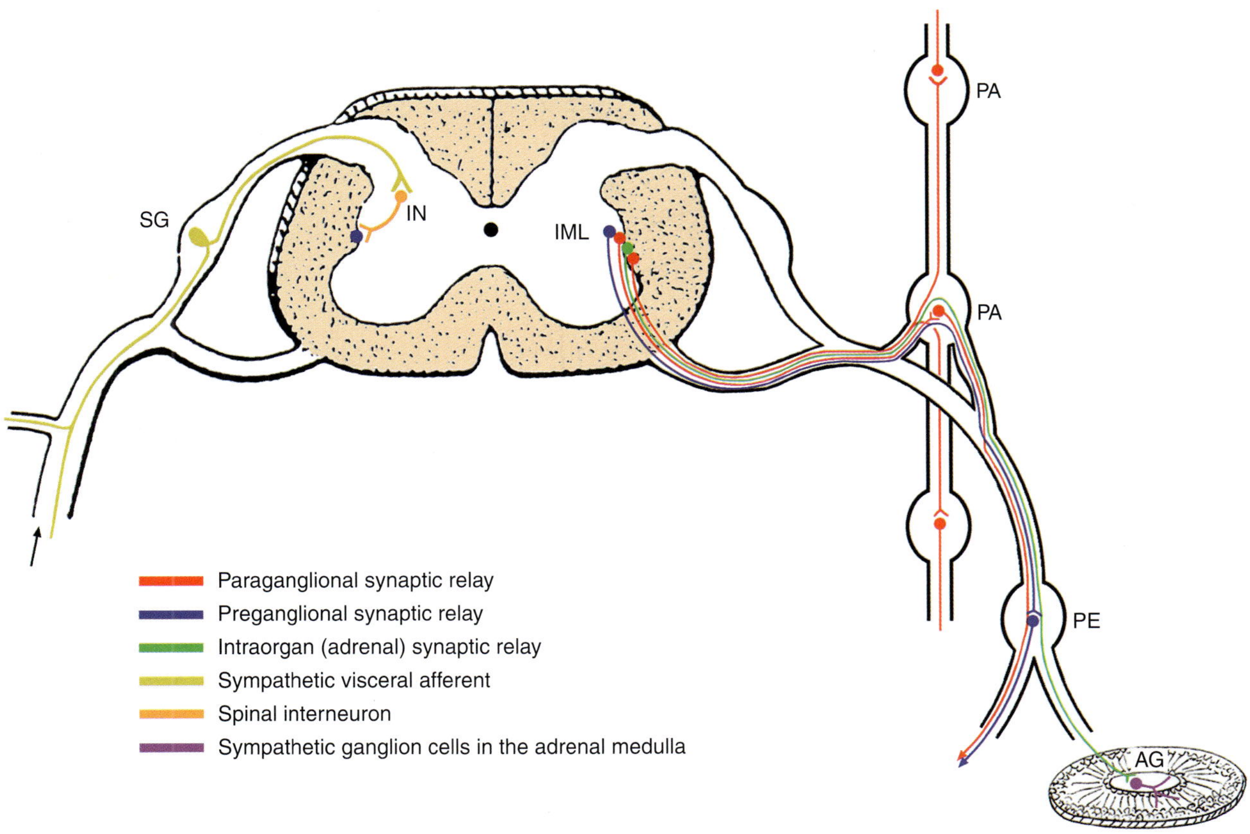

Figure 2 Viscerosensory inputs to the sympathetic preganglionic neurons (left) and the organization of pre- and postganglionic fibers in the sympathoadrenal and sympathoneural systems (right). AG, adrenomedullary ganglion cells; IML, intermediolateral cell column; IN, interneurons in the dorsal horn; PA, paravertebral ganglion; PE, prevertebral ganglion; SG, sympathetic ganglion.

the adrenal medullary chromaffin cells synthesize and release epinephrine (EPI) into the circulation. EPI in the plasma is exclusively of adrenomedullary origin. Neurons in the sympathetic ganglia project to a variety of peripheral targets in which norepinephrine (NE) is stored and released from the postganglionic sympathetic nerve endings, called varicosities. Almost all NE in the plasma originates from these nerve endings.

Activation of the sympathetic nervous system is accompanied by an increase in the outflow of both NE and EPI. Variation in the sensitivity and the number of pre- and postsynaptic receptors in the sympathetic nervous system may account for regional and functional differences in sympathetic activation, especially in response to different stressors.

Sympathetic Preganglionic Neurons

The sympathetic preganglionic neurons provide the anatomical substrate through which selective regulation of sympathetic nervous system targets is accomplished. The adrenal medulla and the sympathetic ganglion cells are directly innervated by sympathetic preganglionic neurons (**Figure 3**).

The sympathetic preganglionic neurons are cholinergic and form a longitudinal cell line, the intermediolateral cell column (IML), in the lateral portion of the spinal central gray matter, between the first thoracic (T1) and the second lumbar (L2) segments of the spinal cord. Within the IML, the sympathetic preganglionic neurons are topographically organized with respect to their tissue/organ targets. The adrenal medullary sympathetic preganglionic neurons (neurons that selectively project to the adrenal medulla, also called sympathoadrenergic cells) occupy the IML in segments T5–T8, whereas the sympathoneural sympathetic preganglionic neurons occupy, with some overlap, the IML in the other segments. In addition to the IML, scattered sympathetic preganglionic neurons are found in the nucleus intermediomedialis (called the central autonomic area) and in the lateral funiculus, immediately lateral to the IML.

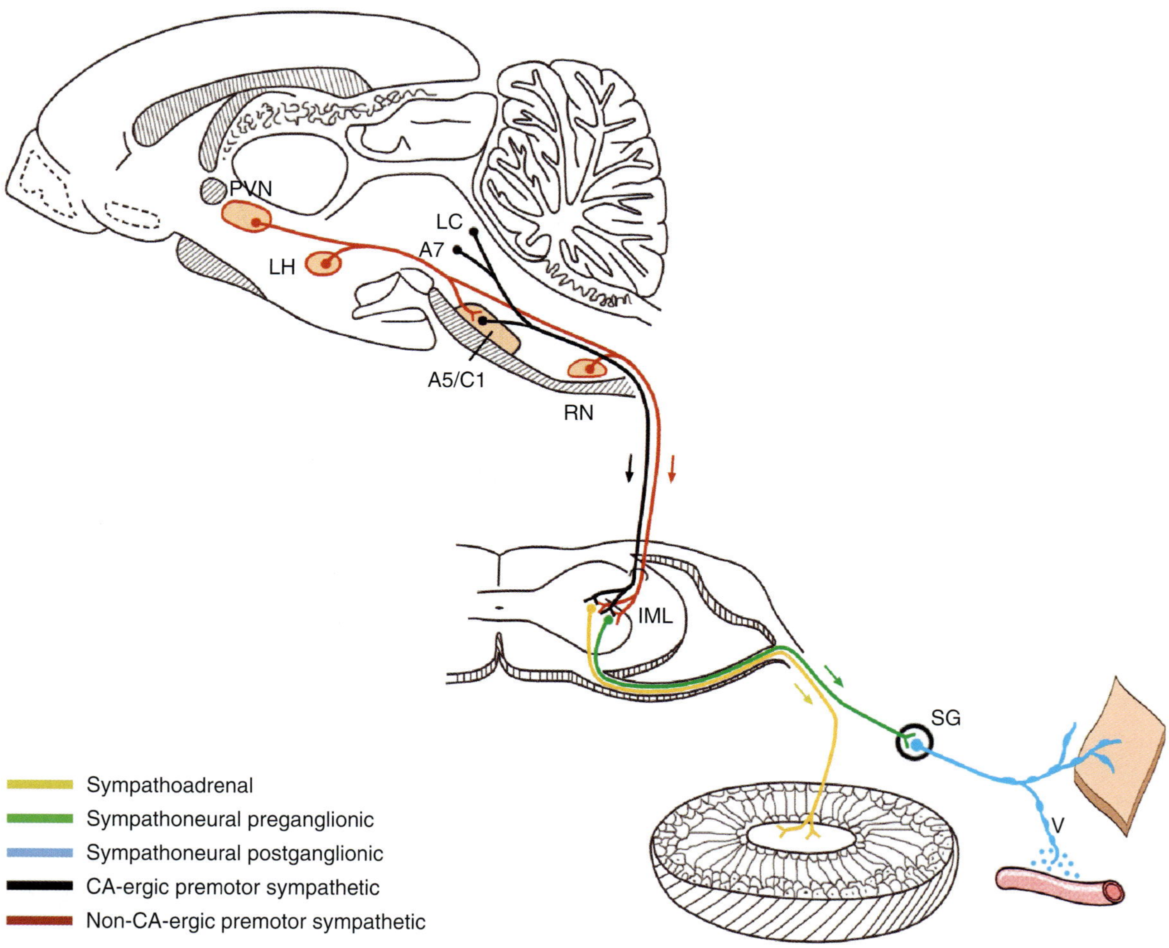

Figure 3 Afferent and efferent projections of spinal sympathetic preganglionic neurons. A5, A5 noradrenergic cell group; A7, A7 noradrenergic cell group; C1, C1 adrenergic cell group; IML, intermediolateral cell column; LC, locus coeruleus; LH, lateral hypothalamic area; RN, medullary raphe nuclei; PVN, paraventricular nucleus; SG, sympathetic ganglion; V, varicosities.

Axons of the sympathetic preganglionic neurons leave the spinal cord through the ventral roots, at the level where their perikarya are located, and initially they run together with somatomotor axons within the spinal nerve. After a short distance, they separate from the spinal nerve and travel in small bundles, called white rami communicantes, to the paravertebral sympathetic chain (**Figure 2**). The sympathetic chain extends from the base of the skull down to the sacrum, on the two sides of the vertebral column. Some of the sympathetic preganglionic fibers form synaptic contact with ganglion cells within the chain (i.e., in paravertebral sympathetic ganglia). A group of the sympathetic preganglionic fibers establish synaptic contacts with ganglion cells at the same level where they enter the chain, whereas others travel upward or downward in the chain and terminate on paravertebral ganglion cells at more rostral or caudal levels (**Figure 2**). The vast majority of the ascending presynaptic sympathetic fibers in the sympathetic chain terminate in the cervical paravertebral sympathetic (superior and inferior (stellate)) ganglia.

The other portion of the sympathetic preganglionic fibers pass the chain without establishing synaptic contacts with any of the paravertebral ganglion cells. They enter some of the branches of the sympathetic chain and terminate on ganglion cells in one of the prevertebral ganglion in the abdomen, such as the celiac/superior mesenteric or inferior mesenteric ganglion (**Figure 2**). The sympathetic preganglionic neurons with synaptic contacts with either para- or prevertebral ganglion cells constitute the SNS.

A group of the sympathetic preganglionic fibers may pass the sympathetic chain, as well as the para- and prevertebral ganglia, without establishing synaptic contacts with ganglion cells (**Figure 2**). These presynaptic fibers leave the sympathetic chain for the splanchnic nerves; they enter the adrenal gland and terminate directly on the chromaffin cells in the adrenal medulla. They constitute the SAS.

The Sympathoadrenal System

The SAS is composed of sympathetic preganglionic neurons and the chromaffin cells of the adrenal medulla. Chromaffin cells, like principal sympathetic ganglion cells, are members of the sympathoadrenal lineage derived from the neural crest. They share a common precursor, the sympathoadrenal progenitor cells. The sympathetic preganglionic neurons that innervate chromaffin cells are located in the IML of the thoracic spinal cord, mainly between segments T5 and T9. These neurons are cholinergic; acetylcholine is released from their terminals. Stimulation of the adrenal medulla leads to release of EPI and NE into the blood.

Two populations of adrenal chromaffin cells have been identified: EPI and NE secreting cells. The ratio of EPI- to NE-synthesizing chromaffin cells is approximately 4:1 in humans and slightly different in mammals. Although this ratio varies among species, EPI-synthesizing chromaffin cells predominate in the adrenal medulla. Note that a small number of chromaffin cells are also localized extra-adrenally, inside or around the sympathetic ganglia (paraganglia).

Each chromaffin cell contains approximately 10 000 chromaffin granules, in which EPI or NE are stored. They are secreted via exocytosis, carried by capillaries that drain from the adrenal medulla into the adrenal vein. Then, EPI and NE are transported throughout the body and exert their effects on most of the major regulatory systems. Besides catecholamines, the chromaffin granules contain numerous other transmitters, granins, and neuropeptides, which are co-localized and co-released with catecholamines.

The NE-synthesizing chromaffin cells possess the full repertoire of functions of EPI-synthesizing cells except the capacity to synthesize EPI. The two types of chromaffin cells are innervated by different sympathetic preganglionic fibers. This arrangement provides a basis for distinct sympathetic circuits underlying the differential regulation of EPI and NE secretion from the adrenal medulla in response to physiological challenges and stressful stimuli.

In addition to chromaffin cells, the adrenal medulla contains a small number of ganglion cells, which synthesize NE. Like chromaffin cells, these ganglion cells are also innervated by sympathetic preganglionic fibers (**Figure 2**), but they contribute little to NE content in plasma and do not synthesize EPI. Their postganglionic axons distribute in the adrenal and terminate both in the medulla and in the adrenal cortex. Thus, ganglion cells in the adrenal medulla have similar characteristics as ganglion cells in the pre- or paravertebral ganglia, neverthelen they are embedded in the innervated organ, that is, in the adrenal gland. Despite their location, the adrenal medullary ganglion cells functionally belong to the SNS rather than the SAS.

The Sympathoneural System

Neuroanatomically, the SNS is organized in a two-neuron chain. The first neuron (as in the SAS) is referred to as the sympathetic preganglionic neuron, whereas the second neuron is called the ganglionic (or, frequently, postganglionic) neuron, which projects a so-called postganglionic axon. The preganglionic neurons in the IML are cholinergic and innervate the sympathetic ganglion cells by release of acetylcholine as the primary neurotransmitter that acts on nicotinic and, to a lesser extent, muscarinic receptors. Various biologically active neuropeptides, such as substance P, vasoactive intestinal polypeptide, and enkephalins, are co-localized with acetylcholine within the sympathetic preganglionic terminals. They may act as neuromodulators of cholinergic transmission.

The ganglion cells reside in sympathetic paravertebral (superior cervical, stellate ganglia, and ganglion cells in the sympathetic chain) and prevertebral (celiac and superior and inferior mesenteric) ganglia (**Figure 2**). With terminal branches, a single sympathetic preganglionic axon terminates on several para- or prevertebral ganglion cells. The divergence ratio of the pre- and postsynaptic neurons, depending on the species, is between 20:1 and 5:1. This divergence permits coordinated activity in sympathetic neurons at several different spinal levels. In contrast, ganglion cells establish synaptic contacts with more than one sympathetic preganglionic neuron. Therefore, a substantial convergence of synaptic inputs exists on each ganglion cell.

The sympathetic postganglionic nerve originating from either a pre- or paravertebral ganglion cell establishes a plexus of terminal fibers within a short distance to the target tissue/organ (**Figure 2**). The length of a terminal fiber may be several millimeters. The postganglionic fibers show a beaded appearance due to local swellings called varicosities. The varicosities are specialized structures involved in the storage and release of NE. They contain a high concentration of large and small granular vesicles that store mainly NE. A single postganglionic fiber may contain more than 20 000 varicosities with more than 1000 granular vesicles in each. Each granule stores approximately 15 000 molecules of NE. The varicosities do not display synaptic junction; NE is released to the extracellular space by exocytosis and diffuses over a large territory of the target area or is drained directly into the blood. Almost all of the NE in the plasma originates from the varicosities of the postganglionic fibers. In certain conditions, the nerve endings may take up and store a significant amount of NE from the extracellular space. The process of synthesis, storage, and release of NE from the varicosities is under the control of the sympathetic preganglionic neurons. In addition to the para- and prevertebral sympathetic ganglia, sympathetic neurons are also found in a small number in ganglia in or near the pelvic organs (pelvic ganglia).

NE is not the sole neurotransmitter in the sympathetic ganglion cells; they express other cotransmitters and neuropeptides, such as neuropeptide Y and galanin. The co-expression and the selective outflow of one or more neurotransmitters or neuropeptides from the sympathetic postganglionic nerve terminals allow the organism to differentiate between sympathetic activities and responses at the level of the target organ.

In addition to ganglion cells, sympathetic ganglia contain small granular cells called intensely fluorescent (SIF) cells. These cells express and store predominantly dopamine, and some of them also express and store EPI. SIF cells, like the sympathetic ganglion cells and the chromaffin cells, are members of the sympathoadrenal lineage derived from the neural crest.

Premotor Sympathetic Neurons

Neurons at multiple levels of the neuraxis, ranging from the lower brain stem to the forebrain, regulate the sympathetic outflow. These neurons, called premotor sympathetic neurons, innervate the sympathetic preganglionic neurons in the IML (**Figure 3**). Neurotransmitters that regulate the preganglionic neurons include NE, EPI, dopamine, serotonin, and neuropeptides. Thus, sympathetic activities elicited by the activation of sympathetic preganglionic neurons are controlled by distinct neuronal circuits and probably by distinct neurotransmitters. Accordingly, the premotor sympathetic neurons used to be classified as catecholaminergic and noncatecholaminergic (**Figure 1**).

The hypothalamus is regarded as the principal brain region of central autonomic regulation. Most of the forebrain regions, such as the amygdala, hippocampus, and limbic cortical areas, are involved in the control of the autonomic nervous system outflow. They do not directly innervate the IML; rather, they exert their influence on preganglionic sympathetic neurons by way of the hypothalamus. Hypothalamic neurons projecting to the IML of the thoracic spinal cord reside mainly in the paraventricular nucleus, but some reside in the lateral hypothalamic area and the arcuate nucleus (**Figure 3**). The hypothalamic premotor sympathetic neurons are peptidergic. Serotoninergic neurons in the rostral ventromedial medulla and the caudal raphe nuclei also project to sympathetic preganglionic neurons. These cells, together with the hypothalamic neurons, represent the noncatecholaminergic premotor sympathetic neurons (**Figure 1**).

In the lower brain stem, catecholaminergic neurons in the rostral ventrolateral medulla (in the A5 noradrenergic and C1 adrenergic cell groups) constitute the major portion of the catecholaminergic premotor sympathetic neurons that preferentially terminate on the sympathetic preganglionic neurons (**Figure 3**). In addition, neurons of the A7 noradrenergic cell group in the pons and neurons in the caudal portion of the locus coeruleus belong to this system. The distribution of the descending premotor sympathetic axons in the IML is topographically and functionally organized: The target-specific IML neurons are selectively innervated by different catecholamine premotor neurons. The NE or EPI nerve terminals establish conventional synaptic contacts with sympathetic preganglionic neurons, especially in the segments T5–T9, where the sympathoadrenergic preganglionic cells are located. The IML cell column also receives dopamine innervations, mainly from the A11 dopamine cell group in the posterior diencephalon.

In certain conditions, the two premotor sympathetic systems may act synergistically: Hypothalamic neurons that project to the IML send axon collaterals to catecholaminergic neurons in the lower brain stem (**Figure 3**).

Sensory Arms of the Sympathetic Nervous System

To maintain homeostasis, the sympathetic nervous system responds to several different types of sensory inputs. Some of these inputs are somatosensory, including nociceptive signals, whereas others – viscerosensory inputs – arise from interoceptors in the internal organs. They may reach spinal and supraspinal receptors by neural or humoral ways. Inputs which influence the activity of the sympathetic preganglionic or premotor sympathetic neurons (**Figure 1**) are called sympathetic sensory afferents. They represent the sensory (also called ascending or afferent) arm of the sympathetic regulatory circuit.

The sympathetic visceral afferent fibers enter the dorsal horn of the spinal cord through the dorsal roots and innervate the sympathetic preganglionic neurons in the IML via interneurons located in lamina V and lamina VII of the spinal cord (**Figure 2**). Some sensory fibers that project to the spinal cord also send a branch to sympathetic ganglia forming reflex circuits that may control some visceral autonomic functions.

Viscerosensory signals to supraspinal premotor sympathetic neurons are relayed in the nucleus of the solitary tract (NTS), which represents the primary viscerosensory center in the central nervous system. Viscerosensory fibers travel in cranial nerves (mainly in the trigeminal, glossopharyngeal, and vagal nerves) or in ascending spinal fibers (spino-solitary tract) and terminate in the NTS. The sensory afferents terminate in a topographically and functionally organized manner in the different subdivisions of the nucleus. The ascending fibers from the NTS may reach both the catecholaminergic and the noncatecholaminergic premotor sympathetic neurons in the brain stem and the hypothalamus. Some of them influence the activity of limbic and cortical structures that may respond to these signals through the activation of hypothalamic or brain stem premotor sympathetic neurons.

Sympathetic Nervous System in the Organization of Stress Response

The sympathetic nervous system helps to maintain homeostasis during exposure to stressors. Activation of the sympathetic nervous system leads to the outflow of catecholamines from the adrenal medulla and from the varicosities of the sympathetic postganglionic axons. These two systems constitute the final compartments of the effector loop of the sympathetic nervous system that participate in the organization of stress response.

Under resting conditions, low levels of EPI and NE are released into the blood flow from the adrenal medulla and sympathetic postganglionic nerve terminals, respectively. During stressful situations, large amounts of EPI and NE are released. Depending on the nature, intensity, and duration of stressful stimuli, levels of NE and EPI in the plasma may increase 10- to 100-fold (or even higher) within a very short period of time after the stressful stimuli occur. The tissue levels of NE measured in various organs are reduced in acute stress since approximately 70% or more of the circulating NE is derived from the varicosities of the postganglionic sympathetic nerve fibers, which provide the sympathetic innervations of the organs. Similarly, levels of NE and EPI are reduced in the adrenal medulla, depending on the intensity and the duration of acute stressors. After long-term or repeated stress exposure, adrenal medullary catecholamine stores are increased in the chromaffin cells. In this situation, the increased catecholamine synthesis, as a consequence of the stress-induced marked elevation of gene expression of catecholamine-synthesizing enzymes (tyrosine hydroxylase, dopamine β-hydroxylase, and phenylethanolamine *N*-methyltransferase (PNMT)) in the adrenal medulla, exceeds the release of NE and EPI.

Based on measurements of plasma levels of EPI, NE, catecholamine precursors, and metabolites in stress, it is generally accepted that SAS and SNS are specifically, and somewhat independently, activated by different stressors. Exposures to cold evoke a selective activation of SNS, as indicated by elevated plasma NE levels, whereas insulin-induced glucoprivation or emotional stressors activate SAS, as indicated by plasma EPI responses. Other stressors, such as restraint or formalin-induced pain, activate both systems. Immobilization represents a severe stress that elicits an extremely large increase in plasma NE and EPI. Results from a variety of studies indicate that not only the peripheral but also the central catecholamine system and the hypothalamic–pituitary–adrenal (HPA) axis respond specifically to different stressful stimuli. An intact HPA axis is essential for the activity of PNMT, the enzyme responsible for EPI synthesis in the adrenal medulla. Thus, depending on the nature and the target sites of various stressors, SAS and SNS may be regulated by different central pathways. For example, a single subcutaneous formalin injection, which strongly increases EPI levels in the plasma in intact animals, may reduce the immobilization-induced high EPI levels whether it was injected before or during immobilization.

Whereas our knowledge of the stress-related activity of SAS is continuously increasing, SNS has been much less studied than the adrenal medulla and relatively little is known about the mechanisms of gene expression of catecholamine biosynthetic enzymes in sympathetic ganglion cells following stressful stimulation.

See Also the Following Articles

Chronic (Repeated) Stress: Consequences, Adaptations; Norepinephrine: CNS Pathways and Neurophysiology; Stress: Definition and History; Sympathetic Noradrenergic and Adrenomedullary Hormonal Systems in Stress and Distress.

Further Reading

Björklund, A., Hökfelt, T. and Owman, C. (eds.) (1988). *Handbook of Chemical Neuroanatomy, Vol. 6: The Peripheral Nervous System.* Amsterdam: Elsevier.

Burnstock, G. and Hoyle C. H. V. (eds.) (1995). *The Autonomic Nervous System, Vol. 1: Autonomic Neuroeffector Mechanisms.* London: Harwood Academic.

Elfvin, L. G., Lindh, B. and Hökfelt, T. (1993). The chemical neuroanatomy of sympathetic ganglia. *Annual Review of Neuroscience* **16**, 471–507.

Gabella, G. (1995). Autonomic nervous system. In: Paxinos, G. (ed.) *Rat Nervous System* (2nd edn., pp. 81–103). San Dieg, CA: Academic Press.

Goldstein, D. S. (2001). *The Autonomic Nervous System in Health and Disease.* Oxford: Oxford University Press.

Kandel, E. R., Schwartz, J. H. and Jessell, T. M. (2000). *Principles of Neural Science* (3rd edn., pp. 961–981. New York: McGraw-Hill.

Langley, K. and Grant, N. J. (1999). Molecular markers of sympathoadrenal cells. *Cell and Tissue Research* **298**, 185–206.

Loewy, A. D. and Spyer K. M. (eds.) (1990). *Central Regulation of Autonomic Function.* New York: Oxford University Press.

Pacak, K. and Palkovits, M. (2001). Stressor specificity of central neuroendocrine responses: Implications for stress-related disorders. *Endocrine Reviews* **22**, 502–548.

Palkovits, M. (1999). Interconnections between the neuroendocrine hypothalamus and the central autonomic system. *Frontiers in Neuroendocrinology* **20**, 270–295.

Strack, A. M., Sawyer, W. B., Platt, K. B. and Loewy, A. D. (1989). CNS cell groups regulating the sympathetic outflow to adrenal gland as revealed by transneuronal cell body labelling with pseudorabies virus. *Brain Research* **491**, 274–296.

Sun, M. K. (1995). Central neural organization and control of sympathetic nervous system in mammals. *Progress in Neurobiology* **47**, 157–233.

Sympathetic Nervous System

D S Goldstein
National Institute of Neurological Disorders and Stroke, Bethesda, MD, USA

Published by Elsevier Inc.

Glossary

Sympathetic nervous system	A major component of the autonomic nervous system. The main sympathetic neurotransmitter for cardiovascular regulation is norepinephrine. The main sympathetic neurotransmitter for sweating is acetylcholine.
Adrenomedullary hormonal system	The hormonal component of the autonomic nervous system.
Norepinephrine	The main sympathetic neurotransmitter for cardiovascular regulation.
Epinephrine	The main hormone of the adrenomedullary hormonal system.
Norepinephrine	The sympathetic neurotransmitter.

Historical and Conceptual Overview

The term sympathetic nervous system originates in the second-century teaching of Galen that the peripheral nerves, conduits for distributing the animal spirit in the body, enable concerted, coordinated (i.e., sympathetic) functioning of body organs. The notion of the sympathetic nervous system, therefore, antedated by approximately 14 centuries Harvey's demonstration of the circulation of the blood.

The sympathetic nervous system is a major component of the autonomic nervous system. In the late nineteenth century, Langley introduced the phrase autonomic nervous system to refer to nerves emanating from cell bodies in ganglia alongside the spinal column and in the gastrointestinal-tract walls. Langley defined three components: sympathetic, with preganglionic cells in the thoracolumbar spinal cord; parasympathetic (a word he coined), with preganglionic cells in the brain stem or sacral spinal cord; and enteric, with preganglionic cells near or in the target organs. The nerves of these systems were thought to differ from those of the somatic nervous system, not only in terms of anatomy but also in terms of function. Somatic nerves mediate conscious, observable changes in skeletal muscle contraction and therefore movement, whereas autonomic nerves mediate unconscious, largely unobservable changes in smooth muscle contraction independently (autonomously) of the central nervous system.

The early-twentieth century American physiologist Walter B. Cannon introduced the word homeostasis. Cannon added a hormonal component to the autonomic nervous system when he theorized that the sympathetic nervous system and the adrenal gland worked together as a unit to maintain homeostasis in emergencies. In the 1930s, he even formally proposed that the sympathetic nervous system used the same chemical messenger – adrenaline – as did the adrenal gland (in 1946, von Euler correctly identified the sympathetic neurotransmitter in mammals as norepinephrine). Accumulating evidence supports the independent regulation of the sympathetic nervous and adrenomedullary hormonal systems, refuting the concept of a unitary sympathoadrenal system. Nevertheless, Cannon's views about the unitary function of the neural and hormonal components of the sympathoadrenal system prevail in stress research.

Sweating, whether to control body temperature (thermoregulatory), evoked by eating spicy food (gustatory), or accompanying fear or anxiety (emotional), is mediated by the sympathetic cholinergic system, in which acetylcholine rather than norepinephrine is the chemical messenger. The autonomic nervous system, therefore, can be viewed as having five components: sympathetic noradrenergic, sympathetic cholinergic, parasympathetic cholinergic, adrenomedullary, and enteric.

Role of the Sympathetic Nervous System in Homeostasis

Adjustments in sympathetic nervous activity accompany virtually every human action and reaction and constitute the main means for the acute regulation of cardiovascular function. According to Goldstein's 1995 theory, comparator homeostats use the sympathetic nervous system as an effector for different stress responses. The sympathetic nervous and adrenomedullary hormonal effectors interact in complex ways with many others, including the hypothalamic–pituitary–adrenocortical system, the endogenous opiate system, vasopressin, the parasympathetic nervous system, and the renin–angiotensin–aldosterone system, in determining responses to stressors.

The sympathetic nervous system consists of nerve networks. Because the axons come from cells in ganglia rather than directly from the spinal cord or brain stem, sympathetic nerves supplying body organs are mainly postganglionic; however, most sympathetic nerves supplying adrenomedullary chromaffin cells are preganglionic, releasing acetylcholine and thereby stimulating membrane nicotinic receptors.

Stresses associated with sympathetic nervous system activation typically include a component of active movement. Patterned sympathetic nervous system activation during stress produces adaptive shifts in the distribution of blood volume or in glandular secretion (**Figure 1a**). When these changes suffice to maintain homeostasis, the organism does not experience them consciously, but when the brain senses that these responses are not or will not mitigate the effects of the stressor, the situation reaches consciousness and adrenomedullary hormonal system activation ensues (**Figure 1b**). Examples of situations associated with prominent increases in sympathoneural outflows include orthostasis, exercise, the postprandial state, cold exposure, and the performance of nondistressing locomotor tasks.

In response to perceived global metabolic threats from external or internal stimuli, increased neural outflow to the adrenal medulla elicits catecholamine secretion into the adrenal venous drainage. In humans, the predominant catecholamine in the adrenal venous drainage is epinephrine (synonymous with adrenaline). Epinephrine rapidly reaches all cells of the body, with the exception of most of the brain, producing a wide variety of hormonal effects at low blood concentrations. We can comprehend the many effects of epinephrine in terms of the body's countering of acute threats to survival that mammals have perennially faced, such as sudden lack of metabolic fuels, trauma with hemorrhage, intravascular volume depletion and hypotension, and fight-or-flight confrontations. Distress accompanies all these situations, the experience undoubtedly fostering the long-term survival of the individual and the species by motivating avoidance learning, enhancing the registration of the event in long-term memory, and producing signs

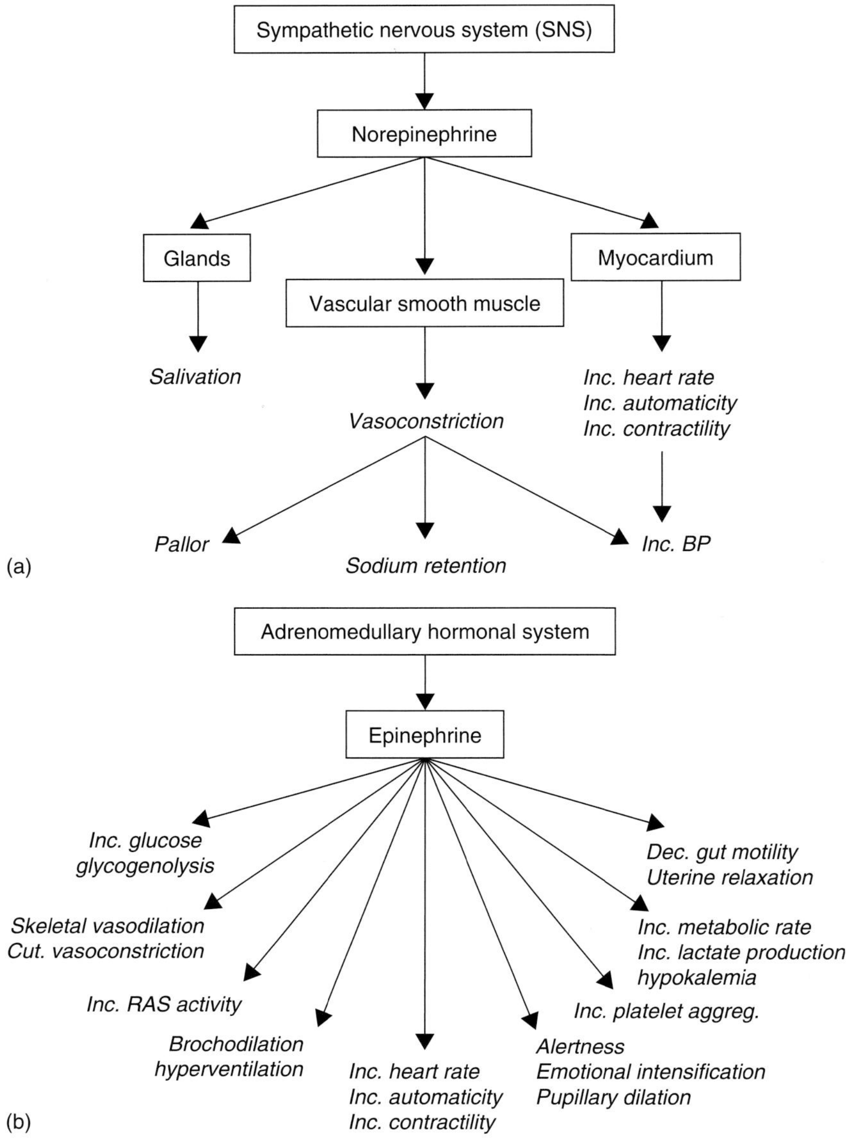

Figure 1 Overview of effects of the activation of (a) the sympathetic nervous system, where norepinephrine acts as the main neurotransmitter, and (b) the adrenomedullary hormonal system, where epinephrine acts as the main hormone. Because the sympathetic nervous system is a neural network, sympathetic nerves to different regions can be activated differentially during stress, producing redistributions of blood flow to body organs. Norepinephrine released from sympathetic nerves generally contracts smooth muscle cells, eliciting glandular secretion, vasoconstriction, and myocardial contraction. Renal vasoconstriction produces an anti-natriuretic effect. Cutaneous vasoconstriction produces pallor. The net effect of systemic vasoconstriction is to increase the total peripheral resistance to blood flow in the body. This, combined with myocardial stimulation, increases blood pressure. In humans, the main hormone released by the adrenal medulla is epinephrine (adrenaline). Epinephrine affects the function of most organs and produces generalized effects such as increased metabolic rate, increased blood glucose levels, hypokalemia, increased lactate production, increased alertness, increased platelet aggregability, and intensification of emotions. Aggreg., aggregation; BP, blood pressure; Cut., cutaneous; Dec., decrease; Inc., increase; RAS, renin–angiotensin–aldosterone system.

universally understood among other members of the species.

Stresses eliciting adrenomedullary hormonal system activation typically also elicit hypothalamic-pituitary-adrenocortical activation, as indicated by high circulating levels of corticotropin or glucocorticoids; increases in release of endogenous opioids, as indicated by high plasma levels of β-endorphin; and vasopressin secretion even when sympathetic nervous system activity declines.

Norepinephrine: The Sympathetic Neurotransmitter

The chemical transmitter at most cardiovascular sympathetic nerve endings is norepinephrine. The binding of norepinephrine to adrenoceptors on cardiovascular smooth muscle cells contracts the cells. The body's myriad arterioles largely determine total resistance to blood flow and therefore contribute in an important way to blood pressure. Sympathetic nerves enmesh blood vessels in latticelike networks in the adventitial outer surface that extend inward to the adventitial-medial border, with the concentration of sympathetic nerves increasing as arterial caliber decreases, so that small arteries and arterioles, the smallest nutrient vessels possessing smooth muscle cells, possess the most intense innervation. The unique architectural association between sympathetic nerves and the vessels that determine peripheral resistance has enticed cardiovascular researchers, particularly in the area of autonomic regulation, for many years. Sympathetic vascular innervation varies widely among vascular beds, with dense innervation of resistance vessels in the gut, kidney, skeletal muscle, and skin. Sympathetic stimulation in these beds produces profound vasoconstriction, whereas stimulation in the coronary, cerebral, and bronchial beds elicits weaker constrictor responses, consistent teleologically with the goal of preserving blood flow to vital organs during stress. Cardiac sympathetic stimulation increases the force and rate of the heartbeat and also augments intracardiac electrical conduction and automaticity.

Norepinephrine released from sympathetic nerve terminals acts mainly locally. Only a small proportion of released norepinephrine reaches the bloodstream. The indirect and distant relationship between plasma norepinephrine levels and sympathetic nerve activity can complicate interpreting plasma norepinephrine levels in response to stressors, pathophysiological situations, and drugs.

Norepinephrine Synthesis

The enzymatic steps in norepinephrine synthesis have been characterized in more detail than those for any other neurotransmitter (**Figure 2**). Catecholamine biosynthesis begins with the uptake of the amino acid tyrosine into the cytoplasm of sympathetic neurons and adrenomedullary cells. Tyrosine hydroxylase catalyzes the conversion of tyrosine to 3,4-dihydroxyphenylalanine (DOPA). This is the enzymatic rate-limiting step in catecholamine synthesis. The enzyme is almost saturated under normal conditions, so alterations in dietary tyrosine intake normally do not affect the rate of catecholamine biosynthesis under baseline conditions. Tetrahydrobiopterin, ionic iron, and molecular oxygen are required for tyrosine hydroxylase activity. Exposure to stressors that increase sympathoadrenal outflows augments the synthesis and concentration of tyrosine hydroxylase by multiple and complex mechanisms. Short-term mechanisms include feedback inhibition and phosphorylation of the enzyme, the latter depending on membrane depolarization, contractile elements, and receptors. Long-term mechanisms include changes in tyrosine hydroxylase synthesis, probably determined by trans-synaptic induction and retrograde transport.

L-aromatic-amino-acid decarboxylase (LAAAD, also called DOPA decarboxylase) in the neuronal cytoplasm catalyzes the rapid conversion of DOPA to dopamine. Many types of tissues contain this enzyme. The activity of the enzyme depends on pyridoxal phosphate, which is vitamin B-6. Although LAAAD metabolizes most of the DOPA formed in catecholamine-synthesizing tissues, some endogenously produced DOPA enters the circulation. This provides the basis for using plasma DOPA levels to examine catecholamine synthesis. By inhibiting the conversion of DOPA to dopamine in the periphery, LAAAD inhibitors such as carbidopa enhance the efficacy of L-DOPA treatment of Parkinson's disease.

Dopamine-β-hydroxylase catalyzes the conversion of dopamine to norepinephrine in tissues that synthesize catecholamines. The enzyme is confined to the vesicles in catecholamine-producing cells. Dopamine-β-hydroxylase contains, and its activity depends on, copper. Because of this dependence, children with Menkes disease, a rare, inherited X-linked recessive disorder of copper metabolism, have neurochemical evidence of decreased conversion of dopamine to norepinephrine and compensatorily increased tyrosine hydroxylation. Dopamine-β-hydroxylase activity also requires ascorbic acid (vitamin C), which provides electrons for the hydroxylation.

Norepinephrine Storage

Vesicles in sympathetic nerves actively remove and trap axoplasmic amines. The vesicular monoamine transporter resembles the neuronal membrane monoamine transporters structurally, but it is relatively nonspecific for catecholamines and serotonin. Magnesium and ATP accelerate vesicular uptake, and reserpine effectively and irreversibly blocks it. Vesicles generated near the Golgi apparatus of the cell bodies travel by axonal transport in the axons to the nerve terminals. Noradrenergic vesicles may also form by endocytosis within the axons. Varicosities in sympathetic nerves contain two types of cytoplasmic vesicles: small dense-core (diameter 40–60 nm) and large dense-core (diameter 80–120 nm). Cores of both types of vesicle contain abundant ATP, the norepinephrine : ATP ratio averaging approximately 1 : 4. The vesicles also contain at least three types of polypeptides: chromogranin A, enkephalins, and neuropeptide Y. The extracellular

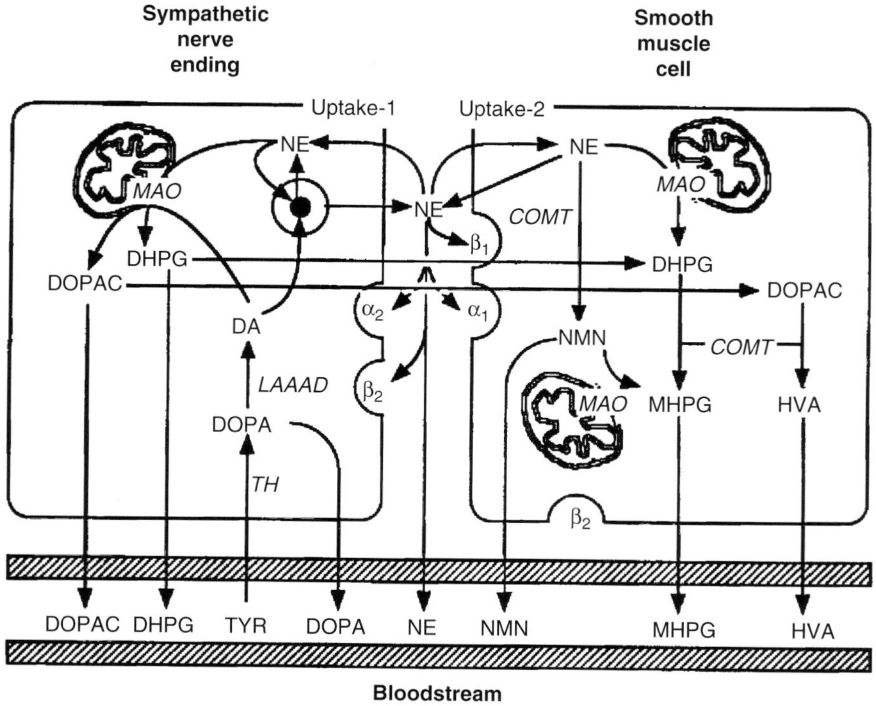

Figure 2 Overview of steps in norepinephrine synthesis, release, reuptake, and metabolism. Hydroxylation of the amino acid tyrosine is the enzymatic rate-limiting step in catecholamine biosynthesis. Tyrosine hydroxylase catalyzes the conversion of tyrosine to DOPA. L-aromatic-amino acid decarboxylase (LAAAD) catalyzes the conversion of DOPA to dopamine. Dopamine-β-hydroxylase is localized to large dense-core vesicles in noradrenergic cells. After uptake of axoplasmic dopamine into the vesicle, dopamine-β-hydroxylase catalyzes the conversion of dopamine to norepinephrine. According to the exocytosis theory, increased transmembrane entry of ionized calcium fosters fusion of the vesicles with the axonal membrane. Endogenously released norepinephrine is taken back up into sympathetic nerve terminals by Uptake-1 and taken up into nonneuronal cells by Uptake-2. Norepinephrine in the axoplasm can be translocated back into the vesicles or converted to dihydroxyphenylglycol by monoamine oxidase (MAO) in the outer mitochondrial membrane. Norepinephrine in nonneuronal cells is converted to normetanephrine by catechol-O-methyltransferase. Dihydroxyphenylglycol can diffuse into the bloodstream or can be taken up by nonneuronal cells and converted to methoxyhydroxyphenylglycol, which is a major end product of norepinephrine metabolism. Dopamine in the axoplasm can be translocated into vesicles and converted to norepinephrine or can be converted to dihydroxyphenylacetic acid by MAO. Dihydroxyphenylacetic acid can diffuse into the bloodstream or can be converted extraneuronally to homovanillic acid, the main end product of dopamine metabolism. The processes of catecholamine uptake and metabolism are generally independent of actions by adrenoceptors on the nerve terminals or nonneuronal cells. COMT, catechol-O-methyltransferase; DA, dopamine; DHPG, dihydroxyphenylglycol; DOPA, 3,4-dihydroxyphenylalanine; DOPAC, dihydroxyphenylacetic acid; HVA, homovanillic acid; LAAAD, L-aromatic-amino acid decarboxylase; MAO, monoamine oxidase; MHPG, methoxyhydroxyphenylglycol; NE, norepinephrine; NMN, normetanephrine; TH, tyrosine hydroxylase; TYR, tyrosine.

fluid levels of each of these compounds have been considered as putative indices of exocytosis.

Norepinephrine Release

According to the exocytotic theory, acetylcholine depolarizes the terminal membranes by increasing membrane permeability to sodium ion. The increased intracellular sodium levels directly or indirectly enhance the transmembrane influx of calcium ion via voltage-gated channels. The increased cytoplasmic calcium concentration evokes a cascade of as yet incompletely defined biomechanical events, resulting in the fusion of the vesicular and axoplasmic membranes. The interior of the vesicle exchanges briefly with the extracellular compartment, and the soluble contents of the vesicles diffuse into the extracellular space. As predicted from this model, manipulations other than the application of acetylcholine that depolarize the cell, such as electrical stimulation or increased potassium ion concentrations in the extracellular fluid, also activate the voltage-gated calcium channels and trigger exocytosis.

During sympathetic neuronal or adrenomedullary chromaffin cell activation, the simultaneous stoichiometric release of soluble vesicular contents – ATP, enkephalins, chromogranins, and dopamine-β-hydroxylase – without a similar release of cytoplasmic macromolecules has provided biochemical support for the exocytosis theory of noradrenergic neurotransmission. Electron micrographs occasionally have shown an omega sign, with an apparent gap in the cell membrane at the site of fusion of vesicle with the axoplasmic membrane. Ultrastructural evidence has suggested the release of the contents of large as well as small dense-core vesicles by exocytosis.

Sympathetic nerve endings can also release norepinephrine by calcium-independent, nonexocytotic mechanisms. One such mechanism probably is reverse transport through the neuronal uptake carrier. The indirectly acting sympathomimetic amine, tyramine, releases norepinephrine nonexocytotically because tyramine releases norepinephrine independently of calcium and does not release dopamine-β-hydroxylase. As predicted from the ionic requirements for neuronal reuptake, increases in intracellular sodium concentrations, such as produced by ouabain, enhance carrier-mediated efflux of norepinephrine. Myocardial ischemic hypoxia evokes the calcium-independent release of norepinephrine. The hydrophilic nature of catecholamines and their ionization at physiological pH probably prevent norepinephrine efflux by simple diffusion.

Pharmacological stimulation of receptors on noradrenergic terminals affects the amount of norepinephrine released during cellular activation. Substantial evidence supports inhibitory presynaptic modulation by norepinephrine itself via α2-adrenoceptors on sympathetic nerves. This modulatory action appears to vary with the vascular bed under study, being prominent in skeletal muscle beds such as the forearm, relatively weak in the kidneys, and virtually absent in the adrenals. In addition to local feedback control of norepinephrine release, reflexive long-distance feedback pathways via arterial and cardiac baroreceptors elicit reflexive changes in sympathoneural impulse activity. Alterations in receptor numbers or of intracellular biomechanical events after receptor activation also affect responses to agonists. These factors therefore regulate norepinephrine release by trans-synaptic local and reflexive long-distance mechanisms.

Norepinephrine Disposition

Unlike acetylcholine, which is inactivated mainly by extracellular enzymes, norepinephrine is inactivated mainly by uptake into cells (**Figure 2**), with subsequent intracellular metabolism or storage. Reuptake into nerve terminals (Uptake-1) is the predominant means of terminating the actions of released norepinephrine. Dopamine is a better substrate than norepinephrine is for uptake via the cell-membrane norepinephrine transporter.

Neuronal uptake absolutely requires intracellular potassium ion and extracellular sodium ion and functions most efficiently when chloride ion accompanies the sodium. Uptake-1 requires energy and is carrier mediated. Transport does not directly require ATP; however, maintaining ionic gradients across cell membranes depends on ATP, and the carrier uses the energy expended in maintaining the transmembrane sodium gradient to cotransport amines with sodium. Many drugs or *in vitro* conditions inhibit Uptake-1, including cocaine and tricyclic antidepressants.

Norepinephrine taken up into the axoplasm by the Uptake-1 transporter is subject to two fates: translocation into storage vesicles and deamination by monoamine oxidase (MAO). The combination of enzymatic breakdown and vesicular uptake constitute an intraneuronal sink, keeping the cytoplasmic concentrations of norepinephrine very low. Reserpine effectively blocks the vesicular transport of amines from the axoplasm into the vesicles. This not only shuts down the conversion of dopamine to norepinephrine but also prevents the conservative recycling of norepinephrine. Reserpine, therefore, rapidly depletes norepinephrine stores.

Neural and nonneural tissues contain MAO, which catalyzes the oxidative deamination of dopamine to form dihydroxyphenylacetic acid and norepinephrine to form dihydroxyphenylglycol. Because of the efficient uptake and reuptake of catecholamines into the axoplasm of catecholaminergic neurons and because of the rapid exchange of amines between the vesicles and axoplasm, the neuronal pool of MAO, located in the outer mitochondrial membrane, figures prominently in the overall functioning of catecholaminergic systems. The isozyme MAO-A predominates in neural tissue, whereas both MAO-A and MAO-B exist in nonneuronal tissue. MAO inhibitors are effective antidepressants. A phenomenon known as the cheese effect limits their clinical use. In patients taking MAO inhibitors, the administration of sympathomimetic amines such as those found in many nonprescription decongestants or the ingestion of foods such as aged cheese, wine, and meat, which contain tyramine, can produce paroxysmal hypertension. Tyramine and other sympathomimetic amines increase the loss of norepinephrine from sympathetic vesicles, and the blockade of MAO augments the bioavailability of ingested tyramine. When given alone, MAO inhibitors usually decrease blood pressure and can produce orthostatic hypotension by unknown mechanisms.

Nonneuronal cells remove norepinephrine actively by a process called Uptake-2, characterized by the ability to transport isoproterenol; susceptibility to blockade by O-methylated catecholamines, corticosteroids, and β-haloalkylamines; and an absence of susceptibility to blockade by Uptake-1 blockers. In contrast with Uptake-1, Uptake-2 functions independently of extracellular sodium. The Uptake-2 carrier has little if any stereoselectivity and has low affinity and specificity for catecholamines. For instance, extraneuronal cells remove imidazolines such as clonidine by Uptake-2. Whereas reverse transport via the Uptake-1 carrier requires special experimental conditions, reverse transport via the Uptake-2 carrier is readily demonstrated. Thus, during the infusion of a catecholamine at a high rate, the catecholamine can accumulate in extraneuronal cells, with reentry of the catecholamine into the extracellular fluid via the Uptake-2 carrier after the infusion ends.

Catechol-O-methyltransferase in nonneuronal cells and adrenomedullary chromaffin cells catalyzes the O-methylation of dihydroxyphenylglycol to form methoxyhydroxyphenylglycol and of dihydroxyphenylacetic acid to form homovanillic acid. Plasma levels of dihydroxyphenylglycol and dihydroxyphenylacetic acid probably mainly reflect neuronal metabolism of norepinephrine and dopamine. Catechol-O-methyltransferase also catalyzes the conversion of norepinephrine to normetanephrine and epinephrine to metanephrine. Uptake-2 and catechol-O-methyltransferase probably act in series to remove and degrade circulating catecholamines. The methyl group donor for the reaction is S-adenosyl methionine. Immunohistochemical studies have indicated extraneuronal localization of catechol-O-methyltransferase in most tissues, such as the liver and kidney. Because of the extraneuronal localization of catechol-O-methyltransferase, recently introduced assay methods for metanephrines have enabled refined assessments of extraneuronal metabolism of catecholamines.

Most of the metabolism of catecholamines takes place within the same cells where the amines are synthesized. This mainly occurs secondary to leakage of catecholamines from vesicular stores into the cytoplasm. The stores exist in a highly dynamic equilibrium, with passive outward leakage counterbalanced by inward active transport controlled by vesicular monoamine transporters.

In catecholaminergic neurons, the presence of MAO-A leads to the formation of reactive catecholaldehydes. The contribution of these toxic aldehydes to neurodegenerative processes depends on the dynamics of vesicular-axoplasmic monoamine exchange and enzyme-catalyzed conversion to inert deaminated acids or alcohols. In sympathetic nerves, the aldehyde produced from norepinephrine is converted to dihydroxyphenylglycol, not dihydroxymandelic acid, as textbooks often indicate. Subsequent extraneuronal O-methylation consequently leads to the production of methoxyhydroxyphenylglycol, not vanillylmandelic acid. Vanillylmandelic acid is instead formed in the liver by the oxidation of methoxyhydroxyphenylglycol catalyzed by alcohol dehydrogenase. Compared to intraneuronal deamination, extraneuronal O-methylation of norepinephrine and epinephrine to metanephrines represent minor pathways of metabolism. The single largest source of metanephrines is the adrenal medulla. Vanillylmandelic acid and methoxyhydroxyphenylglycol, the products of the combined O-methylation and deamination of norepinephrine, are the two main end products of norepinephrine metabolism, vanillylmandelic acid (as just noted) formed mainly in the liver. Adrenomedullary chromaffin cells express catechol-O-methyltransferase, as do pheochromocytomas, which are clinically important chromaffin cell tumors. Pheochromocytoma cells produce large amounts of metanephrines from catecholamines leaking from stores. These metabolites are thus particularly useful for detecting these tumors. The large contribution of intraneuronal deamination to catecholamine turnover, and the dependence of this on the vesicular axoplasmic monoamine exchange process, help explain how synthesis, release, metabolism, turnover, and stores of catecholamines are regulated in a coordinated fashion.

See Also the Following Article

Autonomic Nervous System.

Further Reading

Cannon, W. B. (1939). *The wisdom of the body.* New York: W. W. Norton.

Eisenhofer, G., Kopin, I. J. and Goldstein, D. S. (2004). Catecholamine metabolism: a contemporary view with implications for physiology and medicine. *Pharmacological Reviews* 56, 331–349.

Goldstein, D. S. (1995). *Stress, catecholamines, and cardiovascular disease.* New York: Oxford University Press.

Goldstein, D. S. (2001). *The autonomic nervous system in health and disease.* New York: Marcel Dekker.

Goldstein, D. S., Eisenhofer, G. and Kopin, I. J. (2003). Sources and significance of plasma levels of catechols and their metabolites in humans. *Journal of Pharmacology and Experimental Therapeutics* 305, 800–811.

Pacak, K., Palkovits, M., Yadid, G., et al. (1998). Heterogeneous neuroendocrine responses to various stressors: a test of Selye's doctrine of non-specificity. *American Journal of Physiology* 275, R1247–R1255.

Selye, H. (1950). *The physiology and pathology of exposure to stress: a treatise based on the concepts of the general-adaptation syndrome and the diseases of adaptation.* Montreal: Acta, Inc.

Adrenaline

T M Pollard
Durham University, Durham, UK

This is a revised version of the article by T M Pollard, Encyclopedia of Stress, First edition, volume 1, pp 52–57, © 2000, Elsevier Inc.

Glossary

Adrenal glands Endocrine glands situated above the kidneys, composed of two distinct parts, the adrenal medulla, which secretes adrenaline and noradrenaline, and the adrenal cortex, which secretes corticosteroids.

Adrenergic receptors Receptors that mediate the action of adrenaline. There are two types, α and β receptors.

Atherogenic Encouraging the process of atherosclerosis, which is a change in the lining of arteries consisting of an accumulation of lipids, complex carbohydrates, blood and blood products, fibrous tissue, and calcium deposits.

Catecholamine A group of hormones, including adrenaline, norepinephrine (noradrenaline), and dopamine, which are synthesized from the amino acid tyrosine.

Job strain A construct used to describe work that makes heavy demands but offers little decision latitude for the worker.

Sympathetic tone The basal rate of activity of the sympathetic nervous system.

Adrenaline, also known as epinephrine, is the main catecholamine produced by the adrenal medulla. Its secretion into the adrenal vein is under the control of sympathetic nerves and is the most important indirect pathway of sympathetic activation. Adrenaline plays a major role in the body's physiological response to stress and affects most systems of the body. The axis as a whole is referred to here as the sympathetic adrenal medullary (SAM) axis.

The Effects of Adrenaline

The effects of adrenaline are similar to those of direct sympathetic stimulation, but they last considerably longer. Once in the bloodstream, adrenaline stimulates α and β adrenergic receptors. Through stimulation of cardiac muscle β receptors it causes an increased heart rate, force of contraction, and cardiac output. Its actions on vascular smooth muscle adrenergic receptors cause the shunting of blood away from the skin, mucosa, and kidneys to the coronary arteries, skeletal muscle, and brain. Adrenaline also enhances blood platelet adhesiveness and reduces clotting time. It promotes the role of glucagon in converting glycogen to glucose, leading to an increased secretion of glucose into the bloodstream and production of glucose in the liver. Experimental studies have shown a highly significant increase in glucose levels during infusion of adrenaline. In addition, lipolytic activity in adipose tissues is stimulated, with a resultant increase in levels of plasma free fatty acids, providing another source of energy. There is also an increase in plasma cholesterol levels, including both low-density and high-density fractions, but this effect may be at least partially explained by a reduction in plasma volume. Oxygen supply is improved, as a function of both vascular changes and bronchodilation. As a result, the body is prepared for immediate physical and mental activity, and the response is often referred to as the fight or flight reaction. This emergency function of the adrenal medulla was first identified by Cannon in 1914. At least over a few hours of secretion there appears to be no regulatory mechanism to counteract the effects of adrenaline; that is, these effects are sustained for as long as secretion of the hormone is maintained.

It is thought that repeated adrenaline secretion, or chronically raised levels of adrenaline, are likely to increase risk of cardiovascular disease, partly by changing sympathetic tone and partly by inducing changes that accelerate the process of atherosclerosis. Infusion of adrenaline leads to a sustained rise in blood pressure, and repeated elevation of blood pressure may eventually lead to hypertension via enhanced sympathetic tone and damage to the blood vessels. It is likely that chronic elevation of adrenaline levels may lead to long-term elevation of lipid levels. The free fatty acids whose release is stimulated by adrenaline are used by the liver for the synthesis of very low density lipoproteins, which then become modified to low-density lipoproteins, which are strongly implicated in the atherogenic process. Adrenaline may have a direct role to play in myocardial infarction or cerebrovascular accident through its effects on platelets and clotting time and by the precipitation of cardiac arrhythmias.

Adrenaline can alter a number of aspects of immune function and may well mediate some of the apparent effects of stress on susceptibility to infectious disease and cancers. Studies show that individuals who show large increases in adrenaline in response to laboratory stressors also show the largest immune changes. Furthermore, adrenergic blockers have been demonstrated to prevent stress-induced increases in natural killer cell number and activity. Adrenaline is thought to act on the immune system by altering lymphocyte migration from lymphoid organs such as the spleen.

Measuring Adrenaline Levels

It is possible to determine adrenaline levels in plasma or urine. The main methods used are high-performance liquid chromatography and radioenzymatic assay. The former uses high pressure to separate catecholamines, and this is usually followed by electrochemical detection. The latter relies on radioactive labeling – a radioactive substrate is added together with an enzyme, and the amount of radioactive metabolite formed is measured. Both techniques have been validated and are known to be reliable, but neither is cheap.

Levels of hormone in plasma and urine reflect neuroendocrine activity over different time periods, and it is important to use the appropriate medium. The SAM axis responds to stimuli within a few seconds of their impact, and plasma adrenaline has a half-life of 1 to 2 min, so that levels of hormone in plasma reflect the SAM activity of only the preceding minute or so. Thus, assessment of plasma adrenaline levels is only generally useful for laboratory studies of acute stressors, when an indwelling venous catheter can be used (since venipuncture itself is known to cause an increase in adrenaline levels). Samples must be spun and frozen very shortly after collection.

Levels of excreted free adrenaline or its metabolites can be measured in urine and have been shown to provide an accurate measure of circulating levels. Hormone assayed in urine usually represents a pooling of levels over a period of hours. This is partly because hormone measured in urine is an integration of the hormone excreted into the urine produced by the body since the previous urination, and partly because excreted hormone reflects hormone secreted some time before. Information on the time lag between secretion and excretion is sparse, although some laboratory studies have produced results indicating that urinary adrenaline excretion rate reflects plasma adrenaline levels within an hour. When samples are collected over a few hours, it is important to make some correction for variation in the amount of urine produced during that time. It is also possible to collect all the urine produced in a given 24-h period in order to look at the overall level produced during a day. However, it is not always easy for study participants to comply with the demands of 24-h collection, and some checking for completeness of the sample is often needed, by assessing either total volume or creatinine clearance. Again, degradation and oxidation is a problem, and an antioxidant such as sodium metabisulphite is usually added to urine samples collected for the purpose of catecholamine determination.

Psychosocial Determinants of Adrenaline Variation

Researchers interested in understanding psychosocial determinants of adrenaline variation have investigated changes in hormone levels within individuals as well as differences between individuals. In general, the former approach has been more successful. As we have seen, adrenaline levels respond quickly to changing circumstances, and a lot of information can be gained from examination of changes in hormone levels over time. Comparisons between individuals usually focus on longer-term measures, such as 24-h urinary excretion rates, and thus only make use of averaged information for each subject. Data on within-individual variability is lost, and it is known that adrenaline excretion rates vary as much or more within individuals as they do between them. Furthermore, absolute levels of hormone are influenced by a large number of factors other than stress or the psychosocial environment, so that it is much more useful if each person can be used as his or her own control.

The main findings of studies examining the reasons for variation in adrenaline levels are summarized below, looking first at laboratory studies and then at those that have been conducted in people going about their normal lives.

Laboratory Studies of the Determinants of Adrenaline Secretion

The largest body of research on adrenaline responses in humans has been undertaken in laboratories. In general, the focus of these studies has been measuring the adrenaline response to situations and stimuli that are assumed to be stressful. Mason reviewed the early work in an important article published in 1968. He described situations in which adrenaline levels had been shown to rise in humans. These included watching engaging movies, taking examinations, and performing set tasks such as intelligence tests or mental arithmetic. He concluded from these findings that adrenaline can rise in emotionally arousing situations that are pleasant as well as in those that are unpleasant. Since the 1960s, other workers have reported results that can be interpreted in the same way. As a result of these findings, Frankenhaeuser put forward a model in which the SAM axis was considered to be activated in response to mental or physical effort, regardless of emotional content. These studies provided some indication that adrenaline responses in women are less marked than those in men.

Adrenaline Variation in Everyday Life

Influences of habitual health-related behaviors Adrenaline levels respond to a number of features of human behavior, not just the experience of psychosocial stress. Those that have received the most attention and that are probably most important are the intake of caffeine, nicotine, and alcohol and taking exercise. All have been shown to stimulate adrenaline secretion. Caffeine also appears to potentiate adrenaline responses to stress. In laboratory studies it is possible either to eliminate these influences or to control them. Researchers hoping to isolate the effects of psychosocial stressors outside the controlled laboratory environment have a more difficult task. They have sometimes approached the problem by asking subjects to avoid these influences. However, such an approach can bring problems of its own, perhaps, for example, inducing stress in smokers asked to abstain from cigarettes. Thus, others have asked subjects to keep detailed records of their behavior and included this information in subsequent analyses.

Adrenaline variation across societies Biological anthropologists have examined cross-cultural variation in adrenaline levels and have tried to relate the observed variation to differences in lifestyle. Such cross-sectional data suffer from the problems described previously, but some of the findings are nevertheless suggestive. In general, people living in more urbanized environments appear to excrete higher levels of urinary adrenaline than those engaged in traditional subsistence farming work, despite the lower levels of physical activity characteristic of urbanites. For example, James and colleagues compared urinary adrenaline excretion rates in young Western Samoan men living in villages or the capital, and showed that men living in the city, whether nonmanual workers, students, or laborers, excreted higher levels of urinary adrenaline than villagers on average. Similarly, Tokelauans living on Fakaofo had higher levels of urinary adrenaline than residents of Nukunonu, a nearby island less influenced by the wage economy. Still higher levels were excreted by Tokelauan migrants to New Zealand living in the urban center of Wellington. In both these studies the results were explained largely with respect to working behavior, with the suggestion that engagement in paid work, as opposed to traditional subsistence work, was more stressful.

Adrenaline variation in everyday working life In addition to their laboratory work, Frankenhaeuser and her team also pioneered investigations of the ways in which work-related stress might affect adrenaline levels. Two main kinds of comparisons have been made. The first contrasts hormone levels in people at work and at leisure, usually using a within-subject design; the second compares the effects of different types of work on hormone variation. The comparison of work and leisure addresses the question of whether nonmanual work *per se* causes an increase in adrenaline secretion. It is then relevant to ask what particular aspects of work are associated with elevated adrenaline levels.

There is good evidence that adrenaline levels are higher in men at work than in the same men at leisure. In a particularly large study, researchers in Oxford also found that in a diverse sample of British men, who provided urine samples on a normal working day and on Sunday, a rest day, urinary adrenaline levels were higher on the working day. Women who gave samples as part of the same study also showed significantly raised adrenaline levels on work days. However, there is some suggestion that the effect is not as consistent in women. In another study conducted in the same area, it was found that while men's urinary adrenaline levels were raised on working days, those for women were not, despite the fact that men and women reported experiencing very similar levels of demand.

Taken together, the results of a series of studies can be interpreted to show that workload and time pressure are the key features leading to elevated adrenaline levels at work. For example, increased urinary adrenaline levels in Swedish bus drivers when traffic was heavier were attributed to greater perceived time pressure created by the demands of remaining on schedule. Elevated adrenaline levels have also been seen in sawmill workers operating under time pressure and in people working on conveyer belts.

Efforts have been made to relate variation in adrenaline levels at work to the model of job strain proposed by Karasek and widely tested and applied in studies of workplace stress. Karasek and Theorell suggested that endocrine mechanisms explain the apparent link between job strain and ill health, particularly cardiovascular disease. They proposed that adrenaline is secreted at higher levels in those experiencing job strain due to a heavy workload and lack of decision latitude. However, Karasek acknowledged that adrenaline can also rise with increased workload, whether decision latitude is high or low. There is, then, a general consensus that adrenaline levels are most strongly related to arousal or effort, as in Frankenhaeuser's original model.

Individual Differences in SAM Reactivity

Not all people show the same SAM responsivity to stressors. It has been proposed that more reactive individuals are at greater risk of cardiovascular disease.

Sex Differences

Most early studies of the effects of stress on adrenaline in humans were conducted with only male participants. When researchers began to include women, they found that their responses to stressors were not always the same as men's, as noted previously. It is possible that the high circulating levels of estrogen seen in premenopausal women modify the way in which adrenaline is secreted in response to stress. Evidence for such an effect comes from comparisons of post- and premenopausal women and from studies of women given exogenous estrogen, as, for example, in hormone replacement therapy for postmenopausal women. There is little evidence to support an alternative explanation for increased adrenaline responses in men – that they find exposure to stressors more stressful.

Age

Little is known about the reactivity of the SAM system in normal children. There is evidence that in adults adrenaline secretion in response to acute laboratory stressors declines with age, for example, in 60- to 75-year-old men compared to 20- to 30-year-old men. It is also the case that basal adrenaline secretion from the adrenal medulla declines with age in adults, but because plasma clearance is reduced too, plasma adrenaline concentrations do not decline.

Individuals Experiencing Chronic Stress

In contrast to initial suggestions, recent findings indicate that those experiencing chronic stress (at work, in relationships, or as caregivers) do not show greater adrenaline reactivity to acute laboratory stressors compared to those not experiencing such chronic stressors.

Conclusion

Adrenaline has widespread and important effects on the body, and these effects have clear-cut implications for cardiovascular disease. It is the hormone most consistently shown to respond to stress both in laboratory studies and in people going about their everyday lives. However, adrenaline also responds to experiences not usually considered stressful, since it rises with mental arousal or effort, whether of a negative or a positive connotation. Furthermore, the adrenaline response may not be consistent across all individuals or all stages of the life course.

See Also the Following Articles

Adrenal Medulla; Cardiovascular System and Stress; Sympathetic Nervous System.

Further Reading

Baum, A. and Grunberg, N. (1995). Measurement of stress hormones. In: Cohen, S., Kessler, R. C. & Gordon, L. U. (eds.) *Measuring stress: a guide for health and social scientists*, pp. 175–182. New York: Oxford University Press.

Charmandari, E., Tsigos, C. and Chrousos, G. (2005). Endocrinology of the stress response. *Annual Review of Physiology* **67**, 259–284.

Dimsdale, J. E. and Ziegler, M. G. (1991). What do plasma and urinary measures of catecholamines tell us about human responses to stressors? *Circulation* **22**, II36–II42.

Frankenhaeuser, M. (1989). A biopsychosocial approach to work life issues. *International Journal of Health Services* **19**, 747–758.

Gump, B. B. (1999). Do background stressors influence reactivity to and recovery from acute stressors? *Journal of Applied Social Psychology* **29**, 469–494.

James, G. D. and Brown, D. E. (1997). The biological stress response and lifestyle: catecholamines and blood pressure. *Annual Review of Anthropology* **26**, 313–335.

Mason, J. W. (1968). A review of psychoendocrine research on the sympathetic-adrenal medullary system. *Psychosomatic Medicine* **30**, 631–653.

McKinnon, W., Baum, A. and Morokoff, P. (1988). Neuroendocrine measures of stress. In: Wagner, H. (ed.) *Social psychophysiology theory and emotion: theory and clinical applications*, pp. 43–64. Chichester, UK: Wiley.

Pollard, T. M., Ungpakorn, G., Harrison, G. A., et al. (1996). Epinephrine and cortisol responses to work: a test of the models of Frankenhaeuser and Karasek. *Annals of Behavioral Medicine* **18**, 229–237.

Seals, D. R. and Esler, M. D. (2000). Human ageing and the sympathoadrenal system. *Journal of Physiology* **528**(3), 407–417.

Stoney, C., Davis, M. and Matthews, K. A. (1987). Sex differences in physiological responses to stress and in coronary heart disease. *Psychophysiology* **24**, 127–131.

Ziegler, M. G. (1989). Catecholamine measurement in behavioral research. In: Schneiderman, N., Weiss, S. M. & Kaufman, P. G. (eds.) *Handbook of research methods in cardiovascular behavioral medicine*, pp. 167–184. New York: Plenum Press.

Adrenergic Receptors

J P Hieble
Wayne, PA, USA

Introduction

The adrenoceptors (adrenergic receptors) mediate the diverse effects of the neurotransmitters of the sympathetic nervous system, norepinephrine and epinephrine, at virtually all sites throughout the body. During the past century, the adrenoceptors have been extensively studied by a variety of functional and molecular techniques, and they have been progressively subdivided. Currently, nine adrenoceptors have been cloned, and they have been divided into three major categories – the α_1-adrenoceptors, α_2-adrenoceptors, and β-adrenoceptors. Although there are pharmacological data that suggest the existence of additional adrenoceptor subtypes, it now seems likely that this results from multiple 'affinity states' of a particular adrenoceptor subtype, rather than from a new adrenoceptor protein yet to be cloned. Although the specific receptors involved have not all been identified, norepinephrine-releasing neurons within the central nervous system (CNS) play an important role in psychiatric disorders such as major depression and attention-deficit/hyperactivity disorder (ADHD).

The adrenoceptors belong to the large family of seven transmembrane-spanning, G-protein-coupled receptors, and there is 32–54% amino acid identity between the individual adrenoceptor proteins (**Figure 1**). The most likely sites for interaction of the catecholamines with conserved structural elements of the adrenoceptors have been identified.

α_1-Adrenoceptors

α_1-Adrenoceptors are widely distributed in both central and peripheral sites, and they are activated either by norepinephrine released from sympathetic nerve terminals or by epinephrine released from the adrenal medulla and some central adrenergic neurons. Peripheral α_1-adrenoceptors mediate a variety of functions, including contraction of smooth muscle, cardiac stimulation, cellular proliferation/apoptosis, and activation of hepatic gluconeogenesis and glycogenolysis. α_1-Adrenoceptors are widely distributed within the CNS, where their activation generally results in depolarization and increased neuronal firing. Most of the peripheral actions of α_1-adrenoceptors are mediated through the inositol phosphate pathway, although there is evidence for activation of adenylyl cyclase within the CNS.

Three distinct α_1-adrenoceptor proteins have been cloned; after some confusion in nomenclature, it has been established that these three recombinant α_1-adrenoceptors correspond to the pharmacologically defined α_{1A}, α_{1B}, and α_{1D} adrenoceptors in native tissues. Selective antagonists are available for each of the α_1-adrenoceptor subtypes. Multiple splice variants of the α_{1A}-adrenoceptor have been identified; however, they appear to have identical pharmacological characteristics. The contraction of several vascular and urogenital tissues has distinct pharmacology from other α_{1A}-mediated responses. This was thought to implicate an additional α_1-adrenoceptor, designated as the α_{1L}-adrenoceptor. This receptor was never cloned, and it now seems likely that the α_{1A}-adrenoceptor may have either α_{1A} or α_{1L} pharmacology, depending on the particular assay, tissue, or experimental conditions employed.

α_1-Adrenoceptor subtypes can be differentially distributed in certain tissues. This differential distribution can reflect either expression of receptor protein/message or pharmacological characteristics

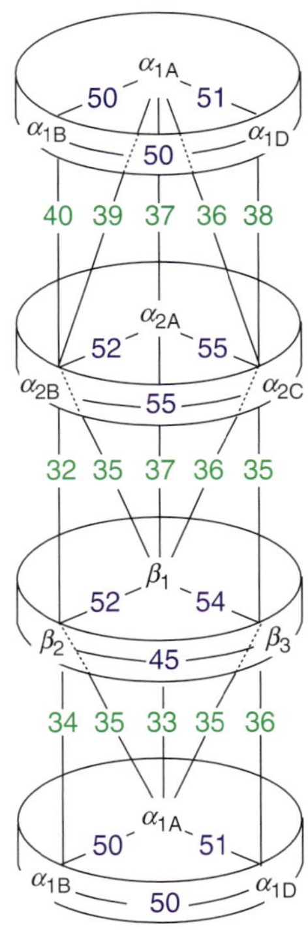

Figure 1 Structural similarity, based on overall amino acid identity, between the nine adrenoceptors. Based on this similarity, the adrenoceptors can be divided into three groups (α_1, α_2, and β), with each group further divided into three subtypes. Structural similarity is higher (45–55% identity) within either of the three groups than between individual members of different groups (33–40% identity).

in functional assays. For example, the predominant α_1-adrenoceptor found in rat spleen is the α_{1B} subtype, and the functional pharmacological profile of α_1-adrenoceptor agonists (i.e., contraction) in this tissue has α_{1B}-adrenoceptor characteristics, as determined by the use of subtype selective antagonists. Although all of the α_1-adrenoceptor subtypes are present in most blood vessels, the pharmacological characteristics of agonist-induced contraction can vary, such that the responses may be α_{1A} (human microvessels and rat caudal artery), α_{1B} (rabbit or canine aorta), or α_{1D} (rat aorta).

Knockout and overexpression experiments have been reported only for the α_{1B}-adrenoceptor subtype. Knockout of the α_{1B}-adrenoceptor results in impaired vascular responsiveness to phenylephrine, demonstrated both in isolated blood vessels and through measurement of blood pressure responses in anesthetized mice. Cardiac-specific overexpression of the α_{1B}-adrenoceptor results in an impairment of cardiac function without cardiomyocyte hypertrophy.

The α_1-adrenoceptor subtypes are differentially distributed within the CNS. Studies in rat brain have shown α_{1B}-adrenoceptor mRNA to be concentrated in cerebral cortex, thalamus, raphe nuclei, cranial and spinal motor neurons, as well as the pineal gland. mRNA for the α_{1D}-adrenoceptor is localized to the olfactory bulb, cerebral cortex, hippocampus, dentate gyrus, reticular thalamic nucleus, motor neurons, and the inferior olivary complex. In the thalamus, the α_{1B}- and α_{1D}-adrenoceptors have a complimentary distribution. Highest levels of α_{1A}-adrenoceptor mRNA are found in regions of the olfactory system, hypothalamic nuclei, and in regions of the brain stem and spinal cord related to motor function. Much less information is available on the distribution of α_1-adrenoceptors in the human brain. Although α_1-adrenoceptors are found in neocortex and dentate gyrus, their distribution differs substantially from that observed in the rat.

Centrally acting α_1-adrenoceptor agonists often potentiate motor stimulation or arousal produced by other pharmacological or behavioral challenges and will increase vigilance when administered alone. α_1-Adrenoceptor agonists can reverse sedation induced by norepinephrine depletion produced by a dopamine β-hydroxylase inhibitor or the cognitive impairment produced by a neurotoxin selective for noradrenergic neurons. Likewise, they can reverse cataplexy in a genetic canine model of narcolepsy. Based on studies in rats and primates, modafinil, currently marketed for the treatment of narcolepsy, may act through the activation of central α_1-adrenoceptors, although based on its structure and peripheral pharmacological effects, this drug would not be expected to be an α-adrenoceptor agonist.

Activation of central α_1-adrenoceptors, presumably in the hypothalamus, stimulates the secretion of several pituitary hormones in human volunteers. A centrally active α_1-adrenoceptor agonist, SDZ NVI-085 (naphtoxazine), improved the performance of patients with Parkinson's disease in some, but not all, tests for attentional deficits. SDZ NVI-085 has shown activity in many of the animal assays for central α_1-adrenoceptor activation.

The functional roles of each α_1-adrenoceptor subtype within the CNS are not completely defined. It has been proposed that both α_{1B}- and α_{2A}-adrenoceptors are present on cell bodies of presympathetic ganglionic neurons in the intermediolateral cell column of the thoracic spinal cord, mediating an excitatory and inhibitory action, respectively. This reciprocal action is consistent with the observation that central α_1-adrenoceptor stimulation will attenuate the sedative actions of an α_2-adrenoceptor agonist in the rat. Mice lacking the α_{1B}-adrenoceptor show different behavioral effects from wild-type mice, in which enhanced reactivity to new situations is observed. Learning behavior in a water maze was impaired, although the ability to escape onto a visible platform was unaffected.

Overexpression of either wild-type or constitutively active α_{1B}-adrenoceptors results in granulovacular neurodegeneration, beginning in the areas of the brain expressing highest levels of the α_{1b}-adrenoceptor (cortex, cerebellum, and hypothalamus) and progressing to other brain areas with age. These mice showed symptoms consistent with neuronal damage, including parkinsonian hindlimb symptoms associated with paralysis and tremor. Grand mal seizures were also observed by 12 months of age. The severity of the seizure disorder was proportional to the level of α_{1B}-adrenoceptor activation, with mice expressing constitutively active receptors being most affected. α_{1B}-Adrenoceptor blockade with terazosin partially reversed the behavioral pathology. However, knockout of the norepinephrine uptake transporter, which results in an increase in central noradrenergic activity, decreases the vulnerability of mice to seizures induced by several convulsant agents.

Correlation of affinity for recombinant α_1-adrenoceptors with their activity in the canine narcolepsy model suggests that the ability of α_1-adrenoceptor agonists to reverse cataplexy in this model results from α_{1B}-adrenoceptor activation. The presence of α_1-adrenoceptors in layers of human hippocampus having a concentration of glutaminergic synapses suggests the possibility for noradrenergic modulation of glutaminergic transmission. Activation of α_1-adrenoceptors in the nucleus tractus solitarius is involved in control of vagal activity to the stomach.

α_2-Adrenoceptors

α_2-Adrenoceptors are also widely distributed throughout the body. Perhaps the most extensively characterized action is the prejunctionally mediated inhibition of neurotransmitter release from many peripheral and central neurons. The demonstration that this effect had a different pharmacologic profile from actions mediated by postjunctional α-adrenoceptors, such as vascular contraction, originally led to the division of α-adrenoceptors into the α_1- and α_2-subtypes. Activation of prejunctional α_2-autoreceptors on sympathetic neurons results in a sympatholytic action. α_2-Adrenoceptors are also present at postjunctional sites, where they mediate actions such as smooth muscle contraction, platelet aggregation, and inhibition of insulin secretion. Many responses produced by α_2-adrenoceptor agonists are mediated through the inhibition of adenylyl cyclase as a consequence of interaction of the agonist–receptor complex with G_i, although other second messengers remain to be characterized.

Three α_2-adrenoceptor proteins have been cloned. These recombinant receptors result in four discrete pharmacological profiles since the α_{2A}-adrenoceptor appears to exist as species orthologs, with those of human, pig, and rabbit having a profile designated as α_{2A}, whereas those of rat, mouse, guinea pig, and cow exhibit pharmacologic profiles designated as α_{2D}. α_{2A}- and α_{2D}-adrenoceptor-mediated responses can be differentiated by the low sensitivity of the α_{2D}-adrenoceptor to blockade by the commonly used antagonists yohimbine and rauwolscine.

Studies in the rat demonstrate the existence of mRNA for all three α_2-adrenoceptor subtypes to be present in the CNS. α_{2A}-Adrenoceptor mRNA is most widely distributed, being found in the cerebral cortex, locus coeruleus, amygdala, hypothalamic paraventricular nucleus, nucleus tractus solitarii, ventrolateral reticular formation, spinal cord, and dorsal root ganglia. Message for the α_{2B}-adrenoceptor is found almost exclusively in the thalamus. The α_{2C}-adrenoceptor is found in olfactory bulb, islands of Calleja, cerebral and cerebellar cortex, hippocampal formation, and dorsal root ganglia. In human brain, radioligand binding assays demonstrate the presence of α_{2A}-adrenoceptor protein in frontal cortex, cerebellum, and hippocampal formation, with another subtype (α_{2B} or α_{2C}) predominant in neostriatum.

α_2-Adrenoceptors within the CNS have long been known to be involved in the antihypertensive action of clonidine and other α_2-adrenoceptor agonists. Although the involvement of a nonadrenergic imidazoline receptor in this action has been postulated, the failure of α_2-adrenoceptor agonists to produce a sympatholytic action in mice where the α_{2A}-adrenoceptor has been knocked out or mutated supports functional experiments in rats and rabbits suggesting an α_2-adrenoceptor-mediated action, at least for systemically administered agonists. In addition to inhibition of sympathetic outflow, the anesthetic and analgesic actions of α_2-adrenoceptor agonists appear to be mediated by the α_{2A}-adrenoceptor. The hypertensive action of α_2-adrenoceptor agonists likely results from activation of vascular α_{2B}-adrenoceptors. Consistent with the apparent role of the α_{2B}-adrenoceptor in the maintenance of vascular tone, mice lacking this receptor subtype failed to develop salt-induced hypertension. Hence, a selective α_{2A}-adrenoceptor agonist may be preferable as a centrally active drug, although sedative and antihypertensive actions can apparently not be dissociated by subtype selectivity. The α_{2A}- or α_{2D}-adrenoceptor subtype (depending on species) appears to be responsible for many other α_2-adrenoceptor-mediated responses, including the major component of prejunctional modulation of sympathetic neurotransmission.

Knockout of the α_{2C}-adrenoceptor has no apparent cardiovascular effect. However, whereas knockout or mutation of the α_{2A}-adrenoceptor subtype produces only partial attenuation of α_2-adrenoceptor-mediated inhibition of transmitter release, elimination of both α_{2A}- and α_{2C}-adrenoceptors results in complete loss of prejunctional modulation of adrenergic neurotransmission and induces pathologic effects related to excess adrenergic tone. Hence, the α_{2C}-adrenoceptor can also participate in prejunctional modulation of neurotransmission. The α_{2C}-adrenoceptor may also participate in cold-induced augmentation of α-adrenoceptor-mediated vasoconstriction.

α_{2C}-Adrenoceptors appear to be involved in the startle reflex and isolation-induced aggression since knockout of α_{2C}-adrenoceptors in mice resulted in an enhanced startle response and shortened attack latency, whereas overexpression of this receptor produced the opposite effect on both parameters. Similarly, the hypothermic response to an α_2-adrenoceptor agonist was attenuated in α_{2C}-adrenoceptor knockout mice, and this response was accentuated by α_{2c}-adrenoceptor overexpression. Behavioral despair in the forced swimming test was enhanced or inhibited by α_{2C}-adrenoceptor overexpression or knockout, respectively. Overexpression of the α_{2C}-adrenoceptor impairs the performance of mice in a water maze.

Despite clinical trials for several indications, no molecule specifically designed to block the α_2-adrenoceptor has been successfully developed as a drug, although α_2-adrenoceptor antagonist activity may play an important role in antidepressants such as mirtazepine. In addition to their use as antihypertensives, selective centrally acting α_2-adrenoceptor agonists are used as adjuncts to general anesthesia in the treatment of opiate withdrawal, ADHD, and Tourette's syndrome. Their ability to alleviate many of the symptoms of opiate withdrawal most likely results from the ability of both opiate agonists and α_2-adrenoceptor agonists to inhibit locus coeruleus firing, although an action at spinal centers may also contribute. Based on data in a rat model, activation of α_2-adenoceptors may contribute to the activity of methylphenidate in ADHD.

β-Adrenoceptors

Important physiological consequences of β-adrenoceptor activation include stimulation of cardiac rate and force; relaxation of vascular, urogenital, and bronchial smooth muscle; stimulation of renin secretion from the juxtaglomerular apparatus; stimulation of insulin and glucagon secretion from the endocrine pancreas; stimulation of glycogenolysis in liver and skeletal muscle; and stimulation of lipolysis in the adipocyte. Prejunctional β-adrenoceptors are present on some central and peripheral nerve terminals, where their activation results in facilitation of stimulation-evoked neurotransmitter release. However, in contrast to the prejunctional α_2-adrenoceptors, these prejunctional receptors do not appear to have major physiologic significance. Most β-adrenoceptor-mediated actions involve stimulation of adenylyl cyclase through the interaction of the agonist–receptor complex with G_s.

Three β-adrenoceptor proteins have been cloned, and the characteristics of these recombinant receptors correspond with those of the three well-characterized β-adrenoceptors on native tissues, designated as β_1, β_2, and β_3. Many useful pharmacological tools are available for β-adrenoceptor characterization. These include agonists capable of selectively activating β_1-, β_2-, or β_3-adrenoceptors, as well as antagonists selective for each of the three subtypes. Although multiple β-adrenoceptor subtypes can participate in the cardiac stimulation produced by the catecholamines, gene knockout experiments demonstrate that the β_1-adrenoceptor subtype plays the major role. Renin release also appears to be mediated by the β_1-adrenoceptor. Bronchodilation is mediated primarily by the β_2-adrenoceptor. The β_3-adrenoceptor is responsible for lipolysis in white adipose tissue and thermogenesis in the brown adipose tissue found in rodents. Species differences appear to be important for the β_3-adrenoceptor since several selective β_3-adrenoceptor agonists can activate rodent, but not human, β_3-adrenoceptors.

In rat brain, mRNA for the β_1-adrenoceptor is widely distributed, whereas message for the β_2-adrenoceptor is concentrated in olfactory bulb, hippocampal formation, piriform cortex, and cerebellar cortex. The β_3-adrenoceptor does not appear to be present in the CNS. Radioligand assays using dissected rat brain have shown that β_1-adrenoceptors are typically associated with forebrain structures (cerebral cortex, striatum, and hippocampus), whereas β_2-adrenoceptors are most dense in the cerebellum. The β-adrenoceptors of rat cerebral cortex may be localized primarily on glial cells.

Central β-adrenoceptors appear to play a role in movement disorders. β-Adrenoceptor antagonists reduce tremor in MPTP-treated monkeys. Studies in human brain show dense β_1-adrenoceptor binding in striatum, which decreases in the late stages of Huntington's chorea. It is well established that chronic treatment with tricyclic antidepressants produces downregulation of central β-adrenoceptors, presumably as a consequence of increased synaptic levels of the catecholamine neurotransmitters as a result of blockade of neuronal reuptake. β-Adrenoceptors may be involved in the antinociceptive activity of the tricyclic antidepressants since β-adrenoceptor antagonists can reverse this activity. Other functions attributed to central β-adrenoceptors include adaptation to stress, memory and learning, control of respiration, and glial proliferation.

Knockouts of β_1-, β_2, and β_3-adrenoceptors have been reported. Mice lacking both β_1- and β_2-adrenoceptors have also been prepared. None of these mice have phenotypic changes reflecting deficits in CNS function, although detailed behavioral studies have not been reported. Knockout of the β_1-adrenoceptor has a marked effect on embryonic viability, although the few homozygous animals surviving appear normal. This effect on viability is not observed with knockout of the β_2- or β_3-adrenoceptor subtypes. Mice lacking the β_1 adrenoceptor fail to respond to the inotropic action of β-adrenoceptor agonists, confirming the importance of this subtype in the control of cardiac contractility. However, maximal exercise capacity is not reduced. Mice lacking the β_2-adrenoceptor have a normal response to exogenous β-adrenoceptor agonists and have even greater exercise capacity than wild-type mice. However, these animals become hypertensive during exercise and have a lower respiratory exchange ratio, suggesting influences of the β_2-adrenoceptor on energy metabolism. Mice lacking both β_1- and β_2-adrenoceptors have normal basal cardiovascular parameters and normal exercise capacity, although the ability of exercise or the administration of exogenous agonists to increase heart rate is blunted. Mice lacking the β_3-adrenoceptor show mild increases in body fat stores and do not show metabolic responses to a selective β_3-adrenoceptor agonist. In several cases, an increased responsiveness to one of the remaining β-adrenoceptors is observed when one of the subtypes is knocked out. Thus, there is increased β_1-adrenoceptor responsiveness in β_3-adrenoceptor knockout animals and enhanced β_3-adrenoceptor responsiveness in β_1/β_2 knockout animals. These observations support the concept that many physiological functions can be mediated by multiple β-adrenoceptor subtypes.

Selective overexpression of β_2-adrenoceptors in airway epithelium or smooth muscle results in decreased sensitivity to methacholine-induced bronchoconstriction and an increased sensitivity to a β-adrenoceptor agonists. Cardiac-directed overexpression of the human β_1-adrenoceptor results in the accumulation of fibrous tissue between cardiac myocytes, myocyte hypertrophy, and myofibrilar disarray. These changes result in cardiac dysfunction in older animals. Overexpression of human β_2-adrenoceptors in mouse heart enhances basal cardiac function due to constitutive activity of the expressed receptors. Fibrotic cardiomyopathy is observed in mice expressing high levels of the β_2-adrenoceptor, with the severity and rate of onset being dependent on the level of receptor expression. Overexpression of cardiac β_2-adrenoceptors exacerbates functional deterioration following pressure overload as a result of aortic stenosis.

Several β-adrenoceptor antagonists have also been evaluated for a variety of CNS applications; perhaps the most convincing results are from the use of these agents in treating anxiety of varying etiology, although it is not clear whether a central or peripheral site of action is involved.

Conclusions

Agonists or antagonists at central or peripheral adrenoceptors have several important therapeutic applications; most of these drugs interact with multiple adrenoceptor subtypes. Newly developed pharmacological tools will help to identify the functional role of specific subtypes. Although an action at multiple adrenoceptors may in some cases be beneficial, drugs interacting selectively with adrenoceptor subtypes could result in either an improvement in therapeutic index or the identification of new therapeutic opportunities.

See Also the Following Articles

Norepinephrine: CNS Pathways and Neurophysiology; Sympathetic Noradrenergic and Adrenomedullary Hormonal Systems in Stress and Distress.

Further Reading

Arnsten, A. F. T. and Dudley, A. G. (2005). Methylphenidate improves prefrontal cortical cognitive function through α_2-adrenoceptor and dopamine D1 receptor actions: Relevance to therapeutic effects in attention deficit hyperactivity disorder. *Behavioral and Brain Functions* **1**, 2.

Bjorklund, M., Sirvio, J., Riekkinen, M., et al. (2000). Overexpression of alpha2C-adrenoceptors impairs water maze navigation. *Neuroscience* **95**, 481–847.

Chotani, M. A., Flavahan, S. A., Mitra, S., Daunt, D. and Flavahan, NA. (2000). Silent α_{2C}-adrenergic receptors enable cold-induced vasoconstriction in cutaneous arteries. *American Journal of Physiology* **278**, H1075–H1083.

Grijalba, B., Callado, L. F., Javier-Meana, J., Garcia-Sevilla, J. A. and Pazos, A. (1996). Alpha-2 adrenoceptor subtypes in human brain. A pharmacological delineation of [^{3}H] RX-821002 binding to membranes and tissue sections. *European Journal of Pharmacology* **310**, 83–93.

Hein, L., Altman, J. D. and Kobilka, B. K. (1999). Two functionally distinct α-adrenergic receptors regulate sympathetic neurotransmission. *Nature* **402**, 181–184.

Hermann, G. E., Nasse, J. S. and Rogers, R. C. (2005). α-1 Adrenergic input to solitary nucleus neurons: Calcium oscillations, excitation and gastric reflex control. *Journal of Physiology* **562**, 553–568.

Hieble, J. P., Bondinell, W. E. and Ruffolo, R. R.,Jr. (1995). α- and β-Adrenoceptors: From the gene to the clinic. 1: Molecular biology and adrenoceptor subclassification. *Journal of Medicinal Chemistry* **38**, 3415–3444.

Koshimizu, T. A., Tanoue, A., Hirasawa, A., Yamauchi, J. and Tsujimoto, G. (2003). Recent advances in α_1-adrenoceptor pharmacology. *Pharmacology and Therapeutics* **98**, 235–244.

Neumeister, A., Charney, D. S., Belfer, I., et al. (2005). Sympathoneural and adrenomedullary functional effects of α_{2C}-adrenoreceptor gene polymorphism in healthy humans. *Pharmacogenetics and Genomics* **15**, 143–149.

Nicholas, A. P., Hökfelt, T. and Pieribone, V. A. (1996). The distribution and significance of CNS adrenoceptors examined with *in situ* hybridization. *Trends in Pharmacological Sciences* **17**, 245–255.

Ruffolo, R. R., Jr., Bondinell, W. E. and Hieble, J. P. (1995). α- and β-Adrenoceptors: From the gene to the clinic. 2: Structure–activity relationships and therapeutic application. *Journal of Medicinal Chemistry* **38**, 3681–3716.

Sallinen, J., Haapalinna, A., MacDonald, E., et al. (1999). Genetic alteration of the α_2-adrenoceptor subtype c in mice affects the development of behavioral despair and stress-induced changes in plasma corticosterone levels. *Molecular Psychiatry* **4**, 443–452.

Spreng, M., Cotecchia, S. and Schenk, F. (2001). A behavioral study of alpha-1b adrenergic receptor knockout mice: Increased reaction to novelty and selectively reduced learning capacities. *Neurobiology of Learning & Memory* **75**, 214–229.

Waeber, C., Rigo, M., Chinaglia, G., Probst, A. and Palacios, J. M. (1991). Beta-adrenergic receptor subtypes in the basal ganglia of patients with Huntington's chorea and Parkinson's disease. *Synapse* **8**, 270–280.

Zujic, M. J., Sands, S., Ros, S. A., et al. (2000). Overexpression of the α_{1B}-adrenergic receptor causes apoptotic neurodegeneration: Multiple system atrophy. *Nature Medicine* **6**, 1388–1394.

Stress and Parasympathetic Control

S W Porges
University of Illinois at Chicago, Chicago, IL, USA

Traditionally, the autonomic nervous system is conceptualized as the paired antagonism between the sympathetic and the parasympathetic nervous system. These components of the autonomic nervous system, based on the region of the brain and spinal cord in which the autonomic nerves (i.e., preganglionic fibers) have their origin, compete functionally by either increasing or decreasing activity of specific target organs. The sympathetic system is defined by the autonomic fibers that exit thoracic and lumbar segments of the spinal cord. The parasympathetic system is defined by the autonomic fibers that exit either the brain stem via the cranial nerves (primarily via the vagus) or the sacral segments of the spinal cord. Since most organs in the viscera receive both sympathetic and vagal input, the regulation of the autonomic nervous system has been modeled as a balance system.

Central nervous system regulation of visceral organs is the focus of several historic publications. For example, in *The Expression of Emotions in Man and Animals*, Darwin described the dynamic neural relationship between the heart and the brain. He stated that

> when the heart is affected it reacts on the brain; and the state of the brain again reacts through the pneumogastric [vagus] nerve on the heart; so that under any excitement there will be much mutual action and reaction between these, the two most important organs of the body.

From Darwin's perspective, the vagus as a cranial nerve was a direct portal to and from the brain. Although Darwin acknowledged the bidirectional communication between the viscera and the brain, the subsequent formal description of the autonomic nervous system minimized the importance of central regulatory structures and afferents. A focus on the peripheral motor nerves with an emphasis on the paired antagonism between sympathetic and parasympathetic efferent pathways on the target visceral organs resulted in a lack of interest in afferent influences to the brain stem areas regulating specific efferent pathways. This early conceptualization of the vagus focused on an undifferentiated efferent pathway that was assumed to modulate 'tone' concurrently to several target organs. Thus, neural circuits regulating the supradiaphragmatic (e.g., myelinated vagal pathways originating in the nucleus ambiguus and terminating primarily above the diaphragm) were not functionally distinguished from the subdiaphragmatic (e.g., unmyelinated vagal pathways originating in the dorsal motor nucleus of the vagus and terminating primarily below the diaphragm). Without this distinction, research and theory focused on the paired antagonism between the parasympathetic and sympathetic innervation to target organs. The consequence of an emphasis on paired antagonism in physiology was an acceptance and use of global constructs focusing on peripheral physiology such as autonomic balance, sympathetic tone, and vagal tone. Ironically, the origin of modern research on stress physiology is often linked to the classical conditioning of autonomic activity, which, as Pavlov demonstrated, requires the involvement of higher brain structures in the modulation of visceral responses.

In the mid-1950s, W Hess proposed that the 'autonomic' nervous system was not solely 'vegetative' and automatic but, rather, was an integrated system with both peripheral and central neurons. In 1949, Hess was awarded the Nobel Prize in Physiology or Medicine. His Nobel lecture was titled 'The central control of activity of internal organs.' In the lecture, Hess acknowledged the importance of the prevailing model of the autonomic nervous system, which emphasized the paired antagonistic innervations of the internal organs and the definition of sympathetic and parasympathetic functions. However, he went well beyond this conceptualization to emphasize the importance of central structures in the regulation of visceral state by describing his studies that demonstrated the influence of the hypothalamus on the autonomic nervous system. By emphasizing the central mechanisms that mediate the dynamic regulation of peripheral organs, Hess anticipated the need for methodologies and technologies to continuously monitor the neural circuits involving both defined brain structures and peripheral nerves in the regulation of visceral function and state and to move from the prevailing conceptualization of autonomic nervous system as a peripheral system. The lecture provides a succinct statement: (1) to emphasize the importance of feedback circuits linking peripheral organs to brain structures and the bidirectionality of these feedback circuits and (2) to acknowledge that, although much can be learned about neural structures and functions via traditional experimental paradigms (e.g., neural blockade, surgery, and electrical stimulation), the dynamic feedback circuits cannot be adequately studied through these paradigms.

Arousal Theory and Stress Responses

For more than a century, researchers have measured autonomic variables (e.g., heart rate and palmar sweat gland activity) as indicators of emotional state related to perceived stress (e.g., fear, mental effort, workload, and anxiety). Historically, arousal theories provided scientists who studied brain–behavior relations with a model that assumed that activation of peripheral physiological measures regulated by the sympathetic branch of the autonomic nervous system provided 'sensitive' indicators of brain 'arousal' or 'activation.' This view was based on a rudimentary understanding of the autonomic nervous system in which changes in easily measured peripheral organs (e.g., sweat glands and heart) were assumed to be accurate indicators of how the brain was processing emotional stimuli. Usually, the emotional states were associated with fight-or-flight behaviors and the sympathetic–adrenal system (e.g., increases in heart rate, sweat gland activity, and circulating catecholamines) initially described by Cannon as well as the increased activity of the hypothalamic–pituitary–adrenal (HPA) axis with an emphasis on cortisol as a dependent variable in stress research as initially described by Selye.

Measures due, in part, to their availability and their neuroanatomical association with the target organs of the sympathetic nervous system (i.e., sweat and heart rate) and with secretions from the adrenal medulla (i.e., epinephrine and norepinephrine) and the adrenal cortex (i.e., cortisol) have become the primary physiological variables used to assess stress. An acceptance of a unitary arousal system created a research environment that neglected several important factors, including an understanding of the brain structures that regulate autonomic function; how these structures evolved from the most primitive vertebrates to mammals; how the autonomic nervous system interacts with the immune system, the HPA axis, and the neuropeptides, oxytocin, and vasopressin; and the co-evolution of stress and coping strategies with the increasing complexity of the autonomic nervous system. Missing from the dialog on stress is the role of the parasympathetic nervous system and especially the vagus with its bi-directional portal between the brain and specific visceral organs.

The Mammalian Nervous System Is a Product of Evolution

Embedded in the mammalian nervous system are neuroanatomical structures related to the expression and experience of stress. Via evolutionary processes, the mammalian nervous system has emerged with specific features that react to the challenge to maintain visceral homeostasis. Stress, simply defined, is the product of demands on the nervous system that result in a deviation from homeostasis. In general, the domains of homeostasis, which have been monitored, have focused on the visceral systems involved in cardiovascular, digestive, reproductive, and immune functions. Adaptive and successful coping to stress results in minimizing the magnitude and duration of this deviation. To survive, mammals must determine friend from foe, when an environment is safe, and communicate with their social unit. These survival-related behaviors limit the extent to which a mammal can be physically approached, whether vocalizations will be understood, and whether coalitions can be established. Moreover, these behavioral strategies, which are used to navigate through the 'stress of life,' form the bedrock on which social behaviors and higher cognitive processes can be developed and expressed. Thus, learning and other expansive mental processes must be structured, manipulated, and studied within the context of how the environment fosters or ameliorates stress-related physiological states.

Table 1 illustrates the phylogenetic differences in the structures that regulate the heart in vertebrates. The heart is selected because the regulation of the heart determines the availability of the metabolic resources required for mobilization as well as for growth and restoration. For example, cardiac output must be regulated to remain calm in safe environments, to mobilize for fight-or-flight behaviors, or to immobilize for death feigning or avoidance behaviors. To regulate cardiac output, several efferent structures have evolved. These structures represent two global and often opposing systems: (1) a sympathetic–catecholamine system including catecholamine-secreting chromaffin tissue and spinal sympathetic nerves and (2) a vagal system (a component of the parasympathetic nervous system)

Table 1 Phylogenetic shifts in vertebrate cardiac control

Group	*CHM*	*DVC*	*SNS*	*AD/m*	*VVC*
Jawless fish	X^+	(X^+)			
Cartilaginous fish	X^+	X^-			
Bony fish	X^+	X^-	X^+		
Amphibians	X^+	X^-	X^+		
Reptiles	X^+	X^-	X^+	X^+	
Mammals	X^+	X^-	X^+	X^+	X^-

CHM, chromaffin tissue; DVC, dorsal vagal complex with vagal efferent pathways originating in the dorsal motor nucleus of the vagus and vagal afferents terminating in the nucleus tractus solitarius; SNS, spinal sympathetic nervous system; AD/m, adrenal medulla; VVC, ventral vagal complex with efferent pathways originating in the nucleus ambiguus that regulate visceral structures (heart, bronchi, and thymus) and striated muscles via special visceral efferents and afferents via the tractus solitarius, trigeminal, and facial nerve.

with branches originating in the medullary source nuclei (i.e., dorsal motor nucleus of the vagus and nucleus ambiguus).

Unlike other vertebrates with a cardioinhibitory vagus, the mammalian vagus contains two branches. One branch originates in the dorsal motor nucleus of the vagus and provides the primary neural regulation of subdiaphragmatic organs such as the digestive tract. However, at the level of the heart and unlike more primitive vertebrates, the efferent vagal pathways that originate in the dorsal motor nucleus of the vagus do not play a major role in the normal dynamic regulation of cardiac output. Rather, during embryological development in mammals, cells from the dorsal motor nucleus of the vagus migrate ventrally and laterally to the nucleus ambiguus. There, they form the cell bodies for the visceromotor myelinated axons that provide potent inhibition of the sinoatrial node, the pacemaker for the heart.

Three principles can be extracted by investigating the phylogeny of the regulation of the vertebrate heart. First, there is a phylogenetic shift in the regulation of the heart from endocrine communication to unmyelinated nerves and, finally, myelinated nerves. Second, there is a development of opposing neural mechanisms of excitation and inhibition to provide rapid regulation of graded metabolic output. Third, with increased cortical development, the cortex exhibits greater control over the brain stem via direct (e.g., corticobulbar) and indirect (e.g., corticoreticular) neural pathways originating in motor cortex and terminating in the source nuclei of the myelinated motor nerves emerging from the brain stem (e.g., specific neural pathways embedded within cranial nerves V, VII, IX, X, and XI), controlling visceromotor structures (i.e., heart, bronchi, and thymus) and somatomotor structures (muscles of the face and head) that results in a neural circuit that functions to facilitate social behavior and to maintain calm behavioral states.

These phylogenetic principles provide a basis for investigating the parasympathetic contribution to stress reactions and recovery. In general, phylogenetic development results in increased neural control of the heart via the myelinated mammalian vagal system, which can promote transitory mobilization and the expression of sympathetic tone without requiring sympathetic or adrenal activation. With this new vagal system, transitory incursions into the environment or withdrawals from a potential predator can be initiated without the severe biological cost of the metabolic excitation associated with sympathetic–adrenal activation. Paralleling this change in neural control of the heart is an enhanced neural control of the face, larynx, and pharynx that enables complex facial gestures and vocalizations associated with social communication. This phylogenetic course results in greater central nervous system regulation of behavior, especially that needed to engage and disengage with environmental challenges.

Polyvagal Theory: Three Phylogenetic Systems Related to Stress Reactivity

The polyvagal theory emphasizes the phylogenetic origins of brain structures that regulate social and defensive behaviors. The polyvagal theory proposes that the evolution of the mammalian autonomic nervous system provides the neurophysiological substrates for emotional experiences, affective processes, and stress responses. The theory proposes that physiological state limits the range of adaptive behaviors and psychological experiences. In this context, the evolution of the nervous system determines the range of emotional expression, the quality of communication, and the ability to regulate bodily and behavioral state including the expression and recovery of stress-related responses. Relevant to adaptive stress responses, the theory makes the following assumptions:

1. Evolution has modified the structures of the autonomic nervous system.
2. The mammalian autonomic nervous system retains vestiges of phylogenetically older autonomic nervous systems.
3. Emotional regulation and social behavior are functional derivatives of structural changes in the autonomic nervous system due to evolutionary processes.
4. In mammals, the autonomic nervous system response strategy to challenge follows a phylogenetic hierarchy, starting with the newest structures and, when all else fails, reverting to the most primitive structural system.
5. The phylogenentic stage of the autonomic nervous system determines the behavioral, physiological, and affective features of stress reactivity.

The polyvagal theory emphasizes and documents the neurophysiological and neuroanatomical distinction between the two branches of the vagus (i.e., the tenth cranial nerve) and proposes that each vagal branch is associated with a different adaptive behavioral and physiological response strategy to stressful events. The theory describes three phylogenetic stages of the development of the mammalian autonomic nervous system (**Table 2**). These stages reflect the emergence of three distinct subsystems, which are phylogenetically ordered and behaviorally linked to communication (e.g., facial expression, vocalization, and listening), mobilization

Table 2 Phylogenetic stages of the neural control of the heart proposed by the polyvagal theory

Stage	*Autonomic nervous system component*	*Behavioral function*	*Lower motor neurons*
III	Myelinated vagus (ventral vagal complex)	Social communication, self-soothing and calming, inhibit 'arousal'	Nucleus ambiguus
II	Sympathetic–adrenal system	Mobilization (active avoidance)	Spinal cord
I	Unmyelinated vagus (dorsal vagal complex)	Immobilization (death feigning, passive avoidance)	Dorsal motor nucleus of the vagus

(e.g., fight-or-flight behaviors), and immobilization (e.g., death feigning, behavioral 'shutdown,' and syncope). The mobilization system is dependent on the functioning of the sympathetic nervous system. The most phylogenetically primitive component, the immobilization system, is dependent on the unmyelinated or 'vegetative' vagus, which is shared with most vertebrates. With increased neural complexity due to phylogenetic development, the organism's behavioral and affective repertoire is enriched. These subsystems provide a framework to study the vagal contribution to the regulation of stress responses.

The mammalian vagus functions as an active vagal brake in which rapid inhibition and disinhibition of vagal tone to the heart can support behavioral mobilization or self-sooth and calm an individual. When the vagal tone to the pacemaker is high, the vagus acts as a restraint or brake limiting heart rate. When vagal tone to the pacemaker is low, there is little or no inhibition of the pacemaker. Due to vagal influences to the sinoatrial node (i.e., the heart's pacemaker), resting heart rate is substantially lower than the intrinsic rate of the pacemaker. In mammals, the primary vagal inhibitory pathways occur through the myelinated vagus originating in the nucleus ambiguus. Consistent with assumptions of the polyvagal theory, the vagal brake contributes to the modulation of cardiac output by decreasing or increasing the inhibitory vagal control of the heart to influence rate and thereby adjust metabolic resources to support either mobilization or social engagement behaviors.

By transitory downregulation of the cardioinhibitory vagal tone to the heart (i.e., removing the vagal brake), the mammal is capable of rapid increases in cardiac output without activating the sympathetic–adrenal system. By engaging this system, rather than the sympathetic–adrenal system, mammals have an opportunity to rapidly increase metabolic output for immediate mobilization. Under prolonged challenge, the sympathetic system may also be activated. By rapidly re-engaging the vagal system, the sympathetic input to the heart is inhibited, resulting in a decrease in metabolic output and a calm behavioral state.

The Vagal Brake: Parasympathetic Regulation of the 'Stress' Response

Due to the tonic vagal influences to the sinoatrial node, resting heart rate is substantially lower than the intrinsic rate of the pacemaker. When the vagal tone to the pacemaker is high, the vagus acts as a brake on the rate at which the heart is beating. When vagal tone to the pacemaker is low, there is little or no inhibition of the pacemaker. Thus, the vagal brake may be used as a construct to describe the functional modulation of heart rate by the myelinated vagal efferent pathways. Neurophysiologically, the vagal brake provides a mechanism to support the metabolic requirements for mobilization and communication behaviors. Functionally, the vagal brake, by modulating visceral state, enables the individual to rapidly engage and disengage with objects and other individuals and to promote self-soothing behaviors and calm behavioral states. Thus, withdrawal of the vagal brake is associated with an adaptive stress response and a reinstatement of the vagal brake with recovery.

Withdrawal of the vagal brake will facilitate the recruitment of other neural mechanisms (e.g., excitation of sympathetic or the unmyelinated vagal pathways) and neural chemical mechanisms (e.g., stimulation of the HPA axis) to regulate physiological state. Thus, consistent with the polyvagal theory, if the vagal brake is not functioning or will not serve the survival needs of the organism, then the phylogenetically 'older' systems (e.g., the sympathetic–adrenal system or unmyelinated vagus originating in the dorsal motor nucleus of the vagus) will be recruited to regulate metabolic output to deal with environmental challenges. For example, if the vagal brake is not functioning, there is the potential for greater dependence on the sympathetic excitation of the cardiovascular system.

The Social Engagement System

Mammals have evolved to have a well-defined neurally mediated social engagement system. Embryologically, components of several cranial nerves develop together (i.e., myelinated vagal pathways from the nucleus ambiguus and special visceral efferent pathways from cranial nerves V, VII, IX, X, and XI) to form the neural substrate of a social engagement system. This system provides the neural gatekeepers for social–emotional interactions. The social engagement system has a control component in the cortex (i.e., upper motor neurons) that regulates brain stem nuclei (i.e., lower motor neurons) to control eyelid opening (e.g., looking), facial muscles (e.g., emotional expression), middle ear muscles (e.g., extracting human voice from background noise), muscles of mastication (e.g., ingestion), laryngeal and pharyngeal muscles (e.g., vocalization and language), and head-turning muscles (e.g., social gesture and orientation). Collectively, these muscles function as filters and control social engagement with the environment. The neural control of these muscles determines social experiences. In addition, the source nuclei (i.e., lower motor neurons) of these nerves, which are located in the brain stem, communicate directly with an inhibitory neural circuit that slows heart rate, lowers blood pressure, and actively reduces arousal to promote calm states consistent with the metabolic demands of growth and restoration of neurophysiological systems. Direct corticobulbar pathways reflect the influence of frontal areas of the cortex (i.e., upper motor neurons) on the regulation of this system. Thus, the social nervous system is intimately related to stress reactivity. In addition, the anatomical structures involved in the social engagement system have neurophysiological interactions with the HPA axis, the neuropeptides of oxytocin and vasopressin, and the immune system. Thus, the social engagement system, as illustrated in **Figure 1**, provides a theoretical model to explain the interactive and stress-related functions of several physiological systems that have central regulatory components but are expressed in the periphery.

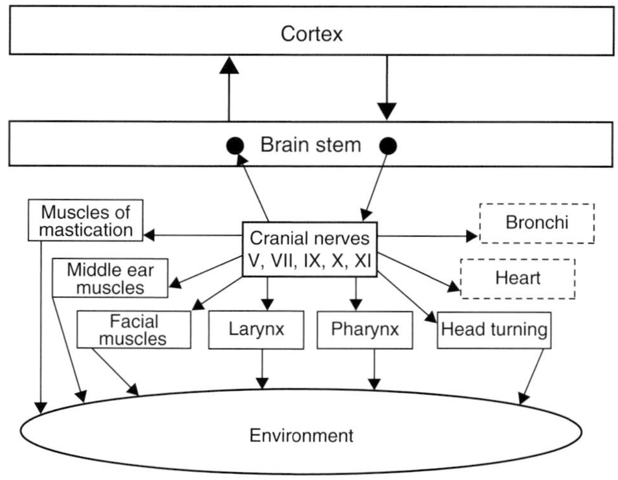

Figure 1 The social engagement system. Social communication is determined by the cortical regulation of medullary nuclei via corticobulbar pathways. The social engagement system consists of a somatomotor component (i.e., special visceral efferent pathways that regulate the striated muscles of the face and head) and a visceromotor component (i.e., the myelinated vagus that regulates the heart and bronchi). Solid rectangles indicate the somatomotor component, and dashed rectangles indicate the visceromotor component.

Vagal Regulation of the HPA Axis

The vagus is involved in the regulation of the HPA axis. Vagal afferents exhibit an inhibitory influence on the HPA axis and reduce cortisol secretion. Studies have demonstrated a covariation between increases in cortisol and decreases in cardiac vagal tone (i.e., measured by the amplitude of respiratory sinus arrhythmia). Thus, there appears to be a coordinated response that functions to promote metabolic activity and mobilization behaviors by withdrawal of vagal tone through the myelinated vagus and increasing both sympathetic activity and activation of the HPA axis. In general, the functioning of the adrenal cortex and the secretion of cortisol appear to be integrated into the mobilization function of the autonomic nervous system by increasing sympathetic activation and circulating catecholamines. These effects suggest that, consistent with the phylogenetic approach described in the polyvagal theory, cortisol secretion may be related to maintenance of mobilization (i.e., the conversion of norepinephrine into epinephrine) for fight-or-flight behaviors and in the recovery from the lactate buildup that may contribute to a functional oxygen debt (i.e., gluconeogenesis).

In addition, reports of dysregulation of the HPA axis, low cortisol, or low cortisol reactivity in disorders such as schizophrenia and posttraumatic stress disorder and also the consequences of neglect and abuse in children may be explained within the context of a phylogenetically ordered response strategy (i.e., polyvagal theory). For example, if mobilization strategies (i.e., fight-or-flight behaviors) are ineffective in removing the individual from the stressor and in modulating the effect of the stress, then the nervous system may degrade to a phylogenetically earlier level of organization. Thus, low cortisol or a hyporesponsive HPA axis may reflect a neural strategy associated with immobilization (i.e., passive avoidance) that would require a reduction in energy resources.

Immune Function

The vagus has been implicated in the immune system. Studies have demonstrated the important role of subdiaphragmatic vagal afferents in conveying information regarding visceral state to the brain. The studies conceptualize the afferent vagus as providing a signal alerting the central structures regulating immune function. A few studies have described motor pathways via the vagus to the thymus. The link between the vagal function and the immune system is not clear. However, it might be plausible to speculate that the neural mediation of the myelinated vagus, via direct influence on thymus and direct inhibition of the sympathetic nervous system, may trigger a physiological state that would promote immune function. Likewise, withdrawal of vagal tone to the heart, increased sympathetic tone, and the release of cortisol have been associated with suppressed immune function.

Oxytocin/Vasopressin

Because the peripheral influences of oxytocin and vasopressin function through feedback, primarily via afferent vagal pathways, the peripheral effects of these peptides are less clear and may be level dependent or differ as a function of acute versus chronic exposure. For example, it is possible that peripheral vasopressin, by stimulating vagal afferents, may trigger massive vagal responses via the dorsal motor nucleus of the vagus. In support of this speculation, it is known that in humans, peripheral vasopressin, and not oxytocin, is related to the nausea experienced during motion sickness. In addition, systemic vasopressin may induce a baroreceptor-mediated bradycardia and a decrease in plasma concentration of norepinephrine.

Based on the polyvagal theory, the mammalian vagus, with myelinated motor fibers originating in the nucleus ambiguus, provides a system for voluntary engagement with the environment, with special features associated with the prosocial behaviors of communication. Paralleling this evolutionary shift in the vagus is a mammalian modification of the hypothalamic regulation of the dorsal vagal complex (i.e., source nucleus of the afferent and efferent pathways of the unmyelinated vagus originating in the dorsal motor nucleus of the vagus and the nucleus of the solitary tract) via both oxytocin and vasopressin. The advent of specific receptors for oxytocin and vasopressin has increased the range of adaptive functions involving the unmyelinated vagus. In mammals, the dorsal motor nucleus of the vagus, the motor component of the dorsal vagal complex, is sensitive to oxytocin and insensitive to vasopressin. In contrast, the sensory components of the vagus, the nucleus of the solitary tract and area postrema, are most sensitive to vasopressin. Although the nucleus of the solitary tract has receptors for oxytocin, area postrema may not be directly influenced by oxytocin. The differential sensitivity of specific components of the dorsal vagal complex to these two neuropeptides (the differential effects of central and systemic release on visceral function and a potential level dependency) results in a wider range of response options, including maximizing mobilization behaviors and the co-opting of the primitive vagal system associated with immobilization to support 'antistress' functions such as social engagement and growth and restoration.

Phylogenetic Approach to the Study of Stress

The phylogenetic orientation focuses our interest on the parasympathetic neural structures and neurobehavioral systems that we share with or have adapted from our phylogenetic ancestry. First, the three response systems proposed in the polyvagal theory (i.e., cranial nerves to regulate the face, sympathetic–adrenal system to increase metabolic output, and an inhibitory vagal system to decrease metabolic output and promote freezing and defecation) are the products of distinct neurophysiological systems. Second, these distinct neurophysiological systems represent a phylogenetically dependent hierarchy, with the use of cranial nerves to regulate facial expression emerging in mammals (well developed in primates); the sympathetic–adrenal system shared with other vertebrates including reptiles; and the inhibitory vagal system shared with more primitive vertebrates, including amphibians, bony fish, and cartilaginous fish. The three systems represent different phylogenetic stages of neural development. This phylogenetic development starts with a primitive behavioral inhibition system, progresses to a fight-or-flight system, and, in humans (and other primates), culminates in a complex facial gesture and vocalization system. Thus, from a phylogenetic perspective, the nervous system of vertebrates evolved to support a greater range of behaviors and physiological states, including states that are often associated with stress.

The physiological responses associated with stress in mammals do not concisely fit into a single neurophysiological system. Although cortisol has often been labeled as the stress hormone, other systems clearly respond to stress. Moreover, there are situations of severe stress in which cortisol is neither responsive nor at a high level. By expanding the phylogenetic model proposed in the polyvagal theory to emphasize the interactions between parasympathetic mechanisms and the HPA axis, the hyporesponsive HPA can be interpreted as reflecting a primitive passive avoidance system. Thus, several systems with target organs at the periphery contribute to the organism's adaptation to challenge and stress. These neurobiological systems are not solely stress systems. Rather, they are intimately involved in the dynamic regulation of homeostasis, growth and restoration, metabolism, and mobilization. These systems form a complex set of mutually interacting neurophysiological pathways that communicate via nerves and neurally active chemicals (e.g., neurotransmitters, neuropeptides, and hormones) to cope with survival challenges.

See Also the Following Articles

Stress: Definition and History; Stress: Homeostasis, Rheostasis, Allostasis and Allostatic Load; Stress Response: Neural and Feedback Regulation of the HPA Axis.

Further Reading

Berlyne, D. E. (1960). *Conflict, Arousal, and Curiosity.* New York: McGraw-Hill.

Bueno, L. M., Gue, M. J., Fargeas, M., et al. (1989). Vagally mediated inhibition of acoustic stress-induced cortisol release by orally administered kappa-opioid substances in dogs. *Endocrinology* **124**, 1788–1793.

Bulloch, K. and Pomerantz, W. (1984). Autonomic nervous system innervation of thymic-related lymphoid tissue in wildtype and nude mice. *Journal of Comparative Neurology* **228**, 58–68.

Cannon, W. B. (1928). The mechanism of emotional disturbance of bodily functions. *New England Journal of Medicine* **198**, 877–884.

Darrow, C. W. (1943). Physiological and clinical tests of autonomic function and autonomic balance. *Physiological Reviews* **23**, 1–36.

Darwin, C. (1872). *The Expression of Emotions in Man and Animals.* New York: Appleton.

Gray, J. A. (1971). *The Psychology of Fear and Stress.* New York: McGraw-Hill.

Hess, W. R. (1954). *Diencephalon, Autonomic and Extrapyramidal Functions.* New York: Grune & Stratton.

Koch, K. L., Summy-Long, J., Bingaman, S., Sperry, N. and Stern, R. M. (1990). Vasopressin and oxytocin responses to illusory self-motion and nausea in man. *Journal of Clinical Endocrinology and Metabolism* **71**, 1269–1275.

Landgraf, R., Mallkinson, T., Horn, T., et al. (1990). Release of vasopressin and oxytocin by paraventricular stimulation in rats. *American Journal of Physiology* **258**, 155–159.

Langley, J. N. (1921). *The Autonomic Nervous System,* ((vol. 1). Cambridge: Heffer and Sons.

Michelini, L. C. (1994). Vasopressin in the nucleus tractus solitarius: A modulator of baroreceptor reflex control of heart rate. *Brazilian Journal of Medical and Biological Research* **27**, 1017–1032.

Morris, J. L. and Nilsson, S. (1994). The circulatory system. In: Nilsson, S. & Holmgren, S. (eds.) *Comparative Physiology and Evolution of the Autonomic Nervous System*, pp. 193–246. Chur, Switzerland: Harwood Academic.

Pavlov, I. P. (1927). *Conditioned Reflexes.* London: Oxford University Press.

Porges, S. W. (1995). Orienting in a defensive world: Mammalian modifications of our evolutionary heritage. A polyvagal theory. *Psychophysiology* **32**, 301–318.

Porges, S. W. (1998). Love: An emergent property of the mammalian autonomic nervous system. *Psychoneuroendocrinology* **23**, 837–861.

Porges, S. W., Doussard-Roosevelt, J. A., Portales, A. L. and Greenspan, S. I. (1996). Infant regulation of the vagal 'brake' predicts child behavior problems: A psychobiological model of social behavior. *Developmental Psychobiology* **29**, 697–712.

Schwaber, J. S. (1986). Neuroanatomical substrates of cardiovascular and emotional–autonomic regulation. In: Magro, W., Osswald, W., Reis, D. & Vanhoutte, P. (eds.) *Central and Peripheral Mechanisms of Cardiovascular Regulation*, pp. 353–384. New York: Plenum.

Selye, H. (1956). *The Stress of Life.* New York: McGraw-Hill.

Vanhoutte, P. M. and Levy, M. N. (1979). Cholinergic inhibition of adrenergic neurotransmission in the cardiovascular system. In: Brooks, CMcC., Koizumi, K. & Sato, A. (eds.) *Integrative Functions of the Autonomic Nervous System*, pp. 159–176. Tokyo: University of Tokyo Press.

Watkins, L. R., Goehler, L. E., Relton, J. K., et al. (1995). Blockade of interleukin-1 induced hyperthermia by subdiaphragmatic vagotomy: Evidence for vagal mediation of immune-brain communication. *Neuroscience Letters* **183**, 27–31.

Electrodermal Activity

G Turpin and T Grandfield
University of Sheffield, Sheffield, UK

This is a revised version of the article by G Turpin and L Harrison, Encyclopedia of Stress, First edition, volume 2, pp 23–27, © 2000, Elsevier Inc.

Glossary

Electrodermal lability An individual difference dimension of electrodermal activity. High labile individuals tend to demonstrate greater rates of nonspecific responses and may also have higher skin conductance levels and slower habituation rates.

Habituation The process whereby the repetition of discrete stimuli leads to the decline in response amplitude or occurrence of electrodermal responses to successive stimulus presentations.

Nonspecific responses Frequency counts of spontaneous or nonspecific responses (e.g., nonspecific skin conductance responses), which occur in the absence of external stimulation. Rates of nonspecific responding are said to reflect individual differences in electrodermal arousal levels and may also be related to task demands for energy mobilization, together with responses to internally mediated thoughts or emotions.

Phasic responses and tonic levels Phasic responses consist of short-lived changes in electrodermal activity (EDA) elicited by discrete external stimuli and are characterized as either skin conductance responses (SCRs) or skin resistance responses (SRRs). Tonic levels are longer-term absolute measures of either skin conductance level (SCL) or skin resistance level (SRL). Typical ranges are 0.05–0.5 μS for SCR and 1–30 $\mu S/cm^2$ for SCL.

Skin conductance (SC) and skin resistance (SR) Units of electrodermal activity, which are expressed in either conductance (microsiemens or micromhos) or resistance (micro-ohms).

Sweat glands Two types of sweat gland are located under the skin surface: the apocrine glands, which are usually associated with the hair follicles and distributed around the axilla and pubic regions, and the eccrine glands, which are widely distributed over the body surface and serve a thermoregulatory function. However, the latter are also more closely distributed (approximately 1000 $glands/cm^2$) on the palms of the hands and the soles of the feet and are sympathetically innervated.

Introduction

At the turn of the nineteenth century, several researchers (e.g., Féré and Tarchanoff) demonstrated changes in the electrical resistance of the skin, which were elicited by either sensory or emotional stimuli. With the advent of electronic amplification and recording equipment in the mid-twentieth century, electrical recording from the skin as a correlate of psychological activity was becoming a common measure within psychological research. Early psychological researchers such as Darrow investigated the mechanisms underlying electrodermal responding, together with its psychological correlates. The use of the galvanic skin response as a measure of classical conditioning or psychological stress and arousal received widespread acceptance within the 1960s. There followed a period of consolidation whereby the appropriate methodologies were standardized and models of electrodermal responding were elucidated. Alongside other noninvasive measures of autonomic activity such as heart rate and blood pressure, electrodermal measures were common place within psychophysiological publications.

Electrodermal responses are frequently interpreted as reflecting changes in attention since they are considered major components of the orienting response. More generally, measures of electrodermal activity (EDA) are considered as reflecting changes in autonomic reactivity elicited by psychosocial events associated with emotion, task demands, motor responding, workload, stress, etc. Although contemporary psychophysiological research tends to rely more on centrally derived measures such as evoked potentials or brain imaging, peripherally recorded autonomic measures such as EDA still have their place as sensitive and noninvasive physiological indices of psychological processes and states. Finally, it should be acknowledged that there are a range of nonelectrical methods for quantifying sweat gland activity. One such method is the Palmar Sweat Index, which consists of taking an imprint of the skin in order that the frequency of active sweat glands can be identified; it has frequently been used by stress researchers.

Methodology

Recording Techniques

There are a number of electronically derived measures of EDA, which can be obtained from the skin surface depending on the design and characteristics of the recording amplifiers. First, endogenous skin potentials (SPs) can be recorded directly using an appropriate amplifier and recording electrodes. This technique is referred to as endosomatic EDA. In contrast, exosomatic EDA consists of changes in an externally applied voltage or current, which is impressed through the skin via a pair of bipolar recording electrodes. The most common techniques rely on direct current (DC) measurement and consist of either measuring changes in conductance by keeping the voltage constant or changes in resistance by keeping the current constant. Alternatively, skin impedance may be measured using alternating current (AC). The most widely accepted technique is the measurement of skin conductance using a constant voltage applied between the electrodes of around 0.5 V. The techniques may also be applied outside of laboratory situations using ambulatory methods. More recently, circuits have been designed to measure EDA concurrently with brain imaging equipment and techniques.

The preparation of the skin surface and placement of electrodes are important methodological considerations. Since only some skin areas contain eccrine sweat glands that are psychologically reactive, EDA tends to be restricted to the palmar surfaces of the hands, and in particular, to the first and second fingers of the nondominant hand. In order to record EDA, specifically prepared electrodes (usually silver/silver chloride) need to be fixed in pairs to the skin and used in conjunction with specially made electrolytes. Researchers wishing to use EDA need to pay particular attention to published accounts of standardized procedures.

The recorded signal, whether it is conductance or resistance, is either displayed using a chart recorder or digitally sampled using an analog-to-digital converter and computer. Care should be taken to ensure that sufficient amplification and digital sampling rates are employed, so that the overall conductance level can be assessed, together with sufficient resolution so that phasic fluctuations can also be discriminated. In the case of traditional amplifiers and chart recorders, this will necessitate the use of a device that backs off a calibrated proportion of the skin conductance level prior to high gain amplification.

It is essential that any research intended for publication and using electrodermal measures strictly conforms to published methodological guidelines.

Quantification

Electrodermal activity is usually expressed in conductance units (microsiemens or micromhos), even if a measure of skin resistance was originally obtained (i.e., conductance = 1/resistance). Researchers usually discriminate between tonic and phasic electrodermal measures. Tonic measures refer to long-term fluctuations in EDA and are best characterized by changes in skin conductance level (SCL) and the frequency of nonspecific or spontaneous fluctuations (see **Figure 1**). They are brief changes in EDA that are not specifically elicited by external stimuli but that arise due to internal thoughts, situational demands, emotional states, and individual differences in electrodermal lability. In contrast, phasic measures are specific skin conductance responses (SCRs), which have been elicited by an identified and usually externally presented stimulus. Phasic SCRs are usually quantified as an amplitude change from a baseline level value (prior to presentation of a stimulus) to

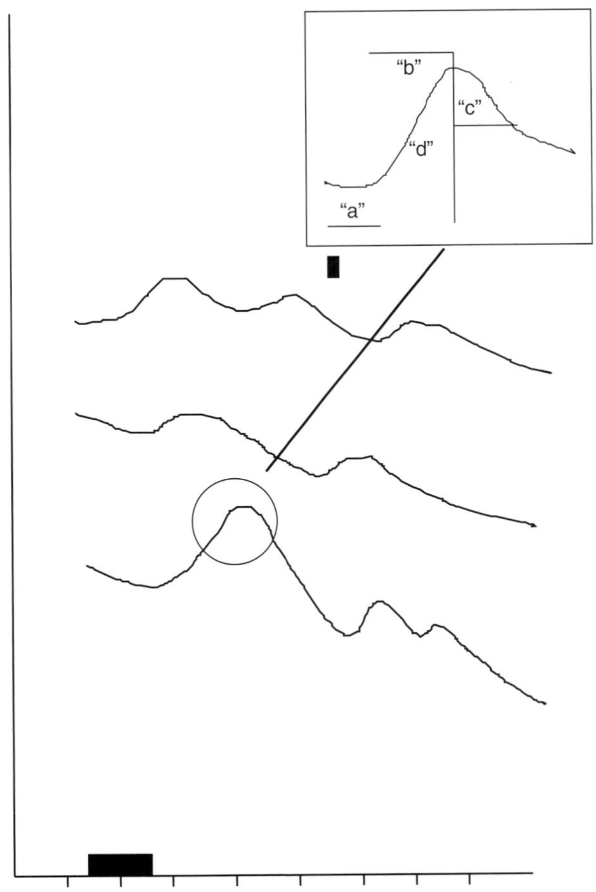

Figure 1 Schematic representation of skin conductance activity. Three individual skin conductance curves are represented with differing skin conductance levels and numbers of nonspecific responses (ns). Inset displays enlarged skin conductance response to specific stimulus (shaded block) and indicates (a) response latency, (b) response rise time, (c) response half-recovery time, and (d) response amplitude.

the peak of the response (see **Figure 1**). In addition to amplitude measures, temporal indices such as response latency, rise time, and half-recovery time may also assessed. Skin conductance responses are frequently obtained within what is known as an habituation paradigm, whereby simple sensory stimuli are presented to the participant and the autonomic responses measured to subsequent repetitions. When habituation paradigms are used, further measures of change in response amplitude across successive trials are also calculated using regression techniques.

Prior to analysis, electrodermal data are frequently transformed in order to achieve more normally distributed samples for parametric statistical analysis. There also exists a statistical dependency between phasic response amplitude and individual differences in tonic levels. Researchers will frequently use a variety of statistical transformations (e.g., log. and ratio measures) and range-correction methods to adjust for this response level dependency, which is sometimes termed the Law of Initial Values.

Biological Mechanisms

Fluctuations in either conductance or resistance have been attributed to variations in sweat gland activity. Essentially, alterations in conductance of the sweat gland are said to arise from a variety of different mechanisms involving changes in both sweat conductivity and physical level of sweat within the duct. The former is said to be associated with an active ionic reabsorption membrane located within the duct wall, and the latter with the mechanical extrusion of sweat from the gland. From a psychological perspective, the most important influence on sweat gland activity is through the autonomic cholinergic innervation to the glands. A variety of brain regions are implicated in the central control of EDA, including the lateral frontal and dorsolateral cortex, together with various cortico-limbic connections including the anterior hypothalamus and anterior limbic and infralimbic cortices. More recently, several brain-imaging studies have been conducted that looked at the functional location of EDA. These studies suggested separate mechanisms for the maintenance of electrodermal level and the activation of responses.

Psychological Applications

Attention and Information Processing

Phasic measures of EDA are frequently adopted as indices of attention and information processing. Skin conductance responses obtained within habituation and classical conditioning paradigms are interpreted in terms of the orienting response. Variations in SCR amplitudes are associated with changes in stimulus intensity, novelty, and significance. According to Ohman, the presence of an SCR indicates that a novel or significant stimulus has been detected by the information processing system and that a call has been made for further controlled processing of the incoming stimulus. The sizes of SCR amplitudes, therefore, are frequently interpreted as measures of attention.

Emotion

Attempts have been made to interpret SCRs with respect to either attentional or emotional responding. Lang and colleagues have argued, however, that whereas other peripheral psychophysiological measures such as heart rate, potentiated startle, and electromyographic activity might distinguish between the positive and negative aspects of emotional experience, SCRs appear sensitive only to the intensity or arousal dimension and not to the direction or valence of the emotion involved.

Stress

Both phasic and tonic measures have been argued to reflect peripheral arousal responses to stressful stimuli. In particular, EDA is said to be sensitive to psychosocial aspects of social interactions, workload, and occupational strain and has also been argued to reflect changes in anxiety. As well as the amplitude of SCRs, increases in the absolute SCL and the frequency of nonspecific response are often interpreted as reflecting increasing response to stress. Indeed, it is argued that a reliable individual difference dimension known as electrodermal lability might moderate the relationship between autonomic arousal and psychosocial influences. Similarly, EDA is frequently assessed in studies of psychopathology and has been widely investigated in clinical populations, including depression, anxiety, schizophrenia, hypertension, and diabetes.

Further Reading

Boucsein, W. (1992). *Electrodermal activity.* New York: Plenum Press.

Critchley, H. (2002). Electrodermal responses: what happens in the brain. *The Neuroscientist* 8, 132–142.

Dawson, M., Schell, A. M. and Filion, D. L. (2000). The electrodermal system. In: Cacioppo, J. T. & Tassinary, L. G. (eds.) *Principles of psychophysiology: physical, social, and inferential elements* (2nd edn., pp. 200–223). New York: Cambridge University Press.

Fowles, D. C., Christie, M. J., Edelberg, R., et al. (1981). Publication guidelines for electrodermal measurement. *Psychophysiology* **18**, 232–239.
Hugdahl, K. (1995). *Psychophysiology: the mind-body perspective.* Cambridge, MA: Harvard University Press.
Jacobs, S. C., Friedman, R. and Parker, J. D. et al. (1994). Use of skin conductance changes during mental stress testing as an index of autonomic arousal in cardiovascular research. *American Heart Journal* **128**, 1170–1177.
Lang, P. J., Greenwald, M. K., Bradley, M. M. and Cuthbert, B. N. Looking at pictures: affective, facial, visceral, and behavioral reactions. *Psychophysiology* **30**, 261–273.
Nagai, Y., Critchley, H. D., Featherstone, E., Trimble, M. R. and Dolan, R. J. (2004). Activity in ventromedial prefrontal cortex covaries with sympathetic skin conductance level (SCL): a physiological account of a "default mode" of brain function. *NeuroImage* **22**, 243–251.
Ravaja, N. (2004). Contributions of psychophysiology to media research: review and recommendations. *Media Psychology* **6**, 193–235.
Schell, A. M., Dawson, M. E., Nuechterlein, K. H., Subotnik, K. L. and Ventura, J. (2002). The temporal stability of electrodermal variables over a one-year period in patients with recent-onset schizophrenia and in normal subjects. *Psychophysiology* **39**, 124–132.
Shastri, A., Lomarev, M., Nelson, S., George, M. S., Hozwarth, M. R. and Bohning, D. E. (2001). A low-cost system for monitoring skin conductance during functional MRI. *Journal of Magnetic Resonance Imaging* **14**, 187–193.
Turpin, G. (1990). Ambulatory clinical psychophysiology: an introduction to techniques and methodological issues. *Journal of Psychophysiology* **4**, 299–304.
Turpin, G. and Clements, K. (1993). Electrodermal activity and psychopathology: the development of the Palmar Sweat Index as an applied measure for clinical settings. In: Roy, J. C., Boucsein, W., Fowles, D. & Gruzelier, J. (eds.) *Advances in electrodermal research*, pp. 49–60. New York: Plenum Press.
Venables, P. H. and Christie, M. J. (1980). Electrodermal activity. In: Martin, I. & Venables, P. H. (eds.) *Techniques in psychophysiology*, pp. 3–67. Chichester: Wiley.
Vetrugno, R., Liguori, R., Cortelli, P. and Montagna, P. (2003). Sympathetic skin response: basic mechanisms and clinical applications. *Clinical Autonomic Research* **13**, 256–270.

Febrile Response

S Gatti McArthur
F. Hoffmann-LaRoche, Basel, Switzerland
T Bartfai
The Scripps Research Institute, CA, USA

This is a revised version of the article by S Gatti McArthur and T Bartfai, Encyclopedia of Stress, First edition, volume 2, pp 116–123, © 2000, Elsevier Inc.

Glossary

Anterior hypothalamus/preoptic area
Hypothalamic area representing the major center of control of the temperature set point of the body.

Basal metabolic rate
The minimal (or steady state) energy use, keeping the body temperature constant under conditions of no net work carried out.

Cytokines and interleukins
Small proteins with regulatory functions produced and secreted mostly by immunocompetent cells.

Endogenous pyrogens
Proinflammatory cytokines or endogenous compounds that function as humoral mediators of fever induction.

Hypothalamic-pituitary-adrenocortical axis
The central and peripheral system sustaining the physiological response to stressors.

Intraperitoneal and intracerebroventricular injections
Usual ways to administer exogenous pyrogens, i.e., lipopolysaccharide or endogenous pyrogens to study their peripheral and central proinflammatory effects.

Lipopolysaccharide
A fraction of the *Escherichia coli* bacterial wall used in different experimental models of gram-negative bacterial infection.

Thermoneutral zone
A range of ambient temperatures compatible with a control of the core body temperature achievable solely by cardiovascular changes in the peripheral compartment of the body.

Introduction

Fever is a transient change of the hypothalamic temperature (HT) set point causing the rise of the core body temperature (BT) of about 2–4°C in humans. This physiological response to inflammatory stimuli is always associated with peripheral and central events:

massive hepatic production of acute-phase proteins, sleep induction, and anorexia, defined globally as the acute-phase response. Fever is triggered by the peripheral and central production of interleukin-1β (IL-1β), tumor necrosis factor α (TNF-α), and interleukin-6 (IL-6) and is caused by the local production of prostaglandins (PGE_2) in the anterior hypothalamus/preoptic area (AH/POA). The rise of the BT during febrile response is achieved by reducing heat loss (vasoconstriction) and by increasing simultaneously the heat production (facultative thermogenesis) via the activation of the sympathetic system. The sudden heat production associated with acute stress, usually described as hyperthermia, is also triggered by the activation of the sympathetic system. It is a common observation that subchronic, chronic, or exhaustive stresses are associated either with fever-like episodes or with an impairment of the whole inflammatory response. Experimental data demonstrate the endogenous production of IL-1β in rat hypothalamus during unescapable stress, pointing to the tight molecular control exerted by glucocorticoids (GCs) and corticotropin-releasing factor (CRF) on the production and effects of pyrogenic cytokines.

Thermal Control in Endotherms

Heat production is a sign of metabolic activity. Heat storage/heat exchange mechanisms are strikingly different in living organisms, resulting from the evolution of specialized systems (e.g., enzymes, organs, and cell types) required to survive and acclimate in different environmental conditions. **Figure 1** shows a summary of the mechanisms controlling thermal balance in endotherms. The core BT is the result of both heat production and heat exchange with the environment under the control of different pools of thermal sensors present in skin, viscera, main cardiovascular districts, spinal cord, and brain. The whole body can be divided in three main compartments (core, periphery, and skin), which regulate the exchange of heat mainly by modifying blood flow in the different districts. Cardiovascular, respiratory, and perspirative effects are always accompanied by behavioral changes in order to obtain an effective increase or drop of the BT. The main metabolic exothermic reactions contributing to heat production are listed in **Figure 1b**. The brown fat tissue (BAT), which is very rich in mitochondria, can produce heat by uncoupling the electron transport/proton gradient in the inner mitochondrial membrane thanks to the presence of uncoupling protein-1 (UCP-1) (nonshivering thermogenesis). Other gene products of the same family, UCP-2 and UCP-3, are expressed in white fat tissue/liver and in the muscular tissue, respectively. The contribution of UCP-2 to thermogenesis during fever is under debate.

Transient (or prolonged) temperature changes, observed during fever, have a deep metabolic impact,

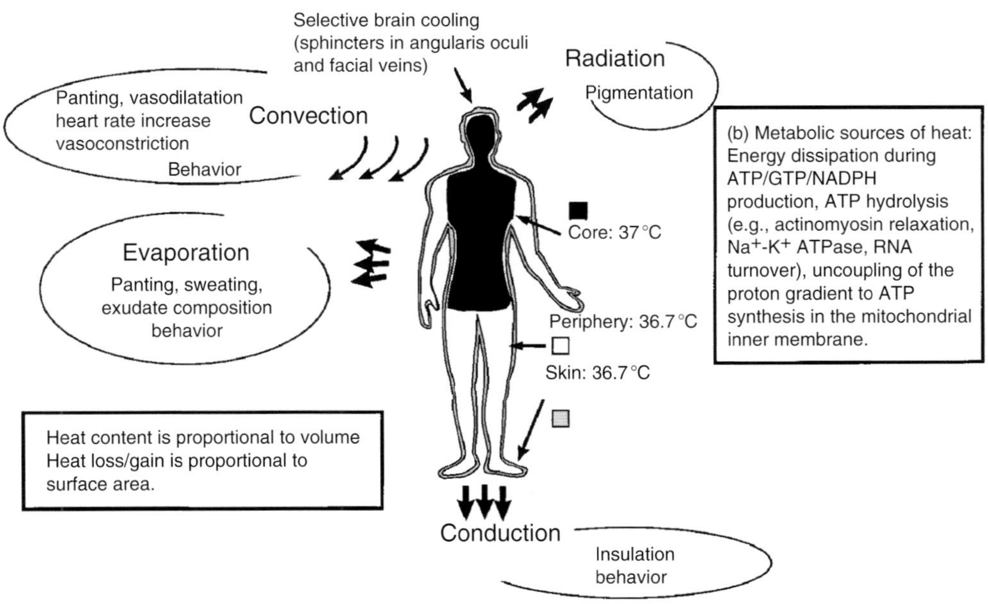

ATP, adenosine triphosphate; GTP, guanosine triphosphate;
NADPH, nicotinamide adenine dinucleotide phosphate; RNA, ribonucleic acid.

Figure 1 Schematic view of the mechanisms of heat production and heat exchange in endotherms. (a) Conduction, convection, radiation, evaporation, and metabolic heat production contribute in an additive manner to the definition of the temperature in the different districts of the body: skin, periphery, and core. The mechanism of selective brain cooling controls the facial venous flow in order to locally control the brain temperature by circulatory means. (b) The main exothermic metabolic reactions.

being associated with kinetic changes in all enzymatic reactions, in membrane conductance, and change of permeability of ionic channels. Furthermore, to actively increase the BT of a human by 1°C within 1 h requires the net heat storage of about 3.48 J kg^{-1} with an energy cost for a human of 70 kg (in thermoneutral conditions) of about 243.6 J. GCs do support the metabolic heat requirements of the febrile response by enhancing several thermogenic reactions. Endogenous pyrogens (EPs) are also responsible for the metabolic changes observed during the acute-phase response. In particular leptin, a protein controlling white fat tissue metabolism and energy expenditure, exerts a necessary role in sustaining facultative thermogenesis during fever. Considering the energy required to mount a febrile response, it becomes understandable why starvation, cachexia, extreme ambient temperature, or other causes of metabolic distress would reduce the magnitude of the febrile response if not abolish it completely.

Temperature Set Point

Figure 2 shows effector systems activated in endotherms to keep the core BT constant while the ambient temperature changes progressively. During cold exposure, shivering is controlled by the activation of the motor system, whereas changes in superficial microcirculation and nonshivering thermogenesis are signs of the activation of the sympathetic system. The energetic requirement of the cold-induced thermal response is reduced progressively as the ambient temperature reaches the thermoneutral zone. Within this narrow range of temperatures, energy requirements to keep the BT constant (in absence of stress and motor activity) are met by the basal metabolic rate (BMR). The response to a warm environment is conversely characterized by vasodilatation, panting, and sweating. Shivering frequency and BMR are inversely correlated on a logarithmic scale with the body mass. Furthermore, the BMR is constantly adapted in different individuals in response to climatic conditions, diet, and motor activity under the control of the thyroid hormones. The BT in the different compartments and the range of temperatures triggering the effector systems in order to increase alternatively heat storage or heat loss are defined by the integration of thermoafferent signals and their comparison with a temperature set point defined in the AH/POA. Among the signals integrated in AH/POA, it is important to point at the local HT, reported by several studies as the stimulus able to overcome peripheral inputs. The local HT cannot fluctuate freely more than 0.1–0.2°C in a narrow range of temperatures that is defining the set point. Whatever change of the local temperature outside the limits of this range would trigger the effector response to a warm or cold environment (**Figure 2**). During fever the hypothalamic set point is shifted upward with a

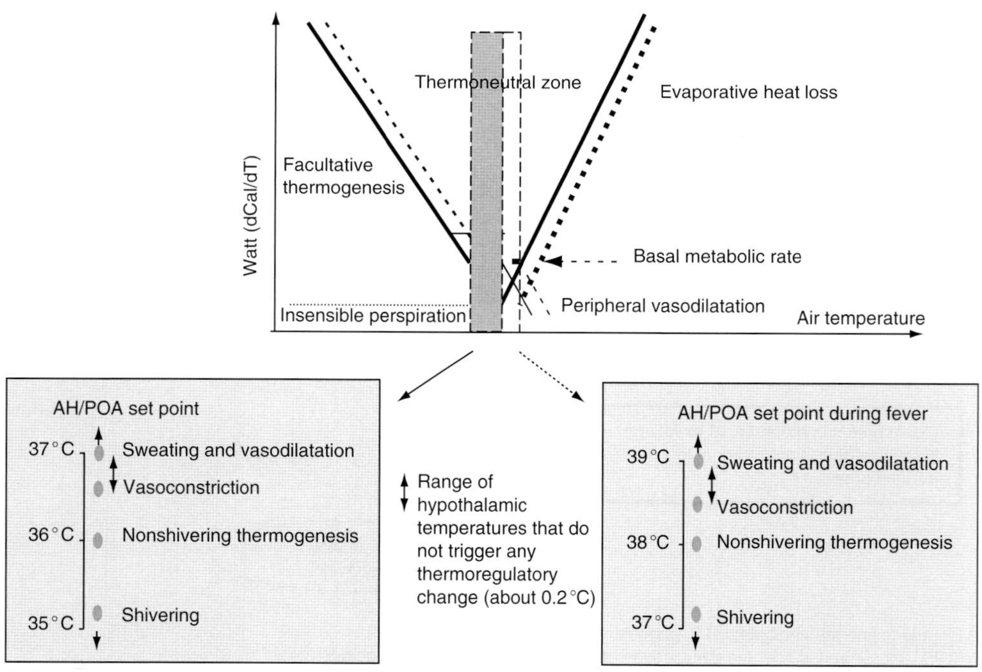

AH/POA, anterior hypothalamus/preoptic area.

Figure 2 Thermal control in endotherms: the sympathetic and parasympathetic systems are alternatively activated by changes of the ambient temperature exceeding the thermoneutral zone in order to keep the core BT constant. The thermoneutral range is defined by the HT set point. The whole system is transiently shifted upward during fever.

reset of the range of HTs triggering the different effector responses. Because the body would need increased heat storage and heat production to reach the new temperature in the different districts, fever, in its initial phase, would cause a thermal response mimicking the normal reaction to a cold environment.

Thermosensitive Neurons

There are no known molecular markers for the neurons involved in the central control of the temperature set point. The only information available about the neuronal populations involved is that they share the common feature of being thermosensitive. Neuronal thermosensitivity (TS) can be characterized by measuring the neuronal firing rate in a paraphysiologic range of temperatures and calculating the thermal coefficient for each cell. The range of thermal sensitivity of AH/POA neurons may vary quite extensively and it is generally linear within a narrow range of temperatures. Two distinct populations of TS neurons have been characterized in the hypothalamus: cold-sensitive and warm-sensitive neurons. Cold-sensitive neurons are less studied, mostly because they represent less than 10% of the TS neurons in AH/POA. Warm sensitivity has been studied quite extensively using hypothalamic slices. These studies demonstrate that TS is an intrinsic cellular property. Warm-sensitive neurons are present in several brain regions: in AH/POA, in lower centers in the brain stem, and in the spinal cord. The presence of TS neurons in different brain regions may suggest temperature differences in the cerebral versus peripheral compartment. However, it has been demonstrated that thermal curves are similar both in time course and in absolute values in the cerebral cortex and the peritoneum under basal conditions, during fever, and pharmacological hypothermia.

Fever and Thermosensitivity

Fever depresses the TS of neurons whose firing rates had been increased previously by local AH/POA warming. Furthermore, local injections in the AH/POA of EPs or prostaglandin E2 (PGE_2) cause a reduction of the tonic firing of warm-sensitive neurons similar to the one observed when lowering locally the HT. The plasticity of warm-sensitive neurons and their responsivity to bath-applied IL-1 or IL-6 has yet to be characterized properly, and moreover, the molecular components of neuronal activity changes in AH/POA during fever have yet to be determined. Few studies reporting intracellular recordings from warm-sensitive neurons are opening up a key path of research in this respect.

Endogenous Pyrogens and Fever Induction

IL-1β was among the first cytokines described, and its biological properties as EP, the leukocytic pyrogen, were described long before the purification of the protein. In general, the concept of a humoral mediator of a fever response is older than the discovery of pro-inflammatory cytokines and was initially related to the observation that bacterial debris lipopolysaccharide (LPS) could cause fever with almost a 2-h delay from the time of the injection. The LPS effect was also characterized by priming and tolerance, further suggesting the presence of endogenous mediators. The progressive discovery of several pyrogenic cytokines present in the plasma only during an inflammatory reaction, and the study of their synergism and production in hypothalamus during a febrile response, further clarified the definition of EP. All EPs cause fever when administered by the intracerebroventricular (ICV) route and in the periphery and they are released into the circulatory system during the fever response to exogenous pyrogens. The magnitude and time course of the fever response could be related to the plasma and hypothalamic levels of the EP only in the case of IL-6. IL-1β or TNF-α seems to trigger the febrile response more than sustaining it because several endogenous antagonistic systems (such as IL-1 receptor antagonist (IL-1ra), in the case of IL-1α and IL-1β) are buffering or suppressing *in vivo* the initial EPs effects both peripherally and centrally (**Figure 3a**). The list of known EPs would then contain interferons (IFN-α, -β, and -γ), IL-1α/β, TNF-α/β, and IL-6. IL-1β is the most potent: a 30-ng kg^{-1} intravenous injection is sufficient to cause fever in humans. IL-6 and chemokines (IL-8, macrophage inflammatory protein-1) would trigger the fever response only when injected centrally into the AH/POA or ICV. The generation of mice carrying null mutations for the different EPs or their receptors has been extremely important in demonstrating the presence of a hierarchy of EP in the generation of the fever response, with IL-6 acting probably downstream of IL-1β and TNFα.

The most relevant results of the studies can be summarized as follows:

- Studies on IL-1 type 1 receptor (IL-1RI) knockout (KO) mice and IL-1R accessory protein (IL-1Rap) KO mice have demonstrated that IL-1RI mediates the fever response induced by an intraperitoneal (IP) injection of IL-1α and IL-1β. The fever response to LPS is rather normal in these animals, suggesting that TNF and other EPs can bypass the IL-1 system in the generation of the febrile response.

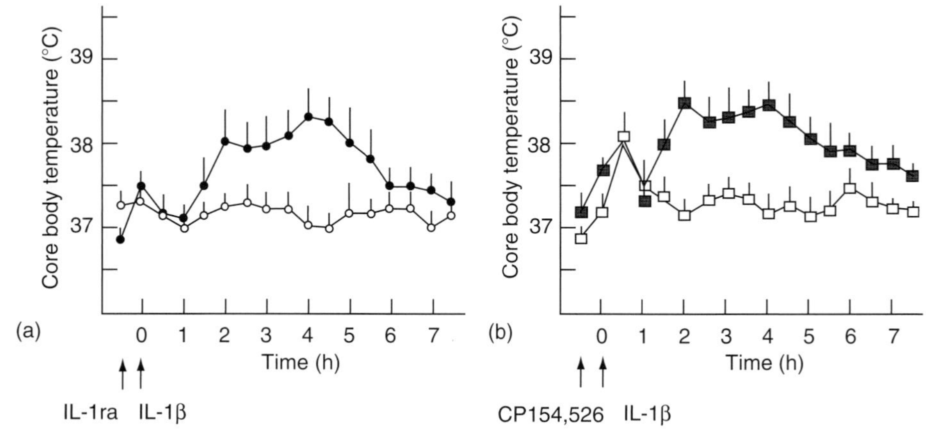

Figure 3 (a) Fever response in rats injected IP with 5 μg kg^{-1} of recombinant human IL-1β.The febrile response is blocked by the injection of recombinant human IL-1ra (2.5 mg kg^{-1}). (b) Fever response in rats injected IP with human recombinant IL-1β (5 μg kg^{-1}). The effect is blocked by the previous injection of the nonpeptidic CRF receptor antagonist CP154,526 (0.16 mg kg^{-1}, IP). Data are means ± standard error means. Data were recorded using a telemetry system and averaged every 30 min. Open circles, IL-1ra plus IL-1β (n = 5), closed circles, IL-1β (n = 3), open squares, CP154 526 plus IL-1β (n = 4), and closed squares, IL-1β (n = 8).

- IL-1β KO mice show hyperresponsive fever mostly in terms of magnitude of the effects in response to IL-1α and IL-1β IP injection.
- IL-6 KO mice are unable to mount a febrile response on injection of IL-1β or LPS in the periphery. Only the parallel co-injection of IL-6 IP seems to restore a sort of fever response to LPS IP injection. Very interesting genetic studies on different autoimmune familiar disorders like Mediterranean fever are pointing future research towards proteins such as pyrin and cryopyrins which are possibly upstream EP production.

Exogenous Pyrogens

The most used experimental model of fever response in the presence of an endogenous stimulus is represented by LPS injection in the periphery. This model mimics a response to gram-negative bacterial infections. Fever is also present during gram-positive bacterial infections because macrophages can produce somnogenic and pyrogenic muramyl peptides during the digestion of staphylococci fractions. Furthermore, agents such as turpentine are broadly used as an experimental model of aseptic inflammation, which is almost uniquely mediated by IL-1β. However, the broadest spectrum of exogenous pyrogens is offered by viral proteins 2 or by the etiological agents of parasitic infections such as schistosomiasis or malaria. In case of viral infections, interferons (IFNs) are the principal responsible of the observed febrile response with IL-1β contributing as EP. EP and Toll-like proteins responsive to exogenous pyrogens are probably present in all vertebrates. Equally ancient from the phylogenetic point of view is the complement cascade of proteins which interact with EPs and EP production mainly via anaphylatoxins.

Expression of Endogenous Pyrogens and their Receptors in the Hypothalamus

IL-1α/β, TNF-α, and IL-6 gene expression can be induced in AH/POA on peripheral immune challenge (with LPS or IL-1β for instance). The peripheral administration of LPS induces IL-1β production in meninges, choroid plexus macrophages, some perivascular cells, and microglial cells shortly after IP injection (1–8 h). Constitutive expression of IL-1β and IL-6/IL-6R in neuronal cell types has been reported by some authors, but the matter is still controversial. Receptors for the different EPs, particularly IL-1RI, are expressed constitutively in AH/POA. Their expression is modulated by GCs and EP, particularly IL-1β. At the same time, pharmacological doses of corticosterone block the LPS-induced fever response and IL-1α/β and TNF-α mRNAs expression in the hypothalamus, suggesting a causal role for the hypothalamic production of cytokines in fever induction. The control by GC and EPs on the expression of EPs/EP receptors is mostly transcriptional. The promoter regions of EP genes contain an unusually high number of GC receptor response elements. In the case of IL-1β and TNF-α, posttranscriptional control of GC at the mRNA and proteic level has been demonstrated to be extremely important in controlling the cellular production of these EPs in immunocompetent cells and the activation/secretion of the mature form of these cytokines.

Humoral Versus Neuronal Mediators of Fever Induction

How does the brain sense EPs? This key question has several answers. In fact, circulating pro-inflammatory cytokines can reach the brain via the interaction with saturable carriers in the plexus chorioideus. However, this mechanism would account for the entrance of a limited amount of protein, eventually able to trigger local cytokine production AH/POA. Several pathologic conditions cause damage to the blood–brain barrier. In this case the amount of circulating EPs reaching the hypothalamus could be higher. There is also a specialized circumventricular organ, the organum vasculosum lamina terminalis (OVLT), located along the margin of the ventricular system that has fenestrated capillaries and, therefore, direct contact with the circulatory system. The role of the OVLT has been demonstrated in the case of peptides such as angiotensin II and cholecystokinin and is probably also essential for the transduction of the plasmatic levels of EPs into central effects. A third mechanism of immune signaling, essential in the case of peritoneal immune challenge, is the peripheral stimulation of sensory nerves, particularly the afferent part of the vagus nerve. IL-1Rs are present in vagal paraganglia, chemosensory bodies, all along the course of the vagal nerve in the cervical region, and in thoracic and abdominal cavities. Subdiafragmatic vagotomy is able to block the central production of IL-1β in response to the IP injection of IL-1β or LPS. The immediate c-fos mRNA induction has been used to trace the neuronal pathway activated in response to the peripheral loading of LPS, and several studies would point to the presence of a selective activation of neurons in the hypothalamus (paraventricular nucleus, ventromedial POA), brain stem (A1 and A2 region), nucleus of the solitary tract, and ventrolateral medulla. In some cases the activated pathways represent antipyretic responses that are initiated during fever, such as the activation of neurons that contain α-melanocyte-stimulating hormone (α-MSH) and arginine-vasopressin.

Role of Prostaglandins in Fever

The role of prostaglandins (PG) of the E series in fever induction was first described by Milton and colleagues in 1970. PGs of the F class can also cause fever. Their effect is, however, mediated by the release of CRF. Both PG series are thus EPs. The fever response triggered by pro-inflammatory cytokines is always mediated by the local production in AH/POA of PGs. In fact, the pyrogenic effect of peripheral LPS and EPs can be blocked by cyclo-oxygenase inhibitors injected locally into AH/POA. A dense distribution of PGE_2-binding sites is present in the anterior wall of the third ventricle surrounding the OVLT in the rat brain. Moreover, a study on mice carrying a null mutation for the different PG receptors demonstrated that receptor EP3 selectively mediates the PGE_2-induced fever response in the presence of IL-1β or LPS. It is important to note that PG synthesis inhibitors are excellent antipyretic agents but have few or no effects on stress. So the picture is not complete. A missing link for fast hypothalamic events triggered by EPs could be the C2-ceramide pathway.

Stress and Fever Induction

Stress-induced fever can be measured using several experimental protocols of stress in rodents, e.g., unescapable stress or restriction. In some cases, it should be noted, however, that the stress response would modify the circadian rhythms of BT and that the results obtained should be normalized considering possible shifts of the circadian rhythm of the BT of the animals. The development of a fever response to certain kinds of stress is also confirmed by the increased expression in the hypothalamus and hippocampus of EPs; particularly IL-1β mRNA and protein. The effects of IL-1β on all the levels of the hypothalamus-pituitary-adrenocortical (HPA) axis are significant and very well characterized by several studies. IL-1β can activate CRF synthesis and release and adrenocorticotropic hormone (ACTH) secretion acting locally at the hypothalamic and pituitary level, respectively. Hence, IL-1β is one of the few known agents able to induce CRF release, although the direct effect of IL-1β on the production/release of GC is still controversial. In contrast, the GC effect on cytokine production is dual and depends on the circulating levels of GC. In fact, physiological levels of GC would support the metabolic requirement of the acute-phase reaction, leading also to increased GC production as the HPA is activated. As a result, the increased GC release during inflammation buffers the pro-inflammatory cytokine effects by restricting their expression. A special note should, however, be taken while discussing the effect of GC on IL-6. In rodents, IL-6 mRNA expression is higher in the hypothalamus after chronic treatment with high doses of corticosterone, and mice overexpressing IL-6 in astrocytes exhibit higher plasmatic levels of corticosterone, reduced ACTH response, and adrenal hyperplasia. This may suggest a direct effect of IL-6 at the level of the adrenal glands. Furthermore, both IL-6 and GC are responsible for the production of different sets of hepatic proteins carrying GC-responsive elements and nuclear factor–IL-6 response elements in the promoter region of their genes, and they are both probably involved in controlling the duration and the magnitude of the acute-phase response. Increased plasmatic cytokine levels during stress have been explained considering the possible bacterial translocation from the gastrointestinal tract to the mesenteric lymph nodes.

The presence of this phenomenon is, however, seldom considered when planning an experimental protocol, and the impact of bacterial translocation on central and peripheral IL-1 production has not yet been characterized clearly. When examining the activation of the HPA axis during fever response, it is important to keep in mind that a central role is played by CRF and vasopressin. Central injection of CRF causes fever in rats and it also activates thermogenesis in the BAT. Furthermore, neutralizing antibodies to CRF or synthetic CRF antagonists block the pyrogenic response associated with IL-1β or TNF injection (**Figure 3b**). CRF plays a necessary but indirect role in the development of the fever response. Vasopressin is an endogenous antipyretic hormone. New synthetic selective antagonists will possibly allow in the future a better understanding of which receptor is mediating fever and HPA-axis effects.

Finally, the role of the sympathetic system in the development of stress or the cytokine-induced thermal response has to be redefined on the basis of the demonstrated presence of the constitutive production of IL-1β and IL-6 in the sympathetic ganglia and in adrenal medulla. *In vivo* during an inflammatory reaction and fever induction, the presence of EP and EP receptors at different levels can ensure a tight control on the activation of the sympathetic system in terms of magnitude and duration of the effect based on the presence of a local or systemic inflammatory reaction.

See Also the Following Articles

Prostaglandins.

Further Reading

Chai, Z., Alheim, K., Lundkvist, J., et al. (1996). Subchronic glucocorticoid pretreatment reversibly attenuates IL-1 beta induced fever in rats; IL-6 mRNA is elevated while IL-1 alpha and IL-1 beta mRNAs are suppressed, in the CNS. *Cytokine* **8**, 227–237.

Dinarello, C. (1998). Interleukin-1, interleukin-1 receptors and interleukin-1 receptor antagonist. *International Review of Immunology* **16**, 457–499.

Elmquist, J., Scammell, T. and Saper, C. (1997). Mechanisms of CNS response to systemic immune challenge: The febrile response. *Trends in Neurosciences* **20**, 565–570.

Kluger, M. (1991). Fever: role of pyrogens and cryogens. *Physiological Reviews* **71**, 93–127.

Lundkvist, J., Chai, Z., Teheranian, R., et al. (1996). A non peptidic corticotropin releasing factor receptor antagonist attenuates fever and exhibits anxiolytic-like activity. *European Journal of Pharmacology* **308**, 195–200.

Nguyen, K. T., Deak, T., Owens, S. M., et al. (1998). Exposure to acute stress induces brain interleukin-1beta protein in the rat. *Journal of Neuroscience* **18**, 2239–2246.

Rolfe, D. and Brown, G. (1997). Cellular energy utilisation and molecular origin of standard metabolic rate in mammals. *Physiological Reviews* **77**, 731–758.

Sanchez-Alavez, M., Tabarean, I. V., Behens, M. M., et al. (2006). Ceramide mediates the rapid phase of febrile response to IL-1beta. *Proceedings of the National Academy of Sciences USA* **103**, 2904–2908.

Schobitz, B., Reul, J. and Holsboer, F. (1994). The role of the hypothalamic-pituitary-adrenocortical system during inflammatory conditions. *Critical Reviews in Neurobiology* **8**, 263–291.

Schonbaum, E. and Lomax, P. (eds.) (1990). *International encyclopedia of pharmacology and therapeutics, sect. 131, Thermoregulation: physiology and biochemistry.* New York: Pergamon Press.

Kluger, M. J., Kozak, W., Leon, L. R., et al. (1998). Fever and antipyresis. In: Sharma, H. S. & Westman, J. (eds.) *Brain function in hot environment. Progress in brain research* (vol. 115), pp. 465–475. Amsterdam: Elsevier Science.

Sundgren-Andersson, A., Gatti, S. and Bartfai, T. (1998). Neurobiological mechanisms of fever. *Neuroscientist* **4**, 113–121.

Sundgren-Andersson, A. K., Ostlund, P. and Bartfai, T. (1998). Simultaneous measurement of brain and core temperature in the rat during fever, hyperthermia, hypothermia and sleep. *Neuroimmunomodulation* **5**, 241–247.

Ting, J. P., Kastner, D. L. and Hoffman, H. M. (2006). CATERPILLERS, pyrin and hereditary immunological disorders. *Nature Reviews Immunology* **6**, 183–195.

Ushikubi, F., Segi, E., Sugimoto, Y., et al. (1998). Impaired febrile response in mice lacking the prostaglandin E receptor subtype EP3. *Nature* **392**, 281–284.

V. INTEGRATIVE ASPECTS OF STRESS RESPONSE

Genetic Polymorphisms in Stress Response

I W Craig
King's College London, London, UK

Glossary

Allele One of two or more possible forms of a gene. An individual may possess two identical or two different alleles, except for the genes on the X-chromosome in males (they possess only a single copy of this chromosome).

Body mass index (BMI) A measure of body fat based on height and weight that applies to both adult men and women.

Case/control studies Comparisons between groups of individuals with particular features or disorders and groups apparently normal for these aspects; often employed to search for differences in the genotype or allele frequencies between the two groups.

Genotype The configuration of alleles at a genetic locus. If both alleles are identical the individual is homozygous; if the two alleles differ the individual is heterozygous.

Haplotype The pattern of alleles at two or more polymorphic sites represented on one of the chromosome homologs.

Intragenic feature A feature located within the conventional boundaries of a gene.

Kilobase (kb) One thousand base pairs.

Linkage disequilibrium The existence of combinations of alleles at two or more polymorphic sites within a region at frequencies greater than expected by random assortment.

Missense mutation A base change in the coding region of the gene that results in the substitution of one amino acid in the encoded protein for another.

Polymorphism The existence at gene locus of more than one allele with the rarest at appreciable frequency (usually assumed to be >1%) in the population.

Promoter The section of DNA that precedes a gene and controls its activity.

Single nucleotide polymorphism (SNP) A polymorphism at a single base position in DNA.

Stressor Stimulus input that creates stress and initiates a response.

Genes and the Stress Responses

The genetic basis for the stress response is complex; nevertheless, the genes involved can be divided into two broad categories: those encoding the autonomic reaction to stressful situations and those involved in the neuroendocrine stress response. The typical rapid reactions to perceived stress are well recognized to be associated with the fight-or-flight response and are mostly mediated by the sympathetic nervous system with the release of norepinephrine from widely distributed synapses and epinephrine from the adrenal medulla. Implicit in this classic description of the rapid stress response is the recognition of the potential violent and aggressive outcomes that stress can engender. A more delayed response is mediated by the release of cortisol, the major glucocorticoid in humans. This is initiated by neural signals to the hypothalamus that releases corticotropin releasing hormone (CRH), which in turn results in the release of adrenocorticotropic hormone (ACTH) from the anterior pituitary, thereby stimulating cortisol production by the adrenal cortex. The production of cortisol assists in restoring homeostasis in response to stress; however, prolonged exposure can be potentially harmful.

Reactions to acute stress are also usually accompanied by perturbations of serotinergic activity, as indicated by altered levels of serotonin (5-HT) or its metabolites. Serotonin is a significant regulator of morphogenetic activities during early central nervous system development, including cell proliferation, migration, and differentiation.

Outcomes following exposure to stress may, therefore, be highly variable depending on a wide range of genetic factors controlling these various aspects. A simplified overview of some of the most important elements of stress response and relevant genes is shown in **Figure 1**. The significance of genetic variation in the better-characterized components of the stress response pathways is considered next. Several case/control studies have examined the association between genes involved in the stress response and somatic or behavioral traits. Some of these are noted; however, it is important to recognize that there are potential confounding factors to such studies and only consistent replication and supporting molecular evidence can establish the formal verification of such links.

Polymorphisms of Genes in the Autonomic Stress Response Pathway

The rapid stress response to stressful stimuli is mediated by the release of norepinephrine in the brain. This leads to the activation of the sympathetic nervous system and the adrenal medulla with release

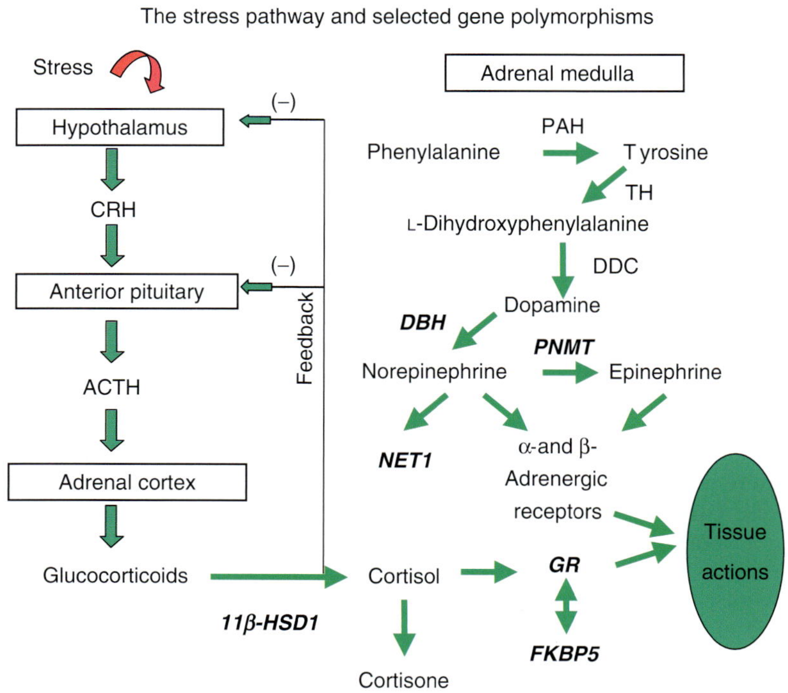

Figure 1 The stress pathway illustrating selected genes (in bold italics). 11β-HSD1, 11-β-hydroxysteroid dehydrogenase enzymes; ACTH, Adrenocorticotropic hormone; GR, glucocorticoid receptor; CRH, corticotropin releasing hormone; DBH, dopamine β-hydroxylase; DDC, DOPA decarboxylase; FKBP5, glucocorticoid receptor co-chaperone; NET1, norepinephrine transporter; PAH, phenylalanine hydroxylase; PNMT, phenylethanolamine *N*-methyl transferase; TH = tyrosine hydroxylase. α- and β-Adrenergic receptors include ADRA1A, ADRA1B, ADRA1D, ADRA2A, ADRA2B, ADRA2C, ADRB1, ADRB2, and ADRB3.

of epinephrine in the blood. Hence, the genes regulating the biogenesis and degradation of both epinephrine and norepinephrine and those encoding their cognate receptors are key players in the primary stress response. The epinephrine and norepinephrine metabolic pathways share components with those for other neurotransmitters. The steps in the synthesis of epinephrine from amino acid precursors are illustrated in **Figure 1**. The last two critical steps are undertaken by the enzymes dopamine β-hydroxylase (DBH) and phenylethanolamine *N*-methyl transferase (PNMT).

Dopamine β-Hydroxylase

The dopamine β-hydroxylase gene (*DBH)* is located on chromosome 9. A SNP in the presumed controlling region of *DBH,* which results in the substitution of a C to T substitution 1021 bp before the transcription start, accounts for up to 50% of the variance in plasma levels of the enzyme. Other variants flanking, or within, the potential promoter region include a polymorphism that depends on the copy number of an intragenic dinucleotide repeat approximately 4 kb upstream of the transcription start and a 19-bp insertion/deletion located 118 bp upstream.

In addition several SNPs have been reported within the coding region. Of these, an arginine to cysteine substitution in exon 11 has been suggested to be the most likely functionally significant variant. Several studies have linked a variation in plasma levels and *DBH* genotypes to various physiological and behavioral disorders, including hypertension, psychosis, depression, migraine, attention deficit hyperactivity disorder, and alcoholism. These reported associations await replication and consolidation.

There are also reports of individuals with undetectable levels of norepinephrine and epinephrine, together with elevated levels of dopamine. Such individuals have low, or absent, circulating DBH enzyme caused by deleterious mutations affecting both copies of the *DBH* gene and manifest a range of symptoms, including orthostatic hypotension.

Although alterations to this key enzyme in the synthetic pathway for norepinephrine and epinephrine are likely to have significant consequences for the stress response, no specific behavioral or physiological features relating to the reactions to stressors *per se* have been reported.

Phenylethanolamine *N*-Methyl Transferase

The gene for PNMT, a key enzyme, is located on chromosome 17. Two SNPs that may affect the regulation of the gene have been identified in the promoter.

When tested in case/control studies, significant association was observed between these and early-onset, but not late-onset, versions of Alzheimer's disease, and there are data suggesting a possible association between these SNPs and hypertension in African American groups. In addition, there is evidence suggesting that a variant of this gene may be associated with blood pressure regulation abnormalities in the stroke-prone, spontaneously hypersensitive rat strain.

Norepinephrine and Epinephrine Receptors

The adrenergic receptors for epinephrine and norepinephrine are divided into two major classes, alpha (subdivided into α1 and α2) and beta (subdivided into β1, β2, and β3). These receptors are targeted by a variety of drugs, including the so-called beta-blockers; hence genetic variation in them may be an important feature for pharmacotherapy. The activation of the β-adrenergic receptors stimulates adenylate cyclase.

α1-Adrenergic receptors The α1-adrenergic receptors are G-coupled trans-membrane receptors that are capable of binding both epinephrine and norepinephrine and thereby mediate some aspects of the sympathetic nervous system. The genes encoding them include *ADRA1A* (formerly known as *ADRA1C*, on chromosome 8), *ADRA1B* (formerly known as *ADRA1*, on chromosome 5) and *ADRA1D* (formerly known as *ADRA1A*, on chromosome 20). Of these, *ADRA1B* is of particular interest because fine mapping with highly polymorphic markers localizes it to a region that also contains the dopamine receptor gene *DRD1A*. Because this chromosome region has been linked to variability in systolic blood pressure, genetic variation in either *ADRA1B* or *DRD1A*, or both, may play an important role in influencing interindividual differences in this feature; however, specific functional variants in these have yet been described.

α2-Adrenergic receptors The release of norepinephrine is controlled by negative feedback from α2-adrenergic receptors, which are located on the presynaptic side of nerve terminals, including nerve muscle junctions. The targets of the released norepinephrine on heart muscle cells (myocytes) are β1-adrenergic receptors. The individual roles of the three highly homologous α2-adrenergic receptors (ADRA2A, ADRA2B, and ADRA2C, encoded by genes located in humans on 10, 2, and 4, respectively) have been studied by gene disruption in mice. Both ADRA2A and ADRA2C subtypes were found to be required for the normal presynaptic control of transmitter release from sympathetic nerves in the heart and from central noradrenergic neurons. In addition, a small deletion (base pairs 322–325) in the *ADRA2C* gene in humans has been shown to decrease function and may act in concert with the beta-receptor gene *ADRB1* as a risk factor for heart attack.

A polymorphism leading to the deletion of three glutamic acid residues from a repeating motif in the third intracellular loop of *ADRA2B* has been associated with variations in basal metabolic rate.

β-Adrenergic receptors β1-Adrenergic receptors encoded by the gene *ADRB1* (also known as *ADRB1R*, located on chromosome 10) are present in heart, and their stimulation causes an increase in heart rate. Many beta-blockers act on these targets (and on β2 receptors to a lesser extent). One variant of the β1-adrenergic receptor gene, which changes an arginine at position 389 in the protein to glycine, has been shown to possess increased function in tissue culture. There is also a polymorphic variant of a small deletion (base pairs 322–325) in the gene for the α2C-adrenergic receptor, *ADRA2C*, that has decreased function. A marked increase in the risk of heart failure among black patients has been observed for those who are homozygous for this and the *ADRB1* variant. This suggests that genotyping of these two genes may be a useful approach for identifying people at risk for heart failure. Further support for an interaction between these two genes has been provided by recent studies indicating that ADRA2A and ADRB1 proteins form heterodimers when expressed in tissue culture cells. In Caucasian women, it has been observed that the arg389 allele of *ADRB1* was associated with greater body weight and BMI.

β2-Adrenergic receptor Several polymorphic variants have been described, the most common and significant of which is a substitution causing a change from glycine to arginine at position 16. β2-Adrenergic receptor agonist drugs are widely employed in the treatment of asthma. It is therefore of interest that an excess of the glycine allele has been observed in nocturnal asthmatics. It appears that this substitution imparts enhanced agonist-promoted downregulation of the receptor.

A second polymorphism is centered on amino acid 27, where a glutamine to glutamic acid replacement is observed. An association with obesity has been reported, with an excess of the glutamine version in nonobese individuals. Possible links of this variant with asthma have also been noted.

A third variant involving a threonine to isoleucine replacement at amino acid 64 exists at lower frequencies. This has a profound functional consequence that results in a fivefold reduction in sensitivity to β2-receptor agonist-mediated vasodilatation. This suggests a mechanistic explanation of decreased survival in patients carrying this variant.

β3-Adrenergic receptor The β3-adrenergic receptor, ADRB3, is located mainly in adipose tissue and for this reason has been studied in relation to obesity. A mutation resulting in the substitution of arginine for tryptophan at amino acid position 64 has been observed at a frequency of approximately 10%. Many studies have examined the relationship of the polymorphism to obesity, BMI, and noninsulin-dependent diabetes mellitus, with some concluding that the locus may have a role in predisposing these phenotypes; but other studies have failed to replicate the observations.

Norepinephrine Transporter

The norepinephrine transporter protein 1 (NET1) is also known as the norepinephrine transporter (NAT1) or the solute carrier family 6, member 2 (SLC6A2). The gene responsible is localized on chromosome 16. Approximately 80% of the reuptake of norepinephrine is mediated at nerve terminal synapses by the norepinephrine transporter. SLC6A2 is a target for the tricyclic antidepressants, including imipramine and desipramine and also for amphetamines and cocaine.

Following a report of SNP in the restriction site for the enzyme *Taq*I, a number of detailed investigations have revealed a range of rare mutations associated with orthostatic intolerance and more than 20 polymorphisms, some of which resulted in missense substitutions; however, no association with behavioral disorders were observed in the case/control studies. An insertion/deletion polymorphism of 4 bp in one of several AAGG repeat motifs in the promoter region at a position overlapping a transcription factor binding site has been reported, and there is some evidence supporting an association between the presence of the insertion and restricting anorexia nervosa. Rare genetic variants encoding a transporter with reduced affinity for norepinephrine have also been described. Carriers have been observed to manifest clinical symptoms (orthostatic intolerance) and metabolic evidence for disordered uptake of norepinephrine.

In summary, studies on the genes implicated in autonomic norepinephrine and epinephrine pathways have demonstrated the potential for a great deal of interindividual diversity. The consequences of this have major impact on a wide variety of disorders, including several with direct or indirect links to stress. Other autonomic pathways are mediated through acetylcholine release and detection.

Polymorphisms of Genes in the Neuroendocrine Stress Response Pathway

Further sources of genetic diversity in individual reactions to stress are the genes implicated in the delayed response of the hypothalamus-pituitary-adrenal (HPA) axis, leading to the release of cortisol from the adrenal cortex initiated by neural signals to the hypothalamus. Other genes are involved in the subsequent mobilization of hypothalamic peptide hormones (including CRH), resulting in the secretion of ACTH from the anterior pituitary and the release of glucocorticoid hormones (cortisol) from the adrenal cortex. Glucocorticoids are produced by the adrenal cortex and restore homeostasis in response to stress; however, prolonged exposure resulting from chronic stressful occurrences is potentially harmful. Cortisol (the most prominent glucocorticoid in humans) or corticosterone (in rats) is largely bound to corticosteroid-binding globulin in the systemic system. It has a classic steroid hormone mode of action via binding to a cognate intracellular receptor (the glucocorticoid receptor) and subsequent migration to the nucleus, where the complex interacts with a specific gene transcription apparatus. The loss or profound diminishment of glucocorticoid secretion leads to a state of deranged metabolism and an inability to deal with stressors, which, if untreated, is fatal. Functional genetic polymorphisms in some important genes of this pathway are recognized.

The Glucocorticoid Receptor

Two specific corticoid receptors are recognized: the glucocorticoid receptor (GR) and the mineralocorticoid receptor (MR). Whereas the latter binds aldosterone and glucocorticoids with similar high affinity, GR is selective for the glucocorticoids. It appears that the main response to raised levels of steroids resulting from stress is mediated primarily by GRs. There have been several polymorphisms described for the *GR* gene, including one in the promoter region. Because there is strong linkage disequilibrium across the gene, there are relatively few different combination of allelic patterns, with four major haplotypes recognized. Knowledge of the haplotype may help determine the response to glucocorticoid treatments. Variants within the coding region include two polymorphisms at adjacent codons for the amino acids 22 and 23 in the protein. Whereas the base change at codon 22 does not change the amino acid (glutamic acid), the polymorphism at codon 23 results in a change from arginine to lysine. Individuals with a specific combination of alleles at the promoter site and the codon 22–23 sites have an associated relative resistance to glucocorticoids. A further polymorphism resulting in a change from asparagine to serine at codon 363 appears to be associated with hypersensitivity to glucocorticoids. A *Bcl*I restriction enzyme polymorphism has also been employed in case/control studies, and there is evidence for an association with hypersensitivity to glucocorticoids that may be related to lower BMI in older individuals.

A wide variety of membrane-bound GRs have been reported in a range of tissues including the liver, lymphocytes, adrenal gland, and pituitary. There is a paucity of information concerning any structural features distinguishing these various forms, and there are no data on how any genetic variation may affect them, other than through changes affecting the GR itself. Significantly, however, the GR function depends on interactions with several components of a large molecular complex. Five co-chaperones of GR are recognized as significant in regulating its activity, and they are encoded by the following genes:

- *BAG1* – BCL2-associated anthanogene 1
- *STUB1* – STIP 1 homologous and U box-containing protein 1
- *TEBP* – Thyroid transcription factor 1 (TITF1)
- *FKBP4* – FK-506 binding protein 4
- *FKBP5* – FK-506 binding protein 5

A recent analysis of SNPs in these genes found three within the *FKBP5* locus to be significantly associated with the increased recurrence of symptom episodes in depressed patients and a rapid response to prescribed antidepressant treatment. Evidence for this apparent association was strengthened by genotyping a range of additional SNPs within and flanking the gene. One marker in particular (rs1360780) seems to track the tightness of the control of glucocorticoid signaling and HPA axis reactivity mediated by the reported interaction of the GR and FKBP5.

11-β-Hydroxysteroid Dehydrogenase Enzymes

Glucocorticoids are metabolized by the 11β-hydroxysteroid dehydrogenase enzymes (11β-HSD1). There are at least two forms of 11β-HSD1: type I (HSD11B1) and type II (HSD11B2). Both catalyze the conversion of cortisol to cortisone; however, the type I enzyme also catalyses the reverse reaction. Both are therefore important in the stress response. The HSD11B2 enzyme inactivates 11-hydroxysteroids in the kidney, the circumventricular organ of the brain, and some other tissues, thus protecting the nonselective MR from occupation by glucocorticoids. A base change confers a restriction-fragment-length polymorphism (detected by the enzyme *Alu*I) in exon 3 of this gene. This variant and a polymorphic microsatellite marker of the *HSD11B2* gene having 12 alleles have been employed to compare salt-sensitive (SS) and salt-resistant (SR) individuals in otherwise nonhypertensive white males. Homozygosity for one of the microsatellite alleles was higher in SS subjects than in SR subjects and the cortisol-to-cortisone ratios were higher in homozygous subjects than in the corresponding control subjects. It is possible that the decreased HSD11B2 activity observed in SS subjects reflects its involvement in the SS blood pressure response in humans and that variants of the gene contribute to different blood pressure responses to salt in humans.

Loci Whose Polymorphisms Interact with Stressful Influences in Mediating Behavioral Outcomes

The Serotonin Transporter

One particularly interesting connection between the perception of stress response and the serotinergic system is through the serotonin transporter, which removes the neurotransmitter from the synaptic cleft. The serotonin transporter (SERT, 5-HTT) plays a pivotal role in brain 5-HT homeostasis. It is also the initial target for both antidepressant drugs and drugs of abuse, some of which are potent neurotoxins. In humans, the gene for the transporter (variously designated as *SERT*, *HTT* or *SLC6A4*) is characterized by functional variants in the promoter region conferring high or low activity in expression of the locus. Several studies have linked variations of the two predominant alleles with anxiety response. Caspi and colleagues were the first to show that it appears that individuals with the low activity are more vulnerable to stressful life events and more likely to become clinically depressed as a result. Glatz and colleagues, in 2003, suggested a possible connection between stress and the serotonin system. They were able to demonstrate that a potent glucocorticosteroid hormone, dexamethasone, stimulates the expression of *SERT* in tissue culture at physiological concentrations. The hormone interacts with the promoter in an allele-specific manner, and this interaction may help to explain the differential vulnerability of individuals who are more susceptible to stressful experiences.

Monoamine Oxidase Type A

A similar picture emerges for variation of another gene involved in the serotonin system, the gene for monoamine oxidase type A, *MAOA*. Although this enzyme also has a role in metabolizing other neurotransmitters, including dopamine, drugs inhibiting its activity have long been employed in the treatment of behavioral disorders (particularly depression) and are thought to work through altering 5-HT levels. There are two major variants in the promoter of this gene that confer either high or low activity. Because the gene is X-linked, males exhibit either one or the other phenotype without complications from the presence of a second allele. There is a consensus view emerging that males who have the low-activity form of the gene are more sensitive to the effects of maltreatment and presumptive stressful environment manifested by their increased risk of antisocial behaviour and aggression. The high-activity form of the gene appears to provide protection against this outcome.

Conclusion

The response of individuals to stress varies considerably and depends on a wide range of environmental experiences, together with cognitive and genetic factors. Considerable progress has been made in characterizing some of the genes in the pathways relevant both to the fight-or-flight response and to those involved in the release and detection of glucocorticoid hormones. Many of the most significant changes to such genes are rare mutations. There are in addition, however, several variants of genes that are widely distributed in the population, and, although their impact may not be directly observable as an altered stress response, they may have important consequences with respect to a range of complex disorders including hypertension and allergic reactions. Furthermore, recent studies have shown common variants in the key enzymes involved in 5-HT metabolism (MAOA and SERT) can interact with stressful life experience to predispose individuals to manifesting antisocial behaviour or depression. Variants in several other related genes have subsequently also demonstrated an interaction with stress in predicting behavioral outcomes.

Further Reading

Caspi, A., McClay, J., Moffitt, T. E., et al. (2002). Role of genotype in the cycle of violence in maltreated children. *Science* **297**, 851–854.

Caspi, A., Sugden, K., Moffitt, T. E., et al. (2003). Influence of life stress on depression: moderation by a polymorphism in the 5-HTT gene. *Science* **301**, 386–389.

Cubells, J. F. and Zabetian, C. P. (2004). Human genetics of plasma dopamine β-hydroxylase activity: applications to research in psychiatry and neurology. *Psychopharmacology* **174**, 463–476.

Dionne, I. J., Garant, M. J., Nolan, A. A., et al. (2002). Association between obesity and a polymorphism in the beta-1-adrenoceptor gene (gly389arg ADRB1) in Caucasian women. *International Journal of Obesity* **26**, 633–639.

Small, K. M., Wagoner, L. E., Levin, A. M., et al. (2002). Synergistic polymorphisms of beta-1- and alpha-2C-adrenergic receptors and the risk of congestive heart failure. *New England Journal of Medicine* **347**, 1135–1142.

Stober, G., Nothen, M. M., Porzgen, P., et al. (1996). Systematic search for variation in the human norepinephrine transporter gene: identification of five naturally occurring missense mutations and a study of association with major psychiatric disorders. *American Journal of Medical Genetics: Neuropsychiatric Genetics* **67**, 523–532.

van Rossum, E. F. C., Koper, J. W., van den Beld, A. W., et al. (2003). Identification of the *Bcl*I polymorphism in the glucocorticoid receptor gene: association with sensitivity to glucocorticoids *in vivo* and body mass index. *Clinical Endocrinology* **59**, 585–592.

van Rossum, E. F. C., Roks, P. H. M., de Jong, F. H., et al. (2004). Characterization of a promoter polymorphism in the glucocorticoid receptor gene and its relationship to three other polymorphisms. *Clinical Endocrinology* **61**, 573–581.

Wüst, S., van Rossum, E. F. C., Federenko, et al. (2004). Common polymorphisms in the glucocorticoid receptor gene are associated with adrenocortical responses to psychosocial stress. *Journal of Clinical Endocrinology and Metabolism* **89**, 565–573.

Relevant Websites

Online Mendelian inheritance in man and Entrez SNP database, http://www.ncbi.nlm.nih.gov.

Hypothalamic–Pituitary–Adrenal (HPA) Axis

N Pecoraro and M F Dallman
University of California at San Francisco, San Francisco, CA, USA

The Hypothalamic–Pituitary–Adrenal Axis

The hypothalamic–pituitary–adrenal (HPA) axis keys reactive and predictive physiological and mental adjustments to environmental demand. Understanding HPA axis complexity requires viewing it as the final common output pathway of diverse inputs – including circadian pattern generators; systems sensitive to metabolic, immune, and nociceptive stimuli; cognitive assessments; and intrahypothalamic networks coordinating neuroendocrine and other motor outflows – and recognizing HPA axis feedback and feed-forward effects on brain.

Motor neurons in the paraventricular nucleus (PVN) of the hypothalamus project to the median eminence and release corticotropin-releasing factor (CRF) into a portal vasculature perfusing anterior pituitary glandular corticotropes that release adrenocorticotropic hormone (ACTH) into the systemic circulation. Systemic ACTH stimulates adrenal cortex to release glucocorticoids (GCs) into the systemic circulation to act on peripheral tissues and organs, and brain regions involved in cognition, memory, motivation, and primary motor outflows, including HPA axis outflow (see **Figure 1**).

The Paraventricular Nucleus of the Hypothalamus

The PVN integrates diverse inputs and contains distinctive neuroendocrine, behavioral, and autonomic cell groups. Neurosecretory regions include parvicellular neurons containing CRF/arginine vasopressin (AVP) peptides that are co-packaged in vesicles, and co-secreted. Synthesis is drive dependent. CRF neurons arc through perifornical hypothalamus exhibiting boutons of passage, sweeping ventrally to the median eminence and anterior pituitary. Magnocellular cells containing oxytocin (OXY) or AVP reside laterally to CRF neurons and project to the neural lobe of the pituitary.

Nonneuroendocrine, descending PVN divisions control behavioral and autonomic outflows. Preautonomic cell groups include the 'dorsal cap,' and a group at the caudolateral tip of the PVN extending caudally into zona incerta. A related retrochiasmatic group participates in a putative pattern generation network (described later).

Pituitary Corticotropes

Proopiomelanocortin (POMC) molecule cleavage products (e.g., ACTH) are stored in intracellular corticotrope vesicles and secreted in response to CRF associating with CRF receptor (CRF_1R) via G-protein/cyclic adenosine monophosphate (c-AMP)-mediated mechanisms. AVP weakly stimulates ACTH secretion, via a receptor ($AVP_{1b}R$)-mediated mechanism, but synergizes with CRF, dramatically increasing ACTH

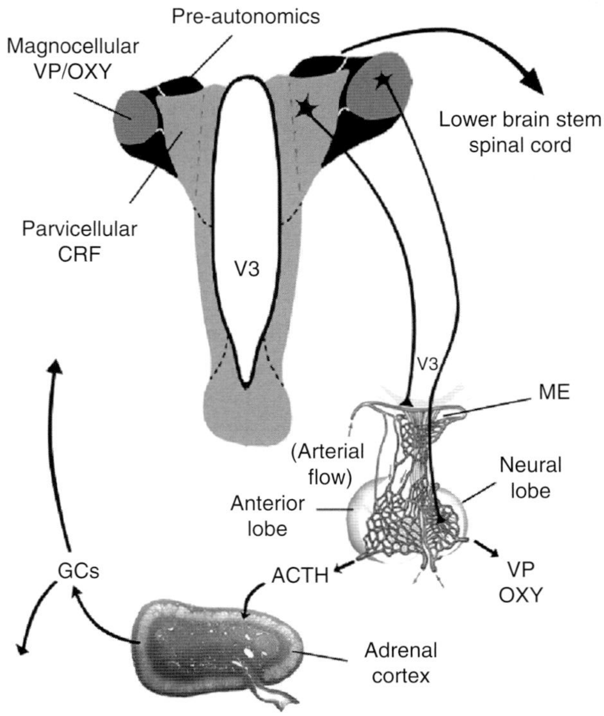

Figure 1 The hypothalamic–pituitary–adrenal axis. The paraventricular nucleus of the hypothalamus is depicted as a bilateral coronal section in an oblique view, with the third ventricle (V3) indicating the midline. The periventricular region (light gray) contains parvicellular neuroendocrine cells with corticotropin-releasing factor (CRF)/arginine vasopressin-containing neurons in the dorsolateral region; these project to the median eminence (ME) and portal vasculature to the anterior pituitary. The magnocellular neuronal division (medium gray) consists of cells containing oxytocin (OXY) and vasopressin (VP); these project directly to the posterior, neural lobe of the pituitary. The descending division of the paraventricular nucleus (black) contains preautonomic neurons projecting to lower brain stem areas and spinal cord, involved in both behavioral and autonomic regulation. CRF/arginine vasopressin release into the portal vasculature of the anterior pituitary stimulates glandular corticotropes to release adrenocorticotropin hormone (ACTH) into the systemic circulation. Plasma ACTH then stimulates adrenocortical cells to synthesize and release glucocorticoids (GC) into the systemic circulation to act on peripheral tissues and organs and the central nervous system.

secretion. Corticotropes contain glucocorticoid receptors (GRs) and corticosteroid-binding globulin (CBG, or transcortin). GR activation inhibits synthesis and secretion of ACTH through a negative glucocorticoid recognition element (GRE) on POMC DNA, but CBG binds GCs with high affinity. Tonic inhibitory action of GCs on corticotropes requires high concentrations, exceeding CBG capacity, making ACTH secretion vulnerable to high doses of exogenous GCs – for example, during treatment of autoimmune diseases, in patients with pituitary ACTH-secreting adenomas (Cushing's disease), or when warding off transplant rejection.

Adrenal Zona Fasciculata

Unlike pituitary corticotropes that store hormone, the adrenal cortex zones synthesize and secrete hormones on ACTH demand. ACTH acts via c-AMP at the rate-limiting step of cholesterol transfer from cytosolic esters to mitochondria, where steroid synthesis begins. ACTH increases other enzymes involved in GC synthesis. All three zones of cortex (zona glomerulosa, zona fasciculata, and, in primates, zona reticularis) respond to ACTH, acting through melanocortin receptors (MCR2). In primates, injection of ACTH stimulates secretion, within minutes, of aldosterone (glomerulosa), cortisol (fasciculata), and dehydroepiandrosterone sulfate (reticularis). The major steroids (cortisol in primates; corticosterone in most rodents) synthesized in the zona fasciculata are most important in HPA function. ACTH transiently stimulates zona glomerulosa cells, but the major role of ACTH is sustained stimulation of GCs.

CBG (Transcortin) Binding

CBG (transcortin), synthesized and secreted from liver, is a high-affinity binding protein for GCs, and, under basal conditions, when adrenal secretion is low, 95–99% of the secreted steroid is bound to CBG without diffusion to targets. CBG–GC is in reversible equilibrium with free GCs. CBG is a saturable reservoir and buffer for biologically active GCs, so that considerable free steroid is able to diffuse to target cells during stress. Because GCs inhibit hepatic CBG synthesis, when tonic GC concentrations are low, circulating CBG is high, and vice versa. Because total GC concentrations in plasma (bound and free) are usually measured, it is worth knowing the history of GC secretion when collecting acute samples.

Inhibition of the HPA Axis by GC

GC elevations inhibit activity in PVN CRF cells and pituitary corticotropes, first by membrane GR-mediated effects, then by GC-associated GR protein–protein interactions altering gene expression. Feedback ensures controlled neuroendocrine responses. Longer term feedback effects exist in both brain and pituitary (e.g., through GC–GR complexes interacting with a negative GRE on POMC in corticotropes). Chronic GCs diminish HPA axis outflow in proportion to exposure, provided no concurrent stress exists, making the axis unresponsive to new stressors and thus explaining the requirement for extra GC coverage during major surgery in patients on chronic GC therapy.

There is rapid inhibitory GC feedback on both CRF and ACTH secretion. In hypothalamic slices *in vitro*, GC alters neuronal activity, including CRF-synthesizing cells, within 3 min. GC stimulates endocannabinoid secretion, presynaptically inhibiting glutamate-stimulated miniature excitatory postsynaptic currents (mEPSCs) via endocannabinoid EC-1 receptors. GCs infused directly into neurons does not have this effect, and rapid GCs actions on pituitary ACTH secretion *in vitro* are not inhibited by exposure to protein or by RNA synthesis inhibitors, suggesting membrane-mediated feedback.

Distinctive HPA Axis Drivers

Distinctive brain systems impinge on HPA axis outflow (**Figure 2**), including two circadian oscillators, brain stem, vasculature, and circumventricular organ systemic networks, cortico-striato-pallidal-brain stem cognitive networks, and an intrahypothalamic network that coordinates other drivers and motor outflows.

Periodic/Circadian Drivers of the HPA Axis

In constant darkness, HPA axis activation exhibits free-running circadian oscillations that entrain to light/dark cycles. Plasma GC concentrations increase at least tenfold around the time of waking. GCs decline throughout the activity phase, propped up by postprandial elevations, before they reach a nadir in early rest. When restricted feeding time is pitted against a light/dark cycle, a separate food-entrainable oscillator allows the HPA axis to separately track mealtimes.

The suprachiasmatic nuclei The suprachiasmatic nuclei (SCN) sit atop the optic chiasm in the basal hypothalamus, serving as the master, light-entrainable oscillator (LEO) in mammals. The SCN receive transduced light stimuli via the retinohypothalamic tract to entrain endogenous pacemaker activities of the SCN, driving the HPA axis and PVN preautonomic neurons. The SCN indirectly influence PVN CRF neurons via substantial projections to the subparaventricular zone, which targets the PVN with γ-aminobutyric acid (GABA)ergic inputs. The SCN project substantially

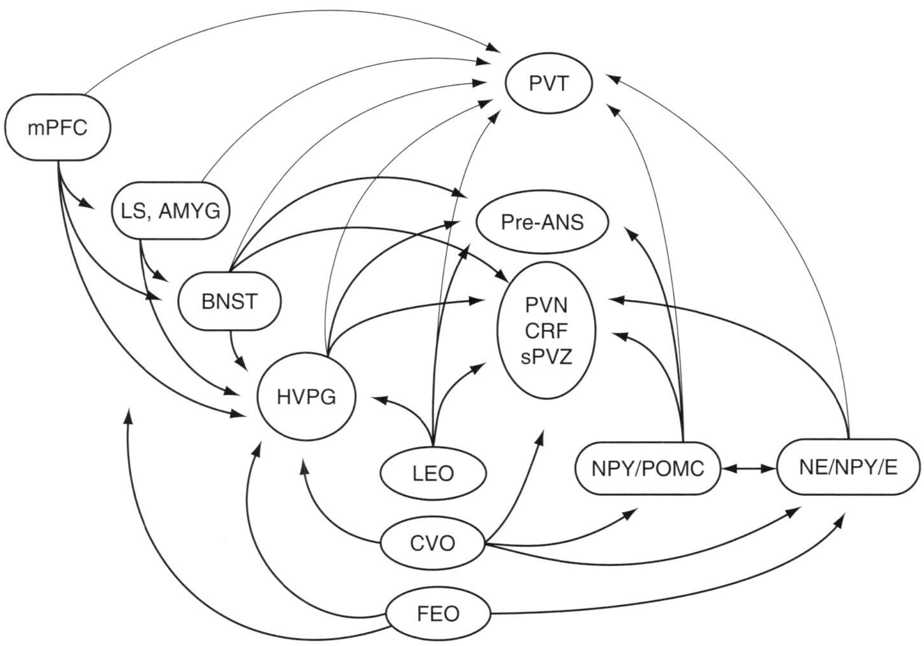

Figure 2 This highly simplified schematic depicts the major drivers of the hypothalamic–pituitary–adrenal (HPA) axis, with some indications of their coordinated drive on the autonomic outflow (pre-ANS; preautonomic nervous system) and on one another. For simplicity, paraventricular nucleus (PVN) corticotropin-releasing factor (CRF)-containing cells are grouped with the heavily interconnected subparaventricular zone (sPVZ). The suprachiasmatic nuclei, the master, light-entrainable oscillator (LEO), provide endogenous circadian drive to the PVN CRF-containing cells, the PVN preautonomics, and the hypothalamic visceromotor pattern generator (HVPG). During restricted, scheduled feedings a second food-entrainable oscillator swings into motion to track mealtimes and entrain food anticipatory rhythms. Systemic threats to homeostasis are signaled through circumventricular organs (CVO), the melanocortin system (NPY/POMC; neuropeptide Y/proopiomelanocortin) in the arcuate nucleus of the hypothalamus, and the ascending medullary catecholaminergic neurons (NPY and NE/E; norepinephrine, epinephrine). Psychogenic drive on the HPA axis is represented by multilayered cortico-striato-pallido-hypothalamic networks, in this case showing the visceromotor medial prefrontal cortex (mPFC) projecting to the lateral septum (LS) and amygdala (AMYG), bed nucleus of the stria terminalis (BNST), and HVPG. Virtually all HPA axis drivers also project to the 'neuroendocrine' paraventricular thalamus (PVT). Also indicated is the food-entrainable oscillator (FEO).

to the dorsomedial hypothalamus (DMH), which also projects to neuroendocrine and preautonomic divisions. AVP levels in and around the PVN vary on a circadian basis, being highest at rest, during basal HPA axis activity. AVP infusions into brain cause rapid decreases in GCs, and lesser decreases in ACTH. The DMH is the most effective infusion site, providing substantial GABAergic inhibitory fibers to CRF neurons. Disinhibition of HPA axis activity by AVP antagonists occurs only in SCN-intact animals, suggesting origination in the SCN. The SCN project to the medial preoptic (MPO) hypothalamus, an area involved in coordination of outflows. Outside hypothalamus, SCN project to the paraventricular thalamus (PVT), a PVN target involved in both acute and chronic stress networks. Pseudorabies virus injected into the adrenals is retrogradely propagated transsynaptically via the intermediolateral column to PVN preautonomics in the SCN. This pathway controls adrenocortical sensitivity to ACTH. In early darkness, bright light inhibits GCs, but not ACTH, secretion, only in SCN-intact rats. Thus, the SCN influence HPA axis output through CRF motor neurons and by neuronally controlling adrenal sensitivity to ACTH.

The food-entrainable oscillator A separate, food-entrainable circadian oscillator (FEO) prevails during restricted, scheduled feedings to entrain activity, feeding, drinking, body temperature, HPA axis activity, and peripheral metabolic rhythms. Entrainment is robust in SCN-lesioned animals that would otherwise be arrhythmic under a light/dark cycle when freely feeding. In intact rats, SCN-coupled rhythms free-run (e.g., 26 h period) in constant dark, but animals can independently and simultaneously anticipate scheduled meals at different periods (e.g., every 24 h) from the free-running rhythms. It takes 3–13 days for anticipatory activity to precede scheduled meals, but evidence suggests that single meals can reset food-entrainable rhythms. Food anticipatory activity continues for several days in the absence of the food zeitgeber prior to damping.

The anatomical locus of the FEO is unknown. Ascending medullary norepinephrine/neuropeptide Y

(NE/NPY) systems entrained by scheduled meals drive prefeeding peaks in HPA axis output and feeding rhythms. Lesions of the ascending ventral noradrenergic bundle (VNAB) prevent food-anticipatory elevations in plasma GCs. Striatal and pallidal inputs to the HPA axis – namely, the central nucleus of the amygdala (CeA) and bed nucleus of the stria terminalis (BNST) – exhibit phase shifts in clock gene expression during food entrainment. Like SCN, both the CeA and the BNST oval (BNST-ov) nucleus exhibit circadian rhythms in the clock gene period2 (per2) that peak at activity onset under *ad libitum* feeding. Restricted feeding forces per2 rhythms in CeA and BNST-ov out of phase relative to SCN. Constant light and free feeding abolish per2 rhythms in all three areas; these are reestablished by restricted feeding, such that peak per2 is in antiphase to feeding. Adrenalectomy (ADX) also abolishes per2 rhythms in limbic regions in a GC-reversible fashion. Lesions of the DMH (or insular cortex) prevent preprandial temperature elevations, and severely damp locomotor activity, pointing to integrated output from the DMH. Both systemic and limbic networks are candidate mediators of HPA axis entrainment by food.

Homeostatic Inflow: Systemically Responsive Networks Driving the HPA Axis

The HPA axis is highly sensitive to energy balance and other systemic threats, such as nociception and immune challenge, which have distinct and shared pathways to the HPA axis.

The arcuate NPY/melanocortin system The melanocortin system (**Figure 2**) includes cell groups in the arcuate nucleus (ARC) of the hypothalamus and the medullary nucleus of the tractus solitarius (NTS) sensitive to energy balance, and expressing POMC (usually co-expressing cocaine and amphetamine-related transcript (CART)) or neuropeptide Y (co-expressing agouti-related peptide (AgRP) in the ARC). POMC neurons mainly reside in the ARC, projecting primarily to stress-sensitive sites, including the PVN, perifornical lateral hypothalamus, NTS, reticular nuclei (RET), lateral parabrachial nucleus, nucleus accumbens (NACC), lateral septal nucleus, BNST, CeA, and medial amygdala (MeA). Tyrosine hydroxylase (TH)-negative POMC-expressing neurons also originate from the NTS. ARC NPY/AgRP neurons have similar projection patterns (e.g., PVN, DMH, PH, PVT, MPO, lateral septal nucleus). Energy balance signals may be transmitted neurally and through proximal circumventricular organs (CVOs).

ARC POMC. ARC POMC cleaves into α-melanocyte-stimulating hormone (α-MSH), a potent agonist at melanocortin-3 and -4 receptors (MCR3 and MCR4). Intracranial administration of leptin activates POMC neurons, suppresses feeding, and increases autonomic outflow. CRF mediates the inhibitory effects of α-MSH on feeding. Like α-MSH, central administration of CART also inhibits feeding, whereas fasting reduces CART mRNA expression. Three populations of CART neurons contribute innervation to the PVN, including medullary and arcuate POMC neurons and a third unknown source.

NPY neurons. NPY neurons directly innervate PVN CRF neurons. Increases in NPY elevate CRF mRNA expression, ACTH and GC secretion, and food intake, and suppress sympathetic outflow to brown fat. In contrast to α-MSH, AgRP is an antagonist at MCRs. Negative energy balance (e.g., low insulin and leptin) activates NPY neurons, including inhibitory GABAergic fibers to POMC neurons. POMC and NPY neurons are 'dueling rheostats' on energy balance.

GC effects on POMC/NPY. POMC/CART and NPY/AgRP neurons in the ARC express GRs. ADX or inhibition of GC synthesis reduces expression of CART mRNA. Though CART appears anorectic, CART-expressing medullary neurons co-express an epinephrine-synthesizing enzyme, phenylethanolamine-*N*-methyltransferase (PNMT), which is involved in feeding responses to glucoprivation. In addition, CART phosphorylation of cAMP response element-binding protein (CREB) in PVN CRF neurons should have additive effects with α-adrenoreceptor activation of CRF expression. Despite opposite signaling functions of CART and GCs, evidence suggests some positive feedback. GCs also stimulate NPY gene expression, peptide synthesis, receptor activity, and NPY-induced feeding. Here, positive feedback biases the system to correct further energetic disturbances. Clear evidence for functional interplay between GC and melanocortin systems exists, but the details require further elucidation.

Systemic threats: The medullary NE/E/NPY system Stimuli signaling actual threats to homeostasis are categorized as systemic stressors; these include including ether, hemorrhage, glucoprivation, and nociception, and are transduced by various lower brain stem NPY/catecholaminergic cell groups, including the dorsomedial medulla (NTS; A2–C2 cell groups) and ventrolateral medulla (A1–C1 cell groups). Ninety percent of all catecholaminergic innervation ascends to the PVN via the ventral noradrenergic bundle (VNAB). Immunostaining for dopamine β-hydroxylase, a marker for epinephrine (E) and norepinephrine (NE), shows extensive innervation of the PVN. NPY immunostaining shows similar, but more extensive, patterns in the PVN. NPY co-localizes in lower brain stem with PNMT in most adrenergic neurons (C1,

C2, C3), but shows less co-localization in noradrenergic A1 neurons, about 60% rostrally and many fewer caudally. Some ascending VNAB fibers arrive at the median eminence rather than at the PVN, possibly controlling exocytosis. Eergic, NEergic, and NPYergic stimulation of the PVN increases HPA axis outflow and feeding. Disrupting ascending inputs through chemical lesions, inhibiting transmitter synthesis in originating neurons, α-1 or β receptor blockade in PVN, or neutralization of CRF neurons, all disrupt HPA axis responses to systemic threats.

Glucoprivation. Acute glucoprivation by peripheral administration of insulin or 2-deoxyglucose (2DG) results in rapid counterregulatory HPA axis and feeding responses. Destruction of medullary Eergic and NEergic neurons via retrograde transport of selective neurotoxins delivered to PVN profoundly blunts counterregulatory responses, but has no effect on HPA responses to psychogenic stress or circadian variations in GCs, thus validating a systemic/psychogenic distinction.

Pain. Nociceptive stimuli (e.g., sharp pinch, thermal, or visceral pain) stimulate the HPA axis through systemic and psychogenic networks. Spinohypothalamic pathways transmit pain stimuli to the lateral hypothalamus (LH), which projects ipsilaterally to PVN CRF neurons. The spinothalamic pathway projects from spine to ventral posterolateral thalamus, then to sensory cortical areas. The spinoreticulothalamic pathway projects from spinal cord to reticular formation, then to midline and intralaminar thalamic nuclei, and on to limbic cortical areas (cingulate, piriform, and entorhinal cortices). Vagal and glossopharyngeal nerves convey visceral pain to the NTS, then to the parabrachial nucleus, thalamus, and visceromotor prefrontal cortex. A2 and C2 cell groups also project to A1 and C1 neurons in the ventrolateral medulla, locus coeruleus, amygdala, and PVN, which shows strong bilateral activation of CRF parvicellular neurons in response to many noxious stimuli. VNAB hemisections reduce PVN activation primarily on the hemisected side. Noncatecholaminergic neurons in the NTS, terminating in the PVN, also express fos after nociceptive stimuli. (Cognitive control of the HPA axis is discussed later.)

Proinflammatory stimuli. Systemic inflammatory responses to immune challenges are powerful stimuli to autonomic outflow and HPA axis activation, which inhibits proinflammatory processes. Proinflammatory molecules include tumor necrosis factor-α (TNF-α), interleukin-1β (IL-1β), and interleukin-6 (IL-6). Brain vasculature expresses receptors for TNF-α, IL-1β, and IL-6 under basal conditions; further induction occurs following immune challenge when plasma cytokine concentrations increase. Activation of cytokine receptors in the blood–brain barrier results in the transcription of various substances, including prostaglandins (PGs) following signaling cascades involving cyclooxygenase-2 (COX-2) and nuclear factor-kappa B (NF-κB). The brain vasculature and irrigation systems are thought to be the primary source of central PGs following systemic cytokine treatment, as COX-2 expression is highly co-expressed in areas staining for von Willebrand factor, a marker for cerebral endothelium. Activation is particularly striking in blood vessels, choroid plexus, and the CVOs.

Prostaglandin E_2 (PGE_2) is involved in neuronal responses to systemic immune challenge. Injection of IL-1 results in PGE2 expression in CVOs, preoptic nuclei, PVN, dorsal hippocampus, and lateral ventricles. Central administration of PGE_2 increases HPA axis and autonomic outflows. Febrile responses may originate in the MPO, whereas HPA axis activation may originate in the PVN, as prostaglandins (PGs) induce CRF mRNA and type 1 receptors in the PVN. Immune challenge activates specific receptors for PGE_2 (subtypes EP1–EP4) in brain regions controlling HPA axis and autonomic outflows. Neurons expressing EP1–EP4 particularly show c-fos activation after systemic IL-1β administration in CVOs and central stress networks, with highest expression in PVN CRF neurons. Central HPA axis and autonomic outflows following systemic immune challenge appear to be coordinated by classic central stress response networks, in part by activation of brain endothelial and leptomeningeal tissues, resulting in signal transduction to neuronal tissues.

Immune signaling may also originate in liver, as hepatic vagotomy eliminates febrile responses, and blunts brain stem c-fos responses, PVN noradrenergic levels, and ACTH responses to endotoxin. Endotoxin-clearing Kupffer cells also release PGE_2 in response to immune challenge stimulating excitatory vagal afferents, relaying signals to regions involved in febrile (MPO) and HPA axis (PVN) responses. Rapid febrile responses to immune challenges occurring prior to cytokine elevations utilize this pathway. Whether the argument holds for rapid HPA axis activation has not been thoroughly tested. Hepatic vagotomy has reduced HPA axis output by about half in response to endotoxin, but had a much smaller effect on responses to IL-6. Unfortunately, HPA axis responses were not measured until 2 h after injections, and not all studies agree on the effects of vagotomy. Inactivating the Kupffer cell phagocytotic activity using gadolinium chloride failed to reduce HPA axis responses to lipopolysaccharide (LPS), but again, ACTH and corticosterone were measured many hours later, long after cytokines were produced and acted in brain.

The Hypothalamic Visceromotor Pattern Generator

Recent anatomical evidence suggests the existence of a hypothalamic visceromotor pattern generator (HVPG) located between hypothalamic neuroendocrine, preautonomic, and behavioral motorneuron pools, involving a DMH 'hub' and five preoptic nuclei. **Figure 3** shows a schematic of connections between the HVPG and the PVN. Core nodes of the HPVG are massively interconnected, with each node idiosyncratically projecting to neuroendocrine and preautonomic cell groups. Notable among the few extrahypothalamic targets are the BNST, lateral septum (LS), periaqueductal gray (PAG), subfornical organ (SFO), and the PVT. The coordination of visceromotor outflow likely includes not only sympathetic, but also parasympathetic, outflow via strong connections between the DMH and parasubthalamic nucleus, which projects heavily to the dorsal vagal complex.

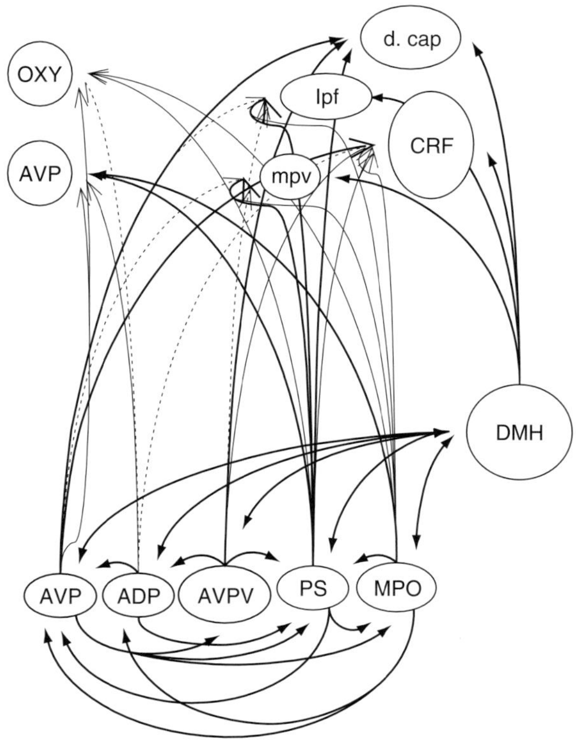

Figure 3 The hypothalamic visceromotor pattern generator. This schematic is based on Thompson's and Swanson's hodological analysis of relations among various hypothalamic nuclei with respect to neuroendocrine and autonomic divisions of the paraventricular hypothalamus. The hypothalamic visceromotor pattern generator consists of the dorsomedial hypothalamus (DMH), its major hub, and five preoptic nuclei, including the anteroventral preoptic (AVP), anterodorsal preoptic (ADP), anteroventral periventricular preoptic (AVPV), parastrial nucleus (PS), and medial preoptic nucleus (MPO). Magnocellular oxytocinergic (OXY) and vasopressinergic (AVP) neurons are shown in the upper left. Parvicellular corticotropin-releasing factor (CRF)-containing neurons are shown in the upper right. The descending division of the paraventricular hypothalamus includes preautonomic neurons in the dorsal cap (d. cap), the caudolateral periforniсal (lpf) paraventricular hypothalamus, and the medial parvicellular (mpv) neurons residing between neuroendocrine cell groups. Heavier projections are indicated by heavier lines. Note the massive interconnectivity between the DMH and preoptic nuclei, and their more idiosyncratic relations to neuroendocrine and autonomic divisions of the paraventricular hypothalamus.

Inputs to the DMH include top-down inputs from cortico-striato-pallidal circuits, including visceromotor cortex (infralimbic), ventral subiculum, LS, MeA, as well as BNST; medial hypothalamic nuclei involved in basic behavioral functions such as reproduction, feeding, and defense; sensory nuclei, such as the parabrachial nucleus, relaying viscerosensory information, and the SFO, relaying humorosensory information; and substantial input from SCN and the subparaventricular zone. Hodological analysis strongly suggests that the HVPG integrates cognitive, systemic, and circadian inputs to coordinate neuroendocrine, autonomic, and some behavioral outflows.

The specific coordinating functions are uncharacterized, but good evidence indicates that the DMH drives the HPA axis and autonomic outflows. Disinhibiting the DMH using $GABA_A$ antagonists (or stimulating the DMH, using excitatory amino acids) increases sympathetic outflow and plasma catecholamines, heart rate, blood pressure, and blood flow to skeletal muscle while reducing blood flow to viscera. Blood pressure increases resulting from DMH stimulation can be blocked by inactivating the rostral ventrolateral medulla (RVLM), whereas tachycardia is likely relayed through descending projections to PAG or raphe pallidus. Lower doses of excitatory amino acids are required to obtain visceromotor outflow in the DMH compared to the PVN. Likewise, the blunting of autonomic and HPA axis outflows to psychogenic stress is greater after DMH than after PVN inactivation by muscimol. Neurons in the DMH expressing c-fos following footshock have been retrogradely labeled from the PVN and are glutamatergic. Muscimol microinfusion into the DMH reduces PVN activation to air-puff stress, but not to hemorrhage, although this should not be interpreted to mean that the DMH plays no role in systemic threats, as hemorrhage is a powerful stimulus.

Psychogenic Networks Driving the HPA Axis

Psychogenic stress is distinct from systemic stress; knife cuts of the ascending VNAB reduce PVN activity after nociception, but not after restraint stress. Top-down pathways to the PVN and surrounding networks consist of excitatory cortical, inhibitory striatal, and disinhibitory pallidal inputs operating both serially and in parallel. Medial prefrontal cortices (mPFCs) are the highest level of motor control over visceromotor outflow. Violations of cortical predictions or changes in the valence of experience alter prefrontal activity and downstream HPA axis and autonomic outflows. Cognitive networks are sensitive to feedback from the visceromotor processes they control, and exhibit stress-dependent plasticity. Hypofunctional cortical states are associated with HPA axis dysregulation.

The mPFC shows substantial immediate early gene activation following stressors, high levels of GR staining, and ADX-reversible glutamate release following a stressor. Inputs to prefrontal cortex include ascending dopaminergic, noradrenergic, and serotonergic inputs, all of which are modulated by HPA axis function. Both dorsal and ventral regions of the mPFC may be involved in HPA axis outflow, but the ventral regions, including infralimbic (IL) cortex and ventral prelimbic cortex, contribute to HPA axis activation and project directly to brain stem preautonomic centers.

After receiving highly processed cortical input, the largely ipsilateral projections of the IL cortex to cerebral nuclei include the CeA, MeA, and LS in the striatum, BNST, and substantia innominata in the pallidum. In hypothalamic brain stem, the IL cortex projects to key nodes of the HVPG, including MPO, lateral preoptic (LPO), DMH, and perifornical LH, all areas projecting to the PVN, but the IL has negligible direct projections to the PVN. In lower brain stem there are moderate to light projections to autonomic areas, such as the parabrachial nucleus (PBN) and PAG, Barrington's nucleus, the DMV, NTS, nucleus ambiguous, and the RVLM. Like nearly every driver of the HPA axis, this also projects substantially to the PVT in the dorsal brain stem. Although some projections to brain stem visceromotor centers may be light, subcortical targets of the IL cortex also project to these centers. Thus, the IL cortex drives a cascade of direct excitatory projections, inhibitory striatal projections, and disinhibitory pallidal projections, layers of stimulation aimed at visceromotor processes.

Chemical, electrical, and lesioning manipulations of mPFC alter HPA axis and autonomic outflows. Corticosterone implants into dorsal mPFC inhibit HPA axis output. Infusions of GABA agonists and *N*-methyl-D-aspartate (NMDA) antagonists into mPFC exaggerate adrenocortical responses to cage-change stress. In contrast, electrical stimulation of IL cortex results in stimulation of the HPA axis, whereas lesions inhibit stress-induced HPA axis activation. It appears that dorsal mPFC tends to inhibit the HPA axis, whereas ventral activation stimulates. Issues of laterality exist, insofar as right hemispheric lesions blunt stress responses, whereas those in the left do not. Unfortunately, large lesions involving dorsal and ventral regions were used.

Subcortically, stimulation of LS or BNST, a pallidal gate of the CeA, also stimulates HPA axis outflow. The BNST also gates input from MeA, as MeA stimulation in anesthetized rats stimulates the HPA axis in intact animals, but not those bearing BNST lesions. The same lesions do not prevent ether-induced HPA responses. BNST and CeA CRF-containing neurons both converge on the PVT, which is involved in changed HPA axis output following chronic stress.

GCs in Central Motive States and Central Plasticity

HPA axis control cannot be viewed without regard for GC effects on brain outside of classical inhibitory feedback mechanisms. GCs also feed forward in brain, facilitating HPA axis outflow, and affect aversive and appetitive motive states, learning and memory, and gross neuronal remodeling, ultimately affecting HPA axis functioning.

Corticotropin-Releasing Factor

Central CRF systems are critical to aversive responding. Although ADX upregulates CRF in the PVN in a GC-reversible fashion, GC pellets implanted in dorsal CeA increase anxiety, stress-induced elevations in CRF mRNA, ACTH and GC secretion, colonic motility, and visceromotor responses to colorectal distension. Chronic stress or GC treatment also increases CRF mRNA in BNST. Chronic intracerebroventricular (icv) infusions of GCs enhance basal and stress-induced HPA outflow. Chronic elevations of GCs in brain upregulate central stress networks and increase HPA, autonomic, and behavioral outflows.

Depolarization of sheep PVN CRF neurons through stress, chemical, or electrical means increases venous cortisol and extracellular amygdalar CRF. Amygdalar CRF response to psychogenic stress exhibits a bimodal pattern: one immediate stressor-related peak, and a second peak resulting from GCs entering the brain. GCs infused intravenously causes one rise in amygdalar CRF following the venous cortisol signal. Repeated activation of amygdalar CRF by GCs causes potentiated acute CRF responses to novel stressors. Exposing sheep once daily to predator stress increases amygdalar CRF upon each exposure. When a novel forelimb shock is later applied, animals show facilitated amygdalar CRF responses, unless daily predator exposures were accompanied by cortisol synthesis inhibition, which prevents GC-mediated facilitation. GC exposure recruits both acute and chronic central stress networks.

Norepinephrine

The ascending dorsal NE system is sensitive to stress and central CRF. Cognitive stressors virtually always activate locus coeruleus (LC) NE neurons, in association with increased NE release in LC targets, such as mPFC and BNST, arousal and anxiety, and HPA axis outflow. Depletion of LC NE blunts HPA axis outflow. CeA and BNST CRF neurons target LC dendrites, and CRF infusions into LC increase LC discharge rates, alter cortical electroencephalogram (EEG), and behavioral, autonomic, and HPA axis responses. CRF effects on LC are dose dependent and are blocked by CRF antagonists. Although tyrosine hydroxylase-immunopositive neurons in LC stain for GRs, the role of GCs in LC is unclear. ADX increases LC discharge rats in a GC-reversible fashion, but also causes metabolic disturbances that disinhibit brain stem TH networks. It is unclear if GC inhibition of LC is due to direct action or to peripheral metabolic corrections.

Dopamine

GCs and CRF target mesocorticolimbic DA systems are associated with multiple appetitive, aversive, and reinforcement mechanisms. GCs stimulate dopamine (DA) efflux in DAergic terminal fields, including nucleus accumbens, prefrontal cortex, BNST, and amygdala. Adrenalectomized rats given low levels of GCs show greatly reduced DA efflux compared to intact rats after tail pinch, cocaine, or morphine treatments. Rapid DA efflux occurs if sufficient GC concentrations are achieved. GR co-localize with D1 receptors in prefrontal pyramidal neurons, substantia nigra, and the ventral tegmental area (VTA). Stress or GCs enhances VTA discharge rates stimulated by excitatory ligands, a GR antagonist-reversible effect. GCs given alone have no effect, suggesting enhanced glutamatergic transmission is required. GC antagonists also block plastic processes in the VTA. Stress-related interactions between prefrontal glutamatergic neurons and VTA DAergic neurons play important roles in stress-related pathologies, including drug abuse. Central CRF systems also target the VTA, and CRF receptors co-localize with DAergic neurons. Like GCs, CRF potentiates excitatory signaling in VTA DAergic neurons, and contributes to neuronal sensitization. Footshock increases CRF and glutamate efflux in the VTA and DA efflux in terminal fields, and promotes reinstatement to drug seeking, a CRF antagonist-reversible effect.

Endogenous Opioid Peptides

Endogenous opioid peptides (EOPs) affect central stress networks state dependently. CRF and AVP both stimulate EOP secretion, and enkephalinergic neurons in the RVLM project to PVN and LC dendrites, overlapping with CRF-containing fibers. The PVN also receives enkephalinergic (ENK) innervation from the MPO and DMH. Stress increases ENK mRNA in the PVN, but downregulates it in the RVLM. Administration of opioid agonists and antagonists can cause both activation and inhibition of the HPA axis. In resting sheep, β-endorphin causes a naloxone-reversible increase in ACTH, whereas in chronically stressed animals it causes a naloxone-reversible inhibition of HPA output. Opioid-induced increases in ACTH are abolished by pretreatment with CRF antiserum. Thus, in a state of stress, opioids may act as a counterregulatory limb of the central stress response, whereas under basal conditions they are stimulatory, as if CRF and EOPs exist as opponent processes, a contention supported by the fact that opioids inhibit LC discharge rates. The effect is again state dependent, as opioid antagonists have no effect on basal LC discharge, but do increase LC discharge under stress, suggesting stress-induced recruitment of opioid signaling. Likewise, excess opioid signaling recruits CRF/NE systems, and dramatic increases in LC discharge rates occur when opioid-dependent animals are given opiate antagonists. Complex sequelae unfold in the HPA axis following intermittent opioid treatment and withdrawal, indicating initial recruitment of HPA axis facilitators leading to HPA axis hyperresponsiveness to stress, followed by recruitment of some mechanism that makes the HPA axis hyporesponsive to stress.

Memory

GCs influence memories of aversive and appetitive events, but the direction of the effect is a structure- and task-dependent event. In the hippocampus, correlates of learning exhibit an inverted-U-shaped dependency on GC concentrations, such that moderate levels promote correlates of learning, whereas absence of or excess GCs degrade them. On the other hand, ADX, GC synthesis inhibition, or selective blockade of GRs all impair memory for aversive tasks, such as inhibitory avoidance. ADX-induced deficits are reversible by GC administration. GCs are most constructive memorially when given immediately posttraining, whereas they impair retrieval when given prior to testing. One locus of positive GC effects is the basolateral amygdala (BLA). GC microinfusions into the BLA, but not its striatal target, the CeA, improve memory consolidation, whereas BLA lesions abolish facilitating effects of high levels of systemic steroid. Improved consolidation is partly mediated by NE, as blockade of β-adrenoreceptors within the BLA prevents the facilitating effects of high steroid levels.

The source of NE may be medullary, as GR agonists-infused into NTS improve memory which is blocked by β-adrenoreceptor blockade in BLA. Posttraining CRF infused into the BLA also improves memory. As the BLA contains CRF receptors, but few CRF-immunopositive fibers, CRF probably diffuses into the BLA from the CeA. Dopamine agonists given simultaneously into the BLA and the accumbens shell region also enhance memory for conditioned fear.

GC-mediated conditioned responses feed back on HPA axis and autonomic outflows. The CeA is essential for expressing behavioral and neuroendocrine measures of conditioned fear, whereas lesions of the LH prevent autonomic but not behavioral components, and lesions of the PAG interfere with behavioral but not autonomic responses. For the HPA axis, lesions of the CeA disrupt conditioned responses to both discrete (e.g., light, tone) and contextual (e.g., room cues) stimuli, whereas lesions of the BNST only disrupt responses to contextual, but not discrete, stimuli, suggesting alternative routes to the HPA axis output, depending on the modality of association.

Neuronal Remodeling

GCs remodel gross brain structure. Acute GC elevations rapidly induce spinogenesis in hippocampal slices in the absence of protein synthesis. Chronic stress, GCs, and ADX inhibit neurogenesis in the dentate gyrus, suggesting that moderate steroid level is permissive to normal structure. Chronic stress reduces dendritic arborization in CA3 fields and total hippocampal volume, effects reversed by stress-free periods. Similar events occur in the mPFC. In contrast, a regimen of repeated immobilization stress increases dendritic length and spinogenesis in the BLA. Acute stress only increases spinogenesis, which increases, rather than decreases, during stress-free periods. The BNST shows some similar effects. Structure-dependent effects of stress on neuronal remodeling are consistent with the direction of correlates of learning in these structures. GCs favor memorial and structural modifications related to emotional processing at the expense of cognitive executive processing.

Conclusion

Although the HPA axis is a relatively simple final common output pathway, its complexity increases when properly viewed in terms of its integration of diverse central drivers and its feedback and feed-forward effects on the brain. Diverse central drivers include two distinct circadian oscillators controlling daily cycles of energy balance, bottom-up inputs controlling systemic homeostatic pressures, such as the melanocortin system and the ascending catecholaminergic system, and top-down cortico-striato-pallido-hypothalamic circuits controlling psychogenic responses, and a putative intrahypothalamic pattern generator that coordinates HPA axis outflow with behavioral and autonomic outflows. In addition, a system of circumventricular organs and perhaps signals from the hepatic vagus allow signaling between the immune system and the HPA axis. GCs enter the brain to have both immediate, membrane-mediated effects on various transmitter and neuromodulatory systems and more delayed, genomically mediated effects. The net effect of GC feedback in brain depends on the parameters of stimulation, such as whether a stressor is acute or chronic, with some effects being time or state dependent. GC actions in brain can lead to both inhibition and facilitation of further HPA axis outflow, affecting other motor outflows and influencing mood, incentive, memorial, and structural systems relevant to adaptation. The HPA axis defends the body against systemic derangements, while sculpting and mounting brain networks to anticipate and avoid further challenge.

See Also the Following Articles

Corticotropin-Releasing Hormone: Integration of Adaptive Responses to Stress; Norepinephrine: CNS Pathways and Neurophysiology; Stress Response: Neural and Feedback Regulation of the HPA Axis.

Further Reading

Antoni, F. A. (1993). Vasopressinergic control of pituitary adrenocorticotropin comes of age. *Frontiers in Neuroendocrinology* **14**, 76–122.

Buijs, R. M. and Van Eden, C. G. (2000). The integration of stress by the hypothalamus, amygdala and prefrontal cortex: Balance between the autonomic nervous system and the neuroendocrine system. *Progress in Brain Research* **126**, 117–132.

Cone, R. D. (2005). Anatomy and regulation of the central melanocortin system. *Nature Neuroscience* **8**(5), 571–578.

Cook, C. J. (2002). Glucocorticoid feedback increases the sensitivity of the limbic system to stress. *Physiology & Behavior* **75**, 455–464.

Dallman, M. F., Akana, S. F., Cascio, C. S., et al. (1987). Regulation of ACTH secretion: Variations on a theme of B. In: Clark, J. H. (ed.) *Recent Progress in Hormone Research*, (vol. 43)), pp. 113–173. Orlando: Academic Press.

Dallman, M. F., Akana, S. F., Jacobson, L., et al. (1987). Characterization of corticosterone feedback regulation of ACTH secretion. *Annals of the New York Academy of Sciences* **512**, 402–414.

Dallman, M. F., Pecoraro, N., Akana, S. F., et al. (2003). Chronic stress and obesity: A new view of 'comfort food.'

Proceedings of the National Academy of Sciences of the United States of America **100**(20), 11696–11701.
De Kloet, E. R., Vreugdenhil, E., Oitzl, M. S., et al. (1998). Brain corticosteroid receptor balance in health and disease. *Endocrine Reviews* **19**(3), 269–301.
Erickson, K., Drevets, W. C. and Schulkin, J. (2003). Glucocorticoid regulation of diverse cognitive functions in normal and pathological emotional states. *Neuroscience & Biobehavioral Reviews* **27**, 233–246.
Lamont, E. W., Robinson, B., Stewart, J., et al. (2005). The central and basolateral nuclei of the amygdala exhibit opposite diurnal rhythms of expression of the clock protein Period2. *Proceedings of the National Academy of Sciences of the United States of America* **102**(11), 4180–4184.
LeDoux, J. (2003). The emotional brain, fear, and the amygdala. *Cellular and Molecular Neurobiology* **23**(4–5), 727–738.
McEwen, B. S. and Magarinos, A. M. (2001). Stress and hippocampal plasticity: Implications for the pathophysiology of affective disorders. *Human Psychopharmacology* **16**(S1), S7–S19.
Mistlberger, R. (1994). Circadian food-anticipatory activity: Formal models and physiological mechanisms. *Neuroscience & Biobehavioral Reviews* **18**(2), 171–195.
Pacak, K. and Palkovits, M. (2001). Stressor specificity of central neuroendocrine responses: Implications for stress-related disorders. *Endocrine Reviews* **22**(4), 502–548.
Perreau-Lenz, S., Pevet, P., Buijs, R. M., et al. (2004). The biological clock: The bodyguard of temporal homeostasis. *Chronobiology International* **21**(1), 1–25.
Piazza, P. V. and LeMoal, M. (1997). Glucocorticoids as a biological substrate of reward: Physiological and pathophysiological implications. *Brain Research Reviews* **25**, 359–372.
Przekop, F., Mateusiak, K., Stupnicka, E., et al. (1990). Suppressive effect of beta-endorphin and naloxone on the secretion of cortisol under stress conditions in sheep. *Experimental and Clinical Endocrinology* **95**(2), 210–216.
Ritter, S., Watts, A. G., Dinh, T. T., et al. (2003). Immunotoxin lesion of hypothalamically projecting norepinephrine and epinephrine neurons differentially affects circadian and stressor-stimulated corticosterone secretion. *Endocrinology* **144**(4), 1357–1367.
Rivest, S. (2001). How circulating cytokines trigger the neural circuits that control the hypothalamic–pituitary–adrenal axis. *Psychoneuroendocrinology* **26**(8), 761–788.
Roozendaal, B. (2003). Systems mediating acute glucocorticoid effects on memory consolidation and retrieval. *Progress in Neuro-Psychopharmacology & Biological Psychiatry* **27**(8), 1213–1223.
Saal, D., Dong, Y., Bonci, A., et al. (2003). Drugs of abuse and stress trigger a common synaptic adaptation in dopamine neurons. *Neuron* **37**, 577–582.
Saper, C. B., Lu, J., Chou, T. C., et al. (2005). The hypothalamic integrator for circadian rhythms. *Trends in Neuroscience* **28**(3), 152–157.
Sullivan, R. M. and Gratton, A. (2002). Prefrontal cortical regulation of hypothalamic–pituitary–adrenal function in the rat and implications for psychopathology: Side matters. *Psychoneuroendocrinology* **27**, 99–114.
Swanson, L. W. (2000). Cerebral hemisphere regulation of motivated behavior. *Brain Research* **886**(1–2), 113–164.
Thompson, R. H. and Swanson, L. W. (2003). Structural characterization of a hypothalamic visceromotor pattern generator network. *Brain Research: Brain Research Reviews* **41**(2–3), 153–202.
Valentino, R. J. and Van Bockstaele, E. J. (2001). Opposing regulation of the locus coeruleus by corticotropin-releasing factor and opioids. *Psychopharmacology* **158**, 331–342.
Vyas, A., Mitra, R., Shankaranarayana Rao, B. S., et al. (2002). Chronic stress induces contrasting patterns of dendritic remodeling in hippocampal and amygdaloid neurons. *Journal of Neuroscience* **22**(15), 6810–6818.
Yoshihara, T., Honma, S. and Honma, K. (1996). Prefeeding release of paraventricular neuropeptide Y is mediated by ascending noradrenergic neurons in rats. *American Journal of Physiology* **270**(4, part 1), E596–E600.

Central Stress Neurocircuits

S Kollack-Walker, H E W Day and H Akil
University of Michigan, Ann Arbor, MI, USA

This is a revised version of the article by S Kollack-Walker, H E W Day, and H Akil, Encyclopedia of Stress, First edition, volume 1, pp 414–422, © 2000, Elsevier Inc.

Glossary

Homeostasis Maintaining constancy of the internal environment of the body.

Stressor Stimulus input that initiates a stress response.

Stress response A nonselective response (endocrine, behavioral, autonomic) that targets multiple tissues and organs in response to, or anticipation of, a challenge to homeostasis.

An understanding of central stress neurocircuits requires knowledge of neuroanatomical pathways that underlie detection of various stimuli leading to a stress state, perception of those inputs as stressful (when appropriate), and mediation of select response outputs. In this article, the basic neurocircuitry involved in regulation of the hypothalamic-pituitary-adrenocortical (HPA) axis is reviewed. The HPA axis mediates secretion of glucocorticoids in response to a variety of stimuli ranging from immune responses to hemorrhaging to social defeat. Thus, it is important to understand how such diverse stimuli can lead to activation of the HPA axis. The stress-induced increases in glucocorticoids act to maintain homeostasis as well as to mobilize energy stores for fight-or-flight reactions. Although these actions can and do occur together, it is possible to isolate homeostatic regulation from the more global defense response. These phenomena can be distinct in terms of arousal, emotional salience, conscious perception, and behavioral responsivity. As a consequence, it is also important to understand how the brain responds to different types of stressful events.

Overview of Stress: Inputs, Outputs, and Evaluative Processes

Stress has been described as a multidimensional concept consisting of three major components: the stimulus input, an evaluative process, and the response output. The stimulus input, or stressor, refers to an event that elicits a nonselective response (endocrine, behavioral, autonomic) that targets multiple tissues and organs in response to, or anticipation of, a challenge to homeostasis. In many cases, the link between stimulus inputs and response outputs requires perception of a given event as stressful. This evaluative process can include not only processing of stimulus-specific information and coding of the stressor's intensity and intermittency, but also comparison of the current situation to previous experiences. In addition, this evaluative process reflects the organism's ability to cope with the stressor (e.g., degree of controllability, real or perceived). The response output, or stress response, is the body's adaptations designed to re-establish physiological or psychological equilibrium. Depending on the particular stimulus input, a specific array of responses may be initiated (**Figure 1**).

This concept of stress has been modified to reflect the notion that some stimulus inputs can lead to a stress response without requiring evaluation. Consequently, various authors in the field have classified stressors in distinct ways: physical versus psychological, or systemic versus neurogenic/processive. The key element associated with such distinctions is the need for a stimulus input to be perceived as stressful. For example, the experience of novelty as a mild stressor requires perception of a situation as different with the potential to encounter threatening stimuli. A novel environment would be classified as processive, involving higher order processing within the central nervous system in order to identify the present situation as unique in comparison to previous experiences. In contrast, other stimulus inputs are thought to elicit a stress response without prior evaluation. For example, hemorrhaging activates various reflexes designed

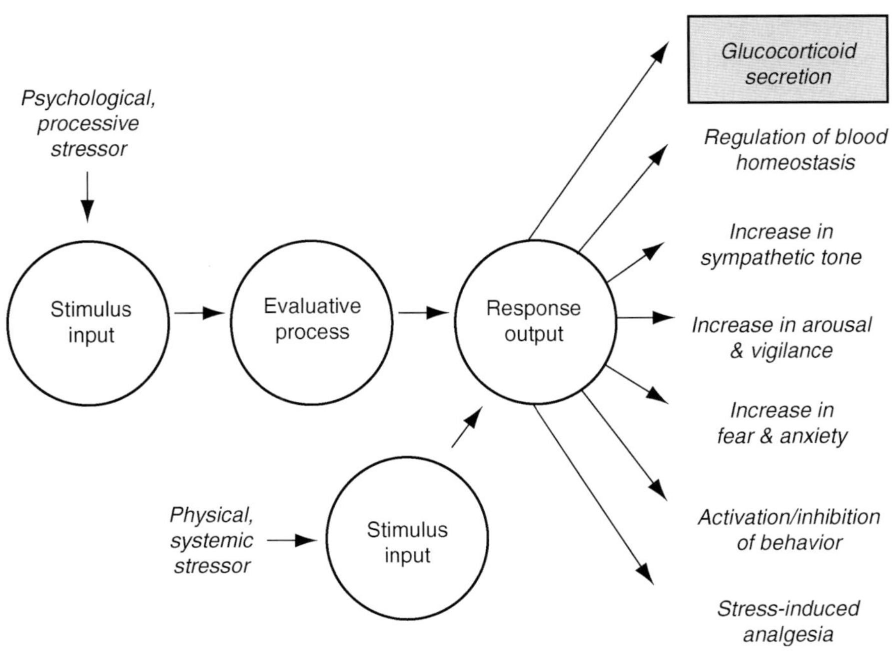

Figure 1 Schematic diagram illustrating the basic relationship between stimulus inputs and response outputs.

to return blood volume to normal values. In this case, it is not necessary to perceive blood loss as stressful – the reaction is automatic. Hemorrhaging would be considered systemic, involving perturbations in homeostasis or a threat to an individual's internal environment.

Although stressors can be distinguished in terms of the type of stimulus input and the need for evaluative processing, a key component of the response output involves activation of the hypothalamic-pituitary-adrenocortical (HPA) axis. The HPA axis mediates release of glucocorticoids from the adrenal cortex, and glucocorticoids play an important role in energy metabolism and the maintenance of homeostasis. In this article, the basic elements of the HPA axis, including a description of specific brain pathways implicated in HPA axis regulation, are reviewed. In this discussion, how the brain responds to two distinct stressors – an immune challenge, as an example of a systemic stressor, and social defeat, as an example of a processive and psychological stressor – is considered. Last, the article considers how a stress response is terminated, a process linked to distinct neurocircuits and stress-induced increases in glucocorticoids.

Hypothalamic-Pituitary-Adrenocortical (HPA) Axis

The HPA axis is involved in control of secretion of glucocorticoids from the adrenal cortex. Neurons within the medial parvocellular subdivision of the paraventricular nucleus of the hypothalamus (mpPVN) synthesize corticotropin-releasing hormone (CRH) and project to the median eminence, releasing CRH into hypophysial portal blood vessels to reach specific cells within the anterior pituitary called corticotrophs. The binding of CRH to its receptor on the corticotroph's cell membrane stimulates a cascade of intracellular events leading to the release of adrenocorticotropic hormone (ACTH) into the general circulation. CRH is the major ACTH secretagogue, although a number of additional molecules have been implicated in facilitating ACTH release (e.g., vasopressin). ACTH acts upon specific receptors in the adrenal cortex to stimulate the synthesis and release of glucocorticoids into the general circulation. Depending upon the species, the major glucocorticoid secreted from the adrenal cortex may be cortisol (human), corticosterone (rat), or both (hamster).

Initiation of the Stress Response

A variety of approaches have been taken to identify brain regions involved in regulation of the HPA axis. Our current state of knowledge is based upon studies that have utilized tract tracing to identify afferent inputs into the mpPVN, expression of immediate early genes to identify activated brain regions, lesions to determine the importance of a given set of inputs for stress-induced glucocorticoid secretion, and pharmacological and biochemical analyses to determine the role of particular neurotransmitters and neuropeptides in HPA axis regulation. Several key findings obtained from these data are summarized in **Figures 2** and **3**.

Is there a common set of pathways within the central nervous system critical for initiating a stress response, or do different stressors activate the HPA axis through distinct neurocircuits? The data collected, thus far, provide evidence in support of both arguments. Indeed, systemic (physical) and processive (neurogenic/psychological) stressors appear to activate the HPA axis largely through distinct pathways, although this does not preclude the possibility that multiple pathways may be involved, especially for complex stressors that have both physical and psychological components. Within the class of processive stressors, similar activation patterns are generally observed, possibly reflecting, at least in part, the activation of core neurocircuits critical for glucocorticoid secretion.

Homeostatic Regulation: Systemic, Physical Stressors

Stressors that are systemic or physical in nature involve a reaction to a threatening stimulus in an individual's internal milieu leading to the activation of regulatory mechanisms that serve to restore homeostasis. A variety of stimulus inputs is under homeostatic control, including body temperature, immune responses, and changes in blood volume and composition. For many of these stimuli, it is absolutely critical that the levels of these variables be maintained within a certain range for survival. Because of this link to survival, systemic stressors are associated with activation of brainstem and circumventricular afferents that have direct projections to mpPVN neurons. In many cases, excitation of the HPA axis is dependent upon ascending catecholaminergic input.

For example, activation of an inflammatory or immune response increases the production and release of various cytokines (e.g., interleukin-1β), which leads to excitation of the HPA axis. This rise in glucocorticoids is an adaptive response that serves to inhibit the immune system, limiting its scope of attack and decreasing the likelihood that the immune system will attack self. **Figure 4** illustrates the general pattern of c-*fos* mRNA expression that occurs within the brain of a male rat 30 min following systemic administration of interleukin-1β (IL-1β). As evident from

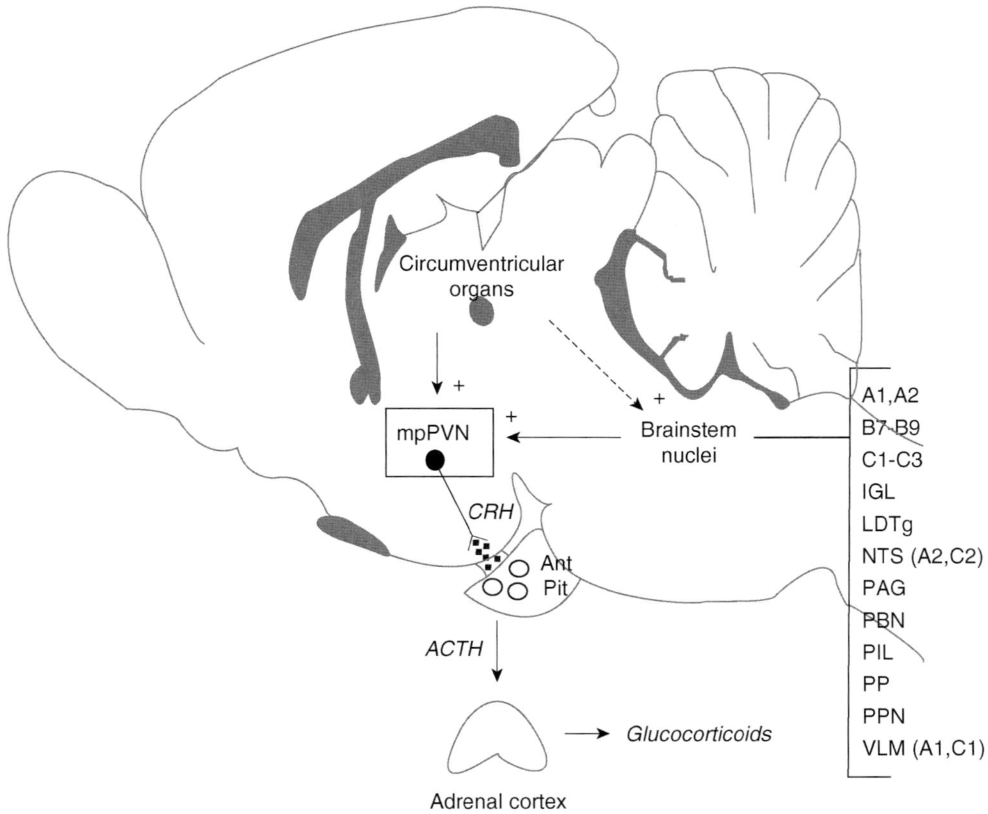

Figure 2 Schematic diagram summarizing the role of brain stem and circumventricular afferents in regulation of the functional activity of mpPVN neurons. This afferent input has been associated with activating the HPA axis in response to systemic and physical stressors.

the photomicrographs, the pattern of neuronal activation is fairly localized, with increased expression of c-*fos* mRNA observed within bed nucleus of the stria terminalis (BST), central amygdaloid nucleus (CeA), mpPVN, parabrachial nucleus (PBN), nucleus of the solitary tract (NTS), circumventricular organs including area postrema (AP), and barrier-related structures including meninges, cerebral vasculature, and choroid plexus. Additional studies have reported activation of neurons within the medial preoptic area (MPOA), supraoptic nucleus of the hypothalamus (SON), magnocellular and autonomic subdivisions of PVN, thalamus, and catecholamine cell groups of the ventrolateral medulla (VLM; A1 and C1 cell groups) and NTS (A2 and C2 cell groups).

Increased expression of c-*fos* mRNA within the PVN presumably reflects excitatory control of the pituitary–adrenocortical axis in response to systemic administration of IL-1β. Catecholaminergic input from the NTS and ventrolateral medulla is critical for activating mpPVN neurons in response to IL-1β, as lesions that destroy these ascending pathways can drastically reduce c-*fos* expression within mpPVN neurons and other measures of HPA axis activity. In accordance, c-*fos* mRNA levels are increased within neurons of the adrenergic (C1, C2) and noradrenergic (A2) cell groups, and retrograde tract-tracing studies have shown that the majority of these activated neurons project to mpPVN. Systemic administration of IL-1β can activate these catecholaminergic cell groups via two main pathways. The NTS receives visceral sensory information carried by the vagus and glossopharyngeal nerves, and there is evidence that these sensory afferents can respond to IL-1β in the periphery. In addition, neurons within the area postrema can transduce IL-1β present in the bloodstream into a neural signal that is then transmitted to neurons within the NTS and VLM. In support of this second pathway, c-*fos* mRNA levels are elevated within the area postrema in response to IL-1β.

The lateral subdivision of the CeA and the dorsolateral or oval nucleus of the BST (BSTov) also show prominent activation following IL-1β administration. Both of these brain regions have been implicated in stress responses, particularly autonomic responses, but it is unclear what their role is in the response to IL-1β administration. They are unlikely to be the primary regions involved in the increase in HPA axis activity for several reasons. First, neurons within the lateral CeA do not project to the PVN, but rather to

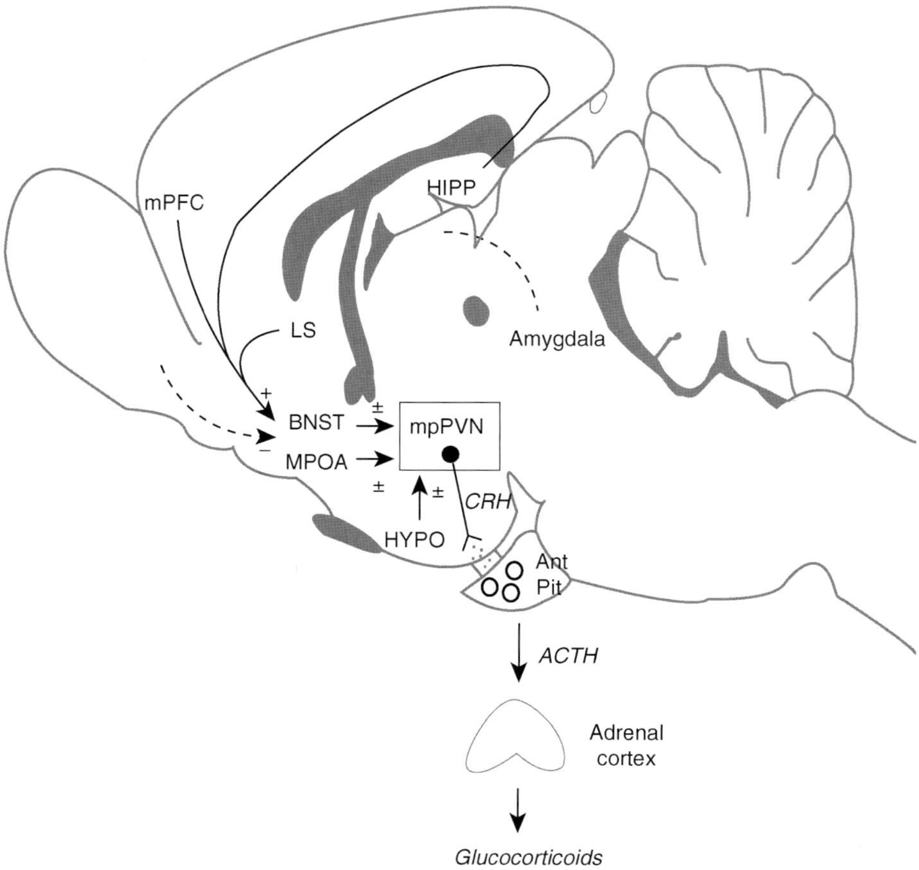

Figure 3 Schematic diagram summarizing the role of BST, MPOA, and hypothalamic and limbic afferents in regulation of the functional activity of mpPVN neurons. The limbic system has been linked to activating the HPA axis in response to processive and psychological stressors.

three main regions – medial CeA, restricted parts of the BST (including the oval nucleus), and the parabrachial nucleus in the pons. Second, while tract-tracing studies show a significant proportion of cells within the NTS and VLM that project to mpPVN and contain Fos protein, a similar finding is not observed for neurons within the CeA or BST. Third, administration of indomethacin, a prostaglandin synthesis inhibitor, blocks the ability of neurons in area postrema to transduce IL-1β into a neural signal. This effect results in decreased activation of neurons within NTS and VLM, leading to decreased activation of mpPVN neurons and a reduction in ACTH release. However, indomethacin administration does not reduce c-*fos* expression within CeA, suggesting that the mechanisms associated with HPA axis regulation in response to IL-1β administration are distinct from those controlling activational processes within CeA. That said, there is some evidence to suggest that the ventral BST modulates the HPA axis response to IL-1β and that the CeA may modulate this BST region.

Fight or Flight Response: Processive, Psychological Stressors

Stressors that are processive and psychological in nature involve a reaction to a real or perceived threatening stimulus in an individual's external environment. Such reactions are associated with increased arousal and vigilance, often eliciting a state of fear (or increased anxiety) and, in many instances, leading to a global response output that has been termed fight or flight. The image conveyed by fight or flight is one of an active state – secretion of glucocorticoids and other neurohormones, activation of the sympathetic division of the autonomic nervous system leading to increases in heart rate, blood pressure, and respiration, and display of behavioral responses designed to effectively cope with the threatening event. A processive stressor requires the processing of exteroceptive signals from multiple sensory modalities that lead to perception of the stimulus input as stressful. This evaluative process may also reflect psychological variables, including predictability and controllability of the stressor as well as coping strategies.

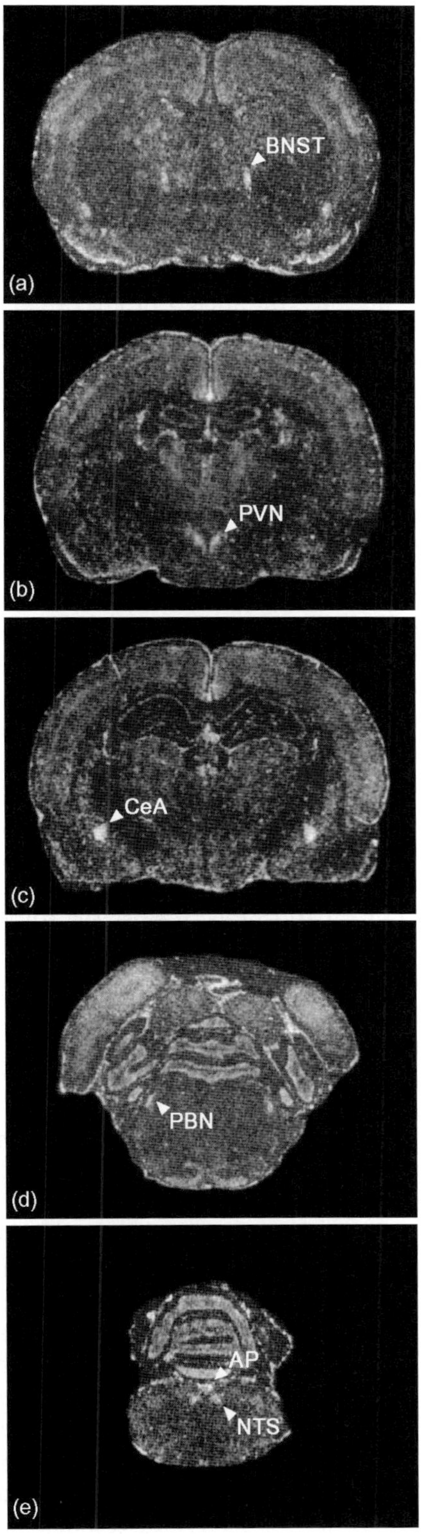

Figure 4 Series of photomicrographs illustrating the location of c-*fos* mRNA within the brain of a male rat following systemic administration of interleukin-1β. Note the selective pattern of neuronal activation with increases in c-*fos* mRNA present within the bed nucleus of the stria terminalis (BST), paraventricular nucleus of the hypothalamus (PVN), central nucleus of the amygdala (CeA), nucleus of the solitary tract (NTS), and area postrema (AP). PBN, parabrachial nucleus.

Because of this need for higher level processing, processive stressors are thought to activate limbic afferents that control HPA axis activity via synaptic connections with the BST, MPOA, and hypothalamus.

The effects of social defeat in the male Syrian hamster have been studied as one model of a processive, psychological stressor. Using a resident-intruder paradigm, the pairing of two isolated male hamsters results in fighting, with one male (dominant) behaving aggressively, attacking and chasing the other male (subordinate), which reacts submissively, defending against attack and displaying flight. The subordinate male is stressed as evidenced by elevated levels of glucocorticoids, while the dominant male is not. **Figure 5** illustrates the general pattern of c-*fos* mRNA expression that occurs within the brain of a socially defeated male 30 min after the onset of fighting. This series of photomicrographs reveals a global pattern of activity encompassing vast regions of the neocortex, septum, amygdala, hypothalamus, and brainstem. By analyzing c-*fos* mRNA expression within different control groups and in dominant and subordinate males, it is possible to identify patterns of neuronal activity associated with handling, fighting, and the stress of defeat. Activation observed in numerous brain regions in handled control, dominant, and subordinate males presumably reflects the detection of exteroceptive signals, leading to an increase in arousal and conscious awareness. In contrast, selective activation of brain regions in subordinate males most likely reflects processes associated with the perception of the stimulus input as threatening and stressful as well as mediation of various response outputs leading to the fight-or-flight response. In subordinate males, c-*fos* mRNA increased selectively within the cingulate cortex (medial prefrontal cortex), lateral septum, BST, MPOA, several hypothalamic nuclei (paraventricular, anterior, ventromedial, arcuate, and supramammillary), CeA, amygdalohippocampal area, periaqueductal gray, dorsal raphe, cuneiform nucleus, and locus coeruleus.

The limbic system plays an important role in regulating HPA axis activity in response to processive and psychological stressors. Following defeat, significant increases in neuronal activation were observed within mPFC, lateral septum, and amygdala. The hippocampus also plays an important role in HPA axis activity, although c-*fos* mRNA levels were not selectively increased within this brain region. This negative finding has been reported following other stress paradigms. The majority of studies have linked mPFC, lateral septum, and hippocampus to inhibition of glucocorticoid secretion (see next section). In contrast, numerous studies have implicated the amygdala in excitatory regulation of the HPA axis.

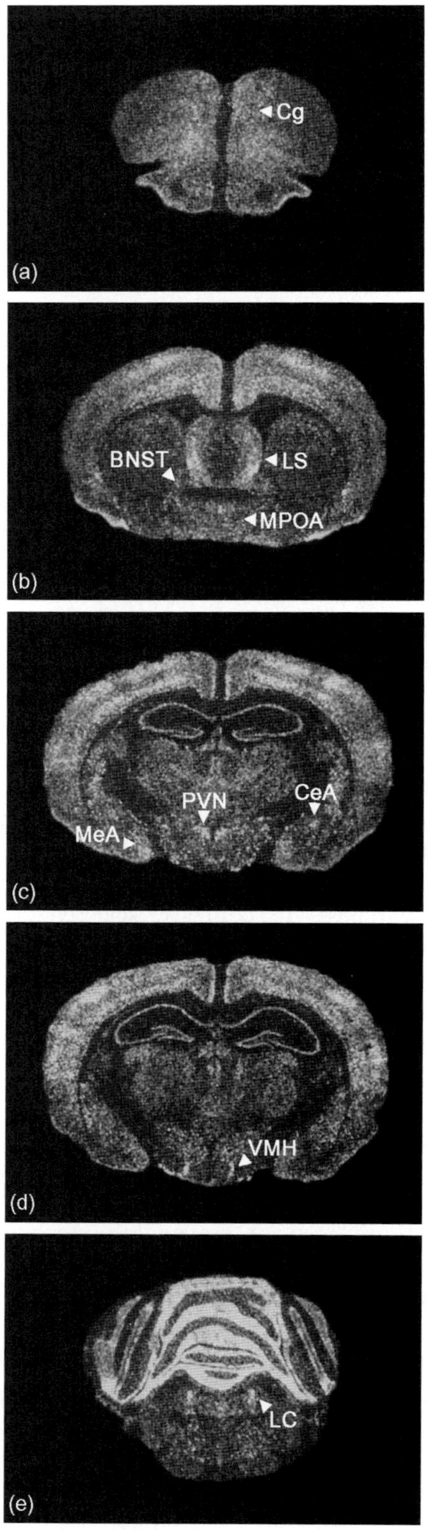

Figure 5 Series of photomicrographs illustrating the location of c-*fos* mRNA within the brain of a male hamster following social defeat. Note the global pattern of brain activity observed throughout the brain. A selective pattern of neuronal activation was observed in the cingulate cortex (Cg), lateral septum (LS), bed nucleus of the stria terminalis (BNST), medial preoptic area (MPOA), paraventricular (PVN) and ventromedial (VMH) nuclei of the hypothalamus (PVN), central nucleus of the amygdala (CeA), and locus coeruleus (LC). MeA, medial nucleus of the amygdala.

For example, electrical stimulation of neurons within the medial, cortical, and central nuclei have all been shown to stimulate glucocorticoid secretion. Furthermore, lesions of the medial and central nuclei can decrease ACTH and corticosterone secretion in response to stress. Following defeat, a significant increase in c-*fos* mRNA expression was observed within CeA. This increase is quite unusual for processive stressors, which in general produce quite meager or no increases in c-*fos* mRNA or Fos protein expression in this area. This is in contrast to systemic stressors such as IL-1β, which cause robust increases of c-*fos* gene products in the CeA. In fact, recent evidence has suggested that many processive stressors, including novelty, loud noise, and restraint, inhibit the neurons in the CeA (and related BSTov). It is possible that brain activity following defeat reflects psychological and physical processes, with increased expression of c-*fos* mRNA within CeA (and dorsolateral BST) synonymous with brain activity observed following systemic or physical stressors (e.g., processing of painful stimuli associated with biting attacks).

Although activated neurons were also detected within the medial and cortical subdivisions of the amygdala, the levels present in subordinate males were not different from those observed in handled control or dominant males. It is at present unclear whether c-*fos* expression within the medial and cortical amygdaloid nuclei following social defeat reflects an increased propensity to stimulate glucocorticoid secretion that is differentially regulated at more central levels (e.g., enhanced in subordinate animals but inhibited in handled control and dominant males). Alternatively, activation within these brain regions may be associated with processes that are not specific to stress, such as coupling sensory cues with behavioral arousal.

While there is some evidence to suggest that the medial and central amygdaloid nuclei can project to the PVN, the input is limited and primarily focused toward autonomic subdivisions of this nucleus. The majority of anatomical studies suggest that the limbic system can influence the HPA axis via synaptic relays within the BST, MPOA, and hypothalamus. Indeed, lesions of neurons within the BST, MPOA, and hypothalamus have been shown to have either excitatory or inhibitory effects on HPA axis activity. Furthermore, tract-tracing studies reveal that many neurons within these three brain areas project directly to the mpPVN. Following defeat, significant increases in c-*fos* expression were observed throughout the BST, MPOA, and hypothalamus. Additional work will be required to identify specific groups of neurons within these brain areas that are activated during defeat and that project to mpPVN.

The global pattern of brain activation seen following defeat is also observed in response to many other processive or psychological stressors, including conditioned fear, audiogenic stress, predator odor stress, footshock, restraint, immobilization, and swim stress. Following many of these stressors, significant increases in neuronal activation can be seen within various components of the limbic system. Several of these areas have been shown to correlate well with ACTH release following audiogenic stress, including the PVN, ventral lateral septum, medial and ventral BST, and medial preoptic area. It remains to be tested whether some or all of these areas form a core neural circuitry mediating the HPA axis response following processive stress.

Termination of the Stress Response

In addition to understanding how the HPA axis is activated during a stressful event, it is equally important to identify the mechanisms involved in terminating or limiting this response. Specific brain regions and stress-induced increases in glucocorticoids play an important role in terminating the stress response.

Neuronal Regulation

Local neurocircuits utilizing γ-aminobutyric acid (GABA) as a neurotransmitter have been implicated in inhibitory regulation of the HPA axis. Lesions placed within the BST, MPOA, or hypothalamus (including the arcuate, ventromedial, and suprachiasmatic nuclei) can increase the levels of ACTH and corticosterone secreted basally and in response to stress. All of these regions contain substantial populations of GABA-containing neurons, and, most recently, it has been shown that mRNA levels of the GABA biosynthetic enzyme glutamic acid decarboxylase increase within these brain areas in response to stress.

In addition, neurons within the lateral septum, mPFC, and hippocampus have also been linked to inhibitory regulation of the HPA axis. For example, lesions placed within any of these brain regions can prolong glucocorticoid secretion in response to stress. In addition, electrical stimulation of the hippocampus has been shown to inhibit glucocorticoid secretion. These data suggest that one function of these limbic brain regions may be to limit or terminate activity within the HPA axis. The major neurotransmitter utilized by neurons within the mPFC and hippocampus is the excitatory neurotransmitter glutamate. It is possible that afferents from the mPFC and hippocampus act to excite GABA neurons within the BST, MPOA, and hypothalamus, leading to increased inhibition of the HPA axis.

Hormonal Regulation

Glucocorticoids act to inhibit the HPA axis at multiple levels: pituitary, PVN, and higher brain centers; and in different time domains: fast, intermediate, and slow (genomic). The genomic, and, to some extent, intermediate forms of inhibition appear to involve the classic mechanism of steroid–receptor-mediated regulation of gene transcription. Elevated levels of glucocorticoids bind to glucocorticoid receptors (GRs), activating the receptor and causing it to translocate to the nucleus where the steroid–receptor complex binds to DNA, leading to decreased transcription of CRH and AVP genes in the hypothalamus and decreased transcription of the POMC gene in the pituitary. The mechanisms that underlie fast feedback inhibition are not well understood. This form of inhibition occurs too rapidly to be explained by changes in gene transcription. It is possible that glucocorticoids act at GRs to mediate nongenomic effects, or, alternatively, glucocorticoids may interact with a different class of glucocorticoid-sensitive receptors (e.g., membrane receptors).

Glucocorticoids are also thought to act at higher brain centers to inhibit the HPA axis. For example, lesions of the hippocampus lead to an increase in the expression of CRH and AVP mRNA within mpPVN neurons, even though basal levels of glucocorticoids are elevated, suggesting that glucocorticoid negative feedback has been reduced following hippocampal damage. Lesions of the hippocampus have also been shown to attenuate the ability of exogenous glucocorticoids to inhibit secretion of stress hormones, although not all studies support this contention. Similarly, implants of glucocorticoids into the mPFC or MPOA have been shown to block restraint-induced secretion of stress hormones. These findings suggest that glucocorticoids interact with neuronal elements to increase inhibitory control over the HPA axis. How this effect is mediated at the level of neurons and neurocircuits is presently unknown.

Concluding Remarks

This article was designed to provide a general understanding of how the brain responds to an acute stress exposure, highlighting important differences in brain activity in response to stressors that are systemic and physical in nature versus those that are processive and psychological. However, the relationship between stress and brain activity may be more complex than simply a reflection of the class of stressor involved. Indeed, how the brain responds to stress can be influenced by a number of associative factors, including the intensity, intermittency, chronicity, and context of the stress exposure as well as the individual's ability to effectively cope with stress. The challenge will be to understand how these more subtle aspects of stress responsiveness are coded within central stress neurocircuits.

See Also the Following Articles

Amygdala; Brain and Brain Regions.

Further Reading

Akil, H. and Morano, M. I. (1996). The biology of stress: from periphery to brain. In: Watson, S. J. (ed.) *Biology of schizophrenia and affective disease*, pp. 15–48. Washington, D.C: American Psychiatric Press.

Burow, A., Day, H. E. W. and Campeau, S. (2006). A detailed characterization of loud noise stress: intensity analysis of hypothalamo-pituitary-adrenocortical axis and brain activation. *Brain Research* **1062**, 63–73.

Campeau, S., Day, H. E. W., Helmreich, D. L., Kollack-Walker, S. and Watson, S. J. (1998). Principles of psychoneuroendocrinology. *Psychiatric Clinics of North America* **21**, 259–276.

Crane, J. W., Buller, K. M. and Day, T. A. (2003). Evidence that the bed nucleus of the stria terminalis contributes to the modulation of hypophysiotropic corticotropin-releasing factor cell responses to systemice interleukin-1β. *Journal of Comparative Neurology* **467**, 232–242.

Cullinan, W. E., Herman, J. P., Helmreich, D. L. and Watson, S. J. (1995). A neuroanatomy of stress. In: Friedman, M. J., Charney, D. S. & Deutch, A. Y. (eds.) *Neurobiological and clinical consequences of stress: from normal adaptation to PTSD*, pp. 3–26. New York: Raven.

Day, H. E. W. and Akil, H. (1996). Differential pattern of c-*fos* mRNA in rat brain following central and systemic administration of interleukin-1-beta: implications for mechanism of action. *Neuroendocrinology* **63**, 207–218.

Day, H. E. W., Badiani, A., Uslaner, J. M., Oates, M. M., Vittoz, N. M., Robinson, T. E., Watson, S. J. and Akil, H. (2001). Environmental novelty differentially affects c-fos mRNA expression induced by amphetamine or cocaine in subregions of the bed nucleus of the stria terminalis and amygdala. *Journal of Neuroscience* **21**, 732–740.

Day, H. E. W., Nebel, S., Sasse, S. K. and Campeau, S. (2005). Inhibition of the central extended amygdala by loud noise and restraint stress. *European Journal of Neuroscience* **21**, 441–454.

Day, T. A. (2005). Defining stress as a prelude to mapping its neurocircuitry: no help from allostasis. *Progress in Neuro-Psychopharmacology and Biological Psychiatry* **29**, 1195–1200.

Herman, J. P. and Cullinan, W. E. (1997). Neurocircuitry of stress: central control of the hypothalamo-pituitary-adrenocortical axis. *Trends in Neuroscience* **20**, 78–84.

Herman, J. P., Ostrander, M. M., Mueller, N. K. and Figueiredo, H. (2005). Limbic system mechanisms of stress regulation: hypothalamo-pituitary-adrenocortical axis. *Progress in Neuro-Psychopharmacology and Biological Psychiatry* **29**, 1201–1213.

Kollack-Walker, S., Watson, S. J. and Akil, H. (1997). Social stress in hamsters: defeat activates specific neurocircuits within the brain. *Journal of Neuroscience* **17**, 8842–8855.

Levine, S. and Ursin, H. (1991). What is stress? In: Brown, M. R., Koob, G. F. & Rivier, C. (eds.) *Stress: neurobiology and neuroendocrinology*, pp. 3–21. New York: Marcel Dekker.

Sawchenko, P. E., Brown, E. R., Chan, R. K. W., Ericsson, A., Li, H.-Y., Roland, B. L. and Kovacs, K. J. (1996). The paraventricular nucleus of the hypothalamus and the functional neuroanatomy of visceromotor responses to stress. *Progress in Brain Research* **107**, 201–222.

Brain and Brain Regions

A G Watts
University of Southern California, Los Angeles, CA, USA

This is a revised version of the article by A G Watts, Encyclopedia of Stress, First edition, volume 1, pp 342–348, © 2000, Elsevier Inc.

Glossary

Catecholamines	Chemical signals (epinephrine, dopamine, and norepinephrine) synthesized from the amino acid tyrosine.
Chromaffin cells	Endocrine cells in the adrenal medulla that release adrenaline (primarily) into the blood on stimulation from sympathetic motor system.
Diencephalon	The part of the forebrain containing the thalamus and hypothalamus (including the preoptic area).
Hypoglycemia	Condition in which blood glucose concentrations fall below 60–75 mg dl^{-1}.
Hypotension	A reduction in blood pressure.
Immediate early gene	A gene whose product (usually a transcription factor) is rapidly produced as a consequence of receptor activation.
Telencephalon	The part of the forebrain containing the cortical regions (including the hippocampus), basal ganglia, bed nucleus of the stria terminalis, amygdala, and septal complex.

Introduction – Stress and the Brain

A wide variety of stimuli evoke motor events that are considered as stress responses. In simple organisms, these are made up of little more than sets of stereotyped reflexes. If the stressor is sufficiently intense or prolonged, these often consist of avoidance responses accompanied by endocrine-mediated alterations in metabolism. However, there is no evidence to suggest that invertebrates can associate emotional affect such as fear or anxiety with particular stressors. Only with the evolution of more complex central nervous systems (CNS) in general, and the telencephalon in particular, do we begin to see this type of associative processing.

In vertebrate species, stress is typically accompanied by endocrine secretions (e.g., from steroidogenic tissue in the interrenal/adrenal glands), autonomic motor events (e.g., piloerection, increased secretion from the chromaffin cell/adrenal medulla system, and alterations in cardiovascular tone), sets of behavioral motor actions (e.g., avoidance responses, changes in defensive behavior, and fear-conditioned freezing), and those attendant emotional percepts generally recognized as being the most characteristic human signatures of stress (e.g., fear and anxiety). From a neural-systems perspective, these examples show that virtually all parts of the CNS can be used to varying degrees for processing the information associated with stress. Here we broadly consider which parts of the CNS are (1) concerned with processing the sensory information used to generate stress responses, (2) responsible for mediating the motor aspects of the stress response, and (3) involved with the integrative mechanisms that control stress responses in the face of influences from, for example, learning and memory mechanisms. To do this we explore concepts that are based on data derived from a number of experimental techniques, including lesions, neuroanatomical tract tracing, and the mapping of immediate early gene expression within the brain and spinal cord.

Many physiological stressors originating in the viscera are addressed by evoking simple reflexes to annul their potentially damaging consequences. Virtually no complex central processing is required and control is often exerted by classic negative feedback (homeostatic) mechanisms from the action of the target. An example of reactive homeostatic components of the stress response is the sympathetic activation evoked to counter the immediate visceral effects of many stressors. For example, if stress-related hypotension or hypoglycemia are prolonged or of sufficient intensity, they are rapidly negated by reactive stress responses that are evolutionarily rather old – sympathetically mediated vasoconstriction and catecholamine secretion by chromaffin cells, respectively (see **Comparative Anatomy and Physiology**).

In contrast, however, most stress responses typically have a more proactive (anticipatory) than a reactive (reflex) character, which involves complex neural processing. With stress activation of the hypothalamic-pituitary-adrenal (HPA) axis, for example, although adrenocorticotropic hormone (ACTH) and corticosterone secretion are obviously triggered by the stressor, they are not motor responses that act to remove the immediate consequences of the stress in a manner similar to the reactive sympathetic responses just described. Instead, the actions of stress-induced increases in circulating corticosterone levels (mediated in part by interactions with leptin, insulin, and the thyroid hormones) anticipate the possibility that the stressor will lead to a debilitating sequence of events, particularly the catabolic effects of negative energy balance, that require the mobilization of energy stores, particularly protein. Understanding the neural complexity required for processing what are effectively anticipatory events provides the framework for explaining why so many neural systems are involved with modulating stress responses.

Brain Regions Concerned with Processing Stress-Related Information

Sensory Processing

Generally speaking, virtually all extero- and viscero- (intero-)sensory modalities are processed along two types of pathway once they enter the CNS (**Figure 1**). The first, path A, is a relatively direct and rapidly effective route that requires little central integrative processing. These types of reflex pathways result in rapid and simply organized (stereotyped) motor responses. Much of the neural processing for these reflexes occurs in the spinal cord (for the behavioral motor components of stress responses), hindbrain (for the autonomic motor aspects of stress responses), and hypothalamus (for the motor output of neuroendocrine stress responses). In path B, the second path, sensory information is also directed to those areas of the brain that provide the additional and often critical modulatory information about arousal state and behavioral planning (timing signals, priorities, etc.), so furnishing the animal with the adaptive plasticity for generating stress responses. Brain regions in the telencephalon (cerebral cortex, amygdala, hippocampus, and septal complex) provide pivotal contributions here, particularly with regard to the neural representations of sensory objects. Collectively, these processes can prioritize stress responses with relation to other behaviors (e.g., placing a higher priority on fleeing a predator than on feeding) and with modulating the organization of stress responses, decreasing or increasing their intensity based on past experience (learning and memory). As a consequence, they are also likely to be involved with generating the detrimental effects of chronic emotional stress. Finally, **Figure 1** shows that the effects of a stress-associated motor event can serve as feedback signals to modulate the motor output of the system, both by reducing the level of sensory input and motor output (simple negative feedback) and by more indirect effects on central integrative processes.

Spinal cord Neurons in the dorsal horn of the spinal cord are the first recipients of nerve afferents from the skin and viscera that process information related to somatosensory modalities (pressure, temperature, and pain). The spinal cord also receives sensory information from muscle spindles related to body position. Dorsal horn neurons are involved with organizing reflexes related to stress responses, but they are not directly involved with generating the more complex motor events usually thought of as stress responses. However, dorsal horn neurons do project much of this sensory information to the hindbrain and thalamus for the higher-order processing (the sensory transduction and processing part of **Figure 1**, path B). Ultimately, higher-order processing can then influence the type of contextual information responsible for generating the stress responses that are accompanied by fear and anxiety. Clearly, because information related to pain can evoke ACTH release, nociceptive information entering the dorsal horn can affect neuroendocrine motor neurons in the hypothalamic paraventricular nucleus (PVH). However, the pathways responsible for this are not entirely clear.

Hindbrain Parts of the hindbrain receive first-order sensory information from the cranial nerves related to the visual (oculomotor) and vestibular systems, as well as somatosensory (the hypoglossal and trigeminal systems) and gustatory (the glossopharyngeal nerve) information from the oropharynx. In many respects how the hindbrain processes this information in a stress-related manner is similar to how exterosensory information is processed bidirectionally by

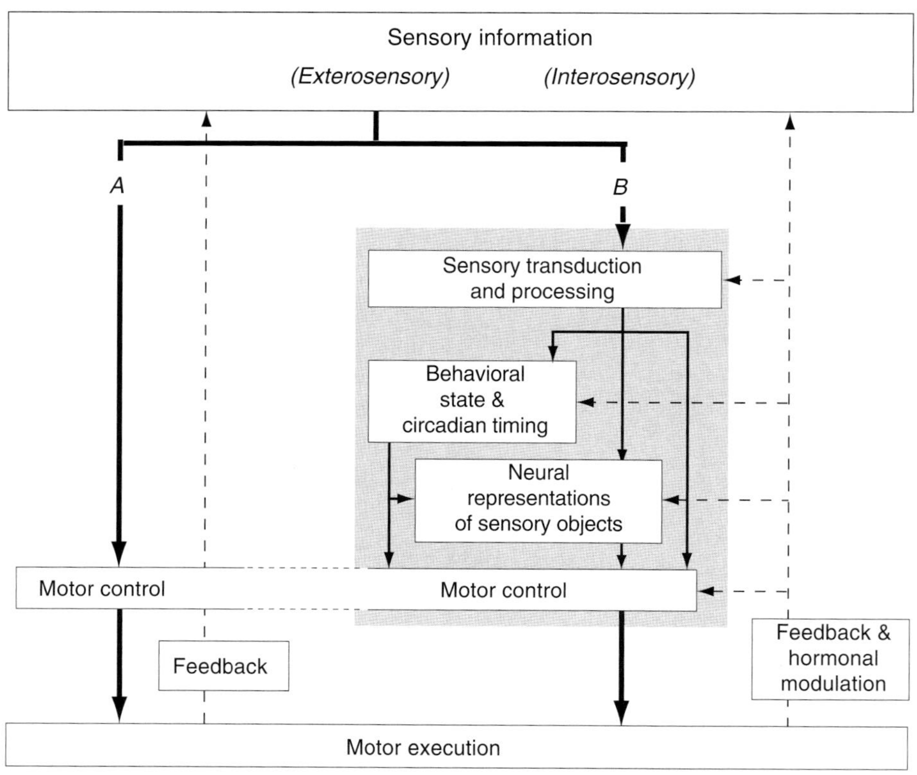

Figure 1 A schematic representation of the two paths along which sensory information is processed in the brain. Path A is a reflex route that does not involve complex central processing and that allows for rapid stereotyped stress responses; path B is a route that allows sensory information to be integrated with other types of information within the brain and that provides stress responses with greater complexity, flexibility, and adaptability. Central neural connections are shown in black, with hormonal and feedback signals shown as dashed lines. The regions that constitute the central control networks in the brain are enclosed within the gray box in path B.

the dorsal horn of the spinal cord (**Figure 1**) – information can initiate reflex loops and it can be passed further into the brain for more sophisticated processing. Projections from the parabrachial nucleus are probably important for projecting pain-related information received from the dorsal horn and cranial nerves that ultimately impact those parts of the hypothalamus regulating the adrenal gland.

The hindbrain is also critical for processing those sensory modalities originating in the internal environment that can generate stress responses. It receives numerous inputs from sensory receptors in the viscera that in general are conveyed to the nucleus of the solitary tract (NTS) by the vagus nerve and spinal cord. In turn, the NTS initiates visceral reflexes such as the baroreceptor reflex that regulates cardiovascular function within a normal range. However, neural projections from the NTS along with other hindbrain regions also project this information to the forebrain (including regions in the hypothalamus such as the PVH) and telencephalon that in turn regulate the HPA axis directly. This explains why many viscerosensory stimuli (e.g., hypoglycemia and hypotension) can evoke robust ACTH and corticosterone secretion.

Thalamus With the exception of olfactory information (which enters the cortex directly and most likely impacts stress-related motor circuits by way of the amygdala and bed nuclei of the stria terminalis (BNST), all exterosensory modalities are processed by the thalamus before being projected to the amygdala and cerebral cortex. Consequently, those specific thalamic regions associated with particular sensory modalities have been implicated in processing stress-related sensory information. For example, the medial geniculate region is thought to contribute to the fear-conditioning evoked by pairing an auditory stimulus with foot shock.

Motor Regions

Spinal cord The spinal cord contains two sets of motor neurons that are directly related to expressing stress responses. First, alpha motor neurons in the ventral horn are the mediators of all behavioral motor system stress responses. And second, the intermediolateral column in the thoracic and upper lumbar spinal cord contains the sympathetic preganglionic neurons that innervate the adrenal medulla and are directly responsible for stimulating adrenaline release during stress. These cholinergic neurons also mediate other components of the sympathetic stress responses and are innervated by a variety of afferents including those from the hypothalamus.

Hindbrain Visceral stress responses are also mediated by sets of preganglionic neurons in the hindbrain. For example, stress-induced modifications to cardiovascular and other visceral functions are mediated through the dorsal motor nucleus of the vagus.

Hypothalamus The hypothalamus is a critical premotor region that can modulate most viscerally directed stress responses. It also contains all the motor neurons used for the neuroendocrine component of the stress response. Foremost among these are the corticotropin releasing hormone (CRH) neurons in the medial parvicellular part of the PVH. The axons of these neurons terminate on the capillaries of hypophysial vasculature in the median eminence and release CRH and arginine vasopressin (AVP) to stimulate ACTH release from corticotropes in the anterior pituitary. The PVH and supraoptic nucleus also contain magnocellular neurons that release oxytocin and AVP during stress events. As with all other motor responses, these neuroendocrine neurons can be activated in relatively simple reflex manner (e.g., by hemodynamic stressors) as well as by inputs from telencephalic regions. In addition, the PVH provides strong projections to sympathetic and parasympathetic preganglionic neurons and is probably a key element in modulating the activity of these systems during stress.

One of the classic functions of the hypothalamus is the generation of motivated behaviors. These include ingestive, reproductive, and defensive behaviors. During the 1940s, Hess demonstrated that electrical stimulation of specific regions of the lateral hypothalamus (LHA) elicit rage or fearful behavior. It is likely that the often inhibitory influences of stress on, for example, feeding and reproductive behaviors are integrated within the hypothalamus with the relevant control networks of these behaviors. The exact mechanisms used for these interactions are not clear, but again they very likely involve inputs from the telencephalon. Finally, it is important to remember that the hypothalamus contains the suprachiasmatic nucleus (SCH). In mammals, this cell group is the circadian clock, which can strongly influence the way stress responses are generated.

Afferents from those brain regions known to regulate the HPA axis and other stress motor functions are organized as two basic projection patterns (**Figure 2**): those that provide inputs directly to the PVH and those that provide indirect inputs, projecting first to other cell groups that in turn then project to the PVH. Neurons with direct inputs to the PVH can be divided into four afferent sets that provide the rich source of

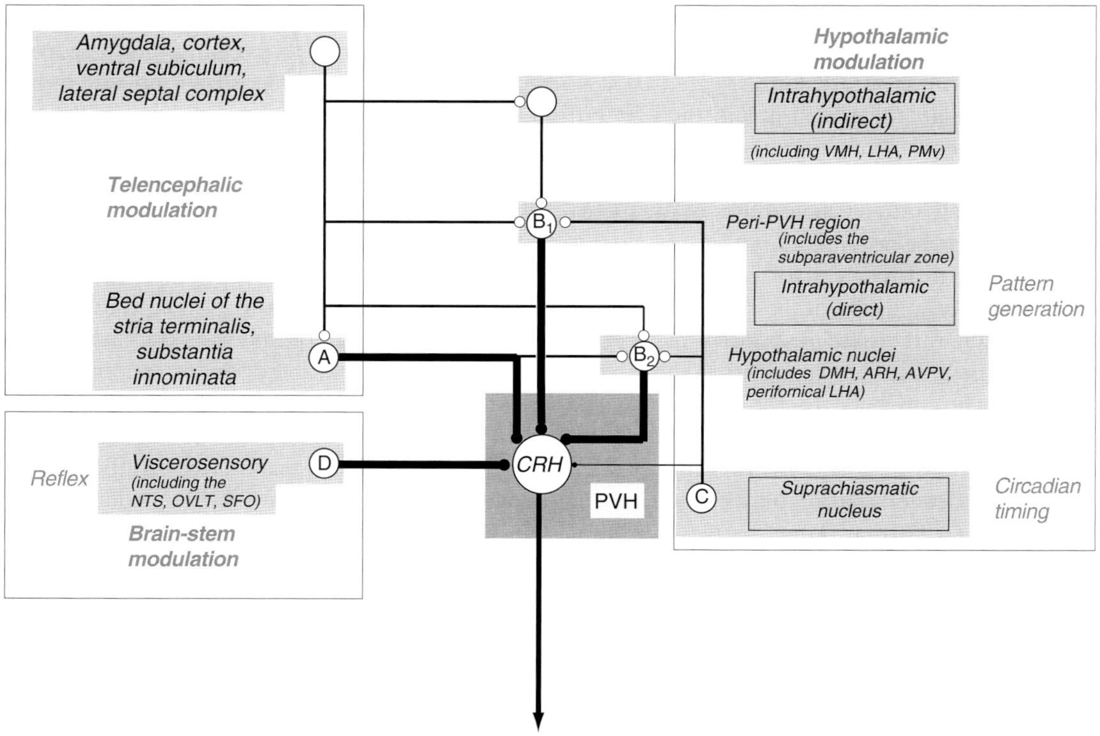

Figure 2 A schematic of the organization of inputs to the paraventricular nucleus of the hypothalamus. This nucleus is a key regulator of neuroendocrine and other autonomic stress responses. However, it receives only a restricted number of direct inputs from the telencephalon, hypothalamus, and hindbrain. Many other hypothalamic and telencephalic regions provide information indirectly by way of these more direct inputs. Finally, circadian timing signals from the suprachiasmatic nucleus impact the PVH directly and, to a greater extent, through other hypothalamic cell nuclei with direct inputs. ARH, arcuate nucleus; AVPV, anteroventral periventricular nucleus; CRH, corticotropin releasing hormone; DMH, dorsomedial nucleus; LHA, lateral hypothalamic area; NTS, nucleus of the solitary tract; OVLT, vascular organ of the lamina terminalis; PMv, ventral premammillary nucleus; PVH, paraventricular nucleus of the hypothalamus; SFO, subfornical organ; VMH, ventromedial nucleus of the hypothalamus.

information for integration by neuroendocrine and pre-autonomic cell groups.

1. The only direct telencephalic inputs to the PVH comes from some of the BNST and the substantia innominata (**Figure 2**, group A).

2. Two groups of direct PVH inputs originate intrahypothalamically (**Figure 2**, group B). First, the PVH is surrounded by local γ-aminobutyric acid (GABA)ergic neurons that are not organized as a distinct hypothalamic nucleus but that electrophysiological and anatomical data suggest form an important group of direct intrahypothalamic inputs (**Figure 2**, group B_1). They receive a major input from the SCH, from the infralimbic cortex, and from other hypothalamic nuclei such as the ventromedial and ventral premammillary nuclei, which in turn receive massive telencephalic inputs. Second, a well-defined group of projections (**Figure 2**, group B_2) originate in the arcuate and dorsomedial nuclei, in the preoptic area (in particular, the median preoptic and anteroventral periventricular nuclei), and the LHA. These nuclei also receive inputs from the telencephalon, including the BNST and lateral septal complex (LS). The overall function of these two groups of direct intrahypothalamic inputs is unclear. However, projections from the arcuate and perhaps the dorsomedial nucleus convey information about peripheral energy status derived from circulating leptin, insulin, and ghrelin, which are important for regulating the stress responses derived from changes to energy balance. Some neurons in this group may also constitute a set of neuroendocrine pattern generators similar in principle to those in the hindbrain and spinal cord that control patterning in the behavioral motor system.

The importance of input sets (1) and (2) to stress responses is that they relay information to the PVH from a host of diencephalic and telencephalic regions (**Figure 2**, groups A, B_1, and B_2). Thus, these areas each receive numerous topographically ordered inputs from the cortex, ventral subiculum (SUBv), amygdala, and LS. Collectively, these inputs are responsible for relaying a great deal of the information critical for controlling stress responses to exterosensory stimuli and under a variety of circumstances that requires complex telencephalic processing.

3. The SCH provides the circadian timing signal that regulates all behaviors and has a critical bearing on the expression of stress responses. Although the SCH provides a small direct PVH projection, its major output (**Figure 2**, group C) is to the subparaventricular zone in the peri-PVH region and the dorsomedial nucleus. Collectively, its efferents to these regions (**Figure 2**, group B_1, B_2, and C) are the likely mediators of circadian influence on the PVH-related stress responses.

4. Afferents from a variety of hindbrain nuclei project topographically within the PVH and convey viscerosensory information derived from the spinal cord, vagus, and glossopharyngeal nerves (**Figure 2**, group B_1). These inputs probably serve two functions; to stimulate patterns of ACTH secretion in response to homeostatic challenges that can generally be described as reflex in nature and to provide the gain control signals required for neuroendocrine CRH neuron function in the basal state. Afferents from the vascular organ of the lamina terminalis and the subfornical organ that provide humoral sensory information about blood osmolality and angiotensin II concentrations, respectively, can also, in terms of function, be included with these direct viscerosensory inputs.

Integrative Regions

Hindbrain The hindbrain contains monoaminergic cell groups that have very wide-ranging connections that in the past have been referred to as the reticular activating system. Included here are the locus ceruleus, the raphe nuclei, parts of the NTS, and pedunculapontine nuclei. Collectively, they receive sensory inputs from the oropharynx and viscera, as well as numerous inputs from the forebrain. They innervate virtually the whole of the neural axis and are thought to regulate behavioral arousal. In some instances (e.g., the locus ceruleus), they are implicated in the stress responses by virtue of their electrophysiological behavior and gene expression. Collectively, however, the precise role of these cell groups in regulating stress responses remains unclear.

Hippocampus It has been known for some time that hippocampal lesions or the severing of hippocampal efferents into the lateral septal complex disrupts ACTH secretion and, thus, glucocorticoid stress responses. The SUBv is the hippocampal subfield most clearly implicated in this context. SUBv lesions increase CRH and AVP gene expression in the neuroendocrine PVH and also elevate plasma ACTH concentrations, suggesting that the SUBv usually provides inhibitory inputs to the PVH. Although specific details about the pathways or the mechanisms involved are not understood, the absence of direct projections from any hippocampal region to the PVH demonstrates that these effects are not mediated directly. The best candidate in this regard is a SUBv-BNST-PVH pathway (**Figure 2**, group A). The most studied overall function of the hippocampus is in learning and memory, particularly regarding short-term spatial memory and animal navigation. However, how this type of information relates to the modulation of stress responses is entirely unknown.

Septal complex The septal complex is a collection of forebrain cell groups that lie directly medial to the lateral ventricles. They are characterized by having bidirectional and topographically organized connections with the hippocampus; the LS receives afferents, and the medial septal complex projects back to the hippocampus. As such the LS is in a position to integrate information from all sensory modalities. By virtue of their efferent connections, the parts of the LS that are most closely associated with regulating endocrine stress responses are located in its rostral (LSr) and ventral (LSv) parts. Although the LSv provides sparse inputs directly into the PVH, it does project strongly to at least two regions that can affect stress responses directly: the peri-PVH region (**Figure 2**, group B_1) and those parts of the hypothalamic preoptic area that then project into the PVH (**Figure 2**, group B_2). In turn, LSv neurons receive topographically ordered projections from the SUBv. In addition to any effects it might have on the HPA axis, the LS probably plays an important role in the expression of defensive behavior and, as such, may well affect the ordering of behavioral priorities during stress events. Certainly, patterns of immediate early gene expression suggest that the LS is somehow concerned with modulating defensive behavior during fear conditioning.

Amygdala The amygdala has long been considered critical for regulating stress responses and their learned components that have fear as the emotional percept. However, the precise role of amygdala is still unclear with regard to its specific contribution. The amygdala is traditionally subdivided into the lateral, basolateral, medial, central, and cortical regions. However, recent debate has challenged the usefulness of the amygdala as a unitary concept, suggesting that a more viable division is first into cortical (with glutamate as a transmitter) and striatal (with GABA as a transmitter) parts, followed by four functional systems based on the segregation of inputs and outputs. In this scheme, the traditionally defined amygdalar nuclei are included into one of these functional systems. For example, the central nucleus of the amygdala is part of the striatal amygdala and, by virtue of its connections to the BNST and parabrachial nucleus, regulates the autonomic aspects of the stress response. Regarding outputs, the hippocampus and BNST are important components in the output structure of the amygdalar nuclei most closely associated with stress responses. Although again, like other parts of the telencephalon, the complex organization of stress responses dictates that all parts of the amygdala are probably involved at some level.

Bed nuclei of the stria terminalis The BNST are a set of numerous, often small, and rather poorly differentiated cell groups located immediately rostral and dorsal to the preoptic area of the hypothalamus. Their precise role has proven difficult to define, mostly because experiments have targeted large regions that encompass a number of nuclei. However, neuroanatomical evidence suggests that each BNST cell group has precise and often distinct connections. As a whole, the BNST receive topographically organized projections from the amygdala and hippocampus and, in turn, project to many parts of the hypothalamus. The importance of the BNST to stress responses is that some of these nuclei receive projections from those parts of the cerebral cortex, amygdala and hippocampus (particularly the ventral hippocampal regions) associated with the overall regulation of the stress responses. Consequently, one of their major functions is to integrate and channel processed telencephalic information directly to the PVH and other parts of the hypothalamus (**Figure 2**, group A).

Cortex Because the cerebral cortex is ultimately involved with formulating and regulating all voluntary behaviors, it must be considered as a major integrative component of stress responses, particularly with respect to behavioral initiation, motor program selection, and prioritization. But as can be imagined, a detailed consideration of its function in this regard is beyond the scope of this article. Regarding cortical influences on neuroendocrine and autonomic motor output, these are generally indirect and are mediated through the LS, BNST, amygdala, and SUBv or through other hypothalamic nuclei that have direct neuroendocrine connections (e.g., **Figure 2**).

See Also the Following Articles

Amygdala; Comparative Anatomy and Physiology; Anatomy of the HPA; Neuroendocrine Systems.

Further Reading

Blessing, W. (1997). *The lower hindbrain in bodily homeostasis.* New York: Oxford University Press.

Herman, J. P., Figueiredo, H., Mueller, N. K., et al. (2003). Central mechanisms of stress integration: hierarchical circuitry controlling hypothalamo-pituitary-adrenocortical responsiveness. *Frontiers in Neuroendocrinology* **24**, 151–180.

LeDoux, J. (1996). *The emotional brain.* New York: Simon & Schuster.

Swanson, L. W. and Petrovich, G. D. (1998). What is the amygdala? *Trends in Neuroscience* **21**, 323–331.

Swanson, L. W. (2000). Cerebral hemisphere regulation of motivated behavior. *Brain Research* **886**, 113–164.

Swanson, L. W. (1987). The hypothalamus. In: Bjorklund, A., Hökfelt, T. & Swanson, L. W. (eds.) *Handbook of chemical neuroanatomy* (vol. 5), pp. 1–124. Amsterdam: Elsevier.

Van de Kar, L. D. and Blair, M. L. (1999). Forebrain pathways mediating stress-induced hormone secretion. *Frontiers in Neuroendocrinology* **20**, 1–48.

Watts, A. G. (2005). Glucocorticoid regulation of peptide genes in neuroendocrine CRH neurons: a complexity beyond negative feedback. *Frontiers in Neuroendocrinology* **26**, 109–130.

Corticotropin-Releasing Hormone: Integration of Adaptive Responses to Stress

P E Sawchenko, Z F Yuan, F Laplante, R A Rissman and J C Bittencourt
Salk Institute for Biological Studies, La Jolla, CA, USA

Introduction

Corticotropin-releasing factor (CRF) is a neuropeptide that was first isolated from the hypothalamus on the basis of its capacity to stimulate the release of adrenocorticotropic hormone (ACTH) from the anterior pituitary gland. Its localization to parvocellular neurosecretory neurons of the paraventricular hypothalamic nucleus (PVH) defined the central limb of the hypothalamic–pituitary–adrenal (HPA) axis. It was recognized early on, however, that the central distribution of CRF is quite broad and includes aspects of the limbic forebrain associated with affective behaviors and brain stem cell groups involved directly in central autonomic control. The subsequent demonstration that the peptide could act within the brain to elicit stresslike behavioral (increased anxiety, arousal, decreased appetite) and autonomic (sympathomimetic) responses gave rise to the hypothesis that the central CRF system may act at multiple levels of the central nervous system to activate, and even integrate, complementary modes of stress adaptation. This notion has provided a dominant unifying framework guiding much contemporary work in the field of stress neurobiology.

The idea that individual signaling molecules may serve similar or complementary functions at diverse sites of expression has been entertained for some time. While this is not a universal generalization, certain catecholamines (epinephrine, norepinephrine) that serve as principal effectors of the sympathoadrenal system in the periphery are also prominently expressed, and situationally active, in aspects of central stress-related circuitry. In addition, there are a number of 'brain–gut peptides' (including CRF) whose expression in the peripheral autonomic and/or enteric nervous systems on one hand, and in the brain on the other, is associated with defined and complementary roles in digestive functions and appetitive control, respectively. Here we consider the functional and anatomical organization of the central CRF system and evaluate evidence bearing on its hypothesized role as an arbiter of multiple modes of stress adaptation.

The CRF Family of Signaling Molecules

CRF exerts its biological activities by binding G-protein-coupled receptors that activate adenylate cyclase. The type 1 receptor (CRFR1) is expressed by anterior pituitary corticotropes and can account for the neuroendocrine actions of the peptide. CRFR1 is expressed widely in brain (**Figure 1**), though its distribution is more suggestive of dominant roles in cortical, cerebellar, and sensory information processing than in the stress-related behavioral and autonomic functions for which CRF is better known. A structurally related type 2 receptor (CRFR2) exists in two principal forms; one variant (CRFR2β) is expressed in the periphery and the choroid plexus, while a second (CRFR2α) is expressed in brain, where its distribution is distinct from, and more limited than, that of CRFR1. The binding affinity of CRF for CRFR2 is relatively low. This information, coupled with the recognition that certain non-mammalian vertebrates express not only obvious CRF homologs but also other structurally related peptides such as sauvagine (from frog) and urotensin I (from fish) prompted an effort to identify new mammalian CRF family members, culminating in the cloning of three novel peptides, termed urocortins (Ucns 1–3). Ucn 1 binds both CRFRs with high affinity, while Ucn 2 and 3 are CRFR2-selective ligands. Each of the Ucns exhibits a distinctive and discrete expression pattern in brain (**Figure 1**), with variable potentials for interacting with cell groups expressing CRFR2 (e.g., Ucn 3) or both receptors (Ucn 1). There is a strong basis for considering these components of the central CRF system as functioning in a unified manner in stress adaptations. Shortly after the identification of Ucn 1, evidence was provided that this peptide can act centrally to mediate some stress-related functions originally attributed to CRF. Moreover, a substantial body of evidence supports an interaction of CRFR1- and CRFR2-dependent mechanisms in sculpting a variety of neuroendocrine, autonomic, and behavioral responses to stress.

In keeping with their binding affinities, a strong general correspondence has been found between the distribution of neurons that are activated in response to central administration of CRF and sites of CRFR1 expression, while central Ucn 1 activates both CRFR1- and CRFR2-bearing targets. The principal exceptions are robust activational responses provoked by either peptide in a set of interconnected cell groups that

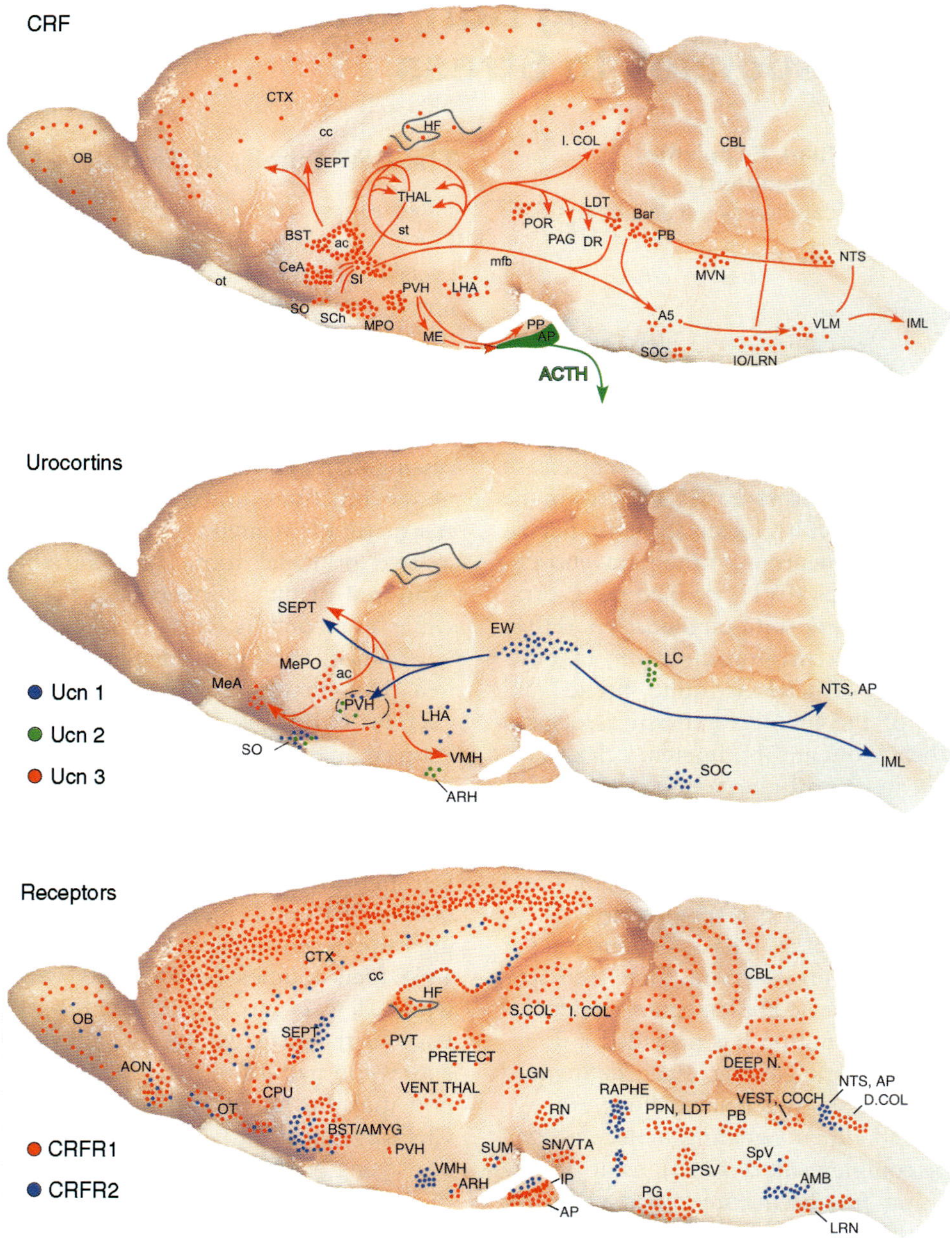

Figure 1 Central distribution of corticotropin-releasing factor (CRF) signaling molecules. Schematic representation on a sagittal view of the rat brain of major sites of cellular expression of CRF-related peptides and receptors; major axonal projections of peptidergic neurons are indicated by arrows. In addition to being expressed by neurosecretory neurons of the paraventricular hypothalamic nucleus (PVH) that comprise the final common path for effecting stress-induced activation of adrenocorticotrophic hormone (ACTH) secretion, CRF (top) is broadly expressed in brain, including in limbic forebrain (BST, CeA) and central autonomic (NTS, VLM, PB, IML) cell groups. The expression of urocortins (Ucn 1–3; middle) is more restricted. The dominant seat of Ucn 1 expression is the Edinger–Westphal nucleus (EW), whose outputs include projections to central autonomic cell groups (PVH and NTS). Ucn 2 is weakly expressed in brain, and axonal projections immunoreactive for this peptide have not been demonstrated. Ucn 3 is expressed in a few discrete forebrain regions that project to some major sites of type 2 CRF receptor expression (medial amygdala, lateral septum and ventromedial hypothalamus). The two known CRF receptor subtypes (CRFR1 and CRFR2, bottom) are differentially distributed, with CRFR1 expression being more widespread. Receptor expression in demonstrated sites of peptide action in eliciting stresslike physiological and behavioral responses is limited mainly to the parabrachial nucleus (CRFR1) and NTS (CRFR2). A5, A5 catecholamine cell group; ac, anterior commissure; AMB, nucleus ambiguus; AMYG, amygdala; AON, anterior olfactory nucleus; AP, area postrema; ARH, arcuate nucleus hypothalamus; Bar, Barrington's nucleus; BST, bed nucleus stria terminalis; CBL, cerebellum; cc, corpus callosum; CeA, central nucleus amygdala; COCH, cochlear nucleus; CPU, caudoputamen; CTX, cerebral cortex; D.COL., dorsal column nuclei; DEEP N., deep nucleus cerebellum; DR, dorsal raphe nucleus; EW, Edinger–Westphal nucleus; HF, hippocampal formation; I. COL, inferior colliculus; IML, intermediolateral column spinal cord; IO, inferior olivary complex; LC, locus coeruleus; LDT, laterodorsal tegmental nucleus; LGN, lateral geniculate nucleus; LHA, lateral hypothalamic area; LRN, lateral reticular nucleus; ME, median eminence; MeA, medial nucleus amygdala; MePO,

comprise a core circuitry for central autonomic and neuroendocrine regulation – responses not readily explicable on the basis of CRFR distributions. These cell groups, collectively termed the central autonomic system (CAS), are of critical importance as most are implicated as principal sites of CRF action in eliciting stress-related responses but have been found to display limited capacity for CRFR expression or CRF binding. These include the central nucleus of the amygdala (CeA), which has been identified repeatedly as a site of CRF action relevant to behavioral (anxiety-like) and autonomic stress responses; the PVH, whose hypophysiotropic CRF neurons receive a CRF-immunoreactive input, defining a substrate for posited feedback and feed-forward effects on the central limb of the HPA axis, and which is otherwise a sensitive site for peptide effects on ingestive behavior and cardiovascular responses; and the nucleus of the solitary tract (NTS) and ventrolateral medulla (VLM), the linchpins of interoceptive information processing in brain and where CRF acts at low doses to elicit sympathomimetic effects on cardiovascular parameters. Many would include among this grouping the locus coeruleus, whose widespread noradrenergic output is thought to set levels of arousal and 'behavioral vigilance' and where unit activity is enhanced by local administration of CRF. Overall, the lack of an apparent basis in CRFR expression for the generalized CAS activation elicited by central peptide injection poses an unresolved challenge to the widely held view of CRF as a common arbiter of multiple modalities of stress responses.

The CAS and Its Role in Adaptive Responses to Stress

The basic organization of circuitry considered to compose the CAS is shown schematically in **Figure 2**. Integral components include aspects of the bed nucleus of the stria terminalis (BST), the PVH, the CeA, the lateral parabrachial nucleus, the A1 and C1 catecholamine cell groups of the VLM, and the medial division of the NTS. The NTS is the pivotal sensory structure in this system as it is the principal central nervous system recipient of primary visceral sensory input carried by the vagus and glossopharyngeal nerves and projects directly to all other components, which, in turn, are extensively interconnected with one another. Both the NTS and the VLM also receive noxious inputs by way of the marginal zone of the spinal dorsal horn, indicating a broader range of sensory control over this circuitry. Major effector arms of the CAS include the main cell groups governing the neural arm (sympathetic preganglionic neurons) and endocrine arm (CRF-expressing neurosecretory neurons) of the stress response. Equally direct access to the limbic forebrain (BST and CeA) provides a basis for invoking mechanisms involved in evaluating the emotional significance of environmental events and in effecting appropriate changes in behavior. Though less elaborately interwoven into this system, the locus coeruleus is considered here along with it as it is interconnected with other CAS components, mediates relevant arousal-like functions, is among the sites at which cellular effects of CRF are best characterized, and, like *bona fide* CAS components, receives a CRF and/or Ucn input that arises from other CAS structures.

The validation of inducible immediate-early genes such as *c-fos* and its protein product, Fos, to serve as markers with which to identify neurons that are activated in response to salient environmental events has enabled substantial progress to be made in unraveling central stress-related circuitry. This work has identified the CAS as being recruited to action in a nearly invariant manner in response to a wide variety of acute stressors, though the extent to which it may mediate adaptive responses may vary as a function of the nature of the challenge. Thus, in so-called physiological stress models (e.g., hemorrhage or immune challenges), core CAS structures are dominant seats of cellular activation, and evidence implicating projections originating from the sensory arm of these pathways in mediating HPA and other adaptive responses in these two models has been provided. Models of the other major, 'emotional' stress category (e.g., restraint, footshock) are also accompanied by widespread CAS activation, though the extent of this activation is variable and less pervasive than that seen in physiological models. The fact that the CAS is so generally called into play in response to diverse challenges is consistent with the view that it may constitute a system for reflexive mediation of generalized alarm responses, in a manner coarsely analogous to the sympathoadrenal system in the periphery. It must be noted, however, that for no emotional stress model

median preoptic nucleus; mfb, medial forebrain bundle; MPO, medial preoptic area; NTS, nucleus solitary tract; OB, olfactory bulb; ot, optic tract; OT, olfactory tubercle; PAG, periaqueductal gray; PB, parabrachial nucleus; PG, pontine gray; POR, perioculomotor raphe; PP, posterior pituitary; PPN, pedunculopontine nucleus; PSV, principal sensory nucleus trigeminal nerve; PVT, paraventricular nucleus thalamus; RAPHE, midbrain raphe nucleus; RN, red nucleus; SCh, suprachiasmatic nucleus; S. COL, superior colliculus; SEPT, septal region; SI, substantia innominata; SN, substantia nigra; SO, supraoptic nucleus; SOC, superior olivary complex; SpV, spinal trigeminal nucleus; st, stria terminalis; SUM, supramamillary nucleus; THAL, thalamus; VENT THAL, ventral thalamus; VEST., vestibular nucleus; VLM, ventrolateral medulla; VMH, ventromedial n, hypothalamus; VTA, ventral tegmental area.

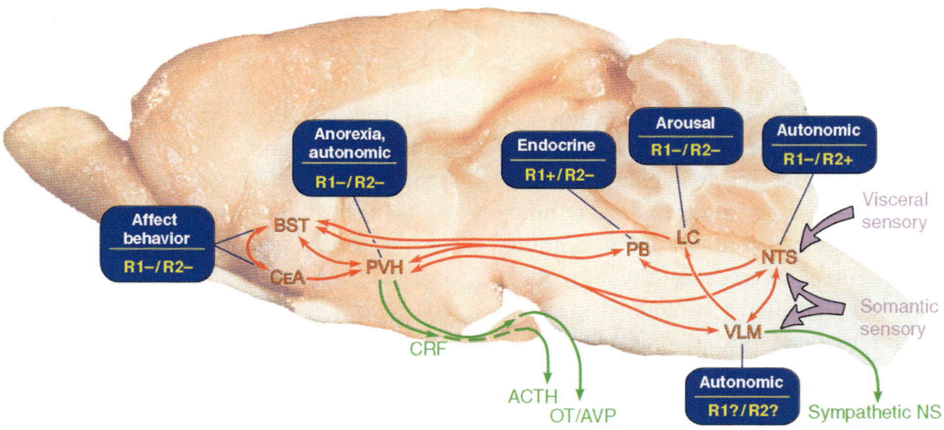

Figure 2 Organization of the central autonomic system in rat brain. Note extensive, often bidirectional interconnections (arrows) among component cell groups. Major sources of sensory input (purple) and motor output (green) are highlighted. The status of each cell group as regards its capacity for CRFR1 (R1) and CRFR2 (R2) messenger RNA expression is indicated, as are some stress-related functions modulated by CRFR agonist/antagonist injections in each. ACTH, adrenocorticotrophic hormone; AVP, arginine vasopressin; BST, bed nucleus stria terminalis; CeA, central nucleus amygdala; CRF, corticotropin-releasing factor; LC, locus coeruleus; NS, nervous system; NTS, nucleus solitary tract; OT, olfactory tubercle; PB, parabrachial nucleus; PVH, paraventricular nucleus; VLM, ventrolateral medulla.

Table 1 Cellular activation profiles elicited by central injection of CRF-related peptides

Peptide	CRFR1-expressing cell groups	CRFR2-expressing cell groups	Central autonomic system cell groups
CRF	+	–	+
Ucn 1	+	+	+
Ucn 2	–	–	+
Ucn 3	–	–	+

Table 2 Effects of CRFR disruption on CRF-induced CNS responses

Disruption	CRFR1-expressing cell groups	CRFR2-expressing cell groups	Central autonomic system cell groups
CRFR antagonist	↓	–	↓
CRFR1 knockout	↓	–	–
CRFR2 knockout	–	–	↑
Double CRFR KO	↓	–	–

has the circuitry underlying CAS activation been identified, and for some such paradigms, the evidence supports a modulatory, rather than a mediating, role.

To what extent does the CRF signaling system participate in the brain's processing of stressful information? Central injections of CRF or Ucn 1 elicit patterns of cellular activation (e.g., Fos induction) that share substantial similarities with those elicited by various stressors, including recruitment of all cell groups of the CAS, as defined here. These responses can be blocked in a dose-related manner by coadministration of nonselective CRFR antagonists. But the evidence supporting an involvement of CRF signaling mechanisms in shaping the brain's response profile in stressful situations is less compelling. Studies involving central administration of CRFR antagonists have reported variable, and generally limited, effectiveness in mitigating stress-induced activation of CAS components. These issues are raised by recent studies of ligand- or stress-induced central nervous system activational profiles in mice genetically engineered to lack functional expression of either or both of the known CRFRs. Thus, central administration of CRF to mice lacking in CRFR1 expression gives rise to markedly reduced activation of cell groups in which CRFR1 is prominently expressed, including cerebral cortex and cerebellum, but CAS responses are unaffected relative to those of genetically intact mice (**Table 1** and **2**). Moreover, CRFR1-deficient animals display no alteration of CAS responses to acute physiological (intravenous endotoxin injection) or emotional (restraint) stressors relative to wild-type controls, while CRFR2-deleted animals showed exaggerated recruitment of some CAS cell groups in

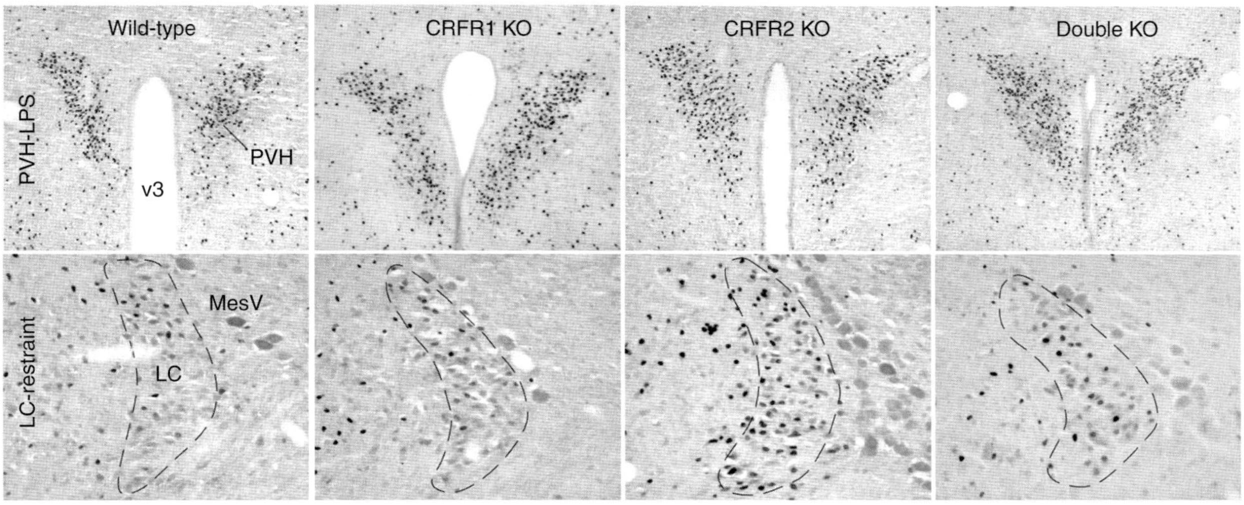

Figure 3 Stress-induced cellular activation of central autonomic cell groups in wild-type and corticotropin-releasing factor receptor (CRFR)-deficient mice. Immunohistochemical localization of Fos protein (a generic marker of neuronal activation) induced in the paraventricular nucleus (PVH; top) in response to a physiological stressor (intravenous lipopolysaccharide (LPS)), and in the locus coeruleus (LC) in response to an emotional stressor (30 min restraint), as a function of CRFR status. None of the CRFR knockouts (KOs) disrupt stress-induced responses in central autonomic system, which are enhanced in the LC of CRFR2 mutants. MesV, mesencephalic trigeminal nucleus; V3, third ventricle.

response to the same challenges (**Figure 3**). Mice lacking both receptors display stress-induced response profiles like those of CRFR1 mutant animals.

These findings define a basic paradox. On one hand, studies employing functional assays strongly support an involvement of the central CRF system in modulating endocrine, autonomic, and behavioral responses to stress and point toward CAS structures as key sites of action in this regard. Yet on the other hand, these cell groups display limited capacity for CRFR expression, and their engagement in response to ligand administration or stress is not critically dependent on the integrity of either or both of the known CRFRs.

Issues in Understanding CAS Activation by Central Peptide Administration and Stress

Questions remain as to the basis for signaling by CRF-related peptides at demonstrated sites of action that are known to exhibit limited expression of cognate ligands and/or receptors and as to how these elements participate in the response of CAS components to central administration of ligand or stress. A number of possible means for reconciling the seemingly pervasive ligand–receptor misalignment in this system may be considered.

CRFR Protein Expression

The lack of a firm understanding of CRFR distributions at the protein level remains a major impediment for work aimed at pinpointing central sites and mechanisms of peptide action. Immunohistochemical studies using a variety of CRFR antisera have been published, but these often describe results at odds with the consensus of analyses at the messenger RNA level, and not one has been conducted to an unimpeachable standard of histochemical rigor. There is abundant evidence to document axonal transport of receptors, which may undergo differential trafficking to assume distinctive intracellular localizations in different cell types. Thus, 'presynaptic' receptor localization may define substrates for reconciling instances of apparent mismatch, such as recent electrophysiological evidence supporting presynaptic CRFR1-mediated effects in the CeA. Moreover, stress-inducible expression of CRFR1 has been described in the PVH, as has a capacity for modulation of CRFR2 expression. The range of sites and conditions under which such capabilities may be manifested as receptor protein expression remains to be determined.

Novel Receptors?

As noted above, CAS activation induced by central peptide injection can be blocked in a dose-related manner by coadministration of CRFR antagonists but is unabated in mice lacking either or both of the known CRFRs. These findings are consistent with the existence of a novel CRFR expressed in one or more CAS components. It may be noted that three distinct CRFRs have been cloned in a catfish species, with all three subtypes exhibiting distinctive distributions, including in brain. Arguing against the existence of a third receptor is the fact that recently isolated receptor isoforms in other G-protein-coupled receptor families have all displayed structural similarities to existing receptors, and searches of human and mouse genome databases for genes related to sequences of various domains of the known CRFRs have failed to identify a gene with significant relatedness to CRFRs or other members of the secretin receptor family.

Receptor Cross-Talk

CAS activation observed in intracerebroventricular injection studies could be a result of interaction of CRF peptides with heterologous receptors. There are precedents for a degree of promiscuity among some subgroups of G-protein-coupled receptors, which may bind more than one structurally related ligand. While there appears to be no precedent for such cross-talk in the CRF system, several members of the secretin receptor family, including receptors for glucagon-like peptide 1, pituitary adenylate cyclase-activating peptide, and vasoactive intestinal polypeptide, are distributed in at least some CAS components and could comprise pharmacologic targets for CRF-related ligands. Further structural characterization of the ligand-binding domains of secretin receptor family members should help define potential participants in such interactions, and their involvement can then be tested using pharmacologic and genetic tools.

Interaction of CRFR- and CRFR2-Dependent Mechanisms

Whether or not the central CRF system proves to be indispensably involved in any given mode of stress adaptation, a growing body of evidence supports an interaction of CRFR1- and CRFR2-dependent mechanisms in shaping such responses. The generally hypo- and hyper-responsive phenotypes of CRFR1 and CRFR2-deficient mice, respectively, may be viewed as indicative of antagonistic interactions. However, there is evidence from both genetic and pharmacologic studies that the two receptors' influences on feeding suppression, anxiety, and HPA axis activation may be cooperative and exerted over distinct time domains. Studies of ligand and stress effects in CRFR-mutant mice provide ample evidence of receptor interplay in CAS sites of action for the above-mentioned responses. The anatomical organization that provides for convergent CRFR influences on a wide range of stress-related endpoints is completely obscure.

Other Ligand-Binding Proteins

A CRF-binding protein (CRF-BP) distinct from CRFRs was isolated as a circulating factor capable of binding and reversibly neutralizing CRF actions, thus preventing inappropriate pituitary–adrenal activation during pregnancy in primates. The CRF-BP is expressed prominently in brain, where its distribution suggests multiple potential sites and modes of interaction with CRF. The question of whether the CRF-BP may serve roles beyond its capacity to passively sequester peptide remains controversial. From synthetic CRF fragments that are bound with high affinity by the CRF-BP, but not either CRFR, evidence has been obtained to support an active role for the BP in signaling. This may be significant as the CRF-BP is more broadly expressed in the CAS than either known CRFR.

In a similar vein, a novel CRFR2α variant has been recently cloned and expressed, and its truncated form predicts that it exists as a soluble receptor (CRFR2α-S). Its abundance in brain rivals that of the membrane-bound form, raising the possibility that CRFR2α-S may serve a role in modulating signaling by CRFR2 agonists. The fact that the reported central distribution of the soluble receptor more closely mimics that of CRFR1 than CRFR2 is ostensibly at odds with this view.

Role of Ucns

Like other CRFR agonists tested to date, central administration of Ucn 2 or 3 strongly activates CAS cell groups; unexpectedly, though, sites of CRFR2 expression are unresponsive. Resolution of this paradox is needed to understand the basis for CRFR2-mediated signaling and its interaction with CRFR1-dependent mechanisms. At least three alternate explanations of this phenomenology may be considered: that CRFR2 activation may be CRFR1-dependent, that the naturally occurring form(s) of Ucn 2 and 3 may differ in activity from those predicted by complementary DNA sequences, and that access of centrally administered CRFR2 agonists may be limited by the actions of CRFR2α-S. Interest in the central functions of Ucns centers about their capacities to elicit stresslike anorexic and anxiolytic behavior, actions originally attributed to CRF, and, as putative endogenous CRFR2 ligands, to modulate a range of CRFR1-mediated activities. Each of the Ucns displays a restricted and unique central distribution (**Figure 2**). Only Ucn 1 pathways have been found to innervate CAS structures (mainly NTS) with any prominence. Ucn 3-containing projections are best aligned with major sites of CRFR2 expression in limbic forebrain (lateral septum, medial amygdala, ventromedial hypothalamus), which have the capacity to influence CAS mechanisms, albeit indirectly.

Significance

A wealth of evidence has implicated the central CRF system in the modulation of neuroendocrine, autonomic, and behavioral responses to stress, and CAS cell groups have been repeatedly implicated as important sites of action in this regard. Studies involving repeated or chronic central administration of CRF have implicated elevated peptide levels in the genesis of stress-related physiological and behavioral disorders. Nevertheless, the relative paucity of evidence for cellular expression of CRFRs within the CAS and the general failure of pharmacologic or genetic disruption of CRFR signaling to mitigate stress-induced CAS activational responses pose stern questions as to mechanisms that provide for CRF system involvement in stress adaptations. Small-molecule CRFR1 antagonists are currently being evaluated in clinical trials for the treatment of major depression, other anxiety-related disorders, and at least one systemic condition, irritable bowel syndrome. Additional applications of drugs that target this signaling system in a range of stress-related illnesses are being explored avidly. Deeper understanding of the sites and mechanisms through which such agents act is essential to exploiting them in an informed and effective manner.

See Also the Following Articles

Chronic (Repeated) Stress: Consequences, Adaptations; Corticotropin-Releasing Hormone and Urocortins: Binding Proteins and Receptors; Stress: Definition and History; Stress: Homeostasis, Rheostasis, Allostasis and Allostatic Load; Stress Response: Neural and Feedback Regulation of the HPA Axis; Sympathetic Noradrenergic and Adrenomedullary Hormonal Systems in Stress and Distress; Sympathoadrenal System: Neural Arm of the Stress Response.

Further Reading

Bakshi, V. P., Smith-Roe, S., Newman, S. M., Grigoriadis, D. E. and Kalin, N. H. (2002). Reduction of stress-induced behavior by antagonism of corticotropin-releasing hormone 2 (CRH2) receptors in lateral septum or CRH1 receptors in amygdala. *Journal of Neuroscience* **22**, 2926–2935.

Bale, T. L. and Vale, W. W. (2004). CRF and CRF receptors: Role in stress responsivity and other behaviors. *Annual Review of Pharmacology and Toxicology* **44**, 525–572.

Bittencourt, J. C. and Sawchenko, P. E. (2000). Do centrally administered neuropeptides access cognate receptors?: An analysis in the central corticotropin-releasing factor system. *Journal of Neuroscience* **20**, 1142–1156.

Chadwick, D. J., Marsh, J. and Ackrill, K. (eds.) (1993). *Corticotropin-Releasing Factor, Ciba Foundation Symposium 172*. London: Wiley.

Dautzenberg, F. M., Kilpatrick, G. J., Hauger, R. L. and Moreau, J-L (2001). Molecular biology of the CRH receptors – in the mood. *Peptides* **22**, 753–760.

De Souza, E. B. and Nemeroff, C. B. (eds.) (1990). *Corticotropin-Releasing Factor: Basic and Clinical Studies of a Neuropeptide*. Boca Raton, FL: CRC Press.

Grammatopoulos, D. K. and Chrousos, G. P. (2002). Functional characteristics of CRH receptors and potential clinical applications of CRH-receptor antagonists. *Trends in Endocrinology and Metabolism* **13**, 436–444.

Herkenham, M. (1987). Mismatches between neurotransmitter and receptor localizations in brain: Observations and implications. *Neuroscience* **23**, 1–38.

Radulovic, J., Ruhmann, A., Liepold, T. and Spiess, J. (1999). Modulation of learning and anxiety by corticotropin-releasing factor (CRF) and stress: Differential roles of CRF receptors 1 and 2. *Journal of Neuroscience* **19**, 5016–5025.

Saper, C. B. (1995). Central autonomic system. In: Paxinos, G. (ed.) *The Rat Nervous System* (2nd edn., pp. 107–128). San Diego, CA: Academic Press.

Spina, M., Merlo-Pich, E., Chan, R. K. W., et al. (1996). Appetite-suppressing effects of urocortin, a CRF-related neuropeptide. *Science* **273**, 1561–1564.

Van Pett, K., Viau, V., Bittencourt, J. C., et al. (2000). Distribution of mRNAs encoding CRF receptors in brain and pituitary of rat and mouse. *Journal of Comparative Neurology* **428**, 191–212.

Vaughan J., Donaldson C., Bittencourt J., et al. (1995) Urocortin, a mammalian neuropeptide related to fish urotensin I and to corticotropin-releasing factor. *Nature* 378: 287–292.

Amygdala

M S Fanselow and R Ponnusamy
University of California, Los Angeles, CA, USA

This is a revised version of the article by M S Fanselow and G D Dale, Encyclopedia of Stress, First edition, volume 1, pp 178–182, © 2000, Elsevier Inc.

Glossary

Central nucleus of the amygdala (CeA)	This striatal-like nucleus is considered the motor interface of the amygdala.
Lateral amygdala (LA) and basolateral amygdala (BLA)	These cortical-like structures are considered the sensory interface for the amygdala's role in fear, anxiety, and stress.
Long-term potentiation (LTP)	A relatively long-lasting form of synaptic plasticity that has been proposed as a mechanism that mediates some forms of learning and memory
Pavlovian fear conditioning	A learning paradigm in which an aversive event is paired with neutral stimuli, resulting in a variety of defensive behavioral and autonomic conditional responses to the previously neutral stimulus. It is the natural way that defensive behavior is controlled but can also contribute to anxiety disorders. In the laboratory it has become a standard way to assess learning and memory.

Introduction

The amygdala, an almond-shaped cluster of interconnected nuclei in the medial temporal lobe, may be the neural structure most intimately tied to emotion. It has long been known that damage to the amygdala produces disturbances in emotional behavior. The linkage is particularly compelling in the case of negative emotions such as fear. In both human and nonhuman animals, fear-related behavior, which is typically analyzed with Pavlovian fear conditioning, depends on the amygdala. Humans with bilateral amygdala damage have difficulty in recognizing the negative emotions in the facial expression of others and as a result may make inappropriate social advances. Rats with lesions of the amygdala lose their fear of cats. Additionally, the ability of emotion to influence declarative memory storage (flash bulb memories) is mediated by the amygdala. The amygdala is well situated for a role in stress and emotion. Features of the environment, initially processed by several different brain regions, converge on the amygdala. Much of this information relates to external and internal stress. Plasticity within certain nuclei of the amygdala allows this structure to connect these stressors with environmental features that predict stress. Therefore, it may also act as a feedforward device that generates behavior in anticipation of stress. This article first reviews the major afferents to the amygdala that bring it this environmental information. Then it turns to the efferents that project to the brain regions that generate behavioral responses to stress. It concludes with a description of the processing that goes on within the amygdala that enables this feedforward regulation of stress.

Multiple Sources of Input: Afferents to Amygdala

Nucleus Tractus Solitarius

The nucleus tractus solitarius (NTS) projects to the amygdala's central nucleus (CeA), both directly and indirectly, via the parabrachial nucleus. A large body of evidence implicates the NTS in stress-related responses. It receives first-order projections from several cranial nerves, including the vagus. These inputs primarily reflect the contribution of visceral sensory information but also convey general somatic input. In addition, ascending pain-related fibers originating from the spinal cord terminate in the NTS. Thus, the NTS can provide the amygdala with visceral sensory, somatosensory, and pain-related information.

Thalamus

The amygdala receives a wide range of sensory information via monosynaptic projections from the thalamus. Considerable functional importance has been attributed to projections from the posterior thalamus to the amygdala. The moderate projection from the paraventricular nucleus terminates in the medial and ventrolateral divisions of the lateral amygdala (LA). Those arising from the medial geniculate provide the LA with auditory information. Pain information represented in the posterior intralaminar nucleus of the thalamus also project to several amygdaloid nuclei. Stimulation of these posterior thalamic projections to the LA can support Pavlovian fear conditioning to an auditory cue. Somatosensory regions of the thalamus are an important route of unconditional stimulus transmission to the amygdala in fear conditioning. However, information about the unconditional somatosensory stimulus is also transmitted from other sources that send fibers through (but do not form essential synapses in) the thalamus en route to the amygdala. The CeA may receive direct thalamic inputs about the conditional stimulus as well as nociceptive stimuli. Furthermore, parts of the ventroposterior medial thalamic nucleus that primarily receive visceral and gustatory information project to the amygdala. These projections may support the amygdala's role in avoidance of novel flavors. In summary, the thalamus is a significant and direct source of information about the internal and external milieu for the amygdala.

Periaqueductal Gray

The midbrain periaqueductal gray (PAG) is the key structure for integrated defensive behavior. While much emphasis has been placed on descending projections from the amygdala to PAG (see later), these projections are largely reciprocal. There are strong projections from PAG to amygdala, particularly to the CeA. In certain situations, lesions of the dorsolateral PAG will enhance conditional fear responses that depend on the amygdala. This has led to the suggestion that the ascending projections from the dorsolateral PAG may exert an inhibitory influence on the amygdala.

Temporal, Insular, and Parietal Cortex

There is a massive exchange of information between the amygdala and the cortex. Along with the sensory projections from the thalamus, the amygdala receives both modality-specific and multimodal neocortical projections. Unimodal projections coding aspects of visual, auditory, and somatosensory information project primarily to the LA and the basolateral nucleus (BLA). Importantly, these projections tend not to originate from the primary sensory cortex. Rather, unimodal sensory information originates from secondary sensory regions. For example, auditory projections arise from Te2 and Te3, and visual information arrives through the perirhinal cortex. The insular cortex, which receives monosynaptic projections from the primary somatosensory cortex, sends substantial projections to both the BLA and LA. It has been suggested that these projections provide the amygdala with nociceptive information that can support fear conditioning.

The hippocampal formation receives some of the most highly preprocessed information in the brain. This component of the temporal cortex projects to the amygdala via sparse projections from the entorhinal cortex, CA1, and subiculum. Fibers from the entorhinal cortex and subiculum pass through the ventral angular bundle, and electrical stimulation of this tract results in a monosynaptic response in the BLA. These projections seems to play an important role in providing contextual or place information for amygdala-dependent behaviors, as lesions of this tract produce deficits in contextual fear conditioning. At least as far as simple emotion-related behaviors are concerned, the thalamo-amygdala and cortico-amygdala circuits appear to have some redundant function and act compensatorily because damage in both pathways appears necessary to eliminate amygdala-dependent behaviors. It is possible that the cortical pathways may allow amygdala-dependent stress responses to be more finely contoured to the specifics of environmental stimulation, but such an analysis has not been performed.

Frontal Cortex

The infralimbic (IL) region of the medial prefrontal cortex strongly projects to the intercalated cells in the amygdala. In turn, intercalated cells project to the CeA. Lesions of IL impair extinction, and electrical stimulation of IL reduces the expression of conditional fear. Therefore, it has been proposed that insufficient inhibition of the amygdala by the medial prefrontal cortex could predispose an individual to develop anxiety disorders. Thus, in terms of cortical information, the amygdala predominately receives highly processed sensory representations that likely play important roles in the coordination of appropriate behavioral responses.

Summary

A diverse array of neural pathways brings the amygdala a wide range of environmental information. Inputs from various functional systems terminate in certain amygdaloid nuclei, and, therefore, different nuclear divisions are exposed to different sets of information. Note that the same divisions might receive inputs from various sources. These interdivisional projections provide a route by which the various kinds of information entering the different portions of amygdala can be associated. In addition to convergence, parallel distribution of information from the same source to multiple amygdaloid areas is another typical feature in the organization of amygdaloid inputs. Most of this sensory information has been highly processed before it arrives at the amygdala. This suggests that the amygdala may provide an information-integrating function in the regulation of stress.

Variegated Outputs: Efferents from Amygdala

In addition to providing reciprocal projections to many of the sensory regions from which it receives input, the amygdala also sends efferent projections to regions responsible for behavioral, autonomic, and endocrine responses to stress. These outputs are organized in a point-to-point manner. It also provides parallel outputs to multifunctional systems, and there are also parallel outputs from various amygdaloid nuclei to the same functional system. These anatomical relationships allow amygdala activity to influence the unconditional response to stress and also to provide substrates by which stimuli predictive of impending stressors can produce anticipatory behavioral adjustments.

Hypothalamus

Physical stress produces a variety of neuroendocrine responses, including increases in plasma adrenocorticotropin (ACTH), corticosterone, norepinephrine, and epinephrine. Control of these responses is mediated in part by a direct action of the hypothalamic paraventricular nucleus on pituitary secretion. The paraventricular hypothalamus has been shown to receive direct projections from the CeA, providing a pathway by which amygdala activity can contribute to endocrine stress responses. A variety of studies have demonstrated a role for the amygdala in the expression of neuroendocrine responses to stress. Lesions of the amygdala attenuate the elevation of plasma epinephrine, norepinephrine, and corticosterone normally observed following footshock, and similarly attenuate the elevation of plasma ACTH produced by immobilization stress but do not completely block these responses. However, given that amygdala lesions do not completely block or alter baseline hormone levels, it is possible that the amygdala lesion-induced attenuation of hormone responses reflects disruption of feedforward amygdala-dependent conditional responses rather than an amygdala control of unconditional endocrine responses.

Projections from the LA and the BLA to the hypothalamus are light and target the lateral hypothalamic area. However, the CeA provides substantial inputs to a larger number of hypothalamic nuclei. Most of the projections originate in the medial division. Moderate to heavy projections are directed to the medial and lateral preoptic area, lateral hypothalamus, and paraventricular nucleus. Lesions of both the CeA of the amygdala and the lateral hypothalamus block the increase in arterial blood pressure caused by a conditional fear stimulus, leading to the suggestion that projections from the amygdala to the lateral hypothalamus mediate this response. Importantly, the hypertension to the shock unconditional response remains intact following hypothalamic lesions. In addition to these direct projections to the hypothalamus, the CeA has strong projections to the bed nuclei of the stria terminalis, which also innervates hypothalamic nuclei. Thus, the lateral hypothalamus seems to mediate conditional sympathetic autonomic arousal to fear stimuli via input from the CeA.

Periaqueductal Gray

The CeA projects heavily to the caudal half of the midbrain PAG. These projections initially innervate more dorsal regions of the PAG, areas that serve active or circa strike defensive behaviors and autonomic arousal. Stimulation of the medial and central amygdala inhibits the behaviors that are generated by stimulation of these dorsal regions of the PAG.

As one moves caudally in the PAG, the CeA projections gradually rotate to innervate the ventral portions of the PAG. These ventral PAG areas are essential for conditional fear-related defenses such as freezing. This area is also critical for the opioid analgesia that accompanies fear. Consistent with this pattern, cells in the caudal ventral PAG express c-fos following fear conditioning. However, this part of the PAG is not critical for the autonomic responses to conditional fear stimuli. The amygdala, predominantly through projection emanating from the CeA, exerts control over species-specific defensive behaviors organized by the PAG.

Brain Stem

The CeA sends projections throughout the brain stem. One function of these projections is to provide control over autonomic function. For example, stimulation of the rabbit's CeA causes a heart rate deceleration mediated by monosynaptic projections to the dorsal motor nucleus of the vagus. This response mimics the bradycardia rabbits show to conditional fear stimuli, which also depends on the CeA. While amygdala lesions block the bradycardiac conditional response to the stimulus paired with electric shock, it is important to note that these lesions do not affect baseline heart rate or the unconditional heart rate orienting response to the conditional stimulus in rabbits. Thus, projections from the CeA to brain stem autonomic nuclei may mediate parasympathetically controlled conditional responses.

Amygdala stimulation enhances reflexes organized in the brain stem such as eyeblink and startle. There are both mono- and disynaptic projections from the CeA to the nucleus reticularis pontis caudalis, which is the part of the brain stem acoustic startle circuit that is modulated by conditional fear stimuli. It has previously been shown in rats, cats, rabbits, and monkeys, using various anterograde tracers, that CeA neurons project to brain stem areas including the NTS. These results provide conclusive evidence for a GABAergic pathway from the CeA to the NTS. Although lesions of the amygdala block the ability of fear stimuli to modulate reflexes, it is important to note that the reflex itself is left intact.

Thus, projections from the CeA to several brain stem regions allow for widespread modulation of autonomic function and reflexive behaviors.

Cortex

In addition to the amygdala receiving substantial cortical projections, recent work suggests that it is in a position to exert widespread influence over cortical activity. Based on anterograde tracer studies, the LA provides strong, topographically organized inputs to the ventral and dorsal perirhinal cortices. The LA also provides a moderate input to the infralimbic cortex as well as to the ventral agranular insula. Projections from the BLA to the frontal cortex are more widespread than those from any other amygdaloid nucleus. The CeA sends substantial ascending projections to the cholinergic basal forebrain, which in turn projects diffusely to virtually all cortical regions. Basal forebrain stimulations produce desynchronization of cortical EEG, as does CeA stimulation. Basal forebrain stimulation supports associative changes in receptive field properties of auditory cortical neurons. Based on these findings, it has been suggested that cholinergic modulation of cortical activity, mediated by amygdala projections to the basal forebrain, is critical for the induction of the stimulus-specific changes in cortical receptive fields observed during Pavlovian fear conditioning.

Hippocampal Formation

In addition to modulating cortical dynamics, the amygdala also exerts a strong influence over hippocampal activity. The hippocampus is considered to be particularly susceptible to chronic stress because it is heavily enriched with corticosteroid receptors and it participates in the termination of stress responses via the glucocorticoid-mediated negative feedback of the hypothalamus-pituitary-adrenocortical (HPA) axis. Because this medial temporal lobe structure is crucial for declarative-explicit memory in humans and spatial-relational memory in rodents, evidence is emerging that stress generally impairs hippocampal-dependent memory tasks in both humans and rats. Lesions of the BLA attenuate the induction of long-term potentiation (LTP) in the dentate gyrus, while BLA stimulation significantly facilitates LTP induction. Recent findings indicate that amygdalar activity is crucially involved in the emergence of stress-induced impairments in hippocampal LTP and hippocampal-dependent spatial memory in rats. The critical period of the amygdalar contribution to stress effects on hippocampal functions was determined by applying muscimol either before or immediately after stress. Results indicate that intra-amygdalar muscimol infusions before restraint tailshock stress effectively blocked stress-induced physiological and behavioral effects. Thus, the amygdala plays a critical role in the induction of cortical- and hippocampal-dependent processes thought to underlie learning and memory.

Summary

The CeA, which receives input from most of the amygdala nuclei, projects to regions responsible for autonomic, hormonal, and behavioral responses. In this way, the amygdala is in a position to muster the full arsenal of the body's responses to stress.

Conclusions and Functions

There are numerous brain structures that are essential components of the neural circuitry mediating stress responses. The amygdala is one of the neural hubs integrating these components and stands in a position to both influence and be influenced by the stress response. Animal models of chronic stress reveal that stress-induced structural plasticity in amygdala neurons provides a candidate cellular substrate for affective disorders.

The amygdala receives a plethora of sensory input from both the environment and the body. Much of this input relates to stressful and threatening events. However, the amygdala also receives both simple and highly processed sensory information that can serve a signaling function. This suggests that the amygdala may integrate these sources of information. An early suggestion was that the amygdala recognizes signals for events with emotional significance. This is perhaps most clear in fear conditioning, in which cues that predict an event come to produce a number of fear-related responses. These behaviors are lost in rats, mice, rabbits, and humans, without an amygdala. There is an LTP of amygdala responses to stimulation of its thalamic, hippocampal, and cortical afferents. Cells in the LA receive both nociceptive somatosensory information and auditory information, and exposure to fear conditioning itself can potentiate the response of these cells. In this manner, stimuli that predict stress can come to activate the amygdala, even if they are not stressful in their own right. Thus, neural plasticity within the amygdala provides the ability for this structure to anticipate stress through learning processes such as Pavlovian fear conditioning. Consistent with such a view, the amygdala projects to most of the brain areas responsible for rapid coping with impending danger.

Under circumstances in which prolonged stress disrupts cognition that is mediated by the hippocampus, it facilitates amygdala-dependent cognition. More specifically, under circumstances in which chronic stress induces dendritic atrophy and debranching in CA3 pyramidal neurons of the hippocampus, it induces hypertrophy of pyramidal and stellate neurons in the LA, the BLA, and the bed nucleus of stria terminalis, an amygdaloid projection site central to anxiety. Chronic unpredictable stress, however, had little effect on pyramidal and stellate neurons and induced atrophy only in BLA bipolar neurons. Thus, stress hormones released as a result of stress-induced amygdala activity can strengthen the excitatory drive within the BLA and thereby influence subsequent information processing by the amygdala and its downstream targets. This suggests that chronic stress could lead to an imbalance in HPA axis function through a gradual gain in excitatory control exerted by the amygdala. In this way, a system that evolved to deal with immediate threats of great evolutionary urgency also has the ability to cause debilitating pathology. The amygdala allows organisms to better cope with future stress by modulating cortical, hippocampal, and striatal circuits involved in declarative memory and motor learning. Through such anticipatory mechanisms, the amygdala provides for the adaptive feedforward regulation of stress. But the amygdala's powerful and adaptive role in short-term emergencies may also leave it open to a role in pathology accompanying chronic stress.

See Also the Following Articles

Brain and Brain Regions.

Further Reading

Aggleton, J. P. (2000). *The amygdala: a functional analysis* (2nd edn). New York: Oxford University Press Inc.

Bechara, A., Tranel, D., Damasio, H., et al. (1995). Double dissociation of conditioning and declarative knowledge relative to the amygdala and hippocampus in humans. *Science* **269**(5227), 1115–1118.

Cahill, L. and McGaugh, J. L. (1998). Mechanisms of emotional arousal and lasting declarative memory. *Trends in Neuroscience* **21**(7), 294–299.

Fanselow, M. S. (1994). Neural organization of the defensive behavior system responsible for fear. *Psychonomic Bulletin and Review* **1**, 429–438.

Fendt, M. and Fanselow, M. S. (1999). The neuroanatomical and neurochemical basis of conditioned fear. *Neuroscience and Biobehavioral Reviews* **23**, 743–760.

Kim, J. J., Koo, J. W., Lee, H. J. and Han, J. S. (2005). Amygdalar inactivation blocks stress-induced impairments in hippocampal long-term potentiation and spatial memory. *Journal of Neuroscience* **25**(6), 1532–1539.

LeDoux, J. E. (1996). *The emotional brain: the mysterious underpinnings of emotional life*. New York: Simon & Schuster.

Maren, S. and Fanselow, M. S. (1995). Synaptic plasticity in the basolateral amygdala induced by hippocampal formation stimulation in vivo. *Journal of Neuroscience* **15**(11), 7548–7564.

Maren, S. and Fanselow, M. S. (1996). The amygdala and fear conditioning: has the nut been cracked? *Neuron* **16**(2), 237–240.

Pare, D., Quirk, G. J. and Ledoux, J. E. (2004). New vistas on amygdala networks in conditioned fear. *Journal of Neurophysiology* **92**(1), 1–9.

Rizvi, T. A., Ennis, M., Behbehani, M. M. and Shipley, M. T. (1991). Connections between the central nucleus of the amygdala and the midbrain periaqueductal gray: topography and reciprocity. *Journal of Comparative Neurology* **303**(1), 121–131.

Roozendaal, B., Koolhaas, J. M. and Bohus, B. (1991). Attenuated cardiovascular, neuroendocrine, and behavioral responses after a single footshock in central amygdaloid lesioned male rats. *Physiology Behavior* **50**(4), 771–775.

Shi, C. and Davis, M. (1999). Pain pathways involved in fear conditioning measured with fear-potentiated startle: lesion studies. *Journal of Neuroscience* **19**(1), 420–430.

Vyas, A., Mitra, R., Shankaranarayana Rao, B. S. and Chattarji, S. (2002). Chronic stress induces contrasting patterns of dendritic remodeling in hippocampal and amygdaloid neurons. *Journal of Neuroscience* **22**(15), 6810–6818.

Walker, D. L., Toufexis, D. J. and Davis, M. (2003). Role of the bed nucleus of the stria terminalis versus the amygdala in fear, stress, and anxiety. *European Journal of Pharmacology* **463**(1-3), 199–216.

Acute Stress Response: Experimental

K Pacak
National Institute of Neurological Disorders and Stroke and National Institute of Child Health and Human Development, National Institutes of Health, Bethesda, MD, USA
R McCarty
University of Virginia, Charlottesville, VA, USA

This article is reproduced from Encyclopedia of Stress, First edition, volume 1, pp 8–16, © 2000, Elsevier Inc.

Glossary

Footshock — A laboratory stressor that involves placing a laboratory rat or mouse into a chamber with a floor of metal rods spaced equally apart. Scrambled electric current of known intensity is passed through the metal rods and this results in a mildly painful stimulus to the animal's footpads. This has been a favored stressor in many laboratories because the intensity, duration, and frequency of the footshocks are under the control of the experimenter.

Hemorrhage — An acute decrease in blood volume. In laboratory studies, hemorrhage has been employed as a physiological stressor and blood is often withdrawn via an arterial or venous catheter.

Hypoglycemia — A reduction in blood glucose levels. This physiological change has been employed as a stressor in laboratory studies and insulin is often administered to effect a reduction in blood glucose.

Immobilization — Often employed as a laboratory stressor, immobilization involves restricting the movement of a laboratory animal (typically a rat or mouse) by taping its limbs to padded metal mounts affixed to a frame. A variation on this approach includes restraint, where an animal's movement is restricted by placing it into a plexiglas cylinder.

Neuroendocrine signature — The concept that exposure to a given stressor elicits a pattern of neuroendocrine responses that is specific to that stressor.

Overview of Acute Stress Responses

Humans and animals respond to exposure to a particular stressor by mobilizing a host of neural, neuroendocrine, endocrine, and metabolic systems. Each stressor produces a specific neurochemical signature, with quantitatively if not qualitatively distinct central and peripheral mechanisms involved. These neurochemical changes occur not in isolation but rather in concert with physiological, behavioral, and even experiential changes. In evolutionary terms, natural selection has favored this pattern of coordinated stress responses by enhancing the survival and propagation of genes. This pattern of stress responsiveness is referred to by Goldstein as "primitive specificity." These and other findings are included in the description of acute stress responses that follows.

A stressor may be viewed as a stimulus that disrupts homeostasis. Stressors may be divided into several groups based upon their character, duration, and intensity. Regarding duration, stressors may be characterized as acute (single, intermittent, and time-limited exposure versus continuous exposure) or chronic (intermittent and prolonged exposure versus continuous exposure).

Physical stressors include cold, heat, intense radiation, noise, vibration, and many others. Chemical stressors include ether, all poisons, and insulin. Pain stress may be elicited by many different chemical and physical agents. Psychological stressors profoundly affect emotional processes and may result in behavioral changes such as anxiety, fear, or frustration. Social stressors include an animal's placement into the territory of a dominant animal and in humans unemployment and marital separation among others. Many stressors used in animal research, however, are mixed and act in concert, such as handling, immobilization, anticipation of a painful stimulus, and hemorrhage with hypotension.

In terms of duration, stressors may be divided into two main categories: acute versus chronic stressors. It should be noted that many stressors differ in their intensity. The adaptive responses that are elicited in response to an acute stressor include the physiological and behavioral processes that are essential to reestablish homeostatic balance. During an acute stress response, physiological processes are important to redirect energy utilization among various organs and selectively inhibit or stimulate various organ systems or their components to mobilize energy reserves and to be prepared for exposure to additional, unpredictable challenges. Thus, upon exposure to metabolic stressors, certain tissues tend to reduce their consumption of energy while others, especially those that are important for locomotor activity, receive sufficient nutrients to function properly. The central nervous system also has priority during metabolic stress responses and preferentially receives a sufficient amount of nutrients from the circulation. The increased supply of energy to crucial organs is achieved preferentially by release of catecholamines and glucocorticoids that in general increase gluconeogenesis and glycogenolysis, inhibit glucose uptake, and enhance proteolysis and lipolysis. The immune system is another essential component of these physiologically adaptive stress responses.

Behavioral adaptation is viewed as a facilitation of adaptive and an inhibition of nonadaptive central and peripheral neural pathways that enable an organism to cope successfully with stressful situations. These behavioral responses include altered cognitive and sensory thresholds, increased alertness, selective memory enhancement, suppression of feeding and reproductive behaviors, and stress-induced analgesia. If physiological or behavioral responses fail to reestablish homeostasis or are excessive and abnormal, diseases of adaptation may be more likely to occur in susceptible individuals. This is apparent upon exposure to chronic or repeated stressors but may happen as well during acute stress reactions in a situation where the intensity of the stressor is abnormally high. Both physiological and behavioral responses are affected by activation of the primary stress effector systems, including the sympathetic nervous system (norepinephrine release), the adrenomedullary system (epinephrine release), the hypothalamic-pituitary-adrenocortical system [adrenocorticotropic hormone (ACTH) and glucocorticoid release], the parasympathetic nervous system (acetylcholine release), and the renin-angiotensin system (renin release from juxtaglomerular cells in the kidney). Several other systems contribute to a reestablishment of homeostasis, including the hypothalamic-pituitary-thyroid axis (e.g., responsive to cold and heat), the hypothalamic-pituitary-gonadal axis (temporary decrease in reproductive function to shift energy to other more important organ systems), release of growth hormone, and changes in immune function. All of these systems act directly by altering the release or the biological effects of many mediators of acute stress responses (e.g., neurotransmitters, hormones, cytokines, etc.) or they act indirectly by altering levels of monitored variables, with consequent reflexive adjustments determined by internal homeostats.

Stress-Responsive Neuroendocrine Systems

Included below are some examples of ways in which the major stress-responsive physiological systems are altered following exposure to acute stressors.

Hypothalamic-Pituitary-Adrenocortical Axis

The hypothalamic-pituitary-adrenocortical axis is one of the main effector systems that is activated in animals upon exposure to an acute stressor. Generally via several feedback mechanisms at different levels, glucocorticoids released from the adrenal cortex regulate their own synthesis and secretion by actions within the adrenal gland (inhibition of glucocorticoid synthesis), the anterior pituitary (inhibition of corticotrophs), and the hypothalamus [inhibition of corticotropin-releasing hormone (CRH) synthesis and secretion] as well as higher brain centers (e.g., hippocampus). Glucocorticoids readily penetrate the blood–brain barrier and suppress acute stress-induced increases in central neural levels of norepinephrine. Norepinephrine is thought to be the most potent stimulator of CRH neurons within the hypothalamic paraventricular nucleus. Thus, central noradrenergic neurons that terminate in the paraventricular nucleus and synapse on CRH neurons are generally believed to be the site of another negative feedback mechanism by which glucocorticoids attenuate neuroendocrine responses to acute stressors.

During an acute stress response, ACTH and glucocorticoids vary depending on the type and intensity of the stressful stimulus. Exposure of animals to cold stress evokes a very modest increase in plasma ACTH, exposure of animals to hemorrhage or hypoglycemia evokes ACTH responses that reflect the intensity of the stimulus, pain elicits moderate ACTH responses, and immobilization for 120 min evokes the greatest increase in plasma levels of ACTH. The correlation between norepinephrine release in the hypothalamic paraventricular nucleus and plasma ACTH responses may demonstrate the participation of paraventricular norepinephrine in stress-induced activation of the hypothalamic-pituitary-adrenocortical axis (**Figure 1**). Although a strong correlation is found between norepinephrine responses in the paraventricular nucleus and plasma ACTH responses during exposure to different stressors, such correlations may not reflect causal interrelationships. During exposure to metabolic stressors such as hypoglycemia or hemorrhage, increments in plasma ACTH are much higher than those of norepinephrine in the paraventricular nucleus, suggesting that some other paraventricular neurotransmitter or extraparaventricular neuromediators participate in the regulation of the hypothalamic-pituitary-adrenocortical axis following exposure to these stressors. Exposure to pain elicited marked norepinephrine responses in the paraventricular nucleus and moderate plasma ACTH responses, suggesting that paraventricular norepinephrine is responsible for the activation of the hypothalamic-pituitary-adrenocortical axis upon

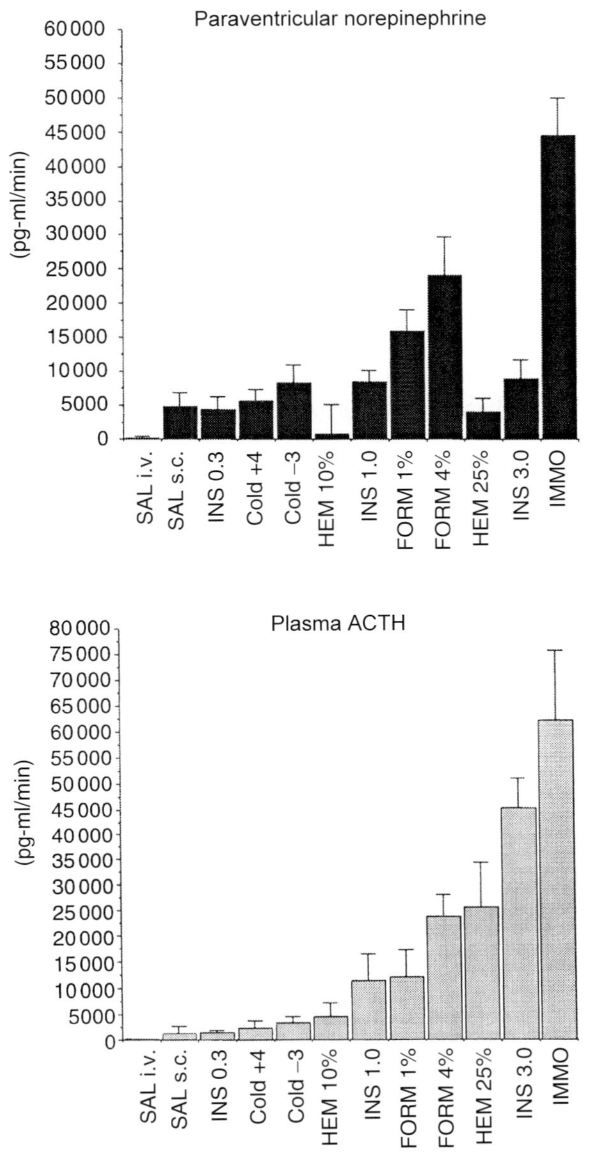

Figure 1 Area under curve measures for microdialysate levels of norepinephrine in the hypothalamic paraventricular nucleus and plasma levels of ACTH from animals exposed to a variety of stressors.

exposure to pain stress. During immobilization stress, the relationship between paraventricular norepinephrine and plasma ACTH was intermediate, suggesting that both paraventricular norepinephrine and other paraventricular and extraparaventricular neuromediators participate in the regulation of the hypothalamic-pituitary-adrenocortical axis during immobilization stress. Cold stress elicited only minimal paraventricular norepinephrine and plasma ACTH responses, suggesting that other neuroendocrine axes (e.g., thyroid axis) participate in the regulation of homeostasis during acute exposure to cold.

Acute activation of the hypothalamic-pituitary-adrenocortical axis is attended by elevations of plasma glucocorticoids that exert many metabolic effects to mobilize energy necessary for survival of the organism and restoration of homeostasis. Regulatory metabolic effects include gluconeogenesis, glycogenolysis, lipolysis, inhibition of lipogenesis, and proteolysis. Other regulatory effects include anti-inflammatory, anti-allergic, and behavioral effects. Permissive effects of glucocorticoids are important for other hormones or factors to function properly (e.g., catecholamine-induced vascular resistance and cardiac performance are decreased in cases of adrenal insufficiency). Generally, permissive effects of glucocorticoids are responsible for maintenance of a basal or resting state, while regulatory effects are seen when glucocorticoids reach abnormally high concentrations such as when an animal is exposed to an acute and extremely intense stressor.

Hypothalamic-Pituitary-Gonadal Axis

Exposure of animals and humans to acute stress is associated with small and often short-lived increases in plasma luteinizing hormone and androgens. In humans, acute stress-induced increases in androgens appear to be caused by an alteration in plasma volume and a decrease in androgen metabolic clearance rather than from a net increase in androgen release. The mechanisms by which luteinizing hormone is increased under stress conditions are not clear but one possibility is that high levels of ACTH may stimulate gonadotropin hormone-releasing hormone neurons in the hypothalamus. Stress-induced responses are also dependent upon estrogen levels. Thus, in female animals during proestrous or in gonadectomized animals there is no increase in luteinizing hormone upon exposure to acute stress, but instead a rapid decrease in circulating luteinizing hormone may be observed. Norepinephrine and serotonin as well as interleukin-1 also participate in the regulation of the hypothalamic-pituitary-gonadal axis during acute stress and most likely exert inhibitory effects on gonadotropin-releasing hormone neurons or luteinizing hormone. Follicle-stimulating hormone may follow the same stress response pattern as luteinizing hormone, but often the changes are very small or do not occur at all. The presence of circulating estradiol may provide some protection against the adverse and inhibitory effects of acute stress on the gonadal axis.

In contrast, upon exposure to chronic stress, there are decreases in reproductive function to conserve and redirect energy for other organ systems that are vital for immediate survival. Such inhibition occurs at all levels, including the hypothalamus (inhibition of gonadotropin hormone-releasing hormone secretion), the anterior pituitary (inhibition of luteinizing hormone release), and the gonads (reduced sex hormone secretion). Stress-induced activation of the hypothalamic-pituitary-adrenocortical axis is one of the main factors contributing to this inhibition of gonadal function since corticotropin-releasing hormone and glucocorticoids are known to inhibit gonadotropin hormone-releasing hormone. In addition, glucocorticoids exert inhibitory effects at the level of the anterior pituitary and the gonads.

Sex differences in stress-induced regulation and in responses of primary stress effector systems exist and the presence of circulating estrogen and androgen has been implicated in these differences. It is postulated that estrogens and androgens are responsible for sex hormone-dependent brain organization that reflects differences in responsiveness to stress. For example, estrogen effects on corticotropin-releasing hormone expression may be related to greater stress-induced hypothalamic-pituitary-adrenocortical responses and for a higher incidence of depression, anxiety, and other disorders in human females exposed to stress. In experimental animals, these sex differences are eliminated following surgical removal of the gonads.

Hypothalamic-Pituitary-Growth Axis

It is well documented that acute exposure to various stressors (e.g., hypoglycemia, exercise, hemorrhage, pain) increases secretion of growth hormone from the pituitary gland. In contrast, other stressors such as cold, handling, hypertonic saline, and electric shock produce marked decreases in plasma growth hormone levels. Acute administration of glucocorticoids also increases growth hormone less concentrations in plasma. Thus, it appears that acute stress responses that are associated with elevations in plasma glucocorticoid levels may increase plasma growth hormone levels through stimulation of the growth hormone gene via glucocorticoid-responsive elements in its promoter region.

In contrast, chronic stress (a state of chronically elevated circulating levels of glucocorticoids) inhibits growth hormone release from the anterior pituitary gland and increases resistance of peripheral tissues to the actions of insulin-like growth factors (e.g., IGF-1). Such inhibition may occur via corticotropin-releasing hormone-induced increases in somatostatin secretion. Thus, dwarfism that occurs in an environment of severe and chronic psychosocial deprivation may reflect a chronically inhibited growth axis.

Little is known about the neural pathways that are involved in stress-induced activation or inhibition of growth hormone secretion. Some evidence suggests that growth hormone responses correlate with changes in catecholamine content in several hypothalamic nuclei, including the paraventricular, dorsomedial, and arcuate nuclei, but more detailed and sophisticated studies are needed to clarify the involvement of catecholamines and other neurotransmitters or neuromodulators in stress-induced growth hormone axis regulation.

Hypothalamic-Pituitary-Thyroid Axis

In contrast to mildly stressful situations, high-intensity stress-induced activation of the hypothalamic-pituitary-adrenocortical axis is associated with inhibition of the thyroid axis. This inhibitory action is reflected by a decrease in release/production of hypothalamic thyrotropin-releasing hormone, decreased production/secretion of thyroid-stimulating hormone, and by inhibition of conversion of thyroxine to the more biological active triiodothyronine in peripheral tissues. The exception to this pattern is exposure to acute cold stress, forced swimming, or noise stress where profound thyroid axis activation occurs. This is not surprising since during cold exposure, an organism needs to generate significant amounts of energy to maintain body temperature and thyroid hormones are known to increase heat production and therefore core temperature. Upon exposure to cold stress, there is increased secretion of hypothalamic thyrotropin-releasing hormone, which leads to increases in release of thyroxine within 15–20 min and triiodothyronine within 1–2 h. The mechanism by which cold-induced activation of thyrotropin-releasing hormone occurs is not fully understood, although catecholamines are thought to participate in this process. It is well known that in a hypothyroid state, plasma catecholamines are elevated and during a hyperthyroid state plasma catecholamines are either unchanged or decreased. In thyroidectomized rats, larger increments in plasma epinephrine and norepinephrine occur during cold exposure, suggesting compensatory activation of catecholamine secretion as a result of the loss of the thyroid gland. The organism is faced with difficulty in maintaining body temperature when the hypothalamic-pituitary-thyroid axis is unable to enhance thermogenesis.

The reason that the thyroid axis is inhibited upon exposure to other stressors is unknown but one possible explanation is that an organism conserves energy necessary for survival and restoration of homeostasis. Corticotropin-releasing hormone, somatostatin, and cytokines (e.g., IL-1 and IL-6) most likely contribute to acute stress-induced inhibition of the thyroid axis.

Prolactin

Prolactin is another anterior pituitary hormone that is increased during exposure of animals to various stressors such as exercise, hypoglycemia, hemorrhage, immobilization, and pain stress. Other situations associated with elevated plasma prolactin levels are nipple stimulation during lactation, chest wall lesions (herpes, incisions), and the acute stress of blood withdrawal. The mechanisms by which acute stressors increase prolactin secretion remain unknown. The physiological consequences of prolactin hypersecretion during stress are not clear, although it is hypothesized that prolactin enhances immune function.

Immune System

The immune system is an important component of acute stress responses although interactions between immune system components and other stress effector systems are very complex and still poorly understood. Upon exposure to various acute stressors, inflammatory cytokines such as tumor necrosis factor and interleukin (IL)-1 and -6 are increased. These substances participate in the maintenance of immunologic homeostasis as well as in regulation of the hypothalamic-pituitary-adrenocortical axis. Interleukin-6 appears to be a very potent stimulator of the hypothalamic-pituitary-adrenocortical axis that most likely occurs via activation of paraventricular CRH neurons. Neuronal pathways participating in interleukin-induced CRH activation are still not well characterized. Stress-induced elevated plasma glucocorticoid levels in turn have profound inhibitory effects on various immune functions. For example, production of cytokines, mediators of inflammation, leukocyte function and traffic, cell-mediated immunity, and suppressor T-cell function are all decreased by stress-induced elevations in glucocorticoid levels.

Immunosuppressive and anti-inflammatory effects of glucocorticoids are essential to prevent harmful infections or unwanted exaggerated immune reactions so as to increase chances for survival. This is well-documented from studies where Lewis rats that are characterized by hyporesponsiveness of the hypothalamic-pituitary-adrenocortical axis (deficient CRH neurons?) have increased susceptibility to inflammatory diseases upon exposure to a variety of stressful stimuli.

Autonomic Nervous System

The sympathoneuronal and adrenomedullary systems are two major stress effector systems. Numerous recent studies have demonstrated differential responses of these two effector systems during exposure to various stressors. In several recent studies, an attempt was made to measure simultaneously release of norepinephrine in the hypothalamic paraventricular nucleus (the most important area in the regulation of the hypothalamic-pituitary-adrenocortical axis and the site where noradrenergic neurons synapse on CRH neurons) using *in vivo* microdialysis and plasma levels of catecholamines and ACTH. These multiple neuroendocrine measures provided an answer to whether stressor-specific noradrenergic activation of the hypothalamic-pituitary-adrenocortical axis and stressor-specific responses of sympathoadrenal and adrenomedullary systems occur. During exposure to any of several stressors, there was a significant correlation between plasma levels of ACTH and paraventricular microdialysate levels of norepinephrine. Although for all stressors levels of norepinephrine in the paraventricular nucleus correlated significantly with plasma ACTH levels, detailed examination of these variables showed differences and not necessarily causal interrelationships. During exposure to metabolic stressors, such as hypoglycemia and hemorrhage, increments of plasma ACTH were much larger than those of norepinephrine in the paraventricular nucleus, suggesting that ACTH release can occur by pathways other than activation of noradrenergic neurons terminating in the paraventricular nucleus. Other intra- or extra-paraventricular non-adrenergic neurons are most likely responsible for stimulating ACTH release during these stressors. In response to pain stress, relatively small ACTH responses were associated with large increases in paraventricular norepinephrine release, suggesting that norepinephrine in this brain region could be a stimulator of CRH neurons. The slope of the relationship

Table 1 Selected behavioral and physiological adaptations designed to restore homeostasis during acute exposure to stressful stimulation

Behavioral adaptation	*Physiological adaptation*
Increased arousal and alertness	Oxygen redirection to CNS and st ress-activated tissues
Euphoria or dysphoria	Nutrients redirected to CNS and stress-activated tissues
Suppression of appetite or feeding behavior	Increased blood pressure and heart rate
Suppression of reproductive behavior	Increased respiratory rate
	Increased gluconeogenesis, glycogenolysis, and lipolysis
	Detoxification of endogenous or exogenous toxic products
	Inhibition of reproductive system
	Inhibition of colonic motility

between paraventricular norepinephrine release and plasma ACTH responses was intermediate during immobilization stress, suggesting that both noradrenergic and nonadrenergic neurons participate in the regulation of the hypothalamic-pituitary-adrenocortical axis in response to the combined psychological and physical stress of immobilization.

These and other findings can be applied to a new concept of stressor-specific neurocircuits in brain and neuroendocrine signatures that are related to specific stressors. The recognition and description of stressor-specific neurocircuits, including mapping of neurotransmitters participating in these neurocircuits, may lead to the development of new therapies for stress-related disorders.

Types of Acute Stressors

Included below are descriptions of the responses to some of the acute stressors that have been employed frequently in laboratory animal studies of stressful stimulation. In the majority of these studies, the focus of attention was directed at the sympathetic-adrenal medullary system or the hypothalamic-pituitary-adrenocortical system. In the former, measures of plasma levels of norepinephrine and epinephrine were reported and in the latter plasma levels of ACTH and/or corticosterone were made.

Hypoglycemia

Hypoglycemia is characterized by a fall in plasma glucose levels under various conditions, including starvation, hepatic dysfunction, administration of insulin, pancreatic B cell tumor, alcohol use, and adrenal insufficiency. Acute decreases in blood glucose levels are associated with increases in circulating levels of epinephrine, ACTH, and cortisol, with little if any concurrent sympathoneuronal system activation as indicated by circulating norepinephrine levels. The selective adrenomedullary activation during hypoglycemia constitutes key evidence for the differential regulation of stress effector systems. Hypoglycemia is characterized by many symptoms associated with neuroglycopenia, including tremulousness, sweating, hunger, palpitations, anxiety, psychotic behavior, seizures, and coma.

The central neuronal circuitry responsible for the elicitation of hunger and eating in response to hypoglycemia remains poorly understood. Stimulation of catechololamine release by insulin-induced hypoglycemia is thought to involve both neurogenic and nonneurogenic mechanisms. Neurogenic mechanisms participate in the initial acute phase (the first 30 min after insulin administration) in which plasma epinephrine levels increase but plasma norepinephrine levels remain unchanged. Glucose-sensitive receptors in the hypothalamus and preganglionic cholinergic nerves that innervate the adrenal medulla are involved in this phase when an absolute fall in plasma glucose levels rather than actual hypoglycemia is an important mechanism to trigger catecholamine responses. Nonneurogenic mechanisms participate in the second phase (30–50 min after insulin administration) and produce increases in both plasma epinephrine and norepinephrine. These responses are independent of a functionally intact nerve supply to the adrenal medulla and can be reversed by glucose administration, suggesting that hypoglycemia is the mechanism that triggers catecholamine responses. However, it should be mentioned that several other studies have not found a biphasic pattern of hypoglycemia-induced catecholamine responses, which may be explained by differing experimental conditions, including the severity of hypoglycemia.

Hemorrhage

Depending upon whether hypotensive or nonhypotensive hemorrhage occurs, various physiological responses are elicited, including activation of the hypothalamic-pituitary-adrenocortical axis, increased vasopressin release, and elevated plasma catecholamine levels. Similar to hypoglycemia, hemorrhage elicits relatively small increases in paraventricular levels of norepinephrine. Activation of all of these systems is an important counterregulatory mechanism to maintain homeostasis.

In clinical studies, acute hypotensive hemorrhage is an extremely dangerous situation since it may lead to shock. Acute hemorrhagic shock is characterized by an activation of all of the main stress effector systems. Clinical symptoms of the former include low energy level, fatigue, a feeling of being cold, dizziness, and sleepiness; clinical signs of the latter include cool or mottled extremities, increased heart rate, low blood pressure, pallor, and altered mental status, ranging from restlessness and agitation to coma. Restoration of blood volume is a high priority, although fluid replacement that is too rapid may be harmful since it may shut down the level of activity of the sympathoadrenal system in the critical period when survival depends on the activity of these stress effector systems.

Hypoxia

Asphyxiation produces the biochemical triad of hypoxemia, hypercarbia, and acute respiratory acidosis. Chemoreceptors, located especially in the carotid bodies adjacent to the carotid sinuses, respond to decreased arterial oxygen concentrations, increased arterial carbon dioxide concentrations, and decreased arterial blood pH. Chemosensitive cells near the ventral surface of the medulla respond to these same stimuli. Acute exposure to hypoxemia and hypercarbic acidosis is associated with increased or unchanged plasma levels of norepinephrine and epinephrine and with increased sympathetic nerve traffic as measured by microneurography. Findings of unchanged plasma norepinephrine levels during acute hypoxemia may be explained by increased nor-epinephrine clearance. The activation of sympathoneuronal and adrenomedullary systems is associated with increases in heart rate, respiration, and vasoconstriction. Sympathectomy decreases and adrenalectomy eliminates increases in heart rate and cardiac output that result from severe hypoxia.

Acute mountain sickness caused by sudden exposure to hypoxia is a frequent cause of morbidity and mortality in people who travel to high altitudes. It is estimated that 30 million people are at risk for altitude-related diseases in the western United States every year. Approximately 20% of tourists who travel to ski resorts in Colorado experience acute mountain sickness. Symptoms of acute mountain sickness include headache, nausea, anorexia, insomnia, cough, difficulties in physical activity, mental changes, seizures, hallucinations, and, finally, in severe cases, coma. All of these symptoms may occur suddenly after a few hours in a high-altitude environment and require immediate medical attention.

Pain

Following exposure of laboratory animals to acute pain induced by formalin administration, only small increments in plasma ACTH levels occur despite large increments in plasma norepinephrine and epinephrine levels. Brainstem centers are the recipients of ascending pathways carrying nociceptive information and are perhaps the most important brain areas in pain mechanisms. Glutamate, aspartate, substance P, and calcitonin gene-related peptide are neurotransmitters that participate in acute pain responses. It is known that behavioral analgesia or inhibition of spinal neurons that respond to painful stimuli may be eliminated by electric stimulation or opiate microinjection into several brainstem regions.

Cold

Cold exposure has been employed as a stressful stimulus in laboratory studies. Several experimental approaches have been taken in these studies. In one such approach, animals are placed in their home cages in a cold environment maintained at a constant temperature and remain there for varying periods of time. Typically the stress session can extend from several hours to multiple days. Alternatively, animals are immersed in water at a given temperature for less than an hour. Exposure to a cold environment at or below 0°C results in dramatic increases in plasma norepinephrine but only modest increases in plasma levels of epinephrine and ACTH. In contrast, placement of laboratory rats in cold water (20–25°C) for as little as 15 min is attended by substantial increases in plasma levels of epinephrine and norepinephrine. The increases in plasma levels of both catecholamines in response to cold swim stress are negatively correlated with water temperature over the range of 20–34°C, with the highest levels of plasma catecholamines at the lowest water temperatures. Indeed, plasma levels of epinephrine during swim stress at 18–20°C are among the highest ever measured for a laboratory stressor.

Footshock

Footshock has been especially valuable as a stressor in studies of neural and endocrine responsiveness. Footshock allows investigators exquisite control over the frequency, intensity, and duration of the stressful stimulus. In addition, footshock is often employed as an aversive stimulus in studies of learning and memory, allowing for studies that link physiological and behavioral responses. Footshock stress activates the sympathetic-adrenal medullary and hypothalamic-pituitary-adrenocortical systems, especially at moderate to high intensity footshock levels (1–2 mA).

Immobilization

For more than 30 years, Kvetnansky and his colleagues have employed immobilization as a consistent feature of their studies on physiological adaptations to stress. Immobilization is a potent stressor and includes physical as well as psychological dimensions. Typically, laboratory rats are fixed to a holder by taping their limbs to padded metal mounts. The stress sessions usually last from 30 to 120 min and may be repeated each day for up to 1 month to assess responses to acute versus repeated stress. A single session of immobilization results in extremely high levels of circulating norepinephrine, epinephrine, ACTH, and corticosterone when compared to other laboratory stressors. Levels of norepinephrine, epinephrine, and ACTH usually peak within the first 30 min of immobilization and then decrease to a stable but highly elevated level for the remainder of the stress session. In contrast, plasma levels of corticosterone peak later in the stress session and remain high for the remainder of the period of immobilization.

Summary and Conclusions

Since its inception, the field of stress research has lacked a strong theoretical foundation upon which investigators could formulate questions, design experiments, and interpret their findings and the work of others. From the beginning of his career, Hans Selye offered a definition of stress that was all encompassing and he advanced a view that exposure to any stressor results in a consistent pattern of physiological responses. Although these concepts are no longer at the forefront of stress research, they have left an indelible imprint.

In the absence of a strong theoretical foundation, much of the effort in the field of stress research has been linked to the development of techniques for measuring biologically active molecules or visualizing substances within various tissues, especially neural tissue. The nature of the stressor in a given study was for a time almost an afterthought. Thus, many laboratories developed their own unique stressors and focused much of their creative energies on assay methodologies. Without a set of consistent stress paradigms, comparisons of research results across laboratories were difficult.

In this overview of acute stress responses, we have provided a brief background on the major stress-responsive neuroendocrine systems. Then we examined the pattern of neuroendocrine responses across some of the commonly used laboratory stressors. After distilling the results of thousands of studies of neuroendocrine activation during acute stress, the case for specificity of physiological responses to different stressors is overwhelming. These neuroendocrine signatures allow an animal to respond to a given stressor with an optimal recruitment of physiological responses to meet the immediate demands of the situation. It is important to keep in mind that most acute stress paradigms present the subject with a great deal of uncertainty and loss of control. The subject has never experienced the stressor before and has no knowledge of how long the stressor will persist, if escape is possible, if stressor intensity will remain constant, and so on. These psychological variables affect central neural circuits that coordinate neural and endocrine activation and must be considered in interpreting the findings of a given acute stress experiment.

Further Reading

Buckingham, J. C., Cowell, A.-M., Gillies, G. E., Herbison, A. E. and Stell, J. H. (1997). The neuroendocrine system: Anatomy, physiology and responses to stress. In: Buckingham, J. C., Gillies, G. E. & Cowell, A.-M. (eds.) *Stress, Stress Hormones and the Immune System*, pp. 9–47. New York: Wiley.

Chrousos, G. P. (1998). Stressors, stress, and neuroendocrine integration of the adaptive response. *Annals of the New York Academy of Sciences* **851**, 311–335.

Goldstein, D. S. (1995). *Stress, Catecholamines, and Cardiovascular Disease*. New York: Oxford University Press.

Johnson, E. O., Kamilaris, T. C., Chrousos, G. P. and Gold, P. W. (1992). Mechanisms of stress: A dynamic overview of hormonal and behavioral homeostasis. *Neuroscience and Biobehavioral Reviews* **16**, 115–130.

McCarty, R. and Gold, P. E. (1996). Catecholamines, stress and disease: A psychobiological perspective. *Psychosomatic Medicine* **58**, 590–597.

Pacak, K., Palkovits, M., Kopin, I. J. and Goldstein, D. S. (1995). Stress-induced norepinephrine release in the hypthalamic paraventricular nucleus and pituitary-adrenocortical and sympathoadrenal activity: *In vivo* microdialy studies. *Frontiers Neuroendocrinology* **16**, 89–150.

Pacak, K., Palkovits, M., Kvetnansky, R., Yadid, G., Kopin, I. J. and Goldstein, D. S. (1995). Effects of various stress on *in vivo* norepinephrine release in the hypothalamic paraventricular nucleus and on the pituitary-adrenocortical axis. *Annals of the New York Academy of Sciences* **771**, 115–130.

Rivier, C. and Rivest, S. (1991). Effect of stress on the activity of the hypothalamic-pituitary-gonadal axis: Peripheral central mechanisms. *Biology of Reproduction* **45**, 523–532.

Chronic (Repeated) Stress: Consequences, Adaptations

M F Dallman
University of California at San Francisco, San Francisco, CA, USA

Chronic Stress

What is important for the organism? Evolutionarily, the answers are, first, survival to achieve and sustain reproductive age and, second, reproductive success. The hypothamic–pituitary–adrenocortical (HPA) axis is intimately involved with the former requirement, and its overactivity may inhibit the latter while taking care of living for the moment. Glucocorticoid (GC) secretion is regulated by the HPA axis and is key to survival after severe insults that threaten the organism. GC modulates energy availability, immune responses, learning, and memory, as well as many behaviors. The consequences of GC secretion reveal an organism that is better fit for survival under conditions of challenges. This is clearly so in the face of punctate, acute stressors that, once finished, do not recur on a regular basis. However, with chronic or repeated stressors that cannot be coped with through behavioral changes, the persistently increased secretion of GC may limit the ultimate longevity of the organism. In the case of chronic or persistent inescapable stressors, mechanisms have evolved that may diminish the HPA response to the unrelieved, or repeated stressor input. This is reflected by the process of habituation of the HPA output to a given stressor, well studied in rats by using shock, restraint, or cold.

A careful look at responses to a new stressor in chronically stressed rats that are habituated to a chronic stressor reveals that the new HPA response is most often facilitated compared with that of a stressor-naïve animal. This demonstrates that, although central mechanisms of habituation are engaged, the brain remains aware of the persistent challenge, and the HPA axis overresponds to a new threat. This article first describes the recruitment of limbic networks accompanying chronic or repeated stressors and then the habituation to repeated or chronic stressors, using repeated restraint as a model, and the brain sites and HPA responses important during habituation. It discusses experimental manipulations of these sites and what they may reveal about the plasticity of brain responses in the face of chronic or repeated stressors. Finally, it briefly recaps the upside and discusses the long-term downside of perpetual challenges to the organism – the wear and tear of life.

Chronic Stress and Recruitment of a Limbic Network That Biases Subsequent Autonomic, Behavioral, and Neuroendocrine Responses to Stressors

The HPA axis is not the only motor system that is affected by chronic or repeated inescapable stressors. Chronic stressors bias autonomic responses toward excessive sympathetic outflow; they bias behaviors toward the fearful- and anxiety-like spectrum; they alter neuroendocrine responses so that the HPA responses to novel stressors are facilitated although those to many known stressors are habituated with repetition. In rats, the somatotropic and thyrotropic axes are inhibited by chronic or repeated stressors; the gonadotropic axis may be either inhibited or facilitated, depending on the stressor that is chronically or repeatedly applied. These effects of chronic stressors may be a consequence of the stimulatory actions of GC on corticotropin-releasing factor (CRF) synthesis and secretion in the central nuclei of the amygdala (CeA). From the CeA, CRF axons innervate and may activate all monoaminergic cell groups that have been shown to be important, and facilitated, after the engagement of the chronic stress network. It is the altered activity of the monoaminergic networks, as well as direct effects of CRF from the CeA, that is responsible for many of the altered autonomic, behavioral, and neuroendocrine responses that accompany activation of the emotional limbic brain during persistent, inescapable stressors.

Habituation of HPA Responses with Time after Inescapable Stressors

What are the HPA characteristics of habituation? Because habituation is measured by comparison of the amplitude and duration of the first HPA response to a given stressor with those of subsequent responses, it is far easier to demonstrate that habituation occurs after the use of mild to moderate stressors that do not saturate the response characteristics of the HPA axis. Habituation has typically been studied in responses to repeated restraint, intermittent or chronic cold, footshock, social stressors, and variable chronic stress paradigms. Although some are top-down, processive stressors and others bottom-up, systemic stressors, the HPA responses more often than not habituate with repetition or time. It seems likely that with both top-down and bottom-up cases, the animal becomes adapted, behaviorally and physiologically, to the repeated or chronic stimuli. Indeed, for restraint, there is evidence, as measured by c-fos expression, that afferent input within the brain is reduced with repetition, whereas with the metabolic challenge of cold, the animal gears up its metabolism and food intake to alter thermogenesis and respond appropriately to the challenge, thus reducing afferent input to the brain. Nonetheless, generally there is evidence that, although habituation may occur with chronicity or repetitions of stressors that are not life-threatening, new central networks have been recruited that allow the animals to hyperrespond to presentation of novel stimuli.

Repeated Restraint

Restraint is probably the most-studied stressor in which the process of habituation has been explored. Restraint, unlike immobilization, simply confines animals in a tube in which they can breathe readily and can move somewhat but in which they cannot turn around. The HPA axis response to an initial bout of restraint is transient. When rats are maintained in a restraining tube for hours, adrenocorticotropin (ACTH) and corticosteroid responses peak at 15–30 min and then return to control concentrations despite continued confinement (**Figure 1**); red lines show responses to restraint during the first encounter with it). It is likely that a portion of the initial response also reflects the stressor of being picked up and placed into the restraining tube. Nonetheless, the HPA response to the stressor seems clearly damped by the adrenal GC feedback signal since in its absence, ACTH concentrations remain high for the full period of restraint. With chronic, repeated restraint, the amplitude of the HPA response decays over days (**Figure 1**; blue lines show responses to restraint during the fifth encounter). All efferent components of the response are diminished and curtailed, and this is reflected by the markedly reduced c-fos response in the hypothalamic paraventricular nuclei (PVN) to restraint on the fifth day compared with the first. Moreover, the CRF cells in the PVN that express c-fos after repeated restraint appear to be located more ventromedially, compared to the dorsomedial neuronal CRF response that occurs to the first episode of restraint. All the downstream responses are shortened, and their amplitude is generally diminished. However, it is characteristic of chronic stressors that HPA responses are still observed, but their magnitude and duration decrease.

Why Habituation?

Familiarity with the stimulus, in part through GC-mediated learning, memory, and recall, perhaps reveals that it is not life-threatening, although it may be boring and uncomfortable, and that it can be endured. Habituation to the much more severe stimulus of immobilization, in which rats are tightly restrained and cannot move even their heads, is much slower, although it, too, occurs eventually. Habituation also occurs with other stimuli, such as cold, mild electrical shock, social stress, and subsequent presentations of a previously experienced stimulus in a variable stimulus paradigm (in which different stressors are presented twice daily for up to a month). However, if stimuli are perceived as life-threatening, subsequent repetitions may produce augmented, rather than habituated, responses, as reported for exposures to predator odor and immune challenge. Again, it seems highly appropriate to have mechanisms (that are still unclear) that allow continued, and even increased responses to potentially life-threatening events.

Where in the Brain Does Habituation to Restraint Occur?

Many sites in brain have been examined for their potential role in habituating HPA responses to repeated restraint. With the use of c-fos messenger RNA, it seems clear that there is decreased responsiveness to recurrent restraint throughout the afferent limbic and cortical brain networks involved in transmission of the signal to the CRF motor zone, the hypothalamic PVN, probably as a consequence of cortical inhibition of these sites.

How Does Habituation Occur?

Although cytotoxic lesions of the posterior paraventricular thalamus do not affect the duration or amplitude of an initial ACTH response, they do block habituation of ACTH to repeated bouts of restraint, suggesting that this structure is important for, perhaps, the memory of prior restraint (**Figure 2**). Moreover, injection of a cocktail of mineralocorticoid receptor and GC receptor (GR) antagonists during each period of repeated restraint also decreases the degree of habituation (**Figure 3**) although they do not affect the initial HPA response to the stressor. Thus, it appears that cells in the posterior paraventricular thalamus that contain GRs (and presumably mineralocorticoid receptors) and that project to both the basolateral amygdala and the prefrontal cortex strongly affect habituation of HPA responses to restraint, although they do not explain the entire habituation response. Similarly, injection of a GR antagonist into the basolateral amygdala, or into the hippocampus, depending on the type of behavior

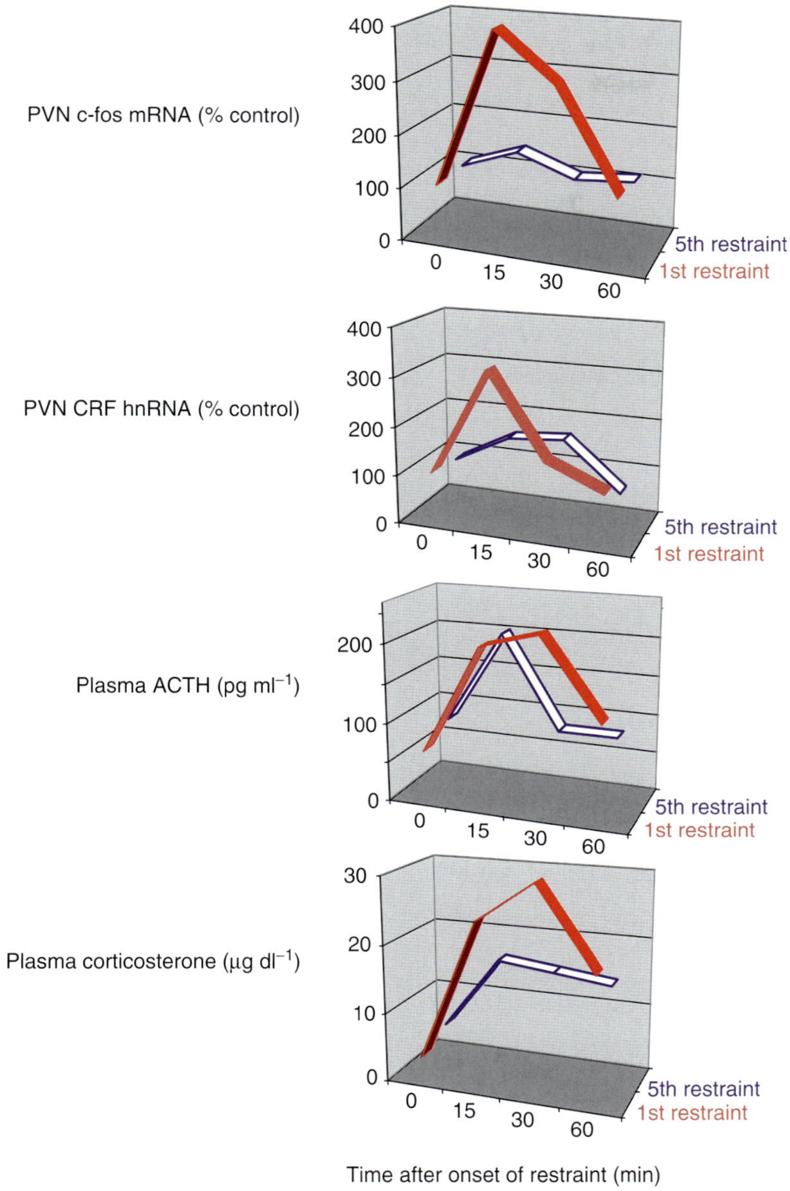

Figure 1 Habituation of HPA responses to restraint: first vs. fifth restraint. ACTH, adrenocorticotropin; CRF, corticotropin-releasing factor; hnRNA, heterogeneous nuclear RNA; mRNA, messenger RNA; PVN, hypothalamic paraventricular nucleus. Redrawn from Girotti M, Pace TWW, Gaylord RI, Rubin BA, Herman JP, and Spencer RL (2006) Habituation to repeated restraint stress is associated with lack of stress-induced c-fos expression in primary sensory processing areas of the rat brain. *Neuroscience* 138: 1067–1081.

examined, can block subsequent behavioral responses to a stressor. It seems clear that the GCs aid learning of and memory for emotionally laden events and that without the GC action, appropriate responses to the events do not occur.

Facilitation to Novel Stimuli Occurs with Chronic Stress

What Does Facilitation Look Like?

Although HPA responses to repeated stimuli dwindle with repetition, it is characteristic of rats undergoing chronic challenge that they exhibit greater-than-normal HPA responses to new stressors. The example provided in **Figure 4** is of rats given intermittent injections of morphine in escalating doses that allow partial withdrawal twice daily, which is an intense stimulus to the HPA axis. However, facilitated responses to novel stressors are characteristic of most chronic challenges and have been observed in rats, mice, sheep, and humans. Facilitated responses are observed at each level (CRF, ACTH, and corticosterone) of the HPA axis in rats. Facilitation of HPA responses to novel challenges, even in an organism undergoing chronic stress with habituated responses,

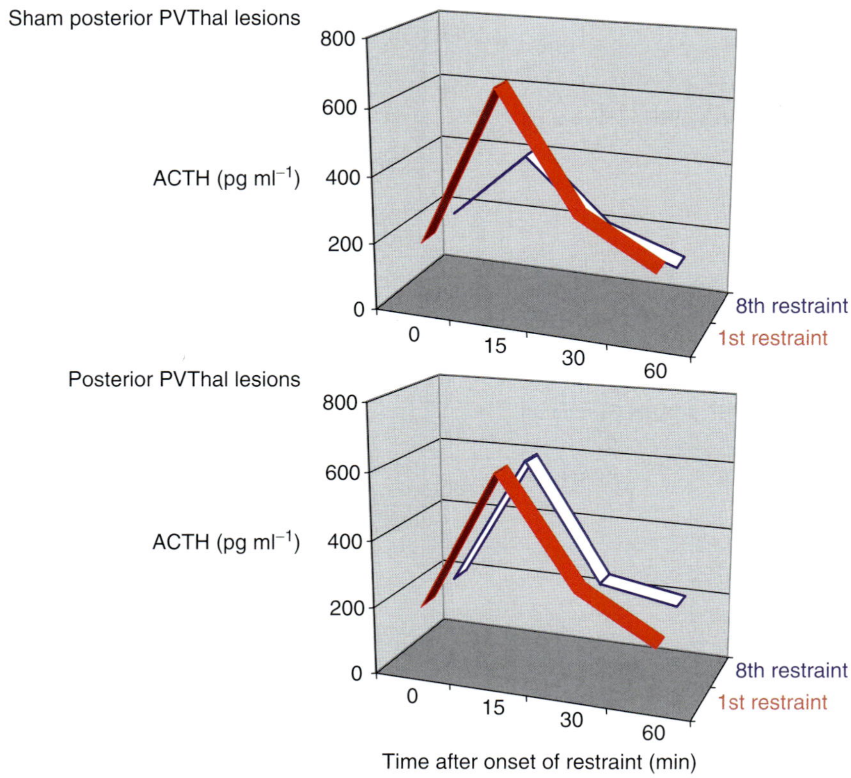

Figure 2 Dishabituation of HPA responses to restraint by lesion of posterior PVThalamus: first vs. eighth restraint. ACTH, adrenocorticotropin; HPA, hypothalamic–pituitary–adrenocortical; PV, paraventricular. Redrawn from Bhatnagar S, Huber R, Nowak N, and Trotter P (2002) Lesions of the paraventricular thalamus block adaptation of hypothalamic–pituitary–adrenal (HPA) responses to repeated restraint. *Journal of Neuroendocrinology* 14: 403–410.

makes a great deal of physiological sense since GC responses of normal magnitude to many stressors are essential for the maintenance of life.

Facilitated Responses Require Sustained or Intermittently Repeated Stressors and Elevated Corticosterone Concentrations

Adrenalectomized rats without GC or with low levels of GC replacement do not exhibit facilitated ACTH responses to novel stimuli under conditions of chronic challenge (**Figure 5**). Although replacement with GC results in normal, monotonic inhibition of ACTH in chronically stressed, compared with control, rats (**Figure 5**, left panel), GC concentrations must be maintained at values above the normal daily mean for intact, unstressed rats for facilitated responses to novel stress to be observable (**Figure 5**, right panel). The corticosterone concentrations that permit facilitation are sufficient to entirely inhibit ACTH responses to novel restraint in control animals that were not chronically challenged. Because GC acts at GRs in the anterior pituitary corticotropes to inhibit both synthesis of proopiomelanocortin, the precursor for ACTH, and secretion of the mature hormone, hypothalamic CRF may increase in response to the acute stimulus, but because of the GC-inhibited corticotrope, ACTH secretion may not occur.

How Does Facilitation Occur?

Facilitation is almost certainly explained by the fact that chronic stressors recruit a limbic network, based on activation of CRF in the central nucleus of the amygdala by GC's acting through GRs. The limbic response network prepares the animal to maintain behavioral, autonomic, and neuroendocrine responsiveness in the face of tonically elevated GC that might otherwise suppress these responses. Facilitated HPA responses to new stimuli are blocked by daily injections with a GR antagonist (RU486) during the period of intermittent challenge. They are also blocked by the injection of a CRF1 receptor antagonist before the novel stimulus is presented. Thus, although the intimate details are still not understood, the stress-induced elevations in GC concentrations promote, not only habituation, but also facilitation, through actions on stressor-recruited limbic structures and on limbic neurons to stimulate CRF synthesis.

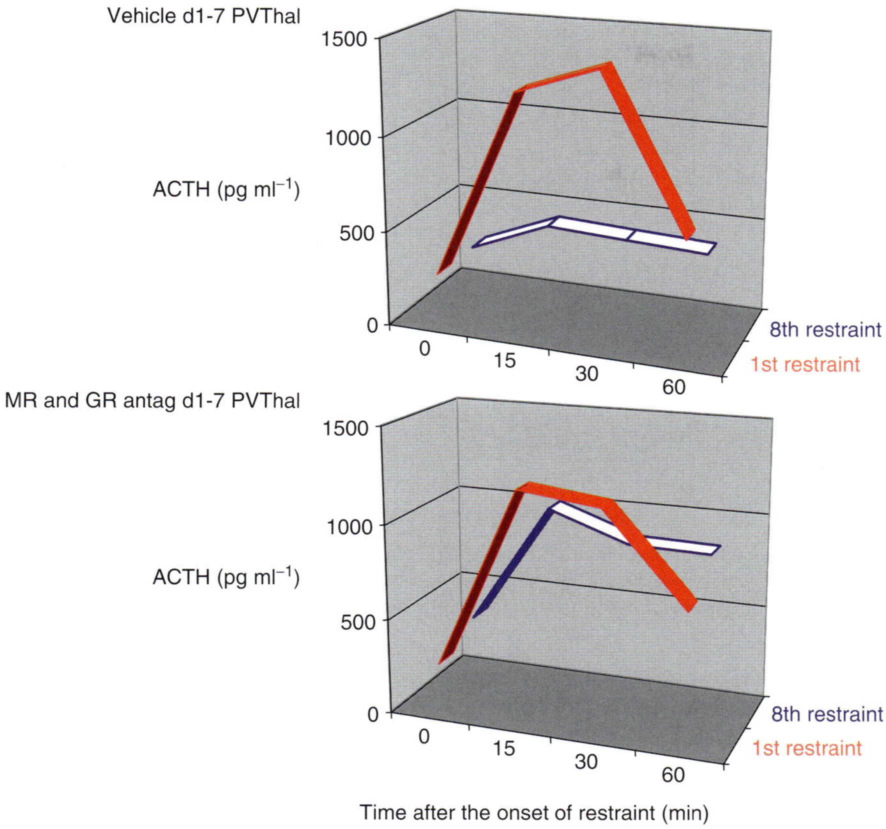

Figure 3 Dishabituation of hypothalamic–pituitary–adrenocortical (HPA) responses to restraint by daily MR and GR antagonists into the posterior PVThalamus: first vs. eighth restraint. ACTH, adrenocorticotropin; GR, glucocorticoid receptor; MR, mineralocorticoid receptor; PV, paraventricular. Redrawn from Jaferi A and Bhatnagar S (2006) Corticosterone can act at the posterior paraventricular thalamus to inhibit hypothalamo–pituitary–adrenal activity in animals that habituate to repeated stress. *Endocrinology* 147: 4917–4930.

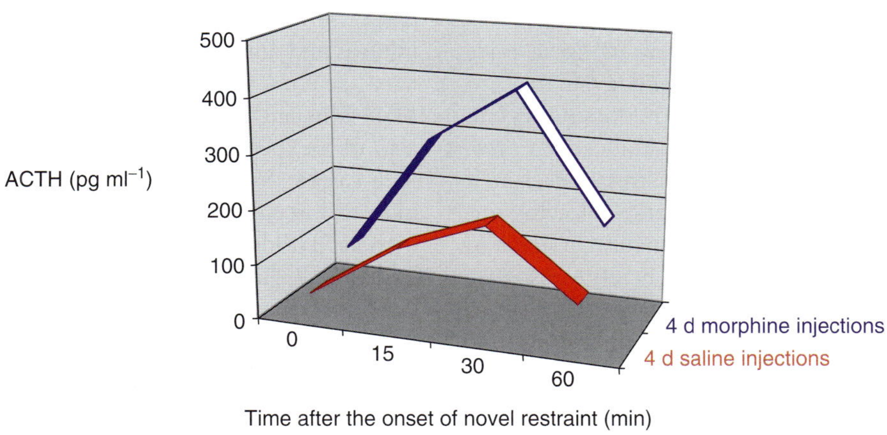

Figure 4 Chronic stress facilitates hypothalamic–pituitary–adrenocortical (HPA) responses to a novel stressor. ACTH, adrenocorticotropin. Redrawn from Houshyar H, Gomez F, Manalo S, Bhargava A, and Dallman MF (2003) Intermittent morphine administration induces dependence and is a chronic stressor in rats. *Neuropsychopharmacology* 28: 1960–1972.

The Up- and Downsides of HPA Responses to Chronic or Repeated Challenge

The Upside

The HPA responses to chronic challenge are essential for maintaining life. Without the GCs, death occurs or metabolism and mentation are not appropriately regeared to meet the challenge. The persistent and overall increases in GC concentrations above basal values that occur during normal physiological responses to chronic stressors sculpt the organism's repertoire to manage the threat flexibly and

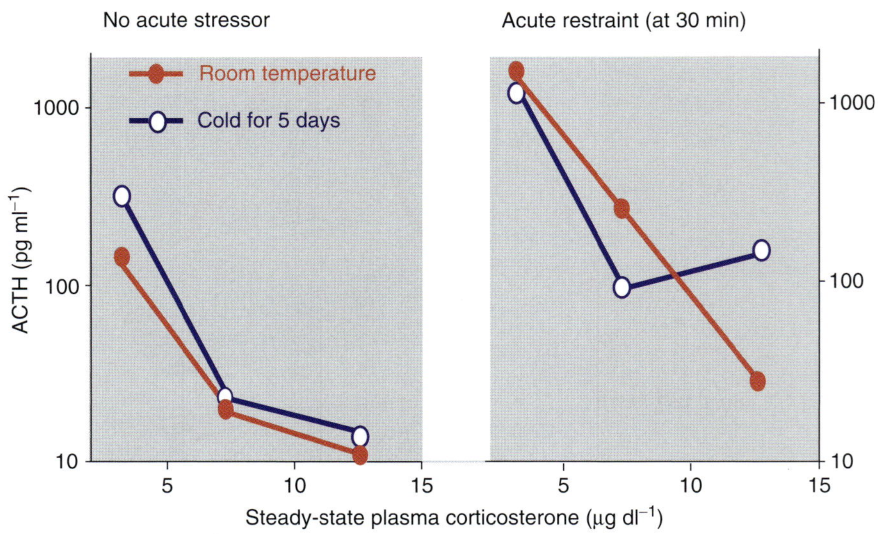

Figure 5 Facilitated ACTH responses to novel restraint require high corticosterone in chronically stressed adrenalectomy (ADX) rats. ACTH, adrenocorticotropin. Redrawn from Akana SF and Dallman MF (1997) Chronic cold in adrenalectomized corticosterone (B)-treated rats: Facilitated corticotropin responses to acute restraint emerge as B increases. *Endocrinology* 138: 3249–3258.

optimally: (1) Metabolic activity is adjusted to produce more gluconeogenesis so that available essential fuel is abundant, drawing on reserves and also rearranging stored metabolic energy toward the center of the animal, where it provides better physical balance for potential escape behaviors. (2) Behaviors are geared more toward fight, flight, anxiety, and ingestive responses, and there is an increased level of arousal that will more accurately pinpoint any new dangers to be assessed. Habituation, mediated at least in part through the GC response, ensures that the HPA response is calibrated and appropriately damped, once the level of the threat is known and evaluated, so that more-than-adequate GC secretion does not occur. Simultaneously, the same challenge-induced GC responses enable full engagement of the stressor-recruited central brain stress-response network, allowing increased responsivity in other central neural systems to ongoing and potential new threats. The HPA response is finely honed to enable and prepare the organism to deal with the ongoing vicissitudes of life.

The Downside

Greatly elevated concentrations of GC, persisting for too long, may exert deleterious effects that will ultimately decrease the life span of the individual. GCs certainly affect learning and memory, and they do so with an inverted U-shaped dose–response relationship. As in the story of Goldilocks and the three bears, the magnitude of the chronic HPA response must be just right, neither too little nor too much. Effects of inappropriately high GC on learning and recall of memory, hippocampal CA3 apical dendritic branching, neurogenesis, and neuronal apoptosis are generally deleterious. As with all things, there is a Janus-like quality to the GCs. They can either augment or inhibit immune responses. During the stressful breeding season, both salmon returning to spawn and the small male Australian marsupial *Antechinus stuartii* die after fertilizing the eggs of the female, and often with evidence of overwhelming infection, probably due to the very high GCs that accompany their efforts. GCs also stimulate not only the learning and memory of high-density palatable calories but also their intake. This is appropriate and plays a large role in seasonal fattening in birds and animals in the wild. However, in industrialized societies, people living under conditions, not only of heightened persistent psychological challenge, but also of inexpensive and readily available, low-quality, high-calorie foods, run into trouble. Stressor-induced increases in palatable food consumption may result in increased abdominal obesity, cardiovascular disease, and type 2 diabetes. All these are known to strongly contribute to morbidity and mortality.

Thus, although they are required for the survival of challenge, the secreted GCs also greatly increase the rate of wear and tear associated with life and may ultimately shorten life span.

See Also the Following Articles

Corticotropin-Releasing Hormone: Integration of Adaptive Responses to Stress; Stress: Definition and History; Stress: Homeostasis, Rheostasis, Allostasis and Allostatic Load; Stress Response: Neural and Feedback Regulation of the HPA Axis; Stress and Parasympathetic Control; Sympathetic Noradrenergic and Adrenomedullary Hormonal Systems in Stress and Distress; Sympathoadrenal System: Neural Arm of the Stress Response.

Further Reading

Akana, S. F. and Dallman, M. F. (1997). Chronic cold in adrenalectomized corticosterone (B)-treated rats: Facilitated corticotropin responses to acute restraint emerge as B increases. *Endocrinology* **138**, 3249–3258.

Bhatnagar, S., Huber, R., Nowak, N. and Trotter, P. (2002). Lesions of the paraventricular thalamus block adaptation of hypothalamic–pituitary–adrenal (HPA) responses to repeated restraint. *Journal of Neuroendocrinology* **14**, 403–410.

Dallman, M., Pecoraro, N. and la Fleur, S. (2005). Chronic stress and comfort foods: Self-medication and abdominal obesity. *Brain, Behavior, and Immunity* **19**, 275–282.

Dallman, M. F., Pecoraro, N. C. and la Fleur, S. E. (2006). Glucocorticoids, chronic stress, and obesity. *Progress in Brain Research* **153**, 75–105.

Dallman, M. F., Viau, V., Bhatnagar, S., Gomez, F., Laugero, K. and Bell, M. E. (2002). Corticotropin-releasing factor (CRF), corticosteroids, stress and sugar: Energy balance the brain and behavior. In: Pfaff, DW. (ed.) *Hormones, Brain and Behavior,* (vol. 1)), pp. 571–631. San Diego, CA: Academic Press.

de Kloet, E. R., Oitzl, M. S. and Joels, M. (1999). Stress and cognition: Are corticosteroids good or bad guys? *Trends in Neurosciences* **22**, 422–426.

Girotti, M., Pace, T. W. W., Gaylord, R. I., Rubin, B. A., Herman, J. P. and Spencer, R. L. (2006). Habituation to repeated restraint stress is associated with lack of stress-induced c-fos expression in primary sensory processing areas of the rat brain. *Neuroscience* **138**, 1067–1081.

Herman, J. and Cullinan, W. (1997). Neurocircuitry of stress: Central control of the hypothalamo–pituitary–adrenocortical axis. *Trends in Neurosciences* **20**, 78–84.

Houshyar, H., Gomez, F., Manalo, S., Bhargava, A. and Dallman, MF. (2003). Intermittent morphine administration induces dependence and is a chronic stressor in rats. *Neuropsychopharmacology* **28**, 1960–1972.

Jaferi, A. and Bhatnagar, S. (2006). Corticosterone can act at the posterior paraventricular thalamus to inhibit hypothalamo–pituitary–adrenal activity in animals that habituate to repeated stress. *Endocrinology* **147**, 4917–4930.

Joels, M., Pu, Z., Wiegert, O., Oitzl, M. S. and Krugers, H. J. (2005). Learning under stress: How does it work? *Trends in Cognitive Sciences* **10**, 152–158.

Lupien, S. J. and Lepage, M. (2001). Stress, memory, and the hippocampus: Can't live with it, can't live without it. *Behavioural Brain Research* **127**, 137–158.

McEwen, B. S. (2005). Glucocorticoids, depression, and mood disorders: Structural remodeling in the brain. *Metabolism: Clinical and Experimental* **54**(supplement 1), 20–23.

Pecoraro, N., Dallman, M. F., Warne, J. P., et al. (2006). From Malthus to motive: How the HPA axis engineers the phenotype, yoking needs to wants. *Progress in Neurobiology* **79**, 247–340.

Sawchenko, P. E., Li, H. and Ericsson, A. (2000). Circuits and mechanisms governing hypothalamic responses to stress: A tale of two paradigms. *Progress in Brain Research* **122**, 61–78.

Schulkin, J., Morgan, M. A. and Rosen, J. B. (2005). A neuroendocrine mechanism for sustaining fear. *Trends in Neurosciences* **28**, 629–635.

Glucocorticoids, Role in Stress

J C Buckingham
Imperial College School of Medicine, London, UK

This article is reproduced from Encyclopedia of Stress, First edition, volume 2, pp 261–269, © 2000, Elsevier Inc.

Glossary

Cell-mediated immunity — The process by which thymus-derived lymphocytes (T cells) respond to specific antigens, undergo clonal expansion, and mount a cytotoxic response.

Humoral immunity — The process by which specific antigens activate bone marrow-derived lymphocytes (B cells), causing cell proliferation and the production and release of specific antibodies; also called antibody-mediated immunity.

Glucocorticoids are steroid hormones produced by the adrenal cortex. Their principal role is to restore homeostasis in conditions of stress. However, prolonged elevations in circulating corticosteroids, which may occur in conditions of chronic or repeated stress, are potentially harmful and may contribute to the pathogenesis of a wide range of disorders.

Secretion in Stress, Delivery to Target Tissues, and Molecular Basis of Action

Secretion of Glucocorticoids in Stress

The glucocorticoids (GCs), cortisol and/or corticosterone, depending on the species, are produced by cells in the zona fasciculata of the adrenal cortex. In normal circumstances, serum GC concentrations are maintained within narrow limits with pronounced excursions occurring only in accord with the well-documented circadian rhythm or in response to physical or emotional stress. Circadian and stress-induced increases in GC secretion are driven by neural and humoral factors that impinge on the hypothalamus to cause the release into the hypothalamo-hypophysial portal vessels of two neuropeptides, corticotropin releasing hormone (CRH) and arginine vasopressin (AVP); these peptides in turn act synergistically on the anterior pituitary gland to initiate the release of adrenocorticotropic hormone (ACTH), the primary trigger of steroidogenesis. The secretion of cortisol/corticosterone is regulated further by a complex servo mechanism through which the steroids themselves negatively regulate the release of ACTH and its hypothalamic-releasing hormones. The hypothalamic-pituitary-adrenocortical (HPA) responses to repeated or sustained stress are complex and depend on both the nature of the stress and the species. For example, in rats the adrenocortical response to cold stress is attenuated progressively with each exposure; that is, the axis becomes tolerant to the stimulus. In contrast, the HPA responses to repeated immune insults are well maintained and may become exaggerated, possibly because the feedback actions of the steroids are overcome.

Delivery of Glucocorticoids to Their Target Cells and Receptors

GCs in the systemic circulation are largely protein-bound (95%), mainly to a specific globulin, termed corticosteroid-binding globulin (CBG, or transcortin). but also to albumin. In principle, only the free steroid has ready access to the corticosteroid receptors, which are located intracellularly in the target cells. However, local mechanisms that release the steroid from its carrier protein(s) appear to exist in at least some target tissues: these include (1) interactions of the carrier protein with cell-surface CBG receptors and (2) enzymatic cleavage of CBG (e.g., by serine proteases in inflamed tissues), a process that lowers the affinity of the binding protein for the steroids. Access of the steroids to their receptors is regulated further within the target cells by 11β-hydroxysteroid dehydrogenase (11β-HSD) enzymes that control the interconversion of cortisol/corticosterone to their inactive counterparts, cortisone/11-dehydrocorticosterone.

Molecular Basis of Glucocorticoid Action

The actions of the GCs are exerted mainly via the classic pathway of steroid action – the free steroid enters the target cells and binds to an intracellular receptor that is subsequently translocated to the nucleus, where it initiates specific changes in DNA transcription and, hence, in protein synthesis. In many instances, the activated steroid–receptor complex induces or represses transcription by binding directly to specific response elements in the promoter region of the gene; in others, however, it may interfere with the activity of other transcription factors, such as activator protein (AP)-1 and nuclear transcription factor (NF)κB. In addition, the activated receptor may regulate posttranscriptional events, including mRNA transcript stability, RNA translation, and posttranslational processing of the protein.

In accord with the intracellular mode of action, the majority of biological responses to GCs are slow to emerge; some, however, are manifested more rapidly; for example, cortisol hyperpolarizes hippocampal neurons and coeliac ganglia within 1–2 min of contact. The mechanisms underlying these rapid action are unknown, but increasing evidence favors a membrane action of the steroids, possibly via a cell surface receptor.

Corticosteroid Receptors

Two distinct subtypes of intracellular corticosteroid receptors have been identified: the mineralocorticoid receptor (MR) and the glucocorticoid receptor (GR). The MR has a high and approximately equal affinity for aldosterone and the endogeneous GCs, corticosterone and cortisol ($K_d \sim$ 1–2 nM). In contrast, the GR is of a lower affinity (K_d cortisol/corticosterone 10–20 nM), is glucocorticoid-selective, and does not bind aldosterone readily; a truncated form of this receptor, termed GR-β, which does not bind ligand but which has the capacity to bind DNA, also exists. MRs in the kidney are protected effectively from cortisol/corticosterone by type 2 11β-HSD (11β-HSD2), which acts primarily as a dehydrogenase and inactivates the steroids rapidly, thus permitting selective access of aldosterone to the receptors. MRs in the brain, however, are not always protected from GCs in this way and in many instances may be almost fully occupied at low physiological concentrations of cortisol/corticosterone. However, the delivery of GCs to GRs in organs such as the liver and white adipose tissues may be facilitated by type 1 11β-HSD (11β-HSD1), which acts primarily as a reductase and thereby regenerates the active steroids from their inactive 11-dehydro metabolites. Although the MR undoubtedly mediates several facets of glucocorticoid activity in nonstress conditions, particularly in the central nervous system (CNS), the responses to the raised levels of the steroids observed in, for example, stress are effected primarily via GRs. These receptors are widely distributed in the body; cell responsiveness depends not only on the presence of GRs, but also the receptor concentration, which is known to fluctuate during development, the cell cycle, following disturbances in endocrine status, and on the activation of 11β-HSD1 enzymes.

Functions of Glucocorticoids in Stress

General Considerations

The concept that corticosteroids play a key role in the body's responses to stress emerged from the work of Selye on the alarm reaction and the general adaptation syndrome. It is now evident that cortisol/corticosterone displays two modes of activity. The first is a permissive or proactive role in which the steroids (1) maintain the basal activity of the HPA axis and set its threshold for responding to stress and (2) normalize the body's response to stress by priming the body's defense mechanisms by, for example, facilitating the effects of catecholamines on lipid and carbohydrate metabolism; upregulating the expression of receptors for inflammatory mediators; and acting centrally to aid processes underlying selection attention, the integration of sensory information, and response selection. The second mode of cortisol/corticosterone action is suppressive or protective and enables the organism to cope with, adapt to, and recover from a stressful insult. Key to this mode are the powerful anti-inflammatory and immunosuppressive actions of the steroids that prevent the host defense mechanisms, which are activated by stress, from overshooting and damaging the organism. Other important protective actions include the ability of the steroids to redirect the metabolism to meet energy demands during stress, to exert important effects within the brain that promote memory processes, and to impair nonessential functions such as growth and reproductive function. The permissive actions of the steroids are evident at low physiological concentrations and are mediated at least partially, although probably not exclusively, by the high-affinity MRs. In contrast, the suppressive actions of the steroids emerge only when cortisol/corticosterone levels are raised by, for example, stress and are effected by the lower-affinity GRs.

The permissive and protective actions of GCs are complementary and enable the organism to mount an appropriate stress response and to maintain homeostasis. Dysregulation of either by genetic or environmental factors is potentially harmful and may predispose the individual to a variety of diseases that, depending on the site of the lesion, may include depression, disorders of the host defense system, osteoporosis, obesity, diabetes mellitus, hypertension, and other cardiovascular diseases. Long-term elevations in GC production that may occur in conditions of chronic stress are particularly hazardous and may have severe deleterious effects on the body. The effects of acute and sustained elevations in serum GCs are compared in **Table 1**.

Glucocorticoids and the Host Defense System

GCs exert multiple effects on the host defense system. In essence, they quench the early and late stages of the inflammatory response; that is, they suppress the initial vasodilation, the infiltration of leukocytes and

Table 1 Response to acute and long-term elevations in serum glucocorticoids

System	*Acute*[a]	*Long-term*
Host defense	Protection from potentially harmful inflammatory mediators	Immunosuppression and vulnerability to infection Poor tissue repair/wound healing
Metabolism	Mobilization of energy stores (↑ glycogen stores, ↑ gluconeogenesis, ↑ blood glucose, ↑ lipolysis, ↑ protein catabolism, ↓ peripheral glucose uptake/utilization)	Insulin-resistant steroid diabetes mellitus Centripetal obesity Protein depletion in muscle, connective, and other tissues Raised serum lipids and cholesterol
Musculoskeletal	Protein catabolism Altered Ca^{2+} homeostatsis	Impaired growth Muscle wasting Loss of connective tissue Osteoporosis and disturbed Ca^{2+} homeostasis
Central nervous system	Improved cognitive function	Mood changes (depression and psychotic episodes) Neurodegeneration
Cardiovascular	Salt and water retention Inhibition of the production of vasoactive inflammatory mediators	Hypertension and other cardiovascular disease
Reproductive	Inhibition of hypothalamic-pituitary-gonadal function	Menstrual irregularities Infertility (male and female)
Gastrointestinal tract	Reduced bicarbonate and mucus production	Increased susceptibility to ulcers

[a]↑, increased; ↓, decreased.

pain, and the subsequent proliferative events associated with wound healing and tissue repair. They also oppose the changes in vascular permeability that occur in inflammation and thus reduce both edema formation and the increased permeability of the blood–brain barrier. In addition, GCs are powerful inhibitors of cell-mediated (i.e., T-cell-dependent) immune responses and may also modulate humoral (B-cell-dependent) responses. Chronic elevations in serum GCs thus induce immunosuppression and render the individual susceptible to infection.

The anti-inflammatory and immunosuppressive actions of the steroids are attributed to their powerful actions on the growth, differentiation, distribution, function, and life span of monocytes, macrophages, polymorphonuclear cells, and lymphocytes. At the cellular level, GCs reduce the number of circulating lymphocytes, monocytes, and eosinophils by causing the cells to be marginated to the lymphoid tissues, mainly the bone marrow. In contrast, blood neutrophil levels rise as the steroids prevent the cells migrating to inflamed tissues by altering the expression of adhesion proteins on their surface and on the endothelium and thereby impairing the adherence and attachment processes. The profile of circulating white cells is also influenced by the fact that GCs also induce the apoptosis (programmed cell death) of thymocytes, mature T cells, and eosinophils, although not of neutrophils.

Several processes contribute to the suppression of cell-mediated immunity invoked by the steroids. These include (1) direction of the development of undifferentiated T helper (Th) cells away from the Th1 phenotype, which is critical to cell-mediated responses, and toward the Th2 phenotype, which facilitates B-lymphocyte-dependent responses; (2) inhibition of the synthesis of interleukin (IL)-1 and IL-2 by antigen-presenting cells and T cells, respectively, and hence the impairment of antigen presentation and T-cell proliferation; and (3) induction of T-cell apoptosis. Very high levels of GCs may also depress the synthesis of the immunokines required for immunoglobulin production and, with time, decrease serum immunoglobulins. However, lesser amounts of the steroids stimulate antibody production, probably because of their positive effect on the differentiation of Th2 cells. Other immune cell functions influenced by GCs include phagocytosis and antigen processing. GCs decrease Fc receptor expression on macrophages and thus prevent the recognition of particulate antigens that are antibody-bound or optimized for subsequent clearance. They also affect mast cell and basophil function in a number of rodent models, inhibiting IgE-dependent degranulation and hence the release of histamine and leukotriene C4.

The diverse effects of GCs on immune/inflammatory cell function are explained at a biochemical level by the striking ability of the steroids to inhibit the synthesis, release, and/or activity of the army of mediators normally produced when these cells are activated. Early studies focused on the powerful inhibitory action of the steroids on the phospholipase A2 (PLA2)-dependent generation of the pro-inflammatory eicosanoids (prostanoids, leukotrienes, and epoxides) and platelet-activating factor (PAF). Several lines of evidence indicate that GCs reduce the expression of the PLA2 subtype (group II) associated with the pathogenesis of inflammation and upregulate the synthesis of PLA2 inhibitory proteins, notably lipocortin 1 (also called annexin 1), which also influences other aspects of the inflammatory response. However, studies have shown that GCs also suppress prostanoid generation by repressing the expression of the inducible isoform of cyclooxygenase (COX II), which is normally expressed in abundance by activated monocytes, macrophages, fibroblasts, and endothelial cells.

GCs also exert profound inhibitory effects on the synthesis of many of the cytokines that are central to the manifestation of immune/inflammatory responses; these include IL-1, IL-2, IL-3, IL-6, IL-8, IL-12, granulocyte colony-stimulating factor (G-CSF), granulocyte–macrophage colony-stimulating factor (GM-CSF), interferon (IFN)-γ, tumor necrosis factor (TNF)-α, and monocyte chemotactic protein. Various mechanisms may contribute to these responses, including the downregulation of gene transcription and acceleration of mRNA degradation, together with effects at the translational and posttranslational levels. The biological actions of the cytokines may also be impaired; this may be explained in part by alterations in receptor expression and, for example, by the IL-2 receptor being downregulated by GCs. However, in many cases (e.g., IL-1, IL-6, and IFN-γ), the repression of cytokine expression is associated with the upregulation of the respective cytokine receptors (**Figure 1**); this phenomenon may help explain the permissive role of the steroids in priming the immune system for action as well as the ineffective responses mounted when GC levels are raised (e.g., by stress) or when adrenal function is impaired.

The release of many other inflammatory mediators may also be prevented by virtue of the powerful regulatory actions of the GCs on the enzymes responsible for their biosynthesis/degradation. For example, GCs suppress the inducible form of nitric oxide (NO) synthase and hence the generation of NO by macrophages. However, they promote the metabolism of nonlipid inflammatory mediators (e.g., bradykinin) by upregulating the enzymes responsible for their metabolism. Further important actions

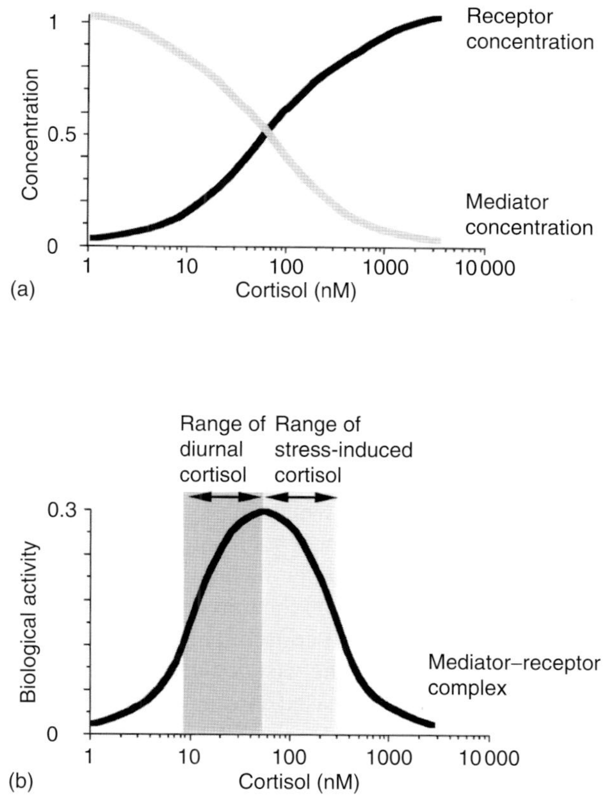

Figure 1 Mathematical model for the permissive and suppressive effects of glucocorticoids over a physiological concentration range. (a), Dose–response curves for a theoretical mediator and its specific receptors; (b), mathematical composite of mediator–receptor complex formation indicating biological activity and suggesting a mechanism by which low cortisol levels could be permissive and stress-induced cortisol surges suppressive in effect. From Munck, A. and Náraj-Fejes-Tóth, A. (1992), The ups and downs of glucocorticoid physiology: permissive and suppressive effects revisited, *Molecular and Cellular Endocrinology* **90**, C1–C4, copyright John Wiley & Sons Limited. Reproduced with permission.

of the GCs include reductions in the serum complement components, in the release of mediators such as 5-hydroxytryptamine (5-HT), and in the production/activity of the proteolytic enzymes (e.g., elastase and collagenase) that are concerned with the late stages of inflammation.

Metabolic Actions of Glucocorticoids

GCs exert complex effects on carbohydrate, lipid, and protein metabolism; their principal actions are catabolic, and they thus mobilize energy stores and oppose the actions of insulin (**Figure 2**).

Carbohydrate metabolism

The principal target is the liver, where GCs increase glycogen storage and gluconeogenesis. The effects of the steroids on glycogen storage reflect an increase in glycogen deposition due to the activation (dephosphorylation) of glycogen synthase and a concomitant decrease in glycogen breakdown due to inactivation of the glycogen-mobilizing enzyme glycogen phosphorylase. The increase in glucose synthesis is explained partly by the upregulation of key enzymes in the gluconeogenic pathway, such as phosphoenolpyruvate carboxykinase (PEPCK). In addition, the catabolic effects of the steroids on protein metabolism in peripheral tissues (e.g., muscle) and lipolysis in adipose tissue increase the availability of substrates (glucogenic amino acids and glycerol), while the fatty acids released with glycerol provide an important energy source for the process. The actions of GCs in the liver are effected by GR, and the delivery of the steroids to the receptors is facilitated by an abundance of 11β-HSD1, which serves mainly as a reductase.

Although much of the glucose formed in the liver in response to GCs is stored locally as glycogen, some is released into the circulation. Blood sugar levels are enhanced further by the actions of GCs in the peripheral tissues, which lead to the downregulation of the glucose transporters and, hence, to decreased glucose uptake and use.

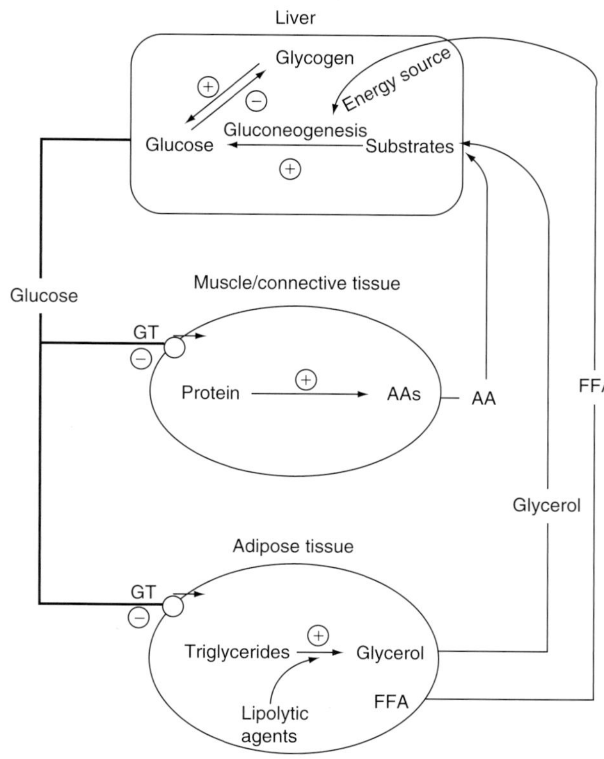

Figure 2 Schematic diagram illustrating the effects of glucocorticoids on carbohydrate, protein, and lipid metabolism. Note that the positive effects of the steroids on lipolysis involve interactions with other lipolytic agents (e.g., growth hormone and catecholamines). ⊕, stimulation; ⊖, inhibition; AA, amino acid; FFA, free fatty acid; GT, glucose transporter.

Lipid metabolism GCs exert a permissive influence on lipid metabolism, producing an acute lipolytic action that appears to reflect an increased responsiveness to catecholamines, growth hormone (GH), and possibly other lipid-mobilizing agents. In the long term, however, GCs produce a striking redistribution of fat, with enhanced deposition in the trunk (centripetal obesity), dorsocervical and subcapsular regions (buffalo hump), and face (moon face), together with a loss of fat in the upper and lower limbs, giving rise to the 'lemon-on-sticks' appearance that is exacerbated by the changes in protein metabolism. Blood lipid and cholesterol levels are also raised. The underlying mechanisms are poorly defined; they may involve alterations in insulin secretion triggered by the changes in glucose homeostasis, and it is interesting to note that white adipose tissue is rich in GRs and 11 β-HSD1. Paradoxically, this pattern of fat redistribution is not seen in experimental animals.

Protein metabolism GCs have a powerfully catabolic effect on protein in muscle and other tissues with the consequent release of amino acids into the circulation, which are converted to glucose in the liver. Long-term elevations in serum GCs may cause severe muscle wasting.

Skeleton and Connective Tissue

Skeleton GCs exert direct and indirect effects on bone, and persistent elevations of serum GCs may lead to osteoporosis. The steroids decrease bone formation by inhibiting (1) the proliferation and differentiation of osteoclasts and (2) the production of type 1 collagen, osteocalcin, and other matrix components such as mucopolysaccharides and sulfate glucoaminoglycans while increasing the expression of collagen. In addition, they exert complex effects on the expression of growth factors and their receptors and reduce Ca^{2+} stores by decreasing intestinal Ca^{2+} absorption, increasing renal Ca^{2+} excretion, and raising serum parathyroid hormone (PTH) levels. GCs also promote bone resorption through mechanisms that are secondary to the rise in PTH and possibly also via direct actions on the bone.

Sustained elevations in serum GCs inhibit linear growth in children and experimental animals. The mechanisms responsible have yet to be defined but are likely to reflect the actions of the steroids on the bone, principally at the site of the epiphyses. Although there are reports to the contrary, the majority of data suggests that the serum levels of GH, insulin-like growth factor (IGF)-1, and IGF-binding proteins are normal in these subjects.

Connective tissue The actions of GCs on connective tissue lead to poor wound healing and tissue repair. The steroids decrease fibroblast proliferation and function; inhibit the production of the matrix proteins, collagen, and hyaluronidate; and augment the production of the matrix-degrading enzymes collagenase, elastase, and hyalurinidase. However, GCs augment the production of fibinonectin, a matrix glycoprotein.

Cardiovascular

Elevations in serum GCs raise blood pressure This may be at least partially explained by mineralocorticoid-like actions of the steroids, which cause increased salt and water retention, and by the anti-inflammatory actions of the steroids, which prevent the release of local vasodilator substances such as prostacyclin and bradykinin. However, other mechanisms also come into play. These include (1) the upregulation of vascular α_1-adrenoceptors and consequent increased sensitivity of the vessels to the vasoconstrictor actions of norepinephrine; (2) increased cardiac output, possibly as a result of increased β1-adrenoceptor expression in the myocardium; and (3) increased production of angiotensinogen and increased sensitivity of the blood vessels to the vasoconstrictor actions of angiotensin II. The endothelium is rich in GRs, and it is conceivable that the steroids also modulate the release/activity of other locally produced vasoactive substances. In addition, reports that GRs are abundant in the brain-stem nuclei raise the possibility that GCs may also act centrally to alter sympathetic outflow.

Mood and Behavior

GCs released in stress may exert significant effects on cognitive function, mood and behavior, and reception of sensory inputs. Subjects whose serum GCs are raised due to either Cushing's disease or exogenous steroids also show marked disturbances in sleep, with a reduction in time spent in the rapid eye movement phase.

Studies on laboratory animals have shown that GCs act in the neocortex and limbic system (hippocampus, septum, and amygdala) to modify learning and memory processes in a context-dependent manner. Thus, an acute rise in GCs may facilitate learning and memory processes but also eliminate learned behavior that is no longer of relevance. The complex actions of the steroids involve both MRs and GRs, with MRs effecting the appraisal of information and response selection and GRs promoting the processes underlying the consolidation of acquired information. The long-term effects of GCs on learning and memory are less well researched and the data available are conflicting, although, when given with neurotoxic agents, learned behavior is impaired by the steroids.

GC levels are raised in some patients with depression, but it remains to be determined whether this is cause or effect; indeed, the effects of GCs on mood appear variable. Thus, approximately one-half of patients with iatrogenic or endogenous Cushing's disease show psychological disturbances; depression is the most common but some subjects show euphoric or manic behavior and, in some cases, overt psychoses. Patients with adrenal insufficiency also frequently experience mood changes; paradoxically, the most common is also depression.

Increasing evidence suggests that sustained elevations in serum GCs, such as those that occur due to chronic stress, may contribute to the processes of neurodegeneration. The toxic actions of the steroids, which have been studied most widely in the hippocampus, are associated with altered glutaminergic transmission, a long-term enhancement of Ca^{2+} influx, and depletion of ATP stores, with a consequent impairment of essential energy-requiring processes such as glucose uptake. The vulnerability of the neurons may be enhanced further by a reduction in neurotrophic capacity because the elevations in serum GCs induced by chronic stress or the administration of exogenous steroids inhibit the expression of brain-derived neurotrophic factor mRNA and also tyrosine kinase, which is required for growth factor action.

Reproductive Function

GCs act at multiple sites within the hypothalamic-pituitary-gonadal axis to impair reproductive function; hence, chronic elevations in serum GCs lead to infertility and menstrual irregularities. An important site of action of the steroids is the hypothalamus. In addition, the steroids exert significant effects at the pituitary level to depress gonadotropin-releasing hormone (GnRH)-driven gonadotropin release and may also exert further regulatory actions within the gonads.

Development

GCs exert both positive and negative effects on cell growth. In addition, they fulfill complex organizational effects pre- and postnatally and thus play a key role in developmental programming. Not surprisingly, the HPA axis is tightly regulated during perinatal life and, in rodents, the stress response is attenuated during a critical phase postnatally. At this time, the developing HPA axis shows a high degree of plasticity, and a growing body of evidence suggests that disturbances in the GC milieu may (1) trigger a plethora of pathologies (e.g., growth retardation or impairment of CNS development) and (2) precipitate abnormalities in GC secretion that persist into adult life and may increase the susceptibility of the individual to conditions as diverse as hypertension, insulin resistance, cognitive and other behavioral disorders, and allergic/inflammatory disease. Perinatal manipulations that alter the expression of GRs (but not MRs) in the brain are particularly hazardous in this regard because, by disrupting the negative feedback mechanisms, they alter the responsivity of the HPA axis to stress throughout the lifetime of the individual. For example, the exposure of neonatal rats to stimuli that raise serum GCs, such as an immune insult (the injection of bacterial lipopolysaccharide) or the administration of exogenous GCs, results in the adult in the downregulation of GRs in the hippocampus and hypothalamus, decreased sensitivity of the HPA axis to the negative feedback actions of the GCs, and exaggerated HPA responses to stress. Similar long-term changes in GR expression occur in rats subjected to prolonged periods of maternal separation; the consequent impairment of the negative feedback system and changes in HPA function are associated with alterations in T-cell antibody responses and in the incidence of age-related neuropathies. In contrast, neonatal handling, which increases hippocampal GR expression by mechanisms involving serotonin, reduces the magnitude and duration of the stress response in the adult; maternal care may therefore help to program events that regulate responses to stress in the adult and thus reduce vulnerability to disease.

Other Actions

GCs inhibit the production of mucus and bicarbonate in the stomach and small intestine by virtue of their ability to block prostaglandin production; sustained elevations in GCs thus increase susceptibility to gastric and duodenal ulcer formation. The steroids also promote Na^+ absorption in the colon by mechanisms that involve MRs and GRs while acting via GRs to augment Na^+ excretion by stimulating the synthesis of atrial natriuretic peptide (ANP) and augmenting the actions of ANP on the kidney, thereby opposing the Na^+-retaining influence exerted via MRs in the distal renal tubule. In addition, GCs may enhance free-water clearance by depressing the synthesis of vasopressin.

See Also the Following Articles

Adrenal Cortex; Cytokines; Glucocorticoids, Effects of Stress on; Glucocorticoids – Adverse Effects on the Nervous System.

Further Reading

Barnes, P. J. (1998). Anti-inflamatory actions of glucocorticoids: molecular mechanisms. *Clinical Science* **94**, 557–572.

Brann, D. W. and Manesh, V. B. (1991). Role of corticosteroids in female reproduction. *FASEB Journal* **5**, 2691–2698.

Buckingham, J. C., Gillies, G. E. and Cowell, A.-M. (1997). *Stress, stress hormones and the immune system.* Chichester, UK: John Wiley.

de Kloet, E. R., Vreugdenhil, E., Oitzl, M. S., et al. (1998). Brain corticosteroid receptor balance in health and disease. *Endocrine Review* **19**, 269–301.

Lukert, B. P. and Raiz, L. G. (1994). Glucocorticoid-induced osteoporosis. *Rheumatic Disease Clinics of North America.*

Munck, A., Guyre, P. M. and Holbrook, N. J. (1984). Physiological functions of glucocorticoids and their relation to pharmacological actions. *Endocrine Review* **51**, 25–44.

Munck, A. and Náraj-Fejes-Tóth, A. (1992). The ups and downs of glucocorticoid physiology: permissive and suppressive effects revisited. *Molecular and Cellular Endocrinology* **90**, C1–C4.

Nestler, J. E. and McClanahan, M. A. (1992). Diabetes and adrenal disease. *Baillière's Clinical Endocrinology and Metabolism* **6**, 829–851.

Pilkis, S. J. and Granner, D. K. (1992). Molecular physiology of the regulation of hepatic gluconeogenesis and glycolysis. *Annual Review of Physiology* **54**, 885–909.

Robinson, I., Gabrielsson, B., Klaus, G., et al. (1995). Glucocorticoids and growth problems. *Acta Paediatrica* **84**, 81–85.

Selye, H. (1952). *The story of the adaptation syndrome.* Montreal: Acta.

Tilders, F. J. and Schmidt, E. D. (1998). Interleukin 1 induced plasticity of hypothalamic CRH neurons and long-term stress hyperresponsiveness. *Annals of the New York Academy of Sciences* **840**, 65–73.

Vinson, G. P. and Anderson, D. C. (1996). *Adrenal glands, vascular system and hypertension.* Bristol, UK: Society for Endocrinology.

Norepinephrine: CNS Pathways and Neurophysiology

G Aston-Jones
Medical University of South Carolina, Charleston, SC, USA
C A Meijas-Aponte
National Institutes of Health, Baltimore, MD, USA
B Waterhouse
Drexel University College of Medicine, Philadelphia, PA, USA

Norepinephrine Cell Groups and Pathways

Locus Coeruleus

The nucleus locus coeruleus (LC) is a dense cluster of noradrenergic neurons in the dorsorostral pons. This nucleus gained prominence in the 1960s when new anatomical approaches revealed it to be the major source of norepinephrine (NE) in brain with projections throughout most central nervous system (CNS) regions. These findings stimulated a great deal of research into this system, resulting in a wealth of knowledge at the cellular, systems, and behavioral levels. Considerable evidence indicates that these neurons are important in a variety of cognitive, affective, arousal, and other behavioral functions, as well as associated clinical dysfunctions.

Locus coeruleus efferent projections As summarized in **Table 1**, LC NE neurons project throughout the neuraxis, including the cerebral cortex, thalamus, cerebellum, midbrain, and spinal cord. In this regard, it is different from other 'typical' brain systems that have very limited projection targets (e.g., thalamo-cortical projections). Despite this high degree of divergence, LC neurons exhibit substantial regional and laminar specificity in their efferent projections. Notably, brain areas in primates that are associated with attentional processing (e.g., parietal cortex, pulvinar nucleus, and superior colliculus) have particularly dense LC projections and NE receptors. Notable areas that receive little or no input from the LC include the caudate putamen and most of the hypothalamus. Ultrastructural evidence indicates that these neurons often make conventional synaptic appositions with postsynaptic targets, although the frequency of such synaptic contacts is controversial. Extrasynaptic (paracrine) release of NE from LC terminals also appears to be possible.

Locus coeruleus afferents A variety of evidence indicates that the LC receives a wealth of different neurotransmitter inputs. This nucleus is densely innervated by fibers that contain opiates, glutamate, γ-aminobutyric acid (GABA), serotonin, epinephrine, histamine, and the peptide orexin/hypocretin. The

Table 1 Organization of the adrenergic system

	Fiber density	Locus coeruleus A4 + A6	Ventral pons and medulla cluster				Dorsal medulla cluster		
			A1	C1	A5	A7	A2	C2	C3
Forebrain									
Cortex	2+	✓							
Hippocampal formation	2–3+	✓							
Amygdala									
Medial	1+		✓				✓		
Central	3+	✓	✓	✓	✓		✓	✓	✓
Basal	3+	✓							
Basal forebrain/septum									
Medial septum	2+	✓	✓	✓			✓	✓	
Medial preoptic area		✓	✓	✓			✓	✓	
Substatia innominata		✓	✓	✓			✓	✓	
Lateral septum	3+	✓	✓	✓			✓		
Bed nucleus stria terminalis	5+	✓	✓	✓	✓		✓	✓	
Ventral pallidum			✓		✓				
Zona incerta			✓	✓	✓				
Subthalamic nucleus		✓			✓				
Nucleus accumbens	1–3+						✓		
Thalamus									
Sensory									
Lateral geniculate nu	3–4+	✓							
Medial geniculate nu	1–2+	✓							
Ventroposterior medial nu		✓							
Ventroposterior lateral mu		✓							
Ventrobasal nu	3–4+	✓							
Ventromedial nu	3+	✓							
Reticular nu	3–4+	✓							
Motor									
Ventrolateral nu	3+	✓							
Ventralanterior nu	3+	✓							
Viscero-limbic									
Anteriormedial nu	4+	✓							
Anteriodorsal nu	3+	✓							
Anterioventral	2+	✓							
Mediodorsal nu	1–2+	✓							
Central medial nu	1+	✓							
Central lateral nu	1–2+	✓							
Reuniens nu	1+	✓							
Parafascicular nu	1+2	✓							
Paraventrivular nu	5+			✓	✓				
Rhomboid nu	2–3+	*							
Epithalamus									
Medial habenulla	5+	*							
Lateral habenulla	4–5+	*							
Hypothalamus									
Periventricular nucleus	5+	✓							
Suprachiamatic nucleus	1–2+	*							
Retrochiasmatic	4+		✓						
Paraventricular nuclues	3–5+	✓	✓	✓	✓		✓		
Supraoptic nuclues	4+		✓				✓		
Dorsomedial	3–5+	✓	✓	✓					
Arcute nuclues	3+	✓	✓	✓			✓		
Medial eminence	2+	✓		✓				✓	
Perifornical area	4+		✓				✓		
Lateral area	3+		✓	✓					
Brain stem									
Sensory									
Main sensory trigeminal nu	2+	✓							

Continued

Table 1 Continued

	Fiber density	Locus coeruleus A4 + A6	Ventral pons and medulla cluster				Dorsal medulla cluster		
			A1	C1	A5	A7	A2	C2	C3
Spinal trigeminal nu	2+	✓							
Mesencephalic trigeminal nu	4+	✓		✓					
Superior olivary complex	1+	✓							
Cochlear nu	2+	✓	✓			✓			
Vestibular nu	0–1+	✓		✓					
Motor									
Oculomotor and trochlear nu	0–1+								
Motor trigeminal nu	4+				✓	✓			
Abducens nu	0–1+								
Facial nu	3–4+				✓	✓			
Hypoglossal nu	2–3+				✓	✓			
Nucleus ambiguus	5+	✓		✓					
Inferior olive	5+	✓	✓		✓				
Red nucleus	1+	✓							
Cerebellum		✓			✓	✓			
Sensorimotor									
Superior colliculus	2+				✓				
Superficial layers		✓							
Deep layers					✓	✓			
Inferior colliculus	2+	✓							
Visceral									
Nucleus of the solitary tract including A2 and C2 areas	5+		✓	✓	✓				
Dorsal motor nucleus of vagus	5+			✓	✓				
Caudal ventrolateral medulla including A1 area	3+			✓	✓				
Rostral ventrolateral medulla including C1 area	3+		✓		✓				
Periaqueductal gray	2+5		✓	✓	✓				
Parabrachial nucleus	4+		✓	✓	✓		✓		
Area postrema	1+		✓	✓			✓		
Modulatory systems									
Substantia nigra, pars compacta	0–1+								
Ventral tegmental area	1+	✓	✓	✓					
Retrorubral field	1+	✓	✓	✓					
Raphe			✓						
Central linear	2+								
Dorsal	2+		✓						
Magnun	3+		✓	✓					
Pallidus	5+		✓	✓					
Obscurus	1+	✓		✓					
Locus coeruleus	2+			✓					✓
A5 area			✓						
Spinal cord									
Intermediolateral cell column				✓	✓	✓			
Dorsal horn		✓							
Ventral horn		**			✓	✓			

This table is based on the organization of LC versus non-LC systems as originally reviewed by Moore and Card in 1984 and published in the *Handbook of Chemical Neuroanatomy*, volume 2. The descriptions of fiber density were obtained from Moore and Card, whereas the information regarding efferent projections was updated based upon a comprehensive survey of research reports available in the literature. The information presented is meant to reflect major efferents of the adrenergic cell groups. Single asterisks indicate structures known to not receive LC afferents but for which the source of adrenergic innervation is unknown. The double asterisk indicates ventral horn innervation by LC, which is dependent upon rat strain.

sources of these various inputs have not been fully elucidated, though some major inputs have been identified. The nucleus paragigantocellularis lateralis (PGi) in the ventrolateral rostral medulla, a major input that strongly excites LC neurons, is a source for glutamate, GABA, enkephalin, corticotropin-releasing hormone (CRH), and epinephrine. A strongly inhibitory GABA and enkephalin input originates from the dorsomedial rostral medulla. Excitatory orexin and histamine inputs originate in the hypothalamus.

The shell of dendrites surrounding the LC nucleus offers additional extensive targets for afferent termination, and indeed it appears that several areas target these extranuclear dendrites more so than the LC nucleus proper. Thus, projections from the periaqueductal gray matter, parabrachial region, preoptic area, amygdala, and medial prefrontal cortex, among other sites, project primarily to the peri-LC region, with relatively little input to the LC proper. Although some of these projections have been shown to contact LC dendrites, additional ultrastructural studies are needed to examine others.

A recent study has extended our understanding of LC afferents to the circuit level. Using transynaptic tracing, lesions, and electrophysiology, Aston-Jones and colleagues determined that the suprachiasmatic nucleus (SCN) indirectly innervates the LC, using the dorsomedial hypothalamus as a relay. Based upon the role of the SCN as the brain's major circadian pacemaker and the role of the LC in arousal and performance (see later), these findings reveal a possible circuit for circadian regulation of arousal and performance.

Recent work by Iba, Aston-Jones, and colleagues reveal that in monkey strong projections to LC originate in cingulate and orbital cortices (**Figure 1**). Given the roles of these prefrontal areas in conflict monitoring, decision making, and other cognitive functions, these projections may be responsible at least in part for the different modes of activity that occur in LC neurons during cognitive performance (described later). Interestingly, these prefrontal projections to LC appear to be stronger in primates than in rats, in concert with the more highly evolved prefrontal cortex and more prominent role of this structure in regulating behavior in primates.

Taken together, these observations indicate that LC is not a relay nucleus for primary sensory or motor information and that it receives highly processed information concerning internal and external sensory stimuli as well as behavioral and affective states. This suggests a highly integrative function for this system.

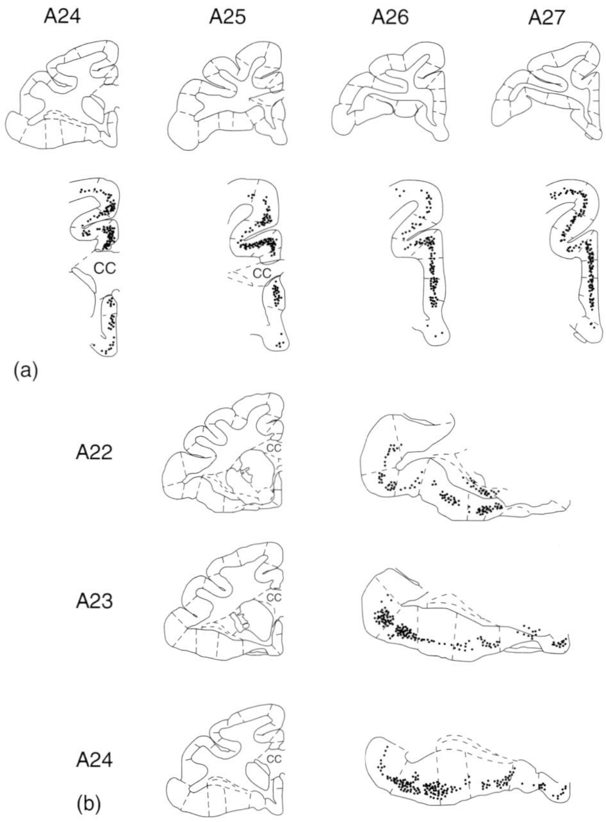

Figure 1 Plots of retrogradely labeled neurons in the nucleus accumbens and orbitofrontal cortex after injections of cholera toxin B into monkey locus coeruleus. (a) Accumbens neurons labeled from the monkey locus ceruleus. Lower sections are high-power views containing plotted cells; upper sections are low-power views to give orientation. (b) Orbitofrontal cortex neurons labeled from the monkey locus coeruleus. Sections on the right are high-power views containing plotted cells; sections on the left are low-power views to give orientation. For both panels, labels A22–A27 refer to distances (in millimeters) from the interaural line. CC, corpus callosum. From Aston-Jones G and Cohen JD (2005) Adaptive gain and the role of the locus coeruleus–norepinephrine system in optimal performance. *Journal of Comparative Neurology* 493: 99–110.

Norepinephrine release Microdialysis methods have recently provided *in vivo* confirmation that certain drugs and behavioral conditions increase or decrease the release of norepinephrine from locus coeruleus axons. For example, reuptake blockers and stress both enhance extracellular NE levels in areas (such as the neocortex) that receive their only NE innervation from the LC. In addition, the amount of NE release in cortex increases in proportion to activity within LC, even at low frequencies (2–4 Hz). Notably, burst stimulation elicits more NE release per impulse than evenly do spaced stimuli. This indicates that phasic LC responses (see later) may be particularly effective in releasing NE in target areas.

Locus coeruleus impulse activity *Sleep and waking.* Spontaneous LC activity in rats, cats, or monkeys varies with the stage of the sleep–wake cycle, with firing being most rapid during wakefulness, slower during slow-wave sleep, and virtually absent during paradoxical sleep. LC neurons are phasically activated by conspicuous unconditioned stimuli. Notably, stimuli that elicit large LC responses in either rats or monkeys also typically disrupt sleep or ongoing behavior, and evoke waking or a behavioral-orienting response. The same stimuli do not disrupt behavior if they elicit small LC responses.

Stress. Other studies have revealed strong activation of LC neurons by stressors. Stimuli such as sciatic nerve activation or other painful events strongly activate LC cells. Other stressors, such as a puff of air in the awake monkey or a variety of environmental or physiological stressors, also activate LC neurons. In addition, LC neurons are activated by corticotropin-releasing hormone, which mediates the response of LC cells to certain physiological stressors such as hypotension.

Locus coeruleus activity during cognitive performance. The preceding results suggest that, in addition to a role in sleep and waking, LC neurons may be involved in behavioral responses to sensory stimuli. Aston-Jones and colleagues tested this by recording impulse activity of LC neurons in monkeys performing a target detection task. These studies indicated that the LC exhibits two modes of impulse activity: a tonic mode in which tonic activity is high but phasic responses to targets are low or absent, and a phasic mode in which LC neurons fire tonically more slowly but exhibit consistent activation shortly following target stimuli. Behaviorally, the tonic mode corresponds to poor task performance with many false alarm errors, whereas the phasic mode is associated with nearly error-free performance. These results indicate that these different modes of LC activity may facilitate either selective, focused attention (phasic mode) or flexible behavior and scanning (tonic mode). Each of these LC and behavioral modes is adaptive, depending on the context.

LC activation at decision completion. Recent studies recording LC neural activity in monkeys performing a forced-choice task revealed that the aforementioned phasic responses described are neither purely sensory nor motor/premotor in nature. As shown in **Figure 2**, these LC responses are more closely linked to behavioral responses (lever releases) than to sensory stimuli that trigger the behavioral responses, but do not occur for lever releases elicited outside of the task context. Finally, the onset of these LC responses occurs at about 200 ms prior to the lever releases, at a time that the decision concerning lever release is being made. Aston-Jones and colleagues concluded from these results that these phasic LC responses reflected completion of a decision process, and that the modulatory gain-enhancing effects of the associated NE release (see later) facilitate brain processes and behaviors called upon by the decision just made. In this way, the LC phasic response supports the current task/goal and facilitates focused performance in that task. The projections to LC from orbital and cingulate cortices (described previously) may mediate these phasic LC responses associated with decision processes.

Non-LC Norepinephrine and Epinephrine Cell Groups

Neurons in other brain nuclei aside from those in the LC constitute 55% of all CNS NE and epinephrine (E) cells. These neurons are clustered in two rostrocaudally aligned columns within the brain stem. One column is located primarily in the ventral aspect of the pons and medulla and contains 44% of all NE/E neurons, whereas the second is situated in the dorsomedial medulla. The individual clusters of non-LC NE/E neurons within these cell columns are further subdivided on the basis of their specific anatomical location and the ability to synthesize E (**Figure 3**).

Non-LC NE/E projections An analysis of projection patterns of LC versus non-LC NE/E neurons reveals similarities and differences (**Table 1**). Non-LC NE neurons project exclusively subcortically and make a preponderance of connections onto motor nuclei in the medulla and spinal cord, and onto structures associated with visceral function. Within the brain stem, targets of non-LC NE/E neurons include cranial motor nuclei such as the dorsal motor vagus, motor trigeminal, motor facial, and the hypoglossal nucleus, as well as visceral–sensory nuclei such as the nucleus of the solitary tract, parabrachial complex, and periaqueductal gray. In the forebrain, non-LC cell clusters provide dense projections to visceral-related structures such as the bed nucleus of the stria terminalis (BNST), central nucleus of the amygdala, and paraventricular hypothalamus. Thalamic and epithalamic targets include the paraventricular nucleus, rhomboid nucleus, and habenula.

Within the different non-LC adrenergic nuclei, there is a preferential innervation of motor systems by A5 and A7 groups, whereas visceral–sensory areas are primarily innervated by medullary A1 and A2 nuclei. The E-containing fibers from C1 neurons innervate both motor and visceral–sensory structures. C1 neurons send collaterals that innervate both spinal cord and brain stem targets. However, most C1 neurons that project to hypothalamus do not project to spinal cord or brain stem structures. In clear contrast

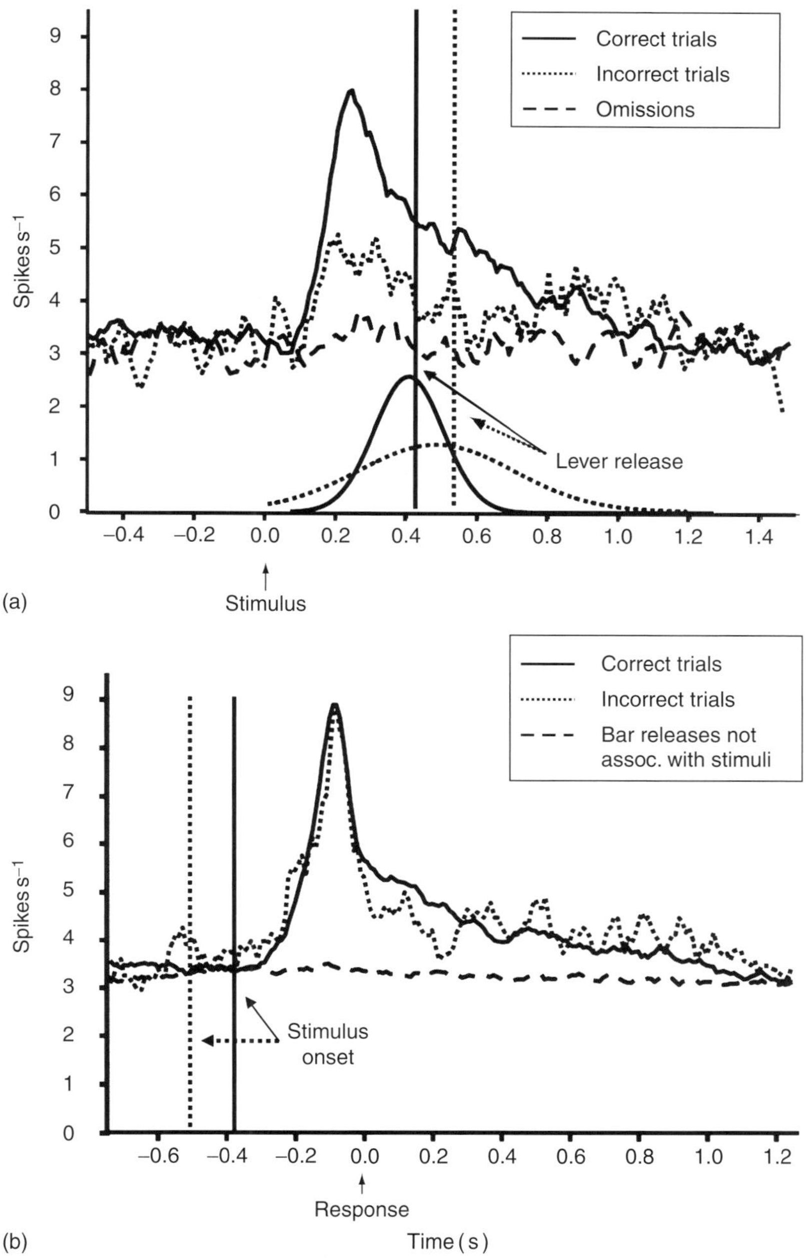

Figure 2 Stimulus- and response-locked population perievent time histograms (PETHs) showing LC responses to cues for trials yielding correct and incorrect behavioral responses. (a) Stimulus-locked population PETHs showing LC response to cues (presented at time 0) for trials yielding correct or incorrect behavioral responses. Note that the LC response peaks sooner and is less prolonged on correct, compared to incorrect, trials in this analysis (17 533 and 1362 trials, respectively). No fluctuation in LC activity was detected on omission trials (dashed line, 1128 trials). Vertical lines indicate the mean behavioral RTs. Curves below PETHs represent the normalized RT distributions for correct and incorrect trials. (b) The difference in the phasic LC response between correct and incorrect trials is no longer evident on response-locked population PETHs. In addition, no LC response occurred prior to or following lever releases not associated with stimulus presentation (dashed line, 3381 trials). Vertical lines indicate the mean stimulus onset times. From Clayton EC, Rajkowski J, Cohen JD, et al. (2004) Phasic activation of monkey locus coeruleus neurons by simple decisions in a forced choice task. *Journal of Neuroscience* 24: 9914–9920.

to this pattern of organization, LC projections to the brain stem and spinal cord are directed almost exclusively to relay sites along ascending sensory pathways, including those associated with somatosensory, auditory, gustatory, and visual systems. This sensory-predominant bias of the LC efferent projection continues to the level of the thalamus and also includes the olfactory system. An overlap between LC and non-LC NE efferent projections to motor structures becomes evident in the cerebellar system, and the

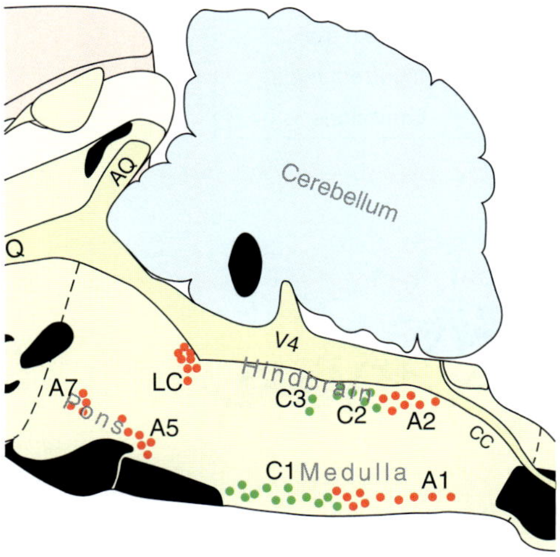

Figure 3 Localization of norepinephrine (red) and epinephrine (green) nuclei in the brain stem. The cell column in the ventral pons and medulla includes A1, C1, A5, and A7 cell groups, whereas the dorsal medulla column includes A2, C2, and C3 cell groups.

LC is the sole source of NE fibers to thalamic motor relay nuclei and motor (as well as sensory) processing regions of the cerebral cortex.

Non-LC impulse activity LC and non-LC neurons have similar electrophysiological signatures but exhibit differing responses to afferents and neurotransmitter systems. They are slow-firing neurons (<5 Hz) with wide action potentials (lasting more than 2 ms). Pharmacologically, both LC and non-LC neurons are inhibited by $\alpha 2$ adrenoceptor agonists, indicating the presence of a functional $\alpha 2$ autoreceptor. Conversely, sciatic nerve stimulation activates LC neurons, and also to a lesser extent A5 neurons, but not A2 neurons, indicating selectivity in the systems that activate the different adrenergic groups. Moreover, morphine strongly inhibits LC neurons but is reported to excite A5 neurons.

The organization of the non-LC adrenergic system and its connection to visceral-related areas prompted many studies of the non-LC adrenergic neurons; the findings indicate a diversity of roles in modulating cardiovascular, respiratory, renal, gastrointestinal, and endocrine functions. For example, the A1 area is involved in hemodynamic regulation by controlling the release of vasopressin, whereas C1 neurons are sensitive to blood pressure and are involved in regulating sodium and water balance. A5 neurons influence the respiratory rhythm generator of the rostral ventrolateral medulla, and A2 cells have a role in the regulation of food intake.

Stress Physiological (cardiovascular, osmotic, and immune challenges) as well as psychological (restraint and intermittent footshock) stressors activate both LC and non-LC NE/E neurons. These stressors also activate major targets of the non-LC system, such as the medial and central nuclei of the amygdala, BNST, and paraventricular hypothalamus, suggesting that non-LC adrenergic neurons are part of a functional stress circuit. A significant difference between LC and non-LC cell groups may be habituation to stressors. Under chronic footshock regimens, LC neurons habituate whereas non-LC cells in A1, C1, A2, and C2 exhibit persistent stress responses. Thus, NE/E transmission in response to acute and persistent stressful conditions is differentially distributed across brain structures according to the unique efferent topographies of the LC and non-LC systems.

Drugs of abuse have profound effects on the activity of NE neurons throughout the brain. The aversiveness of opiate withdrawal is blocked by antagonizing β adrenoceptors in BNST; this NE input largely originates in A1/A2 neurons. A1/A2 neurons also appear to play a particularly prominent role in relapse to drug-seeking induced by stress. Several studies have shown that selective lesions of ascending A1/A2 NE projections, or antagonism of NE receptors in amygdala or BNST, attenuate relapse to drug-seeking induced by footshock stress.

Summary for non-LC systems In summary, several principles of organization emerge from examination of the efferent connections of the central NE/E cell groups. First, the distribution of adrenergic fibers is particularly dense in terminal fields innervated by non-LC adrenergic neurons (**Table 1**). Second, within the brain stem, the LC preferentially innervates primary sensory pathways while non-LC adrenergic nuclei innervate motor and visceral–sensory systems. Third, non-LC forebrain projections target visceral–sensory and autonomic circuits. Fourth, areas that subserve motor integrative functions such as the cerebellar circuit are mainly innervated by LC, with the exception of the inferior olive, which is mainly innervated by the A5 and A7 areas. Fifth, LC is the only source of NE innervation to the cortical mantle. Sixth, although all NE/E neurons have similar electrophysiological properties, LC and non-LC cells may respond differently to the same afferent inputs and neurotransmitter systems. This analysis leads to an appreciation of the complex anatomical relationships and physiological/behavioral properties of the different brain NE/E systems.

Postsynaptic Actions of Norepinephrine

Investigations in the 1960s and 1970s viewed NE as a putative conventional neurotransmitter and set out to determine its ability to increase or decrease the firing rate of target neurons. For the most part, local application of NE by microiontophoresis, or stimulation of LC, suppressed the spontaneous discharge of neurons in cerebellum, cerebral cortex, and elsewhere in the brain. These depressant responses were mimicked and blocked by adrenoceptor agonists and antagonists, respectively. Taken together, these findings support the idea that NE might function primarily as an inhibitory transmitter at central synapses.

Modulatory effects of NE on single neurons In the mid-1970s pioneering studies by Foote et al. in monkey auditory cortex demonstrated a differential depressant effect of microiontophoretically applied NE on single neurons, such that the spontaneous firing rate of recorded cells was suppressed to a greater extent than were stimulus-evoked discharges, thus yielding a net increase in the signal-to-noise ratio. This initial study prompted many other laboratories to investigate the actions of NE in a variety of sensory circuits within the mammalian brain, including olfactory bulb, sensory thalamus, visual, auditory, and somatosensory cortices. In many cases local application of NE was found to enhance extracellular responses of individual sensory neurons to synaptic stimuli; however, mixed effects were observed in other studies, with suppression of stimulus-evoked discharge predominating.

Later work by Waterhouse and colleagues examined NE actions at levels that had minimal or no effect on spontaneous discharge of target neurons. Under these conditions iontophoretic NE frequently produced absolute increases in stimulus-evoked discharge with minimal or no change in baseline firing. In other cases local administration of NE revealed robust cellular responses to otherwise subthreshold synaptic stimuli. The demonstration of NE-induced facilitation of cellular responses to direct iontophoretic application of GABA or glutamate under both normal and low-calcium/high-magnesium conditions argued that such effects were mediated postsynaptically. These findings in cerebral cortex and cerebellum of anesthetized and awake, behaving animals supported the general hypothesis that a prominent physiological function of central noradrenergic pathways is to enhance the efficacy of both excitatory and inhibitory synaptic transmission within target neuronal circuits, rather than to directly suppress cell firing.

Later work by Waterhouse et al. in cat and rat primary visual cortex showed that NE could alter specific receptive field properties (e.g., receptive field size, direction selectivity, velocity tuning) of visually responsive cells (**Figure 4**). Other studies showed that NE was capable of modifying the receptive field structure of cells in somatosensory and auditory cortices and cochlear nuclei. As such, these results go beyond the demonstration of simple monoamine-induced changes in the magnitude of synaptically evoked responses and begin to show that such actions can lead to selective alteration of the feature extraction properties of individual sensory neurons. More recent work by Arnsten, and colleagues indicates that NE and NE agonist drugs can modify the working-memory-related discharge of cells in prefrontal cortex of behaving monkeys. These latter findings suggest that the noradrenergic actions observed in sensory circuits may be generalized across brain regions that serve many different functions.

Additional studies in cortex and elsewhere have determined the pharmacologic specificity and dose dependency of NE-mediated modulatory effects. For example, the magnitude of cellular response to direct glutamate application can be maximally enhanced at a specific level of NE administration, and only moderately or minimally be affected by concentrations above and below this level (**Figure 5(a)**), thus revealing an inverted-U dose–response relationship for this effect of NE. Furthermore, noradrenergic enhancement of neuronal responses to excitatory synaptic stimuli are mimicked and blocked by α1-receptor agonists (**Figure 5(b)**) and antagonists, respectively, whereas the augmentation of inhibitory responses to GABA application (**Figure 6**) or afferent pathway stimulation involves activation of β receptors. Other studies, particularly those in hippocampus, provide data suggesting the opposite (i.e., NE enhancement of excitatory synaptic transmission is dependent upon β-receptor mechanisms and augmentation of synaptic inhibition is mediated by α1-receptor mechanisms). These disparate results have not been reconciled but may reflect unique receptor distributions or second-messenger linkages among neurons within different brain regions. Overall, these observations indicate that within a specified brain circuit an array of noradrenergic modulatory actions is possible, depending upon cellular expression of receptors and levels of NE available for interaction with those receptors.

Cellular mechanisms of NE action Intracellular experiments have demonstrated multiple actions of NE on properties of neuronal membranes. For example, NE-induced blockade of a calcium-activated potassium conductance leads to accommodation block and prolongation of evoked excitatory discharges. It is widely accepted that this effect, in conjunction with a membrane hyperpolarizing action of NE, can account for noradrenergic potentiation or signal-to-noise ratio enhancement of threshold level excitatory

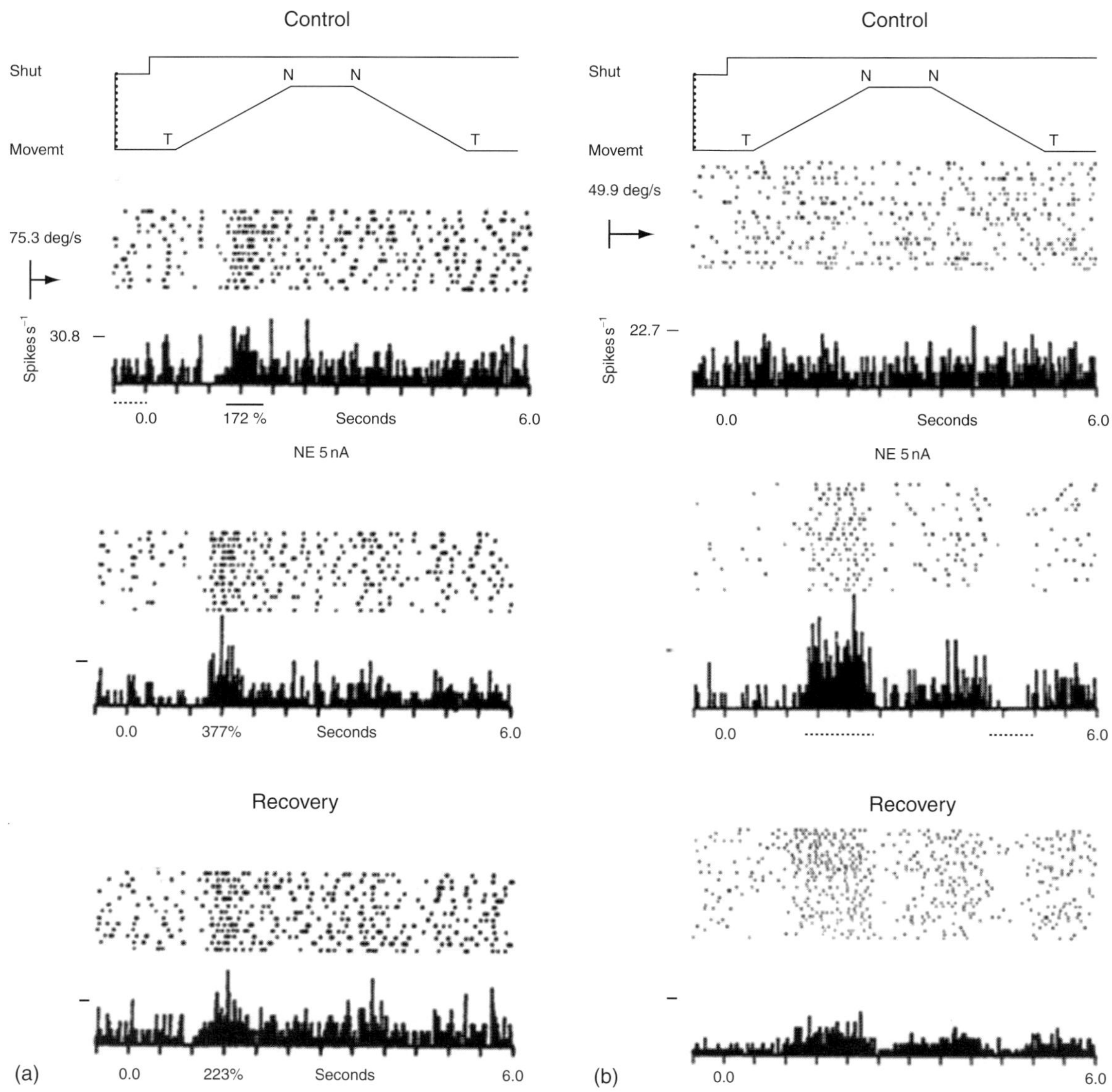

Figure 4 Effects of norepinephrine (NE) on responses of rat visual cortical neurons to visual field stimulation. (a, b) The raster and corresponding perievent histogram records show the extracellularly recorded responses of two single neurons in the rat visual cortex to movements of a vertically oriented (shown on the left) bar of light across the contralateral hemivisual field before, during, and after periods of microiontophoretic administration of NE. For each set of records, the uppermost line depicts the opening (step-up) and closing (step-down) of the shutter controlling the stimulus display. The trapezoid waveform indicates the position of the stimulus in visual space as it moves in the temporal (T) to nasal (N) direction and then back along the same path in the reverse direction. Time is indicated along the horizontal axis of the histogram, and discharge frequency of the cell is indicated along the vertical axis. Stimulus-bound excitatory or inhibitory components of the response were expressed as a percentage increase or decrease, respectively, of background firing rate (dotted line beneath histogram). (a) In the first cell the control response (top) consisted of an excitatory burst (solid bar) preceded by an inhibitory trough as the stimulus moved in the T to N direction, but no significant change in activity as the stimulus moved along the same path in the opposite direction (N to T). The visually evoked excitatory peak represented a 172% increase in firing over the basal level of discharge. Iontophoretic application of NE (5 nA) suppressed basal firing rate but produced an absolute increase in the visually evoked response (middle). Recovery to the control level of response was observed following cessation of NE administration (bottom). Each histogram sums unit activity during 13 trials; bin width = 15 ms. (b) In the second cell, there was no discernible response to the moving bar of light during the control period (top); however, during NE (5 nA) administration (middle) an obvious stimulus-evoked excitation (broken bar beneath histogram) and a stimulus-bound inhibition (dotted line beneath histogram) became evident. After cessation of NE iontophoresis (bottom), the cell gradually lost its sensitivity to the visual stimulus. Control and NE histograms, $n = 22$ trials; recovery histogram, $n = 31$ trials. Bin width = 15 ms.

synaptic responses observed *in vivo*. McCormick and colleagues have found that NE's depolarizing action influences a complex interaction between intrinsic membrane currents in thalamic relay neurons. This interplay moves thalamic neurons back and forth between a non-signal-transmitting oscillatory mode during sleep and a single-spike transmission, or 'relay,' mode during waking.

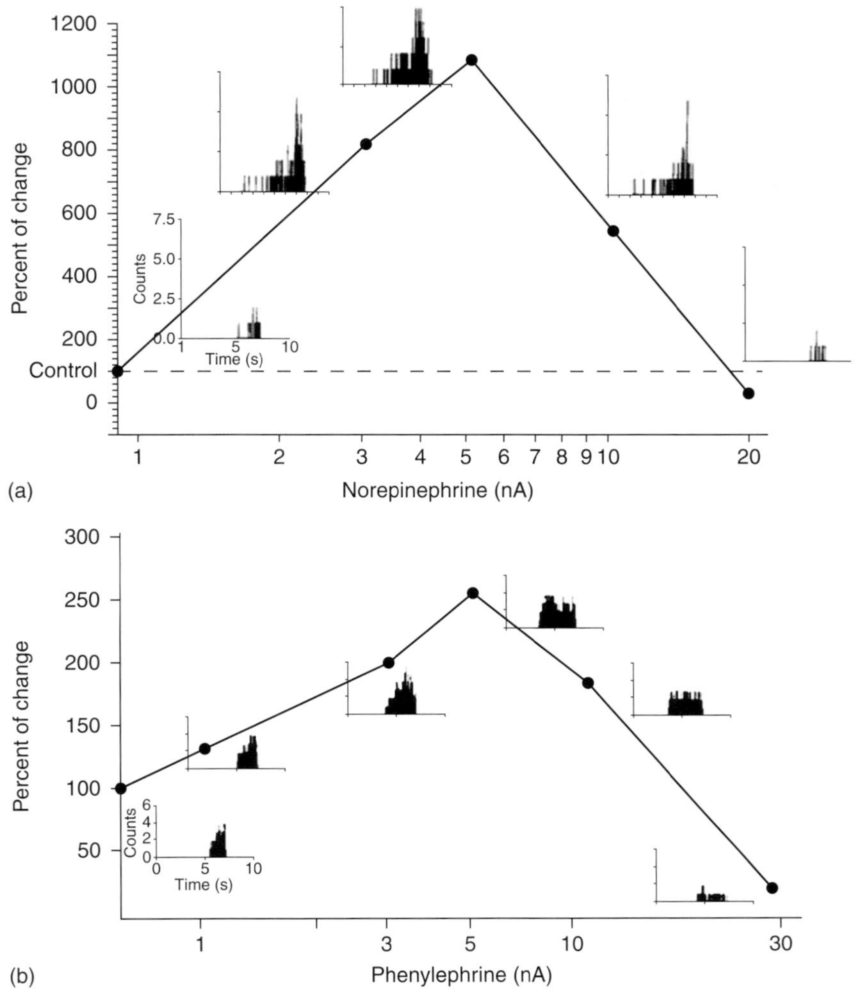

Figure 5 Modulatory actions of ionotphoretically applied norepinephrine and $\alpha 1$ agonist (phenylephrine) on glutamate-evoked discharges in rat barrel field cortical neurons. Responses of individual layer V neurons to iontophoretic pulses of suprathreshold levels of glutamate were quantified by analysis of perievent histograms (shown as insets) that were collected before, during, and after continuous microiontophoretic application of norepinephrine. Responses were then expressed as a percentage change from control (i.e., response to glutamate application alone = 100%) for different iontophoretic doses (nA) of norepinephrine. Each histogram and corresponding point on the graph represents the cell's response to six consecutive glutamate applications. (a) Example of a layer V cortical neuron: its excitatory response to glutamate (28 nA) was progressively increased with increasing levels of norepinephrine (peak at 5 nA) and then progressively suppressed from this optimal value with further increases in norepinephrine ejection current (6–20 nA). (b) Example of a second layer V cortical neuron: its excitatory response to glutamate (40 nA) was likewise progressively increased with increasing levels of phenylephrine (peak at 5 nA) and then progressively suppressed from this peak value with further increases in phenylephrine ejection current (10–30 nA).

Available evidence implicates the β-receptor-linked cyclic AMP system in NE-mediated augmentation of GABA-induced inhibition. For example, *in vivo*, local application of agents that elevate intracellular levels of cyclic AMP mimic or augment NE-mediated enhancement of GABA-induced inhibition of cerebellar Purkinje neurons. Subsequent studies in acutely dissociated cerebellar Purkinje neurons demonstrated augmentation of GABA membrane currents via intracellular diffusion of 8-bromo-cyclic AMP or the catalytic subunit of protein kinase A. And finally, additional investigations found that subunits of the GABA-A receptor can be phosphorylated by protein kinase A. The working hypothesis is that, upon release, NE initiates a cascade of events via postsynaptic β receptors that results in activation of protein kinase A and phosphorylation of GABA-A receptor subunits. In Purkinje neurons this phosphorylation of the receptor leads to enhanced GABA binding capacity or chloride conductance, thus providing for an overall increase in GABA response.

The intracellular events associated with NE-induced enhancement of stimulus-evoked excitatory discharges have not been identified with as much certainty, although work by several laboratories identifies protein kinase A and protein kinase C as candidates for mediating transmitter/modulator effects on synaptically evoked excitation. Elucidating the intracellular

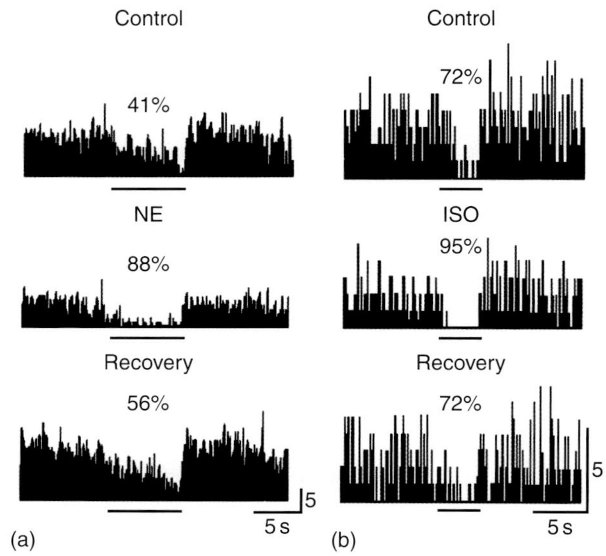

Figure 6 Actions of norepinephrine (NE) and the β agonist isoproterenol (ISO) on γ-aminobutyric acid-induced inhibition of cortical neuron spontaneous discharge. Histogram records show responses of two somatosensory cortical cells (a and b) to regularly spaced, uniform iontophoretic pulses of γ-aminobutyric acid applied before, during, and after NE (a) or ISO (b) administration. Numbers above each histogram indicate the percentage of inhibition of spontaneous firing rate produced by γ-aminobutyric acid application. Each histogram sums unit activity for an equal number of γ-aminobutyric acid pulses, $n = 5$. Both NE (10 nA) and ISO (15 nA) produced a marked enhancement of the γ-aminobutyric acid response relative to a suppression of background firing. Recovery to the control level of response was observed in each case after termination of adrenergic drug application. Calibration: vertical, 5 counts per address; horizontal, 5 s.

events and accompanying physiological actions that underlie NE-induced enhancement of responsiveness to synaptic inputs are major issues for future studies.

Effects of locus coeruleus output on neuronal and neural circuit response properties Studies in anesthetized animals show that stimulation of the LC efferent path elicits NE-like modulatory effects on target neurons in sensory circuits. These findings support the general hypothesis that a major function of the central LC–noradrenergic efferent system is to facilitate the transfer of information through sensory circuits following events that phasically activate the LC nucleus. More recent work in waking animals has shown that phasic and tonic activation of the LC efferent path can enhance the probability of stimulus-evoked spiking in both cortical and thalamic neurons according to an inverted-U function. Thus, as described for iontophoretically applied NE, neuronal responses to afferent stimulation are increased to a maximum at intermediate levels of LC stimulation, and to submaximal levels with LC activation levels above and below this level. As reported for iontophoretically applied NE, activation of the LC efferent pathway can also reveal or 'gate' cellular responses to otherwise subthreshold synaptic inputs. LC stimulation also decreases mean response latency and reduces trial-to-trial variability of response latency for both sensory thalamic and cortical neuron responses to afferent input. Thus, increased output from the LC is capable of altering the magnitude and timing of cellular responses to sensory-driven synaptic input as well as recruiting (gating) additional cells into a response network. These results are important in that they extend observations of LC- and NE-mediated modulatory actions into the waking condition. Further, they show that LC output can simultaneously facilitate stimulus-evoked discharge patterns at multiple levels of an ascending sensory pathway.

The observed effects of LC stimulation on response threshold, response magnitude, and response latency in individual cells suggests that under certain behavioral conditions synaptically released NE can optimize information processing within sensory circuits and provide for a network-wide enhancement of sensory signal transmission. This idea is further supported by recent multineuron recording studies in which LC activation and NE release have been shown to modulate the representation of sensory information across ensembles of functionally related thalamic neurons.

Functional and Clinical Implications

The widespread NE system appears to be functionally multifaceted. On a 24 h timescale it modulates sleep and waking, permitting sleep with inactivity but promoting arousal by becoming active. Recent results for a circuit from the SCN to the LC indicate that this system may contribute to the circadian regulation of arousal and sleep–waking. However, on a much shorter timescale of seconds, this system appears to modulate attention and performance during the waking state. In this domain the LC system regulates behavioral flexibility by promoting either stable selective attention and focused behavioral performance or a scanning type of attention and more flexible behavior.

These findings have implications for the involvement of the LC system in clinical disorders. The role proposed for the LC in attention suggests that dysfunction of this system could contribute to the cognitive and sensory signal-processing deficits that are prominent in schizophrenia, attention-deficit/hyperactivity disorder, and dementia. In regard to dementia, LC neurons have been found to degenerate in both Alzheimer's and Parkinson's diseases.

Many clinical studies have also implicated this system in depression and anxiety. This is consistent with findings that there are substantial projections of NE neurons throughout the limbic system and that the LC system is engaged by novel and alarming stimuli. The high responsiveness of LC neurons to acute and chronic stressors is also consistent with a role for this system in depression. Moreover, many of the drugs used successfully to treat anxiety and depression target the noradrenergic system. There is, as well, a growing body of clinical evidence suggesting a role for the LC–NE system in posttraumatic stress disorder.

There have also been various proposals for a role of the LC in the etiology of sleep disorders. This is consistent with both the close association of activity of these cells with different stages of the sleep–wake cycle and the disrupted sleep patterns that are a hallmark of depression. Recent results indicate that the role of the LC extends to circadian disorders in sleep and performance as well.

Further Reading

Aston-Jones, G., Chen, S., Zhu, Y., et al. (2001). A neural circuit for circadian regulation of arousal. *Nature Neuroscience* 4, 732–738.

Aston-Jones G and Cohen JD (2005) Adaptive gain and the role of the locus coeruleus–norepinephrine system in optimal performance. *Journal of Comparative Neurology* 493: 99–110.

Aston-Jones, G. and Cohen, J. D. (2005). An integrative theory of locus coeruleus–norepinephrine function: Adaptive gain and optimal performance. *Annual Review of Neuroscience* **437**, 556–559.

Berridge, C. W. and Foote, S. L. (1991). Effects of locus coeruleus activation on electroencephalographic activity in the neocortex and hippocampus. *Journal of Neuroscience* **11**, 3135–3145.

Berridge, C. W. and Waterhouse, B. D. (2003). The locus coeruleus–noradrenergic system: Modulation of behavioral state and state-dependent cognitive processes. *Brain Research Reviews* **42**, 33–84.

Clayton EC, Rajkowski J, Cohen JD, et al. (2004) Phasic activation of monkey locus coeruleus neurons by simple decisions in a forced choice task. *Journal of Neuroscience* 24: 9914–9920.

Florin-Lechner, S., Druhan, J., Aston-Jones, G., et al. (1996). Enhanced norepinephrine release in prefrontal cortex with burst stimulation of the locus coeruleus. *Brain Research* **742**, 89–97.

Foote, S. L., Bloom, F. E. and Aston-Jones, G. (1983). Nucleus locus coeruleus: New evidence of anatomical and physiological specificity. *Physiological Reviews* **63**, 844–914.

Guyenet, P. G. (1991). Central noradrenergic neurons: The autonomic connection. *Progress in Brain Research* **88:** 365–380.

Hokfelt, T., Johansson, O. and Goldstein, M. (1984). Central catecholamine neurons are revealed by immunohistochemistry with special reference to adrenergic neurons. In: Bjorklund, A. & Hokfelt, T. (eds.) *Classical Transmitters in the CNS. Part I*, pp. 157–276. Amsterdam: Elsevier.

Moore, R. Y. and Card, J. P. (1984). Noradrenaline-containing neuron systems. In: Bjorklund, A. & Hokfelt, T. (eds.) *Classical Transmitters in the CNS. Part I*, pp. 123–156. Amsterdam: Elsevier.

Ramos, B. P. and Arnsten, A. F. (2007). Adrenergic pharmacology and cognition: Focus on the prefrontal cortex. *Pharmacology & Therapeutics* **113**, 523–536.

Sawchenko, P. E., Li, H. Y. and Ericsson, A. (2000). Circuits and mechanisms governing hypothalamic responses to stress: A tale of two paradigms. *Progress in Brain Research* **122**, 61–78.

Shaham, Y., Shalev, U., Lu, L., et al. (2003). The reinstatement model of drug relapse: History, methodology and major findings. *Psychopharmacology (Berlin)* **168**, 3–20.

Valentino, R. J., Foote, S. L. and Page, M. E. (1993). The locus coeruleus as a site for integrating corticotropin-releasing factor and noradrenergic mediation of stress responses. *Annals of the New York Academy of Sciences* **697**, 173–188.

Woodward, D., Moises, H., Waterhouse, B., et al. (1979). Modulatory actions of norepinephrine in the central nervous system. *Federation Proceedings* **38**, 2109–2116.

Sympathetic Noradrenergic and Adrenomedullary Hormonal Systems in Stress and Distress

D S Goldstein
National Institutes of Health, Bethesda, MD, USA

The body has three peripheral catecholamine systems, corresponding to the three endogenous catecholamines – norepinephrine, epinephrine (synonymous with adrenaline), and dopamine. Each system works differently. Norepinephrine is the main neurotransmitter in sympathetic nervous system regulation of the circulation. In contrast, in the sympathetic cholinergic system, acetylcholine is the neurotransmitter stimulating secretion by sweat glands. In humans, epinephrine is the main hormone of the adrenomedullary hormonal system. Outside the brain, dopamine seems to function as an autocrine–paracrine substance, such as in the kidneys. This article is about the roles of the sympathetic noradrenergic and adrenomedullary hormonal systems in stress and distress. Understanding these roles requires discussion of several concepts – the sympathoadrenal system, stress as a scientific idea, characteristics of distress, allostasis and allostatic load, and scientific integrative medicine. Most of this article is a brief overview of these concepts.

The Sympathoadrenal System

Walter B Cannon proposed that the sympathetic nervous system and the adrenal gland work together as a unit to maintain homeostasis in emergencies – the sympathoadrenal (or sympathoadrenomedullary or sympathico-adrenal) system. This probably was the first suggestion of the existence of an integrated nervous-hormone, or neuroendocrine, system. The notion of a unitary sympathoadrenal system continues in medical thinking, despite evidence for differential changes in sympathetic noradrenergic and adrenomedullary hormonal activities in different forms of stress, as a function of variables such as aging, obesity, and clinical pathophysiologic states.

According to Cannon, in emergencies, rapid activation of the sympathoadrenal system produce compensatory and anticipatory adjustments enhancing the likelihood of survival. Sheltered in a laboratory, with controlled temperature and *ad libitum* water, nutrients, and calories, mammals do not seem to require an intact sympathetic nervous system.

By now it is appreciated that pulse-synchronous bursts of skeletal muscle sympathetic nerve activity and plasma levels of norepinephrine normally are readily detectable even under resting conditions. Norepinephrine continuously enters the venous drainage of most organs. It is also by now clear that continual alterations in sympathetic nervous system outflows attend activities of daily life, such as meal ingestion, changing posture, and locomotion. Each of these activities is associated with a somewhat different set of 'normal' apparent steady states, directed by the brain and determined by coordinated actions of a variety of effector systems. This principle leads directly to the concept of allostasis, discussed below.

Stress and Science

Hans Selye popularized stress as a medical scientific idea. He elaborated a theory based on stress defined as the nonspecific response of the body to any demand, a stereotyped syndrome shared by all organisms in their interaction with the environment. The stress response was nonspecific, meaning that it could be brought on regardless of the stimulus. After specific responses were removed from consideration, the nonspecific syndrome would remain.

Although nonspecific with respect to the inciting agents, the stress response itself was thought to consist of a specific pathological pattern, with three components: enlargement of the adrenal glands, shrinkage of the thymus gland (associated with atrophy of the lymph nodes and inhibition of inflammatory or immune responses), and ulcers or bleeding in the stomach or gastrointestinal tract. The stress response was also thought to have characteristic stages, in a triphasic general adaptation syndrome. The first phase would be a rapid 'alarm' reaction. After an undefined length of time, a longer-lasting stage of resistance would ensue, with increased resistance to the particular stressor but decreased resistance to other stimuli. The stage of resistance would end with depletion of adaptation energy, ushering in the final stage, exhaustion, characterized by resurgence of activity of the adrenal gland, gastrointestinal ulcers, immunological failure, and death. Chrousos and Gold modified the doctrine of nonspecificity by proposing that above a threshold intensity, any stressor elicits the stress syndrome.

More than a half century elapsed before Selye's doctrine of nonspecificity underwent experimental testing, which failed to confirm it. By now, researchers have largely abandoned both Cannon's and Selye's notions of stereotyped, nonspecific neuroendocrine responses regardless of the stressor. More modern theories view stress as a sensed threat to homeostasis, in which the response has a degree of specificity, depending among other things on the particular challenge to homeostasis and the organism's perception of the stressor and ability to cope with it. Nevertheless, Selye's theory figures prominently in current lay literature on stress.

According to the homeostat theory, stress is not an environmental stimulus or a stereotyped response but a condition, in which expectations, whether genetically programmed, established by prior learning, or deduced from circumstances, do not match current or anticipated perceptions of the internal or external environment, and this discrepancy between what is observed or sensed and what is expected or programmed elicits patterned, compensatory responses.

This sensation requires a comparative process, in which the brain compares available information with set points for responding. Central to the homeostat theory is that the body possesses numerous homeostatic comparators, homeostats. Each homeostat compares information with a set point for responding, determined by a regulator. Homeostatic systems typically use multiple effectors to influence values for the monitored variable. The loop is closed by afferent information about the status of the monitored variables. It is the state of sensed discrepancy that defines stress. The organism responds not to the external or internal perturbation itself but to changes in values of the variable that the afferent information actually delivers to the homeostat, usually located in the central nervous system. According to this definition, even a simple homeostatic reflex, such as the baroreflex, can reflect stress, when a perceived discrepancy between a set point for the monitored variable and information about the level of that variable elicits compensatory responses that decrease the discrepancy.

Homeostatic systems of higher organisms always include regulation by negative feedback. This is the key feature that maintains stable levels of the monitored variable. Increases in values of the monitored variable result in changes in effector activity that oppose and thereby buffer changes in the level of that variable. In homeostatic diagrams, a plus sign denotes a stimulatory and a minus sign an inhibitory relationship. Each minus changes the sign of the next relationship in the loop, whereas each plus does not affect the sign of the next relationship. In a system in which the monitored variable is maintained at a plateau level, the loops involving that variable have an odd number of minus signs.

If a loop has only plus relationships and no minus relationships (a positive feedback loop), the system, if otherwise unchecked, would 'explode'; levels of the monitored variable would increase or decrease exponentially. Positive feedback loops are inherently unstable. If a complex system included both a positive feedback loop and a 'nested' negative feedback loop, then the level of the monitored variable would change but to a stable plateau value.

Homeostatic systems use multiple effectors. This redundancy has several consequences. Disabling an effector compensatorily activates the others, enabling at least partial maintenance of the level of the monitored variable. Multiple effectors improve cost efficiency, measured by the energy used to maintain appropriate levels of the monitored variable. By decreasing wear and tear on effectors, having multiple effectors also prolongs the average useful life of the entire system. Finally, having multiple effectors enables patterning of effector responses. Patterning of hormonal, physiological, and behavioral effectors maximizes the likelihood of responses being appropriate for the particular threat to homeostasis.

The body's responses to different forms of stress occur in relatively specific patterns that help maintain appropriate levels of monitored variables such as temperature, blood pressure, blood glucose, and blood oxygen tension. A general theme of these patterns is that they are automatic, involuntary, and unconscious, but once the organism senses that the compensatory adjustments are not maintaining or will not maintain levels of the monitored variables, then the situation may reach consciousness, with the brain directing the adrenal gland to release epinephrine into the bloodstream and the individual experiencing distress, discussed below.

More than one homeostat can regulate activity of the same effector a phenomenon called effector sharing. Examples of effector sharing abound in physiology. For instance, both increased serum osmolality and decreased filling of the heart increase vasopressin secretion, and both decreased delivery of sodium to the kidneys and decreased blood pressure increase activity of the renin–angiotensin–aldosterone system.

Effectors interact with each other, both indirectly, such as via compensatory activation, and directly. Much of physiology research involves studying effector interactions. Examples are effects of adrenocortical steroids on adrenomedullary function and of angiotensin II on sympathetic nervous system outflows.

Disruption of a negative feedback loop, whether by blockade of afferent information, destruction of homeostats, or failure of effectors, increases variability of the monitored variable.

Characteristics of Distress

According to the homeostat theory, distress is a form of stress with the additional characteristics of consciousness, aversiveness, observable signs, and adrenal gland activation. Distress is aversive to the organism, as evidenced by motivation for learning to escape or avoid the stressor.

The homeostat theory does not assume that distress causes disease. In contrast, Selye characterized distress as unpleasant or harmful, without separating these two very different characteristics. He never incorporated the relationship between distress and disease explicitly in his theory. Selye's theory emphasizes the nonspecificity of the stress response, whereas according to the homeostat theory, the experience of distress depends on the character, intensity, and meaning of the stressor as perceived by the organism and on the organism's perceived ability to cope with it. Distress responses, as all stress responses, have a 'purpose,' mitigating effects of a stressor in some way. This applies not only to neuroendocrine aspects of those responses but also to psychological aspects. Distress responses evolved and probably continue to be expressed even in higher organisms, including humans who actually are only rarely exposed to true fight-or-flight agonistic encounters, because of the importance of those responses in instinctive communication. Selye's theory does not consider the communication aspect of distress.

Homeostasis versus Allostasis

Claude Bernard propounded the founding concept of scientific integrative medicine, when he theorized that the overall goal of body systems is to maintain a constant internal cellular environment – the *milieu intérieur.* His *Lectures on the Phenomena of Life Common to Animals and Vegetables*, translated in 1974 from the French publication of 1876, contains one of the most famous passages in the history of physiology: "The constancy of the internal environment is the condition for free and independent life.... All the vital mechanisms, however varied they might be, always have one purpose, that of maintaining the integrity of the conditions of life within the internal environment."

Walter B Cannon coined the word homeostasis. By this, he referred to the stability of the internal environment. The concept of homeostasis was a direct extension from Bernard's *milieu intérieur.* According to Cannon, the brain coordinates body systems, with the aim of maintaining a set of goal values for key variables. Internal or external disturbances threatening homeostasis, by causing large enough deviations from the goal values, arouse nervous and hormone systems, induce emotional and motivational states, and generate externally observable behaviors, all of which have the goal of reestablishing homeostasis. The brain would respond to all emergencies in the same way, by evoking increased secretion of epinephrine.

According to the more recent concept of allostasis, no single set of ideal values exists for levels of internal variables. Allostasis comes from two Greek words that together mean 'other sameness.' The term was used by Sterling and Eyer in 1988, referring to levels of activity required for the individual to "maintain stability through change," that is, to adapt. In terms of the homeostat theory, allostasis is the set of apparent steady states maintained by multiple effectors. In the analogy of the home temperature control system, one can keep temperature at constant but different levels by appropriate use of effectors.

Homeostat resetting redefines the conditions required to maintain homeostasis. Regulation around an altered apparent steady state is the essence of allostasis. An example would be the hyperglycemia of exercise. Even in anticipation of the need for metabolic fuel, by activation of 'central command,' the blood glucose level increases. Resetting alters activities of multiple effector systems required to maintain allostasis, at least for short durations. During stress, short-term changes in homeostatic settings generally enhance the long-term well-being and survival of the organism. Responses during exercise provide an obvious example. When superimposed on a substrate of pathology, however, homeostatic resetting can cause harm. For instance, in the setting of ischemic heart disease, global or patterned increases in sympathetic outflows from homeostat resetting increase cardiac work, the resulting imbalance between oxygen supply and demand precipitating angina pectoris, myocardial infarction, or sudden death.

Allostatic Load and Chronic Disease

It is by way of prolonged activation of effectors to maintain allostasis that chronic stress can contribute to the development of chronic degenerative diseases. Allostatic load refers to effects of prolonged continuous or intermittent activation of effectors involved in allostasis. In the analogy of the home temperature control system, allostatic load increases if a window or door is left open. In this situation, one or more effectors are activated frequently or even continuously. Continued use of the furnace and air conditioner in opposition to one another, an example of an inefficient allostatic state, consumes fuel and contributes to wear and tear on both pieces of equipment. Long-term allostatic load – the wear-and-tear cost of adaptation – provides a conceptual basis for studying long-term health consequences of stress.

Distinct Roles of the Sympathetic Noradrenergic and Adrenomedullary Hormonal Systems

Differences in the extents of activation of the adrenomedullary hormonal and sympathetic noradrenergic systems in different stress responses provide convincing evidence for distinctive neuroendocrine stress response patterns (**Table 1**). This is ironic, because it was Cannon who was so instrumental in describing and studying these components and yet who advocated the combined and undifferentiated activation of the sympathoadrenal system in response to stress.

After adequately sensitive assay methods for plasma levels of norepinephrine and epinephrine became available, evidence rapidly accumulated for different noradrenergic versus adrenergic responses in different situations. A new concept began to emerge, in which the sympathetic noradrenergic system would help distribute blood flows appropriately, such as during orthostasis, cold exposure, mild blood loss, locomotion, exercise, altered salt intake, and water immersion. The adrenomedullary hormonal system would respond to global or metabolic threats, such as hypoglycemia, hemorrhagic hypotension, exercise beyond an anaerobic threshold, asphyxiation, emotional distress, and shock. Evidence also accumulated for an association between norepinephrine and active escape, avoidance, or attack, and an association in

Table 1 Hypothalamic–pituitary–adrenocortical (HPA), adrenomedullary hormonal system (AHS), and sympathetic noradrenergic system (SNS) responses to different stressors

Condition	*HPA*	*AHS*	*SNS*
Active escape/avoidance in rats	+	+	++
Cardiac arrest (or bypass)	+++	++++	++
Cold exposure, hypothermia	+	++	++++
Cold exposure, no hypothermia	0	+	+++
Exercise	+	++	+++
Exercise to exhaustion	++	+++	++++
Fainting	++	++++	0
Glucoprivation	+++	++++	+
Handling in rats	++	++	+
Hemorrhagic hypotension	+++	+++	+
Hemorrhage, no hypotension	+	+	++
Immobilization in rats	++++	++++	++++
Laboratory mental challenge	++	++	+
Pain	++	+++	++
Passive/immobile fear	++	+++	+
Public performance	++	+++	+
Social stress in rhesus monkeys	++	++	++
Surgery	+	+	++

Different intensities are indicated from 0 through ++++. There is a generally closer association between AHS and HPA than between AHS and SNS responses.

epinephrine and passive, immobile fear. **Table 1** provides some examples of different patterns of sympathetic noradrenergic, adrenomedullary hormonal, and hypothalamic–pituitary–adrenocortical responses to different stressors.

Thus, in contrast with the doctrine of nonspecificity, according to the homeostat theory of stress, activities of effector systems are coordinated in relatively specific patterns, including neuroendocrine patterns. These patterns serve different needs, and the sympathetic noradrenergic and adrenomedullary hormonal systems play important roles in many of them. For instance, sympathetic noradrenergic system activation predominates in response to orthostasis, moderate exercise, and exposure to cold, whereas adrenomedullary hormonal system activation predominates in response to glucoprivation and emotional distress (**Table 1**).

In terms of the body's thermostat, studies of humans exposed to cold or with mild core hypothermia have provided support for the notion of primitive specificity of neuroendocrine stress responses. Cold exposure increases plasma norepinephrine levels, with little if any increases in plasma epinephrine levels, consistent with sympathetic neuronal activation and relatively less adrenomedullary hormonal activation. Mild core hypothermia also increases antecubital venous levels of norepinephrine but not epinephrine. Both norepinephrine and epinephrine levels in arterial plasma increase in this setting, but with larger norepinephrine responses. These findings make sense, in that one can maintain body temperature effectively by sympathetically mediated cutaneous vasoconstriction, piloerection, and shivering. When these mechanisms give way, and core temperature falls, then high circulating epinephrine levels increase generation of calories, associated with the experience of distress, which motivates escape and avoidance and augments norepinephrine release from sympathetic nerve terminals for a given amount of nerve traffic.

For each stress, neuroendocrine and physiological changes are coupled with behavioral changes. For instance, the regulation of total body water in humans depends on an interplay between behavior (the search for water and drinking), an internal experience or feeling (thirst), and the elicitation of a neurohumoral response pattern (in this case dominated by vasopressin, the antidiuretic hormone, and to a lesser extent angiotensin, a potent stimulator of drinking). Evoked changes in homeostat function often produce not only neuroendocrine and physiological effects but also behavioral responses; however, because of traditional boundaries among physiology, endocrinology, and psychology, interactions producing integrated patterns of response remain incompletely understood.

Scientific Integrative Medicine

Scientific integrative medicine is not a discipline, a group of disorders, or a method of treatment, but an approach, a way of thinking. Scientific integrative medicine uses systems concepts to explain disease processes and develop strategies to treat, prevent, or palliate them. It emphasizes disorders of the multiple interacting systems that regulate the body's "inner world." Scientific integrative medicine asks researchers and clinicians to consider more than one system at a time, as assessed by measuring levels of more than one chemical effector at a time. The scientific integrative medicine approach provides a framework for understanding complex and dynamic challenges to our integrity as organisms.

Scientific integrative medicine builds on systems biology, but it is also distinct in several ways. First, scientific integrative medicine recognizes that in higher organisms, including humans, the brain dominates regulation of the inner world. The brain regulates the many internal monitored variables of the body in parallel – analogous to a computer's multitasking. Second, the brain has plasticity, which enables modifications in the step-by-step instructions for cellular, tissue, organ, and systemic processes – the algorithms of life. According to the concept of allostasis, about which you will learn later in this article, set points and other elements of these algorithms vary, depending on recollections, sensations, and anticipations by the brain. Third, scientific integrative medicine is medical; its overall mission is to understand and rationally treat disorders and diseases. The systems that maintain the stability of the inner world eventually degenerate. Their efficiencies decline, and as they decline, the likelihood of deleterious, self-reinforcing positive feedback loops increases, threatening organismic stability and survival. Clinicians rarely cure; they manage. They exploit negative feedback loops and attempt to forestall or counter positive feedback loops. Finally, the medications and treatments clinicians prescribe interact with their patients' internal systems. Multiple, simultaneous degenerations, combined with multiple effects of multiple drugs and remedies and myriad interactions among those processes and the drug used to treat them, have come to the fore.

What renders scientific integrative medicine new, different, and powerful is the focus on disorders of the multiple, interacting, feedback-controlled systems that regulate the monitored variables of the body. Scientific integrative medicine recognizes that the operating characteristics of internal systems change over time, based on numerous life exposures and experiences that range from carrying out genetic instructions (especially in fetal development through adolescence) to aging-related degenerative disorders and interactions between medications and those disorders.

Integrative medicine has gained popularity recently. The word integrative has been used synonymously with holistic, mind–body, complementary, or alternative. The scientific integrative medicine approach, however, actually fits quite well with conventional, mainstream clinical medicine. Effective clinicians apply such an approach all the time. One such approach is to "exploit the lesion," where a treatment's success depends on an abnormality that occurs as part of the disease process itself. An example would be treatment of angina pectoris by nitroglycerine in patients with coronary artery disease. Nitroglycerine relaxes veins, decreasing venous return to the heart and cardiac stroke volume. Normally, decreased cardiac filling 'unloads' baroreceptors, and heart rate increases reflexively. The work of the heart changes little, because while the heart rate increases, the systolic blood pressure falls from the direct effects of the drug. Patients with angina pectoris from coronary artery disease, however, typically have low baroreflex-cardiovagal gain. When they take nitroglycerine, the drug reduces systolic blood pressure, but because of the low baroreflex-cardiovagal gain, the heart rate increases relatively little. The work of the heart therefore decreases, relieving the angina pectoris.

Another adage of scientific integrative medicine is "treat patients, not numbers." For hyperglycemia in gastrointestinal bleeding, or hyponatremia in heart failure, astute clinicians focus on treating the underlying problem. Appropriate treatment eliminates secondary effects of effector sharing, in these cases of the adrenomedullary hormonal system and vasopressin system, whereas attempting to reverse the abnormal laboratory findings directly can make matters worse.

One can also try to prevent compensatory damages, deleterious effects of reflexive effector activation. For instance, patients awakening from general anesthesia typically have postoperative hypothermia. Sympathetic noradrenergic and adrenomedullary hormonal system activation to counter hypothermia increases myocardial oxygen consumption. This can contribute to the relatively high frequency of morbid events in patients with coronary artery disease during the immediate postoperative period.

The major goal of scientific integrative medicine is to treat effectively or prevent diseases before they become symptomatic. Beyond practices that promote health in general, such as regular exercise, dietary moderation, and refreshing sleep, the rapidly expanding availability of genetic, physiological, and biochemical information enables prevention of allostatic load and timely institution of effective treatments that are specific for the individual.

Induction of a positive feedback loop in a homeostatic system evokes instability. For instance, activation of the renin–angiotensin–aldosterone system in congestive heart failure increases sodium retention and vascular tone, leading to increased cardiac preload and afterload that worsen the congestive heart failure. Therefore, treatment with an angiotensin-converting enzyme inhibitor or angiotensin II receptor blocker can successfully treat congestive heart failure.

The homeostatic theory of stress and the concept of allostasis can help understand chronic as well as acute medical consequences of stress. Chronic activation of allostatic effectors in allostatic states promotes allostatic load. For instance, chronic elevations in adrenomedullary and hypothalamic–pituitary–adrenocortical outflows worsens insulin resistance, and chronic cardiac sympathetic activation accelerates cardiovascular hypertrophy and development of heart failure.

Another application of the homeostatic idea to medical consequences of stress is in terms of the perceived ability to cope. An organism experiences distress upon sensing that the effector responses will not be sufficient to restore or maintain allostasis. In contrast with distress, stress does not imply a conscious experience. Thus, even heavily sedated humans have substantial adrenomedullary stimulation in response to acute glucoprivation. Distress instinctively elicits observable signs and pituitary–adrenocortical and adrenomedullary activation. Via these neuroendocrine changes, distress could worsen pathophysiologic processes. For instance, because of adrenomedullary activation, in a patient with coronary artery stenosis, distress could elicit cardiovascular stimulation and produce an excess of myocardial oxygen consumption over supply, precipitating myocardial infarction or lethal ventricular arrhythmias. Moreover, long-term distress could augment both the risk of a mood disorder and the risk of worsening coronary disease.

Stress is an interdisciplinary topic, and understanding health consequences of stress requires an integrative approach. Research and ideas about stress must move beyond considering only one effector system, such as the pituitary adrenocortical system, and only one monitored variable, such as serum glucose levels, to incorporate multiple effectors that are regulated in parallel by multiple homeostats. They must also move beyond the notion of a single set of ideal values for monitored variables – homeostasis – to incorporate dynamic changes in homeostatic settings – allostasis. Merging of the homeostatic definitions of stress and distress with the concept of allostasis should provide a better understanding of the roles of catecholamine systems in stress, distress, and disease and provide a conceptual basis for the further development of scientific integrative medicine.

Further Reading

Cannon, W. B. (1939). *The Wisdom of the Body.* New York: W.W. Norton.

Chrousos, G. P. and Gold, P. W. (1992). The concepts of stress and stress system disorders. Overview of physical and behavioral homeostasis. *Journal of American Medical Association* **267**, 1244–1252.

Goldstein, D. S. (1995). *Stress, Catecholamines, and Cardiovascular Disease.* New York: Oxford University Press.

Goldstein, D. S. (2001). *The Autonomic Nervous System in Health and Disease.* New York: Marcel Dekker, Inc.

Goldstein, D. S. (2003). Catecholamines and stress. *Endocrine Regulations* **37**(2), 69–80.

Goldstein D.S. (2006). *Adrenaline and the Inner World: An Introduction to Scientific Integrative Medicine.* Baltimore, MD: The Johns Hopkins University Press.

Goldstein, D. S. and McEwen, B. (2002). Allostasis, homeostats, and the nature of stress. *Stress* **5**(1), 55–58.

Kvetnansky, R., Pacak, K., Fukuhara, K., et al. (1995). Sympathoadrenal system in stress. Interaction with the hypothalamic–pituitary–adrenocortical system. *Annals of the New York Academy of Sciences* **771**, 131–158.

McEwen, B. and Stellar, E. (1993). Stress and the individual. Mechanisms leading to disease. *Archives of Internal Medicine* **153**, 2093–2101.

Pacak, K., Palkovits, M., Yadid, G., Kvetnansky, R., Kopin, I. J. and Goldstein, D. S. (1998). Heterogeneous neurochemical responses to different stressors: A test of Selye's doctrine of nonspecificity. *American Journal of Physiology* **275**, R1247–R1255.

Selye, H. (1956). *The Stress of Life.* New York: McGraw-Hill.

Blood–Brain Barrier, Stress and

S N Malaeb and B S Stonestreet
Brown Medical School, Providence, RI, USA

Glossary

Blood–brain barrier	The interface between circulating blood and brain interstitium.
Hypoxia	Deficiency in the amount of oxygen reaching body tissues.
Ischemia	Cessation of blood flow with subsequent deprivation of glucose and oxygen delivery to the tissue.
Neuroinflammation	The activation of the innate inflammatory cascade within the brain parenchyma in response to various insults, cellular damage, and inflammatory molecules.
Neurovascular unit	The histological structure and function forming the blood–brain barrier.
Tight junctions	Protein complexes located at the apical portion of the cell that associate with homologous structures on the adjacent cell to seal the gap between the cells.

Structure and Function

The blood–brain barrier (BBB) serves as an interface between circulating blood and the brain interstitium. Histologically, the BBB corresponds to the neurovascular unit (**Figure 1**), a highly specialized structure composed of specialized brain capillary endothelial cells, astrocytes and astrocyte processes, pericytes, neuronal terminals, and occasional microglial cells. The brain capillary endothelial cells line the interior of the neurovascular unit and differ from systemic endothelial cells by having rare pinocytic vesicles and absent fenestrations. Thus, the main

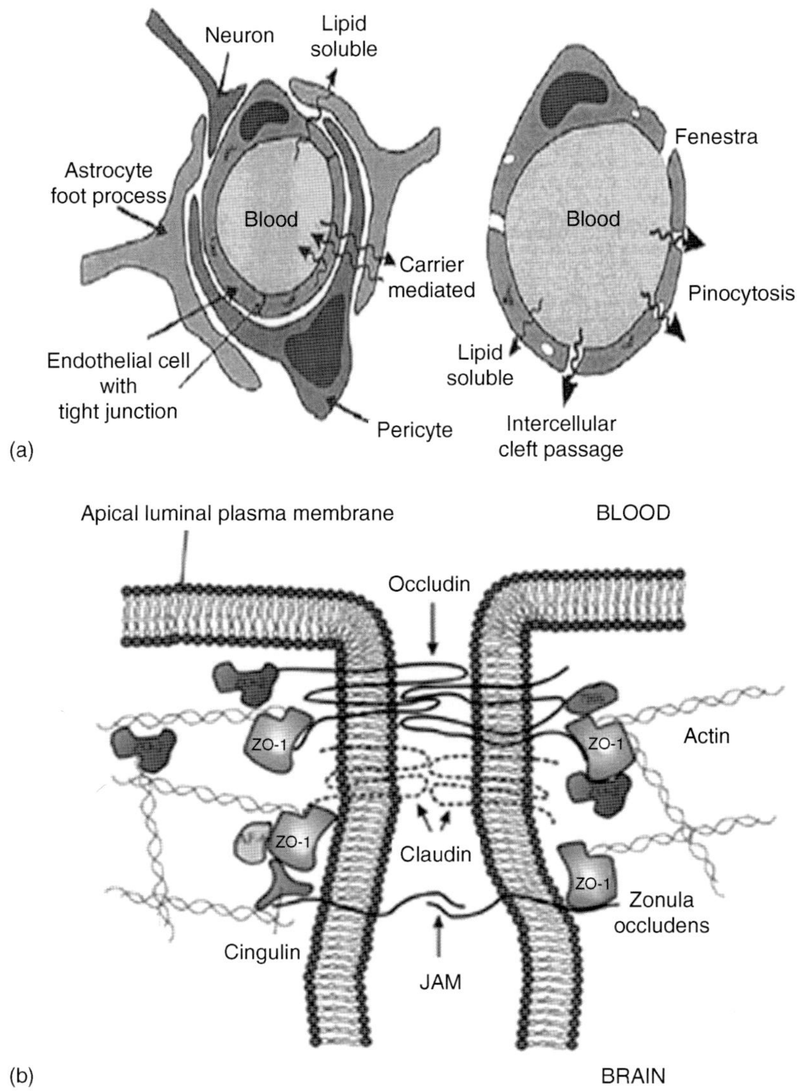

Figure 1 Schematic illustrating specialized features of the neurovascular unit compared to other endothelial vascular beds in the body (a) and the basic structure of tight junctions between endothelial cells at the blood–brain barrier (b). Adapted with permission from Misra (2003) and Hawkins (2005).

gap in the barrier is the space between the cells. These endothelial cells have extensive tight junctions that seal the gap to form the barrier and are held together by strong adherence junctions. Tight junctions are located at the apical portion of the cell and are composed of transmembrane proteins such as occludin, claudins and junctional associated proteins, and intracytoplasmic proteins such as zonula occludens and other proteins that bridge the tight junctions to actin and other proteins of the cytoskeleton. The cells of the neurovascular unit express various transporters that regulate the flux of glucose and other nutrients, metabolites, water, sodium, potassium, and other substances into and out of the brain parenchyma. The BBB also isolates the brain tissues from blood constituents and drugs that could alter neuronal function and provides a large surface area by which the brain can sense alteration in the circulation supplying its various structures. Proper functioning of the BBB is essential to maintain homeostasis of the central nervous system (CNS). Disruption of BBB integrity and alterations in its structure and constitution mediate the pathophysiology of a wide range of CNS disorders and the neurological sequelae of many systemic diseases. The BBB can respond to and be influenced by alterations in the internal and external conditions of the human body as well. This article reviews the pathology of the BBB in various disturbances and stressors intrinsic and extrinsic to the CNS.

Disturbances in Endogenous Stressors

Infection and Inflammation

The BBB integrity and permeability are influenced to a great extent by systemic and local inflammatory mediators acting on the various elements of the neurovascular unit. It has been shown in many experimental models that there is a breakdown in BBB with increased permeability to proteins in conditions of systemic inflammation. These effects are mediated by direct exposure and binding of circulating inflammatory ligands (e.g., lipopolysaccharide) by Toll-like receptors, and of circulating cytokines (e.g., interleukin-1 and tumor necrosis factor-α) and activated complement proteins to their receptors at the BBB and other specialized structures such as the circumventricular organs and the choroid plexus. In addition, increased local production of these factors within the brain parenchyma causes similar effects.

When molecules of the inflammatory cascade bind to their respective response elements on the BBB, nuclear factor-κβ and other inflammatory pathways are induced in the endothelial cells. In addition, other cellular constituents of the neurovascular unit are activated, which induce the activation of nitric oxide synthase (iNOS), cyclooxygenases that release prostanoids, free radicals, histamines, bradykinins, vascular endothelial growth factor, and other paracrine factors. These factors in concert serve to further propagate the inflammatory wave across the BBB and into the brain parenchyma. Propagation of these inflammatory waves also upregulates local matrix metalloproteases (e.g., MMP-9), which will further disrupt the extracellular matrix supporting the structure of the neurovascular unit and the blood vessels in the brain. Cell adhesion molecule (e.g., ICAM-1, VCAM, MCP-1) expression is also increased on endothelial cells. These molecules bind to the endothelial cells and facilitate the trafficking of inflammatory cell across the BBB into the brain parenchyma potentiating the ongoing inflammatory cycles. Increases in P-glycoprotein expression and other molecules also control the transport of inflammatory related substances across the BBB.

The expression, localization, and interaction of proteins that form the tight junctions between endothelial cells of the BBB are altered and disrupted during the inflammatory process described previously. This process serves to weaken the integrity of the BBB and increase the permeability of the barrier to cells, proteins, and smaller molecules normally present in the systemic circulation that would otherwise be excluded from the brain parenchyma by an intact BBB under physiological conditions. The resultant disturbances in CNS homeostasis contribute to the pathophysiology of a number of disease processes affecting the CNS.

Chronic local inflammatory pain in peripheral organs has been associated with increased cell adhesion molecule expression, microglial activation, alterations in tight junction proteins, and increased BBB permeability. These alterations in the BBB are thought to mediate some neurological manifestations of chronic fatigue syndrome and other rheumatic conditions.

Microorganisms can cause systemic illness and, consequently, induce the cascade of inflammatory events described previously. Further, many microorganisms have the ability to gain access into the brain parenchyma by translocating through the BBB. Bacteria (e.g., group B streptococcus, *Escherichia coli*) viruses (HIV), yeast, and prions utilize many of the mechanisms and molecules described previously for inflammation in order to cross the BBB and gain access to the brain. Circumventing the BBB by neurotrophic lentiviral vectors is a major area of interest for gene delivery models in modern neuroscience.

The mechanisms of BBB alteration described for inflammatory conditions are basic not only to inflammatory diseases of the CNS, but also to the pathophysiological processes that underlie brain injury in hypoxia, ischemia, oxidative stress, trauma, tumors, and many other CNS disorders.

Hypoxia/Ischemia Reperfusion Injury

Hypoxia/reoxygenation and ischemia/reperfusion injury alter the permeability and structural properties of the BBB. A large number of *in vitro*, *in vivo*, and magnetic resonance imaging (MRI) studies have documented increased BBB permeability and compromised structural BBB integrity under hypoxic conditions. Both hypoxic and ischemic conditions induce alterations in the expression and localization of a variety of key tight junction proteins, glucose and nutrient transporters, water and electrolyte transporters, and increase in nonspecific transport of blood-borne proteins into the brain parenchyma.

Mechanisms underlying these changes in permeability and structure of the BBB involve the simultaneous activation of a number of second messenger systems that mediate the consequences of hypoxia/reoxygenation, and ischemia/reperfusion injury on the BBB. These include the increases in hypoxia inducible factor, vascular endothelial growth factor, nitric oxide, and the activation of protein kinase C, nuclear factor-κβ, adenylate cyclase, and intracellular calcium pathways. These mechanisms include direct effects of oxygen toxicity and metabolite deprivation, production of oxygen free radicals, cessation of shear blood flow with static leukocytes adhering to the blood vessel walls and invading the neurovascular unit, and the induction of local inflammatory cascades. Local and leukocyte-derived MMP-9 activation mediates BBB breakdown after transient focal cerebral ischemia. During thrombolytic treatment of human stroke and the resulting reperfusion, lipoprotein receptor-mediated induction of MMP by tissue plasminogen activators can predispose a patient to hemorrhagic complications. Higher MMP-9 pretreatment levels have been shown to correlate with more severe hemorrhagic complications after thrombolysis. Biochemical markers of BBB dysfunction and brain ischemia such as elevated S100B values have been shown to be powerful predictors of a poor prognosis for neurological outcomes after cardiac surgery, particularly when elevated levels are associated with other CNS complications.

Hypercapnia and Acidosis

Markers of BBB permeability are increased in the brain parenchyma and cerebrospinal fluid (CSF) under conditions of severe hypercapnia. Hypercapnia-related increases in bilirubin deposition results from increased BBB permeability for bilirubin and is one of the mechanisms by which hypercapnia can predispose newborn subjects to CNS bilirubin toxicity. Other mechanisms include the accumulation of these markers in the brain because decreases in CSF secretion during prolonged hypercapnia could limit the removal of the substances from the CNS via the CSF route. Elevated carbon dioxide levels and the direct effects of acidosis can increase the barrier permeability to molecules in the systemic circulation, which normally are excluded by the intact BBB from the CNS. At relatively low pHs, the resulting changes in the ionic milieu can alter the negatively charged endothelial cell surface sialoglycoproteins and glycolipids, which are integral parts of the BBB. Changes in blood carbon dioxide concentrations, hydrogen ion, and bicarbonate contents also may alter the expression and activity of H^+-ATPase, Na^+/H^+ exchanger, a ubiquitous plasma membrane transport system, and other ion exchangers, which normally regulate the cytoplasmic pH in the cells of the BBB. Such changes in the composition of the BBB contribute to the pathophysiology of acid–base-related disturbances in the CNS.

Osmotic Stress

Exposure to hyperosmotic conditions can disrupt the tightness and integrity of the BBB. Osmotic opening of the BBB is potentially reversible upon cessation of the osmotic stress. Reversible osmotic disruption and reconstitution of the BBB may be due not only to simple mechanical shrinkage of the endothelial cells but also to intracellular Ca^{2+}-activated mechanisms. *In vitro* studies have shown that intracellular Ca^{2+} concentrations increase rapidly, and values peak within 10 s after the application of mannitol and return to the basal levels within 200 s. A specific Na^+/Ca^{2+} exchanger mediates the reconstitution of the BBB at the cellular level. Considering the usefulness of reversible opening for delivery of chemotherapeutic agents across the BBB, manipulations of this exchanger by selective inhibitors may have clinical implications in prolonging the opening phase of the capillary endothelial cells for more efficient drug delivery into the CNS.

During chronic hypertonic conditions such as severe hypernatremia, cells accumulate intracellular organic osmolytes to equilibrate the osmotic gradients. Rapid reduction of extracellular hypertonicity predisposes these cells to excessive swelling and edema. Circulating ions and osmolytes equilibrate slowly across the BBB, and rapid decreases in plasma osmolality can cause major brain fluid shifts resulting in edema and severe cerebral lesions. Rapid correction of chronic hyponatremia can cause osmotic-induced demyelination of the brain. An intact BBB protects oligodendrocytes to a certain extent from the direct exposure to osmotic imbalances. However, disruption of the BBB during an osmotic stress results in massive damage to oligodendrocytes with subsequent development of demyelinating lesions in the brain.

The ability of the brain to exhibit volume regulation when subjected to osmotic stress develops in a region- and age-related fashion. In ovine fetuses, brain volume regulation develops first in the cerebral cortex at 90% of gestation and in the cerebral cortex and cerebellum of newborn lambs, and then it develops in the medulla of the lambs at 20–30 days of age. Therefore, in young subjects, the adverse effects of hyperosmotic stress may vary in an age- and region-specific manner.

Diabetes

The effects of long-standing diabetes on BBB permeability and integrity are region specific and variable. MRI studies in well-controlled diabetics showed increases in signal intensity in the basal ganglia with contrast infusion, indicating increased permeability of the BBB in basal ganglia compared to controls. Other studies suggest that chronic hyperglycemia may induce vascular endothelia growth factor production by glial cells at the blood–retinal barrier. This alters the expression of tight junction proteins such as occludin and ZO-1, and consequently increases capillary endothelial permeability that predisposes to the edema formation in diabetic maculopathy. In contrast, BBB permeability and tight junction protein expression were not altered in the cerebral cortex of diabetic patients. Chronic hyperglycemia decreases the number of glucose transporters available at the BBB. The primary mechanism underlying this downregulation is a posttranscriptional inhibition of glucose transporter mRNA translation. Such an adaptation could decrease the net flux of glucose into the brain during sustained hyperglycemia. The downregulation of glucose transporters during chronic hyperglycemia also contributes to the alarming sensitivity to hypoglycemia in diabetic patients. Diabetic ketoacidosis is associated with a life-threatening development of cerebral edema immediately after the recovery from ketoacidosis. Accumulation of weak acids such as ketoacids and free fatty acids in the cytoplasm of brain cells lowers the intracellular pH, resulting in activation of the Na^+/H^+ exchanger, leading to cellular swelling and cerebral edema.

Hypertension

Studies on the effects of chronic hypertension on BBB permeability indicate a regional predilection for CNS lesions compared with permeability under normotensive conditions. Focal increases in the rate of BBB transfer for small molecules have been reported to increase up to two to seven times the normal rate of transfer. Particularly susceptible regions include the hippocampus, hypothalamus, blood–retinal barrier, and the blood–CSF barrier at the choroid plexus. Acute hypertensive crises have been associated with disruptions in the BBB integrity, when systolic blood pressures reach a certain threshold, or when the BBB has been weakened by other conditions such as in diabetes. These disruptions in the BBB during acute hypertension are more pronounced to neutrally charged molecules than to negatively charged molecules.

Disturbances in Exogenous Stressors

Smoking

Smoking is one of the major risk factors for stroke in humans. *In vitro* stroke models studying bovine brain microvessel endothelial cell cultures under hypoxic/aglycemic conditions demonstrated that BBB K^+ transport mechanisms by the abluminal Na,K,2Cl-cotransporter are downregulated after exposure to nicotine and cotinine at concentrations comparable to plasma levels seen in smokers, and these changes could influence ischemic brain K^+ homeostasis in crucial times of neuronal recovery after stroke.

Alcohol

Alcohol increases BBB permeability in a dose-dependent fashion. Ethanol-induced activation of myosin light chain kinase (MLCK) in the endothelial cells of the BBB leads to phosphorylation of MLCK, occludin, and claudin-5 with resultant cytoskeletal alterations and tight junction changes that facilitate monocyte migration across the BBB. In addition, alcohol predisposes to oxidative stress in brain endothelial cells, causing BBB dysfunction and aggravation of neuroinflammatory disorders of the CNS.

Immobilization and Restraint Stress

Immobilization and restraint stress have been associated with increased BBB permeability in the hypothalamus, midbrain reticular formation, and the cerebellum. Activation of mast cells that preferentially populate these regions of the brain and possible activation of serotonergic pathways have been speculated as possible mechanisms. The resultant oxidative stress and BBB breakdown have been associated with increased circulating levels of S100B protein. Interestingly, biting suppresses oxidative stress induced by restraint stress, and the antistress effect of masticatory motor activity movements, such as biting or chewing, may be important for reducing the adverse effects associated with exposure to psychological stressors.

Steroids

Exogenous corticosteroid administration has been shown to decrease BBB permeability in many *in vitro* and *in vivo* studies of adult and fetal models. Other studies suggest that corticosteroid administration promotes tightening of the BBB during adverse events such as focal cerebral ischemia. Glucocorticoids may act by suppressing inflammation and by directly affecting phosphorylation, organization, and upregulation of tight junction proteins in endothelial cells. However, glucocorticoids also can inhibit glucose transport in cultured hippocampal neurons and glia, and may reduce nutrient delivery to the brain during critical periods of hypoxia and ischemia. Pretreatment with antenatal dexamethasone did not reduce the extent of pathological brain injury following ischemia/reperfusion in an ovine fetal model. Estradiols have also been shown to attenuate BBB disruption induced by cerebral ischemia/reperfusion injury in female rats and to enhance brain glucose uptake by upregulation of glucose transporter-1 expression in the BBB. Thus, estradiols may have advantages over corticosteroids in this regard.

Endogenous corticosteroid production by the hypothalamic-pituitary-adrenocortical axis under stressful conditions, such as systemic inflammation and cerebral ischemia, provides an endogenous negative feedback loop to reduce the extent of ongoing neuroinflammation and BBB disruption secondary to these insults. Blocking this mechanism by corticosteroid antagonists markedly exaggerates the damage secondary to ischemic brain injury.

Thermal Stress: Hypothermia, Hyperthermia, and Ultrasound Waves

Hypothermia, when initiated early on, can attenuate the development of the BBB opening to various insults. In an ischemia/reperfusion model, whole body cooling to 31.5–32.5°C attenuated the increase in BBB permeability when cooling was initiated early during reperfusion. Hypothermia also has been effective in attenuating BBB disruption by hyperosmolar infusions. This suggests that there are direct effects of hypothermia on the elements of the neurovascular unit, in addition to its role in the reduction of inflammatory cascades accompanying ischemia/reperfusion injury.

Hyperthermia has detrimental effects on ischemic infarct volumes both during and after the induction of ischemia. Many studies have found increases in BBB permeability along with disruptions in the integrity of tight junctions and decreased expression of ZO-1 after hyperthermia. The pathophysiology of hyperthermic brain injury and BBB disruption is complex, with many factors such as NOS, histamines, prostaglandins, and other pathways contributing to the hyperthermic-related injury. These changes are more pronounced in younger subects than in adult subjects and may be implicated in the pathophysiology of febrile seizures in younger children.

Local opening of the BBB by mild hyperthermia induced by ultrasound waves is gaining interest as a novel approach to increase drug uptake in brain microvascular endothelial cells. High-intensity focused ultrasound is capable of reversible BBB disruption in a targeted region of interest by opening capillary endothelial cell tight junctions; this opening reverses after 72 h. Sometimes ultrasound-induced hyperthermia can damage tissues in a small volume within the region of BBB opening. Newer techniques are being studied to achieve local and reversible BBB disruption without damaging neurons by the use of noninvasive focused ultrasound at frequencies suitable for trans-skull sonications applied to cavitate special lipid-coated microbubbles within the cerebral microvasculature for delivery of both low- and high-molecular-weight therapeutic compounds to the brain.

Other Stressors

Effects of long-term mobile communication microwave exposure and electromagnetic radiation on the vascular permeability in the brain has been a public health concern. Current evidence suggest that most of the reported effects are negligible as long as the radiation intensity remains in the nonthermal range. BBB dysfunction has been speculated in the pathophysiology of high altitude cerebral edema and acute mountain sickness and diving and decompression sickness, probably due to circulatory microbubble-induced damage of the BBB.

BBB and Aging

Senescence is associated with changes in BBB function. Conditions associated with aging, such as hypertension and cerebrovascular ischemia, aggravate the age-related alterations in BBB function, and the barrier becomes more susceptible to disruption with aging. Such alterations appear to be region specific. More profound changes have been associated with Alzheimer's disease, and the BBB is now thought to have an important role in this disorder. Common age-related changes in the neurovascular unit include loss of capillary endothelial cells, elongation of the remaining endothelial cells, decreased capillary diameter, and a decrease in the number of mitochondria in endothelial cells. The aging BBB shows alterations in carrier-mediated transport systems, including a decrease in transport of choline, glucose, butyrate, and triiodothyronine.

Implications and Clinical Correlations

BBB dysfunction plays a major role in the pathogenesis of a large number of neurological disorders including stroke, multiple sclerosis, Alzheimer's disease, Parkinson's disease, cerebral palsy, leukoencephalopathies, and cerebral hemorrhages. Impairment of BBB function contributes significantly to the neurological sequelae resulting from or associated with many systemic stresses and disorders. A thorough understanding of the pathophysiology of the BBB and of the factors influencing its structure, function, and integrity is essential for the development of targeted drug delivery strategies and safer and more effective therapies in the management of many diseases of the CNS.

See Also the Following Articles

Infection; Inflammation.

Further Reading

Abbott, N. J. (2000). Inflammatory mediators and modulation of blood–brain barrier permeability. *Cellular and Molecular Neurobiology* **20**(2), 131–147.

Abbruscato, T. J., Lopez, S. P., Roder, K. and Paulson, J. R. (2004). Regulation of blood–brain barrier Na,K,2Cl-cotransporter through phosphorylation during *in vitro* stroke conditions and nicotine exposure. *Journal of Pharmacological and Experimental Therapy* **310**(2), 459–468.

Haorah, J., Heilman, D., Knipe, B., et al. (2005). Ethanol-induced activation of myosin light chain kinase leads to dysfunction of tight junctions and blood–brain barrier compromise. *Alcoholism: Clinical and Experimental Research* **29**(6), 999–1009.

Hawkins, B. T. and Davis, T. P. (2005). The blood–brain barrier/neurovascular unit in health and disease. *Pharmacology Reviews* **57**(2), 173–185.

Hynynen, K., McDannold, N., Sheikov, N. A., Jolesz, F. A. and Vykhodtseva, N. (2005). Local and reversible blood–brain barrier disruption by noninvasive focused ultrasound at frequencies suitable for trans-skull sonications. *Neuroimage* **24**(1), 12–20.

Johnsson, P., Backstrom, M., Bergh, C., Jonsson, H., Luhrs, C. and Alling, C. (2003). Increased S100B in blood after cardiac surgery is a powerful predictor of late mortality. *Annals of Thoracic Surgery* **75**(1), 162–168.

Misra, A., Ganesh, S., Shahiwala, A. and Shah, S. P. (2003). Drug delivery to the central nervous system: a review. *Journal of Pharmaceutical Sciences* **6**(2), 252–273.

Montaner, J., Molina, C. A., Monasterio, J., et al. (2003). Matrix metalloproteinase-9 pretreatment level predicts intracranial hemorrhagic complications after thrombolysis in human stroke. *Circulation* **107**(4), 598–603.

Rapoport, S. I. (2000). Osmotic opening of the blood–brain barrier: principles, mechanism, and therapeutic applications. *Cellular and Molecular Neurobiology* **20**(2), 217–230.

Rivest, S., Lacroix, S., Vallieres, L., Nadeau, S., Zhang, J. and Laflamme, N. (2000). How the blood talks to the brain parenchyma and the paraventricular nucleus of the hypothalamus during systemic inflammatory and infectious stimuli. *Proceedings of the Society for Experimental Biology and Medicine* **223**(1), 22–38.

Stonestreet, B. S., Sadowska, G. B., McKnight, A. J., Patlak, C. and Petersson, K. H. (2000). Exogenous and endogenous corticosteroids modulate blood–brain barrier development in the ovine fetus. *American Journal of Physiology: Regulatory, Integrative, and Comparative Physiology* **279**(2), R468–R477.

Unger, E. C., Unger, E. C., Porter, T., et al. (2004). Therapeutic applications of lipid-coated microbubbles. *Advanced Drug Delivery Reviews* **56**(9), 1291–1314.

Vannucci, S. J., Seaman, L. B. and Vannucci, R. C. (1996). Effects of hypoxia-ischemia on GLUT1 and GLUT3 glucose transporters in immature rat brain. *Journal of Cerebral Blood Flow and Metabolism* **16**(1), 77–81.

Witt, K. A., Mark, K. S., Hom, S. and Davis, T. P. (2003). Effects of hypoxia-reoxygenation on rat blood–brain barrier permeability and tight junctional protein expression. *American Journal of Physiology: Heart and Circulatory Physiology* **285**(6), H2820–H2831.

Multi Drug Resistance P Glycoprotein and other Transporters

E C M de Lange
Leiden University, Leiden, Netherlands

Glossary

ATP-binding cassette (ABC) transporters — A large and multifunctional family of structurally related membrane proteins. ABC transporters use the energy of ATP hydrolysis to pump substrates across cell membranes and are involved in the transmembrane transport of various substances.

Multidrug resistance (MDR) — The ability of cells to develop resistance to a broad range of structurally and functionally unrelated drugs after being exposed to (one of) these drugs. The mechanism is that the efflux transport by these proteins leads to lower intracellular concentrations, thereby protecting the cells and tissues from potential toxic compounds from the external milieu.

Multidrug resistance-related proteins (MRPs) — A group of MDR ABC transporters that are structurally related to but distinct from P-glycoproteins; mainly transports anionic derivatives of drugs when conjugated to glutathione/glucuronide. This family of MRP proteins comprises nine members in humans, designated MRP1–MRP6.

P glycoprotein (Pgp) — The first discovered MDR transporter and most well-known ABC transporter; has been shown to transport a variety of structurally unrelated compounds across cellular membranes.

ATP-Binding Cassette Transporter Superfamily

The ABC transporters comprise a large and multifunctional family of structurally related membrane proteins that are located in the plasma membrane of the cells or in the membrane of various cellular organelles. ABC transporter proteins use the energy of ATP hydrolysis to translocate various molecules across these barriers, and some other ABC transporters use ATP to form specific membrane channels. The ABC transporters serve a variety of physiological roles, and also some inherited diseases appear to be linked to mutations in the genes encoding for the ABC transporters.

At present, approximately 50 ABC transporters are known. Many synonyms exist for these transporters due to their history of discovery. Recently, a consistent nomenclature has been introduced on the basis of the organization of domains and amino acid homology of these ABC transporters. In the new nomenclature, the ABC transporters are divided into seven distinct subfamilies: ABCA, ABCB, ABCC, ABCD, ABCE, ABCF, and ABCG. **Table 1** presents the classification of these

Table 1 ATP binding cassette transporter families and members[a]

Family	*Member (synonyms); most common name*	*Tissue expression*	*Physiological substrates; other substrates;[b] inhibitors/modulators*	*Function*	*Genetic mutations related to human disease*
ABCA	ABCA1 (ABC1, TGD, HDLDT1, CERP)	Ubiquitous (plasma membrane)	Phospholipids, cholesterol	Removal of phospholipids and cholesterol on to high-density lipopotein particles	Tangier disease, artherosclerosis
	ABCA2 (ABC2)	Brain, kidney, lung, heart, lysosomal membrane	*Estramustine*?	Steroid transport?	
	ABCA3 (ABC3, ABCC)	Lung			
	ABCA4 (ABCR, ABC10, STGD)	Retina (rod photoreceptors)	*N-retinylidene-phosphatidyl-ethanolamine, retinaldehyde*		Stargardt disease, retinitis pigmentosa, macular dystrophy, cone–rod dystrophy
	ABCA5	Muscle, heart, testes			
	ABCA6	Liver			
	ABCA7	Spleen, thymus			
	ABCA8 (ABCR)	Ovary			
	ABCA9	Heart			
	ABCA10	Muscle, heart			
	ABCA11	Stomach			
	ABCA12	Low in all tissues			
ABCB	ABCB1 (MDR1, PGP, PGY1, GP170) P-Glycoprotein	Epithelial cells of kidney, liver, choroid plexus, intestine; endothelial cells of brain capillaries	IL-2, IL-4, IFN-γ, amyloid β-40, amyloid β-42, glucosylceramide, platelet-activating factor *Actinomycine D, aldosteron, amprenavir, bisantrene, calcein-M, citalopram, colchicine, corticosterone, cortisol, cyclosporin A, dexamethasone, digoxin, domperidone, doxorubicin, daunorubicin, enaminonen, erythromycine, etoposide, FK506, indinavir, loperamide, lovastatin, morphine, nelfinavir, ondansetron, paclitaxel (taxol), phenytoin, prednisolone, quinidine, rifampin, ritonavir, sanquinavir, sparfloxacin, teniposide, terfenadine, (99m)-Tc-tetrofosfine, valspodar (PSC833), verapamil, vinblastine, vincristine* *Inhibitors:* Agosterol A, amiodarone, amitryptilin, amprenavir, biricodar (VX-710), chlorpromazin, cyclosporin A, diltiazem, dipyridamol, fluphenazin, GF120918, gramicidine D, LY335979, mefipriston, midazolam, nelfinavir, pimozin, pluronic L61, progesterone, promethazin, propafenone, propanolol, quinidine, reserpine, ritonavir, saquinavir, spironolactone, staurosporin, tamoxifen, trifluoperazin, triflupromazin, V-104, valinomycine, valspodar (PSC 833), verapamil	Multidrug resistance	

	ABCB2 (TAP1, PSF1, RING4, ABC17)	Ubiquitous (ER)	Peptides	Peptide transport (into the ER)	Juvenile-onset psoriasis; immune deficiency
	ABCB3 (TAP2, PSF2, RING11, ABC18)	Ubiquitous (ER)	Peptides	Peptide transport (into the ER)	Immune deficiency
	ABCB4 (PGP3, MDR3(2), PFIC-3)	Liver (hepatocytes)	Long-chain phosphatidyl-choline	Phosphatidylcholine transport	Progressive familial intrahepatic cholestasis-3, intrahepatic cholestasis of pregnancy
	ABCB5 (MTABC3)	Ubiquitous			
	ABCB6 (ABC14, UMAT, MTCA3)	Ubiquitous in mitochondria	Iron?	Iron transport	
	ABCB7 (ABC7, ATMIP, ASAT)	Ubiquitous in mitochondria	Iron?	Fe/S cluster transport	Sideroblastic anemia with ataxia
	ABCB8 (MABC1)	Mitochondria	Intermediates in heme/biosynthesis?		
	ABCB9	Lysosomes			
	ABCB10 (MTABC2)	Mitochondria			
	ABCB11 (sPGP, BSEP, PGY4)	Liver (hepatocytes)	Bile salts (e.g., taurocholate) *Paclitaxel (taxol)*	Bile salt transport	Progressive familial intrahepatic cholestasis-2
ABCC	ABCC1 (MRP1, MRP) Multidrug resistance related protein	Ubiquitous in normal tissues (mainly lung and choroid plexus epithelial cells) and brain capillary endothelial cells	17-β-glucuronyl estradiol, S-glutathionyl prostaglandin A2, glutathione disulfide, 4-hydroxynonenol-GS, leukotriene C4 (LTC4)-GS, leukotriene D4 (LTD4)-GS, leukotriene E4 (LTE4)-GS, NNAL-O-glucuronide lipid peroxidation products, nitroquinoline 1-oxide-GS *Aflatoxin B1-epoxide-GS, arsenite, arsenate (sodium), BCECF, calcein, chlorambucil-GS, colchicine, CPT-14, daunorubicin, DHEAS, 2,4-dinitrophenyl-GS doxorubicin, epirubicin, ethacrunic acid-GS, etoposide, fluorescein, flutamide, hydroxyflutamide, glucuronosyl etoposide, herbicides, heavy metals, indomethacin (-GS), melphalan-GS , methotrexate, rhodamine, ritonavir, sequinavir, ^{99}Tc-Sestambi, SN-38, SN-38-GS, SNARF, tobacco nitrosamines, ^{99}Tc-tetrofosmin, vinblastine, vincristine* *Inhibitors:* Agosterol A, benzbromarone, budesonide, biricodar (VX-710), cyclosporin A, indomethacin, probenecid, genistein, quercetin, sulfinylpyrazone, verapamil	Drug resistance, ubiquitous GS-X pump, immune response involving cysteneyl leukotrienes	

Continued

Table 1 Continued

Family	*Member (synonyms); most common name*	*Tissue expression*	*Physiological substrates; other substrates;[b] inhibitors/modulators*	*Function*	*Genetic mutations related to human disease*
	ABCC2 (MRP2, cMOAT)	Liver, intestine, kidney, brain endothelail cells (plasma membrane)	Bilirubin-glucuronides, GSSH, GSH, including cotransport, estradiol-17-β-D-glucuronide, acidic bile salts *Anionic drug conjugates, cisplatin, doxorubicin, epirubicin, etoposide, indinavir, phenytoin, ritonavir, saquinavir, sulfinpyrazome, vinblastine* *Inhibitors/modulators*: Leukotriene C4, probenecid	Organic anion efflux, hepatobiliary extrusion of amphiphatic ions	Dubin–Johnson syndrome
	ABCC3 (MRP3, cMOAT-2)	Liver, bile ducts, gut, adrenal cortex of kidney, intestine, placenta	Bile salts, leukotriene C4 *Anionic drug conjugates, acetaminophen glucuronide methotrexate, etoposide, teniposide* *Inhibitors/modulators:* Probenecid	Drug resistance	
	ABCC4 (MRP4, MOAT-B)	Many tissues (plasma membrane)	Cyclic nucleotides, conjugated steroïds and bile acids, DHEAS nucleotide analogs, 9-(2-phosphophenyl methoxylethyl)-adenine, prostaglandins, taurolithocholate 3-sulfate, thiopurine monophosphates *Nucleotide analogs, organic anions, nucleosides, monophosphates, zidovudin, other antiretroviral agents* *Inhibitors/modulators* Probenecid	Nucleoside transport	
	ABCC5 (MRP5, MOAT-C)	Ubiquitous	Cyclic nucleotides, nucleotide analogs, 9-(2-phosphono-methoxyethyl) adenine, thiopurine monophosphates *Nucleotide analogs, organic anions nucleoside monophosphates, mitoxantrone, topotecan, doxorubici* *Inhibitors/modulators:* Probenecid fumitremorgin C, GF120918	Nucleoside transport	
	ABCC6 (MRP6)	Kidney, liver (plasma membrane)	*BQ-123? (acidic peptide)*	Elastic tissue homeostasis	Pseudo-xanthoma elasticum
	ABCC7 (CFTR)	Exocrine tissues		Cystic fibrosis transmembrane conductance regulator (cAMP-dependent chloride channel)	Cystic fibrosis, CBAVD, pancreatitis, bronchiectasis
	ABCC8 (SUR1)	Pancreas		K(ATP) channel regulation	Familial persistent hyperinsulinemia hypoglycemia of infancy
	ABCC9 (SUR2)	Heart, muscle		Sulfonurea receptor	Dilated cardiomyopathy
	ABCC10 (MRP7)	Ubiquitous (low)			
	ABCC11 (MRP8)	Testis and breast, lower in all other tissues			
	ABCC12 (MRP9)	Brain and testis, lower in all other tissues			

ABCD	ABCD1 (ALD, ALDP)	Many tissues (peroxisomes)	VLCFA	VLCFA transport regulation	
	ABCD2 (ALD1, ALDR)	Many tissues (peroxisomes)	VLCFA		Adrenoleukodystrophy
	ABCD3 (PMP70, PXMP1)	Many tissues (peroxisomes)	VLCFA		
	ABCD4 (PMP69, P70R)	Many tissues (peroxisomes)	VLCFA		
ABCE	ABCE1 (OABP)	Ovary, testes, spleen		Oligoadenylate-binding protein	
ABCF	ABCF1	Ubiquitous			
	ABCF2 (ABC50)	Ubiquitous			
	ABCF3	Ubiquitous			
ABCG	ABCG1 (ABC8, human white)	Ubiquitous		Cholesterol transport	
	ABCG2 (ABCP, MXR, BCRP)	Mainly in liver, placenta, small intestine; also in heart, lung, skeletal muscle, kidney, spleen, thymus, brain capillaries	Heme, porphyrins, flavanoids, pheophorbide, sulfated estrogens	Drug resistance, stem-cell differentiation, survival of stem cells (under hypoxic conditions).	HIV treatment?
	Breast cancer resistance protein		*Anthracyclines, bisantrene, diflomotecan, etoposide, flavopiridol, imatinib mesylate (STI-571, Gleevec), imatrib, irinotecan, SN-38, methotrexate, mitoxantrone, lamivudine, rhodamine 123, teniposide, topotecan, zidovudine,* *Inhibitors/modulators* CI1033, futremorgirin C, GF120918, hammerhead ribozyme, HIV protease inhibitors, imatinib (STI-571, Gleevec) pantoprazole, prazosin, reserpine, ZD1839 (Iressa)		
	ABCG4 (white2)	Liver			
	ABCG5 (steroline 1)	Liver, intestine		Sterol transport, biliary cholesterol secretion/ absorption	Sitosterolemia, sterol accumulation, artherosclerosis
	ABCG8 (steroline 2)	Liver, intestine		Sterol transport, biliary cholesterol secretion/ absorption	Sitosterolemia, sterol accumulation, artherosclerosis

[a]BCECF, 2',7'-bis(carboxyethyl)-5(6)-carboxyfluorescein; CBAVD, congenital bilateral absence of the vas deferens; CFTR, cystic fibrosis transmembrane conductance regulator; DHEAS, dehydroepiandrosterone; ER, endoplasmic reticulum; GSH, glutathione; GSSH, glutathione persulfide; GS-X, GSH conjugate; HIV, human immunodeficiency virus; IFN, interferon; IL, interleukin; PMEA, 9-(2-phosphophenyl methoxylethyl)-adenine; VLCFA, very long-chain saturated fatty-acyl-CoA.
[b]Other substrates appear in italics.

families and their members (including the synonyms), together with their expression, endogenous and exogenous substrates, functions, and relation to human disorders. It is clear that the ABC transporters govern the kinetics of chemical communication in the body, which makes the knowledge of their specific actions in homeostatic and feedback mechanisms extremely important for further insight into the body's functioning at the molecular level under normal and challenged (stress) conditions.

Multidrug Resistance Transporter Proteins

ABC transporters have been the subject of intense scrutiny as potential mediators of clinical drug resistance. The identification of the MDR1-encoded P-glycoprotein (Pgp) approximately 20 years ago, allowed us to recognize that reduced intracellular accumulation of anticancer agents can result in significant degrees of drug resistance. Over the years, Pgp has become the prototype of the MDR transporters. Among the ABC transporters, two other major groups can be identified as being involved in intrinsic and/or acquired MDR of cells: the multidrug resistance-related protein (MRP) family and the breast cancer resistance protein (BCRP). Many drugs that have been developed for the treatment of human diseases are substrates for these multidrug transporters. Because of that, the degree of expression and the functionality of these transporters can directly affect the therapeutic effectiveness of such agents. Treatment failure due to MDR was first found in connection with cancer, but later in time it was also found in connection with other conditions such as some autoimmune disorders and infectious diseases (**Table 1**).

P-Glycoprotein

Pgp is the most well-known of the ABC transporters and was the first to be identified in humans, in which it plays a critical role in drug resistance in the treatment of cancers. Numerous investigations with many drugs have demonstrated that Pgp has an important role in determining the concentration–time profiles of Pgp substrates in the different parts of the body. In general, Pgp preferentially extrudes large hydrophobic, positively charged molecules. This transporter also is involved in the transport of certain cytokines. Pgp may even play a role in allograft rejection and in the inhibition of apoptosis. Another possible role of Pgp lies in the pathogenesis of Alzheimer's disease by the direct interaction of Pgp on amyloid-β40 and amyloid-β42 or by Pgp's influencing the accumulation of these proteins. Also, an interesting role for Pgp is indicated in the neuroendocrine functioning and regulation of the hypothalamic-pituitary-adrenocortical (HPA) axis because Pgp is involved in the efflux of certain natural and synthetic glucocorticoids from the brain.

Multidrug Resistance-Related Protein Family

The MRPs (or the ABCCs) have a broad tissue distribution and are able to extrude negatively charged anionic drugs and neutral drugs conjugated to glutathione, glucuronate, or sulfate. Some MRPs are able to transport neutral drugs if co-transported with glutathione. The total MRP family now includes MRP1–MRP9 (and ABCC7 and ABCC8). MRP1 was the first to be discovered and is actually a prototype glutathion conjugate pump that transports a variety of drugs conjugated to glutathione, sulfate, or glucuronate; anionic drugs and dyes; neutral-basic amphiphatic drugs; and even oxyanions. The most important substrate of MRP1 is the endogenous leukotriene LTC4. MRP1 also contributes to the blood–cerebrospinal fluid (CSF) barrier at the level of the choroid epithelial cells. MRP2 and MRP3 have overlapping substrate specificities with MRP1 but different tissue distributions, and they appear also to exhibit drug resistance. MRP4 and MRP5 broaden the spectrum of drug resistance to nucleotide analog drugs; MRP6 plays a role in elastic tissue homeostasis. The functions of MRP7–MRP9 are largely unknown.

Breast Cancer Resistance Protein

BCRP (or ABCG2) is an ABC half transporter that displays drug resistance. In general, the BCRP transporter preferentially extrudes large hydrophobic, positively charged molecules. BCRP is involved in MDR in cancer, especially with regard to acute myeloid leukemia. Also, it plays a role in the survival of stem cells under hypoxic conditions and might play a role in regulating stem-cell differentiation.

Multidrug Resistance Transporter Proteins and Pharmacokinetics

Both the absorption and body distribution of drugs depend on their passage through diverse barriers. A number of MDR transporters limit the absorption of drugs via the gastrointestinal tract and the distribution of drugs into the brain via the blood–brain barrier; excretion is also governed by these transporters.

Oral Absorption

Efflux transporters such as Pgp and the MRPs in the intestinal may form the rate-limiting barrier to oral drug absorption. The poor bioavailability characteristics of many chemotherapeutic agents for cancer and human immunodeficiency virus (HIV) protease inhibitors may be explained by the fact that those drugs are among the best substrates for these transporters. The co-administration of the relevant substrates with the inhibitors/modulators of these transporters is a possible route to enhancing bioavailability. Of interest is the systematic site-specific expression of Pgp and MRPs along the various parts of the gastrointestinal tract.

Brain Distribution

The brain is the tissue most frequently targeted by drugs. To be effective, drugs must be transported to the site of action. The interface between the blood and brain is composed of the blood–brain barrier (brain capillary endothelial cells) and the blood–CSF barrier (choroid plexus epithelial cells).

The presence of these efflux transporters at the blood–brain/CSF barriers explains the fact that many drugs exhibit poor brain distribution despite their favorable lipophilic character; the barriers are substrates for the efflux transporters. Thus, in many studies Pgp, especially (expressed at the luminal face of the brain capillary endothelial cells), has been shown to be responsible for lowering the brain distribution of many drugs. MRP1 is more specifically localized in the basolateral membrane of the choroid epithelial cells, preventing CSF penetration of its substrates. Pgp is also expressed at the choroid epithelial cells, but in a manner that governs influx transport. Other ABC transporters, such as MRP2 and BCRP, have also been implicated in protecting the brain tissue against exogenous compounds.

Drug Excretion

The liver and kidneys play an important role in the excretion of drugs, the main routes being through the biliary tract and renal proximal tubule, respectively. In both the liver and kidneys, Pgp and other multidrug transporter proteins are variably expressed in the different suborgan structures and cell linings.

Functional Genetic Polymorphism

In addition, functional genetic polymorphisms, as have been identified for the Pgp gene, may influence the absorption, distribution, and excretion of the transporters substrates.

Other Physiological Functions of Multidrug Resistance and Other ATP-Binding Cassette Transporters

The ABC transporters govern a broad spectrum of physiological functions because they are involved in the transmembrane transport of various substances that exhibit a wide variety of chemical structures; examples are endogenous compounds such as ions, amino acids, peptides, sugars, vitamins, steroid hormones, bile acids, and phospholipids and also many exogenous compounds. Next we briefly describe a number of these physiological roles.

Defense against Oxidative Stress, Cancer, and Inflammation

Adequate glutathione (GSH) levels are essential to life and needed to fight infections and cancer cells. The MRPs that have been functionally characterized so far act as ATP-dependent export pumps for conjugates with glutathione, glucuronate, or sulfate. The most important substrate of MRP1 is the endogenous glucuronide conjugate leukotriene C4 (LTC4), a *de novo* synthesized mediator of inflammation. MRP1 and MRP2 also mediate the co-transport of unconjugated amphiphilic compounds, together with free glutathione. MRP3 preferentially transports glucuronides but not glutathione S-conjugates or free GSH. In addition, MRP1 and MRP2 contribute to the control of the intracellular glutathione disulfide levels and may thereby play an essential role in the response to oxidative stress when the activity of glutathione disulfide reductase becomes rate limiting. Thus, the members of the MRP family serve as export pumps that prevent the accumulation of anionic conjugates and glutathione disulfide in the cytoplasm, and they therefore play an essential role in detoxification and defense against oxidative stress.

Lipid Metabolism

The transport of specific molecules across lipid membranes is also an essential factor in the physiology of all living organisms, and a large number of specific transporters have evolved to carry out this function. Many ABC genes play a role in the maintenance of the lipid bilayer and in the transport of fatty acids and sterols within the body. Actually, the ABCA1 transporter is responsible for delivering cholesterol to nascent high-density lipoprotein (HDL) particles, a process known as reverse cholesterol transport. Enhancing ABCA1 activity, either through changes in gene expression or activity, is a plausible therapeutic strategy for increasing HDL levels. Dietary cholesterol is the primary contributor to the risk of developing cardiovascular disease for a subset of patients. The half-transporters ABCG5 and ABCG8 form a heterodimer responsible for regulating intestinal cholesterol absorption and the excretion of cholesterol in the liver. Increasing ABCG5/G8 expression or activity is a viable strategy for reducing dietary cholesterol.

The expression of a large number of ABC transporters in monocytes/macrophages and their regulation by cholesterol flux indicate that these transporter molecules are potentially critical players in chronic inflammatory diseases such as atherosclerosis.

Antigen Presentation

The transporter associated with antigen processing 1 (TAP1; ABCB2) and TAP2 (ABCB3) are half-transporters that serve to transport peptides into the endoplasmatic reticulum. At that site, they can be complexed with class I human leukocyte antigen (HLA) molecules for presentation on the cell surface. TAP expression is required for the stable expression of the HLA class I proteins. The TAP complex transports amino acid peptides with a preference for Phe, Leu, Arg, and Tyr at the C-terminus, similar to the specificity of the HLA class I proteins. Several DNA viruses such as herpes simplex virus express molecules that interfere with antigen expression by disrupting the function of the TAP complex. TAP2 (ABCB3) functions as a heterodimer with TAP1.

Regulation of Insulin Secretion

Mutations in ABCC8 may result in familial persistent hyperinsulinemic hypoglycemia of infancy, demonstrating its role in the regulation of insulin secretion. Actually ABCC8 forms ATP-sensitive potassium channel together with an inwardly rectifying potassium channel. The closure of ATP-sensitive potassium channels in pancreatic islet β-cells initiates a cascade of events that leads to insulin secretion. ABCC8 therefore seems to be responsible for regulating glucose metabolism by insulin secretion.

Chloride Secretion

Chloride is the most abundant anion and the predominant permeating species. The chloride channels are crucial for transepithelial transport and the control of water flow, and they often provide unexpected permeation pathways for a large variety of anions. ABCC7 (CFTR, cystic fibrosis transmembrane) is a cAMP-dependent chloride channel and is responsible for chloride secretion in the gastrointestinal mucosa. The major toxins that cause secretory diarrheas act by increasing the levels of cAMP or cGMP. This results in a secondary increase in active chloride secretion through ABCC7, whereas sodium and water follow passively. Compounds that inhibit ABCC7 appear to be well suited as treatments for both secretory diarrhea and cholera.

Potassium Channel Regulation

ATP-sensitive potassium (KATP) channels, as inhibited by intracellular ATP, play key physiological roles in many tissues. KATP channels set membrane excitability in response to stress challenge and preserve cellular energy-dependent functions. ABCC9, together with an inwardly rectifying potassium channel, forms a KATP channel. This complex may have a vital role in securing cellular homeostasis under stress. Mutations in ABCC9 may lead to KATP channel dysfunctions and have been related to susceptibility to dilated cardiomyopathy.

Bile Salt Transport

Canalicular bile secretion is the rate-limiting step in bile formation. The canalicular membrane contains ABC proteins that transport biliary compounds against steep concentration gradients across the canicular membrane. Pgp excretes hydrophobic cationic compounds, whereas ABCB4 (Pgp3 or MDR3) acts as a phospholipid flippase for phosphatidyl choline. In addition to biliary excretion of phospholipids, bile is also the major pathway for the elimination of cholesterol, mostly derived from HDLs in plasma. ABCC2 (MRP2) is an important (bilirubin) conjugate export pump. A major liver bile-salt transporter in the liver is ABCB11 (BSEP, bile salt export pump). The production of bile is also critically dependent on the coordinated regulation and function of this BSEP. The endothelin antagonist bosentan inhibits BSEP and leads to the intracellular accumulation of cytotoxic bile salts, and bile-salt-induced liver damage. Similarly, troglitazone, an insulin sensitizer, induces cholestasis and hepatotoxicity via competitive inhibition of the BSEP-mediated bile salt transport.

Multidrug Resistance: ATP-Binding Cassette Transporter Modulation and Regulation of Expression

Modulation

MDR modifying agents, which inhibit the function of the MDR transporters by either competitive or noncompetitive mechanisms, are good candidates for the pharmacological modulation of transporter functionality, currently still mostly focused on cancer treatment. The modulators are intended to increase the cytotoxic action of MDR-related drugs by preventing the extrusion of anticancer drugs from the target cells to significantly improve the treatment effectiveness.

To date, three generations of modulators/inhibitors exist, mostly acting on Pgp. The first generation comprises calcium channel blockers (verapamil, diltiazem, and azidopine), quinine derivatives, calmodulin inhibitors (trifluoroperazine and chlorpromazine), and the immunosuppressive agent cyclosporin A. The modulators of the second generation consists of derivatives of the first-generation compounds, for example R-verapamil and PSC-833 (from cyclosporin). Because of differences in the substrate-specificities and inhibitor-sensitivities of the different MDR proteins expressed in different tumor cells, proper therapeutic intervention requires an advanced diagnosis and targeted modulator agents. The third generation of MDR modifiers was devised to specifically interact with a particular MDR transporter. One example is the reversins, which are small hydrophobic peptide derivatives that are supposed to interact with Pgp with high affinity and selectivity; their clinical efficiency has yet to be proven.

Regulation of Expression

A number of environmental stimuli are known to affect the expression of the Pgp (*mdr1*) genes. In humans, it has been suggested that *mdr1* may function as a heat shock gene and its expression may be modulated by the numerous agents that trigger these signaling pathways. It seems likely that cellular stress and Pgp expression are closely linked because this transporter plays a crucial role in the protection of cells from toxic products released during environmental stress. More specifically, it has been found that certain steroid hormones enhance Pgp expression. Enhanced expression does not necessarily lead to enhanced efflux functionality because examples also exist of enhanced expression but decreased functionality.

See Also the Following Articles

Cholesterol and Lipoproteins; Corticosteroids and Stress; Cytokines, Stress and Depression; Hippocampus, Corticosteroid Effects on; Immune Response; Metabolic Syndrome.

Further Reading

Borst, P. and Oude Elferink, R. (2002). Mammalian ABC transporters in health and disease. *Annual Review of Biochemistry* **71**, 537–592.

Dean, M., Rzhetsky, A. and Allikmets, R. (2001). The human ATP-binding cassette (ABC) transporter superfamily. *Genome Research* **11**(7), 1156–1166.

Glavinas, H., Krajcsi, P., Cserepes, J., et al. (2004). The role of ABC transporters in drug resistance, metabolism, and toxicity. *Current Drug Delivery* **1**, 27–42.

Haimeur, A., Conseil, G., Deeley, R. G., et al. (2004). The MRP-related and BCRP/ABCG2 multidrug resistance proteins: biology, substrate specificity and regulation. *Current Drug Metabolism* **5**(1), 21–53.

Kerb, R., Hoffmeyer, S. and Brinkmann, U. (2001). ABC drug transporters: hereditary polymorphisms and pharmacological impact in MDR1, MRP1 and MRP2. *Pharmacogenomics* **2**(1), 51–64.

Liscovitch, M. and Lavie, Y. (2002). Cancer multidrug resistance: a review of recent drug discovery research. *IDrugs* **5**, 349–355.

Meijer, O. C., Karssen, A. M. and de Kloet, E. R. (2003). Cell- and tIssue-specific effects of corticosteroids in relation to glucocorticoid resistance: examples from the brain. *Journal of Endocrinology* **178**(1), 13–18.

Müller, M. B., Keck, M. E., Binder, E. B., et al. (2003). ABCB1 (MDR1)-type P-glycoproteins at the blood-brain barrier modulate the activity of the hypothalamic-pituitary-adrenocortical system: implications for affective disorder. *Neuropsychopharmacology* **28**, 1991–1999.

Renes, J., de Vries, E. G., Jansen, P. L., et al. (2000). The (patho)physiological functions of the MRP family. *Drug Resistance Update* **5**, 289–302.

Schmitz, G. and Kaminski, W. E. (2001). ABC transporters and cholesterol metabolism. *Frontiers in Bioscience* **6**, D505–D514.

Štefkova, J., Poledne, R. and Hubacek, J. A. (2004). ATP-binding cassette (ABC) transporters in human metabolism and diseases. *Physiology Research* **53**, 235–243.

Stein, W. D. (2002). Reversers of the multidrug resistance transporter P-glycoprotein. *Current Opinion in Investigative Drugs* **3**(5), 812–817.

Sukhai, M. and Piquette-Miller, M. (2000). Regulation of the multidrug resistance genes by stress signals. *Journal of Pharmacy and Pharmaceutical Sciences* 268–280.

Tan, B., Piwnica-Worms, D. and Ratner, L. (2000). Multidrug resistance transporters and modulation. *Current Opinion in Oncology* **12**(5), 450–458.

Wijnholds, J., Evers, R., van Leusden, M. R., et al. (1997). Increased sensitivity to anticancer drugs and decreased inflammatory response in mice lacking the multidrug resistance-associated protein. *Nature Medicine* 1275–1279.

Social Stress, Animal Models of

J Bugajski and A Gądek-Michalska
Polish Academy of Sciences, Krakow, Poland
A J Bugajski
Jagiellonian University, Krakow, Poland

This is a revised version of the article by J Bugajski, Encyclopedia of Stress, First edition, volume 3, pp 474–478, © 2000, Elsevier Inc.

Glossary

Adaptation	The situation in which repeated exposure to the same stimulus elicits diminishing responses from the body.
Corticotropin-releasing hormone (CRH)	Neurohormone secreted by the hypothalamus whose functions are related to stress, a primary activator of stress hormones.
Limbic-hypothalamic-pituitary-adrenal (LHPA) axis	The pathway regulating the secretion of stress hormones by brain limbic structures, hypothalamus, pituitary, and adrenal gland and involving release of corticotropin-releasing hormone (CRH) from the hypothalamus, adrenocorticotropic hormone (ACTH) from the pituitary gland, and corticosteroid hormones from the adrenal gland.
Neurotransmitters	Chemical messengers released from different kind of nerve endings involved in the transmission of a nerve impulse.
Social stress	A highly complex set of neuroendocrine changes in response to the immediate social environment of the animal.
Vasopressin (AVP)	Neurohormone secreted by the hypothalamus, a major regulatory peptide, with CRH, for the secretion and synthesis of ACTH; initiates the hypothalamic-pituitary-adrenal (HPA) response to stressors.

Conventional models of physical stressors in laboratory animals show little validity with chronic human psychopathologies. Models of social stress based on the naturalistic events of interactions between conspecifics present a realistic model to include chronic psychosocial stress in animals. Repeated or chronic psychosocial stress induce adaptation of various neurotransmitter and neuropeptide regulatory systems involved in the hypothalamus-pituitary-adrenal (HPA) axis response. Chronic stress impairs the cholinergic and adrenergic system-induced HPA response. The corticotropin-releasing hormone (CRH)- and vasopressin (AVP)-induced activation of the HPA axis follows distinct time courses. Complex transcription factor interactions and mechanisms accompany the activation of these neuropeptides during psychosocial stress.

Social Stress Models

The stress response is usually presented as adaptive physiological and psychological processes activated in animals and humans by various kinds of stressors. It is regarded as an alarm system that is initiated whenever the dynamic equilibrium of the living organism, called homeostasis, is threatened by physical and psychological events that are known as stressors. Current understanding of physiological mechanisms of the central stress response system is based on both clinical data and animal reactions to various physical stressors, such as footshock, forced swim, or immobility, which may elicit behavioral and psychological responses different from those evoked by psychosocial stressors. In socially organized mammals, however, the predominant stressors are not physical events but arise from the immediate social environment of the animal. The majority of stress stimuli in humans is of a psychosocial nature and contributes to the development and expression of disease. In order to study mechanisms involved in the etiology of human affective disorders, various animal models of social stress are used. Apart from genetic factors that predispose for psychopathologies, environmental stress plays an important role in the etiology of these mental diseases.

Common rodent and nonhuman primate models of social stress used in the laboratory with a focus on social hierarchy models contribute in complementary ways to the understanding of social stress. Animal models of social stress involve single, intermittent, or chronic exposure of a subject animal to a conspecific. The most frequently used models for rodents are the social defeat and the social colony models. In the social defeat model, a male intruder is introduced into the territory of another male, the resident conspecific, which attacks and defeats the intruder. The desired outcome of the social conflict is ensured since the resident usually has higher body weight, is familiar with fighting, and frequently belongs to a more aggressive strain than the intruder.

In a social colony, male and female rats are living together in seminatural conditions and a social structure develops, with a single male being the dominant rat and the others subordinates. Social defeat stress induces major functional and structural changes in subregions of the hippocampal formation. Defeated or subordinate animals have an increased activation of HPA axis, demonstrated by an increase in blood adrenocorticotropic hormone (ACTH) and corticosterone levels. Consequently, animal models that involve natural social context seem to be more appropriate because they represent situations that individuals may encounter in their everyday lives.

Crowding typically induces a social stress reaction with prominent psychosocial components, avoiding the physical components present in most typically used stressors and mimicking emotional state alterations. Randomly selected animals are placed together in housing cages such that each has less than a standard amount of space. In crowded rats, no agonistic interactions leading to dominance or subordination are encountered. The prototypical marker of the presence and magnitude of social stress is the activity of the HPA axis. Many responses to social stress appear to be quite consistent across various animal models, with only a few exceptions that may depend on the paradigm or species studied. Psychological stress is a good animal model for investigating the various behavioral and neurohormonal changes related to stressful circumstances.

Psychological stressors are associated with the activation of the sympathetic and adrenomedullary system and the HPA axis. These systems respond to psychological stress with increased output of noradrenaline from the locus coeruleus (LC) and noradrenaline and adrenaline from the adrenal medulla. The hypothalamus produces CRH, which activates the anterior pituitary gland to secrete ACTH, which in turn stimulates the adrenal cortex to secrete corticosteroids, primarily cortisol in humans and corticosterone in rodents. Negative emotional responses disturb the regulation of the HPA system. Relatively pronounced HPA activation is common in depression, with episodes of cortisol secretion being more frequent and persistent among the depressed than among other psychiatric patients and normal subjects. Chronic stress may induce a state of hyporesponsiveness of the HPA axis whereby cortisol secretion is attenuated.

Limbic Stress Processive Pathways

Psychological and neurogenic stressors requiring higher-order sensory processing of signals prior to initiation of a stress response recruit the limbic stress processive pathway. These processive stressors constitute stimuli that become stressful only by comparison with previous experience. Different types of emotional experience may involve different pathways and arise from activity initiated as a result of thoughts and memories in the cortex or as a result of activity initiated in the hypothalamus. The components of the limbic-sensitive pathways include prefrontal cortex, septum, extended amygdala, hippocampus, and hypothalamic nuclei. In contrast, the limbic-insensitive pathway is recruited by stressors that represent an immediate threat to homeostasis and does not require limbic structures. The amygdala and the hippocampus normally inhibit hypothalamic activity, but stress blocks this circuitry and thus leads to stimulation of hypothalamic releasing hormones such as the stress peptide. Both the hippocampus and the medial prefrontal cortex (mPFC) play an important role in the negative feedback regulation of HPA activity during physiological and behavioral stress. Chronic restraint and psychosocial stress can induce atrophy of hippocampal apical dendrites of CA3 pyramidal neurons, depletion of synaptic vesicles in mossy fiber terminals in CA3, and impairment of hippocampal-dependent learning tasks. Chronic elevations in corticosterone also induce a suppression in synaptic plasticity in the CA1 hippocampal field.

The amygdala is also a major extrahypothalamic source of CRH-containing neurons with high expression levels for the CRH-1 and CRH-2 receptors. Psychological stressors can activate the amygdala CRH system without evident activation of the hypothalamic CRH system; the amygdala CRH system is much more sensitive to psychological stressors than the hypothalamic paraventricular nucleus (PVN). The amygdala, in concert with other extrahypothalamic limbic regions, manifests the behavioral responses to stress, while the hypothalamic CRH system is important for modulating neuroendocrine responses to stress. The hippocampus is an important target of circulating adrenal cortical hormones that act on their receptors and are abundant in this structure. Stress affects glucocorticoid receptor and mineralocorticoid receptor gene expression in the hippocampus in a stressor- and gender-specific manner. Chronic exposure to high corticosteroid levels, during prolonged stress, can have a detrimental effect on hippocampal integrity and function and its excitation and plasticity.

Adaptation to Stress

Adaptation of a response to given challenge is one of the key features of the normal ability of an organism to cope with the external world. Social factors, as unavoidable real life events, are powerful modulators of the stress response. Adaptation to stressful challenges involves activation of neural, neuroendocrine, and neuroendocrine-immune mechanisms. The ability of the body to increase or decrease vital functions to a new state is termed allostasis, or stability through change. Allostasis actively maintains homeostasis and promotes adaptation. When the stress response is inadequate or excessive and the cost of restitution of homeostasis is too high, the resulting condition has been termed by McEven allostatic load.

Physiological stress responses are accepted as beneficial in the short term but can be detrimental if overactivated or prolonged. Stress modulators regulate the extent, duration, and long-term impact of acute stress responses. Stress hormones are crucial mediators of both adaptive and maladaptive responses. Chronic stress induces changes in neuroendocrine and neuronal systems at several levels: in morphology of brain nuclei and neurons and in neurotransmitter and second messenger systems including single molecules. This also takes place in limbic brain structures that are under the influence of stress-activated systems. Within the limbic-hypothalamic-pituitary-adrenal (LHPA) system, chronic stress impairs the feedback-control mechanisms associated with decreased gene expression of corticosteroid receptors and structural alterations in the hippocampal formation. Prolonged stress reduces the inhibitory feedback exerted by the hippocampus over the hypothalamic CRH-producing PVN and consequently results in hypersecretion. Sustained stress leads to adrenal hyperactivity. LHPA axis alterations develop in all stressed animals independently of their position in the social hierarchy, whether dominants, subordinates, residents, or intruders, indicating that the HPA axis is more sensitive to the stressful nature of the situation and less modulated by the individual differences in the appraisal of the situation. Dysfunction of systems regulating CRH activity in the central nervous system (CNS) and LHPA axis dysregulation often contributes to the etiology of several psychiatric disorders, such as anxiety, panic disorder, posttraumatic stress disorder, and depression.

Challenging signals from the environment are communicated to the final cellular level of adaptation to stress to turn cascades of gene expression. Genes turned on by stress transcribe the information in their DNA code into messenger RNA (mRNA), which then is translated into proteins making up the structure and adaptive functions of the brain and body. Proteins regulate the structural and energy dynamics of the cell, as well as the neurotransmitters, hormones, and signals of the psychoneuroendocrine system in mind–body medicine. A significant number of the genes in the human genome can be spliced together in different ways to generate alternative sets of proteins that modulate physiological adaptation in response to challenge and stress from purely physical to psychosocial levels.

Transmitter Systems Adaptation

Cholinergic System

Acute stress activates not only the HPA axis but also the septohippocampal cholinergic system in male rats. In the brain, acetylcholine (ACh) is one of the neurotransmitters clearly involved in the stimulation of hypothalamic release of CRH. Acute stress of immobilization increases the synthesis, binding, and release of ACh in the hippocampus and limbic structures. Chronic stress induces reduction of choline uptake and an increase in the number of muscarinic binding sites in the septohippocampal cholinergic system, which is involved in the pituitary-adrenal response to stressful stimuli. The social stress of crowding (21 rats placed in a cage designed for 7) for 3, 7, and 14 days considerably reduces the secretion of corticosterone induced by ICV stimulation of cholinergic muscarinic receptors. The reduced responsiveness of the HPA axis may be caused by a homologous desensitization and downregulation of central muscarinic receptors by an increased secretion of ACh during crowding stress. Homologous desensitization of muscarinic receptor may be regulated by β-adrenergic receptor-like kinase.

The function of the cholinergic system depends on the ACh gene, which codes for ACh and the acetylcholinesterase gene, which codes for the enzyme that hydrolyzes ACh and terminates the function of ACh excitatory neurotransmission in the CNS. Psychosocial stress can alter the cholinergic gene expression or splicing to generate alternative proteins that are involved in a variety of normal mind–body functions, as well as pathologies. Such stress-induced alternative gene splicing may constitute a major pathway in the modulation of gene expression by creative psychological and social processes.

Monoaminergic System under Stress

An important component of the stress response in the brain is the activation of monoaminergic systems. The LHPA axis interacts with a variety of monoaminergic systems, including brain stem noradrenergic and serotonergic systems. Endocrine and central brain stem monoaminergic responses to stress appear to be precisely coordinated to facilitate adaptive physiological responses. Stress-induced stimulation of the noradrenergic/adrenergic, the serotonergic, and the dopaminergic system enables the brain to flexibly respond to challenges by reorganizing its neuronal networks. Acute stress stimulates noradrenaline (NA) release from terminal neurons in the LC, leading to depletion of NA, but repeated or prolonged stress restitutes NA levels in the brain.

Stress raises activity of phenylethanolamine-N-methyltransferase (PNMT), a specific enzyme that converts NA into adrenaline and accelerates turnover of brain NA and adrenaline.

In addition, stress-induced increased expression of the tyrosine hydroxylase gene may elevate NA concentrations. The release of catecholamines in the response to stressors is followed by an increase in the expression of genes that encode catecholamine-synthesizing enzymes by transcriptional mechanisms in the LC and the adrenal medulla. The persistence of transcriptional activation depends on the duration and severity of the stress. In response to an acute stressor, catecholamines stimulate some limbic regions, such as the hippocampus, amygdala, and hypothalamus, whereas the higher cognitive centers in the prefrontal cortex are inactivated. During stress, high concentrations of NA and/or adrenaline cause a decrease in a number of adrenergic receptors, termed downregulation, and low agonist concentrations upregulate adrenergic receptors. Adrenoreceptor (AR) downregulation may result from reduced expression of the receptor gene or proteolytic degradation of receptor molecules. A reduced number of functional receptors results in desensitization of the respective receptor system and impairs its biological response to an agonist. Receptor molecules may be desensitized by phosphorylation through protein kinases, rapid uncoupling from its effector unit, sequestration from the cellular membrane, and internalization into the cytoplasm and intracellular vesicles. Chronic psychosocial stress reduces the number of adrenergic receptors in brain regions that regulate emotional behavior depending on the duration of the stress period and brain regions. In the LC, α_2-AR binding is already reduced 2 days after the onset of the stress and remains at a low level. Diminished autoreceptor activity impairs feedback inhibition of NA release and, consequently, higher levels of the neurotransmitter in projecting regions of the LC. During chronic psychosocial stress, α_2-AR expression alters from initial downregulation to later upregulation, inducing first high and then low levels of NA.

Stress-induced downregulation of brain β-ARs is regarded as an important mechanism of adaptation to stress. Repeated or chronic stress induces high levels of endogenous agonist NA, and adrenaline causes rapid β-AR internalization into the cells and their functional desensitization. This is considered one of the biochemical mechanisms in receptor adaptation performed in order to prevent dangerous effects of the persisting stress-induced high levels of catecholamines. The psychosocial stress of crowding for 3–7 days considerably reduces the secretion of corticosterone elicited by ICV β-adrenergic receptor agonist and evokes progressively lesser diminution of that response after 14 and 21 days of crowding. In brain cortex α_2-ARs are temporarily downregulated after 2 days of stress but upregulated after 4 weeks. Stress rapidly desensitizes the β-AR system via receptor sequestration and internalization, but some of these changes are only transient since internalized β-ARs can reinsert into the plasma membrane and restore normal receptor numbers. Social crowding stress only moderately diminishes the secretion of corticosterone evoked by ICV α_1-adrenergic agonist. Adrenergic receptors, like the cholinergic muscarinic receptor, are linked to G-protein and are regulated by phosphorylation, which regulates desensitization of receptors to their agonists. Phosphorylation of the β-adrenergic receptor by cAMP-dependent kinase and protein kinase C (PKC) during stress is intimately involved in the desensitization of the receptor. The brain, and specifically the hippocampus, have large neuronal plasticity for a successful adaptation to a stressful situation that occurred previously. Changes that occur in the hippocampus are accompanied by alterations in the other brain regions functionally related to the hippocampus. Reacting and changing neurotransmitter systems in brain areas interact in a coordinated fashion aimed at maintaining stability through change in physiological coping mechanisms during stress.

CRH Systems Adaptation

The most well-known hypothalamic peptide whose functions are related to stress is the CRH, which may be regarded as a primary activator of the LHPA system. Produced by many neurons throughout the brain, CRH functions as neurotransmitter. CRH and noradrenergic neurons of the central nervous stress system innervate and stimulate each other in a positive feedback mechanism. CRH given ICV in rats activates the HPA axis and the sympathetic nervous system. Stress activates hypothalamic as well as extrahypothalamic CRH neuronal pathways. In response to a stressful stimulus, CRH is released into the hypophysial-portal blood from neurons in the PVN of the hypothalamus, the site of convergence for stress signals in the brain. Hypothalamic CRH acts as a major mediator of the mammalian stress response by stimulating pituitary pro-opiomelanocortin (POMC) gene expression and ACTH secretion that, in turn, stimulates release of glucocorticoid from the adrenal gland. CRH stimulates POMC gene transcription in pituitary corticotrops by several transcription factors. The transcriptional activation of the pituitary POMC gene by CRH is associated with inhibition of nuclear transcription factor NF-κB DNA-binding activity and with activation of the activator protein-1 (AP-1) factor. CRH activates target pituitary cells and neurons via distinct genes encoding membrane CRH-R1 and CRH-R2 receptors. Stress causes marked increases in the expression and cell content of CRH-R1 receptors, which predominantly mediate the CRH-induced hormonal response to stress. CRH released within the PVN increases cAMP levels, and sequentially facilitates CRH transcription, via cAMP response-element binding protein (CREB) phosphorylation and later limits the transcription via induction of the inducible cAMP early repressor (ICER). Fine modulation of CRH expression depends on a complex balance between activation by phospho-CREB and repression by ICER late during stress. Induction of ICER could serve as a protective mechanism to limit transcription of hypothalamic CRH and avoid pathological consequences of excessive expression of neuropeptide in response to stress.

Precise regulation of circulating glucocorticoids is critical for preserving homeostasis under stress conditions. Excessive CRH production may lead to HPA axis dysfunction and psychiatric disturbances. The inhibitory isoforms of CRE modulator induced during stress contribute to the decline in CRH gene transcription during persistent stimulation.

Vasopressin Systems Adaptation

In the initiation and modulation of the HPA axis response to acute and psychosocial stress both CRH and AVP are involved. These two major regulatory peptides for the secretion and/or synthesis of ACTH are colocalized in the parvocellular neurons in the PVN in both humans and rodents. These peptides, colocalized in the same secretory granules at the nerve endings of the median eminence and coreleased into the portal circulation, exert synergistic effects on ACTH secretion from the anterior pituitary. Apart from presence in the hypothalamus, CRH and AVP are localized in several other limbic and brain structures. A variety of acute and chronic stressors alters their concentrations in the hypothalamus and several other brain regions.

In pituitary corticotrops, the vasopressin V1b receptor isoform is specifically expressed and plays a crucial role in regulating HPA axis activity during stress and in resting conditions. Under stress conditions, both the hypothalamic AVP/V1bR and the CRH/CRH R1 system are required to maintain normal HPA axis regulation. Acute stress results in a rapid increase of CRH heterogeneous nuclear RNA (hnRNA) at the time of maximal ACTH secretory response. The stress-induced AVP hnRNA response in the parvocellular neurons is slower in onset than that of primary CRH transcript, with a maximum at 2 h after challenge. Differences in timing of CRH and AVP hnRNA responses indicate distinct mechanisms underlying stress-induced activation of these genes. Physical or psychological stressors activate the CRH and AVP in the parvocellular neurons of the PVN, the major regulators of ACTH secretion. The AVP gene is upregulated by cAMP. The promoter of the AVP gene contains cAMP response element (CRE), and the promoter activates of transfected AVP gene are upregulated with cAMP. The dual CRH/AVP regulatory system may benefit the organism in coping with various stressful events. The release of CRH and AVP peptides is regulated differently depending on the nature and the duration of the imposed stress. Prolonged stressors induce a gradual shift from a CRH-predominant stress response to an AVP-predominant response after chronic stress. These adaptational changes could partly depend on glucocorticoid receptor changes induced by repeated stress in the PVN and the hippocampus and the greater responsivity of AVP than CRH to chronic stimulatory inputs. CRH and AVP regulate MR and GR in the hippocampus and anterior pituitary, structures with the highest levels of MR and GR mRNA and receptor protein in the CNS. These GRs have an important role in the regulation of the LHPA axis and stress adaptation and the pathophysiology of stress-related disorders.

AVP and CRH bind to specific pituitary corticotrop membrane receptors that activate different second messengers. The rat pituitary AVP receptor is coupled to phospholipase C, and the CRH receptor to an adenylate cyclase. Repeated stress induces rapid adaptation of the CRH mRNA response and desensitization of the pituitary ACTH response, which may be caused by negative feedback mechanisms, as well as depletion of the releasable ACTH pool or down-regulation of pituitary CRH receptors. On the other hand, chronic stress or repeated exposure to identical short-term stressors may induce an increased pituitary responsiveness due to sensitization of pituitary corticotrops to CRH. The social stress of crowding for 3 days facilitates the ACTH response to CRH and corticosterone response remains unaffected, indicating that the HPA system is fully sensitive or even hyperactive. This may reflect predominantly moderate upregulation of pituitary CRH system. Crowding stress considerably reduces the AVP-induced ACTH and corticosterone response. This results from desensitization and/or decrease in the number of AVP receptors in the anterior pituitary corticotrops or from desensitization of the AVP-stimulated intracellular inositol triphosphate and the PKC signaling pathway. AVP plays a primary role in the regulation of the pituitary adrenal axis during adaptation to stress. Chronic stress increases the expression of AVP in parvicellular neurons of the PVN, and secretion of AVP but not CRH into the pituitary portal circulation. Changes in density and sensitivity of pituitary AVP receptors may play a major role in adaptation of the HPA axis to crowding stress, as with adaptation to chronic psychosocial stress.

Further Reading

Barr, C. S., Newman, T. K., Shannon, C., et al. (2004). Rearing condition and rh5-HTTLPR interact to influence limbic-hypothalamic-pituitary-adrenal axis response to stress in infant macaques. *Biological Psychiatry* **55**, 733–738.

Bartolomucci, A., Palanza, P., Sacerdote, P., et al. (2005). Social factors and individual vulnerability to chronic stress exposure. *Neuroscience and Biobehavioral Reviews* **29**, 67–81.

Blanchard, R. J., McKittrick, C. R. and Blanchard, D. C. (2001). Animal models of social stress: effects on behavior and brain neurochemical systems. *Physiology and Behavior* **73**, 261–271.

Bugajski, J. (2000). Social stress. In: Fink, G. (ed.) *Encyclopedia of Stress* (Vol. 3), pp. 474–478. San Diego, CA: Academic Press.

Bugajski, J., Borycz, J., Głód, R., et al. (1995). Crowding stress impairs the pituitary-adrenocortical responsiveness to the vasopressin but not corticotropin-releasing hormone stimulation. *Brain Research* **681**, 223–228.

Buwalda, B., Kole, M. H. P., Veenema, A. H., et al. (2005). Long-term effects of social stress on brain and behavior: a focus on hippocampal functioning. *Neuroscience and Biobehavioral Reviews* **29**, 83–97.

Flugge, G., van Kampen, M. and Mijnster, M. J. (2003). Perturbations in brain monoamine systems during stress. *Cell Tissue Research* **315**, 1–14.

Fuchs, E. and Flugge, G. (2003). Chronic social stress: effects on limbic brain structures. *Physiology and Behavior* **79**, 417–427.

McEwen, B. S. (1998). Stress, adaptation, and disease. Allostasis and allostatic load. *Annals of the New York Academy of Sciences* **840**, 33–44.

McEwen, B. S. (2000). The neurobiology of stress: from serendipity to clinical relevance. *Brain Research* **886**, 172–189.

Rossi, E. L. (2004). Stress-induced alternative gene splicing in mind-body medicine. *Advances in Mind-Body Medicine* **20**, 12–19.

Sabban, E. L. and Kvetnansky, R. (2001). Stress-triggered activation of gene expression in catecholaminergic systems: dynamics of transcriptional events. *Trends in Neuroscience* **24**, 91–98.

Tamashiro, K. L. K., Nguyen, M. M. N. and Saki, R. R. (2005). Social stress: from rodents to primates. *Frontiers in Neuroendocrinology* **26**, 27–40.

Tanoue, A., Ito, S., Honda, K., et al. (2004). The vasopressin V1b receptor critically regulates hypothalamic-pituitary-adrenal axis activity under both stress and resting conditions. *The Journal of Clinical Investigation* **113**, 302–309.

Watanabe, Y., McKittrick, C. R., Blanchard, D. C., et al. (1995). Effects of chronic social stress on tyrosine hydroxylase mRNA and protein levels. *Molecular Brain Research* **32**, 176–180.

VI. CIRCADIAN AND SEASONAL RHYTHMS

Cortisol Awakening Response

A Steptoe
University College London, London, UK

Glossary

Area under the curve — A method of estimating aggregate cortisol output from a series of timed samples. It is typically calculated by assuming that the secretion rate is uniform across the time period. For example, if the salivary cortisol level is 18.0 nmol/liter at T_1, 22.0 at T_2 (14 min later), and 26.0 at T_3 (20 min after T_2), the area under the curve is calculated as $(((18.0 + 22.0) / 2) \cdot 14) + (((22.0 + 26.0) / 2) \cdot 20) = 760.0$.

Carotid intima-media thickness — The depth of the intima-medial layer of the wall of the carotid arteries, assessed noninvasively using duplex ultrasonography. This is an index of subclinical atherosclerosis and correlates with coronary artery disease.

Cortisol awakening response (CAR) — The increase in cortisol during the first hour after waking up, typically peaking at 20–40 min after waking.

Definition

The CAR is the change in cortisol concentration that occurs during the first hour after waking from sleep. The CAR has been studied in detail only over the past decade, following the introduction of salivary cortisol sampling. This has allowed people to collect samples noninvasively under normal life conditions at home instead of under the contrived conditions of the sleep or endocrinological laboratory. The CAR is now a topic of intense investigation.

Cortisol levels are low in the night but rise in the early hours before waking. After waking up, most people show a further rise, the concentration peaking 20–40 min later. This is followed by a progressive reduction of cortisol during the day. There are several reasons why the CAR has become an important research topic. First, there is evidence that the CAR is under somewhat independent control from cortisol output during the remainder of the day. Several studies have shown little association between the CAR and cortisol levels during the rest of the day or the slope of cortisol concentration decline into the evening. Second, twin studies have documented a genetic influence on the CAR that is distinct from the heritability of daytime cortisol levels. Third, the CAR is associated with stress and health in potentially significant ways, suggesting that it is a useful marker of hypothalamic-pituitary-adrenocortical (HPA) function.

A number of different measures of the CAR have been devised, depending on how many saliva samples are obtained over the first hour after waking. Serial sampling suggests that that peak CAR is observed around 30 min after waking, so the simplest method of assessment involves measures at two time points: immediately after waking and 30 min later; the CAR is then defined as a simple difference score. More elaborate assessments involve measurements of several time points, such as immediately after waking and 15, 30, 45, and 60 min later; under these circumstances, the area under the curve can be computed to estimate total cortisol output. Difference scores and area under the curve measures are consistently intercorrelated.

Origins of the Cortisol Awakening Response

The secretion of cortisol is pulsatile, and it has been estimated that each secretory burst induces an increase in salivary free cortisol of approximately 2.5 nmol liter^{-1}. The CAR is a result of one to four secretory bursts over the period following waking. It is consistent across days under stable environmental conditions, but changes in magnitude when conditions vary.

The CAR is sensitive to light in the environment and can be enhanced by augmented light exposure early in the day. It has been proposed that this effect is mediated by the suprachiasmatic nucleus of hypothalamus, which is light sensitive and is involved in circadian regulation. Direct neural connections between the suprachiasmatic nucleus and the adrenal cortex have been identified and may modulate the sensitivity of the adrenal gland to adrenocorticotropic hormone.

The functional role of the CAR has not been established. It may be important metabolically in mobilizing the organism during the transition from sleep to waking. However, no association between the CAR and blood glucose levels has been observed. A role in immunological regulation has also been suggested, but direct evidence is lacking at present. The relevance of psychological factors is apparent from some studies, and it is further endorsed by the observation that the CAR is abolished in individuals with global amnesia, even though the remainder of the circadian rhythm of cortisol output is retained. This hints at the possibility that the CAR may depend either on recent life experiences or on anticipation of the activities and events of the forthcoming day.

Measurement of the Cortisol Awakening Response

Participants in CAR studies are instructed to take saliva samples immediately after waking and then at later defined intervals. Saliva is collected using cotton rolls or by directly spitting into test tubes, and participants are instructed not to brush their teeth, eat, drink, or smoke throughout the sampling period because these factors can influence cortisol values. Because the CAR is dynamic, accurate timing is critical, and failure to adhere to the sampling schedule may confound studies and produce misleading results. If the waking sample is delayed, the CAR may already have commenced, leading to an apparent diminution in the magnitude of the rise of the next 20–30 min. Similarly, if later samples are mistimed, then the magnitude of the CAR will not be assessed correctly.

The significance of timing errors has been demonstrated using saliva collection devices that are time-stamped. One study showed that more than 50% of community volunteers failed to take the 30-min post-waking sample at the correct time. Noncompliant participants produced smaller CARs. The impact of delays in collecting the waking sample is illustrated in **Figure 1**. This figure compares salivary cortisol profiles during the first hour of the day in elderly (65- to 80-year-old) volunteers who reported no delay in taking the first sample after waking and those who admitted delaying for 10 min or more. The no delay group showed a typical CAR with increases from waking to 30 min, whereas a decrease during same period was found in the delay group.

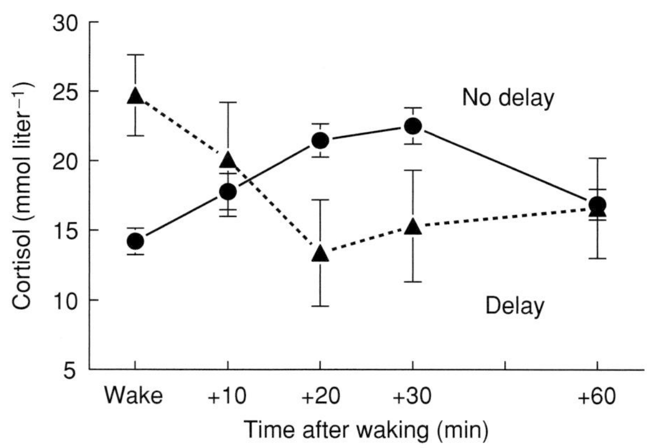

Figure 1 Mean salivary cortisol levels immediately after waking and at 10, 20, 30 and 60 minutes after waking in elderly volunteers who delayed (dashed line) and did not delay (solid line) saliva sampling after waking in the morning. Error bars are standard errors of the mean. From Wright, C. E., & Steptoe, A. (2005). Subjective socioeconomic position, gender and cortisol responses to waking in an elderly population. *Psychoneuroendocrinology, 30*, 582–590. Used with permission.

Several methods of improving the accuracy and reliability of CAR measurement have been proposed. Electronically time-tagged saliva collection methods provide data about the intervals between measurements, but information about the timing of waking up is still provided by the participants. Asking participants to record when they wake and when they take each sample provides a check and limits can be set on acceptable delays, but this method again depends on self-reports. The measurement of waking time using actigraphy is being explored. Another approach is to check for consistency across days and to exclude individuals who show widely discrepant CAR patterns on different days.

Factors Affecting the Cortisol Awakening Response

A wide range of factors potentially affect the CAR. In this section, other factors other than stress that affect the magnitude of the CAR are briefly described.

Gender and Age

Several investigations have shown that the CAR is greater in women than men. Results have not been completely consistent and may depend on whether measures are taken on a work or leisure day. The greater CAR in women may also be affected by the stressful demands they often encounter early in the day. Women are frequently responsible for preparing not only themselves for the day ahead but also children and for doing household chores as well. Most studies of the CAR have shown little association with age in adult populations.

Time of Waking

There has been controversy about the association between time of waking and the CAR. Several studies have shown that the CAR is greater in people who wake up early than in those who wake later, but no association with time of waking has also been reported in a number of large-scale investigations. The issue is complicated by two factors. First, people who say they wake up late in the morning may in fact have woken earlier and have subsequently dozed. Their CAR may therefore have partly taken place prior to the reported waking time. Second, waking early may be a reflection of greater stress, worry, or work demands, which themselves influence the CAR. In one study, the greater CAR recorded in people waking before starting an early work shift was no longer significant once concomitant stress had been taken into account.

Sleep Duration and Quality

The majority of studies to date have not shown any association between sleep duration or time of going to bed and the CAR. Experiments in which healthy participants were deliberately disturbed during the night showed no change in the CAR when they later woke in the morning. The CAR is also unaffected by whether the person wakes spontaneously or with an alarm clock. On the other hand, a negative relationship between cortisol levels on waking and sleep quality has been described, and cortisol levels on waking are lower in individuals diagnosed with primary insomnia.

Smoking

Data relating smoking with the CAR are mixed, but it has recently been shown that the CAR is greater in smokers than in nonsmokers, even when they have not smoked during the early morning period.

Significance of Cortisol Awakening Response for Stress Research

The relationship between the CAR and stress-related processes is intriguing. The early studies of the CAR indicated greater responses in people under chronic stress due to work or other demands, suggesting that the CAR might be a convenient stress measure. The CAR is also greater on work than on leisure days, indicating that the stressfulness of the forthcoming day may be significant. This is illustrated in **Figure 2**, which shows CAR results from a sample of working men and women measured on work and leisure days. It is evident that cortisol levels on waking did not differ between the two days. However, the CAR was substantially greater on work days than on weekend days. In addition, this study found a larger CAR in women than men on work days but not on weekend days.

Subsequent studies have identified several conditions in which the CAR is apparently reduced, indicating that stress-related processes may both accentuate and inhibit the CAR. **Table 1** summarizes the evidence to date. An enhanced CAR has consistently been found to relate to work stress and to measures such as job strain, work overload, and overcommitment to work. Both clinical depression and depressive symptoms within the nonpsychiatric population are characterized by a heightened CAR. By contrast, a diminished CAR has been recorded in people suffering from posttraumatic stress disorder and chronic fatigue and in those who have experienced early life adversity. Other types of chronic strain, such as caring for a demented relative, have been associated with a heightened CAR, while the effects of early life adversity have been variable. Research on socioeconomic status has shown inconsistent results, with elevated CAR in some studies and reduced CAR in others. The literature on burnout is also mixed, with most studies showing clinically defined burnout problems to have no effect on the CAR.

Nearly all of these effects are cross-sectional, so the causal significance of associations is unclear. However, one recent study assessed changes in financial strain over a 3-year period and demonstrated that a reduction in financial strain was accompanied by a decrease in the CAR, indicating a parallel between changes in chronic stress and the magnitude of the CAR.

The explanation for these variations among studies is not clear. They may reflect genuine differences between the patterning of the CAR in relation to different types of stressful experience. But it should be noted that several of these studies did not control rigorously for the timing of sampling. It is conceivable that in some conditions of chronic stress, people are less reliable in the timing of measurements, leading to an apparent diminution in the CAR.

Relationship with Health Outcomes

The CAR has not been studied extensively in relation to health to date. One study divided respondents into people who did and did not report any health problem or chronic disease and showed a smaller CAR in the less healthy group. There have been a number of other interesting observations suggesting that associations may exist with physical health risk. For example, the CAR has been positively associated with waist/hip ratio in men, suggesting that it may relate to HPA dysfunction in abdominal adiposity. Another study assessed relationships with the rate of healing

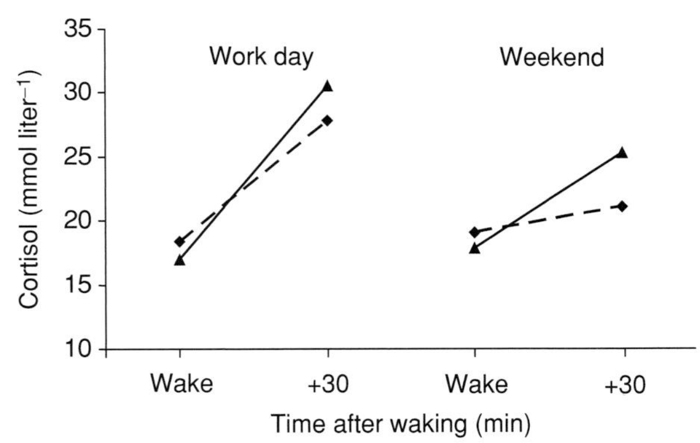

Figure 2 Mean salivary cortisol on waking (Wake) and 30 minutes later (+30) on a work day and weekend day in men (solid lines) and women (dashed lines). Error bars are standard errors of the mean. From Kunz-Ebrecht, S. R., Kirschbaum, C., Marmot, M., & Steptoe, A. (2004). Differences in cortisol awakening response on work days and weekends in women and men from the Whitehall II cohort. *Psychoneuroendocrinology, 29*, 516–528. Used with permission.

Table 1 Psychosocial factors and the cortisol awakening response

Factors associated with increased CAR	*Factors associated with reduced CAR*	*Inconsistent effects*
Work vs. leisure days	Posttraumatic stress disorder	Socioeconomic status
Chronic stress, work overload	Chronic fatigue	Burnout
Job strain, overcommitment to work		Early life adversity
Depression and depressive symptoms		
Financial strain		
Loneliness		
Neuroticism		
Caregiving		

of a wound imposed experimentally on healthy volunteers. Wound healing was slower in people reporting high levels of subjective stress and in those with a larger CAR, indicating that stress may impair wound healing in part through disturbances in cortisol regulation. Another indication of the health relevance of the CAR is the observation that in women a greater CAR was positively associated with progression in carotid intima-media thickness and so correlated with the development of atherosclerosis. Other studies have not measured the CAR directly but, rather, assessed the cortisol level in the early morning. The values recorded in these studies may reflect the peak CAR or some time point soon afterward. Notably, the early morning cortisol level is positively associated with risk of future clinical depression in prospective studies of adolescents and adults and with cardiovascular disease risk factors.

Conclusion

The CAR has only begun to be studied in recent years in stress research, but it is already providing valuable information about the relationship among HPA function, psychosocial factors, and health risk.

See Also the Following Articles

Corticosteroids and Stress.

Further Reading

Backhaus, J., Junghanns, K. and Hohagen, F. (2004). Sleep disturbances are correlated with decreased morning awakening salivary cortisol. *Psychoneuroendocrinology* **29**, 1184–1191.

Clow, A., Thorn, L., Evans, P., et al. (2004). The awakening cortisol response: methodological issues and significance. *Stress* **7**, 29–37.

Goodyer, I. M., Herbert, J., Tamplin, A., et al. (2000). Recent life events, cortisol, dehydroepiandrosterone and the onset of major depression in high-risk adolescents. *British Journal of Psychiatry* **177**, 499–504.

Ebrecht, M., Hextall, J., Kirtley, L. G., et al. (2004). Perceived stress and cortisol levels predict speed of wound healing in healthy male adults. *Psychoneuroendocrinology* **29**, 798–809.

Eller, N. H., Netterstrom, B. and Allerup, P. (2005). Progression in intima media thickness – the significance of hormonal biomarkers of chronic stress. *Psychoneuroendocrinology* **30**, 715–723.

Harris, T. O., Borsanyi, S., Messari, S., et al. (2000). Morning cortisol as a risk factor for subsequent major depressive disorder in adult women. *British Journal of Psychiatry* **177**, 505–510.

Kudielka, B. M., Broderick, J. E. and Kirschbaum, C. (2003). Compliance with saliva sampling protocols: electronic monitoring reveals invalid cortisol daytime profiles in noncompliant subjects. *Psychosomatic Medicine* **65**, 313–319.

Kunz-Ebrecht, S. R., Kirschbaum, C., Marmot, M., et al. (2004). Differences in cortisol awakening response on work days and weekends in women and men from the Whitehall II cohort. *Psychoneuroendocrinology* **29**, 516–528.

Pruessner, M., Hellhammer, D. H., Pruessner, J. C., et al. (2003). Self-reported depressive symptoms and stress levels in healthy young men: associations with the cortisol response to awakening. *Psychosomatic Medicine* **65**, 92–99.

Steptoe, A., Kunz-Ebrecht, S. R., Brydon, L., et al. (2004). Central adiposity and cortisol responses to waking in middle-aged men and women. *International Journal of Obesity and Related Metabolic Disorders* **28**, 1168–1173.

Steptoe, A., Brydon, L. and Kunz-Ebrecht, S. (2005). Changes in financial strain over three years, ambulatory blood pressure, and cortisol responses to awakening. *Psychosomatic Medicine* **67**, 281–287.

Wolf, O. T., Fujiwara, E., Luwinski, G., et al. (2005). No morning cortisol response in patients with severe global amnesia. *Psychoneuroendocrinology* **30**, 101–105.

Wright, C. E. and Steptoe, A. (2005). Subjective socioeconomic position, gender and cortisol responses to waking in an elderly population. *Psychoneuroendocrinology* **30**, 582–590.

Wüst, S., Wolf, J., Hellhammer, D. H., et al. (2000). The cortisol awakening response – normal values and confounds. *Noise and Health* **7**, 77–85.

Circadian Rhythms, Genetics of

F W Turek and M H Vitaterna
Northwestern University, Evanston, IL, USA

This is a revised version of the article by F W Turek and M H Vitaterna, Encyclopedia of Stress, First edition, volume 1, pp 471–477, © 2000, Elsevier Inc.

Glossary

Circadian clock	An internal timing mechanism that regulates the expression of circadian rhythms. In mammals, a master circadian clock is located in the hypothalamic suprachiasmatic nucleus (SCN), although recent findings indicate that most if not all tissues of the body contain circadian clocks that are directly or indirectly regulated by the clock in the SCN.
Circadian clock genes and clock-controlled genes	While only a small number of genes and their protein products appear to be involved in the transcriptional/translational feedback loop that makes up the molecular core of the circadian clock, this molecular clock in turn appears to regulate the expression of hundreds of downstream clock-controlled genes.
Circadian rhythms	Biochemical, physiological, and behavioral events that reoccur in a cyclic fashion with a period of about 24 h.
Entrainment	Process by which an internal circadian clock is entrained or synchronized to the period of an external stimulus that usually has a period of about 24 h. In nature, the light–dark cycle is the primary external environmental signal that entrains the circadian clock to the 24-h period of the day that is due to the rotation of the earth on its axis.
Free-running	Term used to describe circadian rhythms persisting in the absence of any 24-h synchronizing information from the external environment. The expression of free-running circadian rhythms with a period close to (e.g., 23–24 h) but rarely exactly 24 h demonstrates the endogenous nature of the circadian clock underlying the expression of circadian rhythms.
Period	The length of a cycle of the rhythm. The period of a free-running rhythm is considered a fundamental property of the circadian clock.
Phase	The timing of the rhythm. During entrainment, the timing of a phase reference point (such as activity onset) relative to the external time cue (such as lights on) should be stable. This relative timing is referred to as the phase angle of entrainment. The rhythm-resetting response to a perturbation such as a brief light exposure is measured as a phase shift.

The Molecular Circadian Clock

Early studies in invertebrates demonstrated that the period of the circadian clock was clearly under genetic control since 24-h rhythms developed in organisms never experiencing any 24-h changes in the physical environment. Furthermore, rearing mice on non-24-h cycles as extreme as 20 or 28 h has only small (i.e., on the order of a few minutes) and transient effects on the free-running period of the circadian clock when animals are subsequently housed under conditions of constant darkness (i.e., the free-running period remains within a few minutes of 24 h). Until recently, evidence that genetic differences define the characteristics of the circadian clock system in mammals has been determined primarily by comparing properties of circadian rhythms between different inbred strains of the same species.

With the discovery of the first mammalian circadian clock gene (named *Clock*) in 1997, a new era opened for discovering how the mammalian circadian clock ticks. The *Clock* gene was initially identified through a behavioral phenotypic screen of mice that were the offspring of mutagenized animals. Vitaterna et al. identified a mutant animal that demonstrated a lengthened circadian period under free-running conditions (constant darkness). Descendants of this mutant with two copies of the mutant gene initially showed a free-running period of about 27–28 h in constant darkness, with subsequent breakdown in circadian rhythmicity. Next, the *Clock* gene was cloned and found to encode a member of the bHLH-PAS (basic helix-loop-helix, Per-Arnt-Sim domain) family of transcription factors. The role of the putative *Clock* gene was confirmed by creating transgenic mice in which the altered phenotype of *Clock* mutants was rescued by insertion of the wild-type *Clock* gene.

Other key clock genes in mammals have since been characterized. Three murine homologs of the *Drosophila period* gene, *mPer1*, *mPer2*, and *mPer3* have been identified. While double-knockout animals lacking *mPer1* and *mPer2* show behavioral arrhythmicity when placed in constant conditions, there appears to be partial redundancy of function between *mPer* family members. Moreover, *mPer3* does not appear to have an essential function in the core clock mechanism.

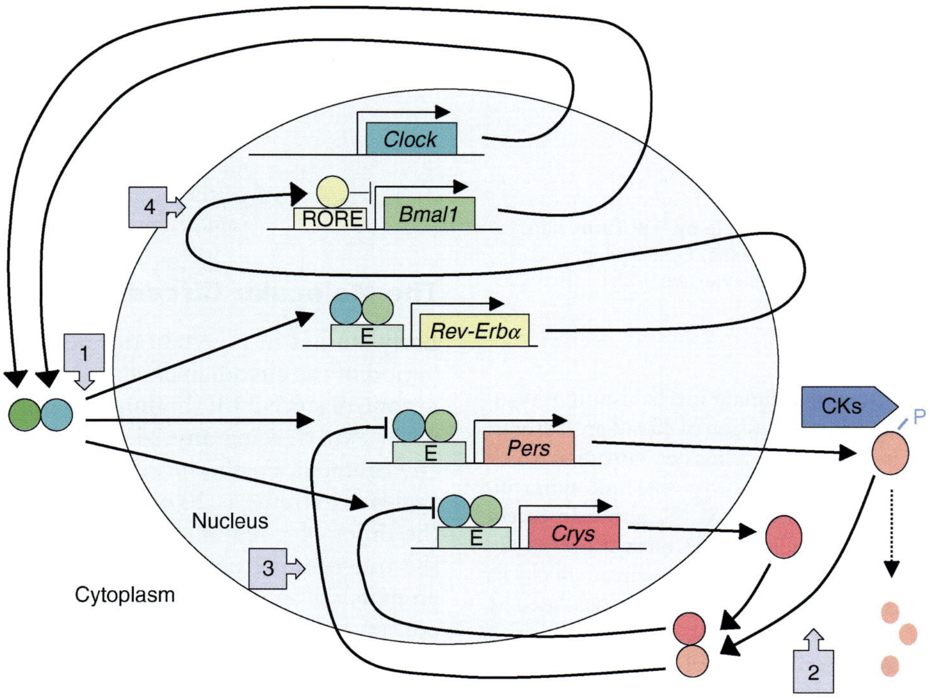

Figure 1 See text for explanation of figure.

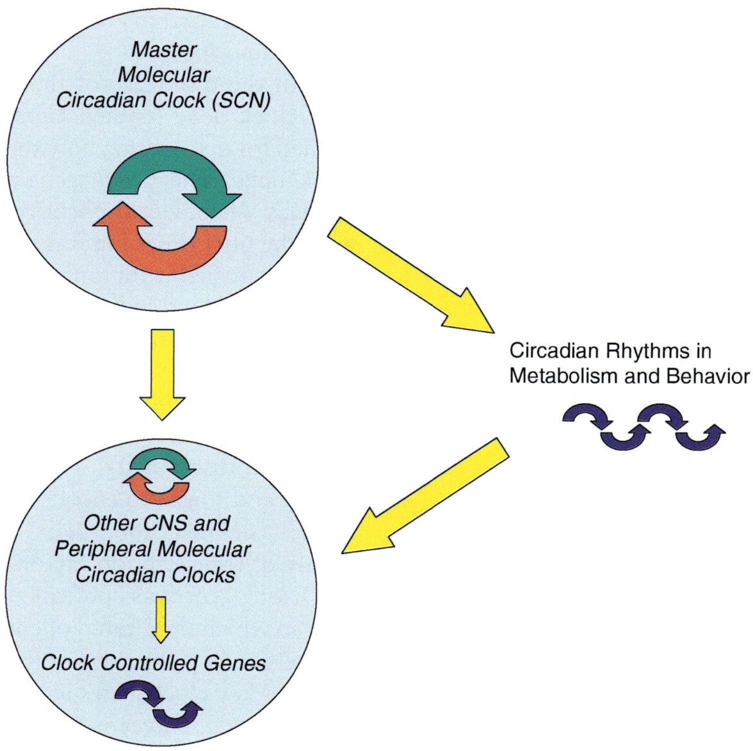

Figure 2 See text for explanation of figure.

A second bHLH-PAS transcription factor, BMAL1, has been identified and shown to be a core circadian clock gene. *In vitro*, CLOCK-BMAL1 dimers activate transcription of *mPer*, and the *Clock* mutation described previously is associated with reduced expression of *mPer1*, *mPer2*, and *mPer3* in the suprachiasmatic nucleus (SCN). These data support a role for CLOCK (and the CLOCK-BMAL1 dimer) in activation of transcription of all three *mPer* homologs.

Two cryptochrome genes, *Cry1* and *Cry2*, also appear to be components of the core circadian system. *Cry2* null mutants exhibit lengthened circadian periods, while *Cry1* null mutants exhibit shortened circadian periods. In *Cry* double-knockout mice, animals are completely arrhythmic immediately after the introduction of constant darkness. CRY1 and CRY2 are both synthesized in the SCN, where at least *Cry1* exhibits rhythmic expression. These proteins inhibit CLOCK-BMAL1-driven transcription, most probably due to binding of CRY1 and CRY2 to clock components. Importantly, CRY1 and CRY2 are able to translocate *per* gene products to the nucleus.

Posttranslational modification of clock proteins seems to be important in the modulation of circadian rhythm. Casein kinase Iε (CKIε), which phosphorylates CRY1, CRY2, PER1, PER2, and BMAL1, is defective in the *tau* mutant in Syrian hamsters, in which the free-running period in constant darkness is 22 h and 20 h in heterozygous and homozygous animals, respectively. In this mutant, CKIε has a lower rate of phosphorylation. Recent data also suggest that a second kinase, CKIδ, is important for the mammalian clock.

The current concept of the core clock is a system of interacting transcriptional/translational feedback loops (**Figure 1**). The two transcription factors, CLOCK and BMAL1, form dimers that bind to DNA and promote rhythmic transcription of three *Per* genes, two *Cry* genes, and the *Rev-Erbα* gene (step 1). The proteins encoded by *mPer1* and *mPer2* bind to the proteins encoded by *Cry1* and *Cry2*, forming complexes with casein kinases (step 2). These translocate into the nucleus, where CRY and PER proteins act as negative regulators, directly inhibiting CLOCK/BMAL1 activity and indirectly the transcription of *mPers*, *Crys*, and *Rev-Erbα* (step 3). Positive feedback is mediated by rhythmic modulation of *Bmal1* transcription. Thus, the REV-ERBα protein, whose synthesis is increased by binding of CLOCK/BMAL1 dimers to DNA, inhibits the transcription of *Bmal1* (step 4).

Recent studies indicating that other genes involved in the posttranslational modification of circadian clock proteins can alter the circadian clock suggest that many other genes may be found that can modify the core genes/protein products of the molecular clock and alter its periodicity.

The Molecular Clock Is Not Confined to the SCN

With the establishment of the bilaterally paired SCN of the hypothalamus as the site of the circadian clock in mammals, considerable attention was focused on how the SCN can generate circadian rhythms at the neural as well as molecular levels. However, once the core components of the molecular circadian clock were identified, a surprising discovery was made: the clock genes not only are expressed in the SCN, but also are rhythmically expressed in the SCN and peripheral tissues throughout the body, including the liver, heart, lungs, and muscle. Furthermore, these circadian oscillations in the peripheral tissues can persist for many cycles *in vitro*, revealing the endogenous nature of tissue-specific circadian rhythmicity. Most importantly, not only are the clock genes oscillating in various tissues, but also they appear to be regulating the transcription of hundreds of downstream clock-controlled genes. In a simplistic form, our understanding of the circadian clock system is as follows (**Figure 2**): 1. The circadian clock genes and their protein products compose a transcriptional/translational molecular feedback loop (with posttranslational components) that can generate precise circadian timing in the master circadian clock in the SCN.

2. The SCN communicates circadian information to other central and peripheral tissues via neural and/or neurohormonal transmission vectors.

3. Non-SCN circadian clocks appear to consist of a molecular core, as does the SCN. Thus, the molecular clock in the SCN (which is itself entrained by the light–dark cycle) somehow entrains a similar molecular clock in other CNS and peripheral tissues. This entrainment may be direct or indirect via the SCN control of metabolic and behavioral rhythms (e.g., feeding, sleep–wake cycle, body temperature).

This simple three-step process does not rule out the possibility that downstream (from SCN) circadian oscillators will not persist on their own (e.g., in SCN-lesioned animals). Nor does it exclude the possibility that they can be entrained by environmental factors (e.g., when feeding occurs out of phase with the normal SCN-timed control of feeding). However, under normal entrained conditions, it appears that the SCN serves as the conductor of an orchestra in regulating the timing, directly or indirectly, of hundreds of downstream oscillators, which in turn are regulating the timing and expression of hundreds, if not thousands, of clock-controlled genes. Such intricate and diverse timing raises profound questions about the role of such timing in health and disease at many levels of organization.

Disruption of Molecular Clock Leads to Tissue and Organismal Dysfunction

A foundation of the field of biological rhythms is that the circadian clock system has evolved to allow organisms to maintain two different kinds of synchronization. One type of synchronization, referred to as external synchronization, enables the organisms to maintain synchrony with the external 24-h environment. Thus, the animal, or plant, is doing the right thing at the right time of the day or night such that optimum survival and reproductive success are ensured. A second, and less visible but no less important, type of synchrony imposed by the circadian clock is referred to as internal synchronization. In internal synchrony, the vast array of internal cellular, metabolic, physiological, endocrine, and behavioral rhythmic processes are maintained in temporal relationships to allow for life processes to be carried out at optimal efficiency. Until recently, this concept of internal synchrony was more often applied to the functioning of the organism as a whole. That is, in the case of mammals, the SCN was seen as the master circadian clock regulating the timing of the various organ systems and behavior of the animal to ensure optimal internal synchrony for survival and reproductive fitness. In the case of humans engaged in shift work or experiencing jet lag, the internal synchrony would be perturbed (i.e., internal desynchronization), leading to less than optimal organ/behavioral performance. However, with the discovery that most if not all tissues and organ systems of the body have their own circadian molecular core machinery, the concept of internal synchrony takes on new meaning. One can now talk about internal desynchronization at the local cellular or tissue level. Such a paradigm shift in thinking about the meaning of internal synchronization has profound implications for health and disease.

The fact that the expression of hundreds of genes is under local (i.e., cellular) circadian control argues that the phase relationship between the rhythmic expression of these genes has functional significance at the cellular and/or tissue level. Just as a breakdown of internal synchrony at the macro-level (i.e., organ system/whole organism) is disruptive to health and well-being, one can expect that a similar breakdown at the micro-level (cellular/tissue) could lead to dysfunction at the local level. Thus, we may have a perfectly functioning circadian clock system at the macro-level, but still have a dysfunctional system at a local tissue level. Age-related diseases are often associated with tissue (CNS or peripheral) dysfunction due to age-related breakdown (e.g., due to oxidative stress, DNA repair dysfunction, accumulated protein/DNA damage) in cellular processes. However, the newly discovered circadian molecular clock machinery and its overall importance for cellular/tissue timing raises the intriguing possibility that many age-related diseases may have at their core a breakdown in the timing or internal temporal organization. Many diseases are due to malfunction of a particular tissue, organ, or organ system, whether due to external or internal factors, and death is often associated with whatever vital system breaks down first. An intriguing offshoot of this concept is that disease may be due to temporal disorganization at the cellular or tissue level, whether due to external or internal factors, and death may be due to the abnormal timing at the molecular/genetic level in specific tissue/organ systems whose normal function is critical for the survival of the organism. The recent finding that a mutation of a canonical circadian clock gene, *Clock*, can lead to a major disruption at tissue and behavioral levels in energy balance, as well as obesity and the metabolic syndrome, may be an example whereby temporal disorganization leads to disease conditions at the macro and micro organizational levels.

See Also the Following Articles

Circadian Clock Genes as Modulators of Sensitivity to Genotoxic Stress; Seasonal Changes in Stress Responses; Seasonal Rhythms.

Further Reading

Akashi, M., Tsuchiya, Y., Yoshino, T. and Nishida, E. (2002). Control of intracellular dynamics of mammalian period proteins by casein kinase I epsilon (CKIepsilon) and CKIdelta in cultured cells. *Molecular and Cellular Biology* **22**(6), 1693–1703.

Albrecht, U., Sun, Z. S., Eichele, G. and Lee, C. C. (1997). A differential response of two putative mammalian circadian regulators, mper1 and mper2, to light. *Cell* **91**, 1055–1064.

Antoch, M. P., Song, E., Chang, A., et al. (1997). Functional identification of the mouse circadian Clock gene by transgenic BAC rescue. *Cell* **89**, 655–667.

Bunger, M. K., Wilsbacher, L. D., Moran, S. M., et al. (2000). Mop3 is an essential component of the master circadian pacemaker in mammals. *Cell* **103**(7), 1009–1017.

Cardone, L., Hirayama, J., Giordano, F., et al. (2005). Circadian clock control by SUMOylation of BMAL1. *Science* **309**(5739), 1390–1394.

Eide, E. J., Vielhaber, E. L., Hinz, W. A. and Virshup, D. M. (2002). The circadian regulatory proteins BMAL1 and cryptochromes are substrates of casein kinase Iepsilon. *Journal of Biological Chemistry* **277**(19), 17248–17254.

Gekakis, N., Staknis, D., Nguyen, H. B., et al. (1998). Role of the CLOCK protein in the mammalian circadian mechanism. *Science* **280**, 1564–1569.

Griffin, E. A., Jr., Staknis, D. and Weitz, C. J. (1999). Light-independent role of CRY1 and CRY2 in the mammalian circadian clock. *Science* **286**(5440), 768–771.

Iitaka, C., Miyazaki, K., Akaike, T. and Ishida, N. (2005). A role for glycogen synthase kinase-3beta in the mammalian circadian clock. *Journal of Biological Chemistry* **280** (33), 29397–29402.

Jin, X., Shearman, L., Weaver, D., et al. (1999). A molecular mechanism regulating output from the suprachiasmatic circadian clock. *Cell* **96**, 57–68.

King, D. P., Zhao, Y., Sangoram, A. M., Wilsbacher, L. D., et al. (1997). Positional cloning of the mouse circadian Clock gene. *Cell* **89**, 641–653.

Kume, K., Zylka, M. J., Sriram, S., et al. (1999). mCRY1 and mCRY2 are essential components of the negative limb of the circadian clock feedback loop. *Cell* **98**(2), 193–205.

Lowrey, P. L. and Takahshi, J. S. (2000). Genetics of the mammalian circadian system: photic entrainment, circadian pacemaker mechanisms and posttranslational regulation. *Annual Review of Genetics* **34**, 533–562.

Lowrey, P. L., Shimomura, K., Antoch, M. P., et al. (2000). Positional syntenic cloning and functional characterization of the mammalian circadian mutation tau. *Science* **288**(5465), 483–492.

Miyamoto, Y. and Sancar, A. (1998). Vitamin B2-based blue-light photoreceptors in the retinohypothalamic tract as the photoactive pigments for setting the circadian clock in mammals. *Proceedings of the National Academy of Sciences of the USA* **95**(11), 6097–6102.

Panda, S., Antoch, M. P., Miller, B. H., et al. (2002). Coordinated transcription of key pathways in the mouse by the circadian clock. *Cell* **109**(3), 307–320.

Reppert, S. M. and Weaver, D. R. (2002). Coordination of circadian timing in mammals. *Nature* **418**(6901), 935–941.

Shearman, L. P., Zylka, M. J., Weaver, D. R., Kolakowski, L. F. J. and Reppert, S. M. (1997). Two period homologs: circadian expression and photic regulation in the suprachiasmatic nuclei. *Neuron* **19**, 1261–1269.

Shearman, L. P., Jin, X., Lee, C., Reppert, S. M. and Weaver, D. R. (2000). Targeted disruption of the mPer3 gene: subtle effects on circadian clock function. *Molecular and Cellular Biology* **20**(17), 6269–6275.

Sun, Z. S., Albrecht, U., Zhuchenko, O., et al. (1997). RIGUI, a putative mammalian ortholog of the Drosophila period gene. *Cell* **90**, 1003–1011.

Takumi, T., Taguchi, K., Miyake, S., et al. (1998). A light-independent oscillatory gene mPer3 in mouse SCN and OVLT. *EMBO Journal* **17**, 4753–4759.

Tei, H., Okamura, H., Shigeyoshi, Y., et al. (1997). Circadian oscillation of a mammalian homologue of the Drosophila period gene. *Nature* **389**, 512–516.

Turek, F. W., Joshu, C., Kohsaka, A., et al. (2005). Obesity and metabolic syndrome in circadian Clock mutant mice. *Science* **308**(5724), 1043–1045.

Van der Horst, G. T. J., Muijtjens, M., Kobayashi, K., et al. (1999). Mammalian Cry1 and Cry2 are essential for maintenance of circadian rhythms. *Nature* **398**, 627–630.

Vitaterna, M. H., King, D. P., Chang, A.-M., et al. (1994). Mutagenesis and mapping of a mouse gene, Clock, essential for circadian behavior. *Science* **264**, 719–725.

Vitaterna, M. H., Selby, C. P., Todo, T., et al. (1999). Differential regulation of mammalian period genes and circadian rhythmicity by cryptochromes 1 and 2. *Proceedings of the National Academy of Sciences of the USA* **96**(21), 12114–12119.

Vitaterna, M. H., Pinto, L. H. and Turek, F. W. (2005). Molecular genetic basis for mammalian circadian rhythms. In: Kryger, M. H., Roth, T. & Dement, W. C. (eds.) *Principles and practice of sleep medicine*, pp. 363–374. New York: W.B. Saunders.

Yoo, S. H., Yamazaki, S., Lowrey, P. L., et al. (2004). PERIOD2::LUCIFERASE real-time reporting of circadian dynamics reveals persistent circadian oscillations in mouse peripheral tissues. *Proceedings of the National Academy of Sciences of the USA* **101**(15), 5339–5346.

Zylka, M. J., Shearman, L. P., Weaver, D. R. and Reppert, S. M. (1998). Three period homologs in mammals: differential light responses in the suprachiasmatic circadian clock and oscillating transcripts outside of brain. *Neuron* **20**, 1103–1110.

Food Shift Effect

F K Stephan
Florida State University, Tallahassee, FL, USA

This article is reproduced from Encyclopedia of Stress, First edition, volume 2, pp 167–169, © 2000, Elsevier Inc.

Glossary

Circadian rhythm	A cycle with a period of approximately 24 h.
Entrainment	A zeitgeber forcing its period and phase on a rhythm.
Phase	A point in the circadian cycle.
Zeitgeber	A periodic external cue that entrains circadian clocks.

Endogenous Circadian Clocks

In 1972, the neural substrate responsible for the generation and entrainment of circadian rhythms by light was identified. Lesions of this small structure, the suprachiasmatic nucleus (SCN) of the hypothalamus, appeared to abolish circadian rhythms in behavior and physiology. However, despite such lesions, rats were still able to anticipate one meal per day by increased activity, a rise in core temperature and serum corticosterone, and other physiological changes that occurred approximately 2–4 h prior to meal access. There is now compelling evidence that these functions are mediated by an endogenous circadian clock: (1) meal anticipation occurs only if the interval between meals is in the

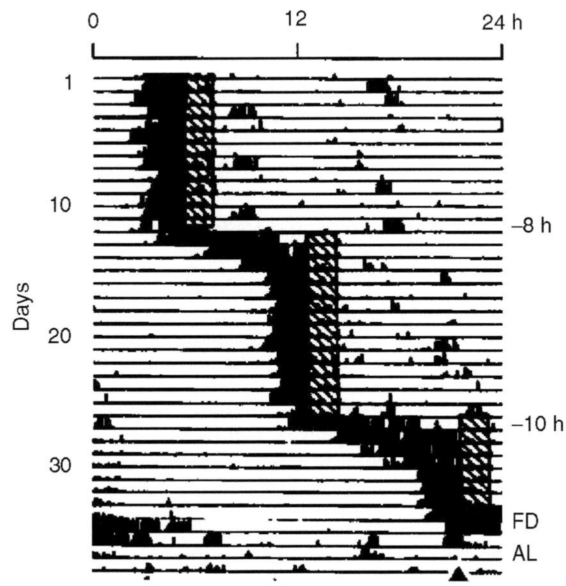

Figure 1 Anticipatory wheel running from a rat with a lesion of the suprachiasmatic nucleus (arrhythmic when fed *ad libitum*). Food is available for 2 h day^{-1}, indicated by the vertical cross-hatched bars. Most wheel running occurs approximately 3 h before meal time. When the meal time is delayed by 8 or 10 h, anticipatory activity takes 3 or 4 days to reentrain to the phase-shifted meal. The activity persists during food deprivation (FD), but is not observed during *ad libitum* (AL) feeding.

circadian range (~22–30 h), (2) anticipatory activity persists for several days when rats are food-deprived or the activity free runs (in some rats) if meals are presented outside the circadian range, and (3) phase shifts of meal-time result in transients, that is, gradual daily adjustments until the activity reentrains to the new meal time (see **Figure 1**). Despite many efforts, this feeding-entrained oscillator (FEO) has not yet been localized. Nevertheless, most mammals, as well as some inframammalian species, are now known to have the capacity to anticipate daily meals, and it would be surprising if humans lacked such a circadian clock. It is well known that hunger sensations arise around the customary meal time. What has been difficult to explain from a purely homeostatic view is that the omission of a meal does not produce monotonically increasing feelings of hunger; instead, hunger subsides until the next customary meal time. However, this makes sense if hunger sensations are based in part on an internal timing signal and not entirely on an energy-deficit signal.

Physiological Correlates of Entrainment by Meals

Before addressing the potentially adverse effects of changes in meal time or meal omission, a brief summary of the main effects of feeding one meal per day on the rat's digestive physiology is in order. As mentioned earlier, serum corticosterone levels rise prior to expected meals. Corticosterone is both a metabolic and a stress hormone, and the brain has receptors for this steroid. Perhaps most surprising is the observation that disaccharidases (enzymes for digesting sugars) in the duodenum also increase before the meal is available. In addition, several aspects of liver function, cell division in the gastrointestinal tract, and intestinal motility become entrained to periodic meals. The increase in core temperature also may facilitate digestion. The general inference to be drawn from these observations is that the digestive physiology is not simply reactive to ingested nutrients but is capable of anticipating and preparing for meals, most likely under the influence of the circadian FEO. If the expected meal is displaced in time, these efforts are for naught and for several days these preparatory responses are out of synchrony with actual food consumption.

Shift Work and Jet Lag

Gastrointestinal malaise is a common complaint of shift workers and travelers across time zones. Along with impaired performance and other complaints, this has been attributed to the desynchronization of SCN-controlled rhythms (e.g., the sleep–wake cycle) from behavior. The discovery of a separate circadian clock raises the possibility that some of these symptoms are caused by forcing the FEO to phase shift to a new time. Unfortunately, the scientific literature regarding the role of meal timing and meal composition in producing jet-lag symptoms in humans is extremely sparse. Only very recently has an attempt been made to assess the consequences of limiting food intake to a single meal. A carbohydrate-rich meal in the morning for 3 consecutive days led to a phase advance of 1 h of the body temperature rhythm, whereas evening meals had no effect. A similar effect has been noted in mice in that the nocturnal activity rhythm is also phase advanced if they are limited to one meal per day. In rats, the FEO is easily phase shifted by a glucose meal, but seems less responsive to a fat meal. A number of other studies indicate that there are interactions between light-entrainable and food-entrainable circadian systems; the period and phase of one has an effect on the other. Thus, there is a possibility that particular meal schedules might facilitate adjustment to temporal shifts in daily routines, but this has not yet been specifically investigated. In an interesting study, patients in a vegetative state (which reduces or eliminates the effects of activity or other external factors) received intraduodenal infusions of a liquid diet continuously, only during the day or only during the night. No consistent temperature rhythms were observed with continuous infusions, whereas day infusions resulted in a peak temperature at 8 p.m. and night infusions resulted in a peak at 4 a.m. Because these peaks occurred at different times relative to meal onset and end, they were probably not entirely due to the thermogenic action of food but may reflect the entrainment of some physiological processes by a circadian oscillator. When humans live in temporal isolation for more than 3 weeks, approximately one-half of the subjects display internal desynchronization. The core body temperature rhythm continues to free run with a period of approximately 25 h, but the sleep–wake cycle assumes a much longer period, between 30 and 48 h. When subjects were asked to eat only two meals per day (breakfast and lunch), the interval between meals was proportional to the wake time. Before internal desynchronization, the average interval between meals was approximately 7.4 h; after internal desynchronization (when the sleep–wake cycle had assumed a period of 35.4 h), the interval increased to 10.4 h. It should be noted that subjects were entirely unaware that their sleep–wake cycle had become abnormally long. It has long been suspected that internal desynchronization is evidence for two separate circadian clocks, but alternative explanations have also been offered. In particular, none of the studies establishes the existence of a separate feeding-entrained circadian clock in humans. Nevertheless, these studies at least suggest a circadian timing component to human hunger. However, in blind humans who have difficulties adhering to a 24-h schedule, regular meals and social routines have not been very effective in forcing entrainment of the sleep–wake cycle.

In other human studies regarding the effect of light or exercise on circadian rhythms, mealtime is either not reported or small meals are given at frequent intervals so that the effects of substantial meals on physiological measures cannot be assessed. Furthermore, temperature data (and other data) are often reported as group means or in other ways that make it impossible to determine even whether temperature or serum cortisol levels in humans rise in anticipation of meals. However, the evidence is quite compelling that such rhythms persist in constant conditions, that is, that they are controlled by one or more endogenous circadian oscillators.

A nearly universal observation is that circadian rhythms adjust more readily to phase delays (e.g., westward flights) than to phase advances (e.g., eastward flights). This asymmetry is even more pronounced in rats with SCN lesions that are entrained to one meal per day. As mentioned earlier, rats can anticipate meals at intervals as long as 30 h, but have difficulty anticipating meals presented at intervals shorter than 22 h, indicating that the FEO slows down more readily than it accelerates. When meals are shifted to a later time, anticipatory activity shifts by 2–4 h day^{-1} until it reaches the new phase position (see **Figure 1**). Conversely, after phase advances of 6 h or more, many rats display delays in anticipatory activity, again of about 3 h day^{-1}, i.e., the oscillator delays by 16–18 h over 5–6 days to catch up with the phase-advanced meal time. It is interesting that some humans also show delaying transients after rotating to an earlier shift (e.g., from the night to afternoon shift).

Conclusion

During the past decades, it has become increasingly clear that the regulation of energy balance is largely proactive rather than reactive. Circadian clocks, such as the FEO, entrain to predictable external events and ready the system for the arrival of nutrients. Phase shifts of mealtime temporarily disrupt these functions and probably account, at least partially, for the symptoms of jet lag or shift-worker malaise. The release of adrenal corticosteroids before meals could be a warning signal to the brain to replenish energy reserves. If food is consumed, serum levels decline, but if the meal is not available, serum levels might remain elevated for many hours. This, as well as other wasted physiological changes that occur in anticipation of meals, is undoubtedly not beneficial. There is no direct evidence as yet (because it has not been studied) that serious harm results from phase shifts of meals; however, it is conceivable that prolonged erratic eating habits contribute to the stress experienced by hectic modern lifestyles.

See Also the Following Articles

Circadian Rhythms, Genetics of.

Further Reading

Aschoff, J. (1998). Human perception of short and long time intervals: its correlation with body temperature and the duration of wake time. *Journal of Biological Rhythms* **13**, 437–442.

Czeisler, C. A. and Megan, E. J. (1990). Human circadian physiology: interaction of the behavioral rest-activity cycle with the output of the endogenous circadian pacemaker. In: Thorpy, M. J. (ed.) *Handbook of sleep disorders*, pp. 117–137. New York: Marcel Dekker.

Krauchi, K., Werth, E., Cajochen, C., et al. (1998). Are carbohydrate-rich meals a zeitgeber in humans? *Society for Research on Biological Rhythms* Abstract 96.

Mills, J. N., Minors, D. S. and Waterhouse, J. M. (1978). Adaptation to abrupt time shifts of the oscillator(s) controlling human circadian rhythms. *Journal of Physiology* **285**, 455–470.

Mistlberger, R. E. (1994). Circadian food-anticipatory activity: formal models and physiological mechanisms. *Neuroscience and Biobehavioral Reviews* **18**, 171–195.

Stephan, F. K. (1992). Resetting of a feeding-entrainable circadian clock in the rat. *Physiology & Behavior* **52**, 985–995.

Stephan, F. K. (1997). Calories affect zeitgeber properties of the feeding entrained circadian oscillator. *Physiology & Behavior* **62**, 995–1002.

Van Cauter, E., Sturis, J., Byrne, M., et al. (1994). Demonstration of rapid light-induced advances and delays of the human circadian clock using hormonal phase markers. *American Journal of Psychiatry* **266**, E953–E963.

Seasonal Changes in Stress Responses

R J Nelson and L B Martin II
Ohio State University, Columbus, OH, USA

This is a revised version of the article by R J Nelson and D L Drazen, Encyclopedia of Stress, First edition, volume 3, pp 402–408, © 2000, Elsevier Inc.

Glossary

Glucocorticoids	A class of steroid hormones secreted from the adrenal cortices that serves to promote energy use. Corticosterone is the glucocorticoid usually secreted by rodents and birds, whereas cortisol is typically secreted by primates.
Melatonin	An indole-amine hormone secreted from the pineal gland at night that is important in the regulation of daily and seasonal biological rhythms.
Photoperiod	Day length or the amount of light per day.
Photoperiodism	The response of plants to the length of day and night, including the ability to determine day length (usually by measuring night length) in both plants and animals; first proposed by botanists Garner and Allard in 1922.
Pineal gland	An endocrine gland that secretes melatonin, usually located between the telencephalon and diencephalon in vertebrates; also called the epiphysis.

Introduction

Stressors are not constant but, rather, vary over time. In addition to daily changes in stress, seasonal changes in the quality and quantity of stress are common. Many energetic adaptations have evolved that attenuate the stress response during the winter when energy shortages may limit the ability of organisms to cope successfully with specific types of stressors. The temporal organization of such stress responses therefore must be considered to obtain a holistic understanding of the mechanisms underlying the stress response.

The main endocrine features of the stress response involve hormones that act to suppress energy storage and promote energy utilization from adipose and liver stores. Epinephrine and the glucocorticoids are the major hormonal components of the stress response. Animals require a relatively steady supply of energy to sustain biological functions. Although these energy demands are somewhat continual, both daily and seasonal fluctuations in energy requirements occur as physiological and behavioral activities wax and wane. Animals typically do not feed continuously to supply energy to cells; rather, adaptations have evolved to allow animals to store and conserve energy when they are engaged in nonfeeding activities. Eventually, however, the chronic need for energy depletes these stores and requires animals to obtain food. In most habitats, significant daily and seasonal fluctuations in food availability occur. For example, outside of the tropics, food availability is generally low during the winter when thermogenic energy demands are typically high. Consequently, energy intake and energy expenditures are never perfectly balanced because of fluctuations in both energy requirements and availability. Whenever a significant imbalance of energy is perceived, a stress response in the form of secreted glucocorticoids ensues.

Reproduction is sufficiently demanding that a stress response is often associated with breeding in terms of elevated glucocorticoid concentrations. That is, glucocorticoids are released to support the energetic needs of reproduction including territorial defense or courtship behaviors. However, when energy is insufficient to support reproduction and thermogenesis or other energetic demands, the stress response becomes prolonged. A chronic stress response results in pathology. Most animals restrict breeding to specific times of the year when food is abundant and survival and reproductive success are most likely. The inhibition of winter breeding is one of the central components of a suite of energy-saving seasonal adaptations evolved among nontropical animals. In addition to the seasonal onset and cessation of reproductive function among nontropical vertebrates, it is also well-established that endocrine, metabolic, growth, neural, immune, and thermogenic processes undergo seasonal changes to promote winter energy conservation. Mechanisms in virtually every physiological and behavioral system have evolved to cope with the winter energetic bottleneck resulting from increased thermogenic energy requirements during periods of low energy availability. Presumably, animals possessing these energy-conserving adaptations enhance their survival and ultimately increase their reproductive success. Generally, glucocorticoid concentrations are higher during the winter than the summer and individuals display more elevated stress responses during the winter than the summer. However, because coping strategies are engaged in anticipation of the winter stressors, many individuals do not show exaggerated stress responses during the winter.

How do animals determine time of year? In most cases, the photoperiod (day length) acts as the principal external cue to determine time of year. Photoperiod measurement is important for organizing the seasonal collapse and regrowth of the reproductive system in mammals and birds from temperate and boreal latitudes. Indeed, changes in day length provide the most error-free signal for predicting favorable conditions. Day length is encoded by the hormone melatonin, which is secreted primarily at night from the pineal gland.

Seasonal Energetic Adaptations

Many aspects of life are energetically challenging, and individuals have evolved timing mechanisms to parse out energetically demanding activities to different times of year. For example, birds engage in predictable cycles of migration, breeding, parenting, molting, and overwintering. These energetically expensive activities generally do not overlap, and, again, all these activities elicit classical stress responses (i.e., elevated activation of the hypothalamic-pituitary-adrenal (HPA) axis).

One 1936 study is particularly informative in understanding the basis of Selye's thinking about stress responses. Rats were housed in low-temperature conditions for 2 days, 2 weeks, or 2 months. After 2 days in these conditions, Selye noted the hypertrophy of the adrenal cortex; reduced eosinophil (a type of immune cell circulating in the blood) numbers; and atrophy of the thymus, spleen, and lymph nodes. In other words, the rats exhibited a classic stress response. After 2 weeks in the low temperatures, it was discovered that rats no longer displayed these symptoms; essentially, they had become cold-adapted and could tolerate low temperatures without exhibiting any further stress responses. After approximately 2 months of exposure to low temperatures, however, the rats lost this acquired resistance to low temperatures and died.

This process of coping with stressors was termed the general adaptation syndrome (GAS), and consists of three stages: (1) the alarm reaction, (2) resistance, and finally, (3) exhaustion. During the alarm reaction, stressors are detected. Coping with the stressor occurs during the resistance stage. The exhaustion stage is characterized by the termination of the stress response and the onset of stress pathology, which in extreme cases can lead to death. Although Selye believed that the exhaustion phase was due to the termination of the stress response, current ideas about stress indicate that the pathological effects of stress are due to the prolonged activation of the stress response. These three stages of the GAS correspond to the response of the rats to low temperatures after 2 days (alarm reaction), 2 weeks (resistance), and 2 months (exhaustion), respectively. If individuals have the opportunity to gradually move to low temperatures or are allowed to prepare for low-temperature conditions by first being housed for 8–10 weeks in short day lengths, then no stress responses occur.

Seasonal Adjustments in Glucocorticoid Secretion

Glucocorticoids are released in response to stressful stimuli and can affect reproduction, digestion, growth, multiple types of immune function, and virtually any other physiological process that requires significant energy. Predictably, seasonal variation in glucocorticosteroid secretion is more often the rule than the exception, probably because of the pivotal role these hormones play in orchestrating the distribution of resources among competing physiological activities.

Most animals studied to date display some seasonal variation in stress responses. For instance, Indian barnacles (*Balanus balanoides*) exhibit elevated antioxidant enzyme activity (a component of this species' stress response) prior to the monsoon season compared with during it. Further, almost all wild amphibians, reptiles, and birds studied to date show marked changes in glucocorticoid concentrations during the year, with maximal values observed during the breeding season. Individuals of most mammalian species exhibit similar basal glucocorticosteroid concentrations year-round in the wild. However, this apparent pattern may reflect the paucity of studies on wild rodents rather than a lack of seasonality of this parameter. Indeed, rodents, such as deer mice (*Peromyscus* sp.), bred and maintained in the lab exhibit high corticosteroid concentrations when kept in long-day (breeding) conditions. Other species, however, such as Siberian hamsters (*Phodopus sungorus*), display elevated glucocorticosteroid concentrations when housed in short photoperiods.

Although it is clear from these studies that stress responses are temporally labile, two questions remain: (1) Is seasonal variation omnipresent within and among species (e.g., over a species' range) and (2) are other aspects of the stress response as seasonally labile as corticosteroid hormone concentrations? In terms of spatial variability, the results are mixed. Presumably, if photoperiod has significant effects on stress responses, then animals living at higher latitudes would exhibit higher circulating corticosteroid concentrations during breeding than animals at low latitudes simply because of the large variation in annual photoperiod. Redpolls (*Carduelis flammea*) are birds that live in the challenging arctic conditions of Alaska. Both males and females showed the typical marked elevation in blood corticosterone concentrations when captured for approximately 1 h, indicating that they responded similarly to many other vertebrates. However, the amount of the elevation in postcapture corticosterone varied across the year; corticosterone concentrations were generally blunted during January and maximal during June when birds were breeding. Generally, birds that had the highest fat stores secreted the lowest amounts of glucocorticoids postcapture. Similar patterns have been reported for other birds living at high latitudes, including the white-crowned sparrows (*Zonotrichia leucophrys gambelii*), snow buntings (*Plectrophenax nivalis*), and Lapland longspurs (*Calcarius lapponicus*). Across latitudes, however, results are mixed. Some species show little variability in circulating glucocorticoid concentrations (e.g., pied flycatchers, *Ficedula hypoleuca,* and mountain chickadees, *Poecile atricapilla*), whereas others (e. g., house sparrows, *Passer domesticus,* and white-crowned sparrows, *Zonotrichia leucophrys*) exhibit spatial variation. In common with spatial variability, the social system of animals can also affect seasonal variation in glucocorticoid responses. A study of greylag geese (*Anser anser*) revealed that social status and physiological stress are not related in the same way in all seasons of the year.

In addition to hormones, other aspects of the glucocorticoid stress response show significant spatial and temporal flexibility. In particular, the HPA axis appears to be substantially malleable among wild songbirds. Individuals of different species can apparently modulate the levels of glucocorticoids they produce at different times of the year by changing the sensitivity of adrenergic tissues to upstream regulatory hormones such as corticotropin releasing hormone (CRH) or adrenocorticotropic hormone (ACTH). Alternatively, some species are capable of modulating steroid-binding globulin levels in their blood across the year instead, although it remains unclear whether these globulins promote or inhibit the actions of the glucocorticosteroids to which they bind. Finally, corticosteroid receptors also appear to be seasonally variable. In house sparrows, membrane corticosteroid receptors are lowest during the nesting season, whereas cytosolic receptors are lowest during winter.

Why Are Stress Responses Seasonally Variable?

Presumably, stress responses help animals prepare for or recover from stressors. Why, then, are stress responses variable during the year when all individuals could benefit from optimal stress responses? Several hypotheses have been proposed. First, glucocorticoid stress responses are expensive and hence may not be affordable at all times of the year. Indeed, pyruvate, a readily usable energy source, blocked the stress-evoked suppression of cell-mediated and humoral immune activity in mice (*Mus musculus*). Second, high corticosterone concentrations, particularly when maintained for extended periods (i.e., chronic), can be immunosuppressive; over the short term, however, glucocorticosteroids can be immunoenhancing. In general, winter survival in small animals is expected to require a positive balance between short-day enhancement of immune defenses and glucocorticoid-induced immunosuppression. Immunosuppression caused by high glucocorticosteroids may be induced by many winter-related factors, including overcrowding, increased competition for scarce resources, low temperatures, reduced food availability, increased predator pressure, and lack of shelter. Moreover, winter breeding, with the potentially concomitant elevation in sex steroid hormones, may also compromise the immune system. Presumably, this explains why winter breeding predominantly occurs when other environmental stressors such as temperature and food availability are not severe. Overall, the balance between enhanced immune function (i.e., to the point where autoimmune disease becomes a danger) and stress-induced immunosuppression (i.e., to the point where opportunistic pathogens and parasites overwhelm the host) must be met for animals to survive and become reproductively successful.

Several studies support this hypothetical construct. For instance, hamsters maintained in short photoperiods (and made to experience short-term stress) show more rapid wound healing and trafficking of leukocytes to the skin compared to unstressed short-day animals (or stressed and unstressed long-day hamsters). In one passerine bird, cutaneous immune responses to a T-cell mitogen (phytohemagglutinin, PHA) were less dramatic in animals induced into breeding than in those in a nonbreeding condition. Moreover, corticosterone appears to be immunosuppressive in the same species only in winter (not summer) conditions. Such immune–endocrine interrelationships are not always uniform between the sexes within a species. For example, acute stress enhances cell-mediated immune activity (delayed-type hypersensitivity to dinitrofluorobenzene) in female, but not male, Siberian hamsters. Indeed, ample evidence indicates that immune activity can vary dramatically between sexes; thus, it is plausible that the glucocorticoid mediators of immune defenses might be labile as well.

One other hormone that is integrally involved in vertebrate photoperiodism, melatonin, can affect the seasonal interplay between corticosterone and immune function. Generally, melatonin enhances immune activity, whereas glucocorticosteroids (at chronically high levels) compromise immune activity. Under certain circumstances, melatonin treatment may ameliorate the immunosuppressive effects of glucocorticosteroids. For instance, Siberian hamsters attenuated the duration of fever during simulated short winter day lengths, presumably to conserve energy. Hamsters housed in long days were injected with saline or melatonin before lights off each day for 1 or 6 weeks; then fever was assessed following injections of bacterial lipopolysaccharide (LPS). The fever duration was attenuated (32%) only in hamsters that decreased body mass, increased glucocorticoid concentrations, and displayed gonadal regression in response to 6 weeks of melatonin. These results suggest that long-term exposure to long-duration melatonin signals induce the physiological changes required for short-day immune responses, perhaps via interactions among hormones downstream from melatonin, such as cortisol and leptin.

In addition to their effects on immune function, corticosteroids can dramatically affect behavior, particularly behaviors associated with reproduction. Generally, stress responses are up- and downregulated across seasons, but the way in which this happens depends on the social and physical environments in which species live. For instance, songbirds living at high latitudes are thought to mount weak corticosterone responses to stress because the abandonment of offspring that it might lead to would be maladaptive given that these species typically only have one opportunity per year to breed. In the tropics, however, corticosterone–behavior relationships may be different because reproductive efforts are generally less constrained by time.

Considered together, both the incidence and responses to stressors vary on a seasonal basis. The environmental regulation of seasonal changes in many traits, including reproduction, metabolism, and immunity, is primarily mediated by photoperiod. From a physiological prospective, the pineal hormone melatonin appears to coordinate seasonal adjustments in stress responses including changes in reproductive, metabolic, and immune function. To what extent the immune-enhancing effects of melatonin are unique to seasonally breeding rodents and whether it is a generalized feature of seasonal adjustments in stress responses among humans remain largely unspecified. Although physiological responses are important mediators of seasonal and photoperiodic changes in stress responses, behavioral alterations might also have an important role in reducing their energetic costs. The careful integration of the behavioral and physiological mechanisms underlying the seasonality of stress responsiveness at both ultimate and proximate levels should provide important and novel insights into the interaction among seasonal environmental factors, stressors, immune function, and the pattern of diseases and mortality. To date, most efforts have not advanced much beyond describing the seasonal changes that occur in responses to stressors. The next step is to identify the cellular and molecular mechanisms that mediate the effects of season and photoperiod on stress responsiveness and link variability in these mechanisms to fitness.

See Also the Following Articles

Circadian Clock Genes as Modulators of Sensitivity to Genotoxic Stress; Glucocorticoids, Role in Stress; Immune Response.

Further Reading

Bilbo, S. D., Dhabhar, F. S., Viswanathan, S. A., et al. (2002). Short day lengths augment stress-induced enhancement of skin immune function. *Proceedings of the National Academy of Sciences USA* **99**, 4067–4072.

Breuner, C. W. and Orchinik, M. (2002). Downstream from corticosterone: seasonality of binding globulins, receptors, and behavior in the avian stress response. In: Dawson, A. (ed.) *Avian endocrinology*, pp. 385–399. New Delhi: Narosa Publishing.

Breuner, C. W., Orchinik, M., Hahn, T. P., et al. (2003). Differential mechanisms for regulation of the stress response across latitudinal gradients. *American Journal of Physiology* **285**, R594–R600.

Martin, L. B., Gilliam, J., Han, P., et al. (2005). Corticosterone suppresses immune function in temperate but not tropical house sparrows (*Passer domesticus*). *General and Comparative Endocrinology* **140**, 126–135.
Neigh, G. N., Bowers, S. L., Pyter, L. M., et al. (2004). Pyruvate prevents restraint-induced immunosuppression via alterations in glucocorticoid responses. *Endocrinology* **145**, 4309–4319.
Nelson, R. J., Demas, G. E., Klein, S. L., et al. (2002). *Seasonal patterns of stress, immune function, and disease*. New York: Cambridge University Press.
Nelson, R. J. (2004). Seasonal immune function and disease responses. *Trends in Immunology* **24**, 187–192.
Niyogi, S., Biswas, S., Sarker, S., et al. (2001). Seasonal variation of antioxidant and biotransformation enzymes in barnacle, *Balanus balanoides*, and their relation with polyaromatic hydrocarbons. *Marine Environmental Research* **52**, 13–26.
Prendergast, B. J., Yellon, S. M., Tran, L. T., et al. (2001). Inhibition of cellular immune function by *in vitro* melatonin is modulated by photoperiodic history in Siberian hamsters. *Journal of Biological Rhythms* **16**, 224–233.
Romero, L. M. (2002). Seasonal changes in plasma glucocorticoid concentrations in free-living vertebrates. *General and Comparative Endocrinology* **128**, 1–24.
Romero, L. M. (2004). Physiological stress in ecology: lessons from biomedical research. *Trends in Ecology and Evolution* **19**, 249–255.
Sapolsky, R. M., Romero, L. M. and Munck, A. (2000). How do glucocorticoids influence stress responses?: integrating permissive, suppressive, stimulatory, and preparative actions. *Endocrine Reviews* **21**, 55–89.
Yellon, S. M., Kim, K., Hadley, A. R., et al. (2005). Time course and role of the pineal gland in photoperiod control of innate immune cell functions in male Siberian hamsters. *Journal of Neuroimmunology* **161**, 137–144.

Seasonal Rhythms

L M Romero
Tufts University, Medford, MA, USA

Glossary

Basal glucocorticoids	Plasma concentrations of glucocorticoids in the absence of a stressor.
Corticotropin-releasing hormone (CRH)	Hormone released by the hypothalamus.
Glucocorticoid-binding globulin (CBG)	Proteins in the plasma that bind glucocorticoids.
Hypothalamic-pituitary-adrenal (HPA) axis	The neuroendocrine pathway leading from the brain to the adrenals that culminates in glucocorticoid release.
Permissive effect	An indirect effect whereby a hormone indirectly allows another system to work better.
Stressor	A stimulus that elicits a release of glucocorticoids.

Evidence for Seasonal Glucocorticoid Rhythms

Glucocorticoid secretion is often considered an obligatory response to stressors. In a laboratory setting, stressors applied in similar circadian, developmental, and psychological contexts within the same species produce remarkably consistent magnitudes of glucocorticoid secretion. Recent evidence, however, indicates that glucocorticoid release is modulated seasonally in the majority of free-living species that have been studied to date. In other words, the magnitudes of both basal and stress-induced glucocorticoid concentrations vary throughout the year. An example, data for white-crowned sparrows (*Zonotrichia leucophrys*), is presented in **Figure 1**.

Many recent studies have measured glucocorticoids in free-living wild animals by directly sampling from freshly caught individuals. Plasma samples collected within a few minutes of capture are assumed to reflect prestress glucocorticoid concentrations because glucocorticoids start to increase 2–3 min after initiation of a stressor. Stress-induced glucocorticoid concentrations then reflect the animal's response to capture, handling, captivity, etc. and are assumed to be a measure of the hypothalamic-pituitary-adrenal (HPA) axis's ability to respond to a stressor.

These studies provide clear evidence that a majority of reptile, amphibian, avian, and mammal species seasonally modulate glucocorticoid concentrations. Males and females sometimes differ in whether they show seasonal rhythms, and occasionally a species will show a seasonal rhythm in basal but not stress-induced glucocorticoid concentrations (or vice versa). However, approximately 90% of all species that have been studied have at least one sex with a seasonal rhythm of glucocorticoid release.

The evidence for an annual glucocorticoid rhythm is generally much stronger for basal concentrations, primarily because more studies have focused on this time point. Furthermore, avian species often show a seasonal rhythm in basal but not stress-induced glucocorticoid concentrations, suggesting that basal and stress-induced glucocorticoid concentrations are regulated differently. Laboratory studies show that basal and stress-induced glucocorticoids have different regulatory mechanisms and serve different physiological functions that are mediated by separate receptors. It is not surprising, therefore, that the HPA axis might be regulated differently under basal and stress conditions, but these regulatory pathways can be further dissociated into different annual cycles.

Of those species that do show a seasonal rhythm, the seasonal peak is usually during the breeding period. There are three notable exceptions. First, the most robust rhythm in birds is a nadir during the prebasic molt when they replace their feathers. This is thought to protect the bird from the protein catabolism effects of glucocorticoids during the protein mobilization of feather replacement. Second, three desert-breeding birds show a seasonal glucocorticoid peak during the rainy season rather than the breeding period, suggesting that seasonal rhythms can be timed to environmental cues as well as seasonal physiological cues. Third, even though most mammal species show a seasonal rhythm, there is no consensus season when mammals tend to have elevated glucocorticoid concentrations.

The capacity of glucocorticoid-binding globulins (CBGs) has also been found to vary seasonally and to be regulated by gonadal testosterone. Because only free steroid is generally considered to be available for diffusion into tissues, free steroid concentrations may be more biologically relevant than total steroid concentrations. When total and free steroid concentrations are compared, the seasonal rhythm in total glucocorticoids often changes or disappears entirely.

Many wild species held in long-term captivity also show seasonal rhythms, but these rhythms do not always match what is found in free-living animals. This likely reflects that both domestication and captivity alter HPA axis function in ways that are different for each species, making it difficult, if not impossible, to ascertain natural annual variation from these populations.

Mechanisms Regulating Annual Rhythms of Glucocorticoids

Progress is just beginning in understanding how HPA axis function is regulated seasonally. What induces these changes, be it photoperiod, temperature, food availability, etc., is currently unknown. Plasma glucocorticoid concentrations often are correlated with adrenal mass, and early studies showed increases in adrenal mass during breeding. Consequently, the ability of adrenal tissue to respond to adrenocorticotropic hormone (ACTH) changes seasonally. A few studies in birds indicate that there are multiple regulatory points in the HPA axis. Some species seasonally regulate glucocorticoid release from the adrenal, others seasonally regulate ACTH release from the pituitary, and still others regulate CRH and arginine vasotocin (the avian congener of arginine vasopressin) release from the hypothalamus. These regulatory control points may be related to how sensitive each species is to adverse environmental conditions.

Glucocorticoids also interact with the gonadal system. Although glucocorticoids inhibit gonadal hormone release, exogenous testosterone elevates glucocorticoids in free-living birds. This suggests a complex interaction between the gonadal and adrenal systems, with glucocorticoids downregulating gonadal androgen release concurrent with gonadal androgens elevating glucocorticoid release. Gonadal androgens, therefore, could potentially be an important physiological regulator of seasonal glucocorticoid rhythms.

Why Do Seasonal Glucocorticoid Rhythms Exist?

Modulation of glucocorticoid release presents an interesting paradox: if glucocorticoid release is so important for survival, then how do animals survive stressors at certain times of the year when they essentially fail to release glucocorticoids? There have been three major hypotheses proposed to explain seasonal glucocorticoid rhythms.

Energy Mobilization Hypothesis

The energy mobilization hypothesis focuses on the metabolic effects of glucocorticoids. Glucocorticoids play an important role in energy mobilization, especially during stress, so glucocorticoid concentrations should be highest during energetically costly times of the year. According to this hypothesis, high glucocorticoid concentrations during breeding result from breeding exerting the highest energetic demands during the year. Females of many species, for example, expend substantial energy during breeding, and breeding males of many species have increased energy costs associated with testosterone and territorial defense. Moreover, increased energy mobilization could explain seasonal peaks during nonbreeding periods

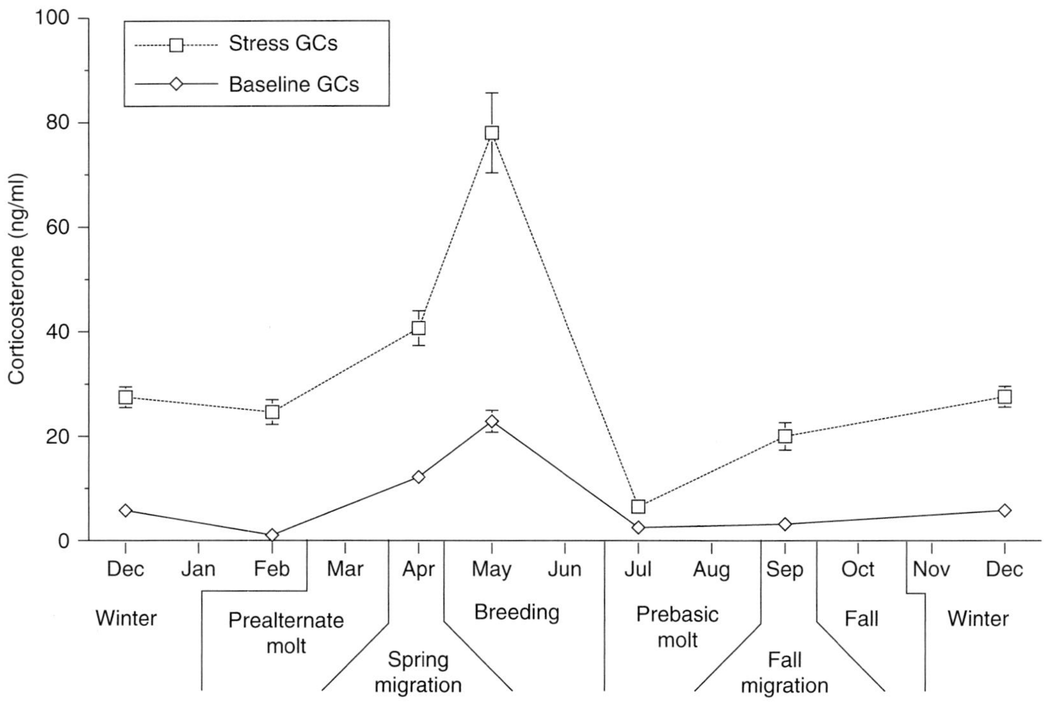

Figure 1 Seasonal rhythm of baseline and stress-induced corticosterone from white-crowned sparrows. Reprinted from Romero, L. M. (2002). Seasonal changes in plasma glucocorticoid concentrations in free-living vertebrates. *General and Comparative Endocrinology* **128,** 1–24 with permission from Elsevier.

if these periods are more energetically costly than breeding.

Two examples, however, mammalian hibernation and avian molt, highlight the insufficiency of the energy mobilization hypothesis in providing a universal explanation for seasonal glucocorticoid rhythms. Hibernating mammals require dramatically increased fat stores to survive the winter, but it is not clear that these energy requirements are greater or less than lactation. Second, feather replacement during molt in birds requires substantial energy expenditure, yet this period is the nadir of the annual rhythm. The energy mobilization hypothesis can be a powerful explanatory mechanism for certain species during some times of the year, but it clearly is insufficient to fully explain seasonal glucocorticoid rhythms.

Behavior Hypothesis

The behavior hypothesis focuses on the behavioral effects of glucocorticoids. It posits that annual glucocorticoid rhythms result from different requirements for expressing (or not expressing) glucocorticoid-mediated behaviors at different times of the year. For example, an important glucocorticoid-mediated behavior in wild animals might be fleeing an area and relocating during storms. This may be an excellent strategy for most of the year, but could be catastrophic for an individual's overall fitness when relocation requires abandoning young. Consequently, the behavior hypothesis suggests that the need to seasonally regulate the expression of those behaviors drives glucocorticoid rhythms.

The behavior hypothesis, however, does not fit a more general annual rhythm in glucocorticoid concentrations. Glucocorticoid concentrations are highest in most species during breeding, exactly when glucocorticoid concentrations should be lowest if seasonal glucocorticoid rhythms were primarily to regulate the behavioral consequences of glucocorticoid release. Consequently, this hypothesis may be useful in explaining modulation of glucocorticoid concentrations within a single season, but not across seasons.

Preparative Hypothesis

The preparative hypothesis focuses on the coordinating aspects of glucocorticoid physiology and posits that seasonal rhythms in glucocorticoid concentrations serve to modulate the priming of other stress pathways during periods with different potential exposure to stressors. Glucocorticoids are only one part of the stress response. Other hormones (especially epinephrine and norepinephrine), neurotransmitters (e.g., 5-HT, CRH), opioid peptides, and cytokines (e.g., IL-6), as well as other brain functions, exert their effects rapidly with the onset of stress without involving the pituitary or adrenals. However, glucocorticoids have a permissive effect on many of these systems and thereby facilitate better performance under stress. Higher basal glucocorticoid concentrations may augment the priming effects on these systems in preparation for further stressors. This is the traditional explanation for timing the circadian peak for the beginning of the active period. These permissive effects may help prepare the organism for subsequent stress responses.

If the preparative hypothesis is correct, higher glucocorticoid concentrations should coincide with seasons in which predictable stressors are more likely. The available data fit this prediction moderately well. The risk of exposure to many stressors in wild animals likely varies seasonally. During the breeding season, for example, predation risk may increase when caring for young; competition for mates, with the risk of frequent fights, increases; and disease may become more prevalent when breeding individuals congregate. Consequently, glucocorticoid concentrations may vary seasonally in order to mediate changes in preparedness in the nonglucocorticoid pathways of the stress response. However, the existence of predictable seasonal increases in stressor risk has not yet been demonstrated.

Adaptive Significance

Proper concentrations of glucocorticoids seem crucial for survival. Too little can result in even mild stressors killing animals, but too much can lead to suppressed gonadal and immune function and ultimately disease. Consequently, a balance must be struck between needing glucocorticoids to survive stressors and modulating glucocorticoid secretion to prevent deleterious exposures. What is becoming clear is that there is a seasonal rhythm in what is the right amount of glucocorticoids. Understanding why the right amount changes seasonally will help us understand why glucocorticoids are released during stress and how they help animals survive. The three explanatory hypotheses presented earlier are derived from different aspects of glucocorticoid physiology. The energy mobilization hypothesis emphasizes glucocorticoid's metabolic effects; the behavior hypothesis emphasizes the desired acute behavioral effects of glucocorticoids; and the preparative hypothesis emphasizes the regulatory role that glucocorticoids have in other stress systems. Integrating these hypotheses into a cohesive physiology will provide the foundation for understanding how elevated glucocorticoid concentrations aid in survival.

See Also the Following Articles

Circadian Clock Genes as Modulators of Sensitivity to Genotoxic Stress; Circadian Rhythms, Genetics of; Corticosteroids and Stress; Cortisol Awakening Response; Corticosteroid Receptors; Gleucocorticoid Negative Feedback.

Further Reading

Guillette, L. J., Cree, A. and Rooney, A. A. (1995). Biology of stress: interactions with reproduction, immunology and intermediary metabolism. In: Warwick, C., Frye, F. & Murphy, J. B. (eds.) *Health and welfare of captive reptiles*, pp. 32–81. London: Chapman & Hall.

Romero, L. M. (2002). Seasonal changes in plasma glucocorticoid concentrations in free-living vertebrates. *General and Comparative Endocrinology* **128**, 1–24.

Sapolsky, R. M., Romero, L. M. and Munck, A. U. (2000). How do glucocorticoids influence stress-responses? Integrating permissive, suppressive, stimulatory, and adaptive actions. *Endocrine Reviews* **21**, 55–89.

Tyrrell, C. L. and Cree, A. (1998). Relationships between corticosterone concentration and season, time of day and confinement in a wild reptile (tuatara, *Sphenodon punctatus*). *General and Comparative Endocrinology* **110**, 97–108.

Wingfield, J. C. (1994). Modulation of the adrenocortical response to stress in birds. In: Davey, K. G., Peter, R. E. & Tobe, S. S. (eds.) *Perspectives in comparative endocrinology*, pp. 520–528. Ottawa: National Research Council of Canada.

Wingfield, J. C. and Romero, L. M. (2001). Adrenocortical responses to stress and their modulation in free-living vertebrates. In: McEwen, B. S. & Goodman, H. M. (eds.) *Handbook of physiology; section 7: The endocrine system; vol. IV: Coping with the environment: neural and endocrine mechanisms*, pp. 211–234. New York: Oxford University Press.

Wingfield, J. C., Hunt, K., Breuner, C., et al. (1997). Environmental stress, field endocrinology, and conservation biology. In: Clemmons, J. R. & Buchholz, R. (eds.) *Behavioral approaches to conservation in the wild*, pp. 95–131. Cambridge, UK: Cambridge University Press.

Circadian Clock Genes as Modulators of Sensitivity to Genotoxic Stress

M P Antoch and R V Kondratov
Lerner Research Institute, Cleveland Clinic Foundation, Cleveland, OH, USA

Glossary

Chronotherapy Timed delivery of therapeutic drugs at empirically established periods of higher efficacy and lower toxicity to the organism.

Circadian rhythms The 24-h periodicities in various biological processes (behavioral, physiological, and biochemical) that have evolved in response to the 24-h periodicity of the Earth's rotation. Controlled by an internal clock mechanism, these rhythms can persist in the absence of environmental cues (for example, in constant darkness), displaying oscillations with periodicities close to 24 h. They can also respond to external stimuli (light, in particular), which coordinate the phases of the internal clock and the light–dark cycle.

Genotoxic stress Condition induced in cells by exposure to different types of external and internal potentially harmful agents, which results in DNA damage and is recognized by the organism's stress response systems.

Molecular circadian oscillator Cell-autonomous oscillator that is formed by the products of core clock genes, which exhibit the 24-h periodicity in their expression/activity.

Peripheral oscillators Circadian oscillators that operate in peripheral (nonneural) tissues and generate rhythmic output in physiology.

Suprachiasmatic nucleus (SCN) The anatomical site of the mammalian circadian master clock. The SCN is composed of ~20 000 neurons residing in the anterior of the hypothalamus. The individual SCN neurons are capable of generating the 24-h periodicities in electrical and metabolic activity and are responsible for synchronization of peripheral circadian oscillators.

Anticancer Therapy and Genotoxic Stress

In the course of their lifetime, all cells, tissues, and entire organisms may be exposed to a variety of harmful agents that cause DNA damage (genotoxic stress). The endogenous sources of DNA-damaging agents result from normal cellular metabolism and include free radicals and peroxides. The most common sources of exogenous genotoxic agents are ultraviolet light, ionizing radiation, oxidative stress, and various chemical mutagens. DNA damage may also result from routine errors in DNA replication and recombination. To prevent detrimental effects on the genome, cells have evolved a response system that induces cell cycle arrest to allow sufficient time to repair the incurred damage, activates the appropriate DNA repair pathway, or, in the case of irreparable damage, induces apoptosis. Thus, response to genotoxic stress is a rather complex process that includes induction of multiple genes associated with cell cycle control, replication, DNA repair, apoptosis, signal transduction, etc. As a result, the cell's fate after genotoxic stress is determined by the superposition of multiple stress response pathways and depends on cell type, cell status, the level of damage, and environmental conditions.

Understanding the molecular mechanisms of cellular response to DNA-damaging agents as well as developing the tools for manipulating stress response have important medical applications, especially in the field of clinical oncology. Thus, two major types of existing anticancer treatments – chemotherapy and radiation – rely on induction of various types of damage to biological macromolecules in tumor cells. Because many of them specifically target DNA, these treatments induce genotoxic stress, which consequently induces the cellular stress response system. Though designed to selectively kill tumor cells, both chemotherapy and radiation are accompanied by nonspecific damage to normal cells and tissues, resulting in undesirable side effects.

One of the approaches that were developed to minimize these side effects was based on the observation that *in vivo* response to various therapies can display significant variation depending on the time of treatment. It has been suggested that these variations may result from differential daily response of both tumor and normal cells, and the final outcome reflects superposition of these effects. While the data on daily variations in therapeutic response of tumors are still sporadic and sometimes inconsistent, daily variations in drug and radiation responses of normal tissues have been studied in more detail. Testing the effect of timed administration of more than 30 anticancer drugs in mice and rats clearly demonstrated that the drug's toxicity varied significantly throughout the day. In addition, several clinical studies indicate that chronomodulated drug administration results in a significant decrease in complications associated with certain types of cancer treatments while maintaining the same therapeutic effect. These variations in the organism's response to anticancer therapy may depend on different parameters: daily variations in the pharmacokinetics of a particular medicine, blood and tissue concentration of various growth factors, cytokines, and hormones, as well as daily variations in the activity of the intracellular genotoxic stress response system. The chronotherapeutic approach takes advantage of natural daily variability in the physiological response of an organism, which, along with many other parameters, is controlled by the circadian clock system.

The Circadian Clock System: A Universal Timing Mechanism

In mammals, various physiological parameters (such as the sleep–wake cycle, endocrine function, blood pressure, energy metabolism, and behavior) show a nearly 24-h rhythm that is controlled by an internal circadian clock system. This system is capable of generating periodicities even in the absence of environmental cues and at the same time responds to various external stimuli to synchronize the phases of the internal clocks with the environment.

The mammalian circadian clock is organized as a hierarchical network of numerous oscillators, with the master clock residing in the neurons of the hypothalamic suprachiasmatic nucleus (SCN). The master clock in the SCN synchronizes the phases of multiple peripheral clocks throughout the body with the natural 24-h light–dark cycle. Importantly, these peripheral clocks can respond to other synchronizing stimuli (for example, the liver's clock can be coordinated with the food intake schedule, thus functioning independently of the SCN). The ubiquitous nature of the clock mechanism and its ability to respond to a variety of external stimuli underscore the important role the circadian clock system plays in controlling different physiological parameters, including the response to genotoxic stress.

Insights on the mechanistic aspects of global circadian regulation were made possible by recent progress in understanding the functional organization of the molecular clock. It is now well established that, at the molecular level, the mammalian circadian clock in all types of cells is formed by interdependent transcription/translation feedback loops (**Figure1**). Two basic helix-loop-helix (bHLH) PAS-domain transcription factors, CLOCK and BMAL1, form the positive elements of the central oscillatory loop. The CLOCK/BMAL1 heterodimer binds to E box elements in the promoters of target genes and drives rhythmic transcription of three *Period* (*Per1*, *Per2*, and *Per3*) and two *Cryptochrome* (*Cry1* and *Cry2*) genes. When PER and CRY proteins are translated, they are translocated to the nucleus, where they act as potent inhibitors of CLOCK/BMAL1-mediated transcription. CLOCK/BMAL1 also controls transcription of *Rev-erbα*, which feeds back to periodically repress expression of *Bmal1*, thus regulating a positive limb of the feedback loop. Positive and negative elements of these regulatory loops function to coordinate transcriptional events at appropriate times to provide 24-h periodicities. In addition, several posttranslational modifications (phosphorylation and sumoylation) play an important role in regulating clock proteins' stability, cellular localization, and functional activity.

The basal transcriptional nature of the core clock mechanism suggests that its control of the output signaling, which translates into daily variations in physiological and metabolic changes, is also transcription based. Indeed, large-scale transcriptional profiling studies have demonstrated that a large number of genes display 24-h periodicities in their mRNA abundance, suggesting that they function under direct (through the E box elements in their promoter regions) or indirect (through the intermediate targets) control of the circadian clock system. Interestingly, circadian transcriptional control demonstrates remarkable tissue specificity, suggesting that additional profiling of drug- and radiation-sensitive tissues may identify critical stress response genes that function under circadian control.

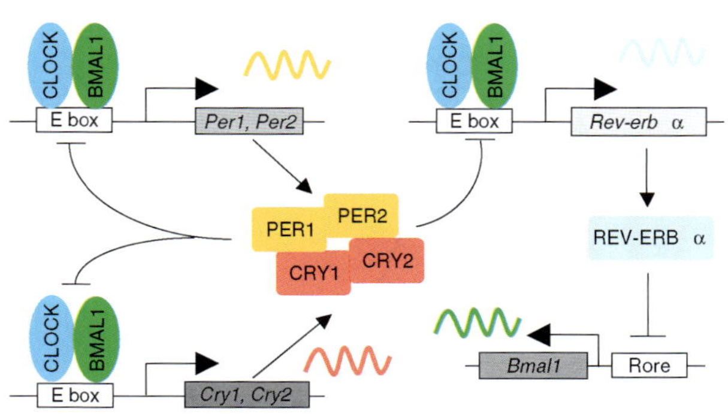

Figure 1 Simplified schematic representation of the mammalian circadian autoregulatory feedback loop. Positive elements of the loop (CLOCK and BMAL1) dimerize to activate rhythmic transcription of *Per* and *Cry* genes through E box enhancer elements. The nuclear-localized CRY and PER proteins interact with CLOCK and BMAL1 to negatively regulate CLOCK/BMAL1-mediated transcription. *Rev-erbα* transcription is regulated by the same components that control *Per* and *Cry* transcription, and the resulting circadian accumulation of REV-ERB α leads to periodic repression of *Bmal1* transcription.

Circadian Clock System Modulates *in Vivo* Response to Genotoxic Treatments

The establishment of the functional link between the circadian and stress response systems was made possible by the availability of various circadian mutant mouse models. All circadian mutant mice display a common phenotype manifested by behavioral arrhythmicity and disrupted rhythmic gene expression. However, at the molecular level they represent two extreme states of circadian clock function in regard to CLOCK/BMAL1 transcriptional activity. The *Clock* mutant and *Bmal1*-deficient mice are characterized by constant low levels of CLOCK/BMAL1 transcriptional activity, while mice with a deficiency of both CRYs contain CLOCK/BMAL1 in its maximally active state. The comparison of the sensitivity of these three types of mutant mice to the anticancer drug cyclophosphamide has shown a direct correlation of survival with the CLOCK/BMAL1 functional status. Thus, when compared to wild-type animals, mice with a deficiency in the positive components of the circadian transcriptional loop (CLOCK and BMAL1) are more sensitive to drug-induced genotoxic stress, while animals with a deficiency in negative elements (CRY1 and CRY2) are more resistant. At the same time, wild-type animals demonstrate daily variations in sensitivity to cyclophosphamide-induced genotoxic stress, which also correlates with normal daily variation in CLOCK/BMAL1 activity (**Figure 2**). The fact that these arrhythmic mutants display opposite phenotypes suggests that sensitivity to genotoxic stress does not depend on persistence of rhythmicity per se, but rather is guided by the activity of the major circadian transactivation complex.

Mutants with a deficiency of the PERIOD protein represent another example of the functional link between the circadian and genotoxic stress response systems. These mice display higher sensitivity *in vivo* to long-term effects of low doses of ionizing radiation, while the primary thymocytes from these animals are more resistant to high doses of radiation in short-term experiments. Taken together, these data suggest that circadian variations in an organism's sensitivity to various types of genotoxic treatments

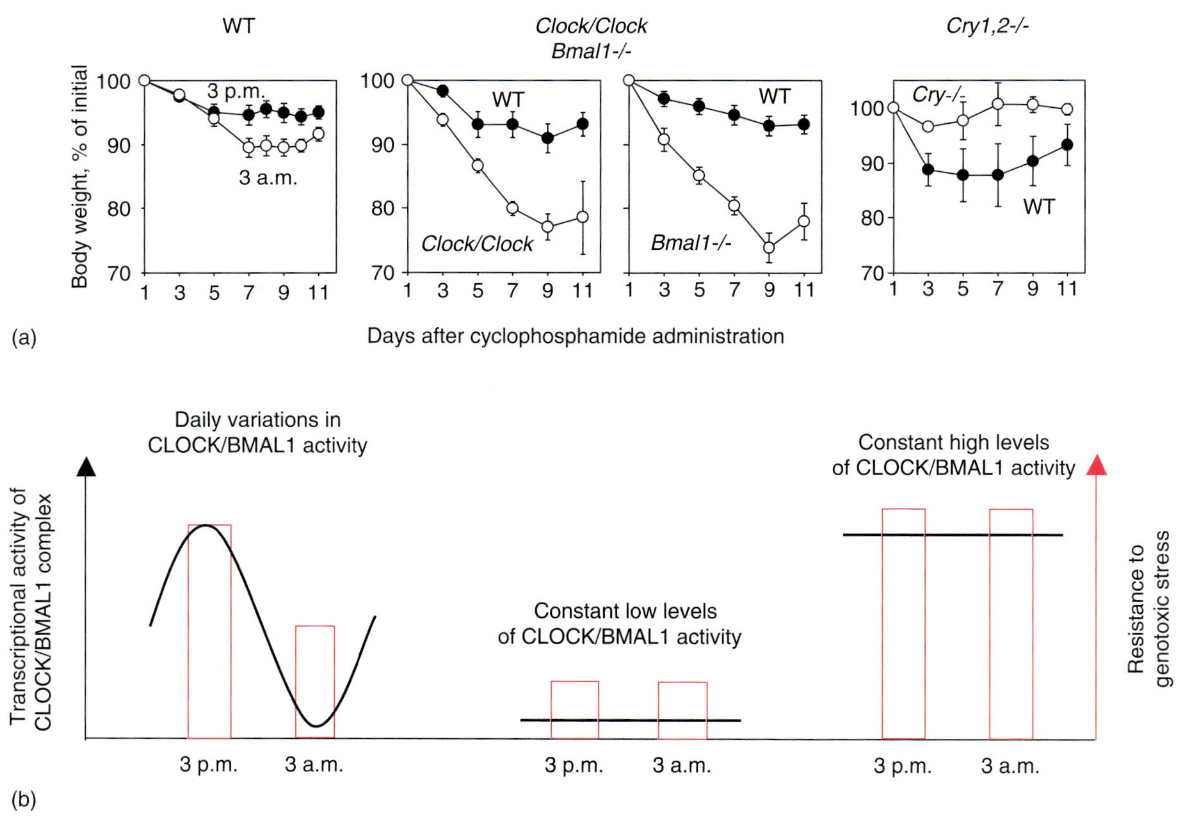

Figure 2 Animals' *in vivo* sensitivity to genotoxic stress correlates with the functional activity of CLOCK/BMAL1 transcriptional complex. (a) Body weight loss of the wild-type and circadian mutant mice after cyclophosphamide treatment. Wild-type animals injected at 3 a.m. demonstrate greater sensitivity to the drug-induced toxicity compared to their littermates injected at 3 p.m. *Clock/Clock* and *Bmal1-/-* animals demonstrate greater sensitivity to cyclophosphamide at all times tested. *Cry1-/-Cry2-/-* mice are more resistant to the treatment. (b) Schematic representation of the correlation between daily or locus-specific variations in CLOCK/BMAL1 functional activity (black line) and resistance to the treatment (red bars) in animals of various circadian genotypes.

are determined by the rhythms in expression and activity of the core circadian proteins.

How can rhythms in the activity of circadian proteins modulate response to genotoxic stress? It is well known that different types of cellular stress lead to induction of multiple transcription factors (i.e., p53, NF-κB or AP1 induction by radiation, induction of NF-κB during the immune response, or HIF1α in response to hypoxia). They in turn activate downstream transcriptional targets, encoding factors important for cell death or survival. The balance of these factors will determine the cellular and organism response to genotoxic treatments. Since the circadian clock controls the output at the transcriptional level, some of the responsive genes may be direct targets of CLOCK/BMAL1. Although not yet confirmed, this view is supported by the fact that the CLOCK/BMAL1 complex directly controls such important regulators of transcription as DBP, REV-ERBα, and RORα. In addition, the CLOCK/BMAL1 complex may display dual transcriptional activity, acting both as transcriptional activator and transcriptional repressor, depending on its interaction with CRYs. Importantly, while functioning as a repressor, it could interfere with the ability of other transcription factors to activate the same promoter. Thus, those genes that are controlled by both the circadian and stress response systems will be induced in response to genotoxic treatments only at those times of day when CLOCK/BMAL1 is functioning as an activator and will be attenuated at the times when it functions as a repressor. As a result, the balance between pro-death and pro-survival pathways will vary depending on the status of the circadian transcriptional complex. Importantly, these recent findings identify CLOCK/BMAL1 as a potential target for a rational search for pharmacological modulators of the organism's response to genotoxic stress that may potentially be used in clinical practice to minimize the side effects of cancer treatment.

See Also the Following Articles

Circadian Rhythms, Genetics of.

Further Reading

Antoch, M., Kondratov, R. and Takahashi, J. (2005). Circadian clock genes as modulators of sensitivity to genotoxic stress. *Cell Cycle* **4**, 901–907.

Fu, L., Pelicano, H., Liu, J., Huang, P. and Lee, C. (2002). The circadian gene Period2 plays an important role in tumor suppression and DNA damage response in vivo. *Cell* **111**, 41–50.

Gorbacheva, V., Kondratov, R., Zhang, R., et al. (2005). Circadian sensitivity to the chemotherapeutic agent cyclophosphamide depends on the functional status of the CLOCK/BMAL1 transactivation complex. *Proceedings of the National Academy of Sciences USA* **102**, 3407–3412.

Hrushevsky, W. J. M. (1994). *Circadian cancer therapy.* Boca Raton, FL: CRC Press, Inc.

Levi, F. (2006). Chronotherapeutics: the relevance of timing in cancer therapy. *Cancer Causes Control* **17**, 611–621.

Matsuo, T., Yamaguchi, S., Mitsui, S., Emi, A., Shimoda, F. and Okamura, H. (2003). Control mechanism of the circadian clock for timing of cell division in vivo. *Science* **302**, 255–259.

Panda, S., Antoch, M. P., Miller, B. H., et al. Coordinated transcription of key pathways in the mouse by the circadian clock. *Cell* **109**, 307–320.

Sehgal, A. (2003). *Molecular biology of circadian rhythms.* Hoboken, NJ: John Wiley & Sons, Inc.

VII. NEURONAL PLASTICITY - MEMORY

Stress and Neuronal Plasticity

B S McEwen
The Rockefeller University, New York, NY, USA

Introduction

The brain is the key organ of the stress response insofar as it processes information and determines whether an event or situation is threatening. Moreover, the outputs of the brain include regulation of autonomic, neuroendocrine and immune function, and behavioral responses that can be health promoting or health damaging. The brain is an adaptable organ, and both acute and chronic stress produce structural as well as neurochemical alterations that are, for the most part, reversible. Yet, severe insults such as seizures, strokes, and head trauma cause permanent damage, and there is also reason to believe that severe and prolonged stress, as well as disorders such as major depression, may also lead to permanent neural damage if they go on for a very long time.

Animal models have provided clues as to how the brain adapts to acute and repeated stress, and the hippocampus is the best-studied brain region. The hippocampus, which is an important brain structure for spatial, contextual, and declarative memory contains receptors for adrenal steroids, which regulate excitability and the morphological changes together with glutamate as well as other neurotransmitters and a host of endogenous neurochemicals.

This article first discusses the hippocampus and then turns to two other stress-sensitive brain structures, namely, the amygdala and prefrontal cortex. It then considers the behavioral consequences of remodeling of neural connections by stress and whether the remodeling increases or decreases the vulnerability of the brain to permanent damage. Finally, the relevance of the structural changes to the mood and anxiety disorders is discussed.

Adaptive Structural Plasticity

One of the ways that stress hormones modulate function within the brain is by changing the structure of neurons. Within the hippocampus, the input from the entorhinal cortex to the dentate gyrus is ramified by the connections between the dentate gyrus and the CA3 pyramidal neurons. One granule neuron innervates, on average, 12 CA3 neurons, and each CA3 neuron innervates, on average, 50 other CA3 neurons via axon collaterals, as well as 25 inhibitory cells via other axon collaterals. The net result is a 600-fold amplification of excitation, as well as a 300-fold amplification of inhibition, that provides some degree of control of the system.

As to why this type of circuitry exists, the dentate gyrus-CA3 system is believed to play a role in the memory of sequences of events, although long-term storage of memory occurs in other brain regions. But, because the DG-CA3 system is so delicately balanced in its function and vulnerability to damage, there is also adaptive structural plasticity, in that new neurons continue to be produced in the dentate gyrus throughout adult life, and CA3 pyramidal cells undergo a reversible remodeling of their dendrites in conditions such as hibernation and chronic stress. The role of this plasticity may be to protect against permanent damage.

Neurogenesis in the Dentate Gyrus

The subgranular layer of the dentate gyrus contains cells that have some properties of astrocytes (e.g., expression of glial fibrillary acidic protein) and which give rise to granule neurons. After bromodeoxyuridine (BrdU) administration to label DNA of dividing cells, these newly born cells appear as clusters in the inner part of the granule cell layer, where a substantial number of them will go on to differentiate into granule neurons within as little as 7 days. In the adult rat, 9000 new neurons are born per day and survive with a half-life of 28 days.

There are many hormonal, neurochemical, and behavioral modulators of neurogenesis and cell survival in the dentate gyrus including estradiol, insulin-like growth factor-1 (IGF-1), antidepressants, voluntary exercise, and hippocampal-dependent learning. With respect to stress, certain types of acute stress and many chronic stressors suppress neurogenesis or cell survival in the dentate gyrus, and the mediators of these inhibitory effects include excitatory amino acids acting via *N*-methyl-D-aspartate (NMDA) receptors and endogenous opioids.

Remodeling of Dendrites

Another form of structural plasticity is the remodeling of dendrites in the hippocampus. Chronic restraint stress causes retraction and simplification of dendrites in the CA3 region of the hippocampus.

Such dendritic reorganization is found in both dominant and subordinate rats undergoing adaptation of psychosocial stress in the visible burrow system and it is independent of adrenal size.

What this result emphasizes is that it is not adrenal size or presumed amount of physiological stress *per se* that determines dendritic remodeling but a complex set of other factors that modulate neuronal structure. Indeed, in species of mammals that hibernate, dendritic remodeling is a reversible process and occurs within hours of the onset of hibernation in European hamsters and ground squirrels, and it is also reversible within hours of wakening of the animals from torpor. This implies that reorganization of the cytoskeleton is taking place rapidly and reversibly and that changes in dendrite length and branching are not 'damage' but a form of structural plasticity.

Mechanisms of Structural Remodeling

Adrenal steroids are important mediators of remodeling of hippocampal neurons during repeated stress, and exogenous adrenal steroids can also cause remodeling in the absence of an external stressor. The role of adrenal steroids may involve interactions with neurochemical systems in the hippocampus, including serotonin, γ-aminobutyric acid (GABA), and excitatory amino acids. Probably the most important interactions are those with excitatory amino acids such as glutamate. Excitatory amino acids released by the mossy fiber pathway play a key role in the remodeling of the CA3 region of the hippocampus, and regulation of glutamate release by adrenal steroids may play an important role.

Among the consequences of restraint stress is the elevation of extracellular glutamate levels, leading to induction of glial glutamate transporters as well as increased activation of the nuclear transcription factor, phosphoCREB. Moreover, 21d chronic restraint stress (21d CRS) leads to depletion of clear vesicles from mossy fiber terminals and increased expression of presynaptic proteins involved in vesicle release. Taken together with the fact that vesicles that remain in the mossy fiber terminal are near active synaptic zones, this implies that CRS increases the release of glutamate.

Extracellular molecules play a role in remodeling. Neural cell adhesion molecule (NCAM) and its polysialated-NCAM (PSA-NCAM) as well as L1 are expressed in the dentate gyrus and CA3 region and the expression of both NCAM, L1, and PSA-NCAM are regulated by 21d CRS. Tissue plasminogen activator (tPA) is an extracellular protease and signaling molecule that is released with neural activity and is required for chronic stress-induced loss of spines and NMDA receptor subunits on CA1 neurons.

Within the neuronal cytoskeleton, the remodeling of hippocampal neurons by chronic stress and hibernation alters the acetylation of microtubule subunits that is consistent with a more stable cytoskeleton and alters microtubule associated proteins, including the phosphorylation of a soluble form of tau, which is increased in hiberation and reversed when hibernation is terminated.

Neurotrophic factors also play a role in dendritic branching and length in that brain-derived neurotrophic factor (BDNF)+/− mice show a less branched dendritic tree and do not show a further reduction of CA3 dendrite length with chronic stress, whereas wild-type mice show reduced dendritic branching. However, there is contradictory information thus far concerning whether CRS reduces BDNF mRNA levels, some reporting a decrease and other studies reporting no change. This may reflect the balance of two opposing forces, namely, that stress triggers increased BDNF synthesis to replace depletion of BDNF caused by stress. BDNF and corticosteroids appear to oppose each other – with BDNF reversing reduced excitability in hippocampal neurons induced by stress levels of corticosterone.

Corticotrophin releasing factor (CRF) is a key mediator of many aspects related to stress. CRF in the paraventricular nucleus regulates adrenocorticotropin (ACTH) release from the anterior pituitary gland, whereas CRF in the central amygdala is involved in control of behavioral and autonomic responses to stress including the release of tPA that is an essential part of stress-induced anxiety and structural plasticity in the medial amygdala. CRF in the hippocampus is expressed in a subset of GABA neurons (Cajal-Retzius cells) in the developing hippocampus, and early life stress produces a delayed effect that reduces cognitive function and the number of CA3 neurons, as well as decreased branching of hippocampal pyramidal neurons. Indeed, CRH inhibits dendritic branching in hippocampal cultures *in vitro*.

What about Permanent Damage as a Result of Stress?

There is always concern that severe and prolonged stress may damage the brain. In the case of depressive illness, there is a high degree of life-time recurrence of major depression, which suggests that an underlying pathophysiological process is involved. What is being learned from animal models of stress and trauma effects in the hippocampus is that the remodeling of the hippocampus in response to stress is largely reversible if chronic stress is terminated at the end of 3 weeks. Yet, it is well established that glucocorticoids exacerbate damage to the hippocampus caused by ischemia and seizures. Nevertheless, the brain protects itself, as for example, in the phenomenon of ischemia preconditioning: that is, prior stimulation of the hippocampus by a small ischemic event can induce a protective mechanism that may reduce the damage produced by a full-scale ischemic event. It is not clear if the same mechanisms might be operative when stress is applied, although there is evidence that 21d CRS increases the vulnerability to excitotoxic damage by ibotenic acid applied directly into the hippocampus. The unanswered question is whether the damage would have been worse if the dendritic retraction that occurs after 21d CRS had not occurred.

We do know that in the hippocampus there is a delicate balance between the generation of damage and destruction and the mechanisms that lead to dendrite retraction during more gradual repetitive stimulation, which may be a protective response that reduces the excitatory input without totally disconnecting the circuit functionally.

Stress-Induced Changes in the Prefrontal Cortex and Amygdala

Repeated stress also causes changes in other brain regions such as the prefrontal cortex and amygdala. Repeated stress causes dendritic shortening in medial prefrontal cortex but produces dendritic growth in neurons in amygdala, as well as in orbitofrontal cortex. Along with many other brain regions, the amygdala and prefrontal cortex also contain adrenal steroid receptors; however, the role of adrenal steroids, excitatory amino acids, and other mediators has not yet been studied in these brain regions. Nevertheless, in the amygdala, there is some evidence regarding mechanism, in that tPA is required for acute stress not only to activate indices of structural plasticity but also to enhance anxiety. These effects occur in the medial and central amygdala and not in basolateral amygdala, and the release of CRH acting via CRH1 receptors appears to be responsible.

Behavioral Effects of Acute and Chronic Stress

Acute stress induces spine synapses in CA1 region of hippocampus and chronic stress also increases spine synapse formation in amygdala but decreases it in hippocampus. Moreover, chronic stress for 21 days or longer impairs hippocampal-dependent cognitive function and enhances amygdala-dependent unlearned fear and fear conditioning, which are consistent with the opposite effects of stress on hippocampal and amygdala structure. Chronic stress also increases aggression between animals living in the same cage, and this is likely to reflect another aspect of hyperactivity of the amygdala. Behavioral correlates of remodeling in the prefrontal cortex include impairment in attention set shifting, possibly reflecting structural remodeling in the medial prefrontal cortex.

Relationship to Anxiety and Mood Disorders

Life events are known to precipitate depressive illness in individuals with certain genetic predispositions. Moreover, brain regions such as the hippocampus, amygdala, and prefrontal cortex show altered patterns of activity in positron emission tomography (PET) and functional magnetic resonance imaging (fMRI) and also demonstrate changes in volume of these structures with recurrent depression: decreased volume of hippocampus and prefrontal cortex and amygdala. Interestingly, amygdala volume has been reported to increase in the first episode of depression, whereas hippocampal volume is not decreased. It has been known for some time that stress hormones such as cortisol are involved in psychopathology, reflecting emotional arousal and psychic disorganization rather than the specific disorder *per se*. We now know that adrenocortical hormones enter the brain and produce a wide range of effects upon it.

In Cushing's disease, there are depressive symptoms that can be relieved by surgical correction of the hypercortisolemia. Both major depression and Cushing's disease are associated with chronic elevation of cortisol that results in gradual loss of minerals from bone and abdominal obesity. In major depressive illness, as well as in Cushing's disease, the duration of the illness and not the age of the subjects predicts a progressive reduction in volume of the hippocampus, determined by structural magnetic resonance imaging. Moreover, there are a variety of other anxiety-related disorders, such as posttraumatic stress disorder (PTSD) and borderline personality disorder, in which atrophy of the hippocampus has been reported, suggesting that this is a common process reflecting chronic imbalance in the activity of adaptive systems, such as the hypothalamic–pitutary–adrenal (HPA) axis, but also including endogenous neurotransmitters, such as glutamate.

Conclusion

Animal stress models not only suggest how the human brain may change under repeated stress, but they also provide mechanistic clues about stress-induced anxiety and behavioral depression, which are relevant to human mood and anxiety disorders. For example, psychosocial stress in an animal model of depressive illness, resident-intruder stress in the tree shrew, suppresses neurogenesis and causes dendritic shrinkage in hippocampus.

Translational studies of brain changes in major mood and anxiety disorders (such as unipolar and bipolar depression and PTSD) show that changes in volume of structures (such as hippocampus, prefrontal cortex, and amygdala) must be considered as part of the neurobiological consequences of these illnesses. Structural remodeling in these brain regions is important for human psychiatric disorders because the altered circuitry is likely to contribute to impaired cognitive function and affect regulation. Moreover, stress is widely acknowledged as a predisposing and precipitating factor in psychiatric illness. Thus, animal models are relevant to human psychiatric disorders by showing the delicate balance between protection and damage and by providing mechanisms that raise the hopeful possibility that brain changes, in at least some major psychiatric disorders, may be treatable if we can find the right agents or therapies and intervene in time.

Acknowledgments

Research support has come from the National Institute of Mental Health Grants MH41256 and MH58911.

See Also the Following Articles

Chronic (Repeated) Stress: Consequences, Adaptations.

Further Reading

Chen, Y., Bender, R. A., Brunson, K. L., et al. (2004). Modulation of dendritic differentiation by corticotropin-releasing factor in the developing hippocampus. *Proceedings of the National Academy of Sciences of the United States of America* **101**, 15782–15787.

Conrad, C. D. (2006). What is the functional significance of chronic stress-induced CA3 dendritic retraction within the hippocampus? *Behavioral and Cognitive Neuroscience Review* 5, 41–60.

Czeh, B., Michaelis, T., Watanabe, T., et al. (2001). Stress-induced changes in cerebral metabolites, hippocampal volume, and cell proliferation are prevented by antidepressant treatment with tianeptine. *Proceedings of the National Academy of Sciences of the United States of America* **98**, 12796–12801.

Isgor, C., Kabbaj, M., Akil, H. and Watson, S. J. (2004). Delayed effects of chronic variable stress during peripubertal-juvenile period on hippocampal morphology and on cognitive and stress axis functions in rats. *Hippocampus* **14**, 636–648.

Leuner, B., Gould, E. and Shors, T. J. (2006). Is there a link between adult neurogenesis and learning? *Hippocampus* **26**, 216–224.

Liston, C., Miller, M. M., Goldwater, D. S., et al. (2006). Stress-induced alterations in prefrontal cortical dendritic morphology predict selective impairments in perceptual attentional set-shifting. *Journal of Neuroscience* **26**, 7870–7874.

Malberg, J. E., Eisch, A. J., Nestler, E. J. and Duman, R. S. (2000). Chronic antidepressant treatment increases neurogenesis in adult rat hippocampus. *Journal of Neuroscience* **20**, 9104–9110.

McEwen, B. S. (1999). Stress and hippocampal plasticity. *Annual Review of Neuroscience* **22**, 105–122.

Pawlak, R., Magarinos, A. M., Melchor, J., McEwen, B. and Strickland, S. (2003). Tissue plasminogen activator in the amygdala is critical for stress-induced anxiety-like behavior. *Nature Neuroscience* **6**, 168–174.

Sandi, C. (2004). Stress, cognitive impairment and cell adhesion molecules. *Nature Review/Neuroscience* **5**, 917–930.

Sapolsky, R. (1992). *Stress, the Aging Brain and the Mechanisms of Neuron Death* ((vol. 1). Cambridge: MIT Press.

Sheline, Y. I. (2003). Neuroimaging studies of mood disorder effects on the brain. *Biological Psychiatry* **54**, 338–352.

Sousa, N., Lukoyanov, N. V., Madeira, M. D., Almeida, O. F. X. and Paula-Barbosa, M. M. (2000). Reorganization of the morphology of hippocampal neurites and synapses after stress-induced damage correlates with behavioral improvement. *Neuroscience* **97**, 253–266.

Vyas, A., Mitra, R., Rao, B. S. S. and Chattarji, S. (2002). Chronic stress induces contrasting patterns of dendritic remodeling in hippocampal and amygdaloid neurons. *Journal of Neuroscience* **22**, 6810–6818.

Wellman, C. L. (2001). Dendritic reorganization in pyramidal neurons in medial prefrontal cortex after chronic corticosterone administration. *Journal of Neurobiology* **49**, 245–253.

Plasticity, and Activity-Dependent Regulation of Gene Expression

M R Mayford
The Scripps Research Institute, La Jolla, CA, USA

Introduction

While we can think of plasticity in the nervous system in two broad domains, neuronal and behavioral, the two are inexorably linked in that any behavioral plasticity must arise from underlying forms of neuronal plasticity. The initial suggestion of a role for new or induced gene expression in plasticity derives from the behavioral domain. Beginning with studies in the early 1960s on the effects of pharmacological inhibitors of protein synthesis on learning and memory, it has become clear that long-lasting forms of plasticity require gene expression. The primary finding, which has been replicated in species as diverse as *Drosophila*, *Aplysia*, and mice, is that when an inhibitor of protein synthesis, such as anisomycin, is administered during the initial learning, the animals develop normal memory recall 1 h after training, but the memory is dramatically reduced when measured at 24 h. The amnestic effects of protein synthesis inhibitors have led to the suggestion that initial learning involves changes in preexisting proteins, but that the stabilization of these molecular changes over 24 h requires the synthesis of new proteins. These new proteins are presumed to be induced during the initial learning and to exert their effects of over a period of hours to consolidate the initial, transient, cellular changes that underlie short-term memory into a long-lasting or permanent form. This is supported by the fact that inhibition of protein synthesis at the later, 24 h, time point does not impact memory. The process by which short-term memories are stabilized into long-term memories, in a protein synthesis-dependent manner, is often referred to as memory consolidation, or molecular memory consolidation, to distinguish it from the more prolonged changes in the anatomy of memory that involve hippocampal function.

A number of basic questions arise from the initial observation that new gene expression is required for memory consolidation: What are the specific genes induced during synaptic or behavioral plasticity? What are the cellular mechanisms for regulating induced gene expression? What are the cellular plasticity processes that these genes act on to stabilize long-term memories? Are these induced genes required for the consolidation of long-term memory? Advances in molecular and genetic technology over the past two decades have allowed these questions to be addressed to some extent. This progress has produced an outline of transcriptional signaling mechanisms linking initial molecular and synaptic events to gene expression, neuronal plasticity, and behavioral memory.

What Are the Specific Genes Induced during Synaptic or Behavioral Plasticity?

Current models of memory formation in the mammalian brain postulate that neuronal activity-dependent forms of synaptic plasticity play a critical role. In order to look for genes that might be induced by neuronal activity, studies in the late 1980s focused on seizure-induced gene expression. The first gene identified as responding to seizure activity was the protooncogene *cfos*. The *cfos* gene is induced within minutes after the onset of seizure activity, but its expression is transient, returning to baseline levels within several hours. Subsequent screening using differential hybridization techniques or, more recently, expression profiling on DNA microarrays has identified approximately 60 genes that show rapid induction in response to high-level neuronal activity. The activity-induced genes represent a wide variety of molecular domains, from transcription factors to growth factors and components of the cytoskeleton. The identity of these genes does not provide any clear insight into common molecular mechanisms that they might subserve.

The activity-dependent genes, such as *cfos*, are induced not only by high-intensity seizure activity but also by artificial electrical stimulation and environmental stimuli. The most widely studied form of synaptic plasticity in the mammalian nervous system is long-term potentiation (LTP). LTP is an activity-dependent form of synaptic strengthening which has many features that make it an attractive candidate as a cellular mechanism of memory. LTP is typically induced by brief bouts of high-frequency stimulation, which have also been shown to effectively induce rapid expression of many of the same genes discovered in seizure screens.

At the behavioral level, many of these activity-regulated genes have been used to map neuronal activation in response to environmental stimuli. *cfos* is perhaps the most widely used marker of neuronal activity, as it has relatively low baseline expression and strong sensitivity to neuronal activity in a wide variety of brain regions. It has replaced, to a large extent, other techniques for mapping brain activation, such as 2-deoxyglucose labeling. Two other seizure-induced genes that have been used widely for mapping activity patterns in the brain are *zif268*, encoding a zinc-finger transcription factor, and *arc*, encoding a cytoskeletal-associated protein. Both of these genes have slightly different anatomical distributions and sensitivity to neuronal activity. The properties of *arc* gene expression have allowed it to be used to assess neuronal activity at two different time points. Experiments using this approach have shown that when animals are exposed repeatedly to the same environmental contingencies they induce *arc* expression in the same neurons, indicating that the gene induction is clearly reporting environmentally relevant neuronal activity rather than nonspecific global activity.

What Are the Cellular Mechanisms for Regulating Activity-Induced Gene Expression?

The cellular mechanisms for induction of gene expression by neuronal activity have been studied extensively. While genes such as *cfos*, *zif268*, and *arc* can be induced by a variety of stimuli using different second-messenger signaling mechanisms, the primary signal in neuronal activity-induced gene expression is Ca^{2+}. The Ca^{2+} can derive from two primary sources, voltage-sensitive Ca^{2+} channels that become active when neurons are depolarized and *N*-methyl-D-aspartate (NMDA)-type glutamate receptors, which require both synaptic activity and membrane depolarization for their activity. In a typical cortical pyramidal neuron during high-frequency firing, both pathways will be active.

The transduction of this Ca^{2+} signal into transcriptional activation is significantly more complex. The majority of studies have been carried out in cell culture using artificial depolarization of neurons and using *cfos* to report gene expression. One of the difficulties in these studies is that a primary Ca^{2+} signal in neurons can activate a wide variety of second-messenger signaling pathways as shown in **Figure 1**. Ca^{2+} increases cAMP levels through stimulation of a Ca^{2+}-dependent form of adenylate cyclase. Ca^{2+} also activates the extracellular signal-regulated kinase/mitogen-activated kinase (ERK/MAPK) signaling pathway through ras

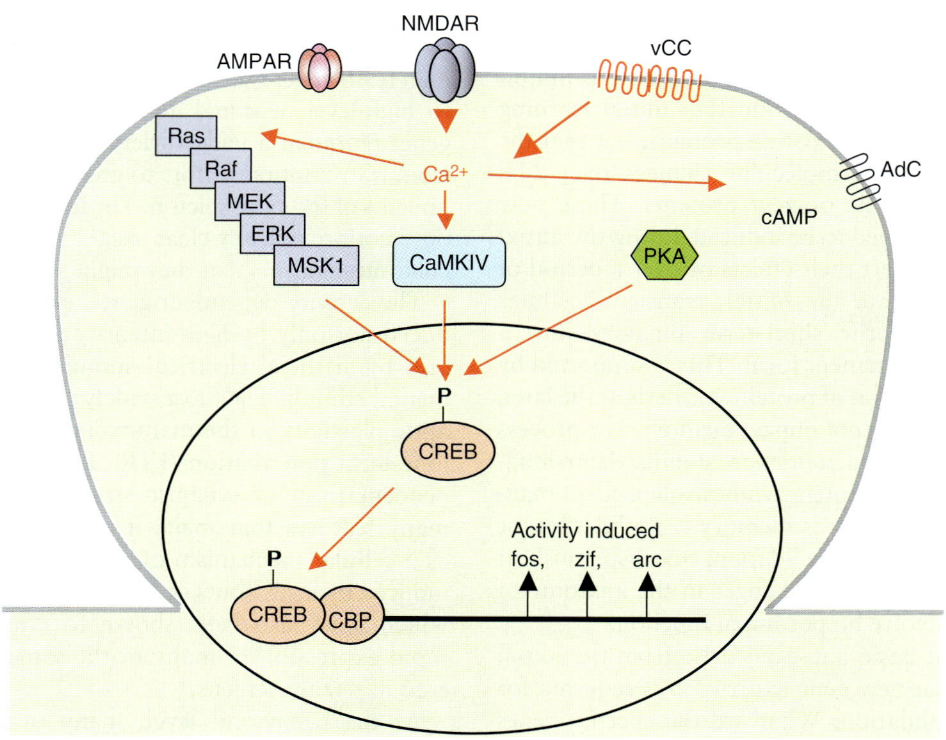

Figure 1 Molecular signaling in activity-dependent gene regulation. Neuronal activity produces an increase in Ca^{2+} primarily through the activation of *N*-methyl-D-aspartate receptors (NMDARs) and voltage-gated Ca^{2+}channels (vCCs). Ca^{2+} can be activated at least in three different second-messenger signaling pathways that converge on the nuclear transcription factor cyclic adenosine monophosphate (cAMP) response element-binding protein (CREB) to induce gene expression. AMPAR, α-amino-3-hydroxy-5-methyl-4-isoxazole propionic acid receptor; AdC, adenylate cyclase; CaMKIV, Ca^{2+}/calmodulin-dependent protein kinase IV; CBP, CREB-binding protein; ERK, extracellular signal-regulated kinase; MSK1, mitogen- and stress-activated kinase 1; PKA, protein kinase A.

activation. Finally, there are protein kinases that are directly activated by Ca^{2+}/calmodulin binding, such as Ca^{2+}/calmodulin-dependent protein kinase II (CaMKII) and CaMKIV. Each of these signaling pathways has been demonstrated to impact, to some degree, the induction of *cfos* by neuronal activity. The relative contribution of each of these signaling pathways to gene expression is likely dependent upon the pattern and time course of the neuronal activity-induced Ca^{2+} signal as well as the subcellular location of that signal. The interaction of these complex signaling mechanisms would in turn control the pattern of gene induction in response to given type of stimulation.

Although there are many transcription factors that respond to the various second-messenger signaling pathways, the cAMP response element-binding protein (CREB) has been studied in the most detail and plays a clear role in activity-induced gene expression. CREB is a transcription factor that was initially discovered based on its response to cAMP. Functional activation of CREB requires phosphorylation at a specific serine residue (Ser133), which can be mediated by the cAMP-responsive protein kinase A (PKA). The same serine residue is a target for phosphorylation by CaMKIV and by a downstream MAPK pathway component, mitogen- and stress-activated kinase 1 (MSK1). In this way multiple different second-messenger signaling pathways that are activated by Ca^{2+} can converge on a single target molecule to regulate transcription. The DNA-binding element for CREB is found in the promoter for the *cfos* gene, as well as in many other genes that are regulated by neuronal activity. This element alone, in a synthetic promoter construct, can confer responsiveness to neuronal activity to cis-linked genes.

What Are the Cellular Processes That These Genes Act on to Stabilize Long-Term Memories?

If new gene expression is required for the consolidation of long-term memories, what might be the cellular processes that underlie its role in memory? This is a component of the larger, and not clearly answered, question of what cellular mechanisms underlie memory. Initial progress on both of these questions has been made in invertebrate model systems such as *Aplysia*. Kandel and his colleagues have analyzed a form of simple learning in this marine mollusk at the behavioral, circuit, cellular, and molecular levels. Sensitization memory in *Aplysia* shows the same dependence on translation, for the conversion from short-term to long-term forms, that is seen in many other species and behavioral paradigms. The underlying cellular changes for this memory appear to be an increase in synaptic efficacy in the specific motor circuit that controls the behavior. In a critical series of experiments, Kandel showed that the synaptic change had the same sensitivity to protein and RNA synthesis inhibitors as did the behavioral memory. That is, when protein synthesis was inhibited during the induction of synaptic plasticity, a short-term form of the plasticity occurred but lasted only a few hours. In the absence of protein synthesis blockade, the synaptic plasticity is stabilized and maintained for more than 24 h. This striking concordance between behavioral memory and a cellular plasticity mechanism suggests that this may be the means by which memory consolidation functions at the cellular level. It also provided the first suggestion that gene expression changes may be critical for neuronal as well as behavioral forms of plasticity.

The cellular plasticity in *Aplysia* is not activity dependent but is mediated by serotonin-induced activation of adenylate cyclase. So while the plasticity in *Aplysia* does not require neuronal activity, it recruits one of the same second-messenger signaling pathways that is activated in the induction of *cfos* by action potential firing in mammalian neurons. *Aplysia* contains CREB homologs that act similarly to mammalian CREB. Blocking CREB-dependent transcription in *Aplysia* neurons produces an effect similar to blocking all transcription or translation, in that the long-lasting synaptic plasticity is inhibited while the short-lasting form is unaffected.

In mammals, the neuronal activity-dependent form of synaptic plasticity, LTP, is commonly studied in the hippocampus, either in the intact brain with implanted electrodes or *in vitro* in brain slices. LTP is induced artificially by high-frequency stimulation, resulting in a prolonged increase in the strength of the stimulated synapses that, in the intact brain, can last for weeks. Most of the molecular and pharmacological studies of LTP have focused on the brain slice preparation. In this preparation, if transcription or translation is pharmacologically blocked during the high-frequency stimulation used for induction, there is an effect similar to that discussed previously for *Aplysia* synaptic plasticity – a short-lasting form of LTP is produced, which then returns to baseline over several hours.

The nature of the transcriptional requirement for LTP has been investigated in an interesting series of experiments by Morris and Frey; their findings suggest that the products of activity-induced gene expression in the nucleus are functionally delivered only to synapses that were recently active. This process is sometimes referred to as 'synaptic tagging' and is supported by the following observations. If synapses are stimulated weakly, this induces a short-lasting potentiation that is not dependent on new gene expression. However, if those same neurons were previously stimulated strongly to induce gene expression, then the short-lasting potentiation is converted into a long-lasting LTP. The suggestion is that the weak stimulation has molecularly altered or tagged the synapses in such a way that they can now make use of activity-induced genes, if the genes are available within the cell. The strong stimulation of the neurons, at a distinct set of synapses, provides that transcriptional signal.

Advances in techniques for genetic manipulation of the mouse, such as gene knockout and transgenesis, have allowed the functional role of specific molecules to be tested in the intact mammalian brain. The role of CREB has been tested using this approach. Mice in which the CREB gene has been deleted or inhibited through expression of a dominant-negative transgene show deficits in long-lasting LTP, while the short-lasting form remains intact. Several of the genes that are rapidly induced by neuronal activity, most notably those for the transcription factor zif268 and the cytoskeletal-associated protein arc, have been knocked out and produce similar LTP phenotypes.

These results demonstrate that in both vertebrate and invertebrate systems, forms of synaptic plasticity that are thought to underlie long-term memory formation show requirements for new gene expression that parallel what is seen at the behavioral level for long-term memory. While this provides a suggestive framework for how one might understand the role of activity-induced gene expression in long-term memory (i.e., the induced genes are necessary to stabilize the synaptic plasticity that in turn stabilizes the memory), this is certainly an oversimplification. It is clear from many studies that there is not a simple relationship between LTP and behavioral memory. LTP is an artificially induced phenomenon of which there are a number of different types, some of which do not require new gene expression. Moreover, there are a number of examples in which transcriptionally dependent forms of LTP can be impaired genetically or pharmacologically while memory remains relatively intact.

Are These Activity-Induced Genes Required for the Stabilization of Long-Term Memory?

The generation of genetically altered mice carrying mutations in the various activity-induced genes or in the signaling molecules important for their induction has allowed the possibility for linking specific genes to behavioral memory. One of the first studies of this type came from *Drosophila*, which, like the other species discussed, shows a requirement for new protein synthesis for the stabilization of long-term memory. Genetic studies in *Drosophila* have identified genes involved in the cAMP signaling pathway in the formation of memory using a simple Pavlovian conditioning paradigm. Using dominant-negative inhibitors of CREB, Tim Tully and his colleagues showed that expression of the CREB inhibitor impaired long-term memory while sparing short-term memory. Strikingly, they went on to show that expression of a CREB activator allowed training paradigms that normally produced only short-term memory to then induce a long-lasting memory. These results suggest that CREB, which, as discussed previously, is a critical mediator of neuronal activity-induced gene expression and long-lasting forms of synaptic plasticity, is also a critical regulator of the conversion of short-term into long-term forms of behavioral memory.

Similar studies have been carried out in mice. Alcino Silva and his colleagues studied a line of mice in which CREB expression was reduced through a genetic manipulation. They found that long-term memory was selectively impaired in these mice. However, the interpretation of phenotypic alterations, particularly behavioral alterations, in genetically modified mice, in which the genetic lesion is present for the entire developmental history of the animal, can be complex. For example, is the phenotype directly due to the loss of the gene of interest or to compensatory changes in the expression of other genes, or in the development of the circuitry underlying the behavior? CREB is a member of a class of related transcription factors and it was found that in the CREB mutant mice there was a compensatory upregulation in other members of this gene family. Was the phenotype indirectly due to this change in the balance of expression in CREB family members?

To address these issue, a number of groups have used inducible genetic manipulations. In this case, the animals can be allowed to develop normally and the genetic change is induced in the adult just prior to behavioral testing. This should preclude any developmental abnormalities and minimize the chances for compensatory changes that could alter or mask the phenotype. This approach was taken for CREB signaling using inducible expression of a dominant-negative transgene that targeted broadly the CREB family of transcription factors. Even when CREB was inhibited as little as 6 h prior to behavioral training, the same pattern of memory impairment, short-term intact/long-term impaired, was observed. Thus, in both *Drosophila* and mammals, using the most precise genetic manipulations available, it appears that the transcription factor CREB is a critical mediator of the stabilization of short-term into long-term memory.

Transcription is not a simple process involving single molecules, but requires the recruitment of many proteins into a complex on the DNA. Transcription is also sensitive to chromatin structure and the covalent modification of DNA and proteins within chromatin. Among the important components of this process are the transcription coactivators, which serve to link specific transcription factors like CREB to the recruitment of the more general transcriptional machinery. In addition, these molecules can serve to alter the structure of chromatin through the covalent modification of histones to a state that facilitates transcription. One of these transcription coactivators is the CREB-binding protein (CBP). The CBP gene has drawn interest since it was identified as the underlying genetic alteration in Rubinstein–Taybi syndrome, a rare disorder in humans that is characterized by both developmental and cognitive abnormalities. Two recent studies examined CBP function in behavior using inducible genetic modification. It was found that even when the gene was inhibited only in adult animals, it caused a deficit in long-term memory similar to that seen with CREB inhibition. This suggests that some of the cognitive phenotypes observed in the human disorder may be due to an acute requirement in the adult for normal CBP function.

In addition to linking CREB to the recruitment of the general transcriptional machinery, CBP functions as an enzyme to modify chromatin structure by acetylating histones. This histone acetylation allows the chromatin to assume an open structure needed for effective transcription. Surprisingly, the behavioral effects of genetic CBP inhibition could be overcome with pharmacological agents that elevate histone acetylation nonspecifically. This demonstrates not only the critical role for chromatin structure modifications in the transcriptional regulation of long-term memory, but also suggests a possible pharmacological intervention in disorders, such as Rubinstein–Taybi, that result from disruption of this process.

The role of CREB-based transcription in the stabilization of long-term synaptic and behavioral plasticity is clear. What of the signaling pathways that activate CREB and the 60 or so activity-induced genes that have their expression mediated by CREB? Here the players are more numerous and the results less clear. Mutant mice have been engineered to disrupt each of the three major upstream signaling pathways to CREB activation (**Figure 1**) – Ca^{2+}-dependent adenylate cyclase, ERK/MAPK, and CaMKIV – with mixed results. Complete elimination of the Ca^{2+}-responsive cyclase leads to a phenotype in both LTP and behavioral memory that is similar to that seen with protein synthesis inhibitors, but not a complete phenocopy. Knockout of CaMKIV leads to a strong reduction in *cfos* inducibility and a deficit in protein synthesis-dependent LTP lasting more than 1 h. Surprisingly, however, the knockout fails to produce similar major changes in long-term behavioral memory. Finally, the ERK/MAPK signaling pathway contains the most components and is the most difficult to dissect. Pharmacological inhibitors of ERK/MAPK signaling have been shown in many studies to disrupt memory and synaptic plasticity. Mutation of an upstream effector of ras function (the neurofibromatosis gene, *NF1*) similarly produces deficits in long-term memory. However, mutations of some of the more downstream effectors have produced conflicting results. This type of complexity is not surprising given the diverse interactions between these very general cellular signaling pathways. As discussed previously, the induction of gene expression likely results from the contribution of each of these signaling pathways, and the impairment of one pathway might be expected to lead to compensation by the others under certain conditions.

The activity-induced genes are numerous and their individual roles in behavioral plasticity have been less well studied. Three of the activity-induced genes that appear to have an influence on memory are the transcription factor gene *zif268*, the brain-derived neurotrophic factor gene *BDNF*, and the cytoskeletal-associated protein gene *arc*. In the case of *zif268* and *arc*, mice carrying a deletion in the gene are viable to adulthood, allowing behavioral testing in which the animals show the selective impairment in long-term memory with sparing of short-term memory that is characteristic of protein synthesis inhibitors. The deletion of the *BDNF* gene produces a severe developmental phenotype. However, one recent study used antisense oligonucleotides to block *BDNF* expression specifically in adult animals and found a similar phenotype. Thus, the individual disruption of three neuronal activity-induced genes, representing distinct categories of molecular function, produces behavioral phenotypes that are similar to that produced with the general blockade of new gene expression.

Summary and Future Directions

A simple framework has been provided for understanding the role of gene expression in neuronal and behavioral plasticity. In summary, the transcription factor CREB plays a critical role, integrating multiple upstream signaling pathways into the increased transcription that is necessary for the stabilization of long-lasting synaptic plasticity and memory. In invertebrates CREB functions primarily by responding to direct cAMP signals. In the mammalian nervous system the critical role of CREB is in integrating multiple molecular signaling pathways that are activated by neuronal activity. Each of these pathways is stimulated by a primary Ca^{2+} signal that occurs when neurons are depolarized, allowing activation of both NMDA receptors and voltage-dependent Ca^{2+} channels. The response to neuronal activity involves the transcriptional activation of about 60 different genes with diverse functions.

The signaling pathways and the molecular and temporal dynamics of activity-induced gene expression are reasonably well understood. The clear deficiency is in understanding the cellular processes on which these genes act. The questions for the future concern how the activity-induced genes effect synapses, how they stabilize synaptic changes, and whether these synaptic changes completely account for their role in long-term behavioral plasticity.

Further Reading

Davis, H. P. and Squire, L. R. (1984). Protein synthesis and memory: A review. *Psychological Bulletin* **96**, 518–559.
Kandel, E. R. (2001). The molecular biology of memory storage: A dialogue between genes and synapses. *Science* **294**, 1030–1038.
Shaywitz, A. J. and Greenberg, M. E. (1999). CREB: A stimulus-induced transcription factor activated by a diverse array of extracellular signals. *Annual Review of Biochemistry* **68**, 821–861.
West, A. E., Griffith, E. C. and Greenberg, M. E. (2002). Regulation of transcription factors by neuronal activity. *Nature Reviews Neuroscience* **3**, 921–931.

Glucocorticoid Effects on Memory: the Positive and the Negative

O T Wolf
University of Bielefeld, Bielefeld, Germany

Glossary

Classical conditioning A form of learning caused by the association (or pairing) of two stimuli.

Declarative memory The conscious (explicit) long-term memory for events or facts, mediated by the medial temporal lobe.

Glucocorticoids (GCs) Steroid hormones secreted from the adrenal cortex in response to stress. Cortisol and corticosterone are naturally occurring GCs in humans and animals.

Meta-analysis A statistical procedure used to pool the results of multiple studies investigating a particular effect. This approach leads to a quantitative summary of a specific field of interest.

Procedural memory Different forms of nonconscious (implicit) long-term memories that express themselves through changes in performance. These forms of memories are largely independent of the medial temporal lobe memory system.

Working memory A system for temporarily (short-term) storing and managing information. This system is dependent on regions of the prefrontal cortex.

Introduction

Everyone has experienced instances of stress influencing his or her memory. There are situations in which we are unable to retrieve prior well-learned information, an example of how stress might interfere with our memory. In contrast, we remember very well specific embarrassing, shameful, or frightening events from the past; this is an example of how stress can enhance our memory. Finally, there are situations of chronic stress or stress associated psychiatric disorders that are characterized by hypo- or hyperamnesia. This article provides a brief and selective overview of what is known about the role of GCs in mediating some of these effects. Advances in the field of psychoneuroendocrinology within the past few years have contributed substantially to a more differentiated and balanced view of the effects of stress hormones on memory in animals and humans.

Interaction with a stressor leads to a cascade of neuroendocrine stress responses designed to facilitate adaptation to the changing demands. The hypothalamic-pituitary-adrenal (HPA) axis, together with the sympathetic nervous system (SNS), is one of the most important systems in this respect. The hypothalamus activates the HPA axis in response to input from several other brain regions. Corticotropin releasing hormone (CRH) and vasopressin reach the pituitary through the portal blood system, which leads to the secretion of adrenocorticotropic hormone (ACTH). In response to ACTH release from the pituitary, the adrenal secretes GCs. In most laboratory rodents (rats and mice) corticosterone dominates, whereas in humans cortisol is the main adrenal GC. GCs, as lipophilic steroid hormones, enter the brain relatively easily and exert multiple effects in regions throughout the brain. These effects are often mediated through the binding to the two receptors for the hormone: the mineralocorticoid receptor (MR) and the glucocorticoid receptor (GR). These two receptors differ in their affinity for cortisol (with the MR having a much higher affinity) and also in their localization in the brain. In addition, GCs can exert rapid nongenomic effects by influencing ion channels or neurotransmitter receptors at the membrane level. We emphasize that CRH, vasopressin, and ACTH can, on their own, influence cognition; the focus of this article, however, is on the effects of GCs on the memory of humans and animals.

To date, there is a substantial, almost overwhelming, literature on stress and memory. A PubMed search conducted with the two search terms stress and memory produced more than 3000 hits. Even a more focused search using glucocorticoids and memory as search terms still resulted in almost 400 hits. In order to provide a structured overview of this large and rapidly growing field, I use the concept of multiple memory systems in the brain to guide the reader through this jungle. Within each discussed memory domain, animal and human data are discussed. Acute stress effects are described, followed by chronic effects.

Effects of Stress on Different Memory Systems

There is a general agreement that there is not a single memory system in the brain but multiple interacting memory systems. Abundant literature exists on this topic, and it is not the goal of the current review to provide an in-depth overview of different models and ideas; the important question of the comparability of different memory systems in different species is not addressed here either. I focus instead on declarative or explicit long-term memory because this domain has been, until now, investigated most intensely with respect to stress effects. In addition, I briefly outline the findings for procedural memory, working memory, and conditioning (or associative learning); these three memory systems have been sparsely investigated, at least in humans.

Declarative Memory

Acute effects Declarative memory is the explicit storage of facts and events, which can later be intentionally retrieved. It is a relational and flexible memory system. This type of memory is tested in the laboratory with word lists, paired associates, or short stories in humans. In animals, spatial maze tasks are used most often, the most famous one being the Morris water maze (MWM). Long-term memory can be further divided into different memory phases: acquisition (or initial learning), consolidation (or storage), and retrieval (or recall). For the successful completion of declarative tasks, an intact medial temporal lobe region (the hippocampus and surrounding cortical structures) is essential for the acquisition of the task. The role of the hippocampus in retrieval is under debate, and it might fulfill a time-limited role only. Especially in humans, it is the prefrontal cortex regions that are of great importance for (effortful) retrieval. The literature regarding the effects of stress on declarative memory is quite diverse and confusing, with groups reporting enhancing as well as impairing effects of GCs on this form of memory. However, it has become apparent that this is largely due to the fact that the different memory phases are modulated by GCs in an opposing fashion.

GCs enhance memory consolidation, and this aspect represents the adaptive and beneficial mode of GCs central nervous system action. **Figure 1a** depicts the chain of events underlying this phenomenon. This process has been conceptualized as the beneficial effects of stress within the learning context or intrinsic stress, emphasizing that a stressful episode is remembered better. This effect is mediated by the action of stress-released GCs on the hippocampal formation, and it is very well documented in animals. Studies by Roozendaal and McGaugh showed that adrenergic activation in the basolateral amygdala (BLA) appears to be a prerequisite for the modulating effects of GCs on other brain regions (e.g., the hippocampus). Lesions of the BLA, as well as β blockade, abolish the enhancing effects of posttraining GC administration.

Although the enhanced memory consolidation is adaptive and beneficial, this process appears to occur at the cost of impaired retrieval (see **Figure 1b**). Using a 24-h delay interval, deQuervain and colleagues were the first to show that stress or GC treatment shortly before retrieval testing impairs memory retrieval in rats in the MWM. Further studies revealed that, again, an intact BLA and adrenergic activation appear to be necessary for the occurrence of this negative GC effect. Roozendaal summarized these findings as indicating that stress puts the brain into a consolidation mode, which is accompanied by impaired retrieval. Such a retrieval reduction might facilitate consolidation by reducing interference.

In humans, the literature on the acute effects of cortisol on declarative memory is somewhat divergent. Few studies reported beneficial effects, some

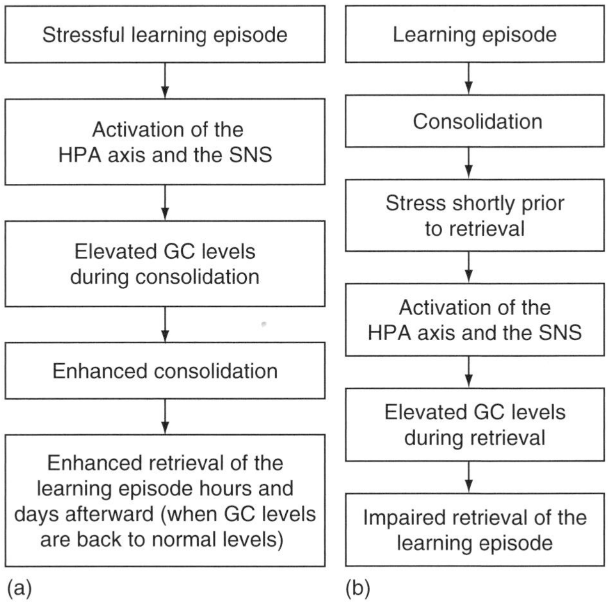

Figure 1 Schematic diagram of the cascade of events underlying the effects of GCs. a, Positive effects on long-term memory consolidation; b, negative effects on long-term memory retrieval. GC, glucocorticoid; HPA, hypothalamic-pituitary adrenal; SNS, sympathetic nervous system.

reported negative effects, and several others found no acute effects. We recently conducted a meta-analysis in order to provide a quantitative summary of the current state of the field. The results supported the model derived from animal studies showing that cortisol impairs memory retrieval. Similar observations have been made in humans who were exposed to a psychosocial laboratory stressor shortly before retrieval testing took place.

To date, the beneficial effects on consolidation could not be clearly established using a meta-analysis, which in part might reflect a power problem. At least some studies, using emotionally arousing learning material and a sufficiently long retention delay in order to assure that GCs can influence consolidation and in addition are back to baseline at the retrieval testing, observed enhanced memory consolidation for emotionally arousing material.

Interestingly, the beneficial effects on consolidation as well as the impairing effects on retrieval in humans are more pronounced for emotionally arousing material. This observation fits nicely with the observation in animals that GCs can exert effects on memory only in the presence of adrenergic activity in the amygdala. This arousal could be the result of specifics of the learning material and/or specifics of the testing conditions.

In the meta-analysis, time of day appeared as a second modulatory factor. Studies that administered cortisol before initial acquisition observed impairing effects on memory when they were conducted in the morning, a time of high endogenous cortisol levels in humans. In contrast, studies in the evening were more likely to observe beneficial effects. This supports an inverted U-shaped function between cortisol levels and memory in humans with both too low and too high levels at the time of acquisition being associated with impairments, especially when retrieval is tested at times when cortisol levels are still elevated.

In sum, studies in animals and humans converge on the idea that GCs acutely enhance memory consolidation of emotional arousing material while impairing memory retrieval. In addition, within this framework, emotional arousal and a nonlinear dose–response relationship are important modulatory variables.

Cortisol also influences declarative memory consolidation during sleep. Here the relationships appear to be different than in the daytime. Low cortisol levels during the first half of the night are a prerequisite for a sleep-induced enhancement of declarative memory consolidation. Moreover, blocking the rise in cortisol levels, which typically occurs during the second part of the night, leads to enhanced emotional memory facilitation.

The interesting issue of individual differences in responsiveness to GCs has received little attention so far. Such differences might be able to account for some of the variance observed within as well as between studies. Individual differences could reflect genetic factors, differences in tissue GC sensitivity, or differences in lifetime cortisol exposure. Attempts to characterize subgroups with high versus low cortisol sensitivity could be one important venue for future research.

Chronic effects The picture is different for more chronic effects as a result of prolonged stress or GC treatment – here negative effects prevail. Chronic stress in animals has repeatedly been shown to result in impaired spatial-memory performance. The neurobiological underpinnings of those effects are still under debate. Stress-induced dendritic atrophy (or dendritic remodeling) in the hippocampus is one possible mechanism for the negative effects of chronic stress on spatial memory in rodents. However, several additional mediators such as reduced neurogenesis and dysregulation of several catecholamines have to be considered. Recent studies demonstrated substantial plasticity in the adult rodent brain. For example, stress-induced dendritic atrophy appears to be reversible.

Interestingly, the negative effect of chronic stress on spatial memory might occur only in male rats and not in females. In fact, similarly, acute stress appears to impair spatial memory only in males. The area of sex differences in response to stress is an important and still relatively neglected field. However, authors who went through the extra effort of studying male and female animals have often observed quite striking sex differences in the effects of stress on a wide range of target systems. These observations in combination with evidence for sex differences in emotional memory lateralization and sex differences in the effects of adrenergic manipulations on emotional memory emphasize that caution should be used when generalizing findings obtained in one sex to predict responses in the opposite sex.

In humans, the effects of chronic long-term GC treatment cannot, of course, be studied experimentally due to ethical considerations. Studies that administered GCs for several (3–10) days observed declarative memory impairments. Moreover, studies of patients receiving GC therapy and studies of hypercortisolemic Morbus Cushing patients observed reduced declarative memory performance, which was associated with hippocampal atrophy. Some treatment studies in Cushing patients suggest that hippocampal atrophy in Cushing is reversible, which fits the observations in rodents previously mentioned.

Aging leads to alterations of HPA activity. Basal activity seems to increase and negative feedback is less efficient. Animal studies have suggested that enhanced HPA activity is associated with poorer memory. In older, otherwise healthy humans, several observational studies also reported associations between elevated or rising cortisol levels and declarative memory impairments. Whether these associations are specific for declarative memory or are, in fact, broader (also including working memory or attention) is currently under debate. Obviously all these human studies do not allow a clear cause and effect interpretation. Moreover, in most of these studies, the acute effects of cortisol cannot be differentiated from the chronic effects. In addition, the possible structural correlate of these hormone-performance associations remains to be firmly established. Hence, the possible association between rising cortisol levels and atrophy of the hippocampus is still not sufficiently understood, and the current empirical situation is somewhat mixed.

Finally, it has to be reiterated that other hormonal influences also might be important. With respect to aging, elevated cortisol levels could be part of the metabolic syndrome. Other aspects of this nonfavorable endocrine condition are impaired glucose tolerance and hypertension. These alterations have also been associated with memory impairment during aging, so future studies on this issue should consider taking a broader set of neuroendocrine measurements.

Procedural (Nondeclarative) Memory

This implicit and automatic form of (long-term) memory is not dependent on the medial temporal lobe. The brain areas involved depend on the specific content of the learning material. The neocortical areas, as well as the cerebellum and the basal ganglia, are involved in procedural memory. This is assessed in the laboratory with priming tasks (e.g., word-stem priming) or with skill-learning tasks (e.g., mirror tracing). In the few studies that used such tasks in the context of stress or GC research, a modulating effect of GCs was not observed, thus supporting the assumption that this memory form is not strongly influenced by GCs.

Working Memory

Working memory refers to the ability to store for the short term and manipulate material. This framework has replaced the older notion of short-term memory and emphasizes the active processing capacity of this system. Neuroanatomically, this function has been linked to the prefrontal cortex (PFC). There are a large number of GRs in the PFC, but, in contrast to the effects of GCs on the hippocampus, the effects on the PFC are less well characterized. Acute impairing effects on working memory have been reported in animals and in some studies in humans, but the results have been somewhat inconsistent.

Regarding the chronic effects of GCs on working memory, impaired performance has been reported in animals and humans. In animals, chronic stress was associated with dendritic atrophy in prefrontal regions, which was reversible. In humans, elevated basal GC levels have been associated in some studies with smaller PFC volumes. The PFC is, of course, not only involved in working memory but also in executive functions. These domains have not been well investigated in humans with respect to GC effects and additional research efforts are still needed.

Classical Conditioning (Associative Learning)

Classical conditioning is one of the most basic forms of learning, and it can be demonstrated in snails, fruit flies, rodents, and humans. The brain regions involved depend on the specific stimuli used and the timing of the conditioned stimulus (CS)–unconditioned stimulus (UCS) association. For example, the cerebellum is involved in simple eyelid conditioning, whereas the amygdala is critical for fear conditioning and the hippocampus is important for contextual conditioning and trace conditioning. In rodents, the effects of stress on conditioning has been studied repeatedly. For eyelid conditioning, Shors and coworkers observed that stress enhanced conditioning in male rats. This was true for delay as well as trace conditioning. Interestingly, they observed the opposite effect in female animals – stress impaired conditioning. These findings are the opposite of the effects of acute stress on spatial memory, in which stress enhanced memory in female rats while impairing it in males. Although the enhancing effects of stress or GCs have been observed for fear conditioning, the issue of sex differences has not been addressed systematically. With respect to chronic stress, enhanced fear conditioning in the presence of hippocampal dentritic atrophy has been detected. In humans, classical conditioning has not been studied intensively in the context of neuroendocrine stress research; however, the available studies also observed sex differences. Because this form of learning and memory is of relevance for several psychiatric disorders, more research appears to be necessary.

Clinical Implications

The basic-science studies discussed thus far are also of substantial clinical relevance. For example, patients with posttraumatic stress disorder (PTSD) have been reported to show reduced basal cortisol levels, which is probably due to an enhanced negative feedback of the system. Recent small-scale clinical studies suggested that cortisol treatment shortly after the trauma might help to prevent PTSD. Moreover, even patients with chronic PTSD appear to benefit from a low-dose cortisol treatment. For such patients, the impaired emotional memory retrieval, in combination with an enhanced and more elaborate (place and time) reconsolidation, might help to reduce the core symptoms of the disorder, illustrating that basic science studies in the field of stress neuroendocrinology can help us to understand and possibly treat major psychiatric disorders.

Summary and Conclusion

Research over the past decade has substantially helped us gain a better understanding of the effects of GCs on memory. It is obvious that a more differentiated picture of stress effects on memory has evolved and that oversimplifications such as “stress impairs memory” are no longer supported by the existing literature. Increases in GCs induced by acute stress enhance memory consolidation but impair memory retrieval. These impairing effects of stress-induced GC secretion might hinder us in performing well in an important exam or at an important job interview. In addition, GCs also appear to reduce the amount of items that can be stored in working memory, but this is less well documented than the effects on declarative long-term memory. Interestingly, there is now convincing evidence that adrenergic activation in the amygdale is a prerequisite for several acute effects of GCs on memory. This activation can be induced either through the cognitive task itself, through the test situation (e.g., novel unfamiliar environment), or through the test material (e.g., emotional slides).

Substantial sex differences have been observed in several animal studies, but evidence in humans is still sparse. The direction of the effect appears to be task-specific. More knowledge about sex differences should, in the long run, help us understand sex differences in stress-associated disorders. Future studies need to investigate whether these sex differences are related to differences in the neuroendocrine stress response or differences in the response of the brain to endocrine stress messengers.

Chronic stress or chronic GC treatment has mostly negative effects on the brain and on the body. These observations are relevant to psychiatric disorders as well as to the aging process. However, it is encouraging that recent research has repeatedly observed evidence for preserved plasticity and structural remodeling once the stress has ceased or GCs return to normal levels.

Especially rewarding for all basic-science research that has been done on stress is that already several clinical applications have been implemented or are on the horizon.

Acknowledgments

The author's work was supported by grants from the German Research Foundation (DFG WO 733/6-1 and WO 733/7-1).

Further Reading

Aerni, A., Traber, R., Hock, C., et al. (2004). Low-dose cortisol for symptoms of posttraumatic stress disorder. *American Journal of Psychiatry* **161**, 1488–1490.

Buchanan, T. W. and Lovallo, W. R. (2001). Enhanced memory for emotional material following stress-level cortisol treatment in humans. *Psychoneuroendocrinology* **26**, 307–317.

Cahill, L. (2003). Sex-related influences on the neurobiology of emotionally influenced memory. *Annals of the New York Academy of Sciences* **985**, 163–173.

Conrad, C. D., Jackson, J. L., Wieczorek, L., et al. (2004). Acute stress impairs spatial memory in male but not female rats: influence of estrous cycle. *Pharmacology Biochemistry & Behavior* **78**, 569–579.

Conrad, C. D., LeDoux, J. E., Magarinos, A. M., et al. (1999). Repeated restraint stress facilitates fear conditioning independently of causing hippocampal CA3 dendritic atrophy. *Behavioral Neuroscience* **113**, 902–913.

Convit, A. (2005). Links between cognitive impairment in insulin resistance: an explanatory model. *Neurobiology of Aging* **26**(supplement1), 31–35.

Croiset, G., Nijsen, M. J. and Kamphuis, P. J. (2000). Role of corticotropin-releasing factor, vasopressin and the autonomic nervous system in learning and memory. *European Journal of Pharmacology* **405**, 225–234.

De Kloet, E. R., Joels, M. and Holsboer, F. (2005). Stress and the brain: from adaptation to disease. *Nature Reviews Neuroscience* **6**, 463–475.

De Kloet, E. R., Oitzl, M. S. and Joels, M. (1999). Stress and cognition: are corticosteroids good or bad guys? *Trends in Neurosciences* **22**, 422–426.

de Quervain, D. J., Roozendaal, B. and McGaugh, J. L. (1998). Stress and glucocorticoids impair retrieval of long-term spatial memory. *Nature* **394**, 787–790.

Het, S., Ramlow, G. and Wolf, O. T. (2005). A meta-analytic review of the effects of acute cortisol administration on human memory. *Psychoneuroendocrinology* **30**, 771–784.

Kuhlmann, S., Piel, M. and Wolf, O. T. (2005). Impaired memory retrieval after psychosocial stress in healthy young men. *Journal of Neuroscience* **25**, 2977–2982.

LaBar, K. S. and Cabeza, R. (2006). Cognitive neuroscience of emotional memory. *Nature Reviews Neuroscience* **7**, 54–64.

Luine, V. (2002). Sex differences in chronic stress effects on memory in rats. *Stress* **5**, 205–216.

Lupien, S. J. and Lepage, M. (2001). Stress, memory, and the hippocampus: can't live with it, can't live without it. *Behavioural Brain Research* **127**, 137–158.

Lupien, S. J., Schwartz, G., Ng, Y. K., et al. (2005). The Douglas Hospital Longitudinal Study of Normal and Pathological Aging: summary of findings. *Journal of Psychiatry & Neuroscience* **30**, 328–334.

MacLullich, A. M., Deary, I. J., Starr, J. M., et al. (2005). Plasma cortisol levels, brain volumes and cognition in healthy elderly men. *Psychoneuroendocrinology* **30**, 505–515.

McEwen, B. S. (2002). Sex, stress and the hippocampus: allostasis, allostatic load and the aging process. *Neurobiology of Aging* **23**, 921–939.

Roozendaal, B. (2000). Glucocorticoids and the regulation of memory consolidation. *Psychoneuroendocrinology* **25**, 213–238.

Roozendaal, B., Okuda, S., de Quervain, D. J., et al. (2006). Glucocorticoids interact with emotion-induced noradrenergic activation in influencing different memory functions. *Neuroscience* **138**(3), 901–910.

Schelling, G., Roozendaal, B. and de Quervain, D. J. (2004). Can posttraumatic stress disorder be prevented with glucocorticoids? *Annals of the New York Academy of Sciences* **1032**, 158–166.

Shors, T. J. (2004). Learning during stressful times. *Learning & Memory* **11**, 137–144.

Squire, L. R. (1992). Memory and the hippocampus: a synthesis from findings with rats, monkeys, and humans. *Psychological Review* **99**, 195–231.

Tulving, E. (2001). Episodic memory and common sense: how far apart? *Philosophical Transactions of the Royal Society of London B Biological Sciences* **356**, 1505–1515.

Wagner, U., Degirmenci, M., Drosopoulos, S., et al. (2005). Effects of cortisol suppression on sleep-associated consolidation of neutral and emotional memory. *Biological Psychiatry* **58**, 885–893.

Wolf, O. T. (2003). HPA axis and memory. *Best Practice & Research: Clinical Endocrinology & Metabolism* **17**, 287–299.

Wolkowitz, O. M., Reus, V. I., Canick, J., et al. (1997). Glucocorticoid medication, memory and steroid psychosis in medical illness. *Annals of the New York Academy of Sciences* **823**, 81–96.

Yehuda, R. (2002). Post-traumatic stress disorder. *New England Journal of Medicine* **346**, 108–114.

Glucocorticoids – Adverse Effects on the Nervous System

R M Sapolsky
Stanford University, Stanford, CA, USA

This is a revised version of the article by R M Sapolsky, Encyclopedia of Stress, First edition, volume 2, pp 238–243, © 2000, Elsevier Inc.

Glossary

Dendritic atrophy — The shrinking of the dendritic processes by which neurons receive excitatory or inhibitory inputs from neighboring neurons.

Glucocorticoids — Steroid hormones released by the adrenal gland basally and in response to virtually all stressors.

Hippocampus — A region of the brain that plays a central role in learning and memory and in the regulation of the adrenocortical axis; it is atypically vulnerable to a number of neurological diseases and has an atypically high concentration of receptors for glucocorticoids.

Neuron death — The death of brain cells that can be due to disease or as part of normal development (i.e., programmed cell death).

It has long been appreciated that prolonged stress or exposure to glucocorticoids (GCs) can have adverse effects throughout the body. In recent decades, it has become clear that these adverse effects can extend to the nervous system, particularly the hippocampus, a brain region critical to learning and memory and with an abundance of corticosteroid receptors. These effects of GCs and stress include (1) reversible atrophy of dendritic processes, (2) inhibition of neurogenesis in the adult hippocampus, (3) compromising of the ability to neurons to survive a variety of insults, and (4) overt neurotoxicity. This article considers the emerging insights as to the cellular and molecular mechanisms underlying these events, as well as the possible clinical implications (including in the realm of normative aging, treatment with exogenous GCs, Cushing's disease, posttraumatic stress disorder, and depression).

Since the time of Walter Cannon, there has been recognition of the critical role of the stress response in maintaining allostatic balance in the face of insult and injury. However, since the time of Hans Selye, there has been the complementary recognition that excessive activation of the stress response can be deleterious, increasing the likelihood of a disease occurring or exacerbating some preexisting disease. The pages of this encyclopedia are filled with ample documentation of the adverse effects of overactivation of the stress response on metabolism, cardiovascular function, reproductive physiology, and so on, and these realms represent the cornerstones of stress pathophysiology. Only more recently has it become clear that excessive activation of the stress response can have deleterious effects on the nervous system.

Background

An array of physiological and psychological stressors causes secretion of catecholamines by the sympathetic nervous system and of glucocorticoids (GCs) by the adrenal cortex. While such peripheral catecholamines do not pass the blood–brain barrier, the steroidal GCs do so readily and appear to be the culprits in damaging the nervous system.

The deleterious effects of GC excess within the nervous system are centered in (but not exclusive to) the hippocampus, the limbic structure that plays a central role in learning and memory. The first hints of such deleterious actions came at a time when it was not yet obvious why the hippocampus should be particularly sensitive to GCs and thus were mostly ignored. This changed in the late 1960s, with the classic work of Bruce McEwen and colleagues, who demonstrated the extremely high levels of receptors for GCs (i.e., corticosteroid receptors) in the hippocampus. Since then, vast numbers of studies have documented the extensive neurochemical and electrophysiological sensitivity of the hippocampus to GCs, and it is basically impossible to think of stress, GCs, and the nervous system without thinking first about the hippocampus.

In the mid-1980s, E. Ron de Kloet and colleagues made the critical observation that there are two types of corticosteroid receptors in the nervous system, with the hippocampus having ample amounts of both. These are the high-affinity, low-capacity mineralocorticoid receptor (MR), and the low-affinity, high-capacity glucocorticoid receptor (GR). The existence of these two receptors, and their possessing such different affinities, clarify a key feature of GC action in the hippocampus. Specifically, mild elevations of GCs, or mild transient stressors, enhance hippocampal-dependent cognition, as well as the synaptic plasticity that mediates such cognition (such long term potentiation [LTP]); this makes sense, in that mild, transient stressors are what we think of as stimulation, something that very much enhances cognition. In contrast, major and/or prolonged stressors or GC exposure has opposite, disruptive effects on cognition. This U-shaped curve of GC effects on hippocampal function (a concept popularized by David Diamond) was explained by the two-receptor system in the hippocampus. Specifically, the high-affinity MRs are mostly occupied basally and are then fully occupied by mild elevation of GC concentrations. Such MRs mediate the salutary effects of GCs upon cognition (i.e., the permissive effects of GCs basally, and the enhancing effects of mild stressors). In contrast, GRs, which are minimally occupied basally and are not heavily occupied until there is a major stressor, mediate the disruptive effects.

GCs and the Function and Structure of Hippocampal Neurons

As just discussed, mild stressors, via MR occupancy, enhance hippocampal-dependent cognition and LTP, whereas major stressors, via GR occupancy, disrupt both. The mechanisms underlying these actions are well understood.

Major stressors and prolonged GC exposure can also cause structural changes in hippocampal neurons. Neurons are highly arborized cells, with information flowing in from neighboring neurons via a dense tree of processes called dendrites, and with information flowing out through a major cable called the axon. The extent of dendritic arborization – the length and complexity of processes – is now recognized to be highly dynamic, being remodeled by a variety of local, systemic, and even experiential influences. Work initiated by McEwen and colleagues has shown that in the rat, sustained exposure to stress or to excessive GC levels over the course of weeks can cause atrophy of dendrites in hippocampal neurons. Reflecting the dynamic nature of dendritic remodeling, the atrophy appears to gradually reverse when the stress or GC overexposure stops. Subsequent work from this group and others has shown that the same atrophy occurs in the nonhuman primate hippocampus as well.

It is the GR receptor that appears to mediate the deleterious GC effects on the dendrites. Moreover, GCs appear to cause the atrophy through the glutamate neurotransmitter system. As evidence, atrophy can be prevented by blocking NMDA glutamate receptors in the hippocampus or by the use of drugs that blunt glutamate release (such as the seizure suppresser phenytoin). Thus, the phenomena of GC-induced dendritic atrophy and of neuroendangerment appear to be linked mechanistically.

What are the consequences of this dendritic atrophy? There are at least three possibilities. First, part of the staggering complexity of the nervous system comes from the multiplicity of synaptic connections between neurons, and a typical neuron can form thousands of synapses with neighbors both near and far. The existence of such neuronal networks is obviously dependent upon an intact dendritic tree, and dendritic atrophy is likely to disrupt and simplify networks within the hippocampus. Stress or GC overexposure on the scale needed to cause dendritic atrophy will also disrupt cognition, and it seems plausible that the two are interrelated. Second, as will be reviewed shortly, GCs and stress can make hippocampal neurons less likely to survive coincident neurological insults. It has been suggested that the dendritic atrophy represents, in effect, a hibernation, of a neuron, an involution that protects it from a coincident insult. Third, in contrast, others have suggested that the atrophy represents a marker of the neuron being made more vulnerable, rather than less, to an insult. While it remains unclear whether the first two models are correct, most existing evidence supports the last.

GCs and the Birth of Hippocampal Neurons

For much of the twentieth century, a central dogma of neuroscience was that the adult mammalian brain did not make new neurons. The 1990s saw an overthrow of this view, with the recognition that a handful of generally ignored pioneering studies in the 1960s disproved this maxim, and the study of adult neurogenesis is now one of the most vibrant fields of neuroscience. Such neurogenesis occurs in only two regions of the brain (the hippocampus being one of them) and is stimulated by environmental enrichment, learning, voluntary exercise, and estrogen. An enormous amount of work has demonstrated that these are, indeed, neurons, that they can migrate some distance from their site of birth, and that they form functional synapses with preexisting neurons. Some of the current issues in the field include (1) whether such neurogenesis occurs in other brain regions as well (particularly the cortex); (2) how much neurogenesis occurs (with estimates ranging from rates that would completely replace certain hippocampal cell fields throughout the lifetime to rates that place the levels orders of magnitude lower); and (3) whether these new neurons are necessary for any aspects of hippocampal function. These issues are quite contentious in this often fractious field.

One of the more consistent findings is that stress and GCs potently and rapidly (over the course of hours) inhibit adult hippocampal neurogenesis, a finding pioneered by Elizabeth Gould and colleagues. The mechanisms underlying this are unclear. As but one example, early reports suggested that neural progenitor cells in the adult hippocampus do not express MRs or GRs, and that the inhibitory effects of GCs had to be through neuron/progenitor interactions; more recent work, using more sensitive assays, suggests that progenitors do indeed possess GRs. Also unclear is how much the effects of GCs on neurogenesis contribute to any of the disruptive effects of GCs upon hippocampal function.

GCs and the Death of Hippocampal Neurons

GC Endangerment

A body of work initiated by Robert Sapolsky and colleagues in the 1980s demonstrated the ability of transient bursts of GC excess to endanger hippocampal neurons, compromising their ability to survive a coincident neurological insult. As such, the greater the GC levels at the time of an insult, the greater the extent of hippocampal damage. Such insults include epileptic seizures, hypoxia-ischemia, hypoglycemia and other metabolic insults, oxidative insults, the β-amyloid peptide (the fragment of the amyloid precursor protein that has been implicated in the neuron death of Alzheimer's disease), and gp120 (the coat protein of the AIDS virus that is thought to play a role in the neurodegeneration seen in AIDS-related dementia). This endangerment is of a considerable magnitude, with stress levels of GCs causing many-fold increases in insult-induced damage in some cases.

Features of this endangerment include the following: (1) it is mediated by GRs, rather than MRs; (2) while most dramatic in the hippocampus, the endangerment can also occur in the cortex and striatum; (3) it is a direct GC effect in the hippocampus (rather than secondary to some peripheral GC action), as the same phenomenon occurs in hippocampal cultures and tissue slices; and (4) it consists of GCs increasing the amount of insult-induced necrotic death, rather than an increase in the amount of apoptotic death (a form of programmed cell death).

In vitro models have made it possible to uncover some of the mechanisms underlying the endangerment. One realm concerns the disruptive effects of GCs upon neuronal energetics. GCs inhibit glucose transport in many peripheral tissues (as part of the strategy to divert energy to exercising muscle during a stressful crisis); this effect is due to a reduction in the number of glucose transporter molecules in the cell membrane. GCs cause a similar inhibition in the hippocampus, leaving neurons energetically vulnerable, thereby worsening insult-induced declines in energy substrates (such as ATP). Such insults cause neurons to release damaging amounts of the excitatory neurotransmitter glutamate. This, in turn, causes a wave of calcium influx in the postsynaptic neuron, which causes an array of calcium-dependent degenerative events; of most significance is the generation of oxygen radicals. It is quite costly for a neuron to contain the excesses of glutamate, calcium, and oxygen radicals, and the mild energetic vulnerability caused by GCs makes each of these steps spiral a bit more out of control, increasing the likelihood of the neuron succumbing.

In addition to these energetic features, GC endangerment probably also arises from the demonstrated abilities of the hormone to increase calcium currents in hippocampal neurons, to decrease the activity of calcium-extrusion mechanisms, to suppress the levels or efficacy of neurotrophins (neuronal growth factors), and to disrupt some of the defenses normally mobilized by neurons during neurological insults.

At present, these data are derived exclusively from rodent and tissue culture studies. Should subsequent work demonstrate GC endangerment in the primate hippocampus, they have a number of disturbing implications. Numerous individuals are administered high-dose GCs to control autoimmune or inflammatory disorders, and this might well exacerbate the damaging effects of some neurological crisis. Plus, GCs are often administered after strokes in order to decrease brain edema (swelling). Most studies show that GCs are less effective at reducing such edema than nonsteroid anti-inflammatory compounds; the present studies suggest that the use of GCs might even worsen the neurological outcome. Finally, stroke, seizure, and cardiac arrest all cause massive GC secretion; such endogenous GC release might add to damage. In effect, what we have learned to view as the typical extent of neurological damage caused by these insults might well reflect the damaging effects of the maladaptive hypersecretion of GCs at that time.

GC Neurotoxicity

Independent of a coincident neurological insult, GCs can directly influence the life and death of a hippocampal neuron. In an unexpected finding, Robert Sloviter and colleagues reported that GCs are required for the survival of dentate gyrus neurons. In the complete absence of the hormone, such neurons undergo apoptosis within days, and very low levels of GCs, via MR occupancy, prevent this effect.

A separate literature showed that truly prolonged exposure to elevated GC levels could directly kill hippocampal neurons. Studies initiated by Phil Landfield and colleagues showed that the loss was centered in the CA3 region of the hippocampus and was highly relevant to hippocampal aging. That region of the hippocampus loses neurons with age, and these studies suggested that it is the cumulative extent of GC exposure over the lifetime that acts as a major determinant of the extent of neuron loss (as well as of hippocampal-dependent memory problems) in old age. As such, stress has the capacity to accelerate hippocampal aging, whereas behavioral or social manipulations that reduce cumulative GC exposure can delay such aging. The finding of GC- and of stress-induced neurotoxicity was replicated by other investigators, including in the nonhuman primate hippocampus.

The mechanisms underlying such neurotoxicity are not well understood. The assumption by most in the field, however, is that it is on a continuum with GC neuroendangerment – in effect, if a day of GC overexposure can compromise the ability of a neuron to survive a massive neurological insult, months of overexposure can compromise its ability to survive the minor metabolic challenges of everyday life, especially during aging. The difficult studies required to test this idea remain to be carried out.

Despite the replication of the finding of GC neurotoxicity, the phenomenon is more controversial than the other adverse GC effects that have been discussed. The disagreements have focused on a number of issues. The basic finding of neuron loss during hippocampal aging has been called into question by some researchers counting neurons with the technique of stereology. Some investigators suggest that overt neurotoxicity can be caused only by massive amounts of ever-shifting stressors (to avoid habituation of the system) or by pharmacological GC exposure, questioning the relevance of the phenomenon to normative aging. GC hypersecretion and hippocampal neuron loss in old age are quite variable among rodents. There appear to be strains in which neither occurs to any dramatic extent. Moreover, dramatic differences in the extent of successful aging can occur within strains. Michael Meaney and colleagues, for example, have shown that remarkably subtle differences in the quality of early maternal care can change the entire trajectory of hippocampal and adrenocortical aging in a rat, in some cases completely avoiding the neuron loss or GC hypersecretion; thus, neither component of that cascade model is an inevitable part of aging. Finally, to the extent that primates and humans hypersecrete GCs in old age, it is a nonlinear phenomenon, emerging only in extreme old age or when coincident with an insult (such as major depression or Alzheimer's disease).

GCs and the Health of the Human Hippocampus

Work in the past decade suggests that these findings regarding the deleterious effects of GCs and stress apply to the human hippocampus. These findings have been most striking in a number of realms.

Cushing's Syndrome

Cushing's syndrome can arise from any of a number of different types of tumors and results in vastly elevated levels of circulating GCs. Magnetic resonance imaging (MRI) studies by Monica Starkman and colleagues of Cushingoid patients have shown selective atrophy of the hippocampus. More strikingly, it is the same patients who have the most severe GC hypersecretion, the most severe hippocampal atrophy, and the most profound cognitive deficits. Post mortem studies to uncover whether this atrophy is due to neuronal loss, atrophy, or compression remain to be carried out. However, when the GC hypersecretion is corrected by removal of the tumor, the hippocampal gradually returns to normal size, in agreement with the model of reversible dendritic atrophy.

Exogenous GC Administration

Synthetic GCs are frequently administered in different realms of clinical medicine. Most cases involve transient exposure to fairly low concentrations, often through routes that do not result in much access of the steroids to the brain. However, there are hundreds of thousands of individuals on long-term, systemic high-dose GC treatment to control various autoimmune or inflammatory diseases. Difficult case-controlled work by Pamela Keenan and colleagues demonstrates that independent of the disease, treatment with such steroids increases hippocampal-dependent cognitive deficits. The mechanisms underlying this effect (e.g., whether it is due to dendritic atrophy, inhibition of neurogenesis, and so on) are unknown.

Clinical Depression

Major clinical depression is an archetypical example of a stress-related disease; as but three pieces of evidence, exogenous GC treatment increases the risk of depression, major stressors do as well, and about half of patients with major depression present with GC hypersecretion. Yvette Sheline and colleagues have observed that a history of prolonged depression is associated with selective hippocampal atrophy on MRI. In this observation, since replicated, the more prolonged the depression, the more atrophy. While the necessary post mortem cell counting has not been carried out, the atrophy appears to be permanent in that it is demonstrable in individuals long after the depressions have resolved; whether this is due to loss of neurons or inhibition of neurons that would otherwise have been born is not clear. Some researchers have suggested a scenario of reverse causality, in which individuals who (for other unrelated reasons) have a smaller than average hippocampus are more at risk for clinical depression. However, such volume loss is not demonstrable shortly after diagnosis, and more prolonged depressions are associated with more volume loss; both findings argue against reverse causality.

Posttraumatic Stress Disorder (PTSD)

Probably the most contentious studies concerning GC effects on the human hippocampus concern PTSD. A large numbers of studies, with the first coming from J. Douglas Bremner and colleagues, demonstrate volume loss in the hippocampi of individuals with PTSD. Furthermore, the more volume loss, the more severe the cognitive impairments, and there is little evidence that either tends to reverse over time. The controversial issues are threefold.

First, are GCs the cause of the volume loss? This question is central to the second issue as well, but the first version of this question focuses on whether GC levels are elevated in PTSD. While it might seem intuitive that this is the case, many (but not all) studies suggest lower than normal levels and that such hyposecretion may even precede and predispose toward succumbing to PTSD. The studies showing hyposecretion, pioneered by Rachel Yehuda and colleagues, also suggest an enhanced sensitivity to GCs in these patients. This would then shift the issue from whether excessive GC levels play a role in the volume loss to whether excessive sensitivity to GCs plays a role.

The second controversy concerns when the volume loss occurs. There are three possibilities: (1) volume loss occurs in response to the trauma itself; (2) volume loss occurs in response to the biology of the prolonged posttraumatic period (i.e., the period of the PTSD); and (3) a small hippocampus (arising for reasons unrelated to stress or GCs) precedes and predisposes toward PTSD. This issue is not resolved, and, at present, there are some striking findings supporting, as well as arguing against, each of these possibilities. One reasonable solution is that from the standpoint of hippocampal neurobiology, PTSD is a heterogeneous disorders, with all three occurring on occasion. Such heterogeneity is certainly seen in the clinical profile of the disorder.

The final issue is whether the volume loss is due to loss of neurons, blockage of birth of new neurons, atrophy of dendritic processes, loss of glia, and so on. As with the other realms of studies of the human hippocampus, resolving this issue requires difficult quantitative postmortem studies.

Obviously, many issues remain to be resolved and are likely to have some important consequences in neurology, psychiatry, and gerontology. Most broadly, the interrelated phenomena of GC neuroendangerment, inhibition of neurogenesis, dendritic atrophy, and neurotoxicity shift the realm of stress-related disease to the nervous system. For nearly 70 years, stress physiology has taught that cardiovascular function, metabolism, and immunity can be sensitive to the adverse effects of stress. This newer literature demonstrates that this vital and fragile portion of our bodies, the brain, can be sensitive to stress as well.

See Also the Following Articles

Corticosteroid Receptors; Cushing's Syndrome, Medical Aspects; Hippocampus, Corticosteroid Effects on.

Further Reading

Gould, E. and Gross, C. (2002). Neurogenesis in adult mammals: some progress and problems. *Journal of Neuroscience* 22, 619–623.

McEwen, B. (2002). Sex, stress and hippocampus: allostasis, allostatic load and the aging process. *Neurobiology of Aging* 23, 921.

Sapolsky, R. (1999). Stress, glucocorticoids and their adverse neurological effects: relevance to aging. *Experimental Gerontology* 34, 721.

Sapolsky, R. (2000). Glucocorticoids and hippocampal atrophy in neuropsychiatric disorders. *Archives of General Psychiatry* 57, 925.

Hippocampus, Corticosteroid Effects on

M Joëls and H Karst
University of Amsterdam, Amsterdam, Netherlands

This is a revised version of the article by M Joëls and H Karst, Encyclopedia of Stress, First edition, volume 2, pp 372–378, © 2000, Elsevier inc.

Glossary

Extracellular recording — A method for recording of electrical activity on the outside of neurons; often applied *in vivo* when recording the collective response of a group of neurons to the stimulation of afferents (i.e., the field response).

Hippocampal slice — A transversal slice of the hippocampal formation (~350 μm thick) kept alive *ex vivo,* in which the main synaptic pathways are still intact.

Intracellular recording — A method for recording of electrical activity in which the cell is impaled with a sharp electrode; generally used to record the potential or resistance over the entire membrane and changes thereof in the presence of neurotransmitters.

Ion currents — Ion fluxes over the neuronal membrane through specific ion channels. The activation of many of these channels depends on the membrane potential. In addition, some channels become inactive in a voltage-dependent manner.

Long-term potentiation (LTP) — Prolonged strengthening of synaptic contacts by patterned stimulation of afferent fibers; thought to play an important role in memory processes.

Long-term depression (LTD) — Prolonged weakening of synaptic contacts by patterned stimulation of afferent fibers; thought to play an important role in memory processes.

Neurotransmitter response — Neurotransmitters change the electrical properties of neurons either through activation of ligand-gated ion channels or G-protein-coupled receptors, which, via the intermediate effects of G-proteins and/or second messengers, act on a specific type of ion channel. Electrophysiological methods record only the final change in electrical activity, (i.e., the neurotransmitter response).

Patch clamp recording — A method in which a very tight seal between an electrode and the cell membrane is established, allowing the recording of currents through single ion channels. If the membrane patch under the electrode is disrupted, the recording of potentials or currents over the whole cell is possible.

Corticosteroid hormones affect cellular and network properties in the hippocampus in a slow but persistent manner. The nature of the effects depends on the relative participation of mineralocorticoid and glucocorticoid receptors.

Mechanism of Corticosteroid Action

Corticosteroid hormones, which are secreted from the adrenal gland in particularly high amounts after stress, enter the brain and bind to specific receptors. Two main types of receptors have been recognized: the high-affinity mineralocorticoid receptor (MR) and the lower-affinity glucocorticoid receptor (GR). Both receptor types are expressed abundantly in the hippocampal formation. In fact, most principal neurons in the hippocampal subfields (**Figure 1a**) coexpress the two receptor types. This has raised the question of how the activation of the two corticosteroid receptor types affects cellular properties in the hippocampus. One of the premises of initial studies was that the activation of MRs may affect hippocampal cell properties in a different way than GR activation. This has proven to be correct.

For neurons that coexpress MRs and GRs, the relative participation of the two receptor types in cellular effects depends on several factors. First, the relative amounts of the two receptor types are important. Even within the hippocampus, the amounts vary among the different subfields. For instance, pyramidal neurons in the CA1 region and granule cells in the dentate gyrus (see **Figure 1a**) express high amounts of both MRs and GRs. Pyramidal neurons in the CA3 region, however, have relatively low amounts of the GR. Second, the affinity of the receptor for the natural ligand, in combination with the availability of the ligand, plays an important role. The bio-availability in the hippocampus is not only determined by adrenal release of corticosterone, but also by factors such as the passage over membranes in which p-glycoproteins play a major role as well as the presence of converting enzymes such as 11β-hydroxysteroid dehydrogenase. Low levels of the ligand activate MRs extensively due to their high affinity, whereas the lower-affinity GRs are only partly occupied. GRs are fully activated only when corticosteroid levels are very high. These two factors are not static entities but are prone to regulation, for example, during prolonged periods of exposure to stress.

Once corticosteroids are bound to their receptor, the steroid–receptor complex dissociates from attached

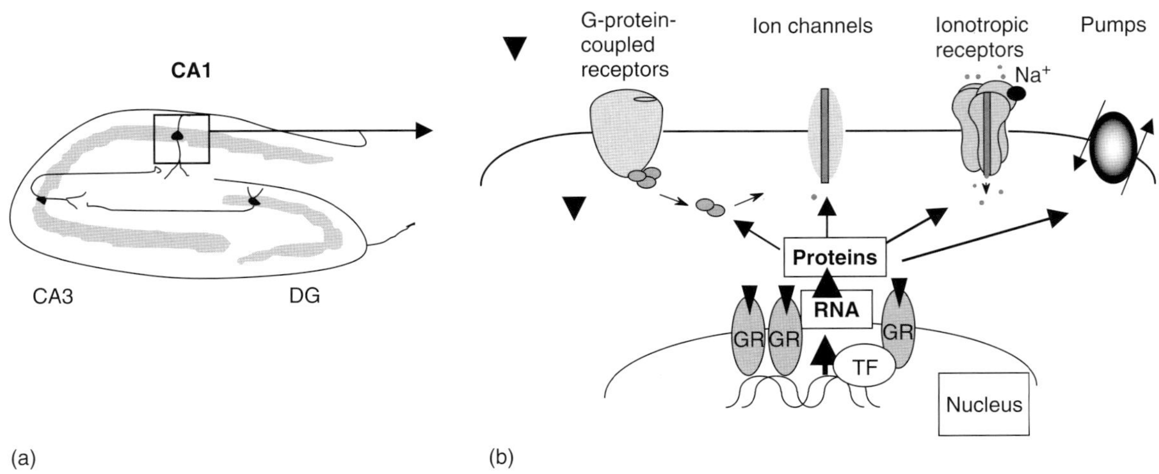

Figure 1 Corticosteroid effects on hippocampal cells. a, Representation of a hippocampal slice showing the main cellular subfields and the synaptic contacts between these subfields; b, Gene-mediated actions of corticosteroid hormones affecting the properties of hippocampal cells, aiming at various targets: ion channels, ionotropic receptors, G-protein-coupled receptors, and ion pumps. Intracellular corticosteroid receptors affect gene transcription either as homodimers binding directly to specific sequences in responsive genes or as monomers interacting with other transcription factors. CA1, cornus ammoni 1; CA3, cornus ammoni 3; DG, dentate gyrus; TF, transcription factor.

proteins and translocates to the nuclear compartment. Rapid cellular effects of corticosteroids that are not gene-mediated have recently been described in hippocampus, but are not discussed here. Classically, it was thought that all gene-mediated corticosteroid actions, including those in the brain, involve binding of receptor homodimers to hormone response elements in the DNA (**Figure 1b**). Indeed, all functional effects studied so far in hippocampal cells appear to require DNA-binding of GR homodimers. However, molecular investigations – including microarray surveys in the hippocampus – indicate that effects can also take place via the interactions of steroid receptor monomers with other transcription factors. A third possible mode of action, via the heterodimerization of MR and GR molecules, has been suggested based on studies in transfected cells in which (among other things) protein–protein interactions were examined. It is still undecided whether MR–GR heterodimers play a major role in the development of corticosteroid actions in the hippocampus.

Over the past years, much more has become known about the genes that form a target for corticosteroid action in the hippocampus, as surveyed with serial analysis of gene expression, microarrays, and single-cell RNA amplification of material from identified hippocampal cells. Thus, MR and GR activation each leads to altered expression of some 70–100 genes, of which roughly 50% was found to be upregulated and one-third were responsive to both receptor types. The hormone coordinates the expression of genes underlying aspects of energy metabolism, cell adhesion, synaptic transmission, oxidative stress, neurogenesis, cell cycle and structural plasticity. These transcriptional effects are likely to underlie cellular changes that have been observed, although the entire pathway has not yet been resolved for any of these. The functional data are in line with the molecular observations and indicate too that steroid-responsive genes may be involved in very diverse aspects of cellular function, such as cell structure and growth, energy metabolism, and membrane properties involved in signal transduction. Part of these cellular effects are summarized next.

Targets for Corticosteroid Action

Ion Channels

Under resting conditions, (passive) membrane properties of hippocampal CA1 and CA3 pyramidal cells are not affected by corticosteroid hormones. However, when the membrane potential of the cells is shifted from its resting level toward more depolarized or hyperpolarized levels (e.g., in response to a neurotransmitter), clear corticosteroid effects can be observed. These effects are generally slow in their onset and very persistent, which is in line with a gene-mediated mechanism of action. Patch clamp and intracellular studies have shown that some, although not all, of the ionic conductances in hippocampal cells are modulated by MR or GR activation. This underlines that the hormone actions are pleiotropic but nevertheless show a distinct degree of selectivity.

Three types of ion conductances have been investigated with regard to corticosteroid sensitivity: potassium (K^+), sodium (Na^+), and calcium (Ca^{2+}). Of these, voltage-dependent Ca^{2+} conductances are clearly most sensitive to corticosteroid receptor activation. It was found that low levels of corticosteroids resulting in a predominant MR activation are associated with small Ca^{2+} currents. If activation of GRs occurs in addition to MRs (e.g., after stress exposure) this results in an increased amplitude of Ca^{2+} currents compared to the situation in which mostly MRs are occupied. Several types of Ca^{2+} channels contribute to the overall Ca^{2+} currents in hippocampal cells. The steroids affect at least L-type Ca^{2+} channels, which cause the sustained current seen with large depolarizations of the cell, such as happen during an action potential. Only the amplitude of the currents and not the kinetic properties or voltage dependency is altered by corticosteroid treatment. Interestingly, in the absence of corticosterone, Ca^{2+} current amplitudes are also large, pointing to a U-shaped corticosteroid dose-dependency (see **Figure 2**). These data indicate that MR activation is necessary to retain Ca^{2+} currents within certain limits (a situation that is preferable for a neuron), whereas GR activation in addition to MR activation increases the Ca^{2+} influx into the hippocampal cells.

Steroid modulation of Ca^{2+} influx indirectly affects the slow Ca^{2+}-dependent K^+ conductance, which is extremely sensitive to the intracellular Ca^{2+} concentration. This conductance is slowly activated when neurons are depolarized for a considerable period of time (>100 ms) and causes accommodation of the firing frequency during depolarization; because the channels are also slowly deactivated, a lingering after-hyperpolarization (AHP) of the membrane is seen after the depolarizing influence is terminated. Both accommodation and AHP suppress the transmission of excitatory input to the hippocampal cells. In agreement with the small Ca^{2+} influx seen with predominant activation of MRs, it was found that accommodation and AHP under those conditions are relatively small, which promotes the transmission of excitatory input. With additional GR activation, accommodation and AHP are increased, leading to a temporary suppression of excitatory signals. Thus, hippocampal CA1 neurons in which mostly MRs are activated effectively transmit excitatory signals without being exposed to large intracellular Ca^{2+} levels. The large Ca^{2+} influx seen with additional GR activation is normally restrained because Ca-dependent K^+ conductances prevent large-scale depolarization. However, when GR activation is associated with extensive depolarization of neurons, such as occurs during epileptic or ischemic insults, cells are at high risk of being exposed to very high Ca^{2+} levels. This may partly explain why hippocampal cells show a more profound loss of function and integrity after hypoxia-ischema or epileptic seizures when corticosteroid levels are persistently elevated.

The K^+ and Na^+ conductances that were investigated appeared to be far less sensitive to corticosteroid receptor activation. Relatively minor effects were observed on the properties of the inwardly rectifying K^+ conductance I_h and on the fast, tetrodoxin (TTX)-sensitive Na^+ conductance. Other K^+ conductances, such as the delayed rectifier or transient A current, showed no steroid dependency at all in the hippocampus. Although the effects on voltage-dependent Na^+ and K^+ conductances are thus relatively small, they could still result in an altered shape of the action potential.

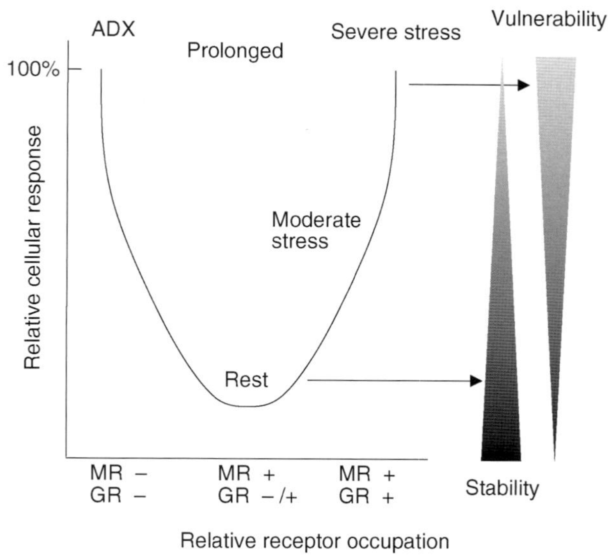

Figure 2 Many hippocampal cell properties, such as calcium currents, are large in the absence of adrenal steroids (adrenalectomy, ADX) or when both corticosteroid receptor types are extensively activated and are small with predominant MR activation. This results in a U-shaped corticosteroid dose-dependency, similar to what has been found for the potency to induce long-term depression versus long-term potentiation in the hippocampus. The relative MR and GR activation is indicated below the dose–response curve. Cellular responses associated with predominant MR occupation induce a situation of stability and resistance to degeneration. Additional GR activation (e.g., after a moderate stress) generally results in a temporary suppression of hippocampal cell activity, in agreement with the adaptive and normalizing role of this receptor in the stress response. The instability linked to GR activation can become deleterious when GR activation occurs concurrently with other challenging situations for the tissue, such as ischemia. Under these conditions, cellular vulnerability is increased if the relative GR to MR activation is high.

Neurotransmitter Responses

Based on chemical structure, three classes of neurotransmitters are recognized that affect the cellular function of hippocampal cells: amino acids, biogenic amines, and neuropeptides. Of these, the responses to biogenic amines appear to be most sensitive to corticosteroid receptor activation. Corticosteroid effects on amino acid-mediated transmission seem to be diverse and only partly gene-mediated. Neuropeptide actions have largely not been investigated in this respect.

The responses to serotonin (5-hydroxytryptamine, 5-HT) are strongly modulated by corticosteroid receptor activation. Serotonin can bind to several types of receptors on CA1 pyramidal neurons, including the 5-HT_{1A} receptor. The activation of this receptor leads, through G-protein-coupling, to the opening of K^+ channels, which results in a hyperpolarization of the membrane. With intracellular recording, it was found that the 5-HT_{1A} receptor-mediated hyperpolarization is small under conditions of predominant MR activation. This may be due to a MR-dependent downregulation of 5-HT_{1A} receptor mRNA expression, as was observed in the dentate gyrus and in some studies also in the CA1 region. The activation of GRs in addition to MRs (e.g., after exposure to a physical stressor) induces large 5-HT_{1A} receptor-mediated responses. The molecular mechanism underlying these large responses is unclear because 5-HT_{1A} receptor expression and binding are not increased after GR activation. Potential targets for steroid modulation downstream of the 5-HT_{1A} receptor are probably also not modulated because steroid actions on the G-protein function or the K^+ channel opened by the G-proteins cannot explain the changes in 5-HT_{1A} response. In addition to modulation of 5-HT_{1A} receptor-mediated responses, corticosteroids also affect responses or expression of 5-HT_4 and 5-HT_7 receptors.

Depolarizing responses mediated via muscarinic acetylcholine receptors appear to have a similar steroid dependency. Because both serotoninergic and cholinergic responses are relatively large in the absence of corticosteroid hormones, there seems to be a U-shaped dose-dependency for the transmitter responses, as in the case of Ca^{2+} conductances (see **Figure 2**). This may signify the existence of a common denominator underlying all these steroid effects. It is possible that corticosteroid receptor activation results in the altered activity of kinases or phosphatases, which affect several membrane components in a comparable way through posttranslational modifications. This does not exclude the development of steroid actions aiming at specific genes. This is supported by the observation that responses to norepinephrine, mediated by β1-adrenoceptors, show an inverse linear steroid dose-dependency rather than the U-shape.

Whereas the steroid modulation of biogenic amine responses is slow in onset, persistent, and requires *de novo* protein synthesis, steroid effects on amino acid-mediated responses seem to have different features. This was mostly investigated by examining the steroid modulation of synaptically evoked responses in the CA1 hippocampal region. The stimulation of Schaffer/commissural fibers in this region leads to a subsequent activation of glutamatergic AMPA and NMDA receptors. It was found that the administration of very high amounts of corticosterone, resulting in concomitant MR and GR occupancy, suppresses field responses mediated by glutamate receptors. With these very high doses of corticosterone a rapid onset of effects is seen and the effects are very prominent when extracellular Ca^{2+} concentrations are high. Moreover, the steroid effects are particularly evident after the repeated stimulation of the afferent pathway. The data suggest that under these circumstances energy-dependent processes in the signal transduction and cellular integrity may be impaired. When glutamate transmission is recorded under more physiological conditions (i.e., comparable to the design used to study effects on ion currents and aminergic responses), a slow GR-mediated enhancement rather than impairment of the responsiveness to synaptic stimulation becomes apparent.

Inhibitory responses mediated by $GABA_A$ receptors are affected only by extreme (and probably physiologically not relevant) doses of corticosterone. $GABA_B$ receptor-mediated responses were found to be stable with predominant MR activation, but declined rapidly with repeated stimulation both in the absence of steroids and in the presence of very high amounts of corticosterone.

Changes in Network Properties

The corticosteroid effects on the properties of individual hippocampal cells or small groups of cells clearly alter the function of hippocampal networks in which these cells participate. In addition, corticosteroid hormones could change network properties that depend critically on the connections and associative contacts between cells in a network.

Examples of processes that depend both on the characteristics of individual hippocampal cells and on the connections between cells are LTP and LTD. The former refers to the situation in which the high-frequency stimulation of afferents results in a prolonged strengthening of synaptic contacts. The fact that LTP is induced rapidly in hippocampal subfields, persists for hours to days, and involves associativity of inputs has led to the hypothesis that LTP may be the neurobiological substrate for learning and memory, although a direct link is still disputed. Stimulating hippocampal pathways at a lower frequency can lead to LTD, the weakening of synaptic contacts. The processes of LTP and LTD each require specific intracellular signaling cascades, phosphorylation targets, and Ca^{2+} levels. In nonstressed animals, LTP can be induced easily with high-frequency stimulation, whereas homosynaptic LTD is relatively hard to obtain.

Many studies over the past decade have demonstrated that MR and GR activation largely affect the likelihood to evoke LTP and LTD. Both in the dentate gyrus and in the CA1 region, conditions that result in the near-complete activation of MRs and only partial activation of GRs are associated with a very efficient induction and maintenance of LTP. When GRs are activated extensively, it becomes hard to evoke LTP, whereas LTD induction is promoted. In the absence of corticosteroid hormones, LTP induction is also suppressed. The degree of potentiation therefore shows an inverted U-shaped steroid dose-dependency, which points to an underlying process that may be common to and perhaps evolve from the steroid actions on Ca^{2+} influx and responses to neurotransmitters such as serotonin.

These observations, generally obtained by administering exogenous corticosterone or selective agonists or antagonists for the corticosteroid receptors, can be extended to behaviorally relevant situations. Thus, several studies have shown that the exposure of animals to stressors that are unpredictable and out of the context of a learning experience suppresses the likelihood of inducing LTP and instead allows the induction of LTD. Even less extreme situations, such as the subjection of animals to a novel environment out of the context of a learning experience, led to a similar suppression of LTP and promotion of LTD. Stress effects on LTP and LTD are sometimes quite rapid in onset and not always associated with extensive changes in GR activation. This indicates that a shift in the likelihood of evoking LTP depends not only on the actual MR–GR occupation but also on other factors, such as the recent history of the postsynaptic cells, which may be influenced by other stress hormones as well, such as norepinephrine and corticotropin releasing hormone (CRH). In the intact organism, the effects of corticosteroids on synaptic plasticity are also determined by the degree to which multiple brain regions, such as the prefrontal cortex and amygdala nuclei, are involved, which in turn depends on the nature of the stressor.

Cellular Effects after Chronic Hypo- or Hypercorticism

The corticosteroid effects on cellular properties and network function described previously, are generally observed over a period of several hours after a change in MR/GR occupation. It is therefore very likely (and this has indeed been demonstrated in several cases) that these effects on hippocampal function take place shortly after exposure to an acute stressful situation. Increased corticosterone levels after stress, resulting in GR activation on top of already activated MRs, evokes an array of effects, most of which temporarily suppress the transmittal of excitatory signals (see **Table 1**). These GR-mediated events may help restore hippocampal function following stress, which is in accordance with the normalizing and adaptive mode by which GRs participate in the stress response.

Although large variations in MR activation probably do not take place under physiological conditions, data nevertheless show that MRs play an important role in hippocampal function. First, MRs seem to be important for the full development of GR-mediated events (and vice versa). Second, MR activation is essential for maintaining a basal level of hippocampal activity (see **Table 1**). And MR activation is even a prerequisite for neuronal viability. This is most evident in granule cells of the dentate gyrus. Dentate granule cells proliferate from progenitor cells even in adulthood and after some time die through apoptosis. There is a continuous balance between the incorporation of newly formed cells and the removal of old cells. When rats are adrenalectomized, this balance is disturbed, so that 3 or more days after adrenalectomy proliferation is increased but also more cells undergo apoptosis. In adrenalectomized rats undergoing apoptosis, the synaptic transmission as well as the plasticity between the entorhinal cortex and the dentate gyrus is impaired. The functional impairment most likely occurs prior to and independent of the change in cell turnover and may in fact form a trigger for an overall synaptic reorganization in the dentate. The impaired synaptic function, as well as the changes in cell turnover, can be prevented by treating animals with MR ligands. The fate of an individual cell also appears to be determined by its

Table 1 Cellular effects observed with predominant MR activation or with concurrent MR and GR activation[a]

	Excitability ↑	*Excitability* ↓
MR activation	Accommodation/AHP ↓ $5\text{-}HT_{1A}$ receptor response ↓ Glutamatergic response ↑ LTP ↑	Carbachol responses ↓
MR + GR activation	$GABA_B$ response ↓ Glutamate release (?)↑ Carbachol responses ↑	Accommodation/AHP ↑ $5\text{-}HT_{1A}$ receptor response ↑ β-Adrenergic response ↓ Glutamate response ↓ LTD ↑, LTP ↓

[a]AHP, after-hyperpolarization; GR, glucocorticoid receptor; LTD, long-term depression; LTP, long-term potentiation; MR, mineralocorticoid receptor.

specific gene expression pattern. The data indicate that relatively young dentate cells can increase the expression of proteins that will help them survive, whereas older cells fail to do so, explaining why destabilizing factors such as enhanced calcium influx or impaired synaptic communication, seen in the absence of corticosterone, can become deleterious. Collectively, normal MR function in the dentate gyrus seems to be important in preserving the delicate balance between viability and cell death.

Although prolonged deprivation of corticosteroids is a threat for dentate granule cell survival, chronic overexposure of the hippocampus to corticosteroid hormones is also potentially harmful. Exposure of rats to 3 weeks of restraint stress causes atrophy of apical dendrites in CA3 pyramidal neurons. Under these conditions, both the presynaptic nerve terminals and the postsynaptic spine density in the CA3 area are altered. Chronic stress also decreases proliferation in the dentate gyrus and in fact may slow down the entire cell cycle for a considerable period of time, possibly by changing the expression of endogenous factors involved in the cell cycle. In addition to (or perhaps related to) the morphological effects, other hippocampal properties are also altered after chronic stress. Glutamate transmission is enhanced both in the CA3 area and dentate gyrus. Conversely, LTP is markedly impaired in all hippocampal subareas. Interestingly, 5-HT_{1A} receptor-mediated responses become gradually attenuated after chronic stress or prolonged overexposure to corticosterone. This may be one explanation for the increased risk of mood disturbances after prolonged hypercortisolemia.

The mechanisms underlying the changes in hippocampal morphology and cell turnover after chronic stress exposure are largely unknown. The observed enhancement in glutamate transmission may be a causative factor, but clearly sequential regulation of many gene targets, including genes encoding for corticosteroid receptors and chaperones, enzymes, structural proteins, cell cycle factors, and growth factors, in concert determines the outcome of the process. Understanding this sequence of events will be one of the challenges for the future. It is already clear that the cellular actions induced by repeated overexposure to corticosterone are not a simple extrapolation of the effects seen after an acute rise in corticosteroid level. Also, in the hippocampus there is no evidence for steroid resistance – generally effects are strongest when chronic stress is combined with an acute rise in the level of corticosterone. Insight into these fundamental processes as well as the potential to intervene with pharmacological treatment (e.g., by applying antiglucocorticoids) will be essential for novel treatment strategies of stress-related disorders involving hippocampal dysfunction.

See Also the Following Articles

Corticosteroid Receptors; Neurogenesis.

Further Reading

Datson, N. A., van der Perk, J., de Kloet, E. R., et al. (2001). Identification of corticosteroid-responsive genes in rat hippocampus using serial analysis of gene expression. *European Journal of Neuroscience* **14**, 675–689.

De Kloet, E. R., Joëls, M. and Holsboer, F. (2005). Stress and the brain: from adaptation to disease. *Nature Reviews Neuroscience* **6**, 463–475.

Gould, E. and Tanapat, P. (1999). Stress and hippocampal neurogenesis. *Biological Psychiatry* **46**, 1472–1479.

Karst, H., Karten, Y. J., Reichardt, H. M., et al. (2000). Corticosteroid actions in hippocampus require DNA binding of glucocorticoid receptor homodimers. *Nature Neuroscience* **3**, 977–978.

Kim, J. J. and Diamond, D. M. (2002). The stressed hippocampus, synaptic plasticity and lost memories. *Nature Reviews Neuroscience* **3**, 453–462.

Kole, M. H., Swan, L. and Fuchs, E. (2002). The antidepressant tianeptine persistently modulates glutamate receptor currents of the hippocampal CA3 commissural associational synapse in chronically stressed rats. *European Journal of Neuroscience* **16**, 807–816.

Korz, V. and Frey, J. U. (2003). Stress-related modulation of hippocampal long-term potentiation in rats: involvement of adrenal steroid receptors. *Journal of Neuroscience* **23**, 7281–7287.

Maroun, M. and Richter-Levin, G. (2003). Exposure to acute stress blocks the induction of long-term potentiation of the amygdala-prefrontal cortex pathway *in vivo*. *Journal of Neuroscience* **23**, 4406–4409.

McEwen, B. S. (1999). Stress and hippocampal plasticity. *Annual Review of Neuroscience* **22**, 105–122.

Shakesby, A. C., Anwyl, R. and Rowan, M. J. (2002). Overcoming the effects of stress on synaptic plasticity in the intact hippocampus: rapid actions of serotonergic and antidepressant agents. *Journal of Neuroscience* **22**, 3638–3644.

Memory and Stress

S J Lupien
McGill University and Geriatric Institute of Montreal, Montreal, Canada
F S Maheu
National Institute of Mental Health, Bethesda, MD, USA

This is a revised version of the article by S J Lupien and S Brière, Encyclopedia of Stress, First edition, volume 2, pp 721–727, © 2000, Elsevier Inc.

Glossary

Acute stress Mental or bodily tension resulting from internal or external factors that tend to alter the existing equilibrium.

Arousal A condition that varies in a continuum from a low point in sleep to a high point represented by intense excitement.

Emotion A state of excited feeling of any kind. Basic emotions presumably are universal, are biologically based, are present from infancy, and have associated facial expressions and primitive action scripts. Basic emotions include love, joy, anger, sadness, and fear.

Stress response The total set of reactions to the stressor.

Stressor Any physical or psychological agent that causes the disequilibrium. Physical stressors are situations that can operate in the absence of consciousness and include disturbances of the internal environment (anoxia, hypoglycemia, etc.), external extremes (heat and cold), and physical strain (exercise or injury). Psychological stressors are situations for which there is a consciously perceived potential for harm and include stimuli that affect emotion and result in fear, anxiety, or frustration.

Emotion, Stress, and Memory

Emotionally arousing and stressful experiences are often cited as the cause of many psychological and physical problems. Many of us have experienced emotionally arousing and stressful experiences at one point or another of our life and have noted that these experiences can have important effects on our memory. Declarative memory, which is the type of memory we refer to during the course of this article, is defined as the conscious or voluntary recollection of previously learned information. We can have forgotten an important meeting or anniversary due to work overload, or else we can have a vivid recollection of a car accident or any other emotionally arousing experience. Because of their impact on our lives, we have a tendency to pay more attention to the negative effects of stress on our memory and to forget that, under certain conditions, emotionally arousing and stressful experiences can also have a positive impact on memory function. The goal of this article is to describe the positive and negative effects of emotionally arousing and stressful experiences on memory function and to delineate the psychological and biological determinants of these effects.

Emotion and Stress: Two Different Entities?

Emotion and stress share many characteristics. A stressful experience will often cause a particular emotion (e.g., surprise, fear, or joy), and particular emotions can create stressful situations (e.g., blushing due to extreme timidity can cause a stressful situation). Moreover, an emotion possesses many of the properties of a stressor. First, it often has an identifiable source. Second, it is usually brief and leads to an intense and conscious experience of short duration. Finally, an emotion creates bodily reactions (e.g., increase in heart rate or perspiration) that are similar to those induced by a stressor, and both states act by increasing arousal. Because of these similarities between emotion and stress, most of the literature on emotion, stress, and memory intermixes the effects of emotion and those of stress on memory function. However, emotion and stress are two different entities. Although a stressful experience will almost always trigger a specific emotion, a particular emotion does not always elicit a stress reaction. As far as laboratory setting is concerned, emotion and stress differ in the way they are induced and, thus, in the way they influence memory in humans. Hence, emotions are usually induced by the presentation of emotional words, films, or pictures, whereas stress is usually induced by putting the individual in a social situation known to create a stress (e.g., public speaking). Because of this important difference between the experimental paradigms used to measure the effects of emotion and stress on memory, different questions have been asked. The induction of emotion has been used to measure memory for emotionally arousing events, whereas the induction of stress has been used to measure the specific effects of stress on subsequent memory function.

Memory for Emotionally Arousing Events

It is well known that what we encode and remember from an event depends primarily on the attention that we devoted to this event and its components. If we do not pay attention to what we are reading right now, there is less chance that we will remember it at a later time than if we gave all our attention to a lecture. This is because the more attention given to an event, the higher the probability that this event will be elaborated (relating the information from this event to other situations and related concepts in memory) at the time of encoding. Research on memory has shown that events that are poorly elaborated (shallow processing) at the time of encoding are remembered less well than events that are deeply elaborated (deep processing) at the time of encoding.

The level of attention devoted to an event at the time of encoding will greatly depend on the emotional salience of this event. Most of us remember what we were doing and with whom we were at the time we learned about the World Trade Center attacks, but the majority of us may have difficulty remembering what we were doing and with whom we were 13 days before or after the attacks. This flashbulb phenomenon may be explained by the fact that the emotion (e.g., surprise or anger) that was triggered by the announcement of the World Trade Center attacks directed the totality of our attention to the event, leading to a deeper elaboration and, thus, to an optimization of our memory for this event.

Memory for Central versus Peripheral Details

Studies of trauma victims have reported how vividly the traumatic event is recalled in the absence of any memory for information surrounding the traumatic event. A closely analogous situation appears in the field of law enforcement and describes the weapon focus phenomenon. Witnesses to violent crimes demonstrate a weapon focus effect in which the weapon captures most of the victim's attention, resulting in a reduced ability to recall other details of the scene and to recognize the assailant at a later time. This phenomenon has been explained by Easterbrook's cue utilization theory, which suggests that emotionally arousing events narrow subjects' attention and lead them to attend only to the center of an event and to exclude more peripheral information. In general, laboratory experiments have confirmed this hypothesis. For example, as reported by Christianson, subjects viewed a series of slides in which the emotional valence of one critical slide in the series was varied. In the neutral version, the critical slide showed a woman riding a bicycle. In the emotional version, the same woman was seen lying injured on the street near the bicycle. In both versions, a peripheral car was seen in the distant background. The results showed that the central detail information (woman and bicycle) was retained better in the emotional condition but that the peripheral information (car in background) was retained better in the neutral event. In general, the pattern of results obtained from various studies shows that the central aspects of an emotional event (those events in the scope of attention) are well retained in memory, whereas memory for peripheral details (out of the scope of attention) are poorly remembered. Recently, Cahill and collaborators pushed this analysis further and reported gender-related influences in the recall of central versus peripheral information from an emotional story. Men and women with high male-related traits on the Bem Sex-Role Inventory show better memory for central aspects of an emotional story, as opposed to peripheral details. On the other hand, women and men with high female-related traits on the Bem Sex-Role Inventory have a better memory for peripheral details of an emotional story, as opposed to central information.

Immediate versus Delayed Memory for Emotional Events

Studies have examined the relation among emotion, retention interval, and memory. What these studies have shown so far is that emotionally arousing events delay forgetting. In a highly cited 1963 study, Kleinsmith and Kaplan presented subjects with pairs of words to learn. Some of the words were neutral, whereas others had a strong emotionally negative component (e.g., rape, mutilation). The memory of the word pairs was tested 2 min or 1 week after presentation. Memory performance tested shortly after learning (i.e., short-term declarative memory) generally refers to consolidation processes occurring within the first 3 h after learning (i.e., early phase), whereas memory performance tested after an extensive delay (i.e., long-term declarative memory) generally refers to the consolidation processes taking place 3 h postlearning (i.e., late phase) and that persist for at least a day and involve gene transcription and protein synthesis. Kleinsmith and Kaplan's study showed that at short intervals memory was poorer for emotional words, but at long intervals memory was better for emotional words. These results have been replicated many times, and the majority of studies have shown enhanced memory for emotionally arousing material, provided that memory is tested at longer retention intervals.

Possible Mechanisms Underlying the Increased Memory for Emotionally Arousing Events

Psychological as well as biological mechanisms have been suggested to explain how emotionally arousing events might enhance memory. At the psychological level, one of the most frequently cited references on the relation between emotionally arousing events and memory is the Yerkes–Dodson law. In a series of studies published in 1908, Yerkes and Dodson reported that arousal improved performance in a linear manner for easy tasks, whereas for difficult tasks they found that an inverted-U-shaped curve related better performance with medium arousal and worse performance with low or high arousal. However, many field and laboratory studies suggest that individuals retain information from high arousing events quite well, a finding that goes against the Yerkes–Dodson law predictions. Thus, Easterbrook nuanced Yerkes–Dodson arousal hypothesis, suggesting the cue utilization theory. According to this theory, increased arousal due to emotionally arousing events acts by narrowing attention to the central details of a scene, leading to better recall of central details compared to peripheral details. Based on this model, Cahill recently suggested that men's ability to better remember central emotional information was attributable to their higher use of the right amygdala when processing emotional material (the right brain hemisphere being biased for a global/holistic analysis of the information). On the other hand, women's remembering more precisely peripheral emotional information was attributable to their higher use of the left amygdala during the processing of emotional material (the left brain hemisphere being biased for local, finer analysis of the information).

Finally, Walker used the arousal hypothesis in conjunction with Hebb's concept of reverberating circuits in order to explain the retention interval effect of emotional memory. He suggested that emotional information, because it creates a high level of arousal at the time of learning, produces a more active consolidation process and leads to a stronger memory trace and better recall at longer intervals. In contrast, because it creates a high level of arousal, emotional information also acts by inhibiting recall at shorter interval due to the fact that the process of consolidation is active (and thus inaccessible) at this time.

Contrary to psychological explanations, biological explanations of memory for emotionally arousing events have presented extensive data indicating that emotionally arousing experiences produce a retrograde enhancement of memory for that experience via a variety of hormones released during these experiences. Hence, during emotionally arousing events, there is a secretion of the peripheral catecholamines epinephrine and norepinephrine by the adrenal medulla, a secretion of central norepinephrine by the locus ceruleus and a secretion of corticosteroids by the adrenal glands. The peripheral catecholamines enhance memory by reaching the vagus nerve, nucleus of the solitary tract, and locus ceruleus. Central norepinephrine is then secreted by the locus ceruleus, activating noradrenergic neurons throughout the brain. Significantly, central norepinephrine is also triggered as soon as an emotionally arousing event occurs, independently of peripheral catecholamines. Corticosteroids, being liposoluble, enhance memory by easily crossing the blood–brain barrier and reaching the brain. Adrenergic hormones and corticosteroids may facilitate memory consolidation for emotional information through their interactions with noradrenergic and corticosteroid receptors located in the amygdala, which, in turn, modulates hippocampal activity and enhances consolidation for emotionally arousing material.

Animal and human studies have confirmed the role of these hormones in the memory-modulating effects of emotionally arousing events. Thus, in rodents postlearning stimulation of the noradrenergic system enhances (but postlearning blockade inhibits) long-term declarative memory of an inhibitory avoidance task. Likewise, posttraining injections of moderate doses of synthetic corticosteroids enhance and pretraining corticosteroid synthesis inhibition impairs long-term expression of inhibitory avoidance in animals. In humans, prelearning blockade of central β-adrenergic receptors or prelearning corticosteroid synthesis inhibition impairs long-term declarative memory for emotionally arousing material, whereas prelearning or postlearning stimulation of the noradrenergic or corticosteroid systems enhances it. Although psychological and biological explanations of the arousal hypothesis were used to explain the positive effects of emotion on memory function, research performed to this day shows that arousal is significant as an intervening variable only when the source of the arousal (in this case, the emotionally arousing event) is directly related to the information to be remembered. As we will see next, when the source of emotion is not directly related to the information to be remembered, other psychological and biological mechanisms come into play and have a stronger impact on memory function than arousal itself.

Memory after Stress

Influences of Acute Stress on Subsequent Memory Function and Possible Psychological Effects Underlying These Influences

Remembering with great accuracy a particular emotionally arousing event is very different from performing various tasks involving memory in a day-to-day situation when we are faced with stress. We may remember with great accuracy the events in our lives surrounding the World Trade Center attacks, but we may also have forgotten the anniversary of a loved one due to work stress. Originally, the effects of a stressor on subsequent declarative memory for material unrelated to the source of stress were studied using noise as a stressor. Indeed, human beings possess a limited amount of attention that can be allocated to a particular task at any one time. Information overload is said to occur when this capacity is exceeded, that is, when there is too much information to process at the same time. When this happens, the individual may have difficulty discriminating between and attending to the relevant and irrelevant information to encode new events in memory. Studies measuring the effects of noise on memory reported that noise impairs the recall of the information encoded at the time of noise stress. This result has been interpreted as showing that noise acts by overloading the limited processing capacity of the individual, leading to impairments in processing task-relevant stimuli because of an increased distraction induced by task-irrelevant stimuli (in this case, noise). Because the individual is unable to discriminate between relevant and irrelevant information when under noise stress, memory impairment appears and is represented by a poorer recall of task-relevant stimuli.

Effects of Acute Stress on Subsequent Memory Function and Possible Physiological Mechanisms Underlying These Effects

In order to better understand the mechanisms by which stress might modulate subsequent memory processing of material unrelated to the source of the stressor, researchers aimed at defining and understanding, more specifically, memory processing, stress-related physiological activation, and the links between these two. Research over the past 40 years revealed that memory is not a unitary and passive process. In the field of cognitive psychology, the individual is viewed as being active, constructive, and organized, not as being a passive recipient of environmental stimulation or overstimulation. Thus, the individual is seen as actively constructing a view of reality, as selectively choosing some aspects of experience for further attention, and as attempting to commit some of that information to memory. Hence, to better understand the influence of stress on subsequent memory processing of information unrelated to the stressor, it is thus necessary to determine the series of stages that make up the given act of memorization and to measure the exact effects of stress on specific components of this information processing system. Declarative memory is temporally defined in three phases; information must first be attended to (arousal and attentional processes) and encoded (short-term/working memory; phase 1) before it is consolidated (phase 2) into long-term memory and recalled (phase 3).

Physiological mechanisms have been suggested to explain the effects of stress on memory phases. The brain is the organ that gives an interpretation to a stressful experience, and it is also responsible for mounting the physiological response to the stressor. Important physiological components of the stress response include the hypothalamic-pituitary-adrenal (HPA) axis (with corticosteroids being the end product), the sympathoadrenal system, and the central noradrenergic system. The HPA axis, along with the sympathoadrenal system, governs metabolic responses to the slings and arrows of everyday life. Both these systems support a range of metabolic responses that serve to ensure the availability of sufficient energy substrates in circulation during periods when there is inevitably increased cellular activity in vital organs and an accompanying increase in the requirement for fuel. The corticosteroid system and the central noradrenergic system have been studied in relation with the memory-modulating effects of stress because these two systems, when activated, can modulate activity in noradrenergic and corticosteroid receptors in the frontal lobes, hippocampus, and amygdala, three brain structures involved in declarative memory processes.

Rodent studies have shown that when a laboratory stressor (e.g., tail shocks, water immersion, or restraint stress) is administered at various times before or after learning, as well as before recall, stress-induced elevations in corticosteroid levels modulate declarative memory according to an inverted-U-shaped function. Optimal declarative memory for material unrelated to the stressor (e.g., inhibitory avoidance protocols or spatial water-maze tasks) occur at moderate levels of stress and stress-induced increases in circulating corticosteroid levels, whereas lower (i.e., boredom or drowsiness) or higher stress levels and stress-induced increases in circulating corticosteroid levels are less effective or may even impair declarative memory performance on these tasks.

In humans, when a laboratory stressor (e.g., a public speaking task combined with a public arithmetic task) is administered before learning or retrieval, high corticosteroid levels following stress are associated with memory impairments for material unrelated to the stressor, such as neutral words lists. Recently, studies measuring the influence of stress on memory for emotional material unrelated to the stressor reported more heterogeneous findings. Thus, when a laboratory stressor was presented before learning or retrieval of emotional and neutral information unrelated to the stressor, high corticosteroid levels following stress were associated with memory impairments for emotional information (whether positive or negative), whereas they had no influence on memory for neutral material. However, two other studies showed that stress administered before or after learning enhanced memory for emotional material, whereas it had no impact or impaired subsequent memory for neutral information.

Altogether, these results show that stress-related elevations in corticosteroids can have different effects on subsequent memory for material unrelated to the stressor. The effects of emotionally arousing and/or stressful events on declarative memory vary according to the nature of the material to be remembered, with elevated levels of corticosteroids enhancing memory for the emotionally arousing event itself but leading, more often than not, to memory impairments for material unrelated to the source of the stressor.

The time of day (morning vs. afternoon) and levels of circulating corticosteroids at the time of testing could also be important factors influencing the effects of stress-related elevations in corticosteroids on subsequent memory for material unrelated to the stressor. Corticosteroid receptors differ in terms of their affinity for circulating levels of corticosteroids. Mineralocorticoid receptors (MRs) have a 6- to 10-time higher affinity for corticosteroids than glucocorticoid receptors (GRs). A wealth of evidence now demonstrates that the activation of MRs is mandatory for the successful acquisition of environmental cues necessary to encode information, whereas the activation of GRs is necessary for the long-term memory consolidation of this information.

Endogenous levels of corticosteroids and, thus, the activation of the MRs and GRs, significantly vary during the day, with higher endogenous levels of corticosteroids in the morning (AM) phase than in the evening (PM) phase. Consequently, the addition of a stressful and emotionally arousing event, which by itself will trigger a significant increase in the endogenous levels of corticosteroids, should have a differential impact on the activation of MRs and GRs as a function of time of day. In the AM phase, most of the MRs and approximately half of the GRs are activated, whereas, in the PM phase, most of the MRs and about one-tenth of the GRs are activated. If we apply a stressor in the AM phase, the endogenous increase in corticosteroid levels will act by saturating GRs, but the same stressor applied in the PM phase will act by activating approximately half of the GRs. Because stress-induced elevations in corticosteroid levels have been shown to modulate declarative memory for material unrelated to the stressor according to an inverted-U-shaped function, the differential activation of MRs and GRs at different times of the day imply that a stressor applied in the morning should impair memory function (right-hand-side of the inverted U-shaped curve), whereas the same stressor applied in the PM phase should increase or have no impact on memory (left-hand-side or top of the inverted-U-shaped curve). Moreover, given that stress has differential effects as a function of the emotional valence of the material to be learned, it can be suggested that the application of a stressor in the AM versus PM phase should have a different effect on memory for emotionally arousing or neutral information unrelated to the source of the stressor.

Individual differences could also be an important factor explaining the discrepancy in the effects of stress-related elevations in corticosteroids on subsequent memory for material unrelated to the stressor. Indeed, high and low corticosteroid responders can show different memory performance following stress. Individual differences could be attributable to genetic factors, corticosteroid sensitivity differences and lifespan cortisol exposure differences, gender, or personality.

Finally, very few studies measured the influence of the central noradrenergic system, activated following stress, on subsequent memory for material unrelated to the stressor. Animal studies reported that stress-induced elevations in norepinephrine levels (following foot shocks) modulate declarative memory according to an inverted-U-shaped function, with optimal levels enhancing (and lower or higher levels of norepinephrine impairing) memory for information unrelated to the source of stress (e.g., passive aversive conditioning). In humans, one recent study showed that the blockade of peripheral and central noradrenergic β receptors before the administration of a stressor did not impair memory for material unrelated to the source of stress. These results suggest that the β-adrenergic system is not implicated in the effects of stress on subsequent declarative memory function, contrasting with the well-established role of this system during the memorization of events that are emotionally arousing in nature. Further studies in humans are needed to determine the exact role played by the central noradrenergic system in the effects of stress on subsequent memory for information unrelated to the stressor.

Conclusion

In sum, important differences in mnemonic performance exist between memory for emotionally arousing events and memory for material unrelated to a stressor that is processed after stress. Interestingly, whether the subject is memorizing the emotionally arousing event itself or material unrelated to the stressor, both the central noradrenergic system and the corticosteroid system are at play, although they seem to act differently in the recall of neutral and emotional information. Experimental factors (e.g., nature of material to remember and time of day) and individual differences (e.g., personality and genetics) are also important components to consider because they can all influence the direction of the effects of emotion and stress on memory. Future studies considering and controlling for these factors and measuring the interactive and/or differential effects of the noradrenergic and corticosteroid systems should prove highly valuable to our understanding of the effects of emotionally arousing and stressful experiences on human declarative memory processes.

See Also the Following Articles

Corticosteroids and Stress; Glucocorticoid Effects on Memory: the Positive and the Negative.

Further Reading

Abercrombie, H. C., Kalin, N. H., Thurow, M. E., et al. (2003). Cortisol variation in humans affects memory for emotionally-laden and neutral information. *Behavioral Neuroscience* **117**, 505–516.

Arnsten, A. F. T. (2000). Through the looking glass: differential noradrenergic modulation of prefrontal cortical function. *Neural Plasticity* **7**, 133–144.

Buchanan, T. W. and Lovallo, W. R. (2001). Enhanced memory for emotional material following stress-level cortisol treatment in humans. *Psychoneuroendocrinology* **26**, 307–317.

Cahill, L. (2003). Sex-related influences on the neurobiology of emotionally influenced memory. *Annals of the New York Academy of Science* **985**, 163–173.

Cahill, L. and Alkire, M. T. (2003). Epinephrine enhancement of human memory consolidation: interaction with arousal at encoding. *Neurobiology of Learning and Memory* **79**, 194–198.

Cahill, L., Gorski, L. and Le, K. (2003). Enhanced human memory consolidation with post-learning stress: interaction with the degree of arousal at encoding. *Learning and Memory* **10**, 270–274.

Cahill, L., Gorski, L., Belcher, A., et al. (2004). The influence of sex versus sex-related traits on long-term memory for gist and detail from an emotional story. *Consciousness and Cognition* **13**, 391–400.

Christianson, S. A. (1992). Emotional stress and eyewitness memory: a critical review. *Psychological Bulletin* **112**, 284–309.

Domes, G., Heinrichs, M., Reichwald, U., et al. (2002). Hypothalamic-pituitary-adrenal axis reactivity to psychological stress and memory in middle-aged women: high responders exhibit enhanced declarative memory performance. *Psychoneuroendo-crinology* **27**, 843–853.

Domes, G., Heinrichs, M., Rimmele, U., et al. (2004). Acute stress impairs recognition for positive words – association with stress-induced cortisol secretion. *Stress* **7**, 173–181.

Easterbrook, J. A. (1959). The effect of emotion on cue utilization and the organization of behavior. *Psychological Review* **66**, 183–201.

Elzinga, B. M., Bakker, A. and Bremner, J. D. (2005). Stress-induced cortisol elevations are associated with impaired delayed, but not immediate recall. *Psychiatry Research* **134**, 211–223.

Golberger, L. and Breznitz, S. (1993). Handbook of Stress: Theoretical and Clinical Aspects (2nd Edition). New York: Free Press.

Jelicic, M., Geraerts, E., Merckelbach, H., et al. (2004). Acute stress enhances memory for emotional words, but impairs memory for neutral words. *International Journal of Neuroscience* **114**, 1343–1351.

Kandel, E. R. (2001). The molecular biology of memory storage: a dialogue between genes and synapses. *Science* **294**, 1030–1038.

Kleinsmith, L. J. and Kaplan, S. (1963). Paired associate learning as a function of arousal and interpolated interval. *Journal of Experimental Psychology* **65**, 190–193.

Kuhlmann, S., Piel, M. and Wolf, O. T. (2005). Impaired memory retrieval after psychological stress in healthy young men. *Journal of Neuroscience* **25**, 2977–2982.

Lupien, S. J., Fiocco, A., Wan, N., et al. (2005). Stress hormones and human memory function across the lifespan. *Psychoneuroendocrinology* **30**, 225–242.

Maheu, F. S., Joober, R., Beaulieu, S., et al. (2004). Differential effects of adrenergic and corticosteroid hormonal systems on human short- and long-term declarative memory for emotionally arousing material. *Behavioral Neuroscience* **118**, 420–428.

Maheu, F. S., Joober, R. and Lupien, S. J. (2005). Declarative memory after stress in humans: differential involvement of the β-adrenergic and corticosteroid systems. *Journal of Clinical Endocrinology and Metabolism* **90**, 1697–1704.

Maheu, F. S., Collicutt, P., Kornik, R., et al. (2005). The perfect time to be stressed: a differential modulation of human memory by stress applied in the morning or in the afternoon. *Progress Neuropsychopharmacology and Biological Psychiatry* **29**(8), 1281–1288.

McGaugh, J. L. (2000). Memory – a century of consolidation. *Science* **287**, 248–251.

Milner, B., Squire, L. R. and Kandel, E. R. (1998). Cognitive neuroscience and the study of memory. *Neuron* **20**, 445–468.

Reul, J. M. H. M. and de Kloet, E. R. (1985). Two receptor systems for corticosterone in rat brain: microdistribution and differential occupation. *Endocrinology* **117**, 2505–2512.

Roozendaal, B. (2002). Stress and memory: opposing effects of glucocorticoids on memory consolidation and memory retrieval. *Neurobiology of Learning and Memory* **78**, 578–595.

Sauro, M. D., Jorgensen, R. S. and Teal Pedlow, C. (2003). Stress, glucocorticoids, and memory: a meta-analytic review. *Stress* **6**, 235–245.
Takahashi, T., Ikeda, K., Ishikawa, M., et al. (2004). Social stress-induced cortisol elevation acutely impairs social memory in humans. *Neuroscience Letters* **363**, 125–130.
Walker, E. L. (1958). Action decrement and its relation to learning. *Psychological Review* **65**, 129–142.
Wolf, O. T., Schommer, N. C., Hellhammer, D. H., et al. (2002). Moderate psychosocial stress appears not to impair recall of words learned 4 weeks prior to stress exposure. *Stress* **5**, 59–64.
Wust, S., Van Rossum, E. F., Federenko, I. S., et al. (2004). Common polymorphisms in the glucocorticoid receptor gene are associated with adrenocortical responses to psychological stress. *Journal of Clinical Endocrinology and Metabolism* **89**, 565–573.
Yerkes, R. M. and Dodson, J. D. (1908). The relation of strength of stimulus to rapidity of habit-information. *Journal of Comparative Neurology and Psychology* **18**, 459–482.

Neurogenesis

P Tanapat and E Gould
Princeton University, Princeton, NJ, USA

This article is reproduced from Encyclopedia of Stress, First edition, volume 3, pp 31–36, © 2000, Elsevier Inc.

Glossary

Bromodeoxyuridine (BrdU) labeling — A nonradioactive method for labeling proliferating cells and their progeny. BrdU is a thymidine analog that is incorporated into cells that are in the DNA synthetic phase of the cell cycle. BrdU incorporation can be visualized using immunocytochemical methods and can be combined with stereological analyses to estimate the total numbers of new cells generated at a given time. Short survival times (e.g., 2 h) can be used to label proliferating cells. When combined with the use of immunohistological markers, longer survival times (e.g., several weeks) can be used to determine the cellular phenotype of the newly generated cells.

Dentate gyrus — A brain region that is part of the hippocampal formation. It consists of the following three major components: (1) the granule cell layer, densely packed with granule cell bodies; (2) the hilus, a region that contains the granule cell axons (mossy fibers), interneurons, and progenitor cells; and (3) the molecular layer, a region that contains the granule cell dendritic trees and interneurons.

Neurogenesis — The process of forming a new neuron. Neurogenesis involves the proliferation of neuronal progenitors and the subsequent differentiation of these cells into neurons.

[^{3}H]Thymidine autoradiography — A method that labels proliferating cells and their progeny with radiolabeled thymidine, a molecule that is incorporated into cells that are in S phase. Cells that have incorporated [^{3}H]thymidine can be visualized with autoradiography. However, because [^{3}H]thymidine autoradiography allows the detection only of labeled cells in the top 3 μm of a section, this technique cannot be used for stereological analyses.

Most neurons in the mammalian brain are produced during the embryonic period. In contrast, the granule cell population of the dentate gyrus of the hippocampal formation is produced during an extended period that begins during gestation and continues well into adulthood. Previously, it was shown that the production of new granule neurons is suppressed by stress. Taken together, these observations suggest that stressful experiences during postnatal development and adulthood have the potential to significantly alter both the structure and function of the hippocampal formation.

Development of the Dentate Gyrus

In most regions of the mammalian brain, the majority of neurons are produced during a discrete part of the embryonic period. In contrast, granule neurons in the dentate gyrus of the hippocampal formation are produced primarily during the postnatal period and throughout adulthood in mammalian species ranging from rodents to primates, including humans. During the embryonic period, the first granule neurons arise from progenitor cells located in the wall of the lateral ventricle that migrate across the hippocampal rudiment

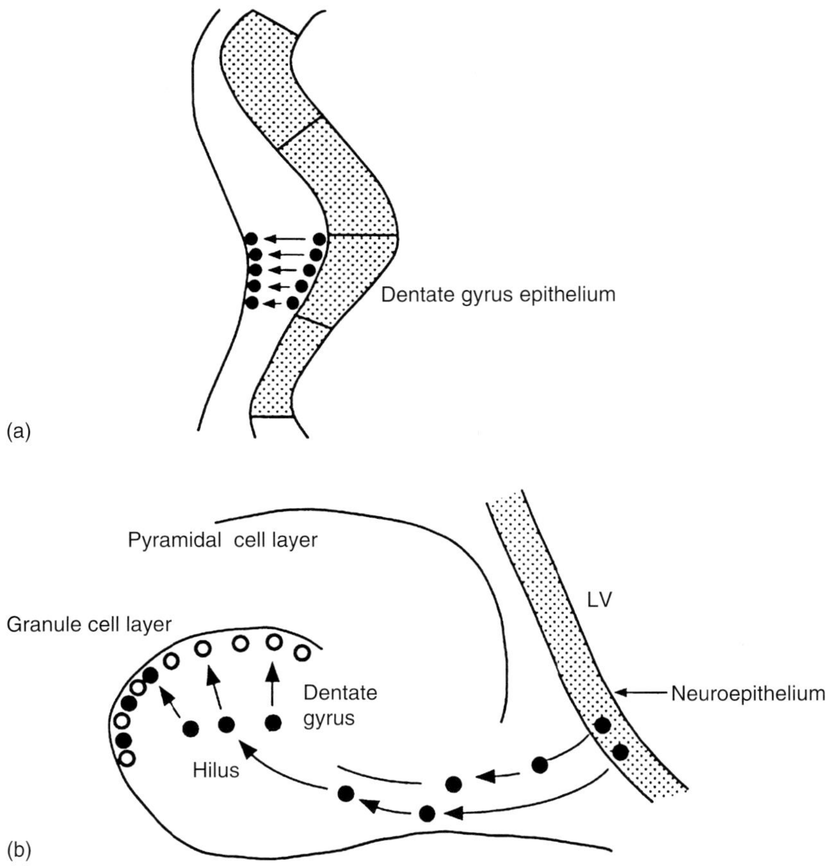

Figure 1 Development of granule cells. a, Embryonic period; b, late embryonic period. During the embryonic period, the first granule neurons arise from progenitor cells located in the wall of the lateral ventricle that migrate across the hippocampal rudiment to reside in the developing granule cell layer. During the late embryonic period and early postnatal development, granule cell precursors in the hilus divide and migrate to the granule cell layer. At the same time, precursor cells in the lateral ventricle continue to migrate into the dentate gyrus. The stippled area represents dentate gyrus neuroepithelium of the lateral ventricle (LV); solid circles represent migrating granule neuron precursors; open circles represent postmitotic immature granule neurons.

to reside in the developing granule cell layer (**Figure 1a**). A subpopulation of these progenitor cells does not undergo final division, is maintained in the hilus and subgranular zone of the dentate gyrus, and continues to give rise to new granule neurons. Inthe rodent, the majority of neurons in the dentate gyrus are produced during the first 2 postnatal weeks from this secondary proliferative zone; cells in the hilus and subgranular zone divide, migrate along radial glial fibers, and ultimately reside in the granule cell layer (**Figure 1b**). In addition, some granule neurons are also produced from cells within the granule cell layer during this period. Following the second postnatal week, cell proliferation and migration decrease and the granule cell layer is formed. In the primate, the formation of the granule cell layer occurs during the prenatal period, but the production of new granule neurons continues postnatally as well.

In both rodents and primates, new neurons are produced throughout adulthood from progenitor cells located in the hilus and subgranular zone (**Figure 2**). Studies using [^{3}H]thymidine or bromodeoxyuridine (BrdU) molecules, which are incorporated by cells during S phase, and various histological markers of cell phenotype have revealed that cells divide, migrate, extend axons, become incorporated into the granule cell layer, and ultimately express the morphological and biochemical characteristics of mature granule neurons. Although the numbers of new cells produced are much fewer than those observed during development, stereological studies have demonstrated that several thousand new cells are produced each day in the adult rodent brain. Because the majority of neurons in the dentate gyrus are produced postnatally, this brain region is particularly sensitive to changes in the environment during both postnatal development and adulthood compared to other brain regions. Thus, factors that regulate the production of granule neurons are capable of exerting significant effects on both the structure and the function of the hippocampal

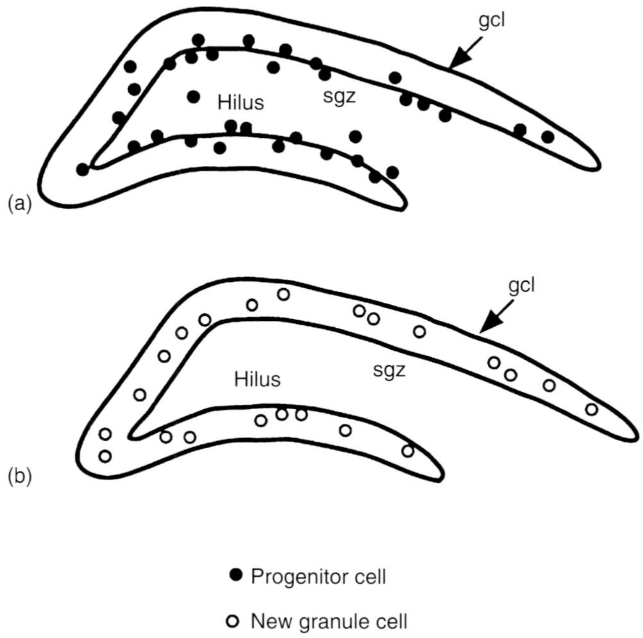

Figure 2 Production of new neurons. a, Progenitor cells; b, incorporation into granule cells. In both rodents and primates, new neurons are produced throughout adulthood from progenitor cells located in the hilus and subgranular zone (sgz). Studies using [^{3}H]thymidine or bromodeoxyuridine, both of which are incorporated by cells during S phase, and various histological markers of cell phenotype have revealed that these cells become incorporated into the granule cell layer (gcl) and ultimately express the morphological and biochemical characteristics of mature granule neurons.

formation, which may extend throughout the life of the organism. The remaining part of this article focuses on the regulation of granule neuron production by stress, the factors likely to mediate this regulation, and the possible functional implications of stress-induced changes in postnatal neuron production.

Stress Effects on Neurogenesis

During the first 2 postnatal weeks, termed the stress hyporesponsive period, rat pups exhibit a diminished response to most stressors that are known to increase circulating levels of adrenal steroids in adulthood. However, male rat pups do exhibit an increase in circulating corticosterone levels following acute exposure to the odor of an unfamiliar adult male (adult males are a natural predator of rat pups). Using this paradigm, it has been shown that a single exposure to the odors of an unfamiliar adult male during the stress hyporesponsive period results in a significant decrease in the proliferation of granule cell precursors in the developing dentate gyrus 24 h following exposure.

Acute stressful experiences also decrease the number of new granule neurons produced during adulthood in a number of different species, including rats, tree shrews (animals considered to be phylogenetically between insectivores and primates), and marmosets. In adult rats, exposure to the odors of natural predators, such as foxes or weasels, elicits a stress response characterized by increased serum corticosterone levels and a characteristic electrophysiological response in the dentate gyrus. A single brief exposure to trimethyl thiazoline, a component of fox feces, rapidly suppresses the proliferation of cells in the dentate gyrus.

Similar observations have been made in studies that have examined the effect of social stress in nonrodent species. In tree shrews, the introduction of two adult same-sex conspecifics immediately results in the establishment of an enduring dominant–subordinate relationship. During this time, the subordinate exhibits a robust stress response characterized by elevated cortisol levels, increased heart rate, hypoactivity, and vigilance. Although able to recover physically on removal from the presence of the dominant, the subordinate exhibits an immediate stress response during subsequent encounters with the dominant. A single brief exposure to a dominant animal, without physical contact, results in a rapid decrease in the number of new cells produced in the dentate gyrus of subordinate tree shrews compared to control animals. Likewise, studies of marmosets using a resident intruder paradigm, a model of psychosocial stress similar to the dominant–subordinate paradigm used with tree shrews, have yielded similar results. In this paradigm, a male marmoset is introduced into the cage of another male. Immediately after being placed in the cage, the intruder exhibits a stress response characterized by elevated mean arterial blood pressure and a dramatically increased heart rate. A single brief exposure to a psychosocial stress in the resident–intruder paradigm results in a rapid decrease in the number of new granule neurons produced in the dentate gyrus compared to naïve control animals.

In addition to exerting an acute impact on granule cell production, stress has also been shown to produce prolonged suppression of this process with repeated exposure. It has been demonstrated that 28 days of exposure to a dominant animal for 1 h each day results in a chronic increase in cortisol levels in adult tree shrews. Furthermore, exposure to chronic stress using this paradigm also results in a decrease in new cell production in the dentate gyrus, which is associated with a decrease in the total volume of the granule cell layer.

Adrenal Steroids Affect Neurogenesis through NMDA Receptors

Although the factors that mediate the stress-induced suppression of granule cell production remain unknown, adrenal steroids are likely to play a significant role in this effect. Several lines of evidence have indicated that adrenal steroids naturally regulate the production of hippocampal granule neurons. First, throughout life, a negative correlation between circulating adrenal steroid levels and the rate of granule neuron production exists. During the late embryonic period, adrenal steroid levels are high and few granule cells are produced. Following parturition, basal levels of glucocorticoids are low during the stress hyporesponsive period. This 2-week period is characterized by a diminished response to stress and maximal rates of neurogenesis. By the third postnatal week and into adulthood, circulating adrenal steroid levels are relatively high and granule production is diminished compared to the levels observed during development. With aging, the levels of glucocorticoids are elevated further and the rate of granule cell production becomes minimal.

Consistent with these natural observations, several studies have demonstrated that the production of neurons can be altered by the experimental manipulation of circulating adrenal steroid levels both during development and adulthood. During the stress hyporesponsive period, the administration of corticosterone results in a significant decrease in the number of granule neurons produced. Similar suppressive effects of adrenal steroids on the proliferation of granule cell precursors have been observed in adulthood as well. The treatment of adult rats with corticosterone results in a decrease in the production of new cells, whereas the removal of adrenal steroids by adrenalectomy results in a rapid increase in the number of new cells produced and, ultimately, in the number of new granule neurons. Despite the dramatic effects of hormone manipulations on cell proliferation in the dentate gyrus, very few granule cell precursors express adrenal steroid receptors, suggesting that adrenal steroids influence neurogenesis indirectly.

In addition to increasing circulating adrenal steroid levels, stressful experiences stimulate hippocampal glutamate release and alter the expression of the NMDA subtype of glutamate receptor in the hippocampal formation. Several lines of evidence suggest that adrenal steroids affect cell proliferation in the dentate gyrus via excitatory input. First, the timing of perforant path development and increased expression of NMDA receptors in the developing dentate gyrus coincides with an observed decrease in granule neuron production. Second, experimental manipulation of NMDA receptor activation during development or adulthood results in rapid changes in the numbers of new granule neurons. The administration of NMDA receptor antagonists increases the proliferation of granule cell precursors and the production of new granule cells during the early postnatal period and in adulthood in rats and tree shrews. It is likely that these effects are mediated by the perforant pathway, inputs that can involve NMDA receptor activation, because lesion of the entorhinal cortex enhances cell proliferation in the dentate gyrus in adulthood.

The regulation of granule cell production by adrenal steroids and NMDA receptor activation occur via a common pathway. Treatment with corticosterone and MK801 during adulthood results in an increase in cell proliferation that is similar to that observed with MK801 treatment alone. Conversely, adrenalectomized rats that are treated with NMDA demonstrate numbers of proliferating cells that are similar to animals treated with NMDA alone; both groups demonstrate a significant decrease in the numbers of proliferating cells compared to control animals. Collectively, these results indicate that adrenal steroids and NMDA receptor activation decrease cell proliferation via a common pathway. In addition, these results indicate that NMDA receptor activation exerts a more proximal effect on cell proliferation, as evidenced by the fact that the experimental manipulation of NMDA receptor activation can block the effects of corticosterone.

Although the mechanism by which adrenal steroids and NMDA receptor activation suppress cell proliferation is not known, it is possible that these factors initiate a cascade of events that result in a lengthening of the cell cycle. *In vitro* studies in nonneuronal systems have shown that glucocorticoids are capable of lengthening the G1 phase or G2/M phases of the cell cycle. Alternatively, these factors may induce changes that prevent precursor cells from progressing through the cell cycle. *In vitro* studies have also demonstrated that glucocorticoids can reversibly halt the progression of the cell cycle in nonneuronal systems. If adrenal steroids do in fact inhibit progenitor cells from dividing, the removal of adrenal steroids may result in the disinhibition of cells that are normally prevented from progressing through the cell cycle. Such an effect could account for the speed and magnitude of the increases in the number of cells in S phase following the removal of adrenal steroids.

Functional Implications of Stress Effects on Neurogenesis

The functional implications of the stress-induced suppression of neurogenesis are not known. However, the suppression of granule cell production during a time when the majority of granule neurons are produced is likely to have a significant effect on the structure of the adult hippocampal formation. The hippocampal formation has been implicated in learning and memory, raising the possibility that decreases in the production of granule neurons during development may have a negative impact on learning and memory in adulthood. Although there is some evidence to support the idea that stressful experience during development is correlated with impaired cognitive function, an involvement of stress-induced changes in granule neuron production has not yet been investigated.

Although the exact functional significance of adult-generated neurons is not known, evidence suggests a relationship between these new cells and hippocampal-dependent learning. Specifically, the survival of adult-generated cells appears to depend on learning hippocampal-dependent tasks at a critical time after their production. Taken together with the observation that stress suppresses the production of granule neurons, the finding that learning enhances the number of granule neurons suggests that stress-induced changes in neurogenesis may have a significant impact on learning. It is important to note that functional changes are not likely to be immediately evident. New cells require time to differentiate and become incorporated into functional circuitry. Thus, the period following stress-induced changes in cell proliferation is most likely to be functionally relevant. In addition, it is important to note that the functional changes attributable to acute changes in cell production are not likely to be of an observable magnitude. For this reason, the impact of stress-induced changes in neuron production is most likely to be of interest when considering conditions of chronic stress. Thus, although previous studies have demonstrated enhancements in learning as a result of conditions of acute stress, the mechanisms that underlie these effects are likely to involve processes other than changes in neuron production, such as changes in synaptic efficacy.

Several studies have demonstrated that chronic stress or corticosterone treatment exerts a significant impact on hippocampal-dependent learning. In addition, later studies have demonstrated that a stress-induced impairment of spatial learning on different tasks can be observed with both a shorter and a longer duration of stress; 8 days of psychosocial stress result in impaired performance on the hole board spatial discrimination task, and exposure to 6 months of psychosocial stress results in impaired performance on the Morris water maze spatial learning task. The stress-induced impairment observed is not permanent; rats that were tested on the radial arm maze 18 days following the termination of stress performed comparably to control rats. This observation is consistent with a possible involvement of adult-generated cells. If adult-generated cells are indeed necessary for normal performance on this task, an impairment may only persist as long as the production of these cells is altered. Once the stress-induced decrease is no longer present, we expect to observe normal levels of performance. However, stress-induced impairments during the early postnatal period, when the granule cell layer is forming, may have lasting effects.

In general, the degree to which the structure of the adult brain can be altered by experience is limited by the fact that neurons in most brain regions are produced during a discrete period of early embryonic development. Thus, the postnatal production of neurons in the dentate gyrus presents an unusual situation in which the experience of an organism may exert dramatic and potentially long-lasting effects on the structure and function of this brain region.

See Also the Following Articles

Glucocorticoid Effects on Memory: the Positive and the Negative; Glucocorticoids – Adverse Effects on the Nervous System; Hippocampus, Corticosteroid Effects on.

Further Reading

Altman, J. and Bayer, S. A. (1990). Migration and distribution of two populations of hippocampal granule cell precursors during the perinatal and postnatal periods. *Journal of Comparative Neurology* **301**, 365–381.

Gould, E. and Cameron, H. A. (1996). Regulation of neuronal birth, migration and death in the rat dentate gyrus. *Developmental Neuroscience* **18**, 22–35.

Gould, E., McEwen, B. S., Tanapat, P., et al. (1997). Neurogenesis in the dentate gyrus of the adult tree shrew is regulated by psychosocial stress and NMDA receptor activation. *Journal of Neuroscience* **17**, 2492–2498.
Gould, E., Tanapat, P., Hastings, N. and Shors, T. J. (1999). Neurogenesis in adulthood: a possible role in learning. *Trends in Cognitive Sciences* **3**, 186–191.
Gould, E., Tanapat, P., McEwen, B. S., et al. (1999). Proliferation of granule cell precursors in the dentate gyrus of adult monkeys is diminished by stress. *Proceedings of the National Academy of Sciences USA* **95**, 3168–3171.
Sapolsky, R. M. and Meaney, M. J. (1986). Maturation of the adrenocortical stress response: neuroendocrine control mechanisms and the stress hyporesponsive period. *Brain Research* **396**, 64–76.
Tanapat, P., Galea, L. A. and Gould, E. (1998). Stress inhibits the proliferation of granule cell precursors in the developing dentate gyrus. *International Journal of Developmental Neuroscience* **16**, 235–239.

Remodelling of Neuronal Networks by Stress

E Fuchs
German Primate Center and Medical School, University of Göttingen, Göttingen, Germany
G Flügge
German Primate Center, Göttingen, Germany

Glossary

BrdU (5-Bromo-2′-deoxyuridine) — A thymidine analog that is incorporated into the DNA of a dividing progenitor cell during the S phase. Fully differentiated neurons do not divide and cannot integrate the label. Depending on the survival time after application, BrdU is a marker of proliferating cells (short survival time) and their progeny (longer survival time). BrdU labeling is a nonisotopic immunocytochemical method.

Early Ideas about the Stress Response

When Selye formulated his stress theory approximately 70 years ago, stress was thought to have a merely endocrine character, and noxious stimuli of physical or chemical nature were the primary stressors discussed. However, subsequent research demonstrated that stress-induced activation of the endocrine system leads to increased release of glucocorticoids (cortisol in primates including humans, corticosterone in rodents) from the adrenal cortex and that these peripheral stress hormones also profoundly influence brain function. Moreover, stress also increases the activity of the sympathetic nervous system to enhance release of norepinephrine from peripheral nerve endings. In addition, stress modulates the activities of, for example, central nervous monoaminergic circuits. These have diverse effects on many brain cells. Great progress has been made in the understanding of the biology of stress reactions and the neurobiological alterations that occur as a consequence of exposure to challenging events in the environment.

Stress Circuits

One of the most intensively investigated stress circuits is the limbic-hypothalamic-pituitary-adrenocortical (LHPA) system, which determines the magnitude and duration of hormonal, neural, and behavioral reactions to stressful experiences. The LHPA system combines both brain and endocrine components and can be regarded as a classic neuroendocrine circuit that integrates cognitive, emotional, neuroendocrine, and autonomic inputs. It consists of the primary brain regions that process emotional information, the limbic system and the hypothalamus, as well as pituitary and adrenal glands as endocrine organs. In concert with other neurohormonal actions such as stimulation of the adrenomedullary system (release of adrenaline from the adrenal medulla), LHPA activation leads to an increased release of corticosteroid hormones from the adrenal cortex into the bloodstream. These steroid hormones are potent modulators of cell physiology, mood, and behavior and serve both to alert the organism to an environmental or physiological challenge and to defend its homeostasis.

Within the LHPA system, the hippocampus plays a central role. This brain structure has a high density of corticosteroid receptors and modulates glucocorticoid release from the adrenal cortex via a negative feedback loop exerting inhibitory effects on the LHPA axis. In addition to its intimate involvement in neuroendocrine regulation, the hippocampus plays an important role in emotional processing and in key aspects of learning and memory. While short-term activation of the LHPA system is essential for vital functions, constant hyperactivity of the circuit results in chronically elevated glucocorticoids, a maladaptive and potentially neuropathological condition. As demonstrated in animal studies, chronic stress leads to an impairment of the negative feedback control mechanism of corticosteroid release from the adrenal cortex, partly because of a reduced expression of hippocampal corticoid receptors.

Activation of Brain Systems

Stress does not have a global effect on all brain areas. Rather, depending on the type of stressor, different neuronal circuits are activated. Limbic brain regions comprising, for example, the hippocampus and amygdala as well as the prefrontal cortex are sensitive to stressors such as restraint or anxiogenic external stimuli, for example, a novel environment. Common to these stressors is the fact that they require, prior to initiation or inhibition of the stress response, a central nervous processing of information coming from different sensory organs. This information processing involves limbic and cortical regions, and its outcome depends on previous experience. In contrast, physiological threats such as exposure to ether result in a direct activation of efferent visceral pathways, in part mediated by the paraventricular nucleus of the hypothalamus. In this case, the rapid activation of brain stem and hypothalamus circumvents cognitive-emotional processing via the higher brain regions.

The intraneuronal communication that finally leads to the stress reaction is brought about by neurotransmitter systems. Rapid neuronal responses to stress are elicited by, for example, glutamate (an excitatory neurotransmitter) and GABA (γ-aminobutyric acid, an inhibitory neurotransmitter). These modulators act on specific receptors and ion channels in neuronal membranes to directly control neuronal firing. This fast neurotransmission is modulated by slow-acting neurotransmitters such as the monoamines (for example, the catecholamines dopamine, norepinephrine, and epinephrine and the indolamine serotonin). Activation of brain monoamine systems is a major component of the stress response, and turnover of monoamines is increased during stressful experiences. Stress-induced alterations in the monoamine system are regarded as the basis for stress-related behavior and are of special interest because the hyperactivity of catecholaminergic and serotonergic neurons that occurs during stress may induce an imbalance between the different neurotransmitter systems. This imbalance may contribute to psychopathologies such as major depression.

Another example of substances that modulate neuronal activity and are involved in mediation of stress responses are neuropeptides, for example corticotropin-releasing hormone (CRH). This is thought to play a major role in the stress response. Neuropeptides as well as monoamines exert their actions via specific receptors located in the membranes of neurons. Some of these receptors are also found in glia cells. Many of these receptors belong to the family of G-protein-coupled receptors (GPCRs) that are linked to intracellular second messenger systems via guanosine 5′-triphosphate (GTP)-binding proteins. The intracellular signal transduction pathways that are regulated by GPCRs bring about many of the short- and long-term effects of stress on neuronal activity and regulate most aspects of neuronal functioning, including metabolism and gene expression. Thus, intracellular signal transduction systems play a key role with respect to stress-mediated regulation of neuronal functioning and structure, and, on the cellular level, they represent the first step of a cascade of events in the brain that leads to changes in neural cells, including alterations in gene transcription and morphology of neurons. Adverse effects of stress are supposed to result partly from (1) sustained activation or inhibition of certain neurotransmitter systems and intracellular pathways and/or (2) chronic exposure to neuroactive substances such as the glucocorticoids. These steroid hormones interact with intracellular receptors, forming complexes that bind to specific sites on DNA to regulate transcription.

Structural Plasticity of the Adult Brain

Approximately a century ago, it was finally established that the brain consists of neurons and glia (neural cells) rather than being a continuous syncytium. Thereafter, a rather static view of the brain prevailed. It was thought that electrical and chemical information was processed by fixed neuronal circuits. Ramon ý Cajal stated that “in adult centers the nerve paths are something fixed, ended, immutable. Everything may die, nothing may be regenerated” (Cajal 1928, p. 750). However, in recent years, this view has been gradually revised on the basis of studies demonstrating that neuronal circuits and connections between cells in the brain are subject to lifelong modifications and reorganizations. An impressive example of the consequences of alterations in sensory inputs and changes in circulating hormones comes from research using ground squirrels. In these hibernating animals, synaptic contacts of mossy fibers with CA3 hippocampal pyramidal neurons are altered in many aspects of their structure during different stages of the torpor–activity cycle. This clearly demonstrates the capacity of the adult brain to adjust its neuronal circuits to altered hormonal and/or sensory input. Based on such findings, it was hypothesized that similar structural modifications may also occur during stressful life events when hormonal levels are altered (for example, elevated glucocorticoids, reduced gonadal steroids) and when sensory input is changed. It has transpired that this view is accurate.

This ability of the brain to perform functionally relevant adaptations following various challenges is called plasticity. Neuronal plasticity is absolutely mandatory for adequate functioning of an individual in a continuously changing environment. The dynamic processes of neuroplasticity are based on the capability of neurons to adapt to alterations in the internal and/or external environment by modifying specific structures and function; they do this by changing their entire cell surfaces, including the synapses, so that the locations of receptors and other molecules imbedded in the plasma membrane are reorganized. Adaptive or experience-dependent plasticity reveals itself in many forms, ranging from changes in gene expression to changes in neurotransmitter release and in behavior. Even under normal or undisturbed conditions, contacts between neurons are continuously replaced and renewed in the adult and differentiated brain. Enhanced axonal outgrowth and collateral sprouting on the presynaptic site may lead to the formation of new synapses, and existing contacts between neurons may be eliminated by terminal retrograde degeneration. The number of postsynaptic sites on a neuron can be increased or decreased by alterations in the size of its dendritic tree or the spine density on the dendrites.

Remodeling of Brain Cells by Stress

Probably the most thoroughly investigated stress-induced change in neuronal morphology is the regression of apical dendrites of pyramidal neurons, which was first demonstrated in the hippocampus. After this finding, dendritic remodeling of CA3 pyramidal neurons has been repeatedly documented after chronic stress as well as after corticosterone administration. Similar shortening of dendritic branches, although to a smaller extent, has been observed in granule cells of the dentate gyrus and in pyramidal cells of the hippocampal region CA1, both in chronically stressed and in corticosterone-treated rats. It is assumed that, as a result of the reduced surface area of the neurons, synaptic contacts are also diminished. Indeed, a significant loss of synapses on CA3 pyramidal cells, as well as profound changes in the morphology of the afferent mossy fibers that terminate on these neurons, was detected in chronically stressed or corticosterone-treated animals. Interestingly, even a brief social defeat stress with a long time delay thereafter can significantly reduce the length of apical dendrites but increase the length and complexity of the primary dendrites at the basis of the pyramidal neurons. These data suggest that a brief social conflict is sufficient to drive a dynamic reorganization of neuronal networks with site-selective elimination as well as *de novo* growth of dendritic branches, changes that persist for several weeks after the acute stress exposure.

Contrary to conclusions from initial studies proposing an impact of chronic stress on the number of pyramidal neurons in the hippocampus, recent stereological investigations failed to detect a statistically significant loss of these neurons following prolonged hypercortisolism resulting from stress exposure, corticosteroid administration, or aging. However, it should be noted that the number of hippocampal interneurons or of neurons in the hilus were not specifically examined in these studies. Recently, evidence was provided that long-term psychosocial stress reduces the number of parvalbumin-immunoreactive neurons that are regarded as GABAergic interneurons. This stress effect was observed in the dentate gyrus and in hippocampal region CA3, whereas subfield CA1 was not affected. Thus, the possibility that long-term stress may induce loss of interneurons without affecting the number of principal cells in the hippocampus cannot be ruled out.

Chronic stress alters dendritic morphology not only in the hippocampus but also in the medial prefrontal cortex (mPFC), which modulates various higher cognitive and emotional functions and contributes to regulation of LHPA system activity. Recent reports demonstrated that 3 weeks of either daily restraint stress or daily corticosterone injections led to changes in pyramidal neurons of the mPFC. Up to 20–35% retraction of the distal dendritic branches was seen, together with a significant (16%) decrease in apical dendritic spine density. Interestingly, even repeated vehicle injections resulted in similar, although less pronounced, changes, indicating that with respect to morphology of neurons, the mPFC is even more sensitive to external influences than the hippocampus.

The amygdala plays a crucial role in regulating fear and anxiety and is essential for the formation of affective memories. Increasing evidence supports a critical role of this brain region in activating the LHPA system. A recent study investigated the impact of chronic stress on the dendritic pattern of amygdaloid neurons. In contrast to findings in the hippocampus, spiny neurons in the basolateral complex of the amygdala exhibited enhanced dendritic branching in response to chronic stress. Examples of stress-induced changes in the brain are summarized in **Figure 1**.

Stress Suppresses Neurogenesis in the Adult Dentate Gyrus

For a long time, a central hypothesis in neuroscience was that in the mammalian brain, the production of neurons occurs only during development and stops before puberty, and new neurons cannot be formed in the adult brain. This widely held belief has been challenged in recent years by extensive evidence from many mammalian species, including nonhuman primates as well as humans, showing that even in the adult brain, certain areas retain the capability to generate new neurons. Adult spontaneous neurogenesis takes place only in certain regions such as the subgranular zone of the dentate gyrus in the hippocampal formation and the subventricular zone at the lateral ventricle. In the dentate gyrus, newly generated cells become incorporated into the granule cell layer and attain the morphological and biochemical characteristics of granule neurons. The neuronal nature of these cells is demonstrated by the formation of synapses on the cell bodies and dendrites, extension of axons into the CA3 region, and generation of action potentials.

These observations on neurogenesis were facilitated by the advent of a novel method for detecting cell proliferation and migration. Using the thymidine analog 5-bromo-2′-deoxyuridine (BrdU), which is incorporated into the DNA of dividing cells during the S phase of mitosis, proliferating cells and their progeny can be labeled. BrdU can be visualized by immunocytochemical techniques, and when used in combination with other specific cell markers, it allows determination of the phenotype of the newly generated cells. Using such methods, it has been demonstrated that the majority of newborn cells in the dentate gyrus differentiate into neurons. In other words, it has been shown that the BrdU-labeled cells express the neuronal marker neuron-specific nuclear protein. A smaller proportion of the newborn cells express markers for glial cells such as glial fibrillary acidic protein. Although the new neurons comprise a minuscule proportion of the total neuronal population, their continuous addition over the entire life span implies considerable structural changes within the neural network. The magnitude and ubiquity of adult neurogenesis across vertebrates suggest that it is functionally significant and not merely a vestige of development.

Stress is a very potent suppressive factor of adult neurogenesis, although a large number of environmental and endogenous parameters also have an impact on the formation of new neurons in the adult brain. The suppression of cell turnover by stress predicts that the age of the cell population, the connectivity of the neurons, and the resulting properties of neuronal circuits in a stressed individual might be substantially different from control situations, with potentially important functional consequences. Several different types of stressful experiences, such as exposure to the odor of a predator, social subordination, or resident–intruder stress, have been shown to inhibit neurogenesis in the dentate gyrus in several species, including nonhuman primates. Furthermore,

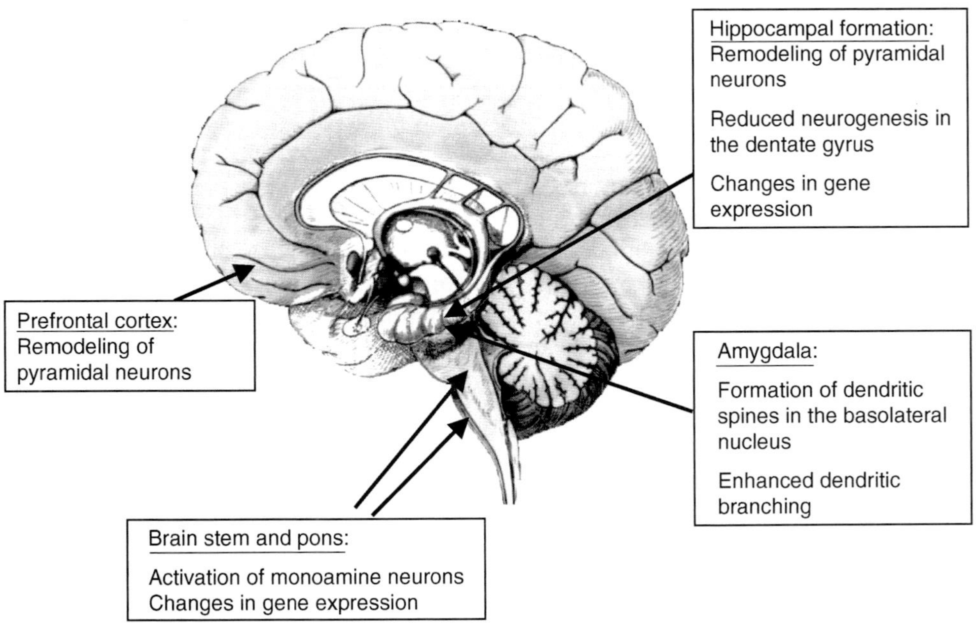

Figure 1 Examples of stress-induced changes in the brain. Hippocampal formation: remodeling of pyramidal neurons characterized by shrinkage of dendrites of pyramidal neurons in region CA3; changes in mRNA and protein reflect that stress regulates expression of genes involved in neuronal differentiation. Prefrontal cortex: remodeling of pyramidal neurons. Amygdala: in the basolateral nucleus, formation of new spines on the dendrites of spiny neurons. Brain stem and pons: activation of monoamine neurons, e.g., those that produce norepinephrine; changes in gene expression.

it appears that the susceptibility of neurogenesis to stress is age dependent in that effects of stress on cell proliferation in the dentate gyrus are more pronounced in old animals than in young ones.

It has become increasingly evident that the antecedents of many illnesses begin in fetal life and, furthermore, that prenatal conditions can have a significant impact on either health or disease in the postpartum period. In a recent study that investigated whether prenatal stress can alter neural, hormonal, and behavioral status in nonhuman primates, pregnant rhesus monkeys were acutely stressed on a daily basis for a quarter of their 24-week gestation using an acoustic startle protocol. At 2 to 3 years of age, hippocampal volume, cytogenesis in the dentate gyrus, and cortisol levels were evaluated in the offspring from stress and control pregnancies. Prenatal stress reduced hippocampal volume and inhibited neurogenesis in the dentate gyrus. These changes were associated with higher cortisol levels in the blood of the monkey offspring, lower levels of exploration, and higher levels of motor behavior. These findings indicate that also in primates, a prenatal environment can alter behavior, may deregulate neuroendocrine systems, and affects the hippocampal structure in a persistent manner.

Plasticity of Astrocytes

The most abundant type of cell within the central nervous system is the glia. In the adult mammalian brain, there are 10 to 50 times more glia cells than neurons. Astrocytes are the most prominent type of glia cells, accounting for about one-third of brain mass. Recent studies have revealed that, in addition to their housekeeping functions, astrocytes are dynamic regulators of synaptogenesis and synaptic strength. These cells control neuronal production, for example, in the adult dentate gyrus. Thus, abnormalities in glial functioning are likely to contribute to the impairment of structural plasticity in the brain. In line with these ideas, it was recently demonstrated that long-term stress significantly decreased both the number and the volume of astroglial somata. In addition, whether antidepressant treatment with the selective serotonin reuptake inhibitor fluoxetine could afford protection from these stress effects was examined. Indeed, fluoxetine prevented a stress-induced decrease in the number of astrocytes but did not counteract shrinkage of the astroglial somata.

Morphological changes in astrocytes most probably have functional significance with respect to neuron–glia interaction, and because this interaction supports neuronal functioning, interneuronal communication will also be affected by the stress-induced changes. The reduced number or weakened activity of astrocytes could change levels of extracellular glutamate, thus leading to high concentrations of this excitatory neurotransmitter that may have excitotoxic effects. An upregulation of the glial glutamate transporter (GLT-1) in the hippocampus has been reported after chronic stress, and it has been suggested that this might be a compensatory mechanism to control for increased extracellular glutamate concentrations caused by stress. Interestingly, a treatment with the antidepressant tianeptine can block the stress-induced upregulation of GLT-1, and tianeptine also reverses stress-induced dendritic remodeling in CA3. Therefore, the modulation of glial GLT-1 expression in hippocampal region CA3 can be considered a regional neurochemical correlate of dendritic remodeling. These changes in the structure and molecular plasticity of astroglia in response to stress and antidepressant treatment support the notion that glial changes may contribute to the pathophysiology of stress-related disorders such as major depression as well as to the cellular actions of antidepressants.

Plastic Changes of Brain Cells Are Reflected by Alterations in Gene Expression

The stress-induced changes in neuronal structure imply that brain cells adjust their biosynthetic pathways to the new requirements. For example, concomitant with retraction of dendrites, there is probably a reduced need for membrane proteins. Related adaptational processes take place partly on the level of gene transcription. Because various methods, namely, cDNA microarrays, serial analysis of gene expression, and subtractive hybridization, are currently used to identify genes that are differentially regulated by stress, such genes still appear rather heterogeneous. However, it is already clear that some observations from gene transcription studies are consistent with what has been found with other methods.

In hippocampal formation, expression of several genes known to be involved in neuronal differentiation was found to be downregulated by chronic social stress. Such genes included those encoding the membrane glycoprotein M6a, the CDC-like kinase 1, and a gene encoding a distinct subunit of certain G-proteins, GNAQ. All these genes are known to be involved in neurite outgrowth and neuronal differentiation, thus supporting the view that alterations in neuronal morphology and/or formation of neurons are primary effects of stress, at least in hippocampal formation. Furthermore, expression of neural cell adhesion molecule (NCAM) was found to be downregulated after chronic restraint stress in the hippocampus. NCAM is known to regulate neurite outgrowth and target recognition in the developing nervous system by mediating cell adhesion and regulating signal transduction.

Neuronal plasticity is accompanied by dynamic changes in elements of the cytoskeleton. Alpha-tubulin, which is the major component of microtubules, can be posttranslationally modified, and tyrosinated and acetylated alpha-tubulin are considered markers of dynamically changing and stable forms of microtubules, respectively. Restraint stress for 4 days decreased the expression of tyrosinated alpha-tubulin and increased expression of the acetylated form in the hippocampus. This is in line with the view that stress alters the morphology of pyramidal neurons.

Plastic changes are not restricted to forebrain areas. In a brain stem region, the rat dorsal raphe nucleus, which contains a large number of serotonergic neurons innervating the forebrain, long-term social stress increased the expression of genes involved in regulation of neurotransmitter release (synaptosomal-associated protein 25 and synaptic vesicle glycoprotein 2b). These data support the view that stress increases activity of neurons in the dorsal raphe nucleus.

Data from mRNA or protein expression studies sometimes appear contradictory. However, when interpreting such data, in which brain region, on which cellular level (neurons versus glia), and in which cellular compartment (neuronal cell body versus area of the dendrites versus axon terminal areas) the stress-induced changes were detected should be considered. Finally, besides the sex and the age of the investigated species, both the type and the duration of the stressor play a crucial role with respect to effects of stress on gene expression.

Structural Changes Are Reversible

As shown in animal studies, apical dendrites of hippocampal pyramid neurons that were shortened by restraint stress or glucocorticoid exposure regained their normal length within 3 weeks after treatment. Several *in vivo* magnetic resonance imaging studies in humans suggest a correlation between hippocampal volume reduction and cumulative glucocorticoid exposure, although exceptions have also been reported. In Cushing's patients who suffer from hypercortisolism, smaller hippocampal volumes returned to normal after successful surgery that led to normal glucocorticoid levels. Thus, up to a certain point, structural changes may be at least partially reversible and may permit restoration of normal functioning. However, it appears that the appropriate intervention should take place within a certain time before the changes become irreversible.

The mechanisms that are responsible for hippocampal volume loss have not yet been identified. Massive neuronal loss following exposure to repeated episodes of hypercortisolemia can be excluded, as no major cell loss was apparent in experimental animals as well as in human postmortem brain tissue. Neurogenesis has been regarded as another mechanism that might affect the volume of the hippocampus. However, hippocampal neurogenesis adds relatively few neurons per day, and those only to the granule cell layer of the dentate gyrus, where an equivalent number of neurons also die. Alternately, hippocampal volume loss might be due to alterations in amounts of thedendritic, axonal, and synaptic components or to changes in levels of glia. Furthermore, stress may induce a shift in fluid balance between the ventricles and brain tissue. This assumption is supported by numerous clinical studies reporting lower volumes of different brain structures in conjunction with enlarged ventricles in patients with affective disorders. However, it remains to be determined whether changes in fluid content cause the aforementioned neuroplastic changes in the neuronal network or just accompany them.

Conclusions

The diverse forms of stress-induced changes in neural cells are of particular interest. They show that even the adult and differentiated brain is a plastic organ. This lifelong plasticity is a prerequisite for the brain to adapt to environmental changes. Plasticity of the neuronal networks is the basis for learning and memory. On the other hand, extensive neuroplastic changes induced by stress may also lead to imbalances in central nervous neural networks. A promising aspect with regard to therapy is that many of these processes appear to be reversible. Reversibility of structural as well as functional plasticity has already been demonstrated, for example, in response to pharmacological treatments. Thus, progress in our understanding of neural plasticity has profound implications for the treatment of a number of neurodegenerative and psychiatric disorders.

See Also the Following Articles

Corticosteroid Receptors; Glucocorticoid Effects on Memory: the Positive and the Negative; Glucocorticoids – Adverse Effects on the Nervous System; Memory and Stress.

Further Reading

Abumaria, N., Rygula, R., Havemann-Reinecke, U., et al. (2006). Identification of genes regulated by chronic social stress in the rat dorsal raphe nucleus. *Cellular and Molecular Neurobiology* **26**, 145–162.

Alfonso, J., Frasch, A. C. and Flügge, G. (2005). Chronic stress, depression and antidepressants: effects on gene transcription in the hippocampus. *Reviews in Neuroscience* **16**, 43–56.

Cajal, S. R. (1928). *Degeneration and regeneration of the nervous system.* London: Oxford University Press.

Czeh, B., Simon, M., van der Hart, M. G., et al. (2005). Chronic stress decreases the number of parvalbumin-immunoreactive interneurons in the hippocampus: prevention by treatment with a substance P receptor (NK1) antagonist. *Neuropsychopharmacology* **30**, 67–79.

Czéh, B., Simon, M., Schmelting, B., Hiemke, C. and Fuchs, E. (2005). Astroglial plasticity in the hippocampus after chronic psychosocial stress and concomitant fluoxetine treatment. *Neuropsychopharmacology,* Dec. 14 [Epub ahead of print].

de Kloet, E. R., Vreugdenhil, E., Oitzl, M. S. and Joëls, M. (1998). Brain corticosteroid receptor balance in health and disease. *Endocrine Reviews* **19**, 269–301.

Flügge, G., van Kampen, M. and Mijnster, M. J. (2004). Perturbations in brain monoamine systems during stress. *Cell and Tissue Research* **315**, 1–14.

Fuchs, E. and Czéh, B. (2005). Adult neurogenesis in rodents and primates: functional implications. In: Steckler, T., Kalin, N. H. & Reul, H. (eds.) *Handbook of stress and the brain Part 1: The neurobiology of stress. Techniques in the behavioral and neural sciences* (Vol. 15), pp. 711–727. Amsterdam: Elsevier.

Fuchs, E., Czéh, B., Kole, M. H. P., Michaelis, T. and Lucassen, P. J. (2004). Alterations of neuroplasticity in depression: the hippocampus and beyond. *European Neuropharmacology* **14**, 481–490.

Herman, J. P. and Cullinan, W. E. (1997). Neurocircuitry of stress: central control of the hypothalamo-pituitary-adrenocortical axis. *Trends in Neuroscience* **20**, 78–84.

Kempermann, G. (2002). Regulation of adult hippocampal neurogenesis – implications for novel theories of major depression. *Bipolar Disorders* **4**, 17–33.

Mason, J. W. (1968). A review of psychoneuroendocrine research on the pituitary-adrenal cortical system. *Psychosomatic Medicine* **30**, 576–609.

McEwen, B. S. (1999). Stress and hippocampal plasticity. *Annual Review of Neuroscience* **20**, 49–70.

Mitra, R., Jadhav, S., Bruce, S., et al. (2005). Stress duration modulates the spatiotemporal patterns of spine formation in the basolateral amygdala. *Proceedings of the National Academy of Sciences USA* **102**, 9371–9376.

Popov, V. I. and Bocharova, L. S. (1992). Hibernation-induced structural changes in synaptic contacts between mossy fibres and hippocampal pyramidal neurons. *Neuroscience* **48**, 53–62.

Reul, J. M., Sutanto, W., van Eekelen, J. A., Rothuizen, J. and de Kloet, E. R. (1990). Central action of adrenal steroids during stress and adaptation. *Advances in Experimental Medicine and Biology* **274**, 243–256.

Sapolsky, R. M. (1999). Glucocorticoids, stress, and their adverse neurological effects: relevance to aging. *Experimental Gerontology* **34**, 721–732.

Selye, H. (1936). A syndrome produced by diverse noxious agents. *Nature London* **138**, 32.

Stanford, S. C. (1993). Monoamines in response and adaptation to stress. In: Stanford, S. C. & Salmon, P. (eds.) *Stress. From synapse to syndrome*, pp. 281–331. London: Academic Press.

Watanabe, Y., Gould, E. and McEwen, B. S. (1992). Stress induces atrophy of apical dendrites of hippocampal CA3 pyramidal neurons. *Brain Research* **588**, 341–345.

Wellman, C. L. (2001). Dendritic reorganization in pyramidal neurons in medial prefrontal cortex after chronic corticosterone administration. *Journal of Neurobiology* **49**, 245–253.

VIII. STRESS - INDUCED/ RELATED PATHOLOGY

A. Immune/Inflammatory Responses

Immune System–Neuroendocrine Interactions

S Rivest
Laval University, Québec City, QC, Canada

Introduction

Inflammation is a general name for reactions occurring after most kinds of tissue injuries or infections or immunologic stimulations as a host defense against foreign or altered endogenous substances. The local inflammatory reaction is characterized by an initial increase in blood flow to the site of injury, enhanced vascular permeability, and selective accumulation of different effector cells from the peripheral blood to injured regions. These cells, mostly circulating neutrophils and monocytes and locally resident macrophages, together mount a rapid inflammatory response that is characterized by the secretion of cytokines, among other features (**Figure 1**). Their secretion into the bloodstream is a key step in triggering the neuronal activity and subsequent neurophysiological responses that take place during systemic and localized tissue insults. Cytokines influence many neuroendocrine systems, the most prominent of which is the hypothalamic–pituitary–adrenal (HPA) axis, activation of which results in the release of adrenocorticotrophic hormone (ACTH) and glucocorticoids. Once present in the bloodstream, these cytokines also have the ability to increase body temperature (fever) and cause symptoms of sickness. The proinflammatory cytokine interleukin-1 (IL-1), especially its β form (IL-1β), is probably the most important molecule capable of modulating cerebral functions during systemic and localized inflammation. Systemic IL-β injection activates the neurons involved in the control of autonomic functions, and neutralizing antibodies or IL-1 receptor antagonists are capable of preventing numerous responses to inflammatory stimuli. Studies in IL-1β-deficient mice have provided solid and compelling evidence supporting the critical role played by this cytokine in neural–immune interaction.

Other cytokines implicated in neuroendocrine and febrile responses include tumor necrosis factor-α (TNF-α) and IL-6. Like IL-1β, intravenous TNF-α injection has a profound influence on the brain, on fever, and on hormones of the HPA axis. In contrast, the role of IL-6 in neuroendocrine and febrile responses is quite controversial. From the observation that IL-6-deficient mice were unable to develop normal fever in response to lipopolysaccharide (LPS) and IL-1β, IL-6 has been defined as one of the principle endogenous pyrogens. It has also been demonstrated that prostaglandins (PGs) mediate IL-6-induced fever and activation of the HPA axis, but IL-6 is unable to stimulate PG formation in the brain. However, a specific antiserum to IL-6, IL-6AS, was able to prevent LPS-induced febrile response, and cyclooxygenase 2 (COX-2)-deficient mice do not develop fever in response to icv IL-6 injection. The mechanisms by which IL-1β and IL-6 activate the autonomic functions are likely to be quite different, and IL-1β is clearly more potent than IL-6 in triggering PGE_2 synthesis in the central nervous system (CNS).

Possible Pathways by Which Circulating IL-1β Signals the Brain

The transport of soluble substances across vascular compartments occurs via either paracellular or transcellular mechanisms. Within the cerebrovasculature, the paracellular route is particularly impermeable because of the blood–brain barrier (BBB). The BBB consists primarily of nonfenestrated endothelial cells that are connected by tight junctions. Furthermore, the large molecular sizes (13–15 kDa) and hydrophilic nature of cytokines preclude their transcellular movement by simple diffusion to any appreciable extent, and early studies concluded that the BBB was impermeable to IL-1β. It is nevertheless possible that endogenous cytokines diffuse across the BBB during extreme periods of fever or in presence of high levels in plasma during a long period of time.

Regions relatively devoid of BBB permit cytokine interaction with the neuronal elements. The circumventricular organs (CVOs) contain capillaries with rather greater permeability than the rest of the CNS, and the vascular density in these regions is extraordinarily high. Therefore, the CVOs have been proposed as potential sites of action, in particular the structure lining the anteroventral third ventricle region, namely the organum vasculosum of the lamina terminalis. The subfornical organ, median eminence, and area postrema are the other potential target CVOs. On the other hand, a medullary group of cells may play an important role in processing visceral sensory information carried out by the vagus and glossopharyngeal nerves. The vagus nerve has indeed been proposed to provide a rapid communication pathway for cytokine signaling between the periphery and brain, but this pathway depends on dosage and route of administration.

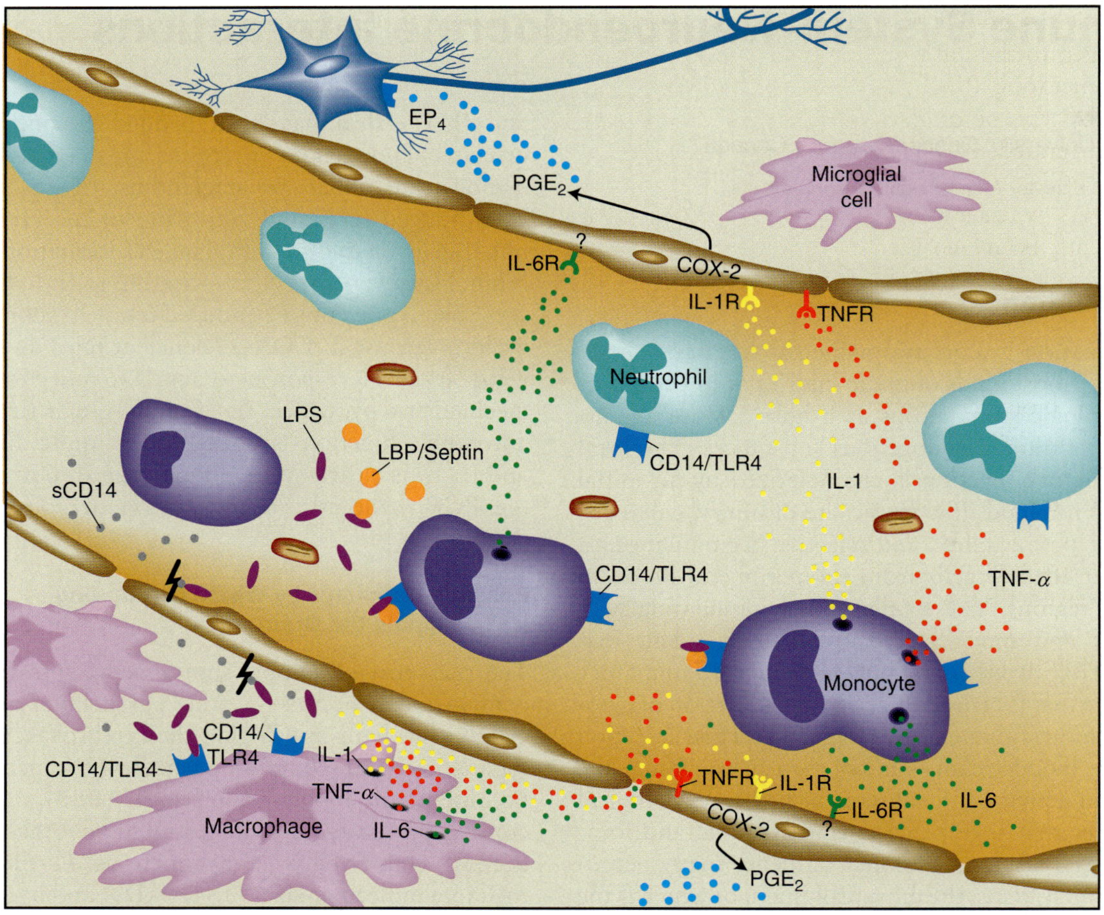

Figure 1 Innate immune response evoked by endotoxic lipopolysaccharide (LPS). LPS is a major component of the outer membranes of Gram-negative bacteria, which is the best-characterized example of innate recognition associated with a robust inflammatory response by phagocytic cells. Secretion of cytokines by circulating monocytes/neutrophils and tissue macrophages by LPS requires a series of mechanisms in cascade, the first step being the binding of the LPS with the serum proteins LPS-binding protein (LBP) or septins. The newly formed complex may then activate different populations of cells by binding to its CD14 receptor and toll-like receptor 4 (TLR4). The latter is the actual signaling receptor for LPS. Two forms of CD14 receptors can be found. The first is present on the surface of myeloid cells (mCD14) and acts as a glycosyl-phosphatidylinositol (GPI)-anchored membrane glycoprotein; the other form is soluble in the serum (sCD14) and lacks the GPI properties, though it can bind LPS to activate cells devoid of mCD14, such as endothelial cells. LBP is not essential for LPS signaling, but the LPS–LBP complex is particularly powerful in activating cells of myeloid origin, that is, neutrophils, monocytes, macrophages, and microglia. One of the well-known consequences of such activation is the production of proinflammatory cytokines, such as interleukin (IL)-1β (IL-1β), tumor necrosis factor alpha (TNF-α), and IL-6. These cytokines may, in turn, bind to their cognate receptors expressed on the surface of cells forming the blood–brain barrier, but they are not essential for mediating the effects of LPS in the central nervous system. LPS is an exogenous ligand for cerebral tissue that expresses both LPS receptors. Such an innate immune/inflammatory response also takes place during tissue injuries and in presence of more complex pathogens (e.g., bacteria and viruses). See text for details. COX-2, cyclooxygenase 2; EP$_4$, a prostaglandin E receptor; PGE2, prostaglandin E$_2$; R, receptor.

On the other hand, a strong body of evidence now supports the concept that cytokines, particularly IL-1, act on the microvasculature, with consequent release of local signaling molecules, namely PGs. Indeed, brain microvessels exhibit constitutive expression levels of IL-1 type 1 receptor transcript, and systemic IL-1β injection causes a rapid and profound transcriptional activation of the gene encoding COX-2 in cells lining the CNS blood vessels. Circulating IL-1 also induces microsomal PGE synthase (mPGES-1), which co-localizes with COX-2 in the perinuclear region of the cerebral endothelium. Of great interest are the data that mPGES-1-deficient mice failed to develop fever in response to either systemic LPS and IL-1, but not to centrally administered PGE$_2$. These data clearly underline the critical role of the PGE$_2$ machinery in the endothelium of the brain's blood vessels to activate the autonomic functions during systemic inflammation.

Biosynthesis of PGs

Prostanoids are a group of 20 carbon-unsaturated fatty acid derivates that are produced via a complex enzymatic cascade. First, COX activity adds molecular oxygen to the unsaturated fatty acid arachidonic acid, generating PGG_2. PGG_2 is then converted to PGH_2 by the peroxidase activity of the enzyme. Once generated, PGH_2 is rapidly converted to PGs (PGD_2, PGE_2, and $PGF_{2\alpha}$), prostacylin, and thromboxane A_2 by tissue-specific synthases. PGE synthase has recently been identified and designated as mPGES and cytosolic PGES (cPGES). These molecules or their derivatives interact with specific receptors to modulate cell function. The diversity of the tissue-specific synthases and receptors gives rise to a wide range of potential biologic functions for the prostanoids. PGG, PGH, prostacyclin, and thromboxane A are chemically unstable and are degraded into inactive products under physiological conditions, with a half-life of 30 s to a few minutes. Other PGs, although chemically stable, are metabolized quickly. It is therefore believed that prostanoids work locally, acting only in the vicinity of the site of production to serve as potent autocrine and paracrine mediators in a wide variety of physiological processes. Although PGE_2 rises in blood promptly after the entry of microorganisms or in response to the endotoxin LPS and cytokines, it is now generally accepted that the PGE_2 detected in the brain is not derived from the blood but rather is produced directly within the CNS.

It is therefore proposed that circulating LPS and cytokines bind to their cognate receptors onto endothelial and/or monocytic cells lining the BBB, which leads to proinflammatory signaling and transcription of the enzymes responsible of the PGE_2 formation in the cerebral tissue. It is interesting to note that systemic inflammatory insults induce COX-2 and mPGES in a rather unspecific manner across the cerebral blood vessels and small capillaries, whereas the neuronal activity is limited to selective nuclei, including the endocrine hypothalamus. It is thus possible that expression of specific PGE_2 receptors within parenchymal cells adjacent to the site of production determines the action of the PG in the brain.

PGE_2 Sites of Action

Classic prostanoid receptors comprise a family of eight encoding transmembrane G-protein-coupled receptors. These receptors are classified on the basis of selective affinities for naturally occurring prostanoids. There are distinct receptors for thromboxane A_2, prostacylin, $PGF_{2\alpha}$, and PGD_2 and four different receptors for PGE_2 (EP_{1-4}). Multiple alternatively spliced isoforms exist for the PGE_2 EP_3 receptor ($EP_{3\alpha}$, $_{3\beta}$, $_{3\gamma}$). They share common extracellular and membrane-spanning regions but differ in intracellular and C-terminal domains. Each receptor is associated with a unique G-protein and consequently a unique second messenger system, namely, elevation of intracellular Ca^{2+} (EP_1) and stimulation (EP_2 and EP_4) or inhibition of (EP_3) of adenylate cyclase. Despite the presence of some conserved sequences, overall homology among the prostanoid receptors is quite limited, ranging from 20–30%. On the other hand, the homology of a given type or subtype of receptor among various species is considerably higher. Each of the eight types and subtypes of receptors shows selective ligand binding specificity that distinguishes it from the others. In addition to transmembrane receptors, the peroxisome proliferator-activated receptor-γ is a member of the nuclear receptor family of transcription factors that can be activated by binding to PGD derivates, such as 15-deoxy-Δ12,14 PG J_2.

In 1988, the distribution of [^{3}H] PGE_2-binding sites, presumably PGE_2 receptors, was first demonstrated in the monkey diencephalon, and more-detailed analysis of [^{3}H] PGE_2-binding sites in rat brain ensued. PGE_2-binding sites were located in a number of discrete brain regions, including thalamic and hypothalamic nuclei, ventral hippocampus, central gray, superior colliculus, parabrachial nucleus, locus coeruleus, raphe nuclei, spinal trigeminal nuclei, and nucleus of the solitary tract (NTS). *In situ* hybridization was thereafter used to determine the exact distribution of each PGE_2 receptor subtype. The hypothalamic paraventricular (PVN) and supraoptic nuclei exhibited EP_1-expressing cells, but a wide distribution was found for the gene encoding the EP_3 subtype. Investigators have reported a very distinct pattern of EP_2- and EP_4-expressing neurons throughout rat brain; that is, EP_2 receptor messenger RNA (mRNA) was detected in the bed nucleus of the stria terminalis, lateral septum, subfornical organ, ventromedial hypothalamic nucleus, central nucleus of the amygdala, locus coeruleus, and area postrema, while EP_4 receptor transcript was located mainly in regions involved in the control of neuroendocrine and autonomic activities. Moderate doses of LPS or IL-1β activate EP_4 neurons, and this activation is prevented when animals are pretreated with COX inhibitors.

All four PGE_2 EP receptor mRNAs are expressed in the anteromedial preoptic region that plays a crucial role in the febrile response. Among these, only EP_4 receptor mRNA is strongly expressed throughout the PGE_2-sensitive regions, including the organum vasculosum of the lamina terminalis, ventromedial preoptic nucleus (VmPO), and median preoptic nucleus. These EP_4-expressing neurons are also activated by systemic inflammation, whereas EP_2- and EP_3-positive neurons do not respond. EP_1 receptor mRNA is present in

PGE_2-sensitive regions, but its expression level is weak. Thus, EP_4 may be the key binding and functional receptor for PGE_2 in the brain to activate the circuits involved in autonomic control.

Nevertheless, pharmacological and genetic mutation experiments suggest otherwise. Drugs with agonist and antagonist properties for each EP receptor have been used in rats. Injection icv of 17-phenyl-ω-trinor-PGE_2 (an EP_1 and $EP_{3\alpha}$ receptor agonist), but not butaprost, M&B28767, or 11-deoxy-PGE_1 (EP_2, $EP_{3\alpha}$, and EP_4 receptor agonists, respectively), induced fever, and SC19220 (an EP_1 receptor antagonist) prevented the febrile response to PGE_2. Another pharmacological study indicated that EP_2 or EP_3 receptor might be the receptors necessary to produce fever. In mice bearing genetic deletions of the EP_{1-4} receptors, only EP_3-knockout animals failed to show the early phase of fever (up to 1 h) after LPS iv or PGE_2 icv. It is important to note, however, that EP_4-deficient mice do not survive and have to be intercrossed in a different background. It is therefore quite difficult to compare them with the other gene-deficient mice, and inducible EP_4 knockout mice will be essential to clearly define the role of this receptor in the brain of mature animals. The relative lack of specificity of EP_4 antagonists and agonists in the species studied may also explain the pharmacological data. It is nevertheless possible that the anatomy and circuits unraveled by functional indices of neuronal activity have little to do with the physiological outcomes, namely, fever and increased activity of the HPA axis.

Functional Circuits by Intraparenchymal PGE_2

Without such anatomical work, however, it is not possible to clarify the exact pathways and groups of neurons involved in neural–immune interaction. Indeed, the final picture is far from complete. The following cascade of events is based on the data described above, but a few steps still remain to be fully validated and should therefore be considered working hypotheses: 1. Endotoxin LPS reaches the bloodstream and binds to the serum protein LPS-binding protein (LBP). The newly formed complex then binds to membrane CD14 and TLR4 receptors located on the surface of myeloid cells, triggering NF-κB signaling, nuclear translocation, and cytokine gene transcription (**Figure 1**). Pro-IL-1β and-TNF-α have to be cleaved by specific cytosolic enzymes before being transported into the extracellular environment. Recent data suggest a critical role of extracellular adenosine triphosphate and the P2X7 receptor in this final secretion process. Once in the bloodstream, both IL-1β and TNF-α can act on distant organs to trigger different physiological responses by binding to their respective type I receptors.

2. The endothelial and perivascular cells are the most obvious target cells in the CNS because they constitutively express numerous cytokine receptors and they are highly sensitive to low circulating levels of proinflammatory molecules. It is important to note that circulating LPS is also a direct ligand for these cells and that the release of circulating cytokines is not a prerequisite for LPS activation of the endothelial and perivascular cells lining the BBB.

3. Circulating LPS/LBP, IL-1, and TNF initiate COX-2 and mPGES transcriptions through a NF-κB and mitogen-activated protein kinase (MAPK) pathway, which is activated within seconds on ligand–receptor interaction. This leads to PGE_2 synthesis and release by the endothelium and pericytes of the brain capillaries. The PG may therefore diffuse across the brain parenchymal elements and bind to specific EP receptors at the surface of the neurons controlling the autonomic functions.

4. Whether one or more EP receptors participate in the neuronal response to PGE_2 is still a matter of great debate, but the neuroanatomy weighs in favor of the EP_4 receptor subtype. This receptor is found in key regions that control fever, HPA axis activity, and other autonomic functions. EP_4-expressing neurons are activated (as revealed by spontaneous induction of the immediate-early gene c-*fos*) in response to centrally injected PGE_2 and systemically administered IL-1 and LPS. Selective and nonselective COX inhibitors have the ability to prevent such functional activation of these neurons. EP_4-expressing neurons display an integrated circuit associated with the control of autonomic functions. The EP_4 receptor is associated with G_s-protein and stimulation of cyclic adenosine monophosphate (cAMP), which is the most potent transduction pathway involved in the release of corticotropin-releasing factor (CRF) from the PVN and increase in HPA axis activity. There is also evidence in support of cAMP signaling in thermosensitive neurons of the VmPO.

5. On the other hand, PGE_2 may inhibit major inhibitory neurons (e.g., γ-aminobutyric acid (GABA)) projecting to the nuclei that control the autonomic circuits. This would explain the data that only EP_3-deficient mice fail to exhibit a febrile response to inflammatory stimuli. This particular receptor is associated with a G_i-coupled protein inhibiting cAMP on its activation, which may take place in GABA neurons that innervate the VmPO and PVN. Obviously, these neurons would not express c-*fos* or other indices of neuronal activation in response to PGE_2. Functional anatomical data supporting this concept are nevertheless lacking, because there are as yet no reliable tools to assess inhibition rather than stimulation *in vivo*. If interaction of PGE_2 with its EP_3 receptor blocks the activity of GABA neurons innervating the VmPO

and PVN, then the spontaneous induction of immediate-early genes in these regions may be indirectly attributable to GABA inhibition rather than to a direct interaction of PGE_2 with its EP_4 receptor. This is a chicken-and-egg problem that will have to be resolved with appropriate tools and animal models.

Alternative Pathways

PGE_2 production in the CNS may rely on two different pathways: (1) a fast transient production in endothelial cells and CVOs dependent on activation (possibly through MAPK p38 phosphorylation) of available constitutive PGE_2 synthesis enzymes ($cPLA_2$, COX-1, cPGES, and mPGES-2), independent of transcription and NF-κB activation (**Figure 2**), or (2) a slow, sustained PGE_2 synthesis in the endothelial cells and perivascular microglia (equipped to respond to cytokines and pathogens) involving the robust induction of the principle enzymes involved in PGE_2 synthesis (especially secretory phospholipase A_2 ($sPLA_2$-IIA), COX-2, and mPGES-1) that are NF-κB- and MAPK-mediated gene products. The slow transcription-mediated response would be massive but could offer a way through which glucocorticoids would then exert their negative feedback on NF-κB activity to shut down the CNS production of PGE_2. The fast response could be involved in priming the later delayed response and prevent drastic changes

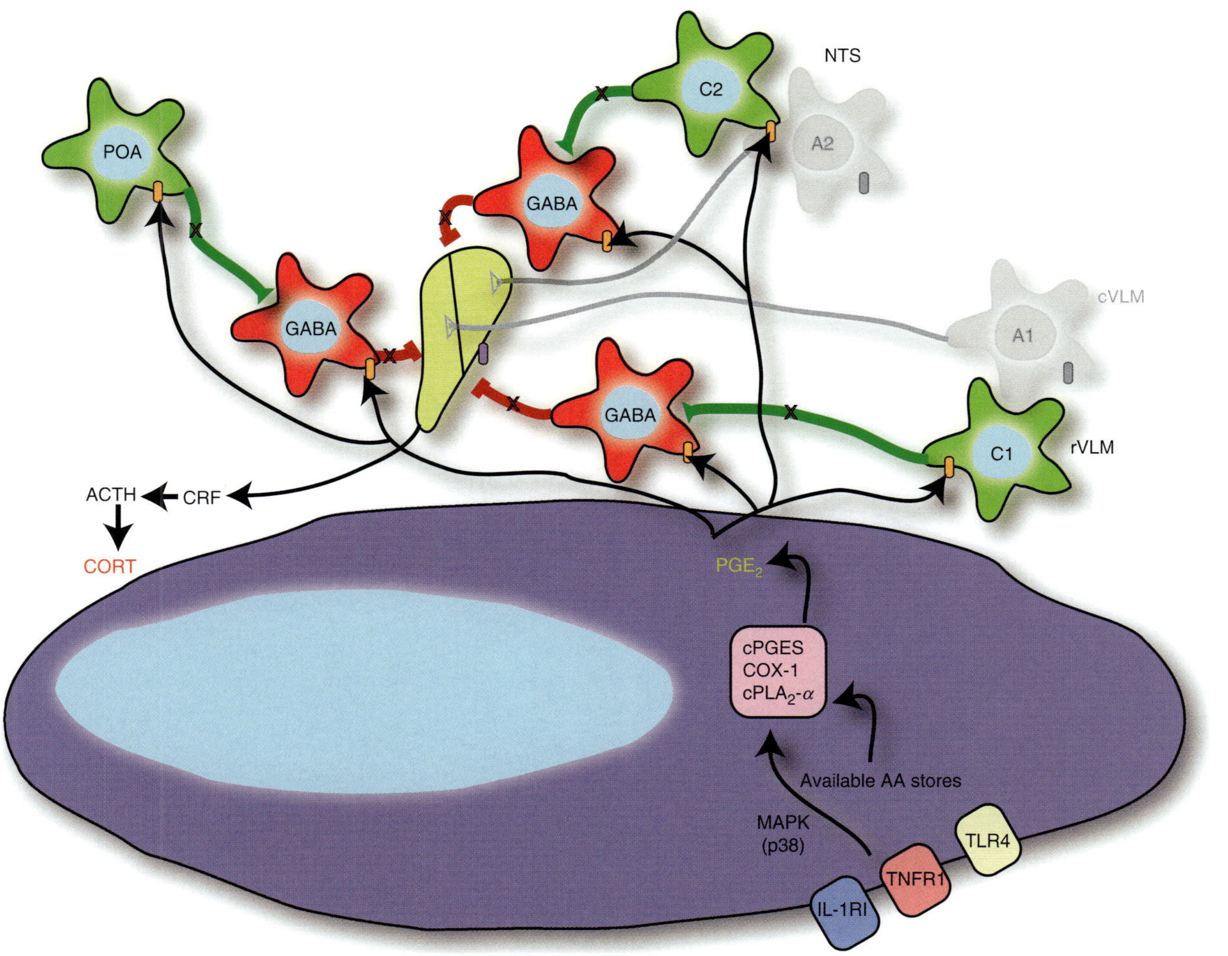

Figure 2 Hypothetical model for the fast prostaglandin E_3 receptor (EP_3)-dependent prostaglandin E_2 (PGE_2) response in the brain. Circulating inflammatory factors (interleukin (IL)-1, tumor necrosis tactor (TNF), lipopolysaccharide (LPS)) bind to their receptors expressed on the surface of endothelial cells of the brain microvasculature. This leads to a rapid use of available constitutive enzymes (cyclooxygenase (COX)-1, cytosolic phospholipase A_2 ($cPLA_2$), cytosolic prostaglandin E synthase (cPGES)) and arachadonic acid (AA) stores to transiently produce and release PGE_2 (possibly through mitogen-activated protein kinase (MAPK) p38 mechanisms). This PGE_2 acts on its EP_3 receptor on γ-aminobutyricacidergic afferences to the hypothalamic paraventricular nucleus, which rapidly turns off the inhibition of the corticotropin releasing factor (CRF)-releasing neurons. A similar scenario may happen at the medial preoptic area (POA), C1 catecholaminergic neurons of the rostral ventrolateral medulla (VLM), and C2 catecholaminergic neurons of the solitary tracts nucleus, where the binding of PGE_2 to the EP_3 receptor inhibits excitation of these GABAergic projections of PVN neurons. ACTH, adrenocorticotropic hormone; CORT, corticosterone; GABA, γ-aminobutyric acid; R, receptor; TLR4, toll-like receptor 4.

to homeostatic processes that the delayed response would have problems overcoming. A study looking at the effects of specific COX-1 and COX-2 inhibitors supports such a role for the COX-1-dependent early response since the ablation of COX-1 activity following LPS administration led to a fast hypothermic response, which could not be overcome by the later COX-2-dependent fever response. This study emphasizes the importance of the coordination between the fast and delayed responses.

The population of cells containing the enzymes responsible for PGE_2 synthesis during systemic inflammation is still debated. Numerous papers have provided clear evidence that both COX-2 and mPGES-1 transcripts and proteins are expressed essentially within the endothelium of the brain blood vessels. On the other hand, few studies have shown that perivascular myeloid cells are responsible to deliver PGE_2 in response to systemic inflammatory stimuli. The action of this PG may therefore be dependent on its cellular source, the endogenous pool of PGE_2 in endothelial cells, and the receptor subtypes expressed on their cellular targets. It has been shown that EP_4 is present on the postsynaptic sites of hypothalamic stimulatory neurons, whereas GABA neurons contain presynaptic EP_3 receptors in their terminals. Activation of both EP_3 and EP_4 receptors is actually involved in the excitatory regulation of supraoptic neurons by PGE_2. These data may suggest that both receptors contribute to the activation of

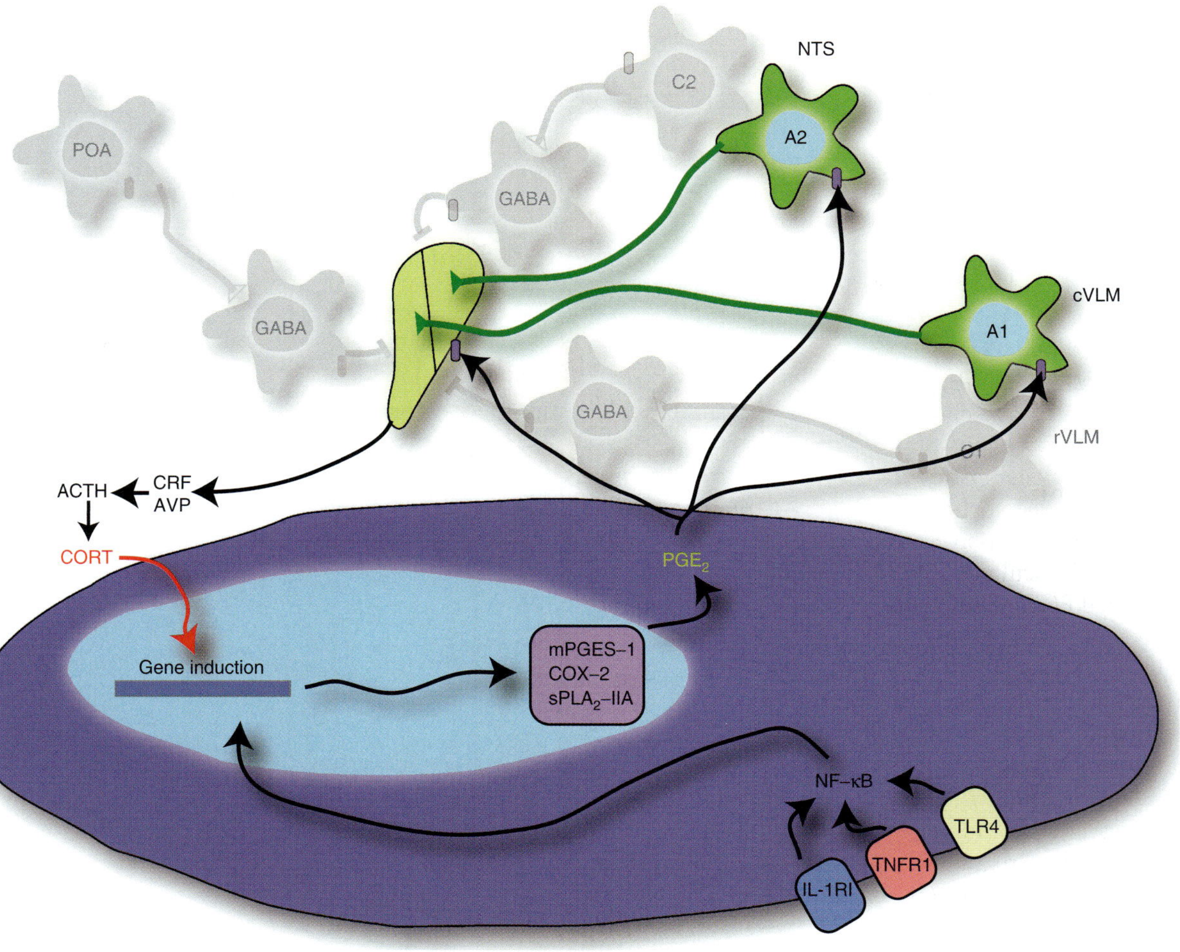

Figure 3 Delayed prostaglandin E_4 (EP_4)-dependent prostaglandin E_2 (PGE_2) response in the brain during systemic immune insults. The delayed PGE_2 response requires transcription of the inducible enzymes (secretory phospholipase A_2 ($sPLA_2$-IIA), cyclooxygenase (COX)-2, microsomal prostaglandin E synthase (mPGES)-1) through nuclear factor-kappa B (NF-κB) and area postrema-1-mediated transcriptional mechanisms. These enzymes permit the massive production of PGE_2 that acts on the EP_4 receptors in the paraventricular nucleus and at the adrenergic A1 region of the caudal ventrolateral medulla (cVLM) and A2 region of the nucleus of the solitary tract (NTS) to enhance corticotropin-releasing factor (CRF) and vasopressin (AVP) release into the infundibular system. This leads to the release of adrenocorticotrophic hormone (ACTH) and subsequently biosynthesis and secretion of corticosterone (CORT) from the adrenal medulla. The latter hormone acts as negative feedback on the transcription of the enzymes responsible for the production of PGE_2 and prevents overproduction of inflammatory molecules during innate immunity. IL-1, interleukin-1; R, receptor; TLR4, toll-like receptor 4; TNF, tumor necrosis factor.

PVN neurons during systemic inflammation, but at different times. Stimulation of the $cPLA_2$–COX-1–cPGES pathway would lead to rapid secretion of PGE_2 from endothelial cells and then cause an immediate activation of the CRF neurons through inhibition of GABA afferents that contain EP_3 receptors (**Figure 2**). The hypothalamic PVN receives robust innervation from GABA neurons that play a critical role in the control of the HPA axis during stress. Inhibition of GABAergic neurons by EP_3 may take place locally at the level of the nerve terminals within the PVN or through distal inhibition of GABA projections originating from different areas, such as the preoptic area, parabrachial nucleus, rVLM, and/or NTS.

PGE_2 synthesis under the control of the $sPLA_2$-IIA–COX-2–mPGES-1 pathway would take the relay and trigger different populations of neurons (**Figure 3**). Enzymes of this pathway are not constitutively present and have to be induced by the proinflammatory signal transduction pathways. It is also possible that both endothelial and microglial cells contribute to the PGE_2 production in the delayed phase. Once secreted, PGE_2 would maintain CRF activity via EP_4 stimulation either directly or through activation of the A1 and A2 catecholaminergic circuits from the caudal ventrolateral medulla and NTS, respectively. These mechanisms fit nicely with the hypothesis of a fast and delayed PGE_2 response, in which the fast phase could be associated with the disinhibition of CRF-releasing neurons of the PVN, without the need for time- and energy-hungry transcription. This response could also prime the PVN to become more receptive to the massive release of PGE_2 by endothelial and perivascular microglial cells with their newly transcribed PGE_2-synthesizing enzymes. In support of this hypothesis is the specific increase in EP_4 mRNA levels in CRF neurons and catecholaminergic afferents to PVN following a systemic immune challenge. The sustained glucocorticoid release provides direct inhibitory feedback on these events at the level of transcriptional machinery, which is the most powerful endogenous immunosuppressive mechanism. This innovative dual regulation of PGE_2 production and action in the brain could have important implications for an appropriate control of fever, HPA axis, and other autonomic functions.

Concluding Remarks

More work is clearly needed to unravel the fine-tuning of the circuits and signal transduction pathways that participate in the neural–immune interface. There is, however, no doubt that PGE_2 plays a determinant role in activating or inhibiting the key populations of neurons that are together involved in engaging the physiological responses necessary for the organism to restore health during illness. An appropriate febrile response and a time-dependent release of glucocorticoids are major phenomena in which the brain has a direct impact on the systemic innate immune system. Imbalances in these two regulatory systems are actually becoming hallmarks of autoimmune diseases and neurodegenerative disorders. Clarifying the exact mechanisms and circuits that allow such fine neurophysiological outcomes will obviously be essential for designing appropriate therapeutic strategies when dysfunction occurs during the acute-phase response. The best guess at this time points to the key kinases controlling the proinflammatory signal transduction pathways in cells of the BBB, PGE_2 biosynthetic machinery and release, and specific EP receptor subtypes expressed on the surface of the neuronal populations that control endocrine and autonomic functions.

See Also the Following Articles

Hypothalamic–Pituitary–Adrenal (HPA) Axis; Stress Response: Neural and Feedback Regulation of the HPA Axis.

Further Reading

Ek, M., Engblom, D., Saha, S., Blomqvist, A., Jakobsson, P. J. and Ericsson-Dahlstrand, A. (2001). Inflammatory response: Pathway across the blood–brain barrier. *Nature* **410**, 430–431.

Elmquist, J. K., Scammell, T. E. and Saper, C. B. (1997). Mechanisms of CNS response to systemic immune challenge: The febrile response. *Trends in Neurosciences* **20**, 565–570.

Engblom, D., Saha, S., Engström, L., et al. (2003). Microsomal prostaglandin E synthase-1 is the central switch during immune-induced pyresis. *Nature Neuroscience* **6**, 1137–1138.

Laflamme, N., Lacroix, S. and Rivest, S. (1999). An essential role of interleukin-1β in mediating NF-κB activity and COX-2 transcription in cells of the blood–brain barrier in response to systemic and localized inflammation, but not during endotoxemia. *Journal of Neuroscience* **19**, 10923–10930.

Narumiya, S., Sugimoto, Y. and Ushikubi, F. (1999). Prostanoid receptors: Structures, properties, and functions. *Physiological Reviews* **79**, 1193–1226.

Nguyen, M. D., Julien, J. P. and Rivest, S. (2002). Innate Immunity: The missing link in neuroprotection and neurodegeneration? *Nature Reviews Neuroscience* **3**, 216–227.

Rivest, S. (1999). What is the cellular source of prostaglandins in the brain in response to systemic inflammation? Facts and controversies. *Molecular Psychiatry* **4**, 501–507.

Schiltz, J. C. and Sawchenko, P. E. (2003). Signaling the brain in systemic inflammation: The role of perivascular cells. *Frontiers in Bioscience* **8**, s1321–s1329.

Turrin, N. P. and Rivest, S. (2004). Unraveling the molecular details involved in the intimate control of the immune and neuroendocrine systems: A revised and innovative hypothesis. *Experimental Biology and Medicine* **229**, 996–1006.
Ushikubi, F., Segi, E., Sugimoto, Y., et al. (1998). Impaired febrile response in mice lacking the prostaglandin E receptor subtype EP3. *Nature* **395**, 281–284.
Yamagata, K., Matsumura, K., Inoue, W., et al. (2001). Coexpression of microsomal-type prostaglandin E synthase with cyclooxygenase-2 in brain endothelial cells of rats during endotoxin-induced fever. *Journal of Neuroscience* **21**, 2669–2677.
Zhang, J. and Rivest, S. (2003). Is survival possible without arachidonate metabolites in the brain during systemic infection? *News in Physiological Sciences* **18**, 137–142.

Immune Response

P J Delves
University College London, London, UK

Glossary

Adaptive (acquired) immune response	Immunity mediated by lymphocytes and characterized by antigen-specificity and memory.
Complement	A group of serum proteins, some of which act in an enzymatic cascade, producing effector molecules involved in inflammation (C3a, C5a), phagocytosis (C3b), and cell lysis (C5b–C9).
Cytokines	Low-molecular-weight proteins that stimulate or inhibit the differentiation, proliferation, or function of immune cells.
Dendritic cell	Refers to an interdigitating dendritic cell which is major histocompatibility complex (MHC) class II-positive, Fc receptor-negative, and presents processed antigens to T cells in the T cell areas of secondary lymphoid tissues.
Granulocyte	Myeloid cells containing cytoplasmic granules (i.e., neutrophils, eosinophils, and basophils).
Innate immune response	Immunity which is not intrinsically affected by prior contact with antigen, i.e., all aspects of immunity not directly mediated by lymphocytes.
Primary immune response	The relatively weak immune response which occurs upon the first encounter of naive lymphocytes with their specific antigen.
Secondary immune response	The much stronger immune response which occurs upon the second encounter of primed lymphocytes with their specific antigen.
Toll-like receptors (TLRs)	A family of pattern recognition receptors involved in the detection of structures associated with pathogens or damaged host tissues.

The immune system has evolved to protect the body from foreign pathogens. It does so using quite a number of different cell types, most of which arise from pluripotent hematopoietic stem cells in the bone marrow and are collectively referred to as leukocytes (white blood cells). These stem cells can enter one of two differentiation pathways, the myeloid pathway which gives rise to monocytes/macrophages, dendritic cells, granulocytes (neutrophils, eosinophils, basophils, and mast cells), erythrocytes, and platelets, and the lymphoid pathway which gives rise to lymphocytes and natural killer (NK) cells (**Figure 1**). The bone marrow is referred to as a primary lymphoid organ and is where many of these cell types, including the B lymphocytes (B cells), reach maturity. However, the precursors of the T lymphocytes (T cells) need to leave the bone marrow and travel to the thymus in order to become fully developed. Given that a thymus is obligatory for the generation of T cells it is also referred to as a primary lymphoid organ. Upon maturation the lymphocytes, together with specialized antigen-presenting dendritic cells, primarily locate to secondary lymphoid organs (mucosa-associated lymphoid tissue (MALT), lymph nodes, and spleen) where the local architecture permits optimal stimulation of the immune response.

In order to become activated, the cells of the immune system need to detect the presence of a pathogen. Structures that can potentially be recognized by the immune system are broadly referred to as antigens and comprise an almost unlimited variety of protein, carbohydrate, lipid, and small molecular moieties. Antigenic structures are therefore associated not only with foreign organisms (viruses, bacteria, fungi, and parasites) and molecules (ingested, inhaled, or absorbed substances) but also the body's own (self) molecules and cells. Despite this capacity of the immune system to recognize an almost infinite variety of antigens, it must avoid making potentially damaging responses against self-antigens and against

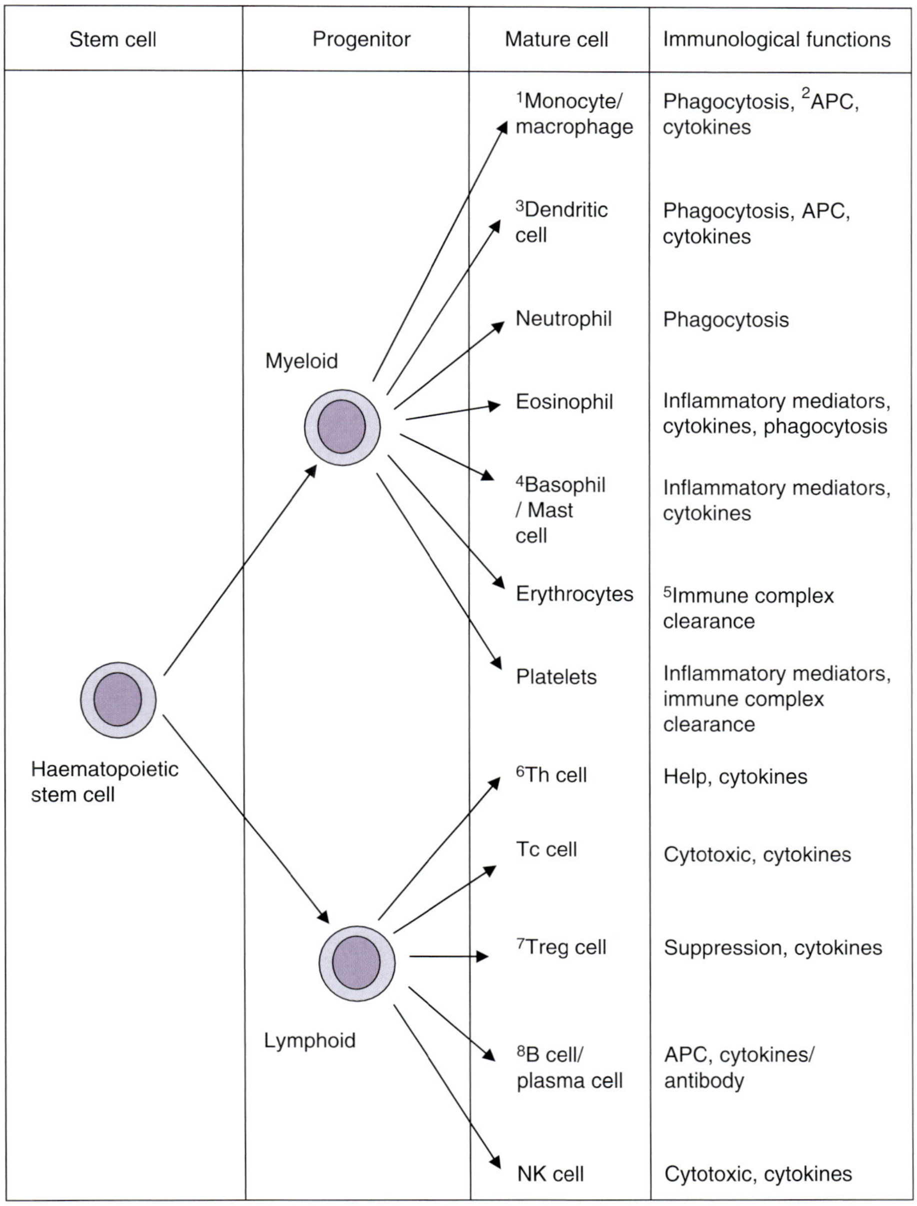

Figure 1 The major players in the immune response derived from hematopoietic stem cells in the bone marrow. Myeloid and lymphoid progenitors differentiate into a number of different cell types that, upon activation, mediate various immunological functions (examples of which are indicated). [1]Monocytes in the blood have functions that generally become more pronounced when these cells enter the tissues and differentiate into macrophages. [2]APC, professional antigen-presenting cell that uses MHC class II molecules to present processed antigen to CD4 (usually helper) T cells. [3]Dendritic cells (DC) come in a variety of forms. In addition to the myeloid dendritic cells, lymphoid dendritic cells (not shown) arise from lymphoid progenitors and have similar immunological functions to those of myeloid DC. Note that DCs are the only cell type that can act as APCs for naive T cells (i.e., T cells that have not previously encountered an antigen). There is also an entirely separate population of cells with a dendritic morphology that are present in secondary lymphoid organs and are referred to as follicular dendritic cells (FDC). FDC are nonphagocytic and lack the MHC class II required of professional APC, but instead present nonprocessed antigen (held on their surface in the form of immune complexes) directly to B cells. [4]Blood basophils and tissue mast cells share functional properties but it is thought that they are independently derived rather than blood basophils giving rise to tissue mast cells. [5]Immune complexes are composed of antigen bound to antibody and also often including complement components. [6]Th cells assist other cells in the immune system partly by secreting immunostimulatory cytokines but also using cell-contact dependent mechanisms. [7]Treg cells are heterogeneous, some inhibit other cells in the immune system by secreting cytokines with immunosuppressive properties while others use cell-contact dependent mechanisms to suppress immune responses. [8]B cells can act as professional APCs for antigen-experienced Th cells, and when activated can themselves secrete cytokines. When B cells differentiate into plasma cells their role is to secrete large amounts of antibody.

beneficial commensal organisms, food antigens, and so on. Thus, the cells of the immune system normally respond when they detect structures associated with pathogenic organisms.

Innate and Adaptive Immune Responses

Most cells of the immune system react with similar vigor however many times they encounter the same pathogen. This type of response is referred to as innate immunity (**Figure 2**) and involves phagocytic cells and NK cells, as well as basophils and mast cells. The phagocytic cells comprise short-lived neutrophils present in both the circulation and in the tissues, blood monocytes which differentiate into the more actively phagocytic macrophage upon entering the tissues, and dendritic cells in the tissues. Eosinophils are also weakly phagocytic but they are more adept at killing organisms that are too large to be engulfed and onto which they release toxic molecules. Basophils in the blood, and the functionally related mast cell in the tissues, release inflammatory mediators such as histamine, prostaglandins, and leukotrienes. The NK cells, present in both the circulation and the tissues, kill infected or malignant cells. Thus, the innate immune response can call upon a number of fundamentally different cell types. In contrast, the adaptive (also referred to as acquired) immune response is mediated by lymphocytes. These cells are exquisitely specific for individual antigens and when they encounter 'their' antigen for the first time they mount a primary immune response that produces not only cells and molecules to deal with the threat at hand but also memory cells. The latter constitute a population of lymphocytes that are expanded in number and have the capacity to generate the qualitatively and quantitatively superior secondary immune response. Of the two main populations of lymphocytes, B lymphocytes (B cells) and T lymphocytes (T cells), it is the B cells that are responsible for producing antibody molecules. T cells can be divided into three main subpopulations. Helper T cells (Th) assist, and regulatory T cells (Treg) can suppress, other cells in the immune response. Cytotoxic T cells (Tc), also referred to as cytotoxic T lymphocytes (CTL), kill infected or foreign eukaryotic cells. Most Th and Treg express a molecule called CD4 on their cell surface, whereas most Tc express CD8 instead.

Recognition of Pathogens and Other Antigens

In order to mount an immune response the cells of the immune system need to detect the presence of a threat. They do this using cell surface receptors which can be grouped into two main types: broadly reactive receptors and antigen-specific receptors.

Broadly Reactive Receptors

The cells involved in innate immune responses have a large number of receptors which are each encoded by entirely separate genes and which recognize structures that are common to many different organisms. These types of receptors are referred to as pattern recognition receptors (PRR) and their ligands designated pathogen-associated molecular patterns (PAMPs). Recently PRRs have been found to also be present on the cells of the adaptive immune response (i.e., lymphocytes), and some PRRs have been shown to recognize certain endogenous (self) ligands as well as recognizing PAMPS. Although the receptors are highly specific for the structures they recognize, their ligands are molecules that are widely distributed amongst many different species of pathogen. Examples include the toll-like receptors (TLRs; such as TLR3 which recognizes viral double-stranded ribonucleic acid (RNA) and TLR5 which detects bacterial flagellin) and the mannose receptor. The latter binds to the terminal mannose structure characteristic of prokaryotes but which is always covered by other sugars in glycoproteins of eukaryotic origin.

Antigen-Specific Receptors

Lymphocytes possess highly antigen-specific receptors on their cell surface. The B-cell receptor for antigen is a transmembrane version of the antibody molecule, while the analogous receptor on T lymphocytes consists of an $\alpha\beta$ or $\gamma\delta$ T-cell receptor (TCR) heterodimer. These receptors contain variable regions which, as their name suggests, vary from one receptor to another and which confer antigen specificity. All the antigen receptors on an individual lymphocyte will possess the same variable region sequence, but those on a different lymphocyte will bear a different variable region and hence specificity for a different antigen. The receptors are generated by a unique gene recombination mechanism in which the nucleotide sequence encoding the variable region of the protein is constructed from more than one gene. Thus, one gene sequence is picked in a fairly random fashion from each of two (for immunoglobulin (Ig) light chains and for TCR α or γ chains) or three (for Ig heavy chains and for TCR β or δ chains) gene pools referred to as variable (V), diversity (D, if utilizing all three gene pools), and joining (J) gene segments and these sequences spliced next to each other (**Figure 3**). The Ig genes undergo recombination in the precursors of B lymphocytes while TCR genes undergo recombination in early T cells. In each lymphocyte a different

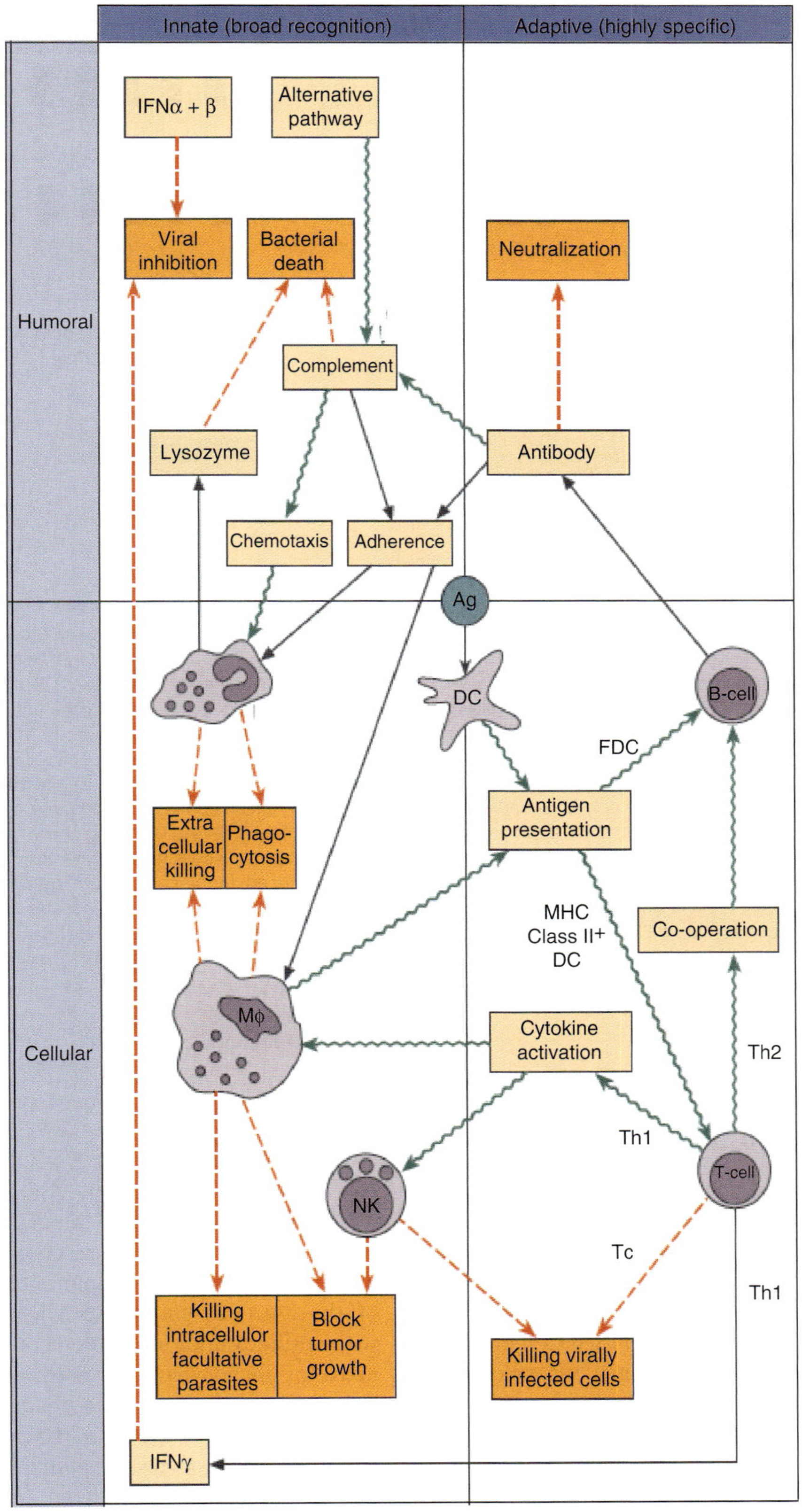

Figure 2 Some innate and adaptive immune responses. Humoral responses are those that are mediated by soluble molecules such as complement and cytokines in the innate response and antibody in the adaptive response. MHC class II$^+$ dendritic cells act as professional APC to present processed antigen to T cells, while the entirely different follicular dendritic cells (FDC) can present native antigen to B cells. Ag, antigen; IFNγ, gamma interferon; Mϕ, macrophage. Green wavy lines indicate processes that activate, whereas red dotted lines indicate processes that inhibit or kill. (Modified with permission from Delves PJ, Martin SJ, Burton, DR, and Roitt IM. (2006). *Roitt's essential immunology*, 11th edn. Oxford: Blackwell Publishers).

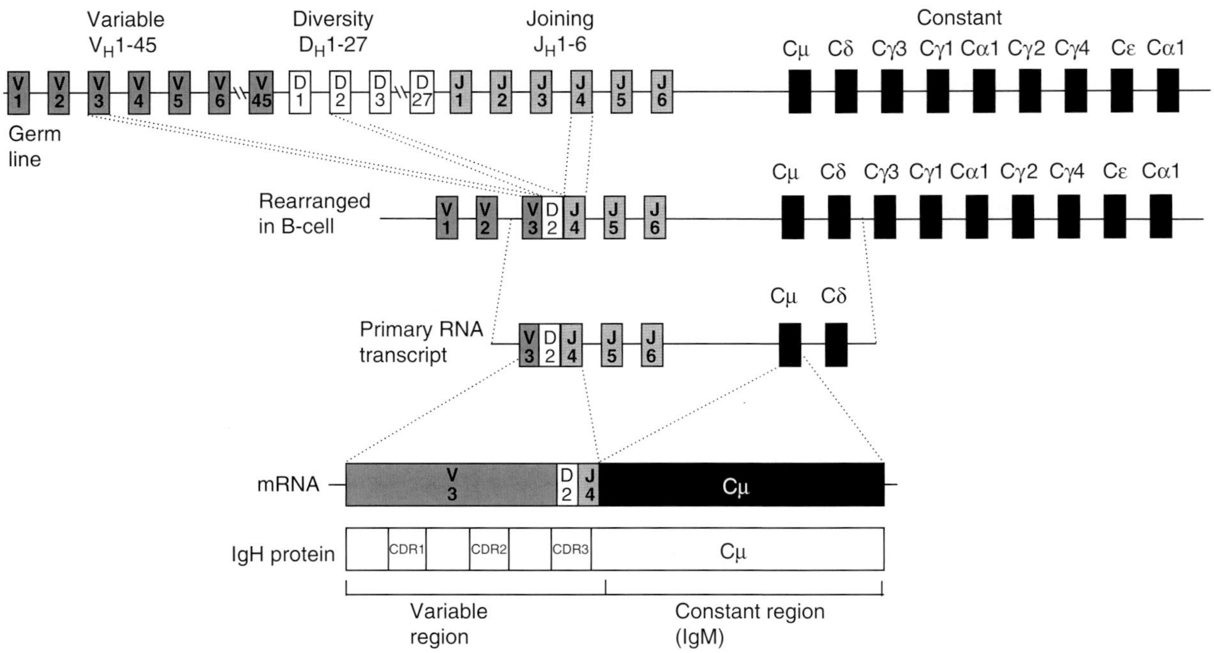

Figure 3 Antigen receptor gene recombination. In this example, immunoglobulin heavy chain (IgH) gene recombination is illustrated, but immunoglobulin light chain genes and the TCR genes undergo similar recombination processes in order to create a large number of different variable region sequences from a relatively small gene pool. Here the B cell has recombined the V3, D2, and J4 immunoglobulin heavy chain gene segments (not drawn to scale) and is utilizing the Cμ constant region gene segment from a primary RNA transcript that also includes Cδ. Alternative splicing of the primary RNA transcript is used to also produce IgD with the same antigen specificity. A different B cell might recombine V42, D16, and J6, etc., and would therefore have a different heavy chain variable region sequence. Recombination to provide variability for the immunoglobulin light chain variable region (not shown) is brought about by similar mechanisms using separate gene loci containing only V, J, and C segments. The heavy chain constant region gene transcription can include transmembrane exons. The heavy and light chain proteins polymerize into the 4 chain (2H + 2L) immunoglobulin molecule, which then sits in the cell surface membrane to function as the antigen-specific B-cell receptor. In plasma cells the transmembrane exons are not utilized and a secreted version of the antibody, with identical antigen-specificity, is produced. In the case of IgM the antibody polymerizes into pentamers prior to secretion. Class switching occurs later in the immune response with Cμ and Cδ usage being replaced with, for example, Cγ1 which specifies the IgG1 subclass of antibody but utilizing the same variable region and thus with the same antigen specificity. The areas of the variable region in both the heavy and the light chain which make contact with the antigen are referred to as complementarity determining regions (CDR).

recombination occurs and, together with a variety of additional molecular mechanisms which further increase diversity, leads to an almost infinite variety of antigen-specific receptors being generated. Therefore one lymphocyte will have antigen receptors that are specific for a particular component of streptococcus, another lymphocyte will be specific for an antigen from staphylococcus, another for a part of the influenza virus, and so on. There will only be a handful of lymphocytes specific for each antigen but collectively all the lymphocytes will provide cover against virtually all antigens that might be encountered.

Generation of the Immune Response

Innate responses are initiated when the PRRs on the surface of phagocytic and other cells detect the presence of PAMPs. Additionally, foreign antigens will very often become coated with proteins that are generated by the complement system, a cascade of molecules activated during immune responses. Later on in the immune response the antigen will additionally be coated with antibody. Among the many different types of molecules on the surface membrane of immune system cells are receptors for complement molecules and for the nonantigen-binding end (Fc) of the antibody molecule. Microorganisms coated with antibody and/or complement are said to be opsonized for phagocytosis, the antibody and complement linking the organism to the phagocyte. Complement carries out other functions; it acts as a chemotactic factor for phagocytes, it stimulates the release of inflammatory mediators from mast cells, and can mediate lysis of certain strains of bacteria.

The response of lymphocytes to an encounter with an antigen is somewhat different to that of the cells of the innate immune response. Whereas the latter go straight ahead with the task required, be it phagocytosis or the release of inflammatory mediators, the lymphocyte undergoes rapid cell division. The clone of lymphocytes with the appropriate antigen-specific receptor thus become greatly amplified in number during the adaptive immune response. T cells (at least the main population of T cells which bear an αβ TCR) cannot recognize antigens directly, but instead see antigen that has been processed and presented. With respect to Th cells which have not previously encountered their specific antigen, i.e., naive T cells, this involves dendritic cells which phagocytose or endocytose antigen, then demolish its protein components using proteases which generate short peptides of around 15 amino acids in length within the endosomal compartment of the cell. While still inside the endosomes these antigenic peptide fragments are combined with major histocompatibility complex (MHC) molecules of the class II type, and the complex of antigen peptide plus MHC class II is transported to the cell surface of the dendritic cell. It is the combination of peptide–MHC that is recognized by the TCR on the T cell, with the dendritic cell also expressing other cell-surface molecules such as CD80 and CD86 which supply the potent co-stimulation obligatory for the activation of naive T cells. Both macrophages and B cells also express peptide-bearing MHC class II molecules on their cell surface but due to their less profound ability to provide high levels of co-stimulation they only activate antigen-experienced T cells. Dendritic cells, macrophages, and B cells are collectively referred to as professional antigen-presenting cells (APC), a euphemism for cells which present antigen to CD4 T cells using MHC class II molecules. However, virtually all cells in the body are able to present peptide antigens using MHC class I molecules. In this case the peptides are usually generated from antigens present within the cytosol of a cell, including foreign antigens such as viruses. Cytosolic proteolysis for subsequent antigen presentation utilizes a modified version of the proteasome enzyme complex that carries out the normal cellular degradative processes. Peptide–MHC class I complexes expressed on the surface of infected cells are recognized by CD8+ Tc cells. Thus CD4+ T cells use their αβ TCR to recognize peptides presented by MHC class II molecules on professional APC whereas CD8+ T cells use their αβ TCR to recognize peptides presented by MHC class I molecules on infected cells.

The MHC is given a different name in different species, in humans it is referred to as human leukocyte antigen (HLA; although present not only on leukocytes) while in mice it is called H-2. In humans there are three main MHC class I gene loci, HLA-A, HLA-B, and HLA-C, and three class II loci, HLA-DP, HLA-DQ, and HLA-DR. In mice the main class I loci are H-2K and H-2D while the class II loci are referred to as I-A and I-E. The MHC molecules are encoded by the most polymorphic of all of the genes in the genome, and thus can vary enormously from individual to individual. It is this MHC polymorphism that is largely responsible for the immune system recognizing and subsequently rejecting organs or tissues from other members of the same species (allografts). The MHC genes are co-dominantly expressed and therefore each individual expresses two polymorphic variants of HLA-A, two of HLA-B, and so on. Certain variants are more common in the population than others and with common variants such as HLA-A2 in Caucasians it is quite frequently the case that an individual will be homozygous at that particular genetic locus.

The Anatomy of the Immune Response

The cells of the innate response such as phagocytic cells can act individually at the site of an infection. They are attracted to such sites by chemotactic factors, and their passage from the circulation out into the tissues is facilitated by the upregulated expression of adhesion molecules on vascular endothelial cells, ligands for which are expressed on the leukocyte cell surface.

As discussed previously, the Th cells of the adaptive response need to interact with professional APC in order to be activated. This requires cell–cell contact as the TCR on the T cell must bind to the peptide–MHC on the APC. The Th cells are also required to be in close proximity with the cells that will receive their help, which is provided by a combination of soluble molecules such as cytokines and by interactions between cell surface molecules on the Th cell and on the cell being helped. There are different subsets of cytokine-producing Th cells (e.g., Th1 cells, Th2 cells) and depending upon which subset is involved, the cytokine-mediated help that is given may facilitate antibody production by B cells, activation of Tc to kill infected cells, or enhancement of macrophage function (**Figure 2**). Given that Th, Tc, and B cells are all antigen-specific, that there are only a handful of cells specific for a given antigen, and that T cells require antigen to be presented to them, there is a need for a meeting place where the relevant cells can get together. This is the role of the secondary lymphoid organs; the spleen, lymph nodes, and MALT. These are the locations in which adaptive immune responses are initiated. Because the majority of pathogens will enter the body by ingestion or inhalation the MALT collectively provides a critical first line of defense against infection and acts as a major effector site for protective immune responses.

Protective Immune Response

The immune response is aimed at destroying foreign pathogens. Engulfment of microorganisms by phagocytes leads to their elimination when a wide variety of microbicidal compounds including toxic metabolites of oxygen such as hydroxyl radicals and enzymes such as lysozyme kill the invader. Eosinophils release toxins to achieve extracellular killing. Mast cells and basophils produce a plethora of molecules which collectively facilitate an acute inflammatory response with recruitment of leukocytes to the site of the infection. Infected cells, and some tumor cells, are dealt with by Tc and NK cells which can both induce apoptotic cell death in the target cell. Many cells in the body are capable of releasing cytokines but Th cells are particularly adept at doing so. In addition to providing help for other cells in the immune system, some cytokines can be directly cytotoxic (e.g., tumor necrosis factor (TNF)). B cells produce antibody molecules which are collectively found in their secreted form at high levels (10–15 mg ml^{-1}) in the circulation and, with the exception of the physically large pentameric IgM, also readily diffuse into the tissues. Antibodies are able to directly neutralize bacterial toxins, prevent viruses binding to cells, agglutinate microorganisms and thereby immobilize them, activate complement, opsonize microorganisms for phagocytosis, and mediate antibody-dependent cellular cytotoxicity (ADCC) in which leukocytes of various types become linked by antibody to infected cells and then kill them.

Avoidance of Harmful Immune Responses

The immune system can potentially react against the body's own components, resulting in immunity to self (autoimmunity). This only becomes a problem if the autoimmune reactions cause pathology, in which case the individual develops an autoimmune disease. Approximately 3–5% of individuals develop autoimmune disease at some time in their life. There are an extremely large number of different diseases in which autoimmune responses are thought to play a role, with the most common including psoriasis, thyroid autoimmune diseases (primarily Hashimoto's thyroiditis and Graves' disease), rheumatoid arthritis, vitiligo, systemic lupus erythematosus, Sjögren's syndrome, celiac disease, Crohn's disease, pernicious anemia, ankylosing spondylitis, type I (insulin-dependent) diabetes, and multiple sclerosis. The fact that the vast majority of individuals do not develop pathogenic autoimmune responses is due to the phenomenon of immunological tolerance. Encounter with self-antigen early on in the development of a lymphocyte leads to its clonal deletion by apoptosis. This occurs in the thymus for T cells and in the bone marrow for B cells. The T cells undergo thymic education involving positive and negative selection events in the thymus. Cells are positively selected if the random rearrangement of their TCR genes generates a receptor capable of recognizing peptides presented by that individual's polymorphic variants of MHC (self-MHC). However, if the TCR recognizes peptides derived from self antigens then a subsequent negative selection step will induce apoptosis of the autoimmune T cell. Thus, the only T cells which leave the thymus are ones that recognize foreign peptides presented by self-MHC. A somewhat similar process of negative selection occurs for B cells in the bone marrow, although their antigen receptor (the antibody molecule) recognizes antigen directly and therefore there is no requirement for positive selection for recognition of self-MHC molecules. The clonal deletion of T and B cells is not foolproof and some of the cells that leave the primary lymphoid organs are self-reactive. Therefore there are backup mechanisms to prevent harmful autoimmunity arising. Pathogenic foreign antigens are normally seen in the context of co-stimulatory activity whereas self-antigens do not provide co-stimulatory signals. When the lymphocyte receives a signal only through its antigen receptor in the absence of co-stimulation the result is not cell activation but rather cell inactivation, a process referred to as anergy. Unlike clonal deletion where the cell is eliminated, this leaves anergic cells which potentially can be re-activated. A further level of control rests with Treg cells that act to suppress any potentially harmful self-reactive cells. There are a number of different types of Treg cells, some of which arise naturally in the thymus and exert their effect via poorly understood cell contact-dependent mechanisms. Other Treg cells are induced to secrete cytokines that can mediate immunosuppressive activity, such as interleukin (IL)-10 and transforming-growth factor-β (TGFβ).

While the avoidance of harmful immune responses to self-antigens is something that operates with a fair degree of success, the capacity of the body to prevent allergic responses to what should be innocuous foreign antigens would appear to be rather less effective. A substantial minority of individuals (estimates vary, but perhaps even as many as 45% of children and 30% of adults) suffer from allergies to varying degrees. This frequently involves atopy, a capacity to produce raised levels of the IgE class of antibody against the allergen. The class of antibody is of paramount importance here because the IgE becomes bound to the surface of mast cells and basophils by virtue of the fact that these cells possess high-affinity receptors for the Fc region of IgE (FcεR). If the IgE has specificity for environmental antigens (allergens) these cross-link the IgE molecules. As a consequence, cross-linking of the FcεRs occurs leading to degranulation of the cells with the release of inflammatory mediators such as histamine.

Neuroendocrine–Immune Interactions

Although immune responses are driven by encounter with antigen and subject to regulation by a variety of cells and molecules which are clearly components of the immune system, it is also known that factors such as nutrition, hormones, and neuropeptides can modify the immune response. Stressors such as exam anxiety, restraint, and noise are known to influence various immune functions including lymphocyte proliferation, IgA secretion, phagocytosis, and the activity of NK cells. Receptors for endorphins, enkaphalins, acetylcholine, β-adrenoceptor agents, corticosteroids, insulin, growth hormone, estradiol, testosterone, and prolactin have all been described on various types of immune cell and their expression presumably infers some functional significance. To give an example, the cytokines IL-1, IL-6, and TNF act via the hypothalamic-pituitary-adrenal (HPA) axis to stimulate the release of glucocorticoids which are then capable of downregulating the activity of both Th1 cells and macrophages. Androgens and glucocorticoids generally suppress, while growth hormone, thyroxine, and insulin generally stimulate, immune responses. Lymphoid tissues, including the thymus, spleen, and lymph nodes, are richly innervated by norepinephrine-releasing sympathetic neurons. There is evidence from studies in knockout mice that in the absence of this neurotransmitter there is impaired production of the Th1-derived cytokines interferon (IFN)γ and TNF in response to challenge with antigen. Dendritic cells bear β-adrenoceptors and it has also been suggested that sympathetic nerves may be involved in controlling the migration of these APCs from the sites of inflammation to the local draining lymph nodes.

See Also the Following Articles

Cytokines; Glucocortoids, Overview; Immune Suppression; Immunity; Infection; Inflammation; Macrophages; Neuroendocrine Systems; Prostaglandins; Vasoactive Peptides.

Further Reading

Abbas, A. K. and Lichtman, A. H. (2006). *Basic immunology: functions and disorders of the immune system* (2nd edn.). Philadelphia, PA: Saunders.

Ader, R. (ed.) (2006). *Psychoneuroimmunology* (4th edn.). San Diego: Academic Press.

Daruna, J. H. (2004). *Introduction to psychoneuroimmunology.* San Diego: Academic Press.

Delves, P. J., Martin, S. J., Burton, D. R., et al. (2006). *Essential immunology* (11th edn.). Oxford: Blackwell Science.

Delves, P. J. (2006). Biology of the immune system. In: Beers, M. H., Porter, R. S., Jones, T. V., et al. (eds.) *The Merck manual* (18th edn, pp. 1320–1331). Whitehouse Station, NJ, USA: Merck.

Goldsby, R. A., Kindt, T. J., Osborne, B. A., et al. (2003). *Immunology* (5th edn.). New York: WH Freeman.

Padgett, D. A. and Glaser, R. (2003). How stress influences the immune response. *Trends in Immunology* **24**, 444–448.

Reiche, E. M., Nunes, S. O. and Morimoto, H. K. (2004). Stress, depression, the immune system, and cancer. *Lancet Oncology* **5**, 617–625.

Rhen, T. and Cidlowski, J. A. (2005). Mechanisms of disease: antiinflammatory action of glucocorticoids – new mechanisms for old drugs. *New England Journal of Medicine* **353**, 1711–1723.

Shepherd, A. J., Downing, J. E. and Miyan, J. A. (2005). Without nerves, immunology remains incomplete – *in vivo* veritas. *Immunology* **116**, 145–163.

Sternberg, E. M. (2006). Neural regulation of innate immunity: a coordinated nonspecific host response to pathogens. *Nature Reviews Immunology* **6**, 318–328.

Vedhara, K. and Irwin, M. (2005). *Human psychoneuroimmunology.* Oxford: Oxford University Press.

Autotolerance

M Durai
Johns Hopkins University School of Medicine, Baltimore, MD, USA
K D Moudgil
University of Maryland School of Medicine, Baltimore, MD, USA

This is a revised version of the article by M E F Melo, K D Moudgil, and E E Sercarz, Encyclopedia of Stress, first edition, volume 1, pp 284–290, © 2000, Elsevier Inc.

Glossary

Autoimmunity The activity of the immune system targeted against body's own (self) components. In a healthy situation, the immune system protects the body against invading pathogens such as bacteria and viruses. However, as a result of a series of orchestrated events involving genetic and environmental factors, there is a break in self-tolerance and the immune system starts attacking the body's own cellular components, which, if uncontrolled, can lead to pathological damage and autoimmune disease.

Autoimmune diseases Diseases caused by autoimmunity; can involve multiple body tissues (systemic) or be restricted to a particular tissue (organ-specific). Examples are multiple sclerosis, rheumatoid arthritis, systemic lupus erythematosus, and thyroiditis.

Heat-shock proteins (Hsps) A group of intracellular proteins whose expression is induced by a variety of environmental stresses such as heat, cold, oxygen deprivation, and other physical and chemical stressors; also called stress proteins. Under normal healthy conditions, Hsps act like chaperones, binding to other cellular proteins and preserving their shape and function, and also participating in their transport within and outside the cell. Under stressful conditions, Hsps protect other cellular proteins from denaturation. Hsps also participate in the display on the cell surface of peptides derived from other proteins for presentation by the MHC molecules to cells of the immune system.

Hypothalamic-pituitary-adrenal (HPA) axis The communication and interplay among the three endocrine tissues via specific chemical mediators secreted by these tissues. The hypothalamus secretes a hormone named corticotropin releasing hormone (CRH) in response to stress. CRH acts on the pituitary gland cells that secrete adrenocorticotropic hormone (ACTH), which in turn acts on the adrenal gland, leading to the secretion of adrenal stress hormones (e.g., cortisol). The adrenal hormones initiate various metabolic events to counter the effect of stress, and they also provide negative regulatory feedback signals to the hypothalamus and the pituitary gland to regulate the secretion of CRH and ACTH. An altered HPA axis activity has been implicated in many diseases, including some autoimmune diseases.

Oxidative stress A state of relative excess of reactive oxygen species (ROS) such as oxygen ions, free radicals, and peroxide within the cell. Oxidative stress is linked to disease processes including aging, atherosclerosis, and Alzheimer's disease.

Reactive oxygen species (ROS) Oxygen species such as oxygen ions, free radicals, and peroxide within the cell. The activity of ROS normally produced during various metabolic processes is controlled by naturally occurring antioxidants; however, in excess ROS are harmful, leading to damage to cellular components such as lipids, DNA, and proteins. Thus, ROS are involved in normal cellular functions, but they also can induce tissue damage leading to mutagenesis and cell death.

Tolerance/self-tolerance/immune tolerance A state of immunological unresponsiveness to a self-antigen without compromising the ability of the immune system to respond to a foreign antigen. Tolerance is effected by the deletion or inactivation of potentially self-reactive T and B cells during their development in the thymus and bone marrow, respectively (central tolerance) as well as by the control of the activity of self-reactive T and B cells in the periphery (peripheral tolerance) via a variety of mechanisms. A state of tolerance against foreign antigens can also be achieved using the appropriate experimental conditions.

Self-Tolerance Is Executed through the Deletion and Regulation of Autoreactive Lymphocytes

Immunological tolerance is the basic property of the immune system that provides for self/nonself-discrimination so that the immune system can protect the host from external pathogens without reacting against itself. Central tolerance is achieved by the clonal deletion of self-reactive lymphocytes expressing receptors with high avidity for self-ligands. Autoreactive lymphocytes that have escaped negative selection in the central lymphoid organs (the thymus and the bone marrow) are present in the peripheral repertoire, but are kept under control by multiple diverse peripheral tolerance mechanisms. These include anergy (functional inactivation) induction in lymphocytes that recognize self-ligands (first signal) in the absence of appropriate costimulation (second signal) on nonprofessional antigen-presenting cells (APCs), activation-induced cell death (AICD), cytokine-mediated regulation and various types of regulatory cells. The failure of tolerogenic mechanisms either within the central lymphoid organs or in the periphery permits the activation and expansion of self-reactive lymphocytes, which in turn can lead to tissue damage and the manifestation of an autoimmune disease. Autoimmune diseases are broadly categorized into systemic and organ-specific disorders. Systemic lupus erythematous (SLE) and multiple sclerosis (MS) are examples of systemic and organ-specific autoimmune diseases, respectively.

In the last several years, there has been increasing realization that the expression of a target autoantigen involved in an organ-specific autoimmune disease is not necessarily restricted to that particular tissue. Instead, the autoantigen is either expressed ubiquitously or also expressed within the thymus (ectopic expression). The latter observation represents a paradigm shift in our understanding of the induction of self-tolerance to tissue-specific antigens. It is now known that many target self-antigens relevant to the pathogenesis of autoimmunity are efficiently expressed within the thymus and that their expression is controlled in part by a transcription factor named autoimmune regulator (aire). Furthermore, both humans and mice deficient in the *AIRE* gene exhibit signs of systemic autoimmunity. The human disorder is referred to as the autoimmune polyendocrinopathy-candidiasis-ectodermal dystrophy syndrome (APECED). In regard to the mechanisms of peripheral tolerance, a deficiency of a subset of T regulatory cells (Treg, $CD4^{+}CD25^{+}$ T cells) also results in autoimmune manifestations. These Treg are characterized by the expression of Foxp3, a unique transcription factor that is a member of the forkhead/winged-helix family of transcriptional regulators. Patients lacking the *FOXP3* gene are deficient in Treg and exhibit features of immune dysregulation, polyendocrinopathy, enteropathy, X-linked (IPEX) syndrome. Thus, in a healthy individual, both central and peripheral tolerogenic mechanisms play critical roles in the induction and maintenance of self-tolerance and, thereby, in the prevention of autoimmunity.

Cells Exposed to Stressful Stimuli Upregulate the Expression of Stress Proteins

Stress proteins (previously known as heat shock proteins; Hsps) are ubiquitous cellular proteins whose expression within cells is upregulated in response to a variety of stressful stimuli, for example, increased temperature, oxidative stress, nutritional deficiency, viral infection, tumor necrosis factor (TNF-)α, endotoxin, adrenergic stimuli, and ultraviolet irradiation. These stimuli may be part of environmental stress or pathological states. The Hsps thus induced protect cells from cellular injury including stress-induced apoptosis. Hsps are highly conserved in prokaryotes as well as eukaryotes, and they are grouped into several families based on their molecular weight (**Table 1**). Hsps are localized in various intracellular compartments and function as molecular chaperones, which take part in the assembly, folding, and translocation of cellular proteins (**Table 2**). Because Hsps are primarily intracellular proteins, their release from necrotic cells into the extracellular environment indicates nonphysiological tissue damage, and such release of Hsps can induce a range of biological responses.

Hsps can influence several functions of the immune system such as antigen processing and presentation, cytokine production, expression of intercellular signaling molecules, lymphocyte trafficking, and target cell lysis (**Table 3**). Hsps also can serve as immunodominant antigens, and one hypothesis underlying the immune alterations induced by Hsps invokes immunological cross-recognition between the mammalian and the microbial homologs.

Tolerance to Stress Proteins Is Incomplete

Despite the existence of several mechanisms for tolerance induction against self-proteins, the presence of self-Hsp-specific T and B lymphocytes in the mature repertoire has been reported in healthy individuals. The presence of self-hsp60-specific T cells was demonstrated in inbred Lewis rats by immunization with mammalian hsp60 using either vaccinia virus or DNA encoding human hsp60 or using rat hsp60 that is 98% homologous to human hsp60. In this context, it has been shown that Hsps are expressed at high levels in the normal thymus. Moreover, the transgenic

Table 1 Mammalian heat shock protein (Hsp) families and their cellular location and function[a]

Hsp family/members	*Localization*	*Functions*
Small Hsps		
Hsp10	Mitochondria	Co-chaperone for Hsp60 activities
αB-crystallin	Cytoplasm	Cytoskeletal stabilization
Hsp27	Nucleus/cytoplasm	Actin dynamics
Hsp32	Cytoplasm	Heme metabolism, antioxidant properties
Hsp40		
Hsp40	Nucleus/cytoplasm	Binds to non-native proteins, regulates the activity of Hsp70
Hsp47	Endoplasmic reticulum	Processing and/or secretion of collagen
Hsp60		
Hsp60	Mitochondria	Both involved in protein folding and assembly
TCP-1	Cytoplasm	
Hsp70		
Hsp70	Nucleus/cytoplasm	Hsp70 regulates HSF-1 activity and Hsp gene transcription
Grp78/Bip	Endoplasmic reticulum	All: Prevent aggregation of unfolded proteins
Grp75	Mitochondria	Bind ATP and show ATPase activity
Hsp90		
Hsp90 (α and β)	Cytoplasm	Bind to other proteins and regulate protein activity Assembly and folding of newly synthesized proteins
Grp94/gp96/Hsp100	Endoplasmic reticulum	Prevent aggregation of refolded proteins
Hsp110		
Hsp110 (human)	Cytoplasm/nucleolus	Thermal tolerance
Apg-1 (mouse)	Cytoplasm	Protein refolding
Hsp105	Cytoplasm	

[a]Apg-1, Autophagy-1, a protein kinase essential for autophagy; ATP, adenosine triphosphate; Bip, immunoglobulin heavy chain binding protein; Grp, glucose-regulated protein; HSF-1, heat-shock factor 1; Hsp, heat shock protein; TCP-1, tailless complex polypeptide.

Table 2 Effects of heat shock proteins on the immune system[a]

Immunological effects	*Hsp involved*	*Specific action and cell types*
Antigen processing and presentation	Hsp70	Peptide loading and antigen processing of MHC class I molecules Interaction with misfolded MHC class II and retention in the ER
	Hsp90	Peptide transport and loading of MHC class I in the ER
	Bip and Calnexin	Assembly of MHC class I and class II molecules in the ER
	gp96	Interaction with misfolded MHC class II and retention in the ER, peptide loading of MHC class II molecules
Expression of intercellular signaling molecules	Mycobacterial Hsp60	ICAM-1 and VCAM-1 expression on vascular endothelial cells
	Chlamydial and human Hsp60	E-selectin, ICAM-1, and VCAM-1 expression on vascular endothelial cells
Cytokine production	Hsp60	Production of IL-1α, IL-6, IL-12, IL-15, nitric oxide, and TNF-α by monocytes and macrophages
	Hsp60 and Hsp70	IFN-γ production by T cells IL-6 production by vascular endothelial cells IL-6 production by smooth muscle cells
Target cell lysis	Hsp70	Tumor cells
Lymphocyte homing	Ubiquitin	Lymphocyte receptor involved in the interaction with high endothelial venules, thereby in lymphocyte homing

[a]Bip, immunoglobulin heavy chain binding protein; ER, endoplasmic reticulum; Hsp, heat shock protein; ICAM-1, intercellular adhesion molecule-1; IL, interleukin; INF, interferon; MHC, major histocompatibility complex; TNF, tumor necrosis factor; VCAM-1, vascular cell adhesion molecule-1.

overexpression of mouse hsp60, in the thymus failed to eliminate T-cell responses to self-hsp60 following hsp60 immunization. Thus, in contrast to other antigens that are tolerogenic at low levels of thymic expression, hsp60 failed to delete antigen-specific T cells even at high levels of expression within the thymus.

Endogenous hsp60 Can Be Processed and Presented to Antigen-Primed T Cells

Although Hsps are intracellular proteins, they can be efficiently expressed on the cell surface as peptide–major histocompatibility complex (MHC)

Table 3 Heat shock proteins and their immunoregulatory effect in autoimmune diseases[a]

Diseases	*Strain/immunogen*	*Hsp involved*
Animal models		
Adjuvant-induced arthritis	Lewis rats/heat-killed *M. tuberculosis*	Mycobacterial Hsp60, Hsp70 and Hsp10 Self (rat) Hsp60 Human Hsp60
	Lewis rats/DDA, a synthetic adjuvant	Mycobacterial Hsp60 Self (rat) Hsp60
Pristane-induced arthritis	Mice/pristane	Mycobacterial Hsp60 Self (mouse) Hsp60
Collagen-induced arthritis	Lewis rats/collagen type II	Mycobacterial Hsp60
	Mice/collagen type II	Mycobacterial Hsp60 and Hsp70
Streptococcal cell wall-induced arthritis	Lewis rats/cell walls of streptococci	Mycobacterial Hsp60
Avridine-induced arthritis		Mycobacterial Hsp60 and Hsp70
Insulin-dependent diabetes mellitus	Nonobese diabetic mice/spontaneous	Mycobacterial Hsp60 Self (mouse) Hsp60 Human Hsp60 and Hsp90
Experimental autoimmune encephalomyelitis	Lewis rats/myelin basic protein	Mycobacterial Hsp60 and Hsp10
Human		
Rheumatoid arthritis	–	Mycobacterial Hsp60 Human Hsp60 and Hsp70 Bip
Juvenile chronic arthritis	–	Human Hsp60
Type I diabetes mellitus	–	Human Hsp60, Hsp70, and Hsp90
Multiple sclerosis	–	Human Hsp60 and Hsp70 αB-crystallin
Systemic lupus erythematosus	–	Human Hsp60 and Hsp90
Hashimoto's thyroiditis	–	Human Hsp60

[a]Bip, immunoglobulin heavy chain binding protein; DDA, dimethyl dioctadecyl ammonium bromide; Hsp, heat shock protein.

complexes. For example, the T cells raised in the Lewis rat against the disease-protective C-terminal epitopes of rat hsp60 can be restimulated *in vitro* in a proliferation assay when cocultured with heat-stressed but not unstressed syngeneic APCs in the absence of exogenous antigen, suggesting that the endogenous hsp60 can both be upregulated and be processed and presented by the APCs to activate antigen-primed T cells. The processing and presentation of hsp60 via class I pathway has also been documented. Cytotoxic T lymphocytes (CTL) specific for mycobacterial hsp60 were shown to recognize stressed macrophages in the absence of exogenously added antigens, suggesting that endogenous self-hsp60 is presented in the context of MHC class I molecules to the CTL. Furthermore, the CTL-mediated lysis of stressed macrophages was suppressed by hsp60-directed antisense oligonucleotides, thereby confirming the specificity of the CTL for hsp60.

The breakdown of self-tolerance leading to the induction of antiself immune response is typically associated with the initiation of autoimmunity. However, studies by different investigators have shown that antiself-hsp60 immunity may be immunosuppressive and beneficial against autoimmunity. Lewis rats immunized with either self-hsp60 (rat hsp60) or its homologous human hsp60 are protected against subsequent induction of adjuvant arthritis (AA). Furthermore, this protection can be adoptively transferred to naïve Lewis rats through the T cells of protected rats. Similarly, other Hsps in addition to hsp60 possess immunoregulatory activity.

Oxidative Stress Influences Several Components of the Immune System Pertaining to Self-Tolerance and Autoimmunity

Oxidative stress results from the increased production of oxidants, reduced generation of antioxidants, or failure to repair an oxidative damage. The damage to cells/tissues is caused by reactive oxygen species (ROS) comprised of free radicals, peroxides, and so forth (e.g., hydroxyl radical, hydrogen peroxide, and peroxynitrite). ROS can be derived from endogenous (e.g., metabolic reactions within the mitochondria or the liver detoxification pathways) or from exogenous (e.g., environmental pollutants or microbial infections) sources. ROS produced during oxidative stress can modulate a wide variety of cellular functions through the regulation of NF-κB. Some of the

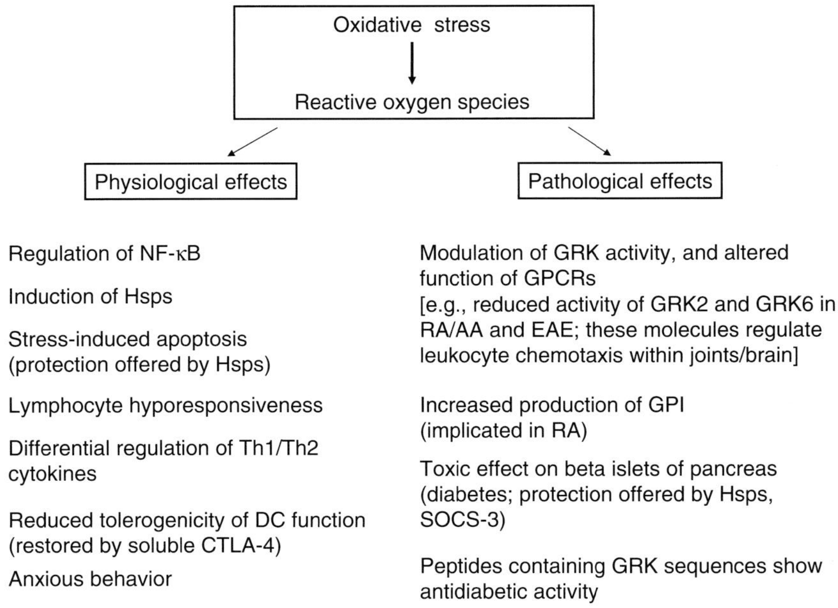

Figure 1 Oxidative stress and its influence on physiological and pathological immune processes. Oxidative stress has been implicated in a large variety of biological reactions. AA, adjuvant arthritis; CTLA-4, cytotoxic T lymphocyte associated-4; DC, dendritic cells; EAE, experimental autoimmune encephalomyelitis; GPCR, G-protein-coupled receptor; GPI, glucose-6-phosphate isomerase; GRK, G-protein-coupled receptor kinase; Hsp, heat-shock protein; NF-κB, nuclear factor kappa B; RA, rheumatoid arthritis; SOCS, suppressor of cytokine signaling; Th1, T helper 1; Th2, T helper 2.

processes influenced by oxidative stress and ROS are summarized in **Figure 1**.

It has been observed that oxidative stress induces hyporesponsiveness in T lymphocytes, which in turn correlates with ROS-dependent protein alterations including structural modification of crucial T-cell receptor (TCR) signaling molecules. Also reported is the inhibition of activated/memory T cells by oxidative stress, which is associated with a block of NF-κB activation. In addition, a predominant decrease in Th1 (but not Th2) cytokine production was observed in the memory/effector subset compared to naïve T cells. ROS can also influence the activity of the major professional APCs such as dendritic cells (DCs). It is known that immature DCs are tolerogenic, whereas mature DCs are immunogenic. In this context, it has been shown that ROS can significantly decrease the tolerogenic activity of DCs. In one study, this inhibitory effect of ROS was shown to be overcome by treatment with soluble CTLA-4. The precise significance of this interrelationship has not yet been fully defined.

Oxidative stress and ROS have been implicated in the pathogenesis of various autoimmune diseases, including arthritis and diabetes mellitus. Oxidative stress can modulate the intracellular levels of G-protein-coupled receptor kinases (GRKs), which in turn influence the activity of G-protein-coupled receptors (GPCRs). It has been observed that the levels of GRK2 and GRK6 are decreased in lymphocytes of patients with rheumatoid arthritis (RA) as well as of rats with AA. Similarly, decreased GRK2 levels have also been found in splenocytes of rats with experimental autoimmune encephalomyelitis (EAE). GRKs are involved in modulating leukocyte chemotaxis into the target organs that constitute the sites of autoimmune inflammation (e.g., the joints in RA and the brain in EAE). Interestingly, peptides containing defined sequences of the kinase-substrate interaction site of GRK2/3 show antidiabetic activity in animal models of type 2 diabetes, supporting the likely therapeutic significance of GRKs in some other diseases as well.

Hypoxia is a characteristic feature of joints observed in both RA patients as well as experimental models of arthritis. Interestingly, it is associated with increased expression of glucose-6-phosphate isomerase (GPI), which has been shown to be one of the target autoantigens in autoimmune arthritis in K/BXN mice. These mice possess a TCR that is transgenic for an epitope within ribonuclease, but it fortuitously cross-reacts with the ubiquitously expressed protein, GPI. An immune response to GPI has been observed in K/BXN mice as well as in RA patients, particularly those with extra-articular complications.

ROS have been shown to have a toxic effect on the β islets of the pancreas, and thereby they have been implicated in the pathogenesis of type 1 diabetes mellitus. Interesting, Hsps can offer protection against ROS-mediated damage to β islets. Another protective pathway in β islets involves the suppressor of cytokine signaling (SOCS-)3. Similarly, SOCS-1 plays a role in the pathogenesis of arthritis, and SOCS-1 deficiency results in severe synovial inflammation and joint destruction. SOCS proteins can be induced by a variety of stimuli, particularly various cytokines, and they regulate cytokine signaling as well as a wide variety of pathways relevant in inflammatory diseases of infectious and autoimmune origin. The pro-inflammatory cytokine interferon (IFN-)γ induces the expression of SOCS-1 and-3.

Oxidative stress may also contribute to an anxious behavior. Furthermore, the levels of two enzymes (glyoxalase 1 and glutathione reductase) that influence oxidative stress also positively correlate with the level of anxiety. Considering the relationship between stress and autoimmunity, this finding provides one of the molecular links between stress and behavior (anxiety) associated with autoimmunity.

Neural Immune Interactions and Their Relevance to Autoimmunity

Several lines of evidence emphasize the interplay between, and cross-regulation of, the activities of the nervous system and the immune system. The nervous system influences the immune system primarily via the hypothalamic-pituitary-adrenal (HPA) axis, the hypothalamic-pituitary-gonadal (HPG) axis, and the chemical mediators of the autonomic nervous system, whereas the immune system modulates the activities of the neural system via cytokines and the vagus nerve. In experimental models of autoimmune diseases and human subjects, an inadequately functioning or blunted HPA axis has been associated with increased susceptibility and/or enhanced severity of autoimmune diseases such as RA and MS. In some cases, the baseline HPA axis activity in the disease-susceptible versus disease-resistant individuals was comparable, but the dysfunction of the HPA axis was manifest on an exposure to the stressful or inflammatory stimuli. Because the stress response intimately involves the components of the HPA and HPG axes, it is apparent that chronic physical and psychosocial stresses constitute one of the factors that have been implicated in the initiation and aggravation of an autoimmune condition.

The underlying hypothesis involving the HPA axis is that susceptibility to autoimmune diseases may be related to inadequate responsiveness of the HPA axis to stressful stimuli such that there is a decreased secretion of cortisol and other biomolecules that are normally required to downregulate the immune responses. Consequently, unchecked immune reactivity leads to the induction of anti-self-directed T cell and/or antibody responses, which if propagated, may eventually lead to autoimmunity. In support of this proposition, studies in the rat model of AA have revealed that susceptible rat strains (e.g., Lewis and DA rats) have impaired HPA axis compared to resistant rat strains (e.g., Fischer F344 and BN rats) that display an aggravated HPA axis response. Interestingly, chemical/pharmacological or surgical manipulations aimed at altering the HPA axis activity in these rats also resulted in a corresponding change in the pattern of susceptibility/resistance to AA. The complementation of the HPA axis activity by the administration of glucocorticoids or transplantation of the hypothalamus from the resistant rat strain into susceptible rat strain led to acquired resistance to AA, whereas interference with HPA axis activity rendered the resistant rat strain susceptible to AA. Such differences in HPA axis activity in response to stress or inflammatory stimuli have also been observed in male versus female rats, with the HPA axis response impaired in female rats relative to male rats. These results suggest that differences in HPA axis responsiveness might contribute to the higher incidence of autoimmune diseases observed in females compared to males. An additional link between gender-related hormones and susceptibility to autoimmunity is provided by the observation that androgens exert a suppressive, anti-inflammatory effect on T-cell and antibody responses, whereas estrogens tend to enhance immune reactivity, particularly antibody responses.

The evidence to support a direct association between HPA axis and autoimmune susceptibility in patients with autoimmune diseases is not as clear as in animal models of these diseases. Nevertheless, clinical histories and the examination of the parameters reflecting HPA axis activity support the idea that HPA axis activity is impaired in diseases such as RA and MS. For example, the decreased secretion of cortisol following HPA axis stimulation, reduced number of glucocorticoid receptors on specific cell types, decreased androgen levels, impaired growth hormone response, and inadequately low ratio of steroid hormones to interleukin (IL-)6 and TNF-α have been observed in RA patients. In addition to the HPA axis, the dysregulated autonomic nervous system is also a critical modifier of autoimmune susceptibility and chronicity of the autoreactive immune response. A cholinergic anti-inflammatory pathway involving the vagus nerve is believed to represent a physiological pathway for the detection of inflammatory stimuli via the afferent vagus and the corresponding regulation of the cytokine (TNF-α) response of macrophages via the efferent vagus. The nicotinic acetylcholine receptor α 7 subunit expressed on the macrophage plays a critical role in this pathway. Taken together, it is evident that other factors in addition to the HPA axis and the autonomic nervous system, such as genetic and environmental factors, also play an important role in determining susceptibility/resistance to autoimmunity.

Immunoregulatory and Therapeutic Approaches Based on Biomolecules and Intracellular Pathways Involved in the Stress Response

1. *Altering the cellular levels of Hsps.* Taking into consideration the chaperone function of Hsps in protecting other proteins from damage in stressed cells as well as the finding that anti-Hsp immunity can be immunoregulatory in nature, the expression of cellular Hsps can be induced physiologically or pharmacologically, or by direct administration of a specific Hsp for a beneficial effect in suppressing autoimmunity. For example, the levels of endogenous Hsps can be increased by hyperthermia, geldanamycin, geranylgeranylacetone, cyclopentenone prostanoids, certain heavy metals, salicylates, or dexamethasone. On the other hand, the expression of Hsps can be decreased by retinoic acid, bioflavinoid compounds, or 15-deoxyspergualin, and this approach may prove useful in augmenting immunity as desired for antitumor immunity.
2. *The use of antioxidants.* A wide variety of synthetic and naturally occurring compounds have been used to counter the cellular effects of oxidative stress and ROS. These compounds possess antioxidant properties. Vitamin E, vitamin C and β-carotenes are well-known antioxidants. The extracts of certain plants have also been found to possess potent antioxidant activity by scavenging free radicals leading to anti-arthritic activity in the rat model of AA. These include pumpkin seed oil, *Semecarpus anacardium*, and *Trewia polycarpa*. In addition, Meloxicam modulates oxidation status and is beneficial in suppressing AA.
3. *Interventions aimed at HPA–HPG axes and the autonomic system.* Pharmacological and surgical procedures have been employed in experimental systems to reconstitute or enhance the activity of the HPA and HPG axes and to alter the activity of the autonomic system and cytokine (TNF-α) secretion by macrophages via the stimulation of the vagus nerve. The administration of androgens to strike a sex hormone balance is another modality that is being exploited for the control of RA, particularly in male patients.
4. *Targeting the stress signaling pathways.* The synovial membrane of arthritic joints is under a variety of stresses: oxidative stress, pro-inflammatory cytokines, heat-stress, and shear stress. Multiple cell surface-resident and intracellular molecules are involved in stress signaling pathways in the milieu of inflammatory synovitis, and these signaling pathways represent novel and promising targets for the control of RA and other autoimmune diseases.

Further Reading

Anis, Y., Leshem, O., Reuveni, H., et al. (2004). Antidiabetic effect of novel modulating peptides of G-protein-coupled kinase in experimental models of diabetes. *Diabetologia* **47**, 1232–1244.

Durai, M., Gupta, R. S. and Moudgil, K. D. (2004). The T cells specific for the carboxyl-terminal determinants of self (rat) heat-shock protein 65 escape tolerance induction and are involved in regulation of autoimmune arthritis. *Journal of Immunology* **172**, 2795–2802.

Eskandari, F., Webster, J. I. and Sternberg, E. M. (2003). Neural immune pathways and their connection to inflammatory diseases. *Arthritis Research and Therapy* **5**, 251–265.

Griffiths, H. R. (2005). ROS as signalling molecules in T cells – evidence for abnormal redox signalling in the autoimmune disease, rheumatoid arthritis. *Redox Report* **10**, 273–280.

Harbuz, M. (2002). Neuroendocrinology of autoimmunity. *International Review of Neurobiology* **52**, 133–161.

Kavelaars, A., Vroon, A., Raatgever, R. P., et al. (2003). Increased acute inflammation, leukotriene B4-induced chemotaxis, and signaling in mice deficient for G protein-coupled receptor kinase 6. *Journal of Immunology* **171**, 6128–6134.

Lombardi, M. S., Kavelaars, A. and Heijnen, C. J. (2002). Role and modulation of G protein-coupled receptor signaling in inflammatory processes. *Critical Reviews in Immunology* **22**, 141–163.

Malmberg, K. J., Arulampalam, V., Ichihara, F., et al. (2001). Inhibition of activated/memory (CD45RO(+)) T cells by oxidative stress associated with block of NF-kappaB activation. *Journal of Immunology* **167**, 2595–2601.

Moseley, P. (2000). Stress proteins and the immune response. *Immunopharmacology* **48**, 299–302.

Moudgil, K. D., Chang, T. T., Eradat, H., et al. (1997). Diversification of T cell responses to carboxy-terminal determinants within the 65-kD heat-shock protein is involved in regulation of autoimmune arthritis. *Journal of Experimental Medicine* **185**, 1307–1316.

Piccirillo, C. A. and Shevach, E. M. (2004). Naturally-occurring CD4+CD25+ immunoregulatory T cells:

central players in the arena of peripheral tolerance. *Seminars in Immunology* **16**, 81–88.
Pockley, A. G. (2003). Heat shock proteins as regulators of the immune response. *Lancet* **362**, 469–476.
Quintana, F. J. and Cohen, I. R. (2005). DNA vaccines coding for heat-shock proteins (HSPs): tools for the activation of HSP-specific regulatory T cells. *Expert Opinion on Biological Therapy* **5**, 545–554.
Steinhoff, U., Brinkmann, V., Klemm, U., et al. (1999). Autoimmune intestinal pathology induced by hsp60-specific CD8 T cells. *Immunity* **11**, 349–358.
van Eden, W., van der Zee, R. and Prakken, B. (2005). Heat-shock proteins induce T-cell regulation of chronic inflammation. *Nature Reviews Immunology* **5**, 318–330.
Venanzi, E. S., Benoist, C. and Mathis, D. (2004). Good riddance: thymocyte clonal deletion prevents autoimmunity. *Current Opinion in Immunology* **16**, 197–202.
Zugel, U. and Kaufmann, S. H. (1999). Role of heat shock proteins in protection from and pathogenesis of infectious diseases. *Clinical Microbiology Reviews* **12**, 19–39.

Macrophages

W P Fehder
New York University, New York, NY, USA
F Tuluc
Children's Hospital of Philadelphia, Philadelphia, PA, USA
W-Z Ho and S D Douglas
Children's Hospital of Philadelphia and University of Pennsylvania Medical School, Philadelphia, PA, USA

This is a revised version of the article by W P Fehder, W–z Ho and S D Douglas, Encyclopedia of Stress, First edition, volume 2, pp 663–668, © 2000, Elsevier Inc.

Glossary

Activated macrophage — A macrophage that has been stimulated either biochemically or immunologically and exhibits an increase in one or more functional activities or the appearance of a new functional activity.

Cytokines — A class of low-molecular-weight soluble protein molecules released by immune cells during the course of immune response that serve to mediate and regulate the amplitude and duration of immune/inflammatory responses in the organism. Cytokines are produced during the effector phases of natural and specific immunity in a brief self-limited event. Many of the same cytokine substances are produced by different cells and may act on many different cell types. Cytokines exert their action by binding to target cell-surface receptors, which may be on the surface of the secreting cell (autocrine action), on the surface of a nearby cell (paracrine action), or on the surface of a cell in a remote location (endocrine action) reached through the bloodstream.

Interleukins (ILs) — Cytokines that are principally synthesized by leukocytes and act primarily on leukocytes.

Macrophages — Large, irregularly shaped white blood cells measuring 25–50 μm in diameter that are the major differentiated cells of the mononuclear phagocyte system.

Mononuclear phagocytes — A class of immune cells that have a common lineage that includes monoblasts, promonocytes, monocytes, and macrophages.

Neurokinin (NK-)1 receptor — A G-protein-coupled receptor that mediates the biological responses to substance P that has been demonstrated on T cells, B lymphocytes, neutrophils, mast cells, and monocytes/macrophages.

Substance P (SP) — An 11-amino-acid peptide present in the central nervous system that is involved in the pathogenesis of nausea/emesis, pain, mood disorders, stress, anxiety, reinforcement, neurotoxicity, and neurogenesis. It is a member of the tachykinin family of neuropeptides. Outside the central nervous system, SP regulates intestinal motility and secretion, causes vasodilation, and serves as a modulator of a number of important immunological functions. Circulating levels of SP become elevated in stressful situations; monocytes stimulated by SP produce and release cytokines such as tumor necrosis factor α, interleukin-1, and interleukin-6.

Tissue macrophages — Members of the monocyte/macrophage family that have migrated from the circulation into a body tissue, remaining adherent for several months and ultimately migrating to nearby draining lymph nodes for disposal at the end of their useful life. Some tissue macrophages may survive for the lifetime of the individual.

Macrophages are a diverse group of leukocytes (white blood cells) that share a common origin in the bone marrow and enter the circulation as incompletely differentiated monocytes. Macrophages are the major differentiated cells of the monocyte/macrophage system.

Origin and Function of Monocytes/ Macrophages

The monocyte/macrophage system comprises bone marrow monoblasts and promonocytes, peripheral blood monocytes, and tissue macrophages. The peripheral blood monocytes differentiate into macrophages that are capable of phagocytosis of particles, cells, bacteria, and fungi; they also have major roles in antigen presentation and cytokine secretion. Monocytes remain in the circulatory system or migrate to different tissues where they increase in size, becoming tissue macrophages. Tissue macrophages become part of the architecture of specific tissues where they may remain, performing specific protective functions and functions unique to the organ. These tissue macrophages are given names according to their location (**Table 1**). Tissue macrophages may be stimulated by chemical messengers to break away from their attachment and migrate along with mobile macrophages and monocytes to areas of inflammation by a process known as chemotaxis. The term monocyte/macrophage system is virtually synonymous with, and has replaced in the nomenclature, the reticuloendothelial system.

Macrophages perform an essential function in the immune system by attacking and destroying invading bacteria, viruses, and other injurious substances, participating in a wide range of physiological and pathological processes. Although many micro-organisms are phagocytized and destroyed with ease by macrophages, certain pathogens such as listeria, salmonella, brucella, mycobacteria, chlamydia, rickettsia, leishmania, toxoplasma, trypanosoma, and legionella are able to parasitize nonactivated macrophages and replicate within them. Only when macrophages have been activated against these specific intracellular pathogens are they able to inhibit or destroy them. Monocytes and macrophages play an active role in the clearance and inactivation of most viral pathogens. Paradoxically, these same cells also represent a major target cell and infectious reservoir for many viruses. The human immunodeficiency virus (HIV-1) infects and replicates within monocytes and macrophages by binding to the CD4 and CCR5 receptors that are present on the macrophage cell membrane.

The macrophages in tissues and body cavities are a cell population that is regularly renewed by the influx of monocytes manufactured in the bone marrow and circulated via the blood. The control of monocyte production, release of monocytes into the blood, monocyte migration and extravasation into tissues, and finally differentiation into tissue macrophages are accomplished by means of soluble chemical factors. These soluble chemical factors are termed cytokines and are themselves influenced by stress-associated factors such as adrenocorticotropic hormone (ACTH), cortisol, adrenergic hormones, and neuropeptides such as substance P (SP), vasoactive intestinal peptide (VIP), and proopiomelanocortin (POMC). Macrophages secrete cytokines that produce effects on other immune cells, as well as receptors for cytokines produced by other immune cells, thereby promoting bidirectional communication. The major cytokines that produce effects on the monocyte/macrophage cells are: interferon (IFN-)γ, IFN-α, IFN-β, and interleukin (IL-)1. Monocyte/macrophages produce and secrete IL-1, IL-6, and tumor necrosis factor (TNF-)α.

Table 1 Tissue-localized macrophage/monocyte cells

Location	*Cell type*
Bone marrow	Monoblasts, promonocytes, monocytes, macrophages
Peripheral blood	Monocytes
Skin	Langerhans cell and histiocyte
Lung	Alveolar macrophage
Bone	Osteoclast
Liver	Kupffer cell
Central nervous system	Microglia
Lymphoid organs	Tissue macrophages, dendritic cells
Spleen	Red-pulp macrophages
Gastrointestinal tract	Tissue macrophages
Serous cavities	Pleural and peritoneal macrophages

Phagocytosis and Microbicidal Functions

The term macrophage was first used more than 100 years ago by Elie Metchnikoff to describe the large mononuclear phagocytic cells he observed in tissues. Through the process of phagocytosis, macrophages are one of the most effective components of nonspecific immunity. Macrophages also play two essential roles in specific immunity, first as professional antigen presenting cells and then, with proper stimulation, as immune effector cells. Once activated by the immune system, macrophages become more powerful than neutrophils in their ability to phagocytize. Macrophages are able to engulf much larger particles such as whole red blood cells and malarial parasites or as many as 100 bacteria. Phagocytized particles are encapsulated and digested by intracellular proteolytic enzymes contained in lysosomes and other cytoplasmic granules. Macrophage lysosomes are unusual in that they contain lipases that aid in the digestion of the thick lipid bacterial membranes. Once the engulfed particles are digested, macrophages can extrude residual products. Macrophages perform many essential roles in the immune response such as the direct killing of damaged cells, bacteria, and viruses and antigen presentation. Macrophages produce and respond to cytokines and other chemicals central to both the inflammatory and the specific immune response. There are populations of macrophages that live throughout the life span of the organism.

Cytokine Mediation of Macrophage Response

Macrophages express major histocompatibility complex (MHC) class II on their surface and are important antigen-presenting cells for both B and T lymphocytes. Macrophages, when activated by cytokines produced by T helper (TH) cells, become effector cells of cell-mediated immunity. Macrophages are the first cells involved in an immune reaction and help orchestrate immune events both by the production of chemical signals (cytokines and SP) and by the processing and presentation of antigens to subsets of T lymphocytes that may either enhance or suppress specific immune responses. Activated macrophages also produce cytokines, such as IL-1, TNF-α, and IL-6, that augment T-cell function, as well as IL-8, macrophage colony-stimulating factor (M-CSF), granulocyte macrophage colony-stimulating factor (GM-CSF), and granulocyte colony-stimulating factor (G-CSF) that stimulate polymorphonuclear neutrophil (PMN) and monocyte activity. The ability of macrophages and lymphocytes to stimulate one another's functions provides an important amplification mechanism for specific immunity. Thus, macrophages play an important and central immunoregulatory role.

Toll-like Receptors

Toll-like receptors, identified in macrophages in mammals, are a relatively new family of membrane receptors able to recognize specific patterns of pathogen components, such as bacterial endotoxins and viral nucleic acids. Toll-like receptor (TLR)-4 is part of a molecular complex that recognizes and mediates intracellular responses to lipopolysaccharide (LPS). Pathogen recognition by TLRs activates the innate immune system through different signaling pathways, causing inflammatory responses such as cytokine production. Impaired adrenal stress response occurs in TLR-2-deficient mice, suggesting that TLR-2 and, possibly, TLR-4 may constitute an important link between the immune and endocrine stress systems at both the central and peripheral levels, particularly during inflammation and sepsis.

Stress and Monocytes/Macrophages

An examination of the role of macrophages in the modulation of immune function by stress is particularly compelling. A representation of the interactions among various stressors and the immune system is provided in **Figure 1**.

Macrophages play a pivotal role in immune responses, first as professional antigen-presenting cells stimulating the expansion of one of two sets of $CD4^+$ T-cell populations (TH1 or TH2) and finally, when activated themselves, functioning as major effector cells in cell-mediated immunity. The TH1 and TH2 responses are highly integrated and contraregulated, relying on two distinctly different profiles of cytokine production. Many of the cytokines produced by one or the other subpopulation have positive effector functions and, in addition, negatively regulate the activity of the alternate subgroup. The negative regulation may be at the level of either T-cell expansion or T-cell effector functions, including macrophage activation. Thus, an immune response in which TH1 cells are stimulated downregulates the co-stimulation of TH2 cells. Conversely, an immune response in which TH2 cells are stimulated downregulates both the co-stimulation of TH1 cells and their effector activity.

TH1 cells produce cytokines associated with aspects of classic cell-mediated immunity, producing IFN-γ, IL-2, IL-3, GM-CSF, TNF-α, and TNF-β, which activate macrophages. IFN-γ induces oxygen burst and nitric oxide production, which are essential for microbicidal reactions. IL-3 activates macrophages, causing increased antigen presentation. IFN-γ and IL-2 both stimulate macrophages to produce TNF-α, which in turn further stimulates macrophage activation in a cascade of events.

TH2 cells produce cytokines (IL-4, IL-5, and IL-6) that are associated with the B-cell responses of humoral immunity. IL-4 acts as a growth factor specific for TH2 cells, acts as an inhibitory factor for the stimulation of TH1 cells by IL-2, and also effectively inhibits IFN-γ activation of macrophages. When appropriately stimulated by TH2 cytokines and antigen, B cells give rise to antibody-secreting plasma cells. The antigen–antibody complex serves as a powerful stimulator of the monocyte/macrophage phagocytosis of these circulating complexes.

In a mouse surgical-sponge model of inflammation, acute restraint-induced stress caused increase in leukocyte trafficking to the site of immune activation. Mice acutely stressed before sponge implantation presented 200–300% higher macrophage, neutrophil, natural killer cell, and T-cell infiltration than did nonstressed animals. Stress-induced increases in

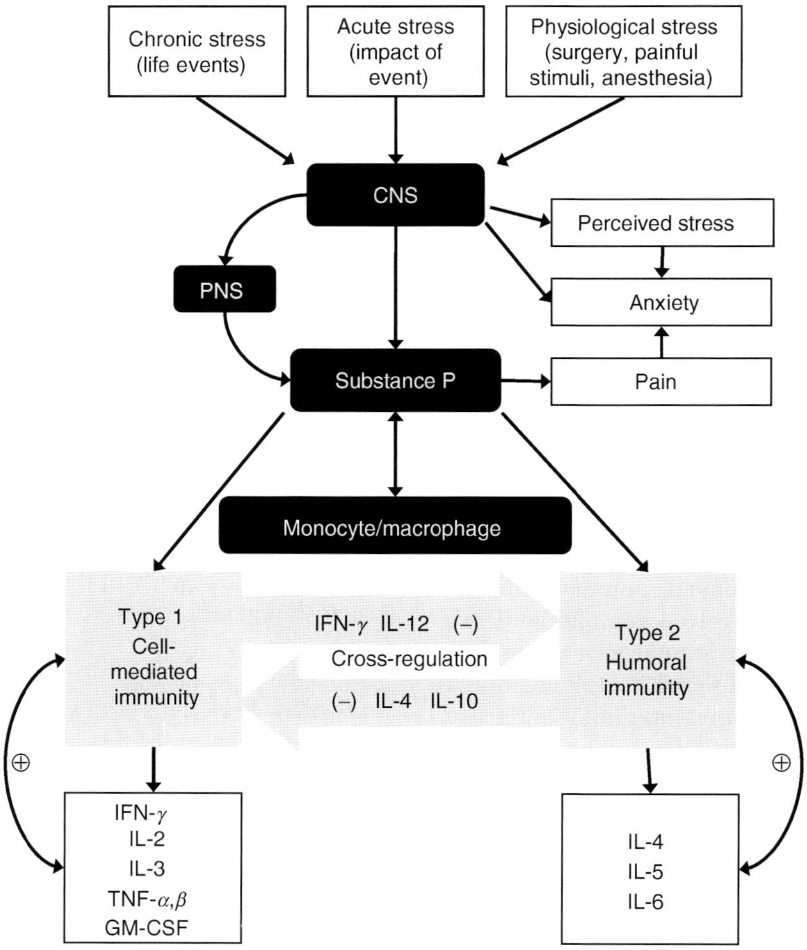

Figure 1 Stress effects on monocyte/macrophages. The effects of stress on the immune system are mediated by the neuropeptide substance P. The cells of the monocyte/macrophage system have receptors for and are able to synthesize and release substance P. Thus, they play a central role in mediating these effects. CNS, central nervous system; GM-CSF, granulocyte macrophage colony-stimulating factor; IFN, interferon; IL, interleukin; PNS, peripheral nervous system; TNF, tumor necrosis factor.

leukocyte trafficking may be responsible for immunoprotection during trauma, surgery, and infection, but it may also exacerbate immunopathological responses during inflammatory diseases, such as arthritis, cardiovascular disease, psoriasis, multiple sclerosis, and gingivitis.

Substance P as a Mediator of Stress Response

A major mediator of the effects of stress on monocyte/macrophage function is the neurotransmitter peptide SP, which is widely distributed in the central, peripheral, and enteric nervous systems. SP may have a major role in several inflammatory disease processes such as rheumatoid arthritis, bullous pemphigus, asthma, and inflammatory bowel diseases such as Crohn's disease and ulcerative colitis, as well as in the transmission of pain. SP may be the chemical messenger of a neurogenic alarm system that serves to communicate stress in a reciprocal manner among the central nervous system (CNS), endocrine system, and immune system. SP is associated with the sympathetic nervous system and is essential to the maintenance of adrenal catecholamine secretion from the adrenal medulla in times of stress.

Studies of surgical patients demonstrate that the stress of surgery shifts the TH1/TH2 cytokine balance toward TH2, suggesting that cell-mediated immunity was downregulated. Furthermore, the highest immune alteration was associated with the most stressful and invasive surgery. Several experimental animal studies indicate an association between stress and levels of SP. Two studies of SP in the brain tissue of rats that had been subjected to stressful stimuli found decreases in SP levels, which the authors attributed to tissue SP depletion following the increased release of SP. Experimental models of induced stress such as restraint stress and sequential removal of group-housed rats were found to be associated with increased levels of SP in the periaqueductal gray area of the brain. Insulin-induced hypoglycemia or mild electric foot shock were shown to increase the release of both catecholamines and SP from rat adrenomedullary cells. The intracerebroventricular administration of SP in conscious rats elicited an integrated cardiovascular, behavioral, and endocrine response in a pattern consistent with an integrated stress response in rodents. Experimental evidence in first-time parachutists and patients undergoing diagnostic procedures demonstrated increased levels of circulating SP associated with acute psychological stress. The high levels of circulating SP remained elevated long after the anxiety associated with the acute stressor diminished.

Macrophages, endothelial cells, eosinophils, and Leydig cells have also been identified as nonneuronal sources of SP. The presence of specific SP receptors on the surface of monocytes and the ability of macrophages to produce SP suggest its role in the autocrine regulation of SP gene expression.

The biological responses to SP are mediated by the NK-1 receptor, a 407-amino-acid G-protein-coupled glycosylated receptor that has been demonstrated on T cells, B lymphocytes, monocytes, macrophages, neutrophils, and mast cells. There is a connection between SP in the peripheral nervous system and the immune system. There is direct innervation of the spleen by SP-containing nerve fibers in splenic areas adjacent to lymphocytes, macrophages, and granulocytes, with evidence of its role in the traffic of lymphocytes from lymph nodes. SP modulates the effector phase of adaptive immunity and serves as a co-stimulator in the activation of monocytes, macrophages, T cells, and B cells, with the subsequent release of regulatory cytokines by these cells.

Effect of Stress on Monocytopoiesis

Macrophages synthesize and release two hematopoietic growth factors, M-CSF and GM-CSF, in response to external stimuli such as particles that are phagocytosed and endotoxin. Furthermore, macrophages release IL-1 and TNF, which in turn can induce fibroblasts and endothelial cells to produce M-CSF and GM-CSF, which stimulate the production of mononuclear phagocytes. The spiral of increased inflammatory response is further magnified by the synthesis of TNF-α by mononuclear phagocytes in response to GM-CSF simulation. Thus, macrophages play a pivotal role in regulating immune response. SP induces the production of hematopoietic growth factors IL-1, IL-6, and TNF-α from human monocytes. Bone marrow is innervated by nerve fibers that release SP in concentrations that induce tissue macrophages resident in bone marrow to release IL-1, IL-3, and GM-CSF.

Furthermore, macrophages express NK-1 receptors and serve as a nonneural source of SP. The release of SP by macrophages serves as a paracrine mechanism (by stimulating nearby macrophages) for amplifying the effect of stress on monocytopoiesis. Thus, stress acting through SP as a mediator may play a physiological role in regulating monocytopoiesis through two mechanisms: stimulation of the direct release of hematopoietic growth factors by monocytes and paracrine amplification.

Effect of Stress on Monocyte/Macrophage Function

The manner and extent to which stress influences immune response is, then, of vital concern. Stress may either enhance or inhibit macrophage function. Experimental evidence shows that SP plays a role in modulating immune response at each of the succeeding levels of response to foreign antigen. SP induces the release of stem cell factor and IL-1 in bone marrow stroma, thereby mediating hematopoesis. A summary of the effects of stress on the monocyte/macrophage system is provided in **Table 2**.

During acute inflammatory reactions, the number of circulating monocytes is increased with enhanced bone marrow production. This is mitigated by the decreased time that the monocytes are in the

Table 2 Effects of stress on monocytes/macrophages

Source	*Model*	*Effect*
Animal (*in vitro*)	Macrophages exposed to salmonella	Increased SP receptors
Animal (*in vivo*)	Mice exposed to salmonella given SP antagonist	Increased mortality
	Mice exposed to cold-water stress	Increased SP; increased IL-6 release by macrophages
	Stressed rats (restraint and sequential removal)	Increased levels of SP in periaqueductal gray area of brain
Human (*in vitro*)	Bone marrow stroma cells exposed to SP	Increased stem cell factor, IL-1
	Monocytes/macrophages exposed to SP	Increased IL-1, IL-6, IL-7, IL-10, IL-12, TNF-α; chemotaxis, and phagocytosis
Human (*in vivo*)	Acute psychological stress in parachutists	Increased SP
	Acute psychological stress in medical diagnostic procedures	Increased SP, $CD8^+$
	Sickle cell patients in vaso-occlusive crisis	Increased SP correlated with pain; increased IL-8

IL, interleukin; SP, substance P; TNF, tumor necrosis factor.

circulation due to efflux into inflammatory exudates. The SP-containing neurons have direct contact with immune and hematopoietic cells in the primary and secondary lymphoid organs. Thus, traffic of lymphocytes may be regulated by the secretion of neuroactive peptides such as SP from nerves.

Macrophages and monocytes increase phagocytosis and increase chemotaxis in response to SP. Increased levels of IL-6 are released by peritoneal macrophages in response to increased levels of SP produced by mice exposed to cold-water stress. Macrophages from humans and guinea pigs have receptors for and respond to SP-releasing cytokines IL-1, IL-6, and TNF-α. Macrophages in mice exposed to oral salmonella doses expressed higher levels of SP receptors and the administration of the SP antagonist spantide II resulted in higher mortality than in non-SP-antagonized mice. Treatment with spantide II was also associated with significantly reduced levels of IL-12 and IFN-γ. Thus, SP serves to amplify ongoing immune reactions and serves as a mediator in stress-induced immune reactions.

See Also the Following Articles

Cytokines; Immune Response; Macrophage Antimycobacterial Activity Effects of Stress on.

Further Reading

Bornstein, S. R., Zacharowski, P., Schumann, R. R., et al. (2004). Impaired adrenal stress response in toll-like receptor 2-deficient mice. *Proceedings of the National Academy of Sciences USA* **101**, 16695–16700.

Chancellor-Freeland, C., Zhu, G., Kage, R., et al. (1995). Substance P and stress-induced changes in macrophages. *Annals of the New York Academy of Sciences* **771**, 472–484.

Douglas, S. and Ho, W. (2006). Morphology of monocytes and macrophages. In: Lichtman, M. A. (ed.) *Williams hematology* (7th edn., pp. 960–970). New York: McGraw Hill.

Hassan, F. and Douglas, S. (1990). Stress-related neuroimmunomodulation of monocyte-macrophage functions in HIV-1 infection. *Clinical Immunology and Immunopathology* **54**, 220–227.

Lewis, C. and McGee, J. (1992). *The macrophage.* Oxford: Oxford University Press.

Ho, W. Z. and Douglas, S. D. (2004). Substance P and neurokinin-1 receptor modulation of HIV. *Journal of Neuroimmunology* **157**, 48–55.

Lai, J. P., Ho, W. Z., Kilpatrick, L. E., et al. (2006). Full-length and truncated neurokinin-1 receptor expression and function during monocyte/macrophage differentiation. *Proceedings of the National Academy of Sciences USA* **103**, 7771–7776.

McGillis, J., Mitsuhashi, M. and Payan, D. (1990). Immunomodulation by tachykinin neuropeptides. *Annals of the New York Academy of Sciences* **594**, 85–94.

Perry, V. (1994). *Macrophages and the nervous system.* Austin, TX: R. G. Landes.

Viswanathan, K. and Dhabhar, F. S. (2005). Stress-induced enhancement of leukocyte trafficking into sites of surgery or immune activation. *Proceedings of the National Academy of Sciences USA* **102**, 5808–5813.

Macrophage Antimycobacterial Activity, Effects of Stress on

C S Boomershine and B S Zwilling
The Ohlo State University, Columbus, OH, USA

This article is reproduced from Encyclopedia of Stress, First edition, volume 2, pp 657–662, © 2000, Elsevier Inc.

Glossary

Nramp — (*natural resistance associated macrophage protein*) A phagolysosomal membrane product encoded by the *Nramp1* gene that confers resistance to mycobacterial growth during the early nonimmune phase of infection. Susceptible mice differ from resistant mice in a nonconservative glycine-to-aspartic acid substitution within a predicted transmembrane domain of Nramp1.

Introduction

Tuberculosis, a worldwide public health problem, has also increased significantly in the United States. The increase in tuberculosis is partly due to depressed cellular immunity associated with HIV infection. However, tuberculosis has also increased independently of

HIV infection. Only since 1997, following mobilization of the public health community, has the incidence of tuberculosis in the United States begun to resume its downward course. Tuberculosis is a highly complex disease with multiple determinants for disease progression and severity. The susceptibility of humans to mycobacterial disease is determined partly by genetic differences. One of the most important genetic factors determining resistance to mycobacterial infection is the ability of host macrophages to control the growth of the tubercle bacilli.

Innate Resistance against Mycobacteria

The innate resistance of macrophages to mycobacterial infection has been studied most thoroughly in mice. The ability of mice to control mycobacterial growth in the spleen, following intravenous injection of *Mycobacterium bovis* BCG, maps to a region on mouse chromosome 1. Mice resistant to mycobacterial growth are termed Bcg^r, whereas those strains in which mycobacteria grow exponentially are termed Bcg^s. The resistance of Bcg^r mice is mediated by the *Nramp1* gene, which has been cloned in both mice and humans. *Nramp1* codes for a phagolysosomal membrane product termed natural resistance associated macrophage protein. Susceptible mice differ from resistant mice in a nonconservative glycine-to-aspartic acid substitution within a predicted transmembrane domain of Nramp1. While the mechanism of Nramp-mediated resistance remains ill defined, work from the authors' laboratory suggests that Nramp1 acts as a transporter of iron into the macrophage phagolysosome.

Although the susceptibility of an individual to mycobacterial disease is influenced strongly by innate immunity, genetic differences alone cannot account for the recent rise in the incidence of tuberculosis. The vast majority (90–95%) of people exposed to pathogenic strains of mycobacteria are able to control the growth of the organism without any disease manifestations. While some macrophages are able to limit mycobacterial growth, they are not sufficient to resolve a primary mycobacterial infection. Fortunately, macrophages are the major antigen-presenting cells of the body. Enzymes in the macrophage phagolysosome digest microorganisms killed by the respiratory burst and some microbial peptides become associated with glycoproteins encoded by genes of the major histocompatibility complex (MHC). Peptides coupled to MHC class II glycoproteins are cycled to the cell surface where they serve as the sole basis for antigen recognition by $CD4^+$ T lymphocytes. These macrophages then travel to regional lymph nodes where they present this processed antigen to T cells.

Specific Immune Response to Mycobacterial Infection

T-cell activation results in the development of cell-mediated immunity and enhanced reactivity to the purified protein derivatives (PPD) of mycobacteria. Activated Th cells then travel to the area of the primary focus and release lymphokines that cause monocytes to migrate into the site and differentiate into specialized histiocytic cells termed epithelioid giant cells. The primary lesion becomes organized into a granuloma, with macrophages containing ingested mycobacteria located centrally surrounded by epithelioid giant cells and activated T cells. The production of interferon (IFN)-γ by activated T cells results in macrophage activation and enhanced antimicrobial activity resulting from the activation of IFN-γ responsive genes. Mycobacteria may persist within macrophages of the granuloma for decades, but in immunocompetent individuals, further multiplication and spread are usually confined. The relative strength of the cell-mediated immunity of the host ultimately determines if resumption in multiplication of the mycobacteria will occur. The consequence of a resumption in the multiplication of bacilli leads to tuberculosis with subsequent tissue destruction, systemic dissemination of disease, and, when left untreated, death. Reactivation of disease has been attributed to several environmental factors, including protein malnutrition associated with chronic alcoholism, immunosenescence associated with aging, and stress.

Stress Influences Mycobacterial Infection

One of the first observations that stressful life events can affect disease pathogenesis was made in studies of tuberculosis by Ishigami. Ishigami found decreased phagocytic cell activity during periods of emotional stress in chronically ill, tuberculous school children. He postulated that the stressful school environment led to the children's immunodepressed state and their increased susceptibility to tuberculosis. Contemporaneous studies have proven that physical and psychological stress can modulate susceptibility to tuberculosis as well as general immune function. Physiologic responses to stressors are mediated by both the hypothalamic–pituitary–adrenal (HPA) axis and the sympathetic nervous system (SNS).

HPA Axis Effects on Mycobacterial Infection

The HPA axis mediates the stress response by producing a cascade of hormones in response to a variety of stimuli, ultimately resulting in the enhanced production of glucocorticoids by the adrenal glands.

Glucocorticoids then enter the circulation and exert their effects through binding to cytoplasmic receptors. Upon binding, the glucocorticoid–receptor complex is internalized and translocated to the nucleus where it binds to glucocorticoid response elements (GREs). The receptor-charged GREs enhance the transcription initiation of glucocorticoid-regulated genes influencing the amount of critical proteins within the cell. Glucocorticoids have been shown to suppress the immune response. Glucocorticoid hormones cause a species- and cell type-specific lysis of lymphocytes. They suppress the inflammatory response by decreasing the number of circulating leukocytes and the migration of tissue leukocytes, inhibiting fibroblast proliferation, and inducing lipocortins that blunt the production of prostaglandins and leukotrienes, which are potent anti-inflammatory molecules.

Mononuclear cells possess high-affinity (type II) glucocorticoid receptors and represent one of the best studied primary target cells for glucocorticoids. Studies have shown that the production of proinflammatory cytokines interleukin (IL)-1, IL-6, and tumor necrosis factor (TNF)-α by activated macrophages is blocked at the transcriptional and posttranscriptional level by glucocorticoids. The downregulation of these potent mediators of inflammation underlies some of the immunosuppressive and anti-inflammatory actions of glucocorticoids, but does not address the effect glucocorticoids have on macrophage–T-cell interactions. Due to the requirement for macrophage MHC class II expression in antigen presentation for the induction of an immune response, the authors began their work by evaluating the effect of restraint stress on the expression of MHC class II glycoprotein expression in murine macrophages.

MHC class II glycoprotein expression is induced in mice following the injection of antigen or microorganisms *in vivo* or by treatment of macrophages with recombinant IFN-γ *in vitro*. It was found that macrophages from resistant strains of mice are able to persistently express MHC class II following infection of the mice with *M. bovis* (strain BCG). It was shown subsequently that the treatment of macrophages from Bcg^r mice with rIFN-γ induced persistent MHC class II expression, whereas macrophages from Bcg^s mice expressed this glycoprotein only transiently. The regulation of MHC class II expression by macrophages from resistant and susceptible mice also differed. Glucocorticoid treatment of macrophages from susceptible mice resulted in decreased MHC class II expression, whereas MHC class II expression by macrophages from resistant mice was unaffected.

The regulation of MHC class II expression by glucocorticoids raised the possibility that stress could modulate class II expression following activation of the HPA axis. This hypothesis was confirmed by demonstrating that restraint stress suppressed MHC class II expression by murine peritoneal macrophages and that this suppression coincided with peak corticosterone levels in plasma. The authors' previous work that showed strain-specific differences in MHC class II glycoprotein expression was extended by showing that the stress-induced suppression of MHC class II expression was limited to certain strains of mice. Bcg^r mice were resistant to the restraint stress-induced decrease in MHC class II glycoprotein expression observed in Bcg^s mice. The resistance of Bcg^r mice was not due to a decrease in HPA axis activation, as corticosterone suppressed the induction of MHC class II by macrophages from both resistant and susceptible mice.

Adrenalectomy ameliorated the suppressive effects of restraint stress on MHC class II expression in Bcg^s mice by abrogating the increase in corticosterone that results from HPA axis activation. Later experiments showed that the difference in MHC class II expression by macrophages from resistant and susceptible mice was due to a difference in MHC class II mRNA stability (**Figure 1**). Cortisterone decreased the stability of

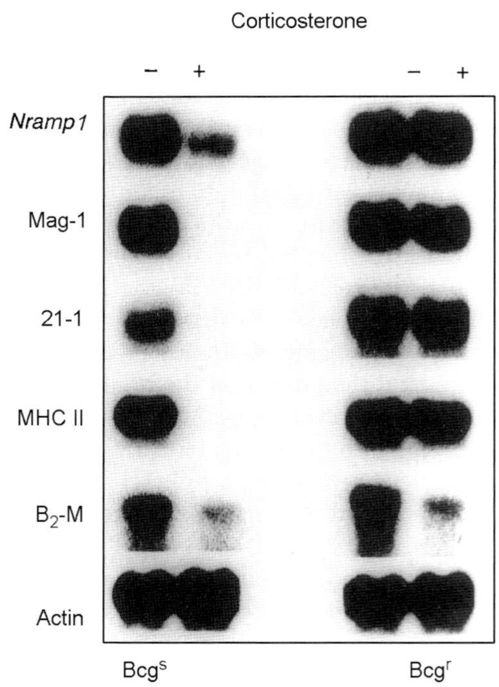

Figure 1 Stabilized expression of mRNA is associated with mycobacterial resistance controlled by *Nramp1*. Splenic macrophages from Bcg^r and Bcg^s mice were stimulated with rIFN-γ for 24 h followed by treatment with corticosterone. After 20 h, total RNA was extracted, and the effect of corticosterone on the expression of rIFN-γ-induced genes was determined by Northern analysis. Copyright 1997 by the American Society for Microbiology. Reprinted with permission from Brown *et al.* (1997).

MHC class II mRNA in macrophages from susceptible mice but not in macrophages from resistant mice. The stability of mRNA of other IFN-γ-induced genes was affected similarly. Thus, the increased mRNA stability of macrophages from Bcg^r mice may account for the pleiotrophic effects that have been attributed to *Nramp1*.

The differential regulation of MHC class II glycoprotein expression by glucocorticoids could account for differences in tuberculosis susceptibility. The role of HPA axis activation in the control of the growth of mycobacteria in humans has been the subject of some discussion. Glucocorticoid treatment of human macrophages suppressed antimicrobial activity markedly. However, Rook and co-workers showed that dexamethasone increased the susceptibility of monocytes from some individuals to mycobacterial growth, but other donor monocytes were unaffected by glucocorticoid treatment.

These studies, together with previous work on MHC class II expression, led the authors to conduct a series of experiments to determine if mycobacterial growth, which is under *Nramp1* control, may also be affected differentially by HPA axis activation. It was found that activation of the HPA axis increased the growth of mycobacteria in susceptible mice but did not affect the ability of resistant mice to limit growth of the bacilli (**Figure 2**). The failure of restraint stress to increase the susceptibility of Bcg^r mice was not due to unresponsiveness of this strain of mouse to HPA axis activation. HPA axis activation resulted in an increase in plasma corticosterone and ACTH levels in both strains of mice. The role of corticosterone in mediating the effects of HPA axis activation was demonstrated in three ways. First, adrenalectomy abolished the effect of HPA activation on mycobacterial growth. Second, treatment of Bcg^s mice with the glucocorticoid receptor antagonist RU 486 abrogated the effects of restraint stress. Finally, the implantation of timed-release pellets that elevated plasma corticosterone levels to those attained by restraint increased the growth of mycobacteria in adrenalectomized susceptible mice. A subsequent *in vitro* study of macrophages from Bcg^r and Bcg^s mice showed that corticosterone addition decreased the antimycobacterial activity of susceptible macrophages, whereas corticosterone had no effect on resistant macrophages (**Figure 3**).

Sympathetic Nervous System Effects on Mycobacterial Infection

Stress results in activation of the HPA axis as well as the SNS. The authors have also reported that epinephrine treatment of peritoneal macrophages suppressed MHC class II expression induced by rIFN-γ. Other observations found that restraint stress also increased epinephrine and norepinephrine levels in the spleen. Numerous other studies have reported that

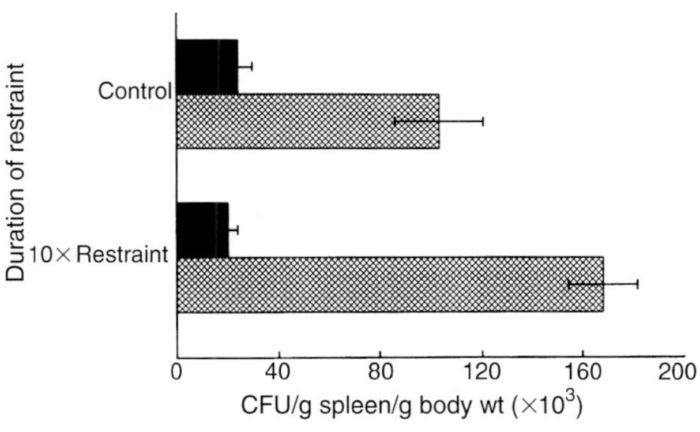

Figure 2 Regulation of mycobacterial growth by the hypothalamic–pituitary–adrenal axis: differential responses of *Mycobacterium bovis* (strain BCG)-resistant and -susceptible mice. Mice were restrained for ten 18-h cycles after infection with 5×10^4 CFU of *M. avium*. The numbers of CFU in the spleens were determined 12 days after infection. Data are the means ± SD for seven animals per group. The difference between growth of mycobacteria in the spleens of Bcg^r (■) mice versus growth in those of Bcg^s (▩) mice was significant ($P < 0.001$). Copyright 1993 by the American Society for Microbiology. Reprinted with permission from Brown *et al.* (1993).

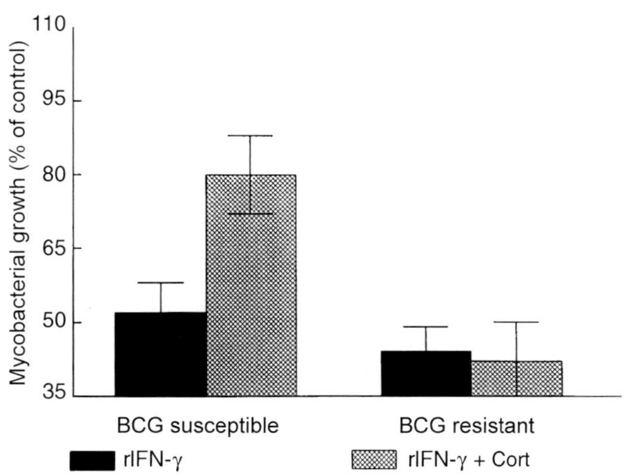

Figure 3 Cytokine-mediated activation of macrophages from *Mycobacterium bovis* (strain BCG)-resistant and -susceptible mice: differential effect of corticosterone on antimycobacterial activity and expression of the *Nramp1* gene. Splenic macrophages were treated with rIFN-γ for 24 h prior to infection with 4×10^5 CFU of *M. avium*. After 24 h to allow for phagocytosis and following removal of unphagocytized bacteria, the cultures were treated with 10^{-6} *M* corticosterone + rIFN-γ or just rIFN-γ for 5 days prior to lysis of the macrophages and pulsing of the bacteria with [^{3}H] uracil. Data are expressed as the percentage of the control value, which represents the amount of radioactivity incorporated by the bacteria after infection of cultures of macrophages treated with rIFN-γ divided by that of cultures not treated with rIFN-γ. The effect of corticosterone on the antimycobacterial activity of rIFN-γ-activated macrophages from Bcg^s mice was significant ($P \leq 0.03$). Copyright 1995 by the American Society for Microbiology. Reprinted with permission from Brown *et al.* (1995).

macrophage function can be suppressed or stimulated by catecholamines. It was found that catecholamine treatment of macrophages infected with mycobacteria inhibited intracellular growth of the bacilli. By using specific adrenoceptor agonists and antagonists, it was shown that this effect of catecholamines was mediated via the α_2-adrenergic receptor. The mechanism that accounts for this stimulation of macrophage functional capacity by catecholamines is under investigation. The use of macrophages harvested from Bcg^s mice in this study demonstrates that susceptible macrophages can be induced to control mycobacterial growth.

It has been reported that epinephrine treatment of *Mycobacterium avium*-infected macrophages increased IL-10 production. This effect was mediated by the β_r-adrenoceptor and could be mimicked by the addition of cAMP. IL-10 is a cytokine produced by a variety of immune cells that has a diverse array of actions. IL-10 production could play a role in tuberculosis by affecting the production of IFN-γ by T cells. IL-10 has been shown to inhibit MHC class II expression on monocytes and to inhibit T-cell proliferation directly. Preliminary studies in the authors' laboratory have also found that catecholamine treatment can inhibit macrophage activity. It has been shown that the addition of catecholamines during the infection of rIFN-γ-primed macrophages reduced reactive nitrogen intermediate production. Studies on the regulation of catecholamine-induced modulation of macrophage function are currently underway.

Summary

Differences in the resistance of certain mouse strains to mycobacterial growth have allowed us to study the effect activation of the HPA axis has on the innate mechanisms of mycobacterial resistance. It has been shown that macrophages from *M. bovis* BCG-resistant and-susceptible mice differ in their susceptibility to HPA axis-mediated effects. MHC class II glycoprotein expression by macrophages from Bcg^s mice decreased in response to increased plasma corticosterone levels induced by restraint. Restraint of Bcg^r mice led to a similar rise in corticosterone levels, but MHC class II expression remained unaffected. Restraint stress also increased mycobacterial growth in susceptible mice but did not affect the ability of resistant mice to limit growth of the bacilli. These results suggest that activation of the HPA axis may account for the increase in susceptibility of Bcg^s mice to mycobacterial growth. This suppression may be particularly apparent in individuals who express the mutation in *Nramp1* that results in susceptibility to mycobacterial disease and may account for the increase in the incidence of active tuberculosis among susceptible populations. Other work in the authors' laboratory has shown that catecholamine treatment of susceptible macrophages increased their ability to inhibit the intracellular growth of mycobacteria. The significance of these findings to mycobacterial disease is under investigation.

See Also the Following Articles

Immune Response; Infection; Macrophages.

Further Reading

Ader, R., Felten, D. L. and Cohen, N. (eds.) (1991). *Psychoneuroimmunology* (2nd edn.). San Diego: Academic Press.

Beato, M. (1989). Gene regulation by steroid hormones. *Cell* **56**, 335.

Blackwell, J. M. (1996). Structure and function of the natural-resistance-associated macrophage protein (Nramp1), a candidate protein for infectious and autoimmune disease susceptibility. *Molecular Medicine Today* **2**, 205–211.

Bloom, B. R. (1992). Tuberculosis, back to the frightening future. *Science* **358**, 538–539.

Brown, D. H., Lafuse, W. P. and Zwilling, B. S. (1995). Cytokine-mediated activation of macrophages from *Mycobacterium bovis* BCG-resistant and -susceptible mice: Differential effects of corticosterone on antimycobacterial activity and expression of the *Bcg* gene (candidate *Nramp*). *Infection and Immunity* **63**, 2983–2988.

Brown, D. H., Lafuse, W. P. and Zwilling, B. S. (1997). Stabilized expression of mRNA is associated with mycobacterial resistance controlled by Nramp1. *Infection and Immunity* **65**, 597–603.

Brown, D. H., Sheridan, J., Pearl, D. and Zwilling, B. S. (1993). Regulation of mycobacterial growth by the hypothalamic-pituitary-adrenal axis: Differential responses of *Mycobacterium bovis* BCG-resistant and -susceptible mice. *Infection and Immunity* **61**, 4793–4800.

Centers for Disease Control and Prevention (1995). Tuberculosis morbidity—United States, 1994. *MMWR Morbidity and Mortality Weekly Report* **44**, 387–389, 395.

Chen, L., Boomershine, C. S., Wang, T., Lafuse, W. P. and Zwilling, B. S. (1999). Synergistic interaction of catecholamine hormones and *Mycobacterium avium* results in the induction of interleukin-10 mRNA expression by murine peritoneal macrophages. *Journal of Neuroimmunology* **93**, 149–155.

Collins, F. M. (1989). Mycobacterial disease: Immunosuppression and acquired immunodeficiency syndrome. *Clinical Microbiology Reviews* **2**, 360–377.

Dannenberg, A. M. (1993). Immunopathogenesis of pulmonary tuberculosis. *Hospital Practice* **1**, 51–58.

Fiorentino, D. F., Bond, M. W. and Mosmann, T. R. (1989). Two types of mouse T helper cells. IV. Th2 clones secrete a factor that inhibits cytokine production by Th1 clones. *Journal of Experimental Medicine* **170**, 2081–2095.

Ishigami, T. (1919). The influence of psychic acts on the progress of pulmonary tuberculosis. *American Review of Tuberculosis* **2**, 470–484.

Kuhn, D. E., Baker, B. D., Lafuse, W. P. and Zwilling, B. S. (1999). Differential iron transport into phagosomes isolated from the RAW264.7 macrophage cell lines transfected with Nramp1^{Gly159} or Nramp1^{Asp169}. *Journal of Leukocyte Biology* **66**, 113–119.

Lalani, I., Bhol, K. and Ahmed, R. (1997). Interleukin-10: Biology, role in inflammation, and autoimmunity. *Annals of Allergy Asthma and Immunology* **79**, 469–481.

Malefyt, R., Haanen, J., Spits, H., et al. (1991). IL-10 and viral IL-10 strongly reduced antigen specific T cell proliferation by diminishing the antigen presenting capacity of monocytes via down regulation of class II major histocompatibility complex expression. *Journal of Experimental Medicine* **174**, 915–924.

Malefyt, T., Yssel, H. and de Vries, J. E. (1993). Direct effects of IL-10 on subsets of human CD4+ T cell clones and resting T cells. *Journal of Immunology* **150**, 4754–4765.

Malo, D., Vogan, K., Vidal, S., et al. (1994). Haplotype mapping and sequence analysis of the mouse Nramp gene predict susceptibility to infection with intracellular parasites. *Genomics* **23**, 51–61.

Miles, B. A., Lafuse, W. P. and Zwilling, B. S. (1996). Binding of alpha-adrenergic receptors stimulates the anti-mycobacterial activity of murine peritoneal macrophages. *Journal of Neuroimmunology* **71**, 19–24.

Rook, G. A. W., Steele, J., Ainsworth, M. and Leveton, C. (1987). A direct effect of glucocorticoid hormones on the ability of human and murine macrophages to control the growth of *M. tuberculosis*. *European Journal of Respiratory Disease* **71**, 286–291.

Safley, S. A. and Ziegler, H. K. (1994). Antigen processing and presentation. In: Zwilling, B. S. & Eisenstein, T. K. (eds.) *Macrophage–Pathogen Interactions*, pp. 115–130. New York: Dekker.

Sheridan, J. F., Dobbs, C., Jung, J., et al. (1998). Stress-induced neuroendocrine modulation of viral pathogenesis and immunity. *Annals of the New York Academy of Sciences* **840**, 803–808.

Stead, W. W. (1992). Genetics and resistance to tuberculosis. *Annals of Internal Medicine* **116**, 937–941.

Vespa, L., Johnson, S. C., Aldrich, W. A. and Zwilling, B. S. (1987). Modulation of macrophage I-A expression: Lack of effect of prostaglandins and glucocorticoids on macrophages that continuously express I-A. *Journal of Leukocyte Biology* **41**, 47–54.

Wiegeshaus, E., Balasubramanian, V. and Smith, D. W. (1989). Immunity to tuberculosis from the perspective of pathogenesis. *Infection and Immunity* **57**, 3671–3676.

Zwilling, B. S. (1994). Neuroimmunomodulation of macrophage function. In: Glaser, R. & Kiecolt-Glaser, J. (eds.) *Handbook of Human Stress and Immunity*, pp. 53–76. New York: Academic Press.

Zwilling, B. S., Brown, D., Christner, R., et al. (1990). Differential effect of restraint stress on MHC class II expression by murine peritoneal macrophages. *Brain Behavior and Immunity* **4**, 330–338.

Zwilling, B. S., Brown, D., Feng, N., Sheridan, J. and Pearl, D. (1993). The effect of adrenalectomy on the restraint stressed induced suppression of MHC class II expression by murine peritoneal macrophages. *Brain Behavior and Immunity* **7**, 29–35.

Zwilling, B. S., Brown, D. and Pearl, D. (1992). Induction of major histocompatibility complex class II glycoproteins by interferon-γ: attenuation of the effects of restraint stress. *Journal of Neuroimmunity* **37**, 115–122.

Zwilling, B. S., Kuhn, D. E., Wikoff, L., Brown, D. and Lafuse, W. (1999). Role of iron in *Nramp1*-mediated inhibition of mycobacterial growth. *Infection and Immunity* **67**, 1386–1392.

Zwilling, B. S., Vespa, L. and Massie, M. (1987). Regulation of I-A expression by murine peritoneal macrophages: differences linked to the Bcg gene. *Journal of Immunology* **138**, 1372–1376.

Immunity

F Chiappelli
UCLA School of Dentistry, Los Angeles, CA, USA

This is a revised version of the article by F Chiappelli and Q N Liu, Encyclopedia of Stress, First edition, volume 2, pp 541–546, © 2000, Elsevier Inc.

Glossary

Immunological synapse
Complex assemblage of rafts that integrates the signaling cascades for the amplification and regulation of T cell activation.

Rafts
Microdomains determined by and anchored to the cytoskeleton of T cells, and important in coordinating the signaling response in T cell-mediated immunity.

Regulatory T cells (Treg)
Characterized phenotypically by the expression of the α chain of the interleukin (IL)-2 receptor, CD25, at the molecular level by the expression of FoxP3, the P3 member of the first forkhead-box (FOX) transcription factor, which functions as a transcriptional repressor at the nuclear factor for activation of T cell (NFAT)/activating protein (AP)-1 sites in cytokine gene promoters, and functionally Treg act to impair proliferative and IL-2 production responses, thus blunting T cell-mediated immunity.

Suppressors of cytokine signaling (SOCS)	A family of seven known cytoplasmic proteins, the suppressor of cytokine signaling, which modulate cytokine-mediated regulation of immunity.

Immunity confers protection of the organism against pathogens. Innate immunity concerns humoral (e.g., complement) and cellular events (e.g., natural killer cells) that do not require priming by antigens. Antigen-specific immunity addresses that branch of cellular (e.g., cytotoxic T lymphocytes and plasma B cells) and humoral immune surveillance (e.g., cytokine patterns, immunoglobulins) that depends upon the phenotypic (e.g., memory CD4+ T cells, CD4+CD45R0+, and B cells) and functional stage maturation of lymphocytes following presentation of the antigen by the major histocompatibility complex (MHC).

Immunity comprises important innate and adaptive immune responses. Viruses, bacteria, or classical parasites all probe the limit of immunity, and of the three basic parameters of immunology – specificity, tolerance, and memory. The practical specificity repertoire of T and B cells is probably in the order of 10^4–10^7 specificities expressed by T cells or by neutralizing antibodies. Tolerance is best defined by rules of reactivity to eliminate infections while avoiding destruction of normal cells by complete elimination of T cells that are specific for antigens persisting in the blood and lymphohemopoietic system. Induction of a T-cell response is the result of antigens newly entering the lymph nodes or the spleen, initially in a local fashion and exhibiting an optimal distribution kinetics within the lymphohemopoietic system. Antigens that stay outside lymphatic tissues are generally immunologically ignored. Immunity is regulated by antigen dose, time, and relative distribution kinetics. Memory relates to the host's resistance following a second exposure to the same agent, and it correlates with antigen-dependent maintenance of circulating antibody titers, and with T-cell responses.

In a previous article, we discussed innate and antigen-dependent immunity in general. Recent research developments have established the central role of T cells in regulating immune surveillance. This article focuses on novel knowledge pertaining to T cell-mediated immunity. The vast domain of autoimmunity is not addressed in this article.

T-Cell Proliferation

T lymphocytes, 70–80% of the peripheral blood mononuclear cells, express the cluster of differentiation (CD)-3, but lack CD14 (i.e., monocyte-specific) and CD20/21 markers (i.e., B cell-specific). CD3 is proximal to the T-cell receptor (TcR), constituted by the α and β chains in circulating T cells, and by the γ and δ chains in the mucosal lymphoid tissue. T cells are stimulated *in vivo* via TcR, and *in vitro* by immobilized anti-CD3 antibody and the CD28 co-stimulus, lest the cells fail to proliferate and enter anergy, a state of stunted cell activation and proliferative capability.

Rafts

Lipids and proteolipids in the T-cell membrane are organized into rafts, microdomains determined by and anchored to the cytoskeleton. Rafts compose the immune synapse, a complex assemblage that integrates the signaling cascades. The synapse amplifies and regulates the activation of T cells. The assembly of the immune synapse at the antigen-presenting site depends on the interactions between rafts and the actin cytoskeleton, which controls the coalescence of smaller raft components into the larger immune synapse complex to integrate cellular responses to diverse signals. Phosphoinositide 1,5 bisphosphate (PIP2) regulates raft cytoskeletal structure by regulating proteins that control actin dynamics. Upon stimulation, PIP2 is converted to PIP3 and diacylglycerol. Ceramide mediates this clustering and insertion into the lipid bilayer by acetylation motifs.

Raft constituents change, define and determine the process of T cell activation, and maturation, as for instance the increase in raft-associated glycosphingolipid GM1. Compared to resting (CD69−CD25−) or naïve T cells (CD45RA+), activated (CD69+CD25+) or memory T cells (CD45R0+) have significantly higher GM1 levels. CD3/CD28 stimulation promotes recruitment into rafts of the Src family kinase lck, which co-localizes in rafts with glycosylphosphatidyl inositol (GPI)-anchored proteins, the adaptor protein LAT and Ras, but not with nonraft membrane proteins (e.g., protein tyrosine phosphatase, CD45). β-endorphin, which is released during stress and which significantly impairs PIP2 metabolism and associated kinase activity during T-cell activation, may alter rafts structure.

Membrane Markers of Cell Activation

T-cell activation results in change of morphology to blast cells with large cytoplasm-to-nucleus ratio, loss of CD62L, the peripheral lymph node homing receptor, expression of the integrin lymphocyte function-associated antigen (LFA)-1, and replacement of CD45RA with the maturation marker CD45R0. Activated T cells express CD69, the activation inducer molecule, a very early activation antigen (MLR-3, Leu-23), several hours before CD25

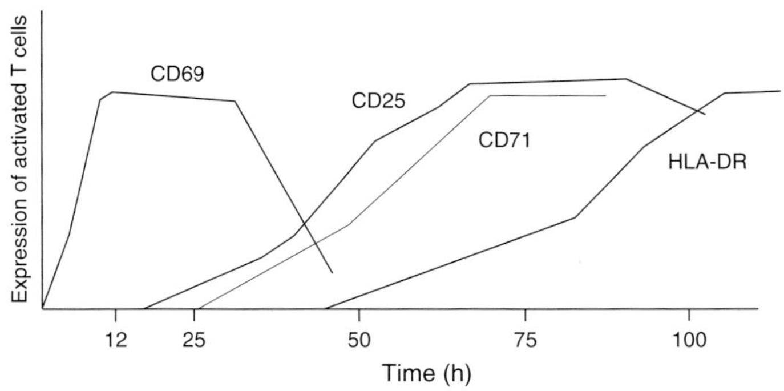

Figure 1 Comparative kinetics of expression of the membrane markers of activation, CD69, CD25, CD71, and human leukocyte antigen (HLA)-DR in activated healthy human adult T cells.

(**Figure 1**). CD69, a member of the natural killer cell family of signal-transducing receptors, is a type II transmembrane glycoprotein with a C-type lectin-binding domain in its extracellular domain. CD69 controls and regulates the expression of the interleukin (IL)-2 gene by its action downstream to the nuclear factor for activation of T cell (NFAT) and activating protein (AP)-1 transcription complexes.

Following expression of CD69, the IL-2 and CD25 genes are activated. CD25, the chain of the IL-2 receptor is expressed in high density on the cell membrane. Rafts regulate immune signaling in part by segregating cytokine receptors. The β chain of the IL-2 and the IL-15 receptors, for example, is enriched in rafts. This enrichment functionally ensures cytokine selectivity and specificity. Rafts thus assist in the recruitment of CD25 to the vicinity of the signaling β chain, and promote formation of the (α,β,γ) high affinity IL-2 receptor complex. Activated T cells express the transferrin receptor, CD71, which is critical for the transport of iron from the extracellular environment into the cell during traversal of the DNA synthesis (S) phase. The expression of these and other membrane activation markers, including the exopeptidase CD26 (dipeptidyl peptidase IV) and CD137, the T cell co-stimulatory molecule (4–1BB) antigen, is transient, and exhibits finely controlled kinetics.

Traversal of the Cell Cycle

Successful traversal of the cell cycle depends on finely regulated biochemical pathways. At each critical juncture that signifies passage from one stage to the next, gatekeeper proteins allow or disallow the activated cell to progress. These molecular regulators are proteins, the cyclins, which associate with their respective kinase enzymes. Cyclin/cyclin-dependent kinase cdk phosphorylate key proteins that directly or indirectly modulate gene transcription and allow the activated T cell to move forward in the cycle.

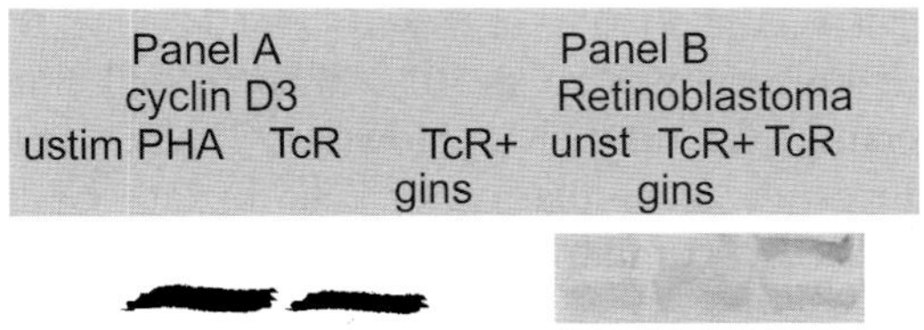

Figure 2 Modulation of cell cycle traversal by ginseng. Normal human T cells were stimulated *in vitro* with immobilized antiCD3/antiCD28 antibody, or the T-cell mitogen phytohemagglutinin, in the presence or the absence of 10^{-9} M ginsenoside Rc (Sigma) for 24 h. Cell extracts were obtained and used for assessment of cyclin D3 (panel A) or retinoblastoma (Rb) protein phosphorylation (panel B) by Western blotting with commercial monoclonal antibodies (Sta Cruz Biochemicals) to measure traversal of G_1. Note: Rb phosphorylation is measured as the ratio between the ratio of the upper, ppRb, and the lower pRb bands. TcR, T-cell receptor; PHA, phytohemagglutinin.

Cyclin D consists of a family whose members contribute to the regulation of G1/S transition. In T cells, cyclin D3 associates with either cdk4 or cdk6 late in Gap1 (G1). Cyclin D3-cdk4/6 kinase phosphorylates the retinoblastoma protein (Rb), which then releases the transcription factor E2F required for entry into the S phase and for DNA replication. For instance, at 10^{-9} M, Panax ginseng (Ginsenoside [20R]-Rg[3]Rc) blunts protein tyrosine kinase activity by 50%, impairs the phosphorylation of the retinoblastoma protein (Rb), and the expression of cyclin D3 (**Figure 2**), and leads to a threefold decrease in IL-2 production in response to CD3/CD28 stimulation. Expression of cyclin D3, and of the proliferating cell nuclear antigen (PCNA), and the phosphorylation of Rb are blunted in T cells by 0.1% ethanol, but enhanced by 12 ng ml^{-1} prolactin. At 10^{-8}–10^{-7} M, the plasma levels of individuals taking ginseng herbal tea, ginseng significantly ($p < 0.05$) stimulates the expression of CD69, and induces a 60% increase in calcium/calmodulin-dependent kinase (CaM kinase) activity. Ion channels are indeed critical in the control of the membrane potential and calcium signaling, and modulate signal transduction pathways following stimulation.

The process and dynamics of cell cycle traversal is monitored by propidium iodine/bromodeoxy uridine (PI/BrdU) immunofluorescent flow cytometry analysis to obtain a timeline sequence monitoring of cells as they traverse G1, S, G2, and mitosis (M). At 10^{-6} M, ginseng has no effect on CD69 expression (4.04 ± 1.34-fold increase versus 4.30 ± 1.70-fold increase), on traversal of the cell cycle by PI/BrdU analysis (**Figure** 3), or on IL-2 production. By contrast, 10^{-6} M mercuric chloride ($HgCl_2$) blunts cell cycle traversal by accumulating activating T cell subpopulations in late S (% cells in S at 48 h, 76.0 ± 13.2 with control versus 91.0 ± 5.0 with $HgCl_2$, $p < 0.07$), which corresponds to a 50% drop in cell number traversing G2 and M. However, 0.2% ethanol produces an accumulation of cells in late G1 (2.5-fold increase, compared to control).

T-Cell Memory – Cytokine Patterns

Monoclonal antibodies against CD45RA can serve to purify naïve T cells from memory T cells (93.94 ± 5.51% pure). Dual fluorescence flow cytometry is then used to monitor the maturation of T cells, i.e., the change in proportion from the naïve (CD45RA+) to the memory phenotype (CD45R0+) following CD3/CD28 stimulation. Kolmogorov-Smirnov analysis quantifies phenotypic T cell maturation. This approach has demonstrated that β-amyloid significantly ($p < 0.05$) blunts the ability of T cells to mature phenotypically.

Cytokines regulate immunity. One aspect of functional maturity of T cells, the variety of cytokines, depends on the initial antigen, and upon the physiological milieu (e.g., modulatory hormones and neuropeptides consequential to the stress response status of the organism). T helper (TH)1 and TH2 patterns of cytokine production are intertwined in terms of both their regulation and their relevance for the overall modulation of immune surveillance in health and disease.

Normal aging and aging-related dementia (e.g., dementia of the Alzheimer's type, DAT) are associated with significant changes in TH1 and TH2 cytokine production by circulating T cells. Intracellular cytokine staining, following stimulation of T cells in the presence of an inhibitor of protein transport thus retaining the cytokines inside the cell, and double-label immunofluorescence flow cytometry, reveals that normal subjects of 55–70 years of age have trace levels of cytoplasmic IL-10, interferon (IFN)γ, or IL-12 in T cells. Cohorts with DAT show significantly ($p < 0.05$) elevated levels of cytoplasmic IL-10 (2.67 ± 1.15 ng ml^{-1}), INFγ (3.25 ± 2.25 ng ml^{-1}), and IL-12 (1.78 ± 19.00 ng ml^{-1}) in T cells. In older (>70 years of age) patients with DAT, these

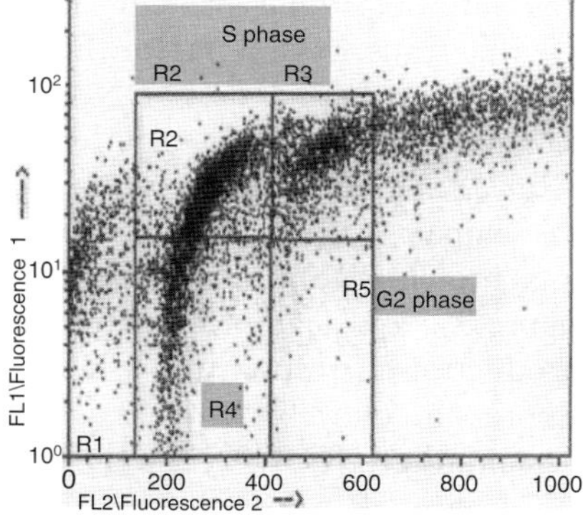

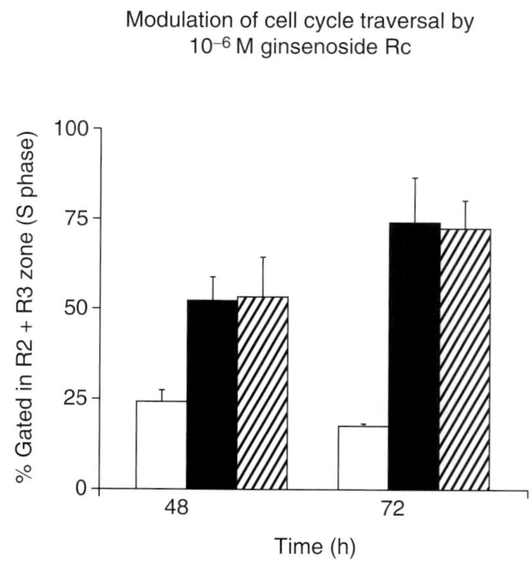

Figure 3 Modulation of cell cycle traversal by ginseng. Normal human T cells were stimulated in the presence or absence of 10^{-6} M ginseng, and the cultures were stained sequentially with propidium iodine (nuclear stain) and bromodeoxyuridine (DNA stain), followed by dual fluorescence flow cytometric analysis. Panel A shows the raw representation of the data from a representative culture, with highlighted the five regions (R1, R2, R3, R4, and R5) that constitute the population of cells traversing the phases of the cell cycle (G_1, S, G_2, and M). Panel B shows summary data of the effect of ginseng on cell cycle traversal as monitored by dual fluorescence propidium iodine/bromodeoxy uridine (PI/BrdU). Open bars, control unstimulated; closed bars, control stimulated; hatched bars, stimulated in the presence of 10^{-6} M ginsenoside.

levels drop to 1.99 ± 0.61 ng ml^{-1}, $p < 0.06$; 1.25 ± 0.05 ng ml^{-1}, $p < 0.09$; 1.04 ± 0.29 ng ml^{-1}, $p < 0.01$ for cytoplasmic IL10, INFγ, and IL-12 in T cells, respectively. In addition, the process of immunological aging is evidently distinct in patients with DAT compared to normal subjects, and cytoplasmic levels of IL-10, IFNγ, and IL-12 in T cells rise to levels similar to their age-cohorts diagnosed with DAT in older normal subjects to 1.99 ± 0.70 ng ml^{-1}, 2.75 ± 1.26 ng ml^{-1}, and 1.33 ± 2.07 ng ml^{-1}, respectively.

These changes can be attributed to a plethora of immunophysiological mechanisms within the context of stress and neuroendocrine immunity. The hypothesis has been put forward that age-associated alterations in immunity are associated with the reduction in hypothalamic dopaminergic tone with aging, related alterations in pituitary hormone, such as the anterior pituitary hormone, prolactin, and interference with the regulation of immunity. For example, 10–15 ng ml^{-1} prolactin increased IL-2 production by stimulated T cells *in vitro* close to twofold (8.15 ± 2.15 ng ml^{-1} versus 4.17 ± 1.22 ng ml^{-1}, respectively, $p < 0.09$). The prolactin effect is specific to Th1 cytokines, and is not obtained with the production of the TH2 cytokine, IL-4.

A third pattern of cytokines refers to the effect of certain growth factors (e.g., granulocyte macrophage colony stimulating factor; GM-CSF) in modulating the increase the production of bone marrow-derived antigen-presenting dendritic cells, and the production of IL-23 by these cells. IL-23 belongs to the IL-12 cytokine family, which shares p40, and binds to the IL12β1/IL-23R receptor complex to play a critical role in end-stage inflammation via signaling of the Janus tyrosine kinases (JAK) and signal transducers and activators of transcription (STAT) (JAK/STAT) pathway. Administration of IL-11 downregulates IL-12. IL-23 augments production of IL-17 by T cells, which becomes the significant cytokine in the involvement of T cells in inflammation. IL-17 leads to decreased neutrophilia in animal models, and *in vitro* administration of IL-17 synergizes the effects of tumor necrosis factor (TNF)-α for GM-CSF induction, for increased intercellular adhesion molecule (ICAM)-1 (CD54) expression by CD34+ progenitors, for increased neutrophil maturation, and for increased proinflammatory IL-6 and prostaglandin (PG)E2 and granulocyte-colony stimulating factor (G-CSF) growth factor production by keratinocytes and endothelial cells. IL-17 also favors increased secretion of the migration-inducing cytokine, IL-8. In human U937 cells, and probably in all lymphoid and myeloid cells, the JAK/STAT signaling pathway is responsible for transducing signals from the IL-17 receptor. Human vascular embryonic cells (HUVEC) express a homolog of IL-17R, as do ductal epithelial cells of human salivary glands, suggesting a significant role for IL-17 in immunity in the oral mucosa. In fact, in inflamed gingival tissue, IL-17 is the predominant cytokine in tissue proximal to 4–5 mm diseased periodontal pockets. IL-17 plays a critical role in immunity and mucosal inflammation, by modulating the effects of GM-CSF and other growth factors.

Migration

Cell migration is critical to immune surveillance. The migration of T cells is brought about by the concerted action of specialized factors and receptors, and is regulated by chemokines. Chemokines belong to three groups: C-X-C, C-C, and C depending on the number and position of cysteine. The first group (C-X-C) contains IL-8, growth-regulated oncogene (GRO)α, and GROβ and other chemokines with chemoattractant properties mainly, but not exclusively, towards neutrophils. The second (C-C) and third (C) groups comprise substances like monocyte chemoattractant protein (MCP)1, MCP2, MCP3, and macrophage inflammatory protein (MIP)1α and MIP1β, which mainly work on macrophages, lymphocytes, and eosinophils.

Recruitment of immune cells generally occurs by upregulating cell-surface adhesion molecule expression, such as endothelial leukocyte adhesion molecule (ELAM)-1 and increased ICAM-1, thereby enhancing cell adherence to the endothelial surface, and facilitating cell diapedesis through endothelial vessel walls. IL-8 mediates the recruitment and activation of immune cells in inflamed tissue, and increases endothelial permeability *in vitro*.

Plasma levels of IL-8 are raised in subjects with chronic alcoholism without liver disease and even more elevated in subjects with alcoholic hepatitis, who also show a rise in C-X-C chemokines. Alcohol abuse is a typical physiological stress that alters the distribution of monocytes and macrophages, and certain T-cell subsets, including a sharp decline in circulating CD4+CD62L+.

Regulation

Healthy human adult peripheral blood T cells express either CD4 or CD8. CD4 allows T cells to adhere by means of TcR to antigen-presenting cells (APC) that expose antigen in association with MHC-class 2. CD8 favors binding of the T cells to APC that present antigen via MHC-class 1. Most CD4+CD3+ cells act as TH cells, but a few CD4+ T cells are endowed with cytotoxic activity. CD8+ T cells are generally cytotoxic T lymphocytes, but they produce cytokines and growth factors that contribute to T cell-mediated immune regulation.

Membrane and Molecular Level

CD4 and CD8 are complexed lck, are members of the immunoglobulin gene superfamily, but are significantly divergent in their structure: CD4 is a monomer, while CD8 consists of two chains and occurs as a homodimer (α/α) or heterodimer (α/β). lck interacts with the CD4's 20 cytoplasmic relatively acidic residues (408–421), and with CD8α's 10 cytoplasmic residues (194–203) via ionic forces and by cysteine residues. The CD8β chain does not bind to lck. T cell stimulation leads to internalization of CD4:lck and its dissociation. The homodimeric form of CD8:lck may be internalized, but does not dissociate. The heterodimeric form of CD8:lck is not internalized, and does not dissociate. That is to say, active lck kinase is released in the cytoplasmic environment only following CD4+ cell activation.

A related src family member, fyn, associates primarily, but not exclusively with CD3, and other peptides generally implicated in the regulation of cell proliferation. The carboxyl domain of src family members exhibits a high degree of homology and contains the catalytic site. The N-terminal is unique to each peptide. The catalytic domain exhibits an adenosine triphosphate (ATP)-binding site at lysine 273, a site for autophosphorylation at tyrosine 394, and a site for tyrosine dephosphorylation mediated by CD45, or other phosphatases.

Related molecular events involved in the regulation of T cell stimulation include AkT (phosphoinositide 3-kinase, protein kinase B, PKB), the tumor suppressor, PTEN (phosphatase and tensin homolog deleted on chromosome 10, which removes phosphates primarily from lipids), Ras, mitogen-activated protein kinase (MAPK)/extracellular signal-regulated kinase (MEK), the dual threonine and tyrosine recognition kinase that phosphorylates and activates MAPK, and the novel tyrosine kinase inhibitor peptide, Tkip, a mimetic of SOCS-1 that binds to the autophosphorylation site of JAK2 and inhibits phosphorylation of STAT1α. Tkip could serve as a potentially important therapeutic target for both constitutive and IL-6-induced STAT3 activation.

Suppressors of cytokine signaling (SOCS) constitute a family of seven known cytoplasmic proteins that regulate the feedback attenuation of cytokine-mediated signal transduction. IL-2 stimulation of T cells induces signaling via JAK/STAT, and SOCS-3 inhibits the JAK/STAT cytokine signaling cascade by directly binding to it, and by preventing access to the signaling complex. IL-2 enhances SOCS-3 messenger ribonucleic acid (mRNA) and protein synthesis, and its phosphorylation on tyosine residues 204 and 221. SOCS-3 blocks the Ras/MEK activation pathway for c-fos and c-jun. Phosphorylation of SOCS-3 destabilizes its bond to proteosomes via elogin B and C, and leads to proteasomal destruction. In the 3T3 fibroblast model, activation of SOCS-1 and SOCS-3 inhibits focal adhesion kinase (FAK) activity *in vitro* and tyrosine phosphorylation of FAK. Activation of SOCS promotes polyubiquitination and degradation of FAK in a SOCS box-dependent manner. Together, these events lead to inhibited FAK-dependent signaling events, including cell motility on fibronectin. Phosphorylation of FAK is an essential regulatory step in T-cell migration.

Another important pathway related to SOCS is the P3 member of the first forkhead-box (FOX) transcription factor (FoxP3). FoxP3 functions as a transcriptional repressor, targeting composite NFAT/AP-1 sites in cytokine gene promoters. The region responsible for NFAT inhibition has now been mapped to the N-terminus of FoxP3. Introduction of FoxP3 into conventional mouse T cells converts these cells to the regulatory T cell (Treg) phenotype (CD4+CD25+).

Cellular Level

Treg are defined phenotypically as CD4+CD25+ T cells. They constitute 7–10% of CD4+ T cells in peripheral blood from healthy donors, and can rise to up to 20% in patients with lymphoma. Depletion of CD4+CD25+ cells significantly ($p < 0.05$) enhances the proliferative response of the remaining CD4+CD25– population, but addition of sorted CD4+CD25+ cells to the CD4+CD25– T cell population blunts proliferative activity. Sorted CD4+CD25+ T cells are susceptible to apoptotic cell death, associated with low Bcl-2 expression, and prevented by IL-2 salvage.

Neuropilin-1 (Nrp1) is a plasma transmembrane receptor (120 kD) involved in axon guidance, angiogenesis, and the activation of T cells. It is a ligand to the class 3 semaphorin subfamily and the heparin-binding forms of vascular endothelial growth factor and placenta growth factor. It acts as another specific surface marker for CD4+CD25+ Treg cells. Nrp1 mediates contacts between the dendritic cells and T cells via homotypic interactions and is essential for the initiation of the primary immune response. It is constitutively expressed on the surface of CD4+CD25+ Treg cells independently of their activation status. Nrp1 is downregulated in naïve CD4+CD25– T cells following TcR stimulation.

Functionally, Treg are endowed with suppressing T-cell activation. Expression of FoxP3, the transcription factor for the scurfin protein product, is a master regulatory gene for the development and function of CD4+CD25+ subset. When transduced into T cells, FoxP3 recapitulates the hyporesponsiveness of naïve T cells, including impaired proliferation and production of cytokines including IL-2 and IL-10 upon TcR stimulation. FoxP3 is less efficient in reprogramming memory T cell subset into Treg cells, and is a reliable marker for functional Treg. Expression on the plasma membrane the glucocorticoid-induced TNF receptor (GITR) by Treg cells strongly suggests an important role for SOCS in neuroendocrine-immune regulation.

Different subsets of Treg cells have been identified. Naïve peripheral CD4+CD25– T cells can be induced *in vitro* into CD25+ anergic/suppressor cells through co-stimulation TcR and TGF-β, which induces Foxp3 gene expression. These TcR-challenged CD4+CD25– naïve can transit toward a regulatory T cell with Treg phenotype and potent immunosuppressive function. Treg are also divided into subsets according to cell-surface expression of CD62L. The suppressive function of the CD62L+ subset is far more potent on a per cell basis, can be expanded far more easily in culture, and is more responsive to chemokine-driven migration, compared to the CD62L– Treg population. Treg cells may be differentiated based on their expression of chemokine receptors, which may contribute to determine their migration properties: e.g., the traffic to and retention in bone marrow of certain Treg cells through CXCR4/CXCL12 signals.

Clinical Implications

Chemokine receptors serve as co-receptors for HIV-1 infection by binding to certain viral envelope proteins. For example, CXCR4 favors X4 HIV-1 strain tropism, and CCR5 favors tropism of R5 strain. Treg from healthy donors that express the HIV-co-receptor CCR5 are highly susceptible to HIV infection and replication. It is not surprising, therefore, that FoxP3-transduced T cells are markedly more susceptible to HIV infection, and that HIV-positive individuals with a low percentage of CD4+ and higher levels of activated T cells have greatly reduced levels of FoxP3+CD4+CD25+ T cells.

CD4+CD25+ T cells expand significantly in peripheral blood of HIV-seropositive patients receiving highly active antiretroviral therapy (HAART), and exhibit phenotypic (e.g., CD25), molecular (e.g., FoxP3), and functional characteristics (e.g., impaired proliferative and IL-2 production responses) of Treg cells. HIV-seropositive patients under HAART treatment supplemented with intermittent IL-2 show an increase of up to 79% (median, 61%) in CD4+CD25+CD69– cells, with a sharp increase in the proportion of cells expressing the CD45R0 memory phenotype, and Ki67 (proliferating cell antigen) expression.

Treg cells suppress Th1 cytokine responses, and ensure polarization of the Th2 pattern of cytokines during infection, such as schistosomiasis. A rat population of constitutive CD4+CD25+ T cells has been described that corresponds to Treg cells described in mice and humans, indicating that Treg phenomena are widespread among mammals.

Treg and T cells in general are critical to the regulation of immunity. We recall that T cells generally express either one of two major subtypes of the TcR. Most T cells in the peripheral blood and in lymphoid organs express the heterodimeric α/β chains TcR. The majority of T cells that express the TcR composed of γ/δ proteins are enriched in epithelial tissues. This distinction is evident to a lesser degree in humans, compared to other mammals (e.g., murine model). Human peripheral blood contains less than 5% of T cells that bear the γ/δ TcR subtype, and in the oro-pharyngo-gastrointestinal mucosa, γ/δ T cells predominate. T cells that express the α/β TcR contribute to the immune surveillance of mucosal tissues. For example, the demonstration that T-cell clones derived from peripheral lymph nodes, and expressing α/β TcR, preferentially home to gingival tissue following infection with the dental plaque microorganism, *Actinobacillus actinomycetemcomitans*. This migration is blocked by anti-very late antigen (VLA)-4 antibodies. Constitutive Treg cells emerge in the peripheral blood from the thymus, and play a critical role in the control of intestinal inflammation. Lymph node-derived Treg cells can effectively counter established, severe, and progressive colitis. Syngeneic Treg cells obtained from spleens and administered to mice with colitis contribute to the resolution of the *lamina propria* inflammation, and to the reappearance of normal intestinal architecture. Treg cells proliferate in the mesenteric lymph nodes and the inflamed colon of mice under treatment. Another plaque-related organism, *Fusobacterium nucleatum*, induces a threefold increase in CD69 expression by CD4 T cells, and hence in the generation of inducible Treg, compared to a 4.15-fold activation in mitogen-stimulated control cultures. $HgCl_2$ at micromolar concentrations suppresses the *F. nucleatum*-mediated stimulation of CD69-expressing Treg by over 90%, and significantly ($p < 0.05$) blunts the production of IL-2. At supramicromolar concentrations (e.g., 10^{-5} M), $HgCl_2$ significantly ($p < 0.05$) increases the expression of CD25 by T cells by almost threefold. Taken together, these observations indicate that Treg from the peripheral and lymphoid system play an important role in the immune surveillance of inflammatory processes of mucosal immunity.

Conclusion

This article has discussed novel mechanisms of the regulation of T cell-mediated immunity. Future research in genomic, proteonomic, interactomic, and molecular cartography in general will elucidate the fundamental pathways in immunity and autoimmunity, and reveal new and improved modes of therapeutic intervention for immune-related diseases.

Acknowledgments

Support for our research efforts was obtained from the National Institutes of Health, the Alzheimer's Foundation, the MacArthur Foundation, the UCLA Psychoneuroimmunololgy program, and the UCLA Schools of Medicine and Dentistry.

Further Reading

Campos, M. and Godson, D. L. (2003). The effectiveness and limitations of immune memory: understanding protective immune responses. *International Journal of Parasitology* **33**, 655–661.

Chen, W., Jin, W., Hardegen, N., et al. (2003). Conversion of peripheral CD4+CD25− naive T cells to CD4+CD25+ regulatory T cells by TGF-β induction of transcription factor Foxp3. *Journal of Experimental Medicine* **198**, 1875–1886.

Chiappelli, F., Kavelaars, A. and Heijnen, C. J. (1992). β-endorphin effects on membrane transduction in human lymphocytes. *Annals of the New York Academy of Sciences* **650**, 211–217.

Chiappelli, F. and Liu, N. Q. (2000). Immunity. In: Fink, G. (ed.) *Encyclopedia of stress* (vol. 2), pp. 541–547. New York: Academic Press.

Chiappelli, F., Kung, M. A., Stefanini, G. F., et al. (2000). Alcohol and immune function. In: Gershwin, M. E., German, J. B. & Keen, C. L. (eds.) *Nutrition and immunology: principles and practice*, Chap. 21, pp. 261–274. New Jersey: Humana Press.

Chiappelli, F., Prolo, P., Iribarren, J., et al. (2006). Alzheimer's disease: new frontiers for the XXI century. In: Welsh, E. M. (ed.) *Advances in psychology research,* pp. 233–258. New York: Nova Science Publisher.

Chiappelli, F., Prolo, P., Fiala, M., et al. (2006). Allostasis in HIV-1 infection and AIDS. In: Minagar, P. A. & Shapshak, P. (eds.) *Neuro-AIDS*. New York: Nova Science Publisher (in press).

Cogoli-Greuter, M., Lovis, P. and Vadrucci, S. (2004). Signal transduction in T cells: an overview. *Journal of Gravitational Physiology* **11**, 53–56.

Crotty, S. and Ahmed, R. (2004). Immunological memory in humans. *Seminars in Immunology* **16**, 197–203.

Eisenlohr, L. C. and Rothstein, J. L. (2005). Antigen processing and presentation. *Cancer Treatment Research* **123**, 3–36.

Esche, C., Stellato, C. and Beck, L. A. (2005). Chemokines: key players in innate and adaptive immunity. *Journal of Investigative Dermatology* **125**, 615–628.

Larsen, L. and Ropke, C. (2002). Suppressors of cytokine signalling: SOCS. *Acta Pathologica, Microbiologica, et Immunologica Scandinavica* **110**, 833–844.

Liu, E., Cote, J. F. and Vuori, K. (2003). Negative regulation of FAK signaling by SOCS proteins. *EMBO Journal* **22**, 5036–5046.

Maffei, A. and Harris, P. E. (1998). Peptides bound to major histocompatibility complex molecules. *Peptides* **19**, 179–198.

Magee, T., Pirinen, N., Adler, J., et al. (2002). Lipid rafts: cell surface platforms for T cell signaling. *Biological Research* **35**, 127–131.

Matsuzaki, J., Tsuji, T., Imazeki, I., et al. (2005). Immunosteroid as a regulator for Th1/Th2 balance: its possible role in autoimmune diseases. *Autoimmunity* **38**, 369–375.

Meiri, K. F. (2004). Membrane/cytoskeleton communication. *Sub-Cellular Biochemistry* **37**, 247–282.

Nishimura, M. I., Roszkowski, J. J., Moore, T. V., et al. (2005). Antigen recognition and T-cell biology. *Cancer Treatment Research* **123**, 37–59.

Piccirillo, C. A. and Shevach, E. M. (2004). Naturally-occurring CD4+CD25+ immunoregulatory T cells: central players in the arena of peripheral tolerance. *Seminars in Immunology* **16**, 81–88.

Reith, W., LeibundGut-Landmann, S. and Waldburger, J. M. (2005). Regulation of MHC class II gene expression by the class II transactivator. *Nature Reviews Immunology* **5**, 793–806.

Romagnani, S. (1992). Human TH1 and TH2 subsets: Regulation of differentiation and role in protection and immunopathology. *International Archives of Allergy and Immunology* **98**, 279–285.

Taams, L. S., Smith, J., Rustin, M. H., et al. (2001). Human anergic/suppressive CD4(+)CD25(+) T cells: a highly differentiated and apoptosis-prone population. *European Journal of Immunology* **31**, 1122–1131.

Trowsdale, J. (2005). HLA genomics in the third millennium. *Current Opinions in Immunology* **17**, 498–504.

van der Merwe, P. A. (2002). Formation and function of the immunological synapse. *Current Opinions in Immunology* **14**, 293–298.

van Seventer, G. A., Salmen, H. J., Law, S. F., et al. (2001). Focal adhesion kinase regulates β1integrin-dependent T cell migration through an HEF1 effector pathway. *European Journal of Immunology* **31**, 1417–1427.

Watford, W. T., Hissong, B. D., Bream, J. H., et al. (2004). Signaling by IL-12 and IL-23 and the immunoregulatory roles of STAT4. *Immunological Reviews* **202**, 139–156.

Weiss, L., Donkova-Petrini, V., Caccavelli, L., et al. (2004). Human immunodeficiency virus-driven expansion of CD4+CD25+ regulatory T cells, which suppress HIV-specific CD4 T-cell responses in HIV-infected patients. *Blood* **104**, 3249–3256.

Yagi, H., Nomura, T., Nakamura, K., et al. (2004). Crucial role of FOXP3 in the development and function of human CD25+CD4+ regulatory T cells. *International Immunology* **16**, 1643–1656.

Zou, L., Barnett, B., Safah, H., et al. (2004). Bone marrow is a reservoir for CD4+CD25+ regulatory T cells that traffic through CXCL12/CXCR4 signals. *Cancer Research* **64**, 8451–8455.

Immune Suppression

P Prolo and F Chiappelli
UCLA School of Dentistry, Los Angeles, CA, USA

This is a revised version of the article by F Chiappelli and D Hodgson, Encyclopedia of Stress, First edition, volume 2, pp 531–535, © 2000, Elsevier Inc.

Glossary

Allostasis Psychobiological process that brings about stability through change of state consequential to stress. The allostatic response encompasses a range of psychobiological outcomes that reflect physiologically important changes in the balance between the psychoneuroendocrine and the immune systems. Allostasis overload leads to statistically significant and clinically relevant damage to the organism due to excessive energy expenditure in the response to stress.

Anergy A state of immune unresponsiveness, induced as soon as the antigen receptor of the T cell is stimulated, which stops T cell responses waiting for second signal from the antigen-presenting cell.

Apoptosis The process of programed cell death needed to eliminate cells that represent a threat to the integrity of the organism.

Circadian A term derived from the Latin *circa diem* meaning about a day, refers to biological rhythms that have a cycle of about 24 hours.

Molecular cartography The science of recognizing and identifying multifaceted and intricate array of gene interaction and gene products that characterize the function of each individual cell in the context of cell–cell interaction, tissue, and organ function.

The renowned XIX century French physiologist, Claude Bernard (1813–78) first proposed that defense of the internal milieu (*le milieu intérieur*, 1856) is fundamental to physiological regulation, from when the phrase homeostasis originated. Walter Cannon (1871–1945) proposed that organisms engage in a dynamic process of adjustment of the physiological balance of the internal milieu in response to changing environmental conditions. Hans Selye (1907–82) established the cardinal points of the generalized stress response in his demonstration of concerted physiological responses to stressful challenges.

The immune response is finely regulated at the molecular, cellular, and physiological levels. Bacteriokines (i.e., bacterial cytokine inducers), produced by infectious pathogens, contribute to the control of the pathological inflammatory response. This article focuses on the homeostasis of the immune response from the perspective of the psychoneuroendocrine and cellular events that contribute to the suppression of immunity in response to stressors.

Allostasis

Allostasis refers to the psychobiological process that brings about stability through change of state consequential to stress. Psychoemotional stress can be defined as a perceived lack of fit of one's perceived abilities and the demands of the environment (i.e., person/environment fit). The perception of stress leads to anxiety, irritability and anger, tension, depressed moods, fatigue, a compendium of symptoms referred to as the sickness behavior (e.g., lethargy, nausea, and fever), and to a set of other bodily manifestations, including perspiration, blushing or blanching of the face, increased heart rate or decreased blood pressure, and intestinal cramps and discomfort, and suppressed immune resistance to antigenic challenges.

Sterling and Eyer (1988) defined allostasis as the set of mind–body systemic events aimed at regulating the recovery from stress. Heterostasis came to describe the situation where the demands upon the organism exceed its physiological capacity.

The process of allostatic regulation signifies the recovery and maintenance of internal balance and viability amidst changing circumstances consequential to stress. It encompasses a range of behavioral and physiological functions that direct the adaptive function of regulating homeostatic systems in response to challenges. The allostatic load refers to the set of physiological, psychological, and pathological side effects of the allostatic process, whereas allostatic overload signifies psychobiological collapse, and is associated with a variety of health outcomes systemically.

Type I and Type II Allostatic Responses

The allostatic response encompasses a range of psychobiological outcomes that reflect changes in the balance between the psychoneuroendocrine and the immune systems. Allostasis overload leads to statistically significant and clinically relevant damage to the organism due to excessive energy expenditure in the response to stress.

Type I

Type I allostasis utilizes stress responses as a mean of self-preservation by means of developing and establishing temporary or permanent adaptation skills. The organism aims at surviving the perturbation in the best condition possible, and at normalizing the normal lifecycle. An example of Type I allostatic response is recurrent aphthous stomatitis (RAS, canker sores), a stress-associated T cell-dependent pathology of the gingival mucosa. RAS lesions are characterized with increased Th1 patterns of cytokine *in situ* (e.g., interleukin (IL)-2). Ongoing work confirms a statistically significant correlation between the clinical incidence of RAS, based on stringent clinical and diagnostic criteria, and scores on a version of the short form-36 health survey questionnaire (SF-36) adapted for dentistry.

Other examples of Type I allostatic response manifested in the oral cavity include teeth grinding: tooth pain that cannot be attributed to carries, cracked tooth syndrome, pulpitis or other circumdental inflammatory process (e.g., gum disease), temporomandibular disorder and pain, and pain at palpation of the masticatory muscles, altered dental anatomy at the coronal surfaces. When the subjects are followed up prospectively, changes in vertical distance of occlusion and the angle of Spee that refers to the curved line that follows the occlusal surface of the posterior teeth of the mandible and is viewed from a sagittal plane are also noted.

Examples of systemic Type I allostatic response include the physiological responses to electromagnetic field. In a paired double-blind study, healthy young adults were exposed to electromagnetic field during controlled sleep. A sharp reduction in secreted melatonin was observed, which was transient and not correlated with any alterations of note in immune responses. The observed twofold increase in IL-2 serum levels failed to alter significantly natural killer cell activity.

Type II

In Type II allostatic load, the stressful challenge is excessive, sustained, or continued, and drives allostasis chronically. An escape response cannot be found. The psychobiological and pathological responses to stress become chronic (e.g., depression, anxiety, hypercortisolemia, and glucocorticoid resistance), with consequential erosion in health and immune surveillance mechanisms.

Oral Lichen Planus

Lichen planus of the oral mucosa (oral lichen planus; OLP) is one example of a Type II allostatic response with evident manifestations of immune suppression in the oral cavity. This form of oral lichenoid lymphocytic mucosal inflammation involves basal cell lysis, and lymphocyte transmigration into the epithelial compartment, and brings about a statistically significant increase in incidence of oral squamous cell carcinoma, which implicates OLP as a premalignant lesion. This chronic inflammatory disorder afflicts 2–3% of the population, and may be in part attributed to aging-associated decrease in the subject's ability to recover from the psychoneuroendocrine-immune changes consequential to stress since OLP is prevalent in individual over 50 years of age. Men are at risk at an earlier age than women (40–49 years with men versus 50–59 years with women). OLP lesions are exacerbated with nonsteroidal anti-inflammatory drugs, antirheumatic drugs, angiotensin-converting enzyme inhibitors, antihypertensive drugs, antibiotics, or β-blockers. These pharmacologic treatments share the commonality of suppressing one or another arm of cellular immunity, suggesting a pathological parallel between OLP lesions and mucositis. The nervous system may play an important role *in vivo* in regulating cellular immune responses in OLP lesions, as suggested by the suggestive alignment of autonomic innervation with lymphocytes (**Figure 1**). Immune suppression is modulated by sympathetic innervation, and by the cholinergic anti-inflammatory pathway, which inhibits proinflammatory cytokine production and secretion. The relationship between OLP and immune suppression is confirmed by the observation that it appears to result from an abnormal immune response to an unidentified causative agent. Over 75%

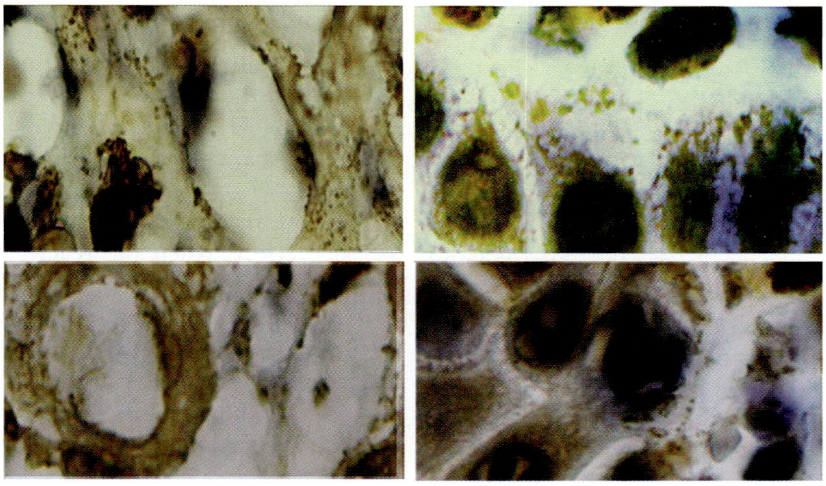

Figure 1 Double-label immunohistochemical staining of erosive OLP lesions with CD3 for T cells, and vesicles of acetylcholine transport (VachT; lower panels) and vesicles for monoamine transport (VAMT; upper panels) for autonomic innervation (magnification ×100, oil immersion).

of invading T cells express the memory phenotype (CD45RO+), the β1 integrin, CD29+, which renders them essentially sessile. A large proportion of the invading cells also appear phenotypically to be activated Treg (CD25+CD69+). Altered antigenicity of cell-surface epithelial cells causes them to be recognized as immunogenic, in a manner akin to an autoimmune disorder. Human hepatitis C virus (HCV) seems to be a predisposing factor for OLP, and comorbidity of HCV infection with OLP is noted in association with the HLA-Dr6 allele. The genetic propensity for OLP is emphasized by the observation that expression of HLA-Bw57 favors OLP, whereas HLA-Dql expression provides resistance against it.

Chronic Pain

A systemic example of Type II allostasis is chronic pain. Patients with fibromyalgia demonstrate altered function of β-adrenoceptors. Activation of G-protein coupled receptors, such as the adrenoceptors, leads to an increase in the intracellular level of cAMP. Levels of cAMP serve to assess, albeit indirectly, the functional state of these receptors in immune cells. Patients with fibromyalgia were compared to sex- and age-matched control subjects, and basal and stimulated intracellular cAMP levels were measured, using the β-agonist, isoproterenol (10^{-3} M–10^{-5} M, following a 5 min preincubation). Basal cAMP levels were shown to be elevated in patients with fibromyalgia (3.02 ± 0.44 pmol/10^6 cells, $P = 0.124$), compared to control subjects (2.26 ± 0.39 pmol/10^6 cells). Stimulation with isoproterenol at 10^{-3} M significantly increased intracellular cAMP in both groups; but isoproterenol at 10^{-5} M failed to produce this outcome in the patient group ($P = 0.74$), compared to the stimulation by isoproterenol obtained in the control group ($P = 0.012$). Taken together, these data show that patients with fibromyalgia harbor diminished adrenoceptor function in circulating immune cells.

Mucositis

Another example of Type 2 allostasis may be the clinical condition of mucositis. Oropharyngeal mucositis is a common and treatment-limiting side effect of cancer therapy. Oral and gastrointestinal mucositis can affect up to 100% of patients undergoing high-dose chemotherapy and hematopoietic stem cell transplantation, 80% of patients with malignancies of the head and neck receiving radiotherapy, and over 50% of patients receiving chemotherapy. Oral mucositis can be so severe as to lead to the need to interrupt or discontinue the therapy protocol, and to hinder cure of the primary disease. Mucositis leads to immune suppression, and to an increased risk of local and systemic infection, opportunistic infections, and mortality due to sepsis. It is a critical condition since in 2004 alone, close to 1.5 million Americans were diagnosed with cancer and received some combination therapies for this disease, including surgery, radiation, chemotherapy, immunotherapy, and/or cell transplantation, and mucositis is the principal oral complication from cancer therapies.

The Allostatic Modulation of Immune Suppression

One important regulatory mechanism in allostasis is the interactive neuroendocrine-immune loop. Stress alters the regulation of both the sympathetic and the parasympathetic branches of the autonomic nervous system, and modulates immune suppression. Autonomic activation, and the elevation of hormones, including those produced by the hypothalamic-pituitary-adrenal axis, play a pivotal role in regulating cell-mediated immune surveillance mechanisms, including the production of cytokines that control inflammatory and healing events.

The experience of stress and of traumatic events leads to the release of glucocorticoids, which regulate cellular immune activity *in vivo* systemically and locally: they block the production of proinflammatory cytokines (e.g., IL-1β, IL-6) and of Th1 cytokines (e.g., IL-2) at the molecular level *in vitro* and *in vivo*, but have little effects upon Th2 cytokines (e.g., IL-4). The activity of the proinflammatory cytokine IL-1β is blocked by IL-1 receptor antagonists (IL-1Ra, sIL-1RII) in combination with the soluble IL-1 accessory protein (IL-1R AcP). This results in a long-term beneficial effect in chronic inflammatory diseases. The net effect of challenging immune cells with glucocorticoids is to suppress immune T cell activation and proliferation, while maintaining antibody production. The secretion of glucocorticoids by the adrenal cortex is under the control of the anterior pituitary adrenocorticotropin hormone (ACTH). Immune challenges release proinflammatory cytokines (e.g., IL-1β, IL-6), which induce hypothalamic secretion of the ACTH inducing corticotropin releasing hormone (CRH). It follows that the consequences of stress are not uniform. The immune-physiological impact of stress may be significantly greater in certain people, compared to others. The impact of stress is dynamic and multifaceted, and the same person may exhibit a variety of manifestations of immune suppression in response to stress with varying degrees of severity at different times. The outcome of stress can be multivalent, and individuals may position themselves along a spectrum of allostatic regulation, somewhere between Type I and Type II allostasis.

Several experimental protocols have been characterized for testing allostasis in animal and human research. Human subjects under stress (e.g., caregivers of elderly patients with dementia and spouses of military personnel in active combat duty) can be subjected to cognitive, sensory, or physiological challenges aimed at studying the allostatic process of immune-physiological adaptation to the challenge in addition to basal states of the stress response.

The Stroop Test

The Stroop color-word interference test is an example of a cognitive challenge that was originally developed in 1935 to examine patterns of cognitive decline. The Stroop challenge is measured as reaction time, and is high in patients with mild to moderate aging-related dementia of the Alzheimer's type (DAT). Patients with more severe dementia show less Stroop interference effect, when the reaction time is adjusted for color naming performance. These observations confirm the need and the importance of partitioning out underlying deficits for the understanding of complex cognitive processes in aging. Principal-components analyses show that disruption of semantic knowledge and speeded verbal processing in certain patients (e.g., patients with neuro-AIDS, patients with DAT) is a major contributor to the incongruent trial. The Stoop challenge is an effective modality for testing the glucocorticoids-cytokine response in healthy young men and women. Two groups of responders can be distinguished based on salivary and plasma glucocorticoids response to the challenge. The bottom 40% of the responders for cortisol responses to the challenge characteristically manifested significantly higher salivary and plasma levels of IL-6, but lower subjective experience of stress, compared to the high-glucocorticoids responders (top 40 percentile). This confirms that individual variations exist in the response of the glucocorticoids-cytokine axis to mild stress, and that these variations can have potentially adverse health outcomes.

An ongoing study is comparing patients with major depression (*Diagnostic and Statistical Manuel of Mental Disorders, 4th edition* (DSM-IV) criteria) with age-, sex-, and ethnicity-matched control subjects for the response on the Stroop test. Preliminary data indicate that the median Raw Color-Word score is 20% higher in the control, compared to the depressed subjects. The median predicted interference score based on Color-Word scores is indistinguishable among healthy and depressed subjects. These data confirm the literature in the substantial differences in percentile position of the median T scores: 66% percentile (depressed patients) versus 42% percentile (healthy control subjects). An important caveat of the Stroop challenge is that color confusion can be inconsistent in certain subgroups of subjects, especially as subjects advanced in age. The Stroop test should not to be used for clinical diagnostic purposes, but rather limited as an experimental tool.

The Cold Pressor Test

Another widely used stress paradigm for testing allostasis in human subjects is the cold pressor challenge.

The physiological mechanism underlying the response to this challenge, which consists in the immersion of the nondominant hand in an ice bath, involves a response temperature as constriction to blood flow of both superficial and deep tissues of the hand, and associated strong perception of pain. This challenge test is an adequate model to study psychobiological responses to stressful discomfort because cold-induced vasospasms are frequently present in syndromes of chronic pain, but it may have adverse effects in subjects with cardiovascular dysfunctions. Pain latency (e.g., length of time of hand immersion) is significantly shorter in certain populations of patients, such as patients with fibromyalgia and secondary concomitant fibromyalgia, compared to healthy control subjects.

This challenge alters the glucocorticoids-cytokine axis responsivity in healthy young adult men and women, and leads to time-dependent patterns of change in the circadian patterns of salivary IL-6. The cold pressor test significantly alters salivary IL-6 in control subjects. IL-6 levels were measured at times t = –5 min, t = 0 min (baseline levels), and t = 1, 31, 61, and 91 min postchallenge. Salivary IL-6 rose two- to threefold during the 90 min after cold pressor test. This effect was more pronounced in female compared to male subjects ($P < 0.05$; **Figure 2**).

The Dexamethasone-Suppression Test

The dexamethasone-suppression test (DST) is a widely used physiological challenge to study the functional response of the glucocorticoids-cytokine axis. Administration of 1–5 mg of dexamethasone (DEX) to healthy subjects in the evening (23.00 h) results in a flattened cortisol plasma level the following morning and day. The cortisol suppression response is an indication of DEX-sensitivity and normal hypothalamic-pituitary-adrenocortical (HPA) response. Significant changes in the migratory properties of circulating CD4+ T cells occur in DEX-sensitive control subjects. The use of the DST challenge is in monitoring the glucocorticoids-cytokine response in a variety of patient populations. In DEX-resistant (i.e., no cortisol suppression following DST) subjects, the migratory properties of circulating CD4+ T cells are not altered. An intimate relationship is evident between the physiological regulation of the neuroendocrine and cellular immune systems *in vivo* in healthy subjects, compared to patient populations. Stress states can lead to enhanced suppression of cortisol by DEX following the DST challenge, although discrepancies exist among reports. Neither low basal cortisol nor enhanced suppression of cortisol are consistent markers of a posttraumatic stress disorder, for instance, major depression, or DAT. The lack of reliability, validity, and specificity of the DST as a diagnostic instrument, however, has not reduced the usefulness of this challenge modality to better understand neuroendocrine-immune interactions and the physiological regulation of immune suppression. Another caveat of this paradigm is that it provides a static challenge to the neuroendocrine-immune system: it leads to a shut-off, albeit temporarily, of glucocorticoids flux by acting on its feedback system. In that respect it presents a reflection of the regulatory response, rather than of the glucocorticoid-cytokine axis potential *per se*, as, for example the CRH stimulation test does. Therefore, the DST challenge is a static challenge of glucocorticoids-cytokine responses.

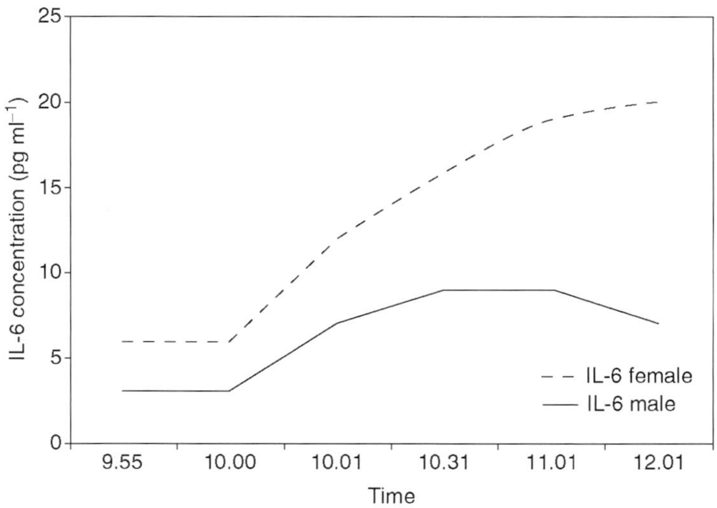

Figure 2 Salivary IL-6 response after cold pressor test applied at 10.00 a.m. on healthy volunteers. IL-6 response to stress was more pronounced in female (dashed line) compared to male subjects (solid line) ($P < 0.05$).

Alcohol and Substance Abuse

Subjects who abuse alcohol or other substances (e.g., cocaine) characteristically exhibit a deregulated pituitary-adrenal axis, elevated cortisol levels, a blunted T cell activation, and consequential immune suppression. Associated is a deregulated distribution of CD4+CD62L+ cells, which upon withdrawal of alcohol or cocaine abuse, normalizes together with plasma cortisol. Indeed, nicotine and ethanol, at concentrations approximating those found in the plasma of smokers and alcohol abusers, decrease immune surveillance of oral carcinoma by interfering with immune cell-mediated clearance of the tumor target. Significant ($P < 0.05$) diminution of migration, binding, activation, and cytotoxic activity by nicotine when coupled with ethanol contributes to the observed immune suppression.

Experimental Findings

Circulating memory CD4+CD45R0+ cells in patients with OLP comprise 66% of the circulating leukocyte population, compared to 49% in healthy control subjects, suggesting an imbalance between naïve and memory T cells. Moreover, serum levels of tumor necrosis factor (TNF)-α and IL-6 are significantly elevated in patients with OLP. These patients also exhibit significant alterations in pituitary-adrenal/cellular immune regulation, as do close to 50% of patients with DAT. In these patients, whole saliva can be used for the reliable assessment of neuroendocrine products and cytokines.

Serum, saliva, and cervicular fluid samples were collected for the determination of IL-6 in healthy age-matched control subjects, in patients with DAT, and in their caregivers. Subjects were assessed by a multidimensional evaluation that included collection of demographic data, cognitive function, level of impairment, and assessment of mood states by means of the profile of moods states. Mean IL-6 levels in both plasma and saliva were higher in the group of patients with DAT, compared to the caregiver and control subjects. Crevicular fluid determinations were unreliable due to the small volume collected. Saliva and plasma IL-6 levels were well correlated. Profiles of moods states scores were significantly higher in the caregiver group (54.80 ± 65.45; –16–166), compared to the patient group with DAT (39.6 ± 50.5; 6–129), and the control subjects (9.4 ± 12.1; –26–2) (Wilcoxon, $P < 0.05$). Caregivers showed lower emotional well-being and more emotional stress than patients and healthy noncaregiver controls.

T Cell Anergy and Apoptosis

T cell activation can lead to the proliferative response. Alternative pathways can attenuate or prevent the response of T cells, and lead to anergy (i.e., absence of response) or apoptosis (i.e., spontaneous programed cell death), and consequential immune suppression.

T cell stimulation by triggering through the T cell receptor (TcR) in the absence of CD28-mediated costimulatory signals induces unresponsiveness to further stimulation in T cells, a phenomenon known as anergy. Anergic T cells do not produce IL-2 when challenged, and are defective in their ability to upregulate protein binding and transactivation at two critical IL-2 DNA enhancer elements: NF-AT (nuclear factor of activated T cells; a sequence that binds a heterotrimeric NFATp, fos, and jun protein complex), activator protein-1 (AP-1; that binds fos and jun heterodimers), the Janus tyrosine kinases (Jak), and the signal transducers and activators of transcription (Stat) act as key regulatory components. The impaired DNA-protein interactions in anergic T cells is related to poor expression of the inducible AP-1 family members c-fos, fosB, and junB, attributable, at least in part, to a selective block in the expression of the AP-1 Fos and Jun family members in anergic T cells. Ligation of CD28 results in its phosphorylation and subsequent recruitment and activation of phosphatidylinositol (PI)3-kinase. Pharmacological and mutational analysis data show that disruption of PI3-kinase association with CD28 is neither necessary nor sufficient for costimulation of IL-2 production. T cell anergy also involves transcription regulators.

Calmodulin

Calmodulin (CaM) is an intracellular Ca^{2+}-binding protein that mediates many of the effects of Ca^{2+}. CaM binds to Fas directly and identifies the CaM-binding site on the cytoplasmic death domain (DD) of Fas. Fas (APO-1/CD95) is a cell-surface receptor that initiates apoptotic pathways, and its cytoplasmic domain interacts with various molecules suggesting that Fas signaling is complex and regulated by multiple proteins. The processes of T cell anergy and apoptosis are intertwined and act together to play critical role in immune suppression.

The Apoptosis Process

The process of apoptosis is a complex network, with different nodes connected by physical interactions of critical domains, including the caspase recruitment domains (CARDs); death effector domains (DEDs); DDs; BIR (baculovirus inhibitor of apoptosis proteins (IAP) repeat) domains of IAPs; Bcl-2 family proteins; caspase protease domains; and endonuclease-associated CIDE (cell death-inducing DNA fragmentation factor (DFF)45like effector) domains. Apoptotic cell death is thus a multifaceted process, whose initial signal is triggered in part by members of the TNF receptor superfamily, including Fas. When Fas interacts with the Fas-ligand, transmembrane signals are initiated through the associated FADD/MORT-1 motif, which interacts with caspase-8. Up to 10 caspases have been identified to date, which have been numbered based upon the chronological order of publication of their respective cDNAs. Active caspases are released from cleavage from the pro-enzyme into a larger peptide (17–22 kD) and a smaller peptide (10–12 kD) that associate to form the active enzyme in cells undergoing apoptosis. Caspase-8 possesses two motifs near the 5′-terminal that associate with FADD, referred to as the death effector domain. Activated caspase-8 in turn activates other caspases, and acts directly on mitochondrial permeability and metabolism.

Mitochondria

Mitochondria are involved in apoptosis through release of soluble molecules, such as bcl-2 that is normally situated in the outer mitochondrial membrane near the inner–outer membrane contact sites where permeability pores form. The action of bcl-2 is to protect against apoptosis by preventing the opening of these pores and release of a 50-kD protease and cytochrome C. Additional events involve changes in the plasma membrane and translocation of phosphatidyl-serine from the inner to the outer aspect of the membrane, which can be reliably detected by its high affinity to the Ca^{2+}-dependent phospholipid-binding protein, Annexin-5 (35–36 kD). Signals reach the nucleus for activation of nucleases and degradation of chromosomes into nucleosomal subunits. These metabolites are detected either as fragments of increasing length on an agarose gel or as cytoplasmic content of nucleosomal proteins.

β-Amyloid

Case in point, the peptide found in the neural plaques that characterize Alzheimer's disease, β-amyloid, significantly modulates T cell-mediated immunity. The 1–42 β-amyloid peptide leads to T cell anergy, and impairs the generation of CD4+CD25+ and CD8+CD25+ Treg by up to 25%. This effect is attributable to the 28–35 portion of the peptide, the same that is responsible for impairing the maturation of T cell *in vitro*. The peptide also induces apoptotic cell death of healthy human T cells, as monitored by augmentation of cytoplasmic oligonucleosomes following treatment with β-amyloid, and a over threefold induction of caspase 3 (**Figure 3**).

A New Strategy: Molecular Cartography

Molecular cartography is the science of recognizing and identifying the multifaceted and intricate array of interacting genes and gene products that characterize

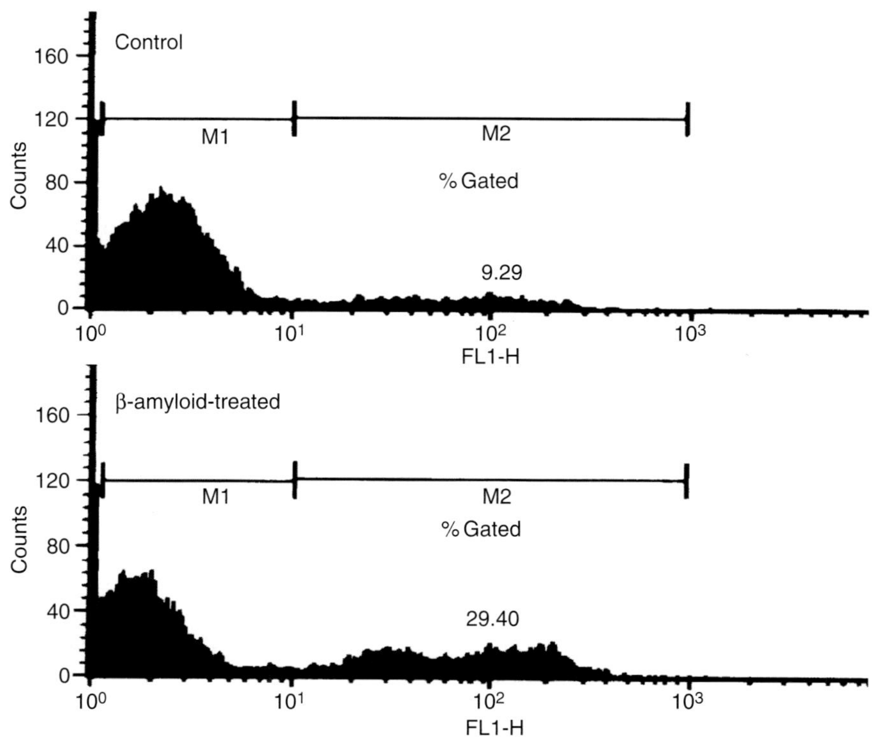

Figure 3 Caspase 3 induction in healthy human T cells exposed to β-amyloid peptide (1–42) for 48 h. Upper panel shows untreated (control) cultures. Lower panel shows β-amyloid-treated cultures. β-amyloid stimulated over threefold induction of caspase 3.

the function and specialization of each individual cell in the context of cell–cell interaction, tissue and organ function. The relevance of molecular cartography pertains to every domain of physiology, including immunity.

Molecular cartography provides the fundamental knowledge and understanding of the genomic, the proteomic, and interactomic processes that regulate the emergence, stability, and function of immune cell populations, and the mechanisms by which the psychoneuroendocrine system regulates immunity. It produces new fundamental knowledge with respect to the processes that regulate immune suppression.

Further Reading

Carli, G., Suman, A. L., Biasi, G., et al. (2002). Reactivity to superficial and deep stimuli in patients with chronic musculoskeletal pain. *Pain* **100**, 259–269.

Chiappelli, F., Kung, M. A., Nguyen, P., et al. (1997). Cellular immune correlates of clinical severity in oral lichen planus: preliminary association with mood states. *Oral Diseases* **3**, 64–70.

Chiappelli, F. (2005). The molecular immunology of mucositis: implications for evidence-based research in alternative and complementary palliative treatments. *Evidence-Based Complementary and Alternative Medicine* **2**, 489–494.

Chiappelli, F. and Cajulis, O. S. (2004). Psychobiological views on "stress-related oral ulcers" *Quintessence International* **35**, 223–227.

Chiappelli, F. and Hodgson, D. (2000). Immune suppression. In: Fink, G. (ed.) *Encyclopedia of stress,* (vol. 2), pp. 531–536. San Diego: Academic Press.

Chiappelli, F., Prolo, P., Fiala, M., et al. (2005). Allostasis in HIV-1 infection and AIDS. In: Minagar, P. A. & Shapshak, P. (eds.) *Neuro-AIDS.* Hauppauge, NY: Nova Science Publisher (in press).

Chiappelli, F., Prolo, P., Iribarren, J., et al. (2006). Alzheimer's disease: new frontiers for the XXI century. In: Welsh, E. M. (ed.) *Trends in Alzheimer's disease research*, pp. 233–258. Hauppauge, NY: Nova Science Publishers.

Czura, C. J., Friedman, S. G. and Tracey, K. J. (2003). Neural inhibition of inflammation: the cholinergic anti-inflammatory pathway. *Journal of Endotoxin Research* **9**, 409–413.

Kunz-Ebrecht, S. R., Mohamed-Ali, V., Feldman, P. J., et al. (2003). Cortisol responses to mild psychological stress are inversely associated with proinflammatory cytokines. *Brain Behavior and Immunology* **17**, 373–383.

Maekawa, K., Twu, C., Lotaif, A., et al. (2003). Function of β-adrenergic receptor on mononuclear cells in female fibromyalgia patient. *Journal of Rheumatology* **30**, 364–368.

McEwen, B. and Wingfield, J. C. (2003). The concept of allostasis in biology and biomedicine. *Hormones and Behavior* **43**, 2–15.

Sterling, P. and Eyer, J. (1988). Allostasis: a new paradigm to explain arousal pathology. In: Fisher, S. & Reason, J. (eds.) *Handbook of life stress, cognition, and health*, pp. 629–645. New York: Wiley.

van der PouwKraan, T. C., Kasperkovitz, P. V., Verbeet, N., et al. (2004). Genomics in the immune system. *Clinical Immunology* **111**, 175–185.

Autoimmunity

B S Rabin
University of Pittsburgh, Pittsburgh, PA, USA

This article is reproduced from Encyclopedia of Stress, First edition, volume 1, pp. 268–274, © 2000, Elsevier Inc.

Glossary

Antibody A protein that combines with the antigen that caused the antibody to be produced. Antibodies have specificity in that they combine most strongly with the particular antigen that stimulated their production. Antibodies are produced by a type of white blood cell called a B lymphocyte. Each B lymphocyte can only produce a single type of antibody, but the B lymphocyte produces thousands of that particular antibody molecule each second. Antibodies bind to antigens that are located outside of tissue cells.

Antigen A substance that activates the immune system to produce a specific response that reacts against the antigen that activated the immune response. An antigen is usually something that is foreign to the body such as an infectious agent.

Autoimmunity An immune reaction that is directed against an individual's own tissue. The immune reaction may damage tissue and cause disease.

Cytokine One of numerous proteins made by a cell which can influence the activity of other cells. Cytokines bind to cytokine receptors on cells with different receptors binding different cytokines. Lymphocytes and antigen-presenting cells produce

	cytokines which, depending on the particular cytokine and the cell that it binds to, may either upregulate or downregulate the activity of other immune cells. Cytokines are also involved in the regulation of endocrine hormone production and contribute to the modulation of activity of the central nervous system.
Lymphocytes	White blood cells responsible for the immune response. Different types of lymphocytes originate from a common stem cell in the bone marrow. Lymphocytes that continue their maturation in the bone marrow become B lymphocytes, which function by producing antibody. Lymphocytes that migrate from the bone marrow to the thymus gland for their maturation become T lymphocytes that function in cell mediated immunity, which is antibody independent.
Tolerance	The specific absence of an immune response to an antigen. This is usually an active process that is related to the deletion of antigen-reactive lymphocytes or a mechanism which suppress the ability of the lymphocytes to respond to antigen. Lymphocytes which have receptors for self-antigen (one's own tissue antigens) are eliminated by the tolerance mechanism(s).

How Can an Autoimmune Disease Be Initiated and How Can Stress Contribute to the Process?

Failure to Eliminate Autoreactive B Lymphocytes

The B lymphocytes are produced and mature in the bone marrow as part of the normal process of B cell maturation. Some B lymphocytes randomly develop immunoglobulin receptors that are reactive to self-antigens. Thus, they have the capability of releasing antibodies that react with self antigens. To prevent the development of autoimmune diseases, the autoreactive B lymphocytes must be eliminated before they can produce harmful reactions. The process of removal of autoreactive lymphocytes is called tolerance. Tolerance may be associated with actual death of the lymphocyte or its functional inactivation. The development of tolerance of newly formed autoreactive B lymphocytes must continue throughout life.

If the process of B cell tolerization were highly effective, no individuals would have autoreactive antibodies in their blood. However, nearly all normal individuals can be found to have low levels of antibodies directed to self-antigens. This suggests that the process of tolerization of newly developed B lymphocytes to self-antigens is not entirely effective.

As there is an epidemiological association of autoimmune disease with stress, it is possible that stress interferes with the tolerization of autoreactive B lymphocytes. Whether this is due to a stress-mediated decrease in the amount of circulating self-antigens which must be present in the marrow for B cell tolerance to develop, a decreased accessibility of self-antigens to the developing B lymphocytes in the marrow, a decreased susceptibility to tolerization of the autoreactive B lymphocytes, or other reasons is undetermined. For example, it is possible that stress hormones alter the kinetics of maturation of B lymphocytes so that there is a shorter window of opportunity for B lymphocytes to become tolerant to self-antigens, alter blood flow to the bone marrow so that there is a decreased concentration of self-antigens present, or alter the release of self-antigens from tissue so that the concentration of these antigens is decreased in the blood.

Failure to Eliminate Autoreactive T Lymphocytes

The T lymphocytes arise in the bone marrow but mature in the thymus gland. Some of the maturing T lymphocytes have receptors on their surface membrane that will combine with self-antigen. It is in the thymus where the autoreactive T lymphocytes undergo the process of tolerization. Similar to autoreactive B lymphocytes, T cell tolerization may involve cell death or functional inactivation.

If all autoreactive T lymphocytes were eliminated in the thymus, there should be no autoimmune diseases. That autoimmune diseases occur indicates that the process is not totally efficient or that there are ways for T cells to escape from tolerance. If the hormonal response to stress alters mechanisms whereby T cell tolerance occurs, stress may increase the likelihood of an autoimmune disease occurring. It is possible that the hormonal response to stress alters the interactions between the cells that are responsible for the induction of tolerance of T lymphocytes. This may result in increased numbers of autoreactive T cells being present in the peripheral lymphoid tissues.

Alteration of Cell Regulation

In the spleen, lymph nodes, and blood, where many immune reactions are initiated, there are a variety of regulatory interactions which occur between cells of the lymphoid system. The mechanism of regulation is likely through the secretion of soluble factors by a particular type of cell that alters the activity of other cells. The hormonal response to stress may alter the function of the regulatory cells which then may predispose to an autoimmune response. Examples included are listed below.

1. Macrophages produce transforming growth factor-β (TGF-β), which inhibits proliferation of T and B lymphocytes. If stress hormones inhibit TGF-β production, activation of autoreactive T or B lymphocytes may be enhanced.
2. The CD4 Th2 lymphocytes produce the cytokines IL-4 and IL-10. These cytokines suppress CD4 Th1 lymphocyte function. Increased Th2 CD4 lymphocyte function, which is associated with a change in the balance between Th1 and Th2 function, has been associated with activation of latent viral infections. Th1 activity is important as it suppresses latent virus activation. An immune reaction against tissue cells expressing viral antigens has been associated with the onset of autoimmune disease. Thus, stressor-induced alteration of the balance of immune function may contribute to the development of autoimmunity through the mechanism of latent virus activation.
3. The CD4 Th1 lymphocytes produce interferon-γ, which suppresses CD4 Th2 lymphocyte function. An increase of Th1 relative to Th2 activity has been associated with tissue damage in autoimmune disease. If the hormonal response to stress suppresses Th2 and increases Th1 CD4 lymphocyte function, an alteration of the course of autoimmune disease may occur.

There is a paucity of basic science studies relating to how an alteration of the balance between the various components of the immune system occurs when different concentrations of stress hormones are present. Such information is required before a determination can be made regarding the biological impact of stressor induced alterations of regulatory immune cell function.

Increased Susceptibility to Infection

Often, an acute stress or the experience of chronic stress decreases the function of the immune system. An increased susceptibility to upper respiratory viral infections and the reactivation of latent viral infections are the best documented indications of a biological effect of stressor-induced immune alterations. However, it is likely that resistance to any infectious agent is impaired by stress.

Infectious agents have been associated with the development of autoimmune diseases. Some infectious agents have antigenic sites that are identical to self-antigens. The presence of self and foreign antigenic sites on a single protein molecule frequently results in the breaking of tolerance to the self-antigen. For example, if infected with a bacteria that has an antigenic component on its surface that is identical to an antigen that is present on one's own tissues, tolerance can be broken. The antibody that is produced has the potential of altering the function of tissue or damaging tissue. Rheumatic fever is caused by this immune mechanism.

When a virus infects a tissue, an immune reaction to the virus kills the infected tissue cell. One of the mechanisms of cell killing is related to the release of enzymes from CD8 lymphocytes, neutrophils, and macrophages. The enzymes may degrade (denature) some of the molecules of self-antigen, resulting in a self-molecule that retains an antigenic site characteristic of the self-tissue and, in addition, has some antigenic sites that differ from self. When this molecule is processed by the cells of the immune system tolerance is broken and an immune response to the self-antigenic determinant results.

If Stress Suppresses Immune Function, How Does Stress Predispose to the Development of Autoimmune Disease?

A logical concern relates to how stress, which is usually associated with a decrease in the function of the immune system, can be associated with diseases which are thought to be caused by increased immune activity. This can occur through alteration of the regulatory components of the immune system, as described above, or through an increased susceptibility to infectious diseases with a subsequent increased risk of an autoimmune response.

Obviously, the relationship between the effects of stress on altering the function of the immune system and the development of an autoimmune disease is complex. Further complications are related to different patients with the same disease having different etiologies to their disease. Eventually, clarification of the factors that contributed to the development of an autoimmune disease in a particular patient depends on identifying the immune pathway that was responsible for the disease in that patient. That allows a more precise characterization of the role of stress in the pathogenesis of autoimmune disease to be identified.

The Relationship of Stress to Specific Autoimmune Diseases

The following presents specific autoimmune diseases that have been shown to have an increased frequency of occurrence or which have an exacerbation at a time of stress. However, there are many unanswered questions in regard to the pathogenesis of autoimmune disease involving onset, remissions, and exacerbations. Many of the studies where stress in a person's life is associated with an autoimmune disease are flawed by the process itself. For example, if an individual who has been diagnosed with an autoimmune disease is asked to recall negative events in their life, that individual may try harder to recall such events or add meaning to events that would seem less important if the individual did not have an autoimmune disease. A person experiencing negative life events may see a physician more frequently just because they are not feeling well emotionally and may be more likely to be diagnosed with a disease at an early stage. It is also possible that early stages of disease that produce metabolic alterations (such as thyroid disease or diabetes) may have behavioral changes due to the altered concentration of endocrine hormones in their blood which increase their likelihood of experiencing negative life events.

Psoriasis

Psoriasis is a skin disease that affects approximately 2% of the population. The involved areas of the skin are a pink color with white flaky scales. The skin lesions frequently undergo remissions and relapses. Psoriasis involves the infiltration of the skin with T lymphocytes and the production of disease-causing cytokines by the lymphocytes. An immune response to infectious agents in the skin may stimulate cytokine release. A hypothetical model can be constructed which supports the possibility that stress participates in the course of psoriasis by releasing neuropeptides from nerves which terminate in the skin. The neuropeptides, particularly substance P, may enhance the migration of lymphocytes into the skin which stimulate localized disease-enhancing cytokine release.

There are numerous published studies indicating that stress is associated with the exacerbation of symptoms in patients with psoriasis. A summary of the literature evaluating stress effects on the course of psoriasis supports the role of stress as a modulator of disease activity and suggests that the severity of the stressor may be associated with more severe disease Additional studies have suggested that relaxation procedures which may produce a psychological relaxation (which would have an effect on the immune system if they decreased sympathetic nervous system activation) are capable of ameliorating the clinical appearance of disease in patients with psoriasis. However, there are many factors which make interpretation of the studies difficult. Usually the number of subjects is low and the stage of disease and the actual pathogenesis of the disease in the subjects may vary. Coping skills (including psychosocial support, physical fitness, optimism, sense of humor, and belief systems) which help to buffer the effects of stress on the immune system may vary. Even whether the subject experienced high levels of stress as a youth or the subject's mother experienced high levels of stress during pregnancy may influence an individual's response to stress.

Rheumatoid Arthritis (RA)

Rheumatoid arthritis is associated with a large accumulation of lymphocytes in the joint spaces. There is destruction of the joint spaces and considerable pain. Systemic manifestations include tendonitis, pericarditis, vasculitis, and subcutaneous nodules pleuritis. The disease frequently has a relapsing and remitting course.

It is usually assumed that the disease is produced by activation of the immune system to an antigen. As identical twins are often discordant for RA it is likely that there is an environmental (antigen) involved in the disease pathogenesis. However, there has not been identification of specific antigen(s) to which the immune response is directed.

If the disease is a response to an antigen the functional competency of the immune system and its modification by stress hormones could modify the disease course. If stress does alter the course of RA, it may be through dysregulation of the normal relationship of the various lymphocyte subpopulations to each other. Reports of the effect of stress on the clinical course of RA have been variable and do not provide an unambiguous understanding regarding whether stress alters the onset or course of disease.

Another approach to evaluating whether stress influences the course of disease in patients with RA is to evaluate the effect of stress reduction interventions. Psychological interventions have suggested that slight clinical improvement can be achieved in patients with RA. Thus, regardless of the difficulty in defining an immunologic etiology in RA or a definitive understanding of the pathogenesis of the disease, there is suggestive evidence for an interaction between stress and the disease process.

There are extensive studies which indicate that psychological intervention programs can decrease the pain perceived by patients with RA. Whether the pain reduction produces an alteration in the amount of opioid produced, both within the CNS and peripherally, and whether there is a subsequent change in immune system function which ameliorates the disease process has not been determined.

Recently diagnosed subjects with RA have a lower activation of the sympathetic nervous system following a mental challenge stress task than control subjects without RA. Those subjects with the greatest amount of pain had the lowest sympathetic activation. The lack of an intact stress response in RA subjects may indicate that the immune pathogenesis of RA differs from the immune pathogenesis of other autoimmune diseases or that RA is more likely to occur in subjects who have an impaired hormonal response to stress.

An impaired hypothalamic-pituitary-adrenal (HPA) axis hormonal response to stress may allow the immune system to become overactivated, promoting an autoimmune process. Indeed, experimental animals which have an increased susceptibility to the induction of arthritis have been found to have functional differences of their HPA axes (susceptible animals have a decreased production of corticosterone) in comparison to experimental animals which are resistant to the induction of arthritis. An abnormal HPA response to immune and inflammatory stimuli has been reported in patients with RA.

Whether humans with RA have an altered response to stress because of modification of CNS function by cytokines or whether there is an innate difference within the CNS that modifies their response to stress has not been defined. However, subjects with another autoimmune disease, multiple sclerosis, have an intact response to the same psychological stressor that produced a diminished response in subjects with RA.

Graves' Thyroid Disease

Graves' hyperthyroidism is associated with weakness, nervousness, weight loss, fatigue, warm and sweaty skin, menstrual irregularities, heat sensitivity, protrusion of the eyes, and an enlarged thyroid gland. The pathogenesis is due to an antibody that binds to a receptor on thyroid epithelial cells that binds thyroid stimulating hormone (TSH). The thyroid stimulating antibody mimics the binding of TSH and stimulates the release of thyroid hormone. However, unlike TSH, which decreases in concentration as the concentration of thyroid hormone increases (reducing the releases of thyroid hormone), there is no inhibition of the physiologic effects of the thyroid stimulating antibody.

There are several studies which found that high levels of stress are more likely to occur in an individual who develops Graves' disease than in individuals who do not develop Graves'. These studies suggest that patients had more negative life events in the months preceding the clinical diagnosis of disease. However, not all studies support an association between prior stress and the onset of Graves'.

It is possible that if thyroid hormones are increased in concentration prior to the clinical diagnosis of disease, behavioral alterations are induced which either contribute to negative life events or the subject's awareness of negative life events. As thyroid hormone measurements are not made in the months preceding the appearance of clinical manifestation of Graves' disease, a possible influence of thyroid hormones on life events cannot be ruled out.

Multiple Sclerosis (MS)

Multiple sclerosis produces weakness, visual dysfunction, and paralysis. Multiple sclerosis lesions develop in the brain and the spinal cord where myelin surrounding nerve fibers is destroyed by lymphocytes and macrophages. There is an infiltrate of CD4 and CD8 lymphocytes, macrophages, and plasma cells. Nerve conduction is impaired. Identical twins have approximately a 50% concordance for MS, indicating that both genetic and environmental factors are involved with the disease pathogenesis.

The exact pathogenesis of MS is uncertain, but there is considerable evidence suggesting participation of the immune system. This includes characteristic changes in the immunoglobulin content of spinal fluid, which suggests an immune reaction occurring within the CNS; the mitogenic responsive of lymphocytes from patients with MS to antigens derived from the CNS; the clinical response to immunosuppressive therapy; and the existence of an experimental model that is induced by immunization with myelin basic protein, an antigen found in myelin.

The studies of stress as a contributor to the etiology of MS are not definitive. They suffer from the faults of small sample size, heterogeneity of the extent and pathogenesis of disease, various stress buffering capabilities of subjects, and concomitant clinical depression having an effect on immune system function. Definition of the exact immune mechanism(s) which produce demyelination is also a hindrance, as without knowing which immune mechanisms are responsible for the tissue damage it is impossible to know which pathway is being altered by stress.

An increase of Th1 lymphocyte function would be compatible with an immune change that could increase the risk for the development of MS. Interestingly, cerebrospinal fluid (CSF) of patients with MS contains cytokines which promote CD4 Th1 lymphocyte activity. An indirect indication of predominant Th1 activity in MS patients is the paucity of IgE-mediated disease in MS patients, as Th1-derived cytokines suppress the Th2 cells that promote B lymphocytes to synthesize IgE. Stress has been found to increase the production of cytokines from Th1 lymphocytes while sparing alteration of cytokine production by Th2 lymphocytes.

There have been many studies which have looked at the association of stress with the clinical course of patients with MS. The studies found that MS patients had significantly more life stress prior to the onset of disease or disease exacerbation than did controls. The most common life events which were related to exacerbation were those involving financial or interpersonal concerns.

An interesting observation regarding stress and disease activity in MS was made during the Persian Gulf war. This study reported a decreased rate of exacerbations of MS during the war. This observation indicates that an intense psychological stressor can have a profound effect on suppressing immune system function and decrease disease activity. However, this is a unique situation that does not argue against less intense life-event stressors having an influence on the exacerbation of the clinical course of MS.

Overall, the clinical observations and the possible stressor-induced immune changes suggest that stress can alter the course of MS. Studies of stress intervention are needed to confirm or refute this hypothesis. Care will have to be directed to the clinical homogeneity of the patient population including HLA characteristics, social support and other buffering systems available to the patient, use by the patient of medications, and how strongly the patient believes in the potential effectiveness of the intervention therapy.

Insulin-Dependent Diabetes Mellitus (IDDM)

A frequent pathogenesis of IDDM is related to immune-mediated destruction of the insulin-producing β-islet cells. Antibodies to insulin and islet cell antigens are present prior to the clinical onset of disease and may indicate a destructive inflammatory process is occurring. Sensitized T lymphocytes that have a cytotoxic effect on islet cells are also present.

The disease is frequently preceded by a viral infection and may be initiated by an immune response to a virus that specifically infects β-islet cells. Indeed, virus has been isolated from the islets of newly diagnosed diabetic subjects and, when the virus is injected into mice, IDDM has occurred with an associated immune-mediated destruction of the β-islet cells. Active viral infection is suggested because of a rising antibody titer in the patient's serum to the isolated virus.

There are several reports associating life-event stressors with the onset of IDDM. Unlike diseases such as rheumatoid arthritis or multiple sclerosis, which have a relapsing and remitting course, IDDM does not remit. Therefore, studies showing an association of stress with alteration of clinical activity are nonexistent, but studies showing an association of stress with disease onset are numerous. Stressor-induced alterations of immune function may contribute to disease onset by (1) suppressing immune function and increasing susceptibility to viral infection and (2) altering the balance of regulatory lymphocyte populations which then allows an autoimmune response to occur.

Early reports linking stressors in an individual's life with an increased susceptibility to the development of IDDM were not rigorously controlled and presented small sample sizes. However, there are studies which suggest that there may be an association between stress and susceptibility to the onset of IDDM. These studies should be considered to be preliminary, as they have not addressed important questions.

Specifically, does stress increase the risk of IDDM onset in all individuals or only those who are HLA-DR3 and/or HLA-DR4 positive? If this association only occurs in HLA-susceptible individuals, should the control group of individuals who do not have high levels of stress be restricted to HLA-DR 3- and/or HLA-DR-4-positive individuals?

The only way to control for genetic differences between subjects is to study identical twins. The concordance for IDDM in identical twins is approximately 50%. Environmental factors are usually designated as explaining the lack of 100% concordance. Environmental factors may include viruses, but may also include stress and the ability of a subject to cope with the stressor. A study conducted in identical twins both concordant and discordant for IDDM where factors such as stress, psychosocial support, physical fitness, belief systems, sense of humor, and being an optimist or a pessimist are considered would make a significant contribution to our understanding of the relationship between stress and susceptibility to autoimmune disease. If identical twins discordant for IDDM experience the same stressors, does the twin who develops IDDM have better coping skills?

Studies which have contributed to the suggestion of an association between stress and the onset of IDDM in children have found that severe emotional stress, usually associated with parental loss, especially occurring early in life, increased the risk for the subsequent development of IDDM.

Summation

Characterization of the potential interrelationship between stress and the development or exacerbation of an autoimmune disease requires knowledge of at least two parameters: (1) What components of the immune system are functionally altered by stress? and (2) How does alteration of the immune system initiate immune-mediated damage to self-tissue? Unfortunately, detailed information regarding each of the two questions is still lacking. However, there is abundant evidence from epidemiological studies that the experience of stress is associated with autoimmune disease onset or exacerbation. Continued studies of stressor-induced immune alteration and the mechanism of onset of autoimmune disease will help to clarify their relationship.

See Also the Following Articles

Cytokines; Immune Suppression.

Further Reading

Anderson, K. O., Bradley, L. A., Young, L. D., McDaniel, L. K. and Wise, C. M. (1985). Rheumatoid arthritis: review of the psychological factors relating to etiology, effects and treatment. *Psychological Bulletin* 98, 358–387.
Hagglof, B., Blom, L., Dahlquist, G., Lonnberg, G. and Sahlin, B. (1991). The Swedish childhood diabetes study: indications of severe psychological stress as a risk factor for type I (insulin-dependent) diabetes mellitus in childhood. *Diabetologia* 34, 579–583.
Herbert, T. B. and Cohen, S. (1993). Stress and immunity in humans: a meta-analytic review. *Psychosomatic Medicine* 55, 364–379.
Kung, A. W. C. (1995). Life events, daily stresses and coping in patients with Graves' disease. *Clinical Endocrinology* 42, 303–308.
Sternberg, E. M. (1995). Neuroendocrine factors in susceptibility to inflammatory disease: focus on the hypothalamic-pituitary-adrenal axis. *Hormone Research* 43, 159–161.
Wilder, R. L. (1995). Neuroendocrine-immune system interactions and autoimmunity. *Annual Review of Immunology* 13, 307–338.

Cytokines

G D Marshall
University of Mississippi Medical Center, Jackson, MS, USA

This is a revised version of the article by G D Marshall, Jr., and J L Rossio, Encyclopedia of Stress, First edition, volume 1, pp 626–632, © 2000, Elsevier Inc.

Glossary

Cytokine — Small molecular weight glycopeptide produced by a variety of cell types that serve to modulate immune and inflammatory responses.

Immunoendocrinology — The study of the impact of soluble products of the immune system on endocrine and neuroendocrine networks as part of the bidirectional communication between the immune and endocrine systems.

Psychoneuroimmunology — The study of the relationships between neurocognitive behaviors, neuroendocrine response, and immune changes occurring in response to stress.

Regulatory T cells — CD4+ (and some CD8+) cells that reside in both the central and peripheral immune systems whose main function is to regulate the intensity and duration of immune responses by inhibiting both cytokine production and effector function.

Stress — Perturbation of homeostatic state by environmental factors demanding an adaptive response from the host.

T helper cell — Lymphocyte that plays a central role in immune modulation by selectively activating various immune and nonimmune cells through the production of specific cytokine combinations.

Relationships between Stress and Immunity

Stress Defined

Stress is best thought of as a psychophysiological process, usually experienced as a negative emotional state. Stressors, defined as events with the potential for posing threat, harm, or challenge to the host, are judged in the context of personal and environmental factors, and if appraised as threatening or challenging, initiate specific physiologic responses directed at reducing or eliminating the stress (fight-or-flight). The field of psychoneuroimmunology seeks to establish the link between behavior, neuroendocrine functions, and immune responses.

Impact of Stress on Health

A common clinical observation is the often adverse relationship between stress and human disease. Various sources have estimated that up to 75% of all visits to physicians' offices are stress-related. This appears to be particularly true in relationship to immune-based dysfunction such as increased susceptibility to infections, autoimmune, allergic, and asthmatic diseases. Stress is also suspected to play a role in morbidity and mortality in other immune-based diseases such as cancer, HIV disease, inflammatory bowel diseases, and even aging. Stress may also cause persistent increases in sympathetic nervous system activity, including increased blood pressure, heart rate, and catecholamine secretion, as well as platelet aggregation which may explain, at least in part, the known association between stress, immune alterations, and cardiovascular disease. Emerging evidence suggests that sleep alterations can modulate the stress–health relationship. Acute stressors and adverse naturalistic events are associated with sleep disruptions as measured by self-report and polysomnography. Poor sleep, in turn, is associated with subsequent decrements in mental health including symptom reporting, incident cases of mood and anxiety disorders, and immune function. Sleep disruptions have also been associated with adverse physical health outcomes, including increased morbidity and mortality compared to populations with adequate patterns and duration of sleep.

Role of Cytokines in the Normal Immune Response

In the normal host, presentation of antigen for a specific protective immune response elicits a complex series of events that results in a mixed cellular and humoral protective response, the intensity and nature of which depends upon the specific inciting antigen. Generally speaking, extracellular parasites (i.e., bacteria) incite primarily a humoral response while intracellular parasites (i.e., virus, fungi, mycobacteria, etc.) elicit a cell-mediated response. Antiviral immunity is particularly complex because both arms are necessary for host resistance – cellular immunity to eliminate the virus-infected host cells and humoral immunity that produces antiviral neutralizing antibodies to prevent reinfection. The host immune response has a variety of mechanisms to direct the immune response into the humoral versus cellular direction, i.e., nature of antigen-presenting cells, major histocompatibility complex (MHC) restriction, and availability of specific T and B cell components. However, the central control of the cellular versus humoral response to an antigenic challenge appears to be via production of specific cytokine milieu.

All cytokines have certain properties in common. They are all small molecular weight peptides or glycopeptides. Many are produced by multiple cell types such as lymphocytes, monocytes/macrophages, mast cells, eosinophils, and even endothelial cells lining blood vessels. Each individual cytokine can have multiple functions depending on the cell that produces it and the target cell(s) on which it acts (called pleiotropism). Also, several different cytokines can have the same biologic function (called redundancy). Physiologically it appears that most cytokines exert their most important effects in a paracrine and/or autocrine rather than endocrine fashion. Their major functions appear to involve host defense or maintenance and repair of the blood elements.

Cytokines are categorized by their major specific function(s) and there are five major categories. Interferons (IFNs) are so named because they interfere with virus replication. There are three major types based upon the source of the IFN. IFN alpha (IFNα) is produced by the buffy coat layer from white blood cells, IFN beta (IFNβ) by fibroblasts, and IFN gamma (IFNγ) by activated T cells, natural killer (NK) cells, and dendritic cells (DC). IFNγ is an important immunoregulatory molecule in determining intracellular versus extracellular host defense responses.

The colony stimulating factors (CSFs) are so named because they support the growth and differentiation of various elements of the bone marrow. Many are named by the specific element they support such as granulocyte colony stimulating factor (G-CSF), macrophage colony stimulating factor (M-CSF), and granulocyte macrophage colony stimulating factor (GM-CSF). Other CSFs include interleukin (IL)-3, which can stimulate a variety of hematopoietic precursors and is being evaluated as a therapy in aplastic anemia and bone marrow transplantation; and c-Kit ligand (stem cell factor) which has been demonstrated as a cytokine necessary to cause the differentiation of bone marrow stem cells into their various precursor elements for eventual differentiation into erythrocytes, white blood cells, and megakaryocytes (platelets).

The tumor necrosis factors (TNFs) are so called because injecting them into animals causes a hemorrhagic necrosis of the animals' tumors. TNF-α is produced by activated macrophages and TNF-β is produced by activated T cells (both T helper (Th) and cytotoxic T lymphocytes (CTL)). These molecules appear to be involved in the pathogenesis of septic shock and much research is aimed at trying to inhibit their activity in septic patients.

The newest group described is the chemokines, small molecular weight proteins that promote chemotaxis and activation of cells to tissue sites experiencing inflammatory reactions. Currently more than 50 human chemokines and 18 receptors have been identified. They appear to be intimately involved in generating selective types of inflammatory cell infiltrates both because of the specific chemokine milieu produced as well as selective expression of particular chemokine receptors on specific inflammatory cell subpopulations. They are categorized into subfamilies (CXC, CC, CX3C, and so on) based on their chemical composition of N-terminal cysteinyl receptors. Examples include RANTES (regulated upon activation, normal T cell expressed and secreted), macrophage inhibitory peptide (MIPs), and eotaxin.

The largest group is the ILs, so named because their fundamental function appears to be communication between (inter-) various populations of white blood cells (leukocytes – leukin). They are produced by a variety of cell types such as monocytes/macrophages, T cells, B cells, and even nonleukocytes such as epithelial cells.

A central source of these cytokines comes from CD4+ helper T cell subpopulations, often referred to as Th1 and Th2 cells. Human Th1 cells secrete a specific cytokine profile including IFNγ and TNF-β. These cytokines are important helper factors in the generation of cellular immune responses including antigen-specific CTL and NK cells. Additionally, IFNγ in particular has an antagonistic activity against Th2 cytokines. IL-12, produced primarily by activated macrophages and other antigen presenting cells (APC), plays a central role in inducing IFNγ production. In contrast, Th2 cells secrete IL-4, IL-5, IL-9, IL-10, and IL-13, which are involved in isotype switching of B cells as well as proliferation and differentiation into antibody-secreting plasma cells. In particular, IL-4 and IL-13 are involved in the isotype switch from immunoglobulin (Ig)M to immunoglobulin (Ig)E, the antibody responsible for classical allergic disease. IL-4 and IL-10 are also regulatory cytokines, antagonizing the activities of Th1 cytokines. In humans, Th cells can have a third cytokine secretory pattern. Th0 cells are capable of secreting all of the above mentioned cytokines and are often thought of as precursors that differentiate into the Th1 or Th2 pathway with antigen challenge. Thus it can be said that the nature, intensity, and duration of a specific immune response depends upon the delicate balance between Th1 and Th2 numbers and/or activities. Since it is now appreciated that many other cell types besides Th cells produce IFNγ, IL-4, IL-5, IL-9, and IL-10, many scientists now refer to these as type 1 and type 2 cytokines, supporting cellular and humoral immune responses, respectively.

Impact of Stress on Neuroendocrine and Immune Function

Extensive research efforts have also examined various psychosocial variables in order to predict patterns of adjustment to stressful situations. These variables include optimism, social support, and coping responses, all of which have been found to buffer the psychological, cardiovascular, endocrine, and immune effects of stress and predict overall adjustment to stressful life events. Further, social support and coping strategies can moderate these effects. There is also research indicating that coping style mediates the effects of social support on distress, such that patients who receive social support may use fewer avoidance coping strategies and therefore have lower overall distress. Similarly, in addition to the direct effects optimism has on adjustment to stressful situations, some researchers have found that the benefits of an optimistic disposition are mediated through its effects on both social support and coping responses. These data lend support to the notion that many of these immune imbalances can be reversed with various forms of stress management.

Impact of Stress and Behavior on Cytokine Expression

It has been suggested that acute versus chronic stress may exert distinct effects on host immunity. Acute stress may initially produce an adaptive immune response that is actually protective of the normal host. NK cell activity, as well as certain potentially antiviral cytokines, increases in normal individuals who undergo acute laboratory stressors. Interestingly, chronic stress exposure appears to result in the opposite effect with decreases in NK function and antiviral cytokines. It has also been reported that acute psychological and/or physiological stresses can be associated with adverse clinical outcomes. It is plausible that chronic stress disrupts the ability of some individuals to generate a protective homeostatic immune response when faced with acute stressful events.

Inflammatory Cytokines

When the host is subjected to infection, trauma, or injury, a series of cellular and molecular events occur to defend against potential invading organisms and initiate tissue repair. Collectively, these events are called inflammation and are of central importance in the maintenance of homeostasis. The normal components of inflammation involve the production of a variety of cytokines that function to recruit and activate the cellular components of inflammation and tissue repair which include neutrophils, mast cells, macrophages, and fibroblasts. This cellular cascade can be initiated by local microbial invasion through production of substances such as endotoxin (lipopolysaccharide – LPS) or the host neuroendocrine system with production of molecules such as substance P. Acute inflammation is characterized by the recruitment of polymorphonuclear (PMN) cells, basophils/mast cells, and the production of fibrinogen to aid in hemostasis. If the inflammatory response continues and becomes chronic, the PMN cells are replaced by mononuclear cells such as lymphocytes and monocytes/macrophages.

Stimulation of neurons can cause localized release of substance P which results in tissue edema from peripheral vasodilatation. Substance P can also stimulate tissue mast cells to become activated and release preformed histamine and other chemical mediators of inflammation including cytokines such as IL-4 and GM-CSF. Augmenting the response, histamine can bind to H1 and H2 receptors located on sensory nerve bodies and axons, further stimulating the release of substance P and thus potentiating the inflammatory reaction.

The major inflammatory cytokines are often considered to be TNF-α, IL-1β, and IL-6. This is accompanied by the production of hepatic proteins collectively known as acute phase reactants (APR) that function to limit the activity and spread of invading microorganisms. Studies have shown the increase in serum inflammatory cytokine levels with certain types of acute stress likely due to mononuclear phagocyte activation. Epinephrine has a similar effect on increasing inflammatory cytokine production *in vitro* and is known to be increased *in situ* during acute stressful events. Acute stress also causes the increased production of substance P which appears to promote upregulation of many cytokines including the primary inflammatory TNF-α and IL-1β. The substance P effect may be direct through stimulation of mononuclear cells or indirect through the induction of increased adrenal catecholamine secretion with stress.

Chronic stress is usually associated with diminished inflammatory response and poor wound healing. The inflammatory cytokine-APR networks can be inhibited by corticosteroids. Chronic stress, through the activation of the hypothalamic-pituitary-adrenocortical (HPA) axis, can increase systemic cortisol levels, thus acting as an inhibitor of inflammation. The increase in inhibitory cytokines, especially IL-10, which accompanies chronic stress may also contribute to the anti-inflammatory activity of stress.

Finally, in certain inflammatory diseases, there appears to be a paradoxical response to chronic stress that results in exacerbation of inflammatory pathways. While the mechanisms have not been established, it appears to involve more the systemic imbalance between pro- and anti-inflammatory cytokines rather than the absolute levels of any specific cytokine. Further, therapeutic interventions for stress reduction have demonstrated a salutary clinical effect in subpopulations of patients identified as having high stress levels. Work is in progress to determine whether this correlates with changes in any cytokine levels.

Immunoregulatory Cytokines

Recent work has demonstrated that the examination of only a single component of an immune response can lead to inaccurate conclusions regarding immunosuppression versus dysregulation. The reporting of a Th1/Th2 cytokine network subsequently expanded to include other cytokine-producing cells helps to explain the observations that an inappropriate humoral response to an antigen that requires a cellular response (and vice versa) is as harmful to the host as is generalized immunosuppression. Cytokines can function in an immunoregulatory fashion, both by upregulating and downregulating the overall immune response as well as directing it toward a cellular, humoral, or mixed response. This is in response to antigen-presenting cells directing a host response to be primarily cellular or humoral against an intracellular versus extracellular parasite invasion.

Stress has been reported to have distinct effects on immunoregulatory cytokine production. A fundamental cytokine for expansion of an ongoing immune response is IL-2. Corticosteroids decrease IL-2 production by T cells. Investigations using rodent models have shown that IL-2 levels and production capability are decreased with various forms of stress. The continuance of diminished IL-2 is observed in adrenalectomized animals and indicates the complex nature of this phenomenon. Similar observations have been made for IFNγ. In rodents, IL-2 and IFNγ are produced by Th1 cells while IL-4, IL-5, and IL-10 are produced by Th2 cells. Several studies in animal and humans have shown the decrease in Th1 (type 1) cytokines with a concomitant rise in Th2 (type 2) cytokines in stress models such as chronic restraint, medical student exams, major depressive disorders, and chronic pain.

In contrast, acute stress in normal animals and humans has been reported to cause at least a transient increase in NK cell activity accompanied by increased IFNγ and decreased IL-10 production. This may represent an innate host immune response for protection against intracellular parasites similar to the demargination of granulocytes for host defense against extracellular parasites in the peripheral blood observed with acute stress. Some studies report that the changes in type 1/type 2 cytokine production are different with acute stress superimposed on a chronically stressed host. This could, at least in part, explain the observations of increased susceptibility to and durations of infections, particularly viral, observed in chronically stressed individuals.

Effector Cytokine Networks

Aside from inflammatory and immunoregulatory activities, cytokines also have direct effector functions. These functions include thermoregulation, antiviral, cytotoxic, and cell trafficking. IL-1, IL-6, and TNF-α have all been described as endogenous pyrogens and function to alter the core temperature as a host defense against invading microorganisms. Antipyretic drugs decrease the sensitivity of the hypothalamus to the effects of these cytokines. IFNγ can have a direct antiviral IFN effect. It also activates macrophages to increase antigen processing of viral particles and CTL and NK cells to kill virally infected target cells. CTL make TNF-β (lymphotoxin) in response to specific antigen challenge that can directly kill the target cell. In order for a host immune response to be protective, the elements of the response must reach and remain at the site of the invading microorganism. This occurs primarily with alterations in leukocyte trafficking through the production of chemokines and adhesion molecules. Specific combinations are critical to insure the proper type, sequence, and duration of inflammatory cell influx.

The effects of stress on these effector networks have not been extensively investigated. Body temperature in situations of acute stress has been reported to increase in both humans and animal models. No significant long-term changes have been reported with chronic stress. As IFNγ levels decrease with chronic stress, it is not surprising that increased incidence, duration, and susceptibility to viral infections occur in these affected populations. This may be the result of decreased CTL and NK cell activity seen with chronic stress. Adhesion molecule expression on lymphocytes and target tissue cells as well as chemokine secretion are both inhibited by glucocorticoids and thus could be expected to diminish in stress environments where HPA axis activity is high.

Impact of Cytokines on Stress and Behavior

It has been appreciated for some time that cytokines can have a direct effect on the central nervous system (CNS) and thus psychological components of the host. This can occur directly through effects on certain parts of the brain that control behavior directly (i.e., hippocampus) or indirectly through the neuroendocrine network involving the hypophyseal-pituitary-adrenal axis. The end result is that cytokine production can affect behavior in both positive and negative ways for host homeostasis.

Effects of Cytokines on the Central Nervous System

This area is only recently emerging as a field of study. Much impetus for study has been as a result of the increased use of recombinant cytokines for the treatment of a variety of diseases. The CNS side effects observed with these agents has led to speculation as to the components of the CNS most affected. Although there is evidence to suggest that recombinant cytokines do not directly cross the blood–brain barrier (BBB), the relationships are none-the-less clear. The patterns with the cytokines are remarkably similar: an acute toxicity (flu-like illness) followed by chronic phase (neurasthenia) with continued cytokine administration. The nature and severity of the chronic symptoms appear to be dose related but occur virtually with all regimens given for more than 2 months. More severe symptoms such as psychomotor and cognitive disorders as well as delirium and coma may develop at any point in the therapeutic regimen and appear to be related to underlying CNS dysfunction (aging, history of brain injury, and concomitant CNS disease).

Natural and recombinant IFNs (α, β, and γ), T cell growth factors (IL-2, IL-4, and IL-12), proinflammatory cytokines (IL-1, IL-6, and TNF-α), and hematopoietins (GM-CSF, IL-3, and stem cell factor) have all been utilized to treat patients with a variety of illnesses. Their biochemistry and receptor bindings are largely unique yet all share similar CNS toxicities suggesting mechanisms based upon common albeit as yet undescribed physiologic activities.

Another area of research that suggests a direct effect of cytokines on CNS activity is pain perception in areas of inflammation. Pain is a protective host response generated in answer to tissue injury. It is mediated by afferent sensory nerves in the midst of tissue injury producing enhanced sensitivity to further noxious (hyperesthesia) as well as innocuous (allodynia) stimuli. The peripheral sensory nerve releases substance P into the injured area which in turn can modulate the production and secretion of inflammatory cytokines (such as TNF-α and IL-1) from resident inflammatory cells which promote the pain response. The effect appears to be indirect through production of nerve growth factor, prostaglandins, etc., since no cytokine receptors have been demonstrated on peripheral nerve cells.

Pain control in peripheral as well as CNS tissue involves endogenous opiate receptors. Corticotropin-releasing hormone (CRH) is part of the HPA axis upregulated in stress responses. It also upregulates the secretion of endogenous opiate precursors in both peripheral and central nervous tissues. IL-1 can potentiate the CRH response. Of note, both IL-1 and CRH receptors are present on lymphocytes and are upregulated during inflammation. Binding of either IL-1 or CRH causes these lymphocytes to secrete β-endorphins. Although IL-1 can mediate hyperesthesia in normal tissue, it appears that IL-1, through upregulation of CRH receptors, can mediate analgesia through inducing the local production of β-endorphin by lymphocytes.

Effects of Cytokines on Neuroendocrine Networks

The effect of HPA as well as sympathetic adrenal medullary (SAM) hormones on immune function has been extensively studied. Much work has been done to characterize the effects of various cytokines on neuroendocrine networks to further define the bidirectional communication between neuroendocrine and immune systems. Research to date strongly suggests that the mechanism for this bidirectional crosstalk involve shared ligands and receptors. While stress is known to effect immunity primarily through its effect on neuroendocrine networks, stimulation of the immune system by invading microorganisms produce a cytokine milieu that can have a direct effect on the neuroendocrine network through CNS receptor binding.

There are multiple neuroendocrine hormones produced by components of the immune system including adrenocorticotropic hormone (ACTH), CRH, thyroid-stimulating hormone (TSH), luteinizing hormone (LH), follicle-stimulating hormone (FSH), prolactin (PRL), growth hormone (GH), and somatostatin (SOM). This explains the observation of various immune activations (including cytokine production) noted *in vitro* after incubation of immune cells with these hormones. The exact physiologic role of these immune cell-derived neuropeptides is still not established.

However, when a microorganism invades the host, immune activation leads to cytokine production that finds its way to the BBB via the peripheral circulation. The cytokines do not pass but bind to neuronal cells in the hypothalamus via their specific cytokine receptors. Although there are many different possible cytokine combinations that may bind CNS tissue, common neuroendocrine effects include upregulation of ACTH and downregulation of TSH release. IL-1, IL-2, IL-6, and TNF-α all activate the adrenal axis through the stimulation CRH and/or ACTH directly. IL-1 and TNF-α inhibit the gonadal axis through downregulation of luteinizing hormone-releasing hormone (LHRH). TNF-α and IFNγ can both inhibit the thyroid axis through downregulating thyrotropin-releasing factor (TRF).

Effects of Cytokines on Behavior

Neurocognitive defects with various cytokines have been described in many of the studies using recombinant cytokine therapy. Further, somnolence, psychoses, depression, and personality changes have all been reported during and after cytokine infusions. Yet it is the so-called sickness behavior (malaise, social withdrawal, somnolence, and hyperesthesia) associated with cytokine release after infection, trauma, or even stress that best demonstrates the effects of cytokines on behavior.

Another condition implicating the relationship between cytokines and behavior is depression. Major depressive disorders commonly occur after stressful episodes and are associated with increased HPA hormone levels. Interestingly, cardinal clinical symptoms of depression (somnolence, anorexia, and diminished libido) can all be induced by cytokines. IL-1, TNF-α, and IFNγ are all soporific when administered systemically. Anorexia is a major clinical sign in both depression and infections. TNF-α, IL-1, and IL6 have all been reported to suppress appetite in both animal models and humans receiving recombinant cytokine therapies. Libido requires an intact hypophysial-pituitary activity to stimulate production of sex hormones. These can also be regulated by the inflammatory cytokines noted above. Of note, several studies report increased IL-1 and IL-6 levels with decreased IL-2 and IFNγ in plasmas from depressed patients.

Summary

The relationships between stress, distress, immunity, and health are now generally accepted but still not fully defined. Cytokines play a central role in immune responses and are quite sensitive to the effects of both acute and chronic stress through the neuroendocrine network. This can be both a physiological protective system as well as pathologically imbalanced or suppressed. Many factors influence the balance between cytokine and neuroendocrine networks and impact host defense mechanisms against infection, hypersensitivity diseases, and cancer. The stressors that influence host defense can be psychological, physiological, or a combination. Cytokines can, in turn, influence neuroendocrine networks, CNS function, and even behavior directly. A better understanding of the cytokine–neuroendocrine crosstalk and the influence of various stressors on that crosstalk offers opportunity for future interventional strategies for stress-related illnesses.

Further Reading

Agarwal, S. K. and Marshall, G. D. (1998). Glucocorticoid-induced type 1/type 2 cytokine alterations in humans: a model for stress-related immune dysfunction. *Journal of Interferon and Cytokine Research* **18**, 1059–1068.

Calcagni, E. and Elenkov, I. (2006). Stress system activity, innate and T helper cytokines, and susceptibility to immune-related diseases. *Annals of the New York Academy of Sciences* **1069**, 62–76.

Cohen, H., Ziv, Y., Cardon, M., et al. (2006). Maladaptation to mental stress mitigated by the adaptive immune system via depletion of naturally occurring regulatory CD4+CD25+ cells. *Journal of Neurobiology* **66**, 552–563.

Glaser, R., Kiecolt-Glaser, J. K., Marucha, P. T., et al. Stress-related changes in proinflammatory cytokine production in wounds. *Archives of General Psychiatry* **56**, 450–456.

Hori, T., Katafuchi, T., Take, S., et al. The autonomic nervous system as a communication channel between the brain and the immune system. *Neuroimmunomodulation* **2**, 203–215.

Ippoliti, F., Santis, W. D., Volterrani, A., et al. (2006). Psychological stress affects response to sublingual immunotherapy in asthmatic children allergic to house dust mite. *Pediatric Allergy and Immunology* **17**, 337–345.

Johnson, J. D., Campisi, J., Sharkey, C. M., et al. (2005). Catecholamines mediate stress-induced increases in peripheral and central inflammatory cytokines. *Neuroscience* **135**, 1295–1307.

Kiecolt-Glaser, J. K., Glaser, R., Gravenstein, S., et al. (1996). Chronic stress alters the immune response to influenza virus vaccine in older adults. *Proceedings of the National Academy of Sciences of the United States of America* **93**, 3043–3047.

Marshall, G. D. Jr., Agarwal, S. K., Lloyd, C., et al. (1998). Cytokine dysregulation associated with exam stress in healthy medical students. *Brain, Behavior, and Immunity* **12**, 297–307.

Marsland, A. L., Cohen, S., Rabin, B. S., et al. (2006). Trait positive affect and antibody response to hepatitis B vaccination. *Brain, Behavior, and Immunity* **20**, 261–269.

Marx, C., Ehrhart-Bornstein, M., Scherbaum, W. A., et al. (1998). Regulation of adrenocortical function by cytokines – relevance for immune-endocrine interaction. *Hormone and Metabolic Research* **30**, 416–420.

Miller, A. H. (1998). Neuroendocrine and immune system interactions in stress and depression. *Psychiatric Clinics of North America* **21**, 443–463.

Moynihan, J. A., Kruszewska, B., Brenner, G. J., et al. (1998). Neural, endocrine, and immune system interactions. Relevance for health and disease. *Advances in Experimental Medicine and Biology* **438**, 541–549.

Myint, A. M., Leonard, B. E., Steinbusch, H. W., et al. (2005). Th1, Th2, and Th3 cytokine alterations in major depression. *Journal of Affective Disorders* **88**, 167–173.

Pucak, M. L. and Kaplin, A. I. (2005). Unkind cytokines: current evidence for the potential role of cytokines in immune-mediated depression. *International Review of Psychiatry* **17**, 477–483.

Redwine, L., Mills, P. J., Sada, M., et al. (2004). Differential immune cell chemotaxis responses to acute psychological stress in Alzheimer caregivers compared to non-caregiver controls. *Psychosomatic Medicine* **66**, 770–775.

Viswanathan, K. and Dhabhar, F. S. (2005). Stress-induced enhancement of leukocyte trafficking into sites of surgery or immune activation. *Proceedings of the National Academy of Sciences of the United States of America* **102**, 5808–5813.

Viveros-Paredes, J. M., Puebla-Perez, A. M., Gutierrez-Coronado, O., et al. (2006). Dysregulation of the Th1/Th2 cytokine profile is associated with immunosuppression induced by hypothalamic-pituitary-adrenal axis activation in mice. *International Immunopharmacology* **6**, 774–781.

Wilson, C. J., Finch, C. E. and Cohen, H. J. (2002). Cytokines and cognition – the case for a head-to-toe inflammatory paradigm. *Journal of the American Geriatrics Society* **50**, 2041–2056.

Yang, E. V. and Glaser, R. (2002). Stress-associated immunomodulation and its implications for responses to vaccination. *Expert Review of Vaccines* **1**, 453–459.

Cytokines, Stress, and Depression

B E Leonard
University of Maastricht, Maastricht, The Netherlands and National University of Ireland, Galway, Ireland
C Song
University of Prince Edward Island, Charlottetown, PE, Canada

This is a revised version of the article by C Song, Encyclopedia of Stress, First edition, volume 1, pp 633–638, © 2000, Elsevier Inc.

Glossary

Corticotropin-releasing hormone (CRH) — Brain peptide that mediates the neural control of adrenocorticotropic hormone (ACTH) release from the anterior pituitary gland. CRH has also been implicated as a central neurotransmitter involved in anxiety and depression.

Cytokines — These are biologically active peptides that elicit responses from the endocrine, immune, and neurotransmitter systems by acting on specific cytokine receptors situated on the cell membrane. Cytokines have a wide range of actions that include cellular differentiation, growth, stimulation of antibody synthesis, and inflammatory changes. Regarding the psychopathology of depression, **pro-inflammatory cytokines** (e.g., interleukin (IL)-1, IL-6, tumor necrosis factor (TNF)-α, and interferon (IFN)) have been shown to increase in the blood and brain where they contribute to the symptoms of depression (such as anhedonia [loss of feeling of pleasure], anorexia, sleep disturbance, and anxiety). Pro-inflammatory cytokines are also thought to increase neuronal apoptosis that could contribute to neurodegeneration. The rise in the pro-inflammatory cytokines in depression is associated with a reduction in the **anti-inflammatory cytokines** (such as IL-4 and IL-10) that normally counteract the effects of the pro-inflammatory cytokines.

General adaptation syndrome Term used by a founder of psychoendocrinology, Hans Seyle, to describe the long-term effects of stressful stimuli that result in hypertrophy of the endocrine and immune organs. Seyle showed that if the stress persists, this eventually leads to complete exhaustion of the animal and death.

Homeostasis Tendency towards the establishment of a stable internal environment. This is usually achieved by biological mechanisms that are activated by a negative feedback mechanism. Thus the rise in the concentration of a hormone, immune regulator, or neurotransmitter triggers an inhibitory mechanism that slows the further release of active molecule.

Hyper-cortisolemia Presence of an excess of adrenocortical hormones (usually cortisol in humans or corticosterone in nonprimates) frequently found in major depression.

Inflammatory mediators Term used to describe the different types of molecules that accumulate in tissues as part of the inflammatory process. In depression, the rise in pro-inflammatory cytokines triggers a cascade of changes that result in the rise in prostaglandin E2 and nitric oxide. Together with the glucocorticoids and pro-inflammatory cytokines, these inflammatory mediators are thought to contribute to the increase in neuronal apoptosis and possible neurodegenerative changes associated with chronic depression.

Negative feedback mechanism This is the mechanism whereby the increase in, for example, circulating glucocorticoid hormones activates the central glucocorticoid receptors that then inhibit the further release of corticotropin-releasing hormone. This reduces the release of adrenocorticotropic hormone from the anterior pituitary gland thereby reducing the further synthesis and release of glucocorticoids from the adrenal gland.

Neurogenesis Term used to describe the proliferation of new neurons in the brain. Experimental evidence shows that stress inhibits the development of new pyramidal cells in the hippocampus due to the reduction in availability of neurotrophic factors such as brain-derived neurotrophic factor (BDNF). Chronic antidepressant treatment has been shown to reverse the effect of stress on the neurogenesis of cells in the hippocampus.

Introduction

The causal relationship between negative emotions and psychological distress on physical health has been confirmed in recent years by epidemiological studies in which an increase in the prevalence of coronary heart disease, osteoporosis, diabetes, and dementia have been associated with chronic stressful life events. Research has largely focused on changes in neurotransmitter function, as well as the endocrine and immune systems, in explaining the basis of the causal relationship between stress and ill-health as these systems provide the main pathways of communication between the brain and the peripheral organs. The anatomical links between the brain, endocrine system, and peripheral nervous system is illustrated in **Figure 1**.

Psychological Stress and Activation of the Endocrine System

It is well established that, in the face of any threat, either real or perceived, an organism mounts a series of co-ordinated and specific hormonal, autonomic, immune, and behavioral responses that allow it to fight, or escape from, the threat. Normally, the characteristics and intensity of the response to the stress matches that posed by the threat and the duration of the response is normally no longer than is necessary to achieve a successful outcome. If the response to the stress is inadequate or excessive then it could give rise to pathological changes.

The scientific basis of adaptation to stress was suggested by Walter Cannon who, in the early part of the twentieth century, introduced the concept of homeostasis. This involved the initiation of the fight or flight response whereby changes in the sympatho-adrenomedullary system co-ordinated the physiological aspects underlying homeostasis. This concept was developed further by Hans Seyle (1936) who stressed the importance of the hypothalamic-pituitary-adrenocortical (HPA) axis in the stress response. Seyle described the general alarm reaction as an early response to a noxious stimulus that was characterized by a nonspecific activation of the endocrine and the sympatho-medullary system. Continued exposure to the same stressful stimulus was proposed to lead to long-term changes in the endocrine and immune

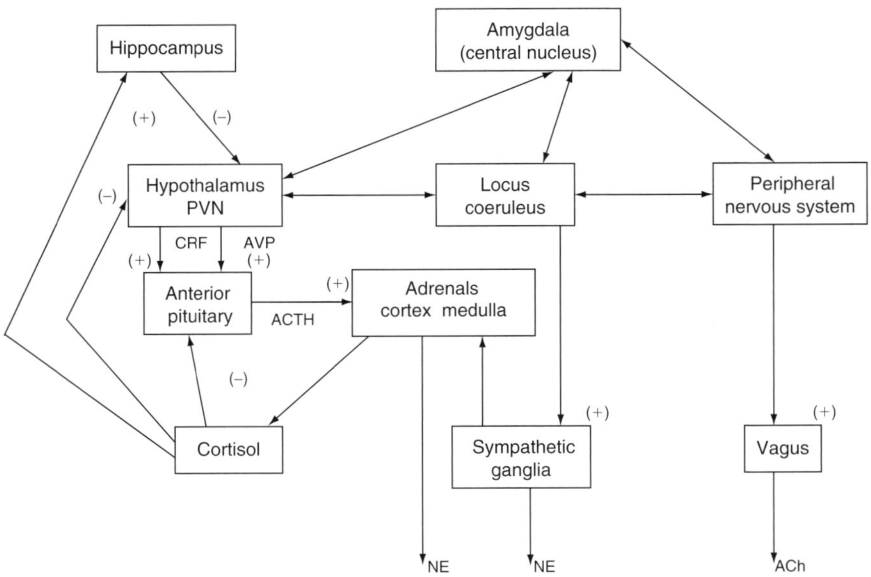

Figure 1 The relationship between stress and neuroendocrine system. (+), positive feedback; (–), negative feedback; ACh, acetylcholine; ACTH, adrenocorticotropic hormone; AVP, arginine vasopressin; NE, norepinephrine; PVN, paraventricular nucleus.

systems. These were characterized by hypertrophy of the pituitary and adrenal glands. Seyle termed this chronic effect of stress the general adaptation syndrome. An organism could recover from the changes once the stressful stimulus was terminated by exhaustion, but death could occur if the stress continued.

The concept of stress being physically and functionally damaging was initially thought to be due to the hypersecretion of glucocorticoids, a concept that was supported by the observation that various diseases of the adrenals and pituitary were associated with psychopathological changes that resolved when the HPA axis was normalized. However, it is now accepted that the stress response is often beneficial in protecting the organism from harmful situations and that adaptation, a learned response, is important in adjusting to future adverse situations. Nevertheless, problems arise when stress becomes repetitive and sustained, and adaptation becomes difficult. This forms the basis of stress-induced ill-health that can result in hypertension, hypercortisolism, abnormal immune function, and ultimately mental ill-health, particularly depression.

Stress and the Role of Corticotropin-Releasing Hormone Receptors

Depression may be interpreted as the result of the sustained hyperactivity of the stress axis that results from the overactivity of the corticotropin-releasing hormone (CRH) pathway, an effect that is correlated with the hyperactivity of the central and peripheral sympatho-adrenal system and the secretion of the glucocorticoids. In addition to the psychological effects of maladaptation to stress, physical damage may also occur as indicated by a loss of bone mass, hippocampal atrophy, and neurodegeneration.

CRH produces its effects by activating CRH-1 and CRH-2 receptors. It is now evident that the fight or flight response involves activation of CRH-1 receptors whereas the much slower response system that promotes recovery and adaption to stress, is activated by urocortin acting on CRH-2 receptors.

The fight or flight response, the fast response, occurs when CRH activates CRH-1 receptors on the paraventricular nucleus (PVN) of the hypothalamus, together with noradrenergic neurons of the locus coeruleus. CRH-1 receptors also occur on the corticotrophs in the anterior pituitary which, on activation, results in the release of the adrenocorticotropic hormone (ACTH).This is followed by the activation of the adrenal cortex by ACTH that leads to the synthesis and release of glucocorticoids.

Epinephrine and norepinephrine are released from the adrenal medulla in response to the stress-induced increase in the activity of the locus coeruleus. The fast response is particularly sensitive to the negative feedback activation of the mineralocorticoid receptors, under conditions of normal stress, or glucocorticoid receptors, under conditions of high stress.

It is now apparent that the slow stress response system is driven by the peptides urocortins 2 and 3, two peptides that are distinct from the CRH family of peptides. The urocortins have been identified as selective, high-affinity ligands for CRH-2 receptors. They are synthesized in the hypothalamus and amygdala and their terminals are located in the hypothalamus and brain stem where the CRH-2 receptors are mainly located. The CRH-2 receptors are thought to facilitate coping and behavioral adaptation. Further, the central administration of these peptides evokes anxiolytic-like responses whereas CRH causes anxiogenic effects in rodents.

The stress response to adverse stimuli is driven not only by CRH but also by arginine vasopressin (AVP), a peptide that is synthesized in a different region of the PVN of the hypothalamus to CRH. Stress increases the proportion of cells that synthesizes AVP. The secretion of CRH is usually accompanied by AVP but whereas AVP usually has a low efficacy for stimulating the release of ACTH compared to CRH, AVP potentiates the effects of CRH thereby enhancing ACTH release. Chronic stress desensitizes the CRH-1 receptors in the pituitary gland but, under these circumstances, the AVP receptors are sensitized thereby sustaining the release of ACTH and the activation of the adrenal cortex.

In addition to its role in stimulating the HPA axis and the central sympathetic system, CRH neurons are activated by different neurotransmitters from several brain regions. Excitatory inputs to the CRH pathways include serotonin, norepinephrine and peptides such as neuropeptide-Y, while the inhibitory inputs include γ-aminobutyric acid (GABA) and the opioids.

Different types of stressful stimuli activate the CRH pathway in different ways. Thus painful stimuli (infections, inflammation, toxic agents, hypoglycemia, and hypo- and hypertension) activate monosynaptic pathways to the CRH neurons. By contrast, stressful, psychological stimuli activate neurons of the limbic-cortical region that subserve nociception, emotional, and cognitive functions. It now appears that these emotional circuits in the central amygdala, frontal cortex, and hippocampus project to a GABAergic network that surrounds the PVN. The effect of this GABAergic system on the function of the hypothalamus varies and can be either disinhibitory to CRH release, when the input is from the amygdala, or inhibitory when the input is from the hippocampus. This pathway functions to process cognitive and emotional aspects of a stressful situation to be assessed.

Depression and the Hypothalamic-Pituitary-Adrenocortical Axis

Some 50 years ago, Board and colleagues (1956) first reported that cortisol was elevated in the plasma of depressed patients but it was Sachar and coworkers (1970) who showed that the hypersecretion of cortisol was accompanied by an altered circadian pattern. They also showed that the frequency, magnitude, and duration of the secretory bursts of cortisol secretion were elevated. More recently, it has been shown that a high morning salivary cortisol concentration is a possible risk factor for depression. The possible link between the hypersecretion of cortisol and the symptoms of depression is also supported by the observation that, therapeutically, glucocorticoids can precipitate depression even in those who were not apparently vulnerable to the condition. Conversely, low doses of glucocorticoids are administered to rodents have rewarding effects, changes that have been attributed to the stimulation of the mesencephalic dopaminergic system. It is possible that this system forms part of the coping strategy to stress whereas chronic, high glucocorticoid concentrations are causally responsible for provoking both anxiety and depression. **Table 1** summarizes the major changes that have been reported in the HPA axis of patients with major depression.

The Chronic Effects of Stress: Depression and Neurotoxicity

Several studies have reported that there is a reduction in the volumes and metabolic activity of the hippocampus, amygdala, and pre-frontal cortex in depressed patients. Such changes could be associated with the cause of depression, or could be a consequence of depression. Whatever the relationship, it is apparent that the shrinkage of the hippocampus could account for the inability of the patient to readily adapt to stressful situations. Whether the decrease in the hippocampal volume is attributable to hypercortisolemia, as is frequently stated, is not certain as patients with posttraumatic stress disorder also have a reduced hippocampal volume but frequently suffer from hypocortisolemia.

The connection between the shrinkage of some of the limbic regions and neuronal atrophy has also been

Table 1 Changes reported to occur in the hypothalamic-pituitary-adrenal axis of patients with major depression

Short-term stress: acute exposure	*Pathophysiological effects: chronic stress*
Energy mobilization	Myopathy, fatigue, steroid-induced diabetes
Control of stress reactions	Hypertension
Increased vascular tone	Osteoporosis
Suppression of growth	Amenorrhea, infertility
Suppression of fertility	Impaired immune function
Anti-inflammatory effects	Affective disorders
	Neurotoxicity

the subject of debate. For example, some investigators have reported no signs of increasing neuronal death in the hippocampus of depressed patients, and while there is evidence that the gray matter and glia numbers are reduced in the prefrontal cortex of depressed patients, there does not appear to be an equivalent loss of neurons. By contrast, animal studies clearly indicate that chronic stress has a profound effect on the structure of hippocampal neurons, changes that are effected through the actions of the glucocorticoids. For example, the dendrites of the pyramidal cells in the CA3 region of the hippocampus retract after an acute stress and become irreversibly damaged if the stress becomes chronic. Other experimental studies have shown that the CA1 neurons of the hippocampus are particularly vulnerable to neurotoxic damage caused by glucocorticoids. Glucocorticoids are known to block glucose uptake by the neurons thereby initiating the excitotoxic cascade of changes caused by the excessive activation of *N*-methyl-D-aspartate (NMDA) receptors. Furthermore, glucocorticoids block the reuptake of glutamate into glia and thereby enhance the concentration of the excitatory amino acid in the vicinity of the neurons. In addition for these changes that could account for glucocorticoid induced neurotoxicity, there is also evidence that stress, and glucocorticoids, suppress neurogenesis. Neurogenesis is enhanced by neurotrophic factors such as brain-derived neurotrophic factor (BDNF) and by the activation of 5-HT1A receptors.

In rodent studies, stress has been shown to increase the turnover of serotonin in the prefrontal cortex, nucleus accumbens, amygdala, and lateral hypothalamus. These effects of stress are mediated through the glucocorticoids, which have major effects on the expression of both the 5-HT1A and 5-HT2A receptors. It is known that the 5-HT1A receptors are under the tonic inhibition by the adrenal steroids, by activation of the type 1 glucocorticoid receptors. Conversely, 5-HT2A receptor expression is increased following chronic stress, or by exogenous glucocorticoid administration, and decreased in response to adrenalectomy. Thus the 5-HT1A and 5-HT2A receptors appear to play an antagonistic role in stress which may help to explain why elevated basal cortisol concentrations are attenuated in depressed patients by the 5-HT1A agonist ipsapirone. These results suggest that the dysfunctional HPA axis in depression results in a glucocorticoid subsensitivity of the postsynaptic 5-HT1A receptors. The link between the serotonergic system, stress, and the effect of stress has been the subject of a recent review.

The results of these experimental studies support the hypothesis that stress and glucocorticoids reduce neurotrophic factor synthesis in the hippocampus, a process that contributes to hippocampal damage. There is evidence that the cellular actions of BDNF and serotonin are interlinked and a reduction in BDNF reduces the density of 5-HT1A receptors and increases that of 5-HT2A receptors in the frontal cortex. This results in increased aggressiveness in BDNF-deficient rodents, a similar situation to that occurring following the drug-induced depletion of serotonin. These changes probably contribute to the reduction in neurogenesis thereby resulting in a reduction in the size of the hippocampus that is reported to occur in patients with chronic depression. Conversely, chronic antidepressant treatment has been shown to increase neurogenesis; this correlates with the attenuation of the symptoms of depression.

It is still uncertain from the results of these studies whether the shrinking of the hippocampus in patients with chronic depression is the cause or the result of stress. If a smaller than normal hippocampus is genetically determined, as seems possible from the results of primate studies, then it seems possible that this could contribute to an increased vulnerability to the effects of stress. For example, this could result in a decreased ability of the patient to cope with stress. It is also possible that while there may not be gross changes in the cytoskeleton, there could be changes in the synaptic plasticity that would not be evident in the imaging studies on patients with depression. Thus, while it is presently uncertain that chronic stress results in increased neuronal apoptosis, partly because of the limited sensitivity of the imaging methods available, experimental studies clearly indicate that persistent high concentrations of glucocorticoids cause atrophy of the hippocampus, prefrontal cortex, amygdala, and other brain regions that are considered to be anatomically associated with depression. The changes in the monoamine neurotransmitters in the brain, which form the basis of the amine hypothesis of depression, are therefore postulated to occur as a consequence of the primary changes in the HPA axis and immune system.

If the vulnerability of the adverse effects of stress is a causative factor in the etiology of depression, it would be anticipated that drugs activating the central glucocorticoid receptors would have antidepressant activity. There is some clinical evidence to support this view. Thus DeBattista and colleagues have reported that the intravenous administration of a high dose of cortisol (15 mg) produces an improvement in the symptoms of depression while in recent controlled studies the glucocorticoid antagonist mifepristone has been shown to have a significant antidepressant effect in patients with psychotic depression. This suggests that the glucocorticoid antagonists block the action of endogenous cortisol on glucocorticoid receptors in afferent pathways. Presumably a very high bolus dose of cortisol acts by desensitizing these receptors. From the results of the experimental and clinical studies, it may be concluded that the overactivity of the CRH system plays a crucial role in the psychophysiology of depression. This could result in long-term structural and functional changes in neurons in the limbic system that may contribute to increased apoptosis. This raises the important question whether the neurodegenerative changes that occur in depression could contribute to the onset of dementia in vulnerable individuals. Hypercortisolemia is a common feature of chronic depression and some types of dementia while qualitatively similar changes have been reported to occur in patients with depression, and also in those suffering from dementia.

Changes in Pro-Inflammatory Cytokines in Depression

The evidence implicating a role for the pro-inflammatory cytokines in the etiology of depression is provided by studies on the changes in the concentrations of interleukin (IL)-1, IL-6, and tumor necrosis factor (TNF)-α in the plasma of depressed patients. Additional evidence is provided by the effects of interferon (IFN)-α on nondepressed patients being treated for hepatitis or malignancy. The results of such studies imply that the pro-inflammatory cytokines are causative factors in the symptoms of major depression. These symptoms include depressed mood, anxiety, cognitive impairment, lack of motivation, loss of libido, sleep disturbance, and deficits in short-term memory. These symptoms usually disappear once the plasma cytokine concentrations normalize. The changes appear to be a consequence of the neurotransmitter and endocrine changes induced by the cytokines rather than the pathological condition for which the treatment has been given. It is perhaps not surprising therefore to find that the symptoms of depression frequently occur in patients who are recovering from a chronic infection, those with multiple sclerosis, allergies, and rheumatoid arthritis. In all these situations, pro-inflammatory cytokines are known to be overexpressed. The initial studies linked depression with an abnormality of the immune system, such as impaired mitogen-stimulated lymphocyte proliferation and reduced natural killer cell activity in untreated depressed patients. These immune changes largely returned to normal once the patient has recovered from the depressive episode.

Some research into the immune changes that occur in depression has concentrated on pro- and anti-inflammatory cytokines, soluble cytokine receptors, and acute-phase proteins. For example, positive acute-phase proteins have been shown to increase, while the negative acute-phase proteins decrease, in depression. These changes are known to be a consequence of the stimulant action of IL-6 on the liver. In addition, Song et al. (1994) showed that complement proteins (C3, C4) and immunoglobulin M are increased in depressed patients. Such changes are evidence that immune activation involves both the inflammatory cytokines and the B cells that are activated by the pro-inflammatory cytokines. Further evidence of immune activation in depressed patients is provided by the studies showing that the plasma concentrations of IL-1, IL-6, IFN, soluble IL-6, and soluble IL-2 receptors, and the soluble IL-1 receptor antagonist, are raised. These changes are correlated with a rise in acute-phase proteins. Effective antidepressant treatments attenuate these immune changes. In addition to the changes in the pro-inflammatory cytokines, there is also evidence of an increased number of T helper, T memory, activated T cells, and B cells that act as a source of plasma cytokines. From these changes, it would appear that in depression there is an imbalance between the inflammatory and anti-inflammatory arms of the immune system, the cytokines from the inflammatory Th-1 pathway (such as IFN-γ) becoming predominant over those of the anti-inflammatory Th-2 pathway (such as IL-10). A recent study has shown that the Th-3 cytokine, transforming growth factor (TGF)-β1, whose function is to re-establish the balance between the Th1 and Th2 pathways, is increased in depressed patients following effective antidepressant treatment. Although TGF is reported to be a regulatory cytokine that maintains the balance between the pro- and anti-inflammatory cytokines, precisely how the changes are established is presently unclear. It is of interest that many clinical and experimental studies show that the chronic administration of antidepressants normalize the immune changes thereby suggesting that antidepressants have an anti-inflammatory action. This suggests that antidepressants may modulate monoaminergic function indirectly as a consequence of their actions on the disturbed immune system and the HPA axis.

Conclusion

Chronic stress, by initiating changes in the HPA axis and the immune system, acts as a trigger for depression. There is experimental and clinical evidence that the rise in the concentrations of pro-inflammatory cytokines and cortisol, which occurs following chronic stress and in depression, contribute to the neurodegenerative changes in the hippocampus, prefrontal cortex, and amygdala. The structural changes in the brain could contribute to the chronicity of depression and be a prelude to dementia. Effective antidepressant treatment attenuates the endocrine and immune changes thereby suggesting that antidepressants have central anti-inflammatory actions that may contribute to their therapeutic efficacy.

Further Reading

Board, F., Persky, H. and Hamburgh, D. A. (1956). Psychological stress and endocrine function. *Psychosomatic Medicine* **18**, 324–333.

Brambilla, F. (2000). Psychoneuroendocrinology: research on the pituitary-adrenal-cortical system. *Psychosomatic Medicine* **30**, 576–607.

Bremner, J. D., Narayan, M., Andersoin, E. R., et al. (2000). Hippocampal volume reduction in major depression. *American Journal of Psychiatry* **157**, 115–118.

Chrousos, G. B. (1998). Stressors, stress and neuroendocrine integration of the adaptive response. *Annals of the New York Academy of Sciences* **750**, 311–335.

Chrousos, G. B. and Gold, P. W. (1998). A healthy body and a healthy mind – and vice versa; the damaging power of uncontrollable stress. *Journal of Clinical Endocrinology and Metabolism* **83**, 1842–1845.

Connor, T. and Leonard, B. E. (1998). Depression, stress and immunological activation: the role of cytokines in depressive disorders. *Life Sciences* **62**, 583–606.

DeBattista, C., Posener, J. A., Kalehzan, B. M. and Schatzberg, A. E. (2000). Acute antidepressant effects of intravenous hydrocortisone and CRH in depressed patients: a doudle-blind, placebo controlled study. *American Journal of Psychiatry* **150**, 656–657.

Duman, R. S., Malberg, J., Nakgawa, S. D., et al. (2000). Neural plasticity in mood disorders. *Biological Psychiatry* **48**, 732–739.

Fuchs, K. C. F. and Gould, E. (2000). Mini-review: *in vivo* neurogenesis in the adult brain: regulation and functional implications. *European Journal of Neuroscience* **12**, 2211–2214.

Leonard, B. E. (2005). The HPA and immune axes in stress: the involvement of the serotonergic system. *European Child and Adolescent Psychiatry* **20**(suppl.3), S302–S306.

Maes, M., Smith, R. and Scharpe, S. (1995). The monocyte T-lymphocyte hypothesis of major depression. *Psychoneuroendocrinology* **20**, 111–116.

McEwan, B. S. (1998). Protective and damaging effects of stress mediators. *New England Journal of Medicine* **338**, 171–179.

Myint, A. -M., Kim, Y. -K., Verkirk, R., et al. (2005). Th1, Th2, and Th3 cytokine alterations in major depression. *Journal of Affective Disorders* **88**, 169–173.

Reul, J. M. H. and Holsboer, F. (2002). CRF receptors 1 and 2 in anxiety and depression. *Current Opinion in Pharmacology* **2**, 23–33.

Sachar, E., Hellman L., Fukushima, D. A. and Gallagher, T. F. (1970). Cortisol production in depressive illness. *Archives of the General and Psychiatrists* **23**, 289–298.

Sapolsky, R. M. (1996). Why stress is bad for your brain. *Science* **273**, 749–750.

Selye, H. (1936). Syndrome produced by diverse noxious agents. *Nature* **138**, 32.

Smith, R. (1991). The macrophage theory of depression. *Medical Hypotheses* **35**, 298–306.

Song, C. and Leonard, B. E. (1995). The effect of olfactory bulbectomy in the rat, alone and in combination with antidepressants and endogenous factors, on immune function. *Human Psychopharmacology* **10**, 7–18.

Song, C., Earley, B. and Leonard, B. E. (1995). Behavioral, neurochemical and immunological response to CRF administration. *Annals of the New York Academy of Sciences* **771**, 55–72.

Watanabe, Y., Sakai, R. R. and McEwan, B. S. (1993). Stress and antidepressant effects on hippocampal and cortical 5HT1A and 5HT2A receptors and transport sites for serotonin. *Brain Research* **615**, 87–94.

Prostaglandins

S Moshonov and U Zor
Weizmann Institute of Science, Rehovot, Israel
Z Naor
Tel Aviv University, Tel Aviv, Israel

This is a revised version of the article by S Moshonov, U Zor and Z Naor, Encyclopedia of Stress, First edition, volume 3, pp 266–272, © 2000, Elsevier Inc.

Glossary

Adrenals — The organs that cap the kidneys. The outer layer, the cortex, synthesizes the corticosteroids, whereas the inner layer, the medulla, synthesizes epinephrine.

Cytokines — Regulatory proteins, such as the interleukins and lymphokines, that are released by cells of the immune system and act as intercellular mediators in the generation of an immune response.

Glucocorticosteroids — Anti-inflammatory steroids; also called glucocorticoids. Cortisol and corticosterone are natural corticosteroids secreted by the adrenal cortex and have strong glucocorticoid activity.

Hypothalamus — A specialized area in the brain that regulates automatic body functions such as

	temperature, sleep, and water balance. It coordinates the endocrine system.
Noradrenergic cells	Nerve cells that release norepinephrine.
Nonsteroidal anti-inflammatory drugs (NSAIDs)	Drugs (e.g. aspirin, indomethacin) that act by inhibition of the cyclo-oxygenases (COX-1 and COX-2) and hence prevent prostaglandin synthesis.
Phospholipids	Lipid (fat) molecules with a nonlipid phosphate head. Phospholipid bilayers are the basic components of cell membranes.
Phosphorylation	The process of adding phosphorus to a dormant enzyme, thereby activating it. Occasionally, phosphorylation deactivates an active enzyme.
Pituitary	The master endocrine gland that lies just beneath and is attached by the pituitary stalk to hypothalamus. The pituitary controls major endocrine systems, growth, body water and electrolytes, lactation and pasturition. The pituitary gland is under central nervous control, which in the case of the anterior pituitary gland is mediated by hypothalamic neurohormones transported from the hypothalamus by the hypohysial portal vessel system.
Prostaglandins (PGs)	A family of hormones whose chemical structure is identical, except for small changes in the pentane ring; these differences provide the distinguishing nomenclature (prostaglandin D, E, F, and I and thromboxane A). The subscript in the name (e.g., PGD_2) refers to the number of unsaturated carbon bonds.
Stressors	Any agent that induces stress in the intact animal or in cell or tissues in culture.

Introduction

Stress, generally classified in terms of emotional or physical, presents a very clear pattern of pathophysiological changes. These are the consequences of stimulation by the many biologically active agents – hormones, neurotransmitters, and cytokines – generated by the nervous, endocrine, and immune systems aroused by stress. To a large extent, the systems are interdependent, and their complex networking is still far from being completely understood. The body maintains its healthy state by continuously readjusting to the changing environment, a process known as homeostasis. Stressors push the homeostatic mechanisms beyond normal limits, and the body enters a new, temporary state called stress.

The participation of the main agents of stress, adrenocorticotropic hormone (ACTH), corticosteroids, and catecholamines (CAs), has been long established. PGs, which are local rather than transported hormones, are not among these main stress hormones that are poured out immediately in response to stress. However, cells from stressed animals produce more PGs than controls do, and PG levels in serum, spinal fluid, and the hypothalamus are elevated during stress. The role of PGs in stress is still largely undefined, but they appear to be involved in at least two stages (**Table 1**): (1) the initiation of the stress response in the brain and (2) the expression of some symptoms of stress.

Characteristics of Prostaglandins

Background

As first reported in the 1930s, PGs were the most powerful, ubiquitous, diversified, and mysterious biological substances yet discovered. Some 30 years later, they were finally unmasked by the Swedish medicinal chemists Süne Bergström and Bengt Samuelsson, who in 1982 were awarded the Nobel Prize in Physiology with the British pharmacologist John Vane. They isolated, identified, and characterized the PG family, establishing unsaturated lipids derived from the cell membrane as an unexpected class of highly sensitive bioactive regulators. Thanks to Vane and colleagues, the mechanism of action of aspirin, the first of the manufactured NSAIDs and one of the most successful drugs ever to be marketed, was now, some 70 years later, finally elucidated, proving to be a specific inhibitor of PG synthesis.

Synthesis of Prostaglandins

Cell membranes, comprising largely phospholipids, are themselves the major source material for PGs and other biologically reactive eicosanoids (20-carbon unsaturated carboxylic acids) such as leukotrienes (LTs).

Phospholipase A_2 Arachidonic acid (AA), an unsaturated fatty acid, is detached from membrane

Table 1 Stages in the response to a stress signal that may be affected by prostaglandins

Stages of stress response	*Prostaglandin link*
Recognition of stress signal	Unclear
Initiation of stress response	Positive
Transmission and modulation of stress response	Possible
Expression of stress symptoms	Positive

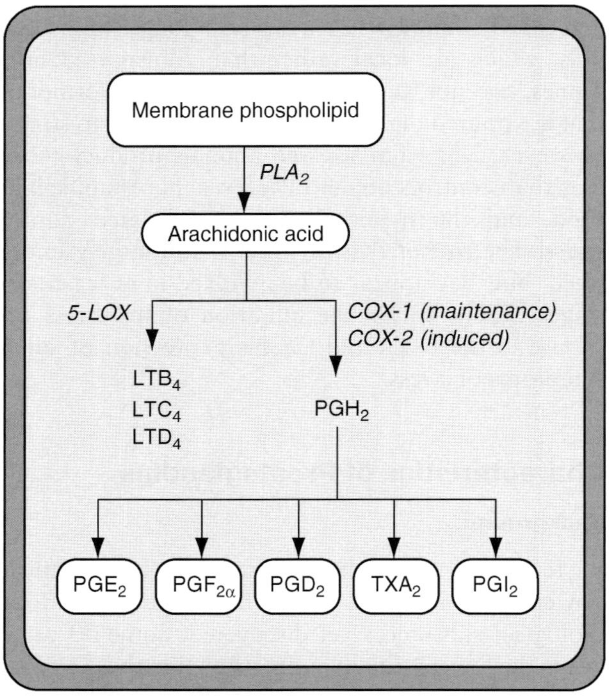

Figure 1 Prostaglandins and their synthesis. COX, cyclo-oxygenase; LOX, lipoxygenase; LT, leukotriene; PG, prostaglandin; PGI_2, prostacyclin; PLA_2, phospholipase A_2; TXA_2, thromboxane A_2.

phospholipids by the enzyme phospholipase A_2 (PLA_2), transformed by cyclo-oxygenases (COXs) into the unstable endoperoxide PGH_2, and then metabolized by the various synthases to PGE_2, $PGF_{2\alpha}$, PGD_2, prostacyclin (PGI_2), or TXA_2 (**Figure 1**). The superfamily of the PLA_2 enzymes consists of 14 groups (I–XIV) and at least 19 members. The low-molecular-mass (~12- to 19-kDa) secretory PLA_2 ($sPLA_2$) proteins are all related evolutionarily, share a common catalytic histidine, and fall into the groups I–III, V, and IX–XIV. A high-molecular-mass (60- to 110-kDa) family of calcium-dependent (requiring micromoles of Ca^{2+} for activation) cytosolic PLA_2 ($cPLA_2$) proteins use a catalytic serine and have a high specificity to AA. Some are activated by Ser505 phosphorylation, use a novel catalytic dyad of Ser228 and Asp549, and are designated group IV (A, B, C or α, β, γ $cPLA_2$). The calcium-independent PLA_2 ($iPLA_2$) (group VI) contains eight ankyrin repeats, has a lipase consensus sequence with an active serine that serves as a nucleophile, plays a role in phospholipids' remodeling and homeostasis via the production of lysophospholipids, and falls into the subgroups (A-1, A-2, and B). Groups VII and VIII PLA_2 are platelet-activating factor (PAF)-acetylhydrolases that cleave PAF to form lyso-PAF and a free acetyl group. mRNA expression of $cPLA_2$ is enhanced by pro-inflammatory cytokines and inhibited by glucocorticoids (GCs).

An alternative and equally important route for AA is metabolism by lipoxygenases (LOXs) to the exceedingly potent LT derivatives (**Figure 1**). Like PGE_2 and $PGF_{2\alpha}$, LTs mediate inflammatory and allergic reactions, but their contribution to stress is largely uncharted. Other branches of the PG–LT family are also not discussed in this article; they appear to be less bioreactive and less is known in general about their contribution to pathophysiological mechanisms.

Cyclo-oxygenases The COX enzyme was first known as PGH_2 synthase (PGHS) because of its ability to catalyze the first two reactions in PG synthesis from arachidonate to PGH_2. COX was first isolated in 1976, and its two isoforms, COX-1 and COX-2, were discovered around 1992. The two isoforms (71 kDa), are encoded by different genes, are structurally similar, are composed of some 600 amino acids, and catalyze the same substrate. The enzymes contain a heme group that binds molecular oxygen. COX-1 is mainly found in the endoplasmic membrane, whereas COX-2 is found also in the nuclear envelope. The active sites of the two enzymes differ, which may explain why the enzymes are inhibited by different drugs. COX-1 is constitutive (i.e., always present in almost all cell types) and is associated with normal physiological PG activities, such as protection of the kidney and the stomach lining from damage and maintenance of vascular homeostasis. However, COX-2 is induced by stimuli, both stressful ones such as inflammatory agents and natural ones such as growth factors; it is also found constitutively in a few organs, one of which is the brain. It is not, however, expressed in nerve cells that synthesize the PGs responsible for stress-induced fever, hyperalgesia, and sleepiness. The origin of this stress-induced COX-2 is the endothelial cells lining the blood vessels in the brain, which are accessed easily by the PG-stimulating blood-borne cytokines. Anti-inflammatory GCs, complexed with their specific receptors, penetrate the nucleus, bind to DNA at the hormone response element sequence, regulate transcription, and preferentially suppress the induction of COX-2.

Nature and Functions of Prostaglandins

Prostaglandins are very potent local hormones that are synthesized rapidly by a wide variety of cells in the body. PGs are released into the extracellular space by specific PG transporters. Once released, PGs bind to their cognate receptors, which belong to the G-protein-coupled receptor (GPCR) superfamily. There are four major receptor subtypes for PGE_2 (EP1, EP2, EP3, and EP4), which are encoded by separate genes. There is a major receptor for $PGF_{2\alpha}$ (FP), for PGD_2 (DP), and for PGI_2 (IP). The various PG receptors differ in their signaling pathways. Sequence homology is found between receptors that share a signaling cascade rather than a ligand. Therefore, the group IP, DP, EP2, and EP4, which act via Gs to elevate cAMP levels, are known as the relaxant receptors because of their common effect on smooth muscle relaxation. The contractile receptors TP, FP, and EP1 mobilize calcium via Gq and induce smooth muscle contraction. PGs, therefore, act in an autocrine/paracrine manner via cognate GPCRs. Within a short time, usually less than 30 min and in the case of thromboxane A_2 (TXA_2) a mere 30 s, PGs are inactivated (90%) to oxidized metabolites when passing through the lungs; very little PG is normally found in the circulation.

Pathological functions of prostaglandins and connections with stress PGs almost always act in the vicinity of their synthesis. The blood-borne, proinflammatory cytokines interleukin (IL)-1, IL-6, and tumor necrosis factor (TNF)-α are released from leukocytes in the blood and macrophages in tissues and are among the agents that locally trigger PG synthesis.

- Inflammation. Traumatic, inflammatory, immune, or other foreign stimuli trigger the activation and recruitment of PGs and LTs. They are part of the inflammatory reaction, promoting leukocyte infiltration, edema, and local vasodilation. Stress generates the same arachidonic AA metabolites and cytokines as inflammation.
- Fever. The elevation of body temperature, but not the maintenance of core temperature, is controlled by PGE_2 in the preoptic area of the hypothalamus. Stress-induced fever is reduced by the prior administration of aspirin-like drugs, such as indomethacin. The stimulation of PGE_2 synthesis in the endothelial cells of hypothalamic blood vessels by stressors such as lipopolysaccharide (LPS), which mimic the symptoms and the stress of bacterial infection in experimental animals, elevates body temperature. Fever also accompanies the stress of surgery (trauma), pain, and cage switching in rats, restraint in pigs, and open field (but not the stress of restraint) in rats or pigs being transported or frustrated by a lack of reward after exhibiting reward-training behavior.
- Hyperalgesia. Heightened sensitivity to pain, or hyperalgesia, is another stress symptom related to PGs. Pain is processed along the spinothalamic tract, reaching the thalamus, limbic system, and frontal cortex before descending through moderating pain-inhibitory nerve pathways. Stress-induced COX-2 is most evident in the spinal cord. Animal models of inflammatory stress and pain, such as carrageenin injected into rat foot pads, show that PGs are generated locally at the sensory nerve endings and in the spinal cord and cause hyperalgesia. COX-2 inhibitors (such as NS398 and DuP 697) and mixed COX-1 and COX-2 inhibitors (such as aspirin and indomethacin), applied directly to the spinal fluid, are analgesic.
- Dysmenorrhea. Dysmenorrhea is a condition with painful menstrual periods with uterine hypercontractility. Increased levels of PGE_2 and $PGF_{2\alpha}$ were found in the menstrual fluid of women with dysmenorrhea, and COX enzyme inhibitors alleviate the pain.
- Endometriosis. Endometriosis occurs when endometrial tissue is found in extrauterine sites; it is associated with pelvic pain and infertility. The increased production of PGE_2 and $PGF_{2\alpha}$ and overexpression of COX-2 are thought to be associated with endometriosis. Estrogen and angiogenic factors, such as vascular endothelial growth factor (VEGF), may be involved in the proliferative responses induced by the PGs in endometriosis.
- Cancer. Various studies have indicated a role for the COX enzymes, PGs, and PG receptors in the pathology of cancers. The overexpression of the COX enzymes and PG receptors and the increased production of PG were found in various cancers. The studies suggested the use of COX enzyme inhibitors in treating some cancers. Because COX-1 is regarded as a constitutive enzyme, whereas COX-2 is the regulated enzyme, attention has been paid to the development of selective COX-2 inhibitors.

Some physiological functions of prostaglandins with connections to stress The various PGs have diverse and frequently opposing actions (**Table 2**). PGs used in nonpathological functions are synthesized mainly by the constitutive (maintenance) enzyme COX-1.

- Blood pressure. PGE_2 and prostacyclin (PGI_2) are vasodilators and have a role in normal blood pressure control. However, TXA_2 is a strong vasoconstrictor. Blood pressure rises in stress and is not affected by PG inhibitors.
- Gastric ulcers. In the gastrointestinal system, PGE_2 and PGI_2 protect the stomach lining by inhibiting gastric acid secretion and promoting the healing of ulcers. Prolonged use of aspirin or other NSAIDs to inhibit PG synthesis. Gastric ulcers are enhanced.
- Preterm birth. The presence of PGE_2 and $PGF_{2\alpha}$, both of which contract the pregnant uterus and are produced by uterine and fetal tissue, is essential for the survival of the fetus. During maternal or fetal stress, these PGs are induced and can lead to preterm birth.

Table 2 Diversity of physiological and pathological effects of the prostaglandins[a]

	PGD_2	PGE_2	$PGF_{2\alpha}$	PGI_2	TXA_2
Blood pressure	Down	Down	No change	Down	Up
Airway	Constrict	Dilate	Constrict	Dilate	Constrict
Uterus (nonpregnant)		Relax	Contract		
Uterus (pregnant)		Contract	Contract		
Kidney (GFR)	Increase	No change		No change	Reduce
Stomach secretions		Inhibit	Stimulate	Inhibit	
Gut motility		Increase	Increase	Increase	Increase
Platelet aggregation			Inhibit		Stimulate
Sleep	Induce				
Fever		Induce			
Pain		Lowers threshold		Lowers threshold	

[a]Chart is not comprehensive.

• Sleep. A central function of PGD_2 is thought to be sleep induction. Its metabolic enzyme PGD_2 synthase is located in the cerebrospinal fluid and the meninges and choroid plexus, nonneuronal cells lining the whole central nervous system (CNS). Sleepiness is a stress response, and PGD_2 could be involved in this process.

Stimulation of Prostaglandin Synthesis in Stress

Most stressors stimulate PG synthesis. Increased plasma (or medium) PGE_2 was induced by heat, pain, trauma (bone fracture), exercise, LPS, restraint, water immersion, and cage switching. A fall in PGE_2, however, was associated with cold stress in rats and captivity in frogs. In these captive frogs, $PGF_{2\alpha}$ increased, as it also did in individuals subjected to the stress of surgery, students taking examinations, and cells that were heat-stressed. PGI_2 was also increased by examination and surgery stresses, and it was removed from the aorta of immobilized rats.

In the brain of stressed animals, IL-1-stimulated PGE_2 releases the corticotropin releasing hormone (CRH) in the hypothalamus, thus activating the hypothalamic-pituitary-adrenal (HPA) axis. Most studies report that PGE_2 is synthesized by the cytokines in the brain; $PGF_{2\alpha}$ and PGD_2 are also mentioned in such studies. PGs induced by IL-1, IL-6, and TNF-α in the preoptic area also bring about fever and cause hyperalgesia via the spinal cord (and at sensory nerve endings), whereas PGD_2 in the cerebrospinal fluid and meninges induces sleep. The sources of these PGs are not necessarily neuronal but, rather, originate from the blood vessels, microglia, or other cells lining the brain.

Assay for Prostaglandins in Stress

Types of stress and measurement of prostaglandins For pharmacological purposes, there is no gross difference between emotional and physical stress. Cell systems galvanized by the body to express and to cope with the stress of, for example, bereavement (emotional or psychological) are ultimately the same ones used in the stress caused by an illness (internal physical) or a supreme athletic effort (external physical). An element of psychological stress generally accompanies a physical stress.

Experimental models of stress have been devised to mimic human stress-provoking situations, in which animals, or cells or tissues in culture, are subjected to one of a number of unpleasant procedures. In these models, stress behavior, in the presence and in the absence of drugs that modify PG synthesis, is observed and the biochemical changes are monitored. Alternatively, tissue samples are assayed for PGs, PLA_2, or COX-2 before and after provoking stress. PGs are commonly assayed using radioimmunoassay techniques, and enzymes are assayed by measuring their activity on labeled substrates or measuring their mRNA levels. Increases in enzyme activity (PLA_2 and COX) and a rise in concentration of a specific PG have been consistently reported in many different stress states.

Inhibitors of prostaglandins Prostaglandin synthesis is inhibited by two groups of anti-inflammatory agents: NSAIDs and GCs (the very same hormones elicited by stress). NSAIDs interfere only with COX activity; the prime example is aspirin, although indomethacin is routinely used in experimental systems. These drugs inhibit COX-1 and COX-2 to varying degrees. COX-2-selective inhibitors (COXibs) such as Celecoxib (Celebrex) and Rofecoxib (Vioxx), developed in the 1990s, are relatively large inhibitors that penetrate the active site of COX-2 but not that of COX-1. They offered much promise when they first appeared on the market, but were found to be associated with a potential risk of myocardial infarction and sudden cardiac death. More recently, attention has been given to the pharmacology of the PG receptors. Efforts are being made to develop receptor-specific antagonists that will inhibit the biological action of the PG rather than their synthesis. GCs, such as dexamethasone, depress the whole AA metabolite network by partial inhibition of PLA_2 synthesis and control stress-induced PGs, in particular by preventing cells from inducing COX-2. The very strong anti-inflammatory action of GCs is due to their wide-ranging anti-inflammatory base. The GC receptor complex interacts directly with and regulates the gene transcription of many inflammatory enzymes and proteins, including COX-2. Inhibitors of PG have been widely employed in the stress models to determine the contribution of PGs to the stress symptoms. This use of PG inhibitors as indirect proof has its limitations because the NSAIDs that can distinguish between the various PGs have not yet been developed and GCs suppress a whole spectrum of agents provoked by stress.

Prostaglandins in the Hypothalamic-Pituitary-Adrenal Axis

Stress Hormone Flow

The perception of distress is instantly transmitted via one or more neural circuits, each with its own neurotransmitter system, to the median eminence (ME) in the hypothalamus. The production of CRH, the major stress hormone released by the hypothalamus, and arginine vasopressin (AVP) is intensified immediately and stimulates the anterior pituitary to release ACTH into the circulation. The adrenal cortex is stimulated by ACTH to produce cortisol and corticosterone, powerful GCs that, by suppressing the production of pro-stress agents, including PGs, keep the sharp stress response from running fatally out of control (**Figure 2**).

The sympathetic nervous system, also activated in stress, releases CAs into the circulation – norepinephrine (NE) and epinephrine (EPI) – setting the body in the stress-alert mode for flight or fight. CAs stimulate PG synthesis in many tissues, including the brain.

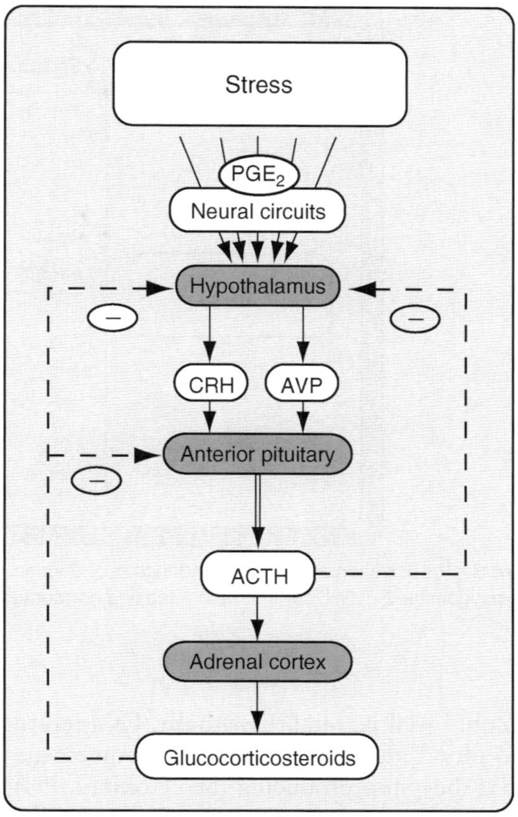

Figure 2 Activation of the hypothalamic-pituitary-adrenal (HPA) axis by stress. Release of adrenocorticotropic hormone (ACTH) is under the negative control (–) of the corticosteroids it induces. Prostaglandin E_2 (PGE_2) stimulates the release of corticotropin releasing hormone (CRH) or arginine vasopressin (AVP) from the hypothalamus and mediates the noradrenergic activation of the HPA axis.

Prostaglandins in the Initiation of Stress Response

Prostaglandin activity has been located in the HPA axis, prior to CRH release. The stress-related PG presence has not been confirmed at other points along the axis. One of the CRH-stimulating neural circuits is noradrenergic. These neurons originate in and/or project to the paraventricular nucleus (PVN) of the hypothalamus and are stimulated by IL-1- and IL-6-induced PGE_2. The rat hypothalamus can synthesize PGE_2, $PGF_{2\alpha}$, PGI_2, and TXA_2, but, at least *in vitro*, only PGE_2 is produced in response to IL-1 and IL-6, although PGD_2, $PGF_{2\alpha}$, and TXA_2 also induce CRH release. The noradrenergic circuit that stimulates the HPA axis can stimulate PG synthesis and is inhibited by indomethacin. PGs also seem to be able to directly induce CRH or AVP release. Thus, PGs may activate the HPA axis through the direct stimulation of CRH or AVP neurons or via noradrenergic neurons in the PVN (**Figure 3**).

Stress and Antistress: Prostaglandins versus Glucocorticosteroids

The stress-induced production of pathological PGs, together with anti-stress GCs, raises the question of their mutual operation during stress. The GC surge elicited by stress effects an inbuilt antistress facet to limit some aspects of the stress response itself. In the absence of GCs, stress responses – high blood pressure, increased heart rate, and fever – are unbridled

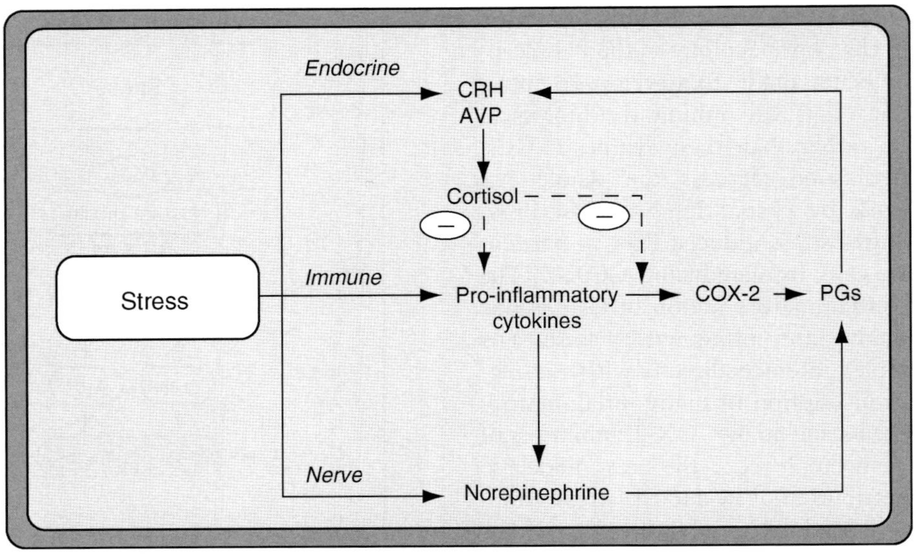

Figure 3 Participation and interdependence of endocrine, immune, and nervous systems in stress. AVP, arginine vasopressin; COX-2, cyclo-oxygenase-2; CRH, corticotropin releasing hormone; PGs, prostaglandins.

and could well be fatal. Essentially, GCs return activated blood and other cells to their quiescent state so that they stop producing the cytokines, PGs, and other inflammatory agents that constitute the host defense mechanism.

Under normal physiological conditions, COX-2 is regulated, among others, by endogenous GCs. Whether the GC surge during stress – a pathophysiological state – affects concomitant PG synthesis has been examined using the rather crude technique of adrenalectomy (ADX) and, more recently, with GC-receptor antagonists such as RU486 (mifepristone). GCs do indeed moderate stress-induced PG production because PG synthesis is elevated in the absence of viable GCs and is reduced again by exogenous dexamethasone, but not by EPI, which is also lacking after ADX.

In the brain, suppression by GCs of PGE_2 along the HPA axis presents an interesting negative feedback response because at least one of the noradrenergic neural circuits leading to ACTH release is mediated via PGE_2. This PGE_2 is stimulated by circulating IL-1, and pro-inflammatory cytokines released into the plasma are also suppressed by GCs. Thus, GCs prevent their own stimulation. The inhibition of IL-1- and PGE_2-induced GCs by GCs could be part of a mechanism for the negative feedback between ACTH and GCs.

In general, and left to themselves, COX-2-stimulated PGs are injurious (they support inflammation allergy). The repression of COX-2 puts GCs into their familiar role of damage control by holding the body's stress response in check and trying to restore homeostasis.

See Also the Following Articles

Congenital Adrenal Hyperplasia (CAH); Corticosteroid-Binding Blobulin (Transcortin); Corticosteroids and Stress; Glucocorticoids – Adverse Effects on the Nervous System.

Further Reading

Bernadini, R., Chiarenza, A., Calogero, A. E., et al. (1989). Arachidonic acid metabolites modulate rat hypothalamic corticotropin-releasing hormone secretion. *Neuroendocrinology* **50**, 708–715.

Brody, T. M., Larner, J. and Minneman, K. P. (1998). *Human pharmacology: molecular to clinical* (3rd edn.). St. Louis, MO: Mosby-Year Book.

Bugajski, J., Olowska, A., Gadek-Michalska, A., et al. (1996). Effect of indomethacin on the CRH- and VP-induced pituitary-adrenocortical response during social stress. *Life Sciences* **58**, 67–72.

Cowell, A. M. and Buckingham, J. C. (1989). Eicosanoids and the hypothalamic-pituitary axis. *Prostaglandins, Leukotrienes and Essential Fatty Acids* **36**, 235–250.

Elmquist, J. K., Scammell, T. E. and Saper, C. B. (1997). Mechanisms of CNS response to systemic immune challenge: the febrile response. *Trends in Neuroscience* **20**, 565–570.

Gether, U. (2000). Uncovering molecular mechanisms involved in activation of G protein-coupled receptors. *Endocrine Review* **21**, 90–113.

Gilman, A. G., Rall, T. W., Nies, A. S. and Taylor, P. (1990). *The pharmacological basis of therapeutics* (8th edn.). New York: Pergamon Press.

Goppelt-Struebe, M. (1997). Molecular mechanisms involved in the regulation of prostaglandin biosynthesis by glucocorticoids. *Biochemical Pharmacology* **53**, 1389–1395.

Graham, D. J., Campen, D., Hui, R., et al. (2005). Risk of acute myocardial infarction and sudden cardiac death in patients treated with cyclooxygenase 2 selective and non-selective non-steroidal anti-inflammtory drugs: nested case-control study. *Lancet* **365**, 475–481.

Hata, A. N. and Breyer, R. M. (2004). Pharmacology and signaling of prostaglandin receptors: multiple roles in inflammation and immune modulation. *Pharmacology and Therapeutics* **103**, 147–166.

Jabbour, H. N. and Sales, K. J. (2004). Prostaglandin receptor signalling and function in human endometrial pathology. *Trends in Endocrinology and Metabolism* **15**, 398–404.

Morimoto, A., Watanabe, T., Morimoto, K., et al. (1991). Possible involvement of prostaglandins in psychological stress-induced responses in rats. *Journal of Physiology* (London) **443**, 421–429.

Narumiya, S., Sugimoto, Y. and Ushikubi, F. (1999). Prostanoid receptors: structures, properties, and functions. *Physiological Reviews* **79**, 1193–1226.

Nasushita, R., Watanobe, H. and Takebe, K. (1997). A comparative study of adrenocorticotropin-releasing activity of prostaglandins E1, E2, F2 alpha and D2 in the rat. *Prostaglandins, Leukotrienes and Essential Fatty Acids* **56**, 165–168.

Oates, J. (1982). The 1982 Nobel Prize in physiology or medicine. *Science* **218**, 765–768.

Rivier, C. (1995). Influence of immune signals on the hypothalamic-pituitary axis of the rodent. *Frontiers in Neuroendocrinology* **16**, 151–182.

Vane, J. R., Bakhle, Y. S. and Botting, R. M. (1998). Cyclooxygenases 1 and 2. *Annual Review of Pharmacology and Toxicology* **38**, 97–120.

Watanabe, T., Morimoto, A., Morimoto, K., et al. (1991). ACTH release induced in rats by norepinephrine is mediated by prostaglandin E2. *Journal of Physiology* (London) **443**, 431–439.

Watanobe, H., Sasaki, S. and Takebe, K. (1995). Role of prostaglandins E1, E2 and F2 alpha in the brain in interleukin 1 beta-induced adrenocorticotropin secretion in the rat. *Cytokine* **7**, 710–720.

Zor, U. (1994). *Lipid mediators in health and disease.* London: Freund.

Infection

H Friedman and S H Pross
University of South Florida College of Medicine, Tampa, FL, USA

This is a revised version of the article by H Friedman and S Specter, Encyclopedia of Stress, First edition, volume 2, pp 570–580, © 2000, Elsevier Inc.

Glossary

Adrenocorticotropic hormone (ACTH)	A secreted serum factor from the adrenal glands that is considered a stress hormone.
Cytotines	Soluble proteins secreted by one type of cell that interacts and activates immune cells.
Legionella pneumophila	An opportunistic bacterium that causes Legionnaire's disease and primarily infects macrophages, a class of immune cells responsible for host resistance to infectious diseases.
Lentiviruses	A retrovirus, such as human immunodeficiency virus, that primarily infects immune cells and can induce acquired immunodeficiency syndrome.
Opportunistic infections	Infections caused by otherwise lowly pathogenic microbes in individuals who have some immunodeficiency.
Respiratory viruses	Small microorganisms that preferentially infect the cells of the respiratory system.

Introduction

Stress is a major factor in the progression of infectious diseases in humans as well as in experimental and domestic animals. In this regard, it is now known that the central nervous system (CNS), the endocrine system, and the immune system are complex systems that interact with one another. In particular, the brain and CNS exert a profound effect on the immune system, including mechanisms necessary for resistance to microbial infection. Stress dysregulates the immune response by affecting the interplay of these systems. New knowledge developed during the last few decades through experimental and clinical studies provide evidence that many immune alterations are due to stressful events that provoke health changes. Stressors, including specific stressful events, can stimulate the activities of the hypothalamic-pituitary-adrenal (HPA) axis as well as the sympathetic nervous system to enhance an individual's ability to adapt physiologically in response to a threat (**Figure 1**). Furthermore, psychological stress ensues when events or environmental demands exceed an individual's perceived ability to cope. Stress can increase susceptibility to infectious agents, influence the severity of infectious diseases, diminish an immune response to a vaccine, reactivate a latent herpesvirus, and in general depress resistance to opportunistic infectious organisms that otherwise should not cause overt disease. Moreover, stressful events and the stress they evoke also may substantially increase the production of pro-inflammatory cytokines associated with a wide range of diseases, especially chronic immune diseases.

Not only the CNS is complex; there is now much new knowledge about the complexity of the immune system, which consists of both cellular and humoral elements. Many immune responses are mediated by soluble factors such as cytokines produced by lymphoid cells and by factors important for control of the CNS, including steroids and various neuropeptides and neurohormones produced by neuronal cells (**Figure 1**). Important mechanisms whereby stress influences susceptibility or the more rapid progression of infectious diseases are becoming clearer because of new experimental and clinical studies by investigators worldwide. Specifically, the current explosion of new knowledge concerning the nature and mechanism of the immune response system has focused attention on the important role of various lymphoid cells for resistance versus susceptibility to microbes, especially intracellular pathogens such as opportunistic bacteria, viruses, fungi, and even parasites. It is now known that the brain and CNS in general have profound effects on immunity. The interaction between the brain and immune system entails a complex series of activities involving responses of many cells to multiple stimuli.

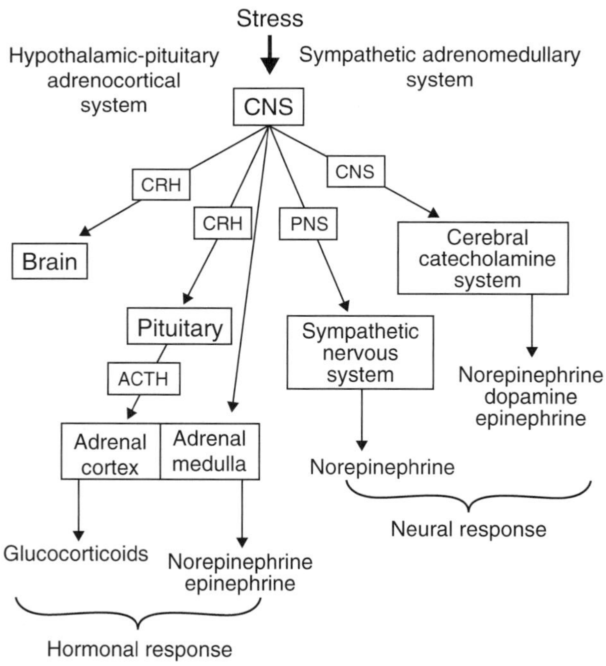

Figure 1 Arrangement of the hypothalamic-pituitary-adrenocortical and sympathetic adrenomedullary systems. The central noradrenergic system is activated in parallel with the peripheral sympathetic nervous system, and it is the central nervous system counterpart. The cerebral catecholamine system (i.e., dopamine and epinephrine) is activated under stress. ACTH, adrenocorticotropic hormone; CNS, central nervous system; CRH, corticotropin releasing hormone; PNS, peripheral nervous system.

Central Nervous–Immune–Endocrine System Interactions

The modulation of the immune response by the CNS is mediated by a complex network of bidirectional interactions between the nervous, endocrine, and immune systems. The HPA axis and autonomic nervous systems provide two key pathways for immune system dysregulation. For example, stress may activate the sympathetic adrenomedullary (SAM), as well as the HPA axis, and thereby result in the release of pituitary and adrenal hormones, including catecholamines (epinephrine and norepinephrine), ACTH, cortisol, growth hormone, and prolactin, which are influenced by stressful events, including negative emotions. Each of these soluble factors results in quantitative and qualitative changes in immune activity. For example, external factors, including stress, increase cortisol levels, which may induce adverse immunological alterations. Immune cells express receptors for one or more factors associated with the HPA and SAM axes, generally called hormones. Immunomodulation by hormones occurs through two pathways: directly, through binding to a specific cell receptor, or indirectly, by the induction of cytokines such as interferon (IFN-)γ, interleukins (ILs), and pro-inflammatory cytokines such as tumor necrosis factor (TNF-)α. Such cytokines interact with various target cells. Furthermore, the interaction between the CNS and the immune system is bidirectional. For example, immune cell-derived ILs such as IL-1 affect the production of corticotropin releasing hormone (CRH) by the hypothalamus in the brain. An increase in stress hormone levels results in the further dysregulation of immune function. Similarly, lymphocytes produce many hormones such as ACTH, prolactin, and growth hormone.

Resistance to microbes, including bacteria, viruses, and parasites, depends on both innate and adaptive immune responses, consisting of a variety of cell types such as T and B lymphocytes; phagocytic monocytic cells, such as dendritic cells and macrophages; neutrophils; and polymorphonuclear cells. Soluble factors produced mainly by lymphoid cells, including ILs, IFNs, and other cytokines, are essential for host resistance. Immune resistance is based on primary and secondary antibody responses and cell-mediated immunity due to T lymphocytes such as Thl effector and Th2 helper cells, as well as Th3 regulatory cells. Such cells produce the many humoral factors important for immunoregulatory and protective pro-inflammatory activity, especially to intracellular opportunistic microbial pathogens.

Stress Hormones and Infections

As already indicated, many types of signals to the brain (e.g., visual, tactile, and emotional) cause the hypothalamus to release CRH, and, in turn, this stimulates the pituitary gland to release ACTH into the circulation, which then stimulates the adrenal cortex to produce glucocorticoids. ACTH inhibits the response of lymphocytes to antigenic or mitogenic stimulation, depresses cytokine responses by lymphocytes, and suppresses natural killer (NK) cell activity and antibody responses to a variety of antigens, including those associated with microorganisms. It is widely recognized that increased glucocorticoid production is by no means the only response to stress. The levels of several neuropeptides, including vasoactive intestinal peptides, substance P, prolactin, and growth hormones are increased, as are catecholamines such as epinephrine and norepinephrine. Localized increases in catecholamine levels probably account for the suppression of lymphocyte responses to mitogens or antigens. The immune system also returns signals to the CNS to close this circle. As previously stated, immune cells synthesize a number of neuropeptide hormones, including ACTH and β-endorphin. Moreover, cytokines produced by lymphocytes and macrophages have effects that are signals to the brain. Various ILs, including TNF-α, stimulate the hypothalamus, resulting in the induction of fever and release of corticosteroid hormones. Receptors for neuropeptides are present on lymphoid cells (**Table 1**), and neuropeptides derived from neural or immune cells stimulate leukocytes (**Tables 2–3**).

Many studies have shown that increases in stress, especially those resulting in increased levels of stress hormones such as corticosteroids, alter the susceptibility of experimental animals to infectious diseases significantly (**Table 4**). The study of effects of neuroendocrine–immune interactions on microbial pathogenesis and immunity during the course of infectious disease is an important area of interdisciplinary research, and various studies showed that physiological stress and psychiatric illness can compromise immune function and alter susceptibility to infectious agents (**Table 5**). It is widely known that patients with psychiatric disorders, including schizophrenia and even depression, are more likely to have infectious diseases. This may be associated with altered HPA activity or physiological dysfunction related to immunomodulation associated with drugs that affect the brain. Unconventional life styles,

Table 1 Receptors for neuropeptide hormones on cells of the immune system[a]

Hormone	*Receptor site*
ACTH	Rat spleen T and B cells
β-Endorphin	Rat spleen T and B cells
Calcitonin gene-related peptide	Rat spleen T and B cells
CRH	Human PBL
Growth hormone	Rodent spleen, thymus, human PBL
Growth hormone-releasing hormone	Rodent spleen, human PBL
Luteinizing hormone-releasing hormone	Rat thymocytes
Prolactin	Human and mouse T and B cells
Somatostatin	Human PBL
Substance P	Mouse T and B cells
Thyrotropin	Human neutrophils, monocytes, B cells

[a]ACTH, adrenocorticotropic hormone; CRH, corticotropin releasing hormone; PBL, peripheral blood leukocytes.

Table 2 Stimuli for leukocyte-derived peptide hormones[a]

Hormone	*Stimulator*
Arginine vasopressin	Unknown
Corticotropin and endorphin	Newcastle disease virus
	Lymphotrophic viruses
	Bacterial lipopolysaccharide
	CRH
	Arginine vasopressin
	IL-1
Follicle-stimulating hormone	Con A
Growth hormone	Growth hormone-releasing hormone
	Growth hormone
Luteinizing hormone	Luteinizing hormone-releasing hormone
Metenkephalin	Con A
Neuropeptide Y	Unknown
Parathyroid hormone-related protein	Human T-cell lymphotrophic virus
Prolactin	Con A
Somatostatin	Hypersensitivity
Substance P	Unknown
Thyrotropin	Staphylococcal enterotoxin A
	Thyrotropin-releasing hormone
Vasoactive intestinal peptide	Histamine liberators
	Hypersensitivity

[a]Con A, concanavalin A; CRH, corticotropin releasing hormone; IL, interleukin.

Table 3 Modulation of immune responses by neuropeptides[a]

Neuropeptide	*Immune response*
Arginine vasopressin	T-cell helper function Functions for IFN-γ production
Corticotropin	Antibody synthesis IFN-γ production B-lymphocyte stimulation
Endorphins	Antibody synthesis Mitogenesis NK-cell activity
Growth hormone	Cytotoxic T-cell activity Mitogenesis
Growth hormone-releasing hormone	Inhibit NK-cell activity Inhibit chemotactic response
Luteinizing hormone	Cytokine formation
Prolactin	IL-2 receptor production
Somatostatin	Reduces IFN-γ production
Substance P	Stimulate chemotaxis Stimulate proliferation Modulate cytokine levels
Thyrotropin	Antibody synthesis Co-mitogen Co-mitogenic with Con A

[a]Con A, concanavalin A; IFN, interferon; NK, natural killer.

Table 4 Effect of glucocorticoids on microbial immunity[a]

Organism	*Glucocorticoid effect*
Bordetella pertussis	Promotes initial protective effect, then promotes microbial survival
Candida albicans	Exacerbates infection
Escherichia coli	Decreases inflammation but not bacterial clearance
Legionella pneumophila	Exacerbates infection
Listeria monocytogenes	Increases susceptibility, impairs monocyte function
Mycobacterium avium	Impairs macrophage function
Mycobacterium leprae	Alters IFN-γ effects on monocytes
Mycobacterium tuberculosis	Increases cellular infiltration, increases bacterial growth
Neisseria gonorrhoeae	Increases infection rate
Plasmodium berghei	Decreases parasitemia
Pneumocystis carinii	Increases susceptibility
Propionibacterium acnes	Exacerbates infection
Pseudomonas aeruginosa	Increases susceptibility
Staphylococcus aureus	Ameliorates IP route infection
Streptococcus faecalis	Increases resistance
Trichinella spiralis	Decreases nematode clearance, cellular infiltration
Yersinia pestis (Pasteurella pestis)	Increases invasive infection, bacteremia

[a]IFN, interferon; IP, intraperitoneal.

eating disorders, poor hygiene, and other factors associated with severe mental health problems may contribute to altered immune function. In this regard, it is now recognized that the recreational use and abuse of illegal drugs such as marijuana, cocaine, heroin, and other opiates, as well as more widely used legal substances such as alcohol and tobacco, have marked effects on the CNS and the immune system. Individuals who use these drugs frequently are more susceptible to opportunistic microorganisms. The detrimental effects of such abused drugs on immunity in both humans and animals have now been extensively studied. These drugs are known to increase corticosteroid levels in both humans and experimental animals, either at the time of addiction or during withdrawal, and this effect has been related to altered immune resistance to microbial infection. Addiction to a psychoactive substance (as in the stimulation of the HPA axis) induces enhanced adrenal corticosteroid secretion, followed by consequential increases in serum glucocorticoids and the activation of the sympathetic nervous system. These responses result in immune dysregulation and increased susceptibility to microbial infections, especially to opportunistic pathogens.

Numerous early clinical observations reported that individuals often become more susceptible to infections following stressful situations. However, the concept of stress was not defined sharply. A stressor was often defined as any type of external or internal challenge, visual, tactile, or emotional, that disrupts the physiological equilibrium or homeostasis of an individual. For example, a number of studies showed that infection by mycobacteria, which cause tuberculosis, is increased by stress.

Alterations in the susceptibility to other opportunistic bacteria, as well as to viruses and parasites in general, have been studied extensively. Increases in infections due to stress occur not only in human populations but also in farm animals and experimental animals. There is now a large body of biomedical literature showing that stress alters susceptibility to infection. The mechanism of the stress includes effects on humoral function such as the production of glucocorticoids. The effects of stresses on two types of infective diseases, bacterial and viral, are discussed next as examples.

Bacterial Infections and Steroids

Legionella pneumophila, an opportunistic ubiquitous bacterium, is the causative agent of Legionnaire's disease. Although almost all individuals are exposed to *Legionella,* only a small percentage of individuals exposed to these organisms are infected clinically. Indeed, when *Legionella* was first discovered in the outbreak of Legionnaire's disease in Philadelphia in the late 1970s, most of the 2500 conventioneers exposed to this organism from the air conditioning system in the Belleview Stratford Hotel developed

Table 5 Effects of stress on microbial immunity

Pathogen	*Animal species*	*Stressor*	*Effect*
Escherichia coli	Chicken	Cold	Increases resistance
	Chicken	Social	Increases resistance
Hymenolepis nana	Mouse	Predator	Increases reinfection rate
Mycobacterium avium	Mouse	Restraint	Increases susceptibility, impairs macrophage function
Mycobacterium tuberculosis	Rabbit	Tumbling	Increases susceptibility
Plasmodium berghei	Mouse	Electric	Increases survival
Salmonella enteritidis	Chicken	Fasting	Decreases antibody response
Salmonella typhimurium	Mouse	Crowding	Increases susceptibility

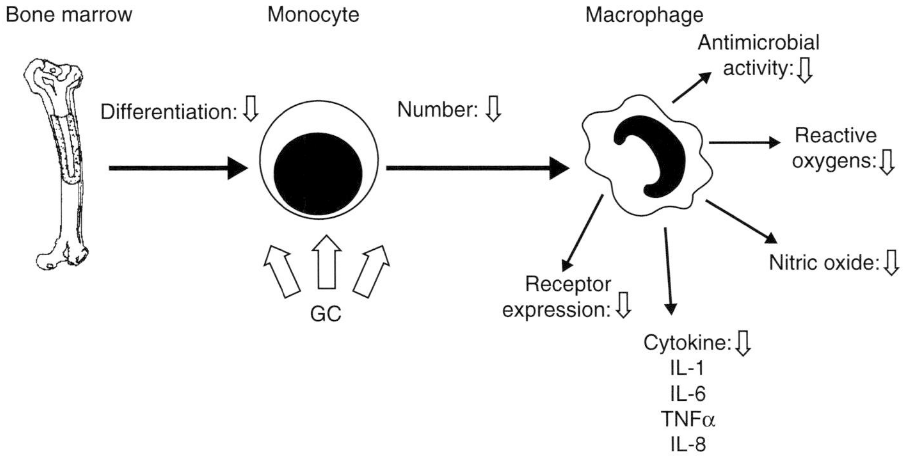

Figure 2 The effect of steroids on macrophages and monocytes. Glucocorticoids have a direct action on the number and function of phagocytic cells, including cytokine production and receptor expression. ⇩, decrease; GC, glucocorticoid; IL, interleukin; TNF, tumor necrosis factor.

significant titers to these bacteria. However, only approximately 200 individuals became clinically ill, and a significant number of these people died. These individuals had certain factors associated with their susceptibility, including increased alcohol consumption, cigarette smoking, (in general) being older, and being more immunocompromised. It is now well recognized that *L. pneumophila* causes clinical infection mainly in immunocompromised individuals, including patients who are treated with immunosuppressive drugs in hospitals for cancer chemotherapy or for organ transplantation.

Increases in susceptibility to infection by *Legionella* associated with steroid use have been studied in detail (**Table 4**). Although steroid therapy for various diseases has had revolutionary therapeutic effects and is widely recognized as constituting a major success for modern medicine, it is often associated with serious side effects; steroids have both beneficial and nonbeneficial features, and these may be inseparable. The anti-inflammatory and immunosuppressive activities of steroids are considered essential for the therapy of certain diseases, including autoimmune diseases, and to prevent organ rejection following transplantation. However, steroids may also result in an increased susceptibility to infections, especially by an opportunistic bacterium such as *L. pneumophila*. Although the spectrum of microbes causing infections in patients during steroid therapy is not completely clear, experimental animal studies showed that steroid treatment is associated with increased infections caused by certain groups of opportunistic bacteria, including *Legionella*. The general consensus concerning the mechanism whereby steroids induce altered susceptibility to bacterial infection is that steroids suppress the immune response system.

The most important host defense mechanism against invading intracellular opportunistic bacteria is phagocytosis by macrophages, followed by intracellular killing and digestion of the microbes. It is now clear that steroids suppress the number and function of macrophages and neutrophils (**Figures 2–3**). For example, experimental studies have shown that peritoneal macrophages from hydrocortisone-treated mice are more susceptible to infection and killing by *L. pneumophila in vitro*. The steroid-involved impairment of antimicrobial activity by macrophages from mice infected with *Legionella* is generally similar to that

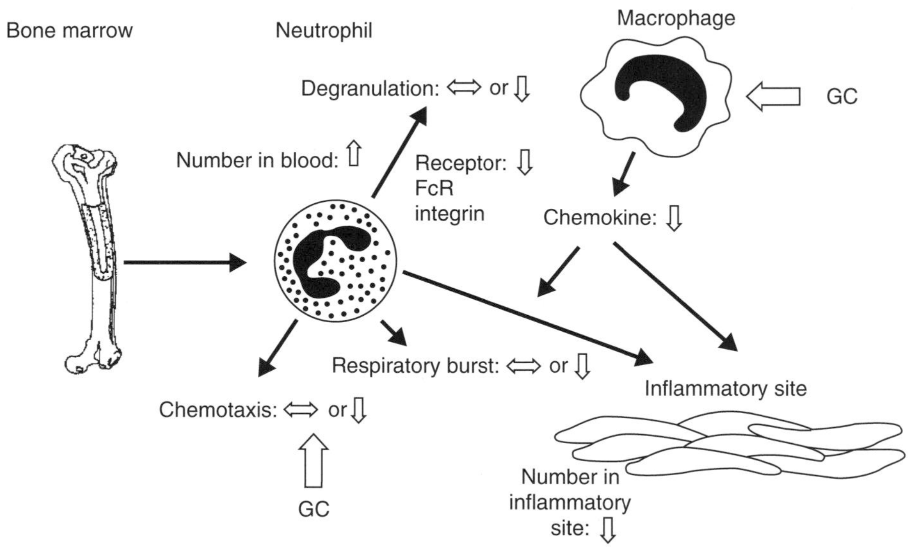

Figure 3 Prevention of neutrophil accumulation at local inflammatory site by steroid treatment. The chemotactic activity of neutrophils from steroid-treated animals or humans was enhanced, inhibited very weakly, or unaffected, except for neutrophils from inflammatory exudates, which showed reduced chemotactic activity. ⇓, decrease; ⇑, increase; ⇔, minimal or no change, FcR, Fc receptor; GC, glucocorticoid.

reported for *Listeria monocytogenes.* For example, *in vivo* treatment of mice with hydrocortisone acetate affects the ability of peritoneal macrophages from the animals to kill *L. pneumophila in vitro,* as well as other microorganisms such as *Listeria monocytogenes, Streptococcus pyogenes, Staphylococcus aureus, Staphylococcus epidermidis, Escherichia coli,* and *Pseudomonas aeruginosa.*

The treatment of macrophages with steroids *in vitro* may affect antimicrobial immunity directly. For example, the ability of macrophages treated with steroids to kill *L. pneumophila* and organisms such as *Staphylococci in vitro* is markedly reduced. The specific mechanisms involved in the steroid impairment of macrophages, however, are unclear. In general, the intracellular killing of bacteria and other microbes by macrophages requires lysosomal migration to and fusion with the microbe-containing phagosome. It is probable that the mechanism of the steroid-induced impairment of antimicrobicidal activity of monocytes or macrophages is associated with the stabilization of lysosomes by steroids, which prevents their fusion with phagosomes. However, the possibility exists that steroids induce the impairment of the antimicrobial activity of macrophages by suppressing the synthesis of one or several specific proteins of the killing system of the phagocytes. Nevertheless, several observations have indicated that macrophages treated with steroids ingest microorganisms at a normal rate and, after phagocytosis, secrete the usual reactive oxygen intermediates and exhibit normal fusion of lysosomes and phagosomes (i.e., the oxidative killing systems). Steroid-treated macrophages react to a cytokine such as IFN and are normally primed to secrete reactive oxygen intermediates on challenge. Thus, there have been reports negating the likelihood there is a direct deleterious effect of steroids on the antimicrobial activity of macrophages.

Virus Infections and Stress

Virus infection can be exacerbated by stress hormones such as cortisone. For example, hydrocortisone-treated mice show an increased susceptibility to challenge with viruses such as influenza virus, Coxsackie virus, or even mouse hepatitis virus. Peritoneal macrophages from cortisone-treated mice are almost 1000 times more susceptible to challenge with the mouse hepatitis virus *in vitro* than are macrophages from untreated mice. Resistant macrophages from normal mice succumb to cytolysis by mouse hepatitis virus when cultured with spleen cells from cortisone-treated mice but not with spleen cells from normal mice, suggesting that a soluble product from lymphoid cells may be involved in increased susceptibility of the macrophages due to steroids.

Various studies have reported the association between naturally occurring stresses and individuals' susceptibility to upper respiratory tract viral infections. Although most of these studies provide some support for the hypothesis that stress is associated with an increased risk of upper respiratory viral infections, it is not yet clear how this occurs. Longitudinal studies performed with large populations of individuals suggest that stress is a significant factor in increasing the susceptibility to viral infection.

A number of studies have been performed testing the possibility that stress is involved in experimentally induced upper respiratory tract viral infections. Psychologically stressed, experimentally infected individuals had significantly higher levels of upper respiratory tract infections, but there were no differences in the incidence of infections or the amount of shed virus in nasal secretions between these and unstressed individuals. Several studies reported that stress precedes the onset of upper respiratory tract viral infection episodes, especially in children; for example, several studies reported a significant increase in minor stresses a few days before the onset of upper respiratory tract infection symptoms. The likelihood exists that the severity of the symptoms of upper respiratory tract infections rather than the incidence of infection may be affected by different types of psychological stress. So far, it is apparent that more clinical studies must be performed before we can fully understand the relationship between stress and upper respiratory tract viral infections in patient populations. In addition, little is known about how the timing of the stressor and viral exposure influences the development of these infections. There is some evidence suggesting that stress occurring after experimental viral exposure may increase susceptibility; however, there are differing published findings, some indicating an increased and some a decreased susceptibility even when stress precedes viral exposure.

Studies have been reported concerning stress and progression of acquired immunodeficiency syndrome (AIDS) in human immunodeficiency virus (HIV)-positive subjects. For example, a study published by investigators from the University of Miami School of Medicine, supported by the National Institute of Mental Health, showed that HIV-positive high-risk subjects had less evidence of progression to clinical AIDS when psychological intervention techniques, such as stress reduction by counseling, music therapy, or exercise, were used. This study supported the view that psychological stress in HIV-positive individuals can result in a more rapid progression to clinical AIDS and that psychological stresses were often related to lack of an effective support system and with the notification of HIV-positive status. Such findings suggested that psychological stress and its intervention may be associated with the progression of chronic life-threatening viral infections, such as HIV.

There are also well-known studies concerning the effects of stress on herpesvirus exacerbation. A landmark study performed at the Ohio State University Medical School reported that medical students taking a routinely scheduled examination had increased psychological stress immediately preceding the examination and that this was associated with decreased immune function and the increased recurrence of herpesvirus titers, indicative of the reactivation of the herpesvirus. The study was particularly well controlled, consisting of medical students who were generally healthy and immunologically mature (i.e., approximately the second decade of life). All the students had normal immune functions, but at the time of the examination they were shown by psychological tests to have a significant stress level and increased serum glucocorticoids. Simultaneously, they showed a decrease in an immune function important in resistance to viral infection, NK cell activity and T-cell levels. Many of the students had an exacerbation of latent herpes shortly after the examination (with its associated stress).

Note that temporal relations often cannot be controlled readily in population studies. Furthermore, little is known about the differential effects of acute (short-term) versus chronic (long-term) or repetitive stressors. The clinical literature suggests that chronic stress may have particularly strong pernicious effects on health. But it is difficult to undertake true experimental studies of stress exposure in human populations because it is difficult to randomly assign subjects to defined stressor conditions. Although challenge viral exposure in experimental studies appears to be relatively controlled, it is often not because of independent variables and because stress is difficult to assess and manipulate. Furthermore, little is known about the biological pathways that may be responsible for the association between stress and increased viral infection in patient populations.

The effect of psychosocial interventions in ameliorating a number of infectious problems in patients with diseases as diverse as cardiovascular disease and cancer is currently being investigated. Many investigators believe that appropriate psychosocial intervention may result in reduced stress and thus reduced viral infections. Nevertheless, most studies to date with patient populations and viral infections suggest only that there is an association between stress and increased susceptibility to infection.

Discussion and Conclusion

It is now widely accepted that stress plays an important role in altering the susceptibility to infectious agents such as bacteria, viruses, and even parasites. Furthermore, stress is also acknowledged to be involved in increasing the susceptibility to the progression of autoimmune diseases and malignancies. Many studies have suggested that the stress hormones, especially cortisone and ACTH, are important in altering the immune mechanisms, especially in the lymphoid cells, which are important in the resistance to opportunistic microorganisms such as intracellular bacteria and viruses.

Various studies showed that a variety of stressors increase the susceptibility of experimental animals to bacterial infections. Some of the most defined studies to date were performed with mycobacteria, organisms that cause tuberculosis in humans and in domestic and experimental animals. Infection by mycobacteria is known to be increased by stress; for example, a number of widely known studies showed that mice that were normally resistant to mycobacterial infection showed increased susceptibility when given certain stressors. This has been related to increases in glucocorticoid levels, which are known to affect lymphoid cell function.

Glucocorticoids produced by the adrenal cortex under the influence of ACTH from the pituitary gland in the brain affect both humoral and cellular immune responses. Mice treated with glucocorticoids often show increased cellular infiltration following infection with mycobacteria and increased growth of the bacteria. Glucocorticoids have been shown to increase the susceptibility of experimental mice to infectious agents such *Listeria monocytogenes* and *Pneumocystis carinii*. However, glucocorticoids promote the survival of *Bordetella pertussis*, the causative agent of whooping cough in humans, although initially this hormone provides some protection against challenge infection. Furthermore, cortisone ameliorates infection by *Staphylococcus aureus* in experimental animals, but has been reported to increase the susceptibility to *Pseudomonas aeruginosa* in humans and animals and also to exacerbate infection by the ubiquitous fungus *Candida albicans*. Thus, there is a marked variability in the effects of corticoids on infection, depending on the organisms involved; the reasons for this remain unknown. For example, various studies showed that infection with *Propionibacterium acnes* is exacerbated by corticosteroids but that infection with *Streptococcus faecalis* is decreased by them. Furthermore, animals infected with *Plasmodium*, the cause of malaria, showed decreased parasitemia due to corticosteroids.

It is clear that corticosteroids decrease the accumulation of neutrophils at a local inflammatory site. Such neutrophil accumulation is important in clearance of or resistance to bacterial infection. It has also been reported that the chemotactic activity of neutrophils from steroid-treated animals or humans can be enhanced, inhibited very weakly, or unaffected; however, most studies showed that neutrophils obtained from inflammatory exudates in steroid-treated mice showed reduced chemotactic activity. Such data indicate that the poor accumulation of neutrophils in inflammatory sites may be mediated by the inhibition of the release of local chemotactic factors rather than a direct effect on neutrophils. This possibility seems likely because steroid treatment does not inhibit neutrophil accumulation induced by the injection of a chemotactic complement component into human skin. It has been demonstrated that the treatment of purified human neutrophils with the synthetic steroid deoxymethasone does not inhibit neutrophil chemotaxis in response to a range of concentrations of known chemoattractants.

There are several mechanisms for gene regulation by the steroid–receptor complex. Glucocorticoid response elements regulate the rate of transcription initiated by promoters of the corresponding glucocorticoid response genes. Another possible regulation mechanism is the interaction with DNA-binding proteins associated with regulatory elements of DNA, such as the glucocorticoid modulatory element protein. Thus, it appears that steroids regulate the transcription of certain genes coding for proteins that augment steroid effects.

The infection of animals with the ubiquitous bacterium *L. pneumophila* is modulated markedly by steroids. Thus, steroid levels are an important factor in the increased susceptibility of organ-transplant patients, who are often immunosuppressed with steroids prior to the transplant and thus may become more susceptible to an opportunistic infection such as *Legionella* in hospitals. Viral infections have also been shown to be exacerbated by stress hormones, including cortisone. It is well known that hydrocortisone-treated mice show an increased susceptibility to challenge with a variety of viruses, including influenza virus, Coxsackie virus, and mouse hepatitis virus. It seems likely that, because stress is often associated with increased corticosteroid levels only, changes in the level of this hormone may be related to the apparent increased susceptibility of individuals to an upper respiratory tract viral infection following a stressful event. Results obtained using animal models show an increased susceptibility to challenge infection with bacteria or viruses, and studies of humans, infected either naturally or experimentally, strongly suggest a relationship between stress-induced immunomodulatory hormones and increased susceptibility to infection.

The complex interrelationship between the nervous and the immune system parallels the association of the susceptibility or resistance to infections by various microorganisms under conditions of stress. This is even more likely because it is known that the immune response is modulated markedly by a wide variety of neuropeptides associated with the CNS, not only corticotropin but also other hormones such as endorphins, prolactin, growth hormone, vasopressin, and somatotrophin. Neuropeptides affect a wide variety of immune responses, including antibody formation, mitogenic responses of lymphocytes, cytotoxicity by T cells, NK cell production and activity, and cytokine production. Thus, neuropeptides, hormones, and their receptors, present not only in the CNS but also on immune cells, are important factors in immunomodulation related to altering the susceptibility to infection by microorganisms, especially intracellular opportunistic bacteria and viruses. However, because of the complexity of both the CNS and the immune system, it is difficult to isolate the various pathways that are important in this altered susceptibility to infection associated with stress. Further studies in numerous laboratories, including those mainly concerned with the neurological system and those concerned with infectious diseases and immunity, will undoubtedly provide a greater understanding of the role of stress in infection.

See Also the Following Articles

Immunity.

Further Reading

Ader, R. and Cohen, N. (1993). Psychoneuroimmunology: conditioning and stress. *Annual Review of Psychology* **44**, 53–71.

Ader, R., Felten, D. and Cohen, N. (1991). *Psychoneuroimmunology* (2nd edn.). San Diego, CA: Academic Press.

Akira, S. and Kishimoto, T. (1992). IL-6 and NFκB in acute phase response and viral infection. *Immunological Reviews* **127**, 26–41.

Baue, A. F. (1989). Neuroendocrine response to severe trauma and sepsis. In: Faist, E., Ninnemann, J. & Green, D. (eds.) *Immune consequences of trauma, shyock and sepsis*, pp. 17. New York: Springer-Verlag.

Bayle, J. E., Guellati, M., Ibos, F., et al. (1991). *Brucella abortus* antigen stimulates the pituitary-adrenal axis through the extra-pituitary B-lymphoid system. *Progress in Neuroendocrinimmunology* **4**, 99–112.

Beisel, W. R. (1975). Metabolic response to infection. *Annual Review of Medicine* **26**, 9–29.

Blalock, I. E. (1992). Production of peptide hormones and neurotransmitters by the immune system. In: Blalock, J. E. (ed.) *Neuroimmunoendocrinology* (2nd edn.). Basel: Karger.

Friedman, H., Klein, T. W. and Friedman, A. L. (1996). *Psychoneuroimmunology, stress and infection.* Boca Raton, FL: CRC Press.

Friedman, H., Klein, T. W. and Specter, S. (1996). *Drugs of abuse, immunity and infections.* Boca Raton, FL: CRC Press.

Friedman, H., Newton, C. and Klein, T. W. (2003). Microbial infection, immunomodulation and drugs of abuse. *Clinical Microbial Reviews* **16**, 209–220.

Glaser, R. and Kiecolt-Glaser, J. K. (2005). Stress-induced immune dysfunction: implications for health. *Nature Reviews Immunology* **5**, 243–252.

Hart, B. L. (1988). Biological basis of the behavior of sick animals. *Neuroscience and Biobehavioral Reviews* **12**, 123–129.

Jefferies, W. M. (1991). Cortisol and immunity. *Medical Hypotheses* **34**, 198–215.

Kass, E. H. and Finland, M. (1958). Corticosteroids and infections. *Advances in Internal Medicine* **9**, 45–61.

Padgett, D. A. and Glaser, R. (2003). How stress influences the immune response. *Trends in Immunology* **24**, 444–453.

Rabin, B. S. (1999). *Stress, immune function, and health: the connection.* New York: Wiley-Liss & Sons.

Schattner, A. and Schaffner, T. (1987). Glucocorticoid-induced impairment of macrophage antimicrobial activity: mechanisms and dependence on the state of activation. *Review of Infectious Diseases* **9**, 5620.

Sheridan, J. F., Dobbs, C., Brown, D., et al. (1994). Psychoneuroimmunology: stress effects on pathogenesis and immunity during infection. *Clinical Microbial Reviews* **7**, 200.

Stone, A. and Bovbjerg, D. (1994). Stress and humoral immunity: a review of human studies. *Advances on Neuroimmunology* **4**, 49.

Stone, E. A. (1975). Stress and catecholamines. In: Friedhoff, A. J. (ed.) *Catecholamines and neuropsychopharmacology*, (vol. 2), p. 31. New York: Plenum Press.

Webster, J. I., Tonelli, L. and Sternberg, E. M. (2002). Neuroendocrine regulation of immunity. *Annual Review of Immunology* **20**, 126–163.

Inflammation

G Z Feuerstein, R R Ruffolo, C Coughlin, J Wang and D Miller
Wyeth Research, Collegeville, PA, USA

Glossary

Apoptosis A process of cell death that results from the activation of specific signaling pathways that lead to the intracellular disruption of mitochondrial integrity, activation of cascade of proteases (e.g., caspases), and cell disintegration while maintaining the cell membrane intact.

Chemokines A family of polypeptides that comprises about 50 members and 20 different receptors. This family of polypeptides is all involved in leukocyte traffic. Their diverse biological actions include interactions with viruses and cell receptors in numerous tissues.

Chemotaxis The orientation and movement of a cell along a specific chemical concentration. Positive chemotaxis denotes movement of the cell toward the high-concentration site of the chemical; negative chemotaxis denotes movement of the cell away from the source of the chemical. Chemotactic properties are prevalent in all forms of leukocytes and in a wide variety of substances released in sites of tissue injury or activated cells.

Complement system The entire functionality of approximately 20 distinct plasma proteins, their receptors, and ancillary/regulatory proteins that are responsible not only for immune cytolysis but also for reactions such as anaphylaxis, phagocytosis, opsonization, and hemolysis. Two major pathways for activation of the complement system are known: the classic pathway in which all components C1–C9 participate in the reaction and the alternative pathway in which only part of the plasma factors participate along with others that are not essential in the classic reaction.

Cytokines Nonantibody peptides and polypeptides that are released by activated cells (e.g., T cells) and transfer signals to other cells. Lymphokines (cytokines produced by lymphocytes) and monokines (cytokines produces by monocytes) are cytokines.

Inflammation A localized protective response elicited by injury or destruction of tissues, which serves to destroy, dilute, or wall off (sequester) both the injurious agent and the injured tissue. It is characterized in the acute form by the classic signs of pain, heat, redness, swelling, and loss of function. Histologically, it involves a complex series of events, including the dilation of the arterioles and capillaries, extravasation of fluids, and migration of plasma proteins and leukocytes into the injured area.

Interleukins (ILs) A generic term for a group of multifunctional cytokines that are produced by a variety of lymphoid and nonlymphoid cells. Originally believed to play a role only in leukocyte biology, ILs are now recognized as the products of diverse nonlymphoid cells that also act on diverse receptors on multiple cells outside the lymphoid system. Over 20 ILs have been identified to date that act via different receptors with large divergent and cross-activation among the IL family members. ILs are involved in many disease processes and are targets for promising drug discovery.

Leukocytes Colorless blood cells capable of ameboid movement; they are capable of moving directionally in response to chemical stimuli (chemotaxis). Leukocytes are divided morphologically into granular cells (basophils, eosinophils, and neutrophils) and nongranular cells (lymphocytes and monocytes). Leukocytes are the primary cells that launch immune and inflammatory reactions. Leukocytes are present in the systemic circulation and in special lymphoid tissue such as the lymph node, bone marrow, and thymus.

Lymphocytes Mostly mononuclear, nonphagocytic leukocytes found in the blood and lymphoid tissue that make up the primary body of immune competent cells. Lymphocytes belong to two primary classes – T cells (thymus dependent) and B cells (Bursa dependent) – but several other subclasses with various functional and biochemical markers are known. Lymphocytes function via direct cell–cell interaction (specialized receptors) and via humoral mediators such as cytokines, interleukins, and chemokines as well as antibodies (a primary B-cell function). T cells are primarily responsible for cell-mediated immunity.

Mast cells	A connective tissue cell that elaborates highly reactive mediators such as cytokines, histamine, and enzymes, which can modulate matrix proteins such as chymotrypsin and tryptase. Mast cells (or mastocytes) are believed to play an important role in allergic rhinitis and asthma and, via enzymes released, to contribute to inflammation and atherosclerosis.
Matrix metalloproteinases (MMPs)	Zinc-dependent endopeptidases known for their ability to cleave one or several constituents of the extracellular matrix. MMPs consist of a large family of proteases that share common structural and functional elements.
Metabolic syndrome	A clinical condition that manifests four or five risk factors for cardiovascular and metabolic disorders. These include obesity, high glucose levels, high blood pressure, and aberrant plasma lipid levels (high triglycerides and low high-density lipoproteins).
Monocytes	Mononuclear phagocytic leukocytes that originate in the bone marrow. Monocytes are the source of tissue macrophages, which are abundant in lung and liver.
Nonsteroidal anti-inflammatory drug (NSAID)	Small organic (synthetic) chemicals that have been developed to suppress inflammation of various mechanisms, locations, and durations. They are commonly compounds that do not act like the steroid hormones (e.g., glucocorticoids). This class of medicines contains primarily inhibitors of the cyclooxygenase enzymes (which produce pro-inflammatory metabolites of the fatty acid arachidonate) and displays various proportional inhibitory capacities toward the cyclooxygenase 1 or 2 enzymes. Many such agents are marketed for pain relief from conditions such as arthritis and other muscular-skeletal conditions.
Sepsis	A condition that results from a harmful or host response to infection. Sepsis is marked by endotoxemia (the presence of bacterial or other toxins in the blood) and the activation of multiple systems such as the immune, cardiovascular, respiratory, coagulation, and complement systems. Sepsis can lead to multiple organ failure and death.

Introduction

Inflammation is a fundamental reaction of the body to injury. It is a complex biological phenomenon that comprises diverse cellular, neural, hormonal, and humoral systems. Inflammation involves the vascular system as well as blood-borne components linked via a complicated network of mediators. Inflammation can be the result of endogenous or exogenous injurious events. Inflammation is fundamentally viewed as a purposeful reaction aimed to repair, salvage, and restore the structure, function. and integrity of the injured tissue, organ, and organism well-being at large.

However, inflammation may also become a destructive or pathological condition that underlies numerous diseases in humans. Such diseases include bone and cartilage diseases (rheumatoid arthritis and osteoarthritis), skin diseases (psoriasis), central nervous system (CNS) diseases (multiple sclerosis and Alzheimer's disease), vascular diseases (atherosclerosis), cardiac diseases (heart failure and myocardial infarction), respiratory diseases (asthma and chronic obstructive pulmonary disease, COPD), gastrointestinal diseases (inflammatory bowel disease and Crohn's disease), and chronic unresolved infectious diseases (e.g., tuberculosis). In recent years, inflammation is increasingly recognized as a fundamental contributing element in many human diseases that have not been traditionally associated with inflammation. Conditions such as obesity, diabetes, metabolic syndrome, stroke, and cancer are all recognized as harboring various immune and inflammatory cells and mediators.

Inflammation is invariably linked to general homeostasis systems (e.g., coagulation and fibrinolysis) as also to the immune, complement, and the nervous system. As such, intervention in or modulation of specific pro-inflammatory mediators might result in broader consequences than the intended anti-inflammatory objective. Moreover, many mediators of inflammation are actually part of the normal physiological repertoire of molecules and cells that secure essential function and health. Therefore, the modulation (blockade or enhancement) of many recognized pro-inflammatory mediators, although potentially to providing medical benefits, could also harm. Thus a fine balance needs to be preserved in many cases so as not to disrupt functionalities that require the same mediators to be at a level context and duration that, if not secured, could lead to pathological conditions on their own.

The advances made in understanding the cellular elements and mediators that initiate, propagate, and amplify various forms of inflammation have already yielded important therapeutics. Nonsteroidal anti-inflammatory drugs (NSAIDs), steroids, and, more recently, ant-cytokines and interleukin mimetics have an important role in the treatment of inflammation. It is, however, important to keep in mind that no anti-inflammatory therapeutic introduced into medical practice is free of adverse effect.

Immune and Inflammatory Cells in Acute Inflammation: Role of Endothelium and Adhesion Molecules

Acute injury to tissues, such as bruises, blunt-force trauma, or infectious agents, elicit a typical inflammatory reaction. The early response consists of local neurovascular reaction and release of preformed mediators that induced vasodilation, microvascular permeability, and extravasation of plasma components into the injured zone. This early stage is followed by the recruitment and migration of leukocytes from the systemic circulation with primary role of the polymorphonuclear (PMN) cells. The PMN cells are followed by monocytes, which together with the PMS cells and tissue macrophages provide the local tissue with the ability to conduct phagocytosis of invading pathogens, engulf cell debris (e.g., necrotic cells), and set the stage for tissue repair. The recruitment of leukocytes into the injury zone is governed by two key processes: chemotaxis and cell adhesion. The directional influx of leukocytes into the injured tissue is dependent on mediators such as chemokines or complement factors, which, along with cytokines and interleukins, also activate the leukocytes. In addition, the endothelium along the microvessels associated with the injury zone express adhesion molecules (in addition to constitutive ones) that enable the interaction with ligands that are expressed on the leukocytes. These cell adhesion molecules act as a cascade of events – from loose rolling, loose adhesion, committed adhesion, and final migration mostly through the endothelium junction. The key adhesion molecules are the. vascular cell adhesion molecule (VCAM-)1; intercellular adhesion molecule (ICAM-)1, selectins (E, P, and L), and platelet-endothelial cells adhesion molecules (PECAMs).

Inflammation, Artherosclerosis, and Cardiovascular Diseases

The major pathological process that underwrites heart attacks, strokes, and peripheral vascular diseases is arteriosclerosis. Although the role of lipids (cholesterol in particular) in initiation and propagation of the arteriosclerotic pathology is well documented, inflammation is considered to be a major pathological feature in the evolution of this vascular disease. Lipid-loaded cells are the hallmark in any vascular atheroma, or plaque, which are macrophages (derived from blood monocytes) that phagocytosed modified cholesterol within lipoproteins particles. This process leads to the activation of the macrophages and release of cytokines, chemokines, interleukins, and other pro-inflammatory mediators such as arachidonic acid metabolites (lipoxygenase and cyclooxygenase). Apoptosis of excessively loaded macrophages (also called foam cells) is believed to release numerous inflammatory mediators that exacerbate the inflammatory process and increase the likelihood of its rupture. Most significantly in this regards are matrix metalloproteinases (MMPs; especially MMP-2 and -9), which are believed to reduce the fibrous cap of the atheroma and enhance plaque rupture, leading to the initiation of thrombosis and vascular occlusion. The atheromatous plaque is also rich in other inflammatory cells such a mast cells and T cells. The vascular inflammation part of the atherosclerosis process is viewed as an important therapeutic target and a component of the efficacy of major anti-atheroslerosis drugs such as the statins.

Inflammation and Cancer

A causal link between cancer and chronic inflammation has been demonstrated in the more than 1 million cancer patients linked to viruses and bacteria. Infection with human papillomaviruses, HCV, HBV; *Helicobacter pylori;* and Epstein–Barr virus are major risk factors for the development of cervical, gastrointestinal (GI), and hepatocellular cancer and lymphoma, respectively. The link between inflammation and cancer is not limited to infectious agents; chronic inflammation from cigarette smoke, asbestos, inflammatory bowel disease, silica, and so on contributes to the development of malignancy in the lungs, bladder, and GI tract. The activation of innate inflammation has been shown to contribute to cancer progression, including tumor necrosis factor (TNF)-α, and nuclear factor (NF)-κB signaling. The disruption of the adaptive (or antigen-specific) immune response to tumors has been shown to be crucial to carcinogenesis. Many studies have documented the anergic antitumor immune responses contrasting with the favorable prognosis conferred by the infiltration of tumors with cytotoxic killer T cells in several malignancies. In contrast, infiltration with supportive immune elements, such as growth-promoting macrophages, confers a worse prognosis in some malignancies. Finally, the association between multiple inflammatory biomarkers, such as interleukin (IL-)8, macrophage inflammatory protein (MIP-)1a, and various chemokines, whose expression levels correlate directly with worse prognosis, underlies the intimate relationship between inflammation and cancer development and progression.

Inflammation and Metabolic Syndrome

Metabolic syndrome emerges as the twenty-first-century epidemic that threatens both developed and less developed nations. Although the original concept defining metabolic syndrome focused on insulin resistance, namely, the poor responsiveness of target cells to insulin's ability to advance glucose metabolism, it has been recently recognized that inflammatory mediators are likely to be causally associated with the state of insulin resistance and, hence, metabolic syndrome. Most notable in this regards are the cytokines TNF-α, and IL-6. These cytokines, and primarily TNF-α, reduce the efficacy of insulin to enhance glucose uptake into the cells, a situation that manifests itself as hyperglycemia, a hallmark of the insulin resistant condition. Obesity, a key feature of the metabolic syndrome, is considered a pro-inflammatory state. Obesity is associated with increased oxidative stress, a biochemical condition prone to activating NF-κB, NADPH, and other factors. Oxidative stress-induced inflammation increases endothelial leukocyte adhesion molecules that enhance leukocyte engagement with the endothelium, a primary step for their entry into the tissue, their activation, and the further release of inflammatory mediators. Excessive caloric intake, from carbohydrates or fats, is considered to significantly contribute to the inflammation state that drives key elements of metabolic syndrome.

Inflammation and Respiratory Diseases

Chronic obstructive pulmonary disease (COPD) is a chronic lung disorder that is mostly the result of smoking and other environmental toxic agents. The disorder is characterized by the accumulation of inflammatory cells such as macrophages and neutrophils, which are activated to release numerous mediators. The inflammation resides within the terminal bronchioles (small airways) and alveoli (small vesicular spaces where oxygen and CO_2 exchange takes place). The persistent inflammation ultimately leads to the destruction of these pulmonary structures and respiratory failure. Prominent in the COPD pathomechanism are the inflammatory products of arachidonic acid and MMPs released by the activated inflammatory cells. MMP-9 and, in particular, MMP-12 play a predominant role in COPD by degrading the matrix proteins such as elastin, a matrix protein that is vital to the recoil of the bronchioles (small airways) and to alveolar health. MMP-12-mediated elastin degradation is believed to lead to emphysema, a state of destruction of the normal architecture of the lung respiratory elements. MMP-12 also plays a role in macrophage recruitment. Promising data emanating from recent research suggest that selective inhibitors of MMP-12 might be useful drugs in the treatment and prevention of COPD.

Bronchial asthma, a disease of lung airway spasm that leads to severe respiratory distress and severe forms to death, has strong inflammatory components. Arachidonic acid metabolites of potent inflammatory properties figure prominently in this disease. Lipoxigenase products called leukotrienes, prostanoids (prostaglandins and thromboxane A2), and isoprostanes have been implicated in this disorder. Indeed, anti-inflammatory agents such as glucocorticosteroids have been a cornerstone of asthma-attack prevention, largely due to their inhibition of inflammatory eicosanoids. In addition, specific inhibitors of cysteinyl leukotriene have proven to serve additional therapeutic efficacy.

Inflammation and Joint Diseases

Several joint and bone diseases, such as rheumatoid arthritis and osteoarthritis, are probably the result of degenerative (the former) or immune and inflammatory (the latter) processes. Rheumatoid arthritis is a chronic systemic disease primarily affecting the joints in which severe chronic inflammation leads to the destruction of the joint structure and, ultimately, functional disability. Misdirected inflammation is the cardinal feature of rheumatological diseases. It involves both the initiation and maintenance phases of the disease, and the processes and players (cells and mediators) involved are similar to that in other diseases. Major cells in the immune system (i.e., neutrophils, macrophages, dendritic cells, B cells, and T cells) are the major culprits in the development and exacerbation of the disease. Although autoimmune mechanisms (including the generation of antibodies against joint tissue components) are believed to play a major causative role, the chronic condition is probably sustained by numerous inflammatory mediators, including cytokines, ILs, chemokines, MMPs, prostanoids, and reactive oxygen radicals. Traditional anti-inflammatory agents such as the NSAIDs have been widely used to alleviate pain in and swelling of the joint, but their efficacy in mitigating the fundamental pathological process remained questionable. Likewise, the more recent class of anti-rheumatoid arthritis drugs, the COX-2 inhibitors, have a proven efficacy, yet at the cost of some increased risk for a cardiovascular adverse event. More recently, disease-modifying anti-arthritis drugs (DMARDs) have been successfully introduced into the medical management of rheumatoid arthritis. Such agents neutralize the cytokine TNF-α. Other cytokines and ILs (e.g., IL-6, IL-1, and IL-18) as well as interferon (IFN)-γ and endothelium leukocyte adhesion molecules (ICAM-1, VCAM-1, and selectins) are also targeted by therapeutic agents, as well as angiogenesis promoters such as vascular endothelium growth factor (VEGF).

The role of inflammation in osteoarthritis is less clear, although many of the cytokines already discussed are believed to play a key role in the destruction of bone and cartilage. Cartilage destruction probably involves cytokine activation of aggrecanase, an enzyme that destroys a major constituent of the normal cartilage.

Inflammation and Sepsis

Sepsis is a complex clinical syndrome that results from the harmful host response to infection; it results from the failure of the innate and acquired immune mechanisms to resolve the infectious condition and the damage induced by the toxins elaborated by the infectious agent. The bacterial toxins activate many of the inflammatory cells (in particular, neutrophils and monocytes/macrophages) but also other cells such as the endothelium. As a result of the toxins' action on the inflammatory cells, numerous preformed and newly elaborated mediators are produced, including oxygen radicals, bioactive lipid mediators, cytokines, chemokines, enzymes, and pro- and anticoagulation factors. Although many of the inflammatory cell products are helpful in confining and eliminating the infectious agent and its toxins, multiple tissues, organs, and system are also affected. Oxygen radical have bactericidal action, yet also affect the vasculature. Chemokines and cytokines modify the endothelium to support the fast recruitment of inflammation cells into the tissue to remove the invading agent while ILs activate and enhance the neutrophils, lymphocytes, and endothelium function. The inflammation cells also play a role in tissue repair and rehabilitation via the generation and release of growth factors that enhance the regeneration of the damaged circulation, the matrix elements, and tissue integrity. The immune and inflammation cells and mediators are the most critical systems that secure defenses in sepsis. The failure of these defenses could lead to organ failure and death.

Summary

Inflammation plays a key role in acute injuries as well as chronic diseases. The immune and inflammatory reactions serve as the major defense mechanism against numerous external injurious events and pathological events that emerge as a result of endogenous aberrant genetic and biochemical imbalances. However, immune and inflammatory reactions can also evolve as a cause of diseases such as autoimmune diseases; granulomatous conditions; cancer; respiratory, joint, and bone diseases; and atherosclerosis. Thus, anti-inflammatory drugs emerge as an important source of novel therapeutics for diverse diseases such as cancer, metabolic syndrome, atherosclerosis, joint and bone diseases, and respiratory tract disorders.

Further Reading

Barish, G. D., Narkar, V. A. and Evans, R. M. (2006). PPARδ: a dagger in the heart of the metabolic syndrome. *Journal of Clinical Investigations* **116**, 590–597.

Bloomgarten, Z. T. (2005). Inflammation, atherosclerosis, and aspects of insulin action. *Diabetes Care* **28**, 2312–2319.

Cohen, J. (2002). The immunopathogenesis of sepsis. *Nature* **420**, 885–891.

Dandona, P., Aljada, A., Chaudhuri, A., et al. (2005). Metabolic syndrome: a comprehensive perspective based on interaction between obesity, diabetes and inflammation. *Circulation* **111**, 1448–1454.

Fontech, A. N. and Wykle, R. L. (2004). Arachidonate remodeling and inflammation. In: Parnham, M. J. (ed.) *Progress in Inflammation*, pp. 1–243. Basel: Birkhauser Verlag.

Lagente, V., Manoury, B., Nenan, S., et al. (2005). Role of matrix metalloproteinases in the development of airway inflammation and remodeling. *Brazilian Journal Medical Biological Research* **38**, 1521–1530.

Libby, P. and Theroux, P. (2005). Pathophysiology of coronary artery disease. *Circulation* **111**, 3481–3488.

Morgan, D. W., Forssmann, U. J. and Nakada, M. T. (2004). Cancer and inflammation. In: Parnham, M. J. (ed.) *Progress in inflammation*, pp. 1–201. Basel: Birkhauser Verlag.

Moser, B., Letts, G. and Neote, K. (2006). Chemokine biology – basic and clinical application. Vol. 1: Immunology of chemokines. In: Parnham, M. J. (ed.) *Progress in inflammation research*, pp. 1–205. Basel: Birkhauser Verlag.

Rolin, S., Masereel, B. and Dogne, J. -M. (2006). Prostanoids as pharmacological targets in COPD and asthma. *European Journal of Pharmacology* **533**, 89–100.

Schottenfeld, D. and Beebe-Dimmer, J. (2006). Chronic inflammation: a common and important factor in the pathogenesis of neoplasia. *Journal of Clinical Investigations* **56**, 69–83.

Simmons, D. L. (2006). What makes a good anti-inflammatory drug target? *Drug Discovery Today* **11** (5–6), 210–219.

Van den Berg, W. B. and Miossec, P. (2004). Cytokines and joint injury. In: Parnham, M. J. (ed.) *Progress in inflammation*, pp. 1–291. Basel: Birkhauser Verlag.

Weizmann, M. N. and Pacifici, R. (2006). Estrogen deficiency and bone loss: an inflammatory tale. *Journal of Clinical Investigations* **116**, 1186–1193.

Zelcer, N. and Tontonoz, P. (2006). Liver X receptors as integrators of metabolic and inflammatory signaling. *Journal of Clinical Investigations* **116**, 607–614.

Sepsis, Acute Respiratory Distress Syndrome, and Glucocorticoid Resistance

G U Meduri
University of Tennessee Health Science Center
Department of Medicine, Memphis, TN USA

Glossary

Hypoxemic respiratory failure A life-threatening reduction in blood oxygenation requiring assisted mechanical ventilation.

Multiple organ dysfunction Systemic inflammation-associated impairments of vital organs: brain, lung, cardiovascular system, renal, liver, and hematopoietic system.

Sepsis Systemic inflammation induced by infection.

Systemic inflammation The release of inflammatory cytokines in the systemic circulation manifesting clinically with fever and increased heart rate, respiratory rate, and white cell blood count.

Introduction

Hundred of thousands of American are affected every year by severe sepsis (700,000) and acute respiratory distress syndrome (ARDS; 190,000) creating a significant short-term and long-term burden on public health and health-care economics. Dysregulated systemic inflammation with persistent elevation of circulating inflammatory cytokines over time is the pathogenetic mechanism for the dysfunction and failure of the vital organs, the leading cause of death in patients with sepsis and ARDS. In sepsis and ARDS, the down-regulation of inflammation is *conditio sine qua non* to their resolution. An improved understanding of the cellular mechanisms that initiate, propagate, and restrict inflammation in sepsis and ARDS is essential to make advances on present treatment modalities and to develop more reliable methods of monitoring disease progression and responses to therapy.

It is now appreciated that at cellular level transcription factors nuclear factor (NF-)-κB, which is activated by inflammatory signals, and the glucocorticoid receptor (GR)α, which is activated by endogenous or exogenous glucocorticoids (GCs), have diametrically opposed functions (stimulatory vs. inhibitory) in regulating inflammation. NF-κB is recognized as the principal driver of the inflammatory response, being responsible for the transcription of more than 100 genes, including tumor necrosis factor (TNF-)α and interleukin(IL-)1β (**Figure 1**). Once activated, NF-κB and GRα can mutually repress one another through a protein–protein interaction that prevents their DNA binding and subsequent transcriptional activity. Known interactions between NF-κB and the activated glucocorticoid receptor (GC-GRα) are depicted in **Figure 1**. The activation of one transcription factor in excess of the binding (inhibitory) capacity of the other shifts cellular responses toward the increased (dysregulated) or decreased (regulated) transcription of inflammatory mediators over time (**Figure 2**). The role of GC supplementation in patients with life-threatening systemic inflammation is undergoing a cyclical reassessment, stirred by a new understanding of the role of GCs in regulating inflammation and the positive results of recent randomized controlled studies.

Acute Respiratory Distress Syndrome

ARDS is a life-threatening form of hypoxemic respiratory failure (mortality of 30–60%) that develops within 12–48 h of a patient's acquiring an acute illness complicated by severe systemic inflammation. The most common condition precipitating ARDS is severe sepsis, and the mortality rate for sepsis-induced ARDS has not significantly decreased in the last 20 years. In ARDS, the evolution (regulated vs. dysregulated) of systemic inflammation in the first week of mechanical ventilation determines the physiological progression of the disease and the final

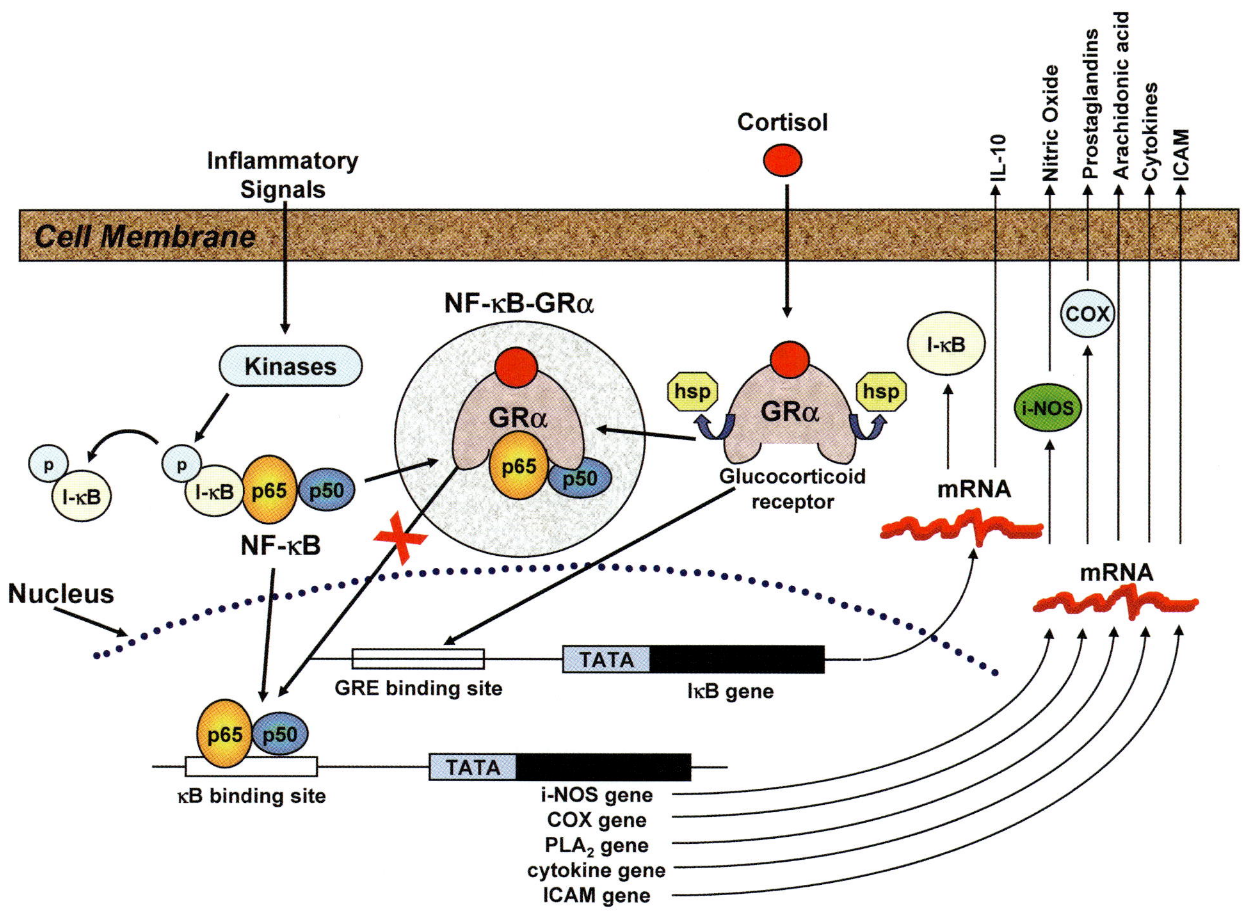

Figure 1 Positive regulatory loop interaction between NF-κB and the activated glucocorticoid receptor (GC-GRα). When cells are stimulated by inflammatory signals, specific kinases phosphorylate the inhibitory protein IκB and cause its rapid degradation. The activated form of NF-κB then moves to the nucleus, initiating the transcription of mRNA of inflammatory cytokines, chemokines, cell adhesion molecules, and inflammation-associated enzymes (cyclooxygenase, phospholipase A2, and inducible nitric oxide). Cortisol or exogenous glucocorticoids freely cross into the cytoplasm and bind to their specific glucocorticoid receptors (GRα) to form GC-GRα. GC-GRα complexes may influence NF-κB activity in five major ways: (1) physically interacting with the p65 subunit to form an inactive (GC-GRα–NF-κB) complex, (2) inducing the synthesis of the inhibitory protein IκBα via interaction with glucocorticoid-responsive element DNA in the promoter of the IκB gene, (3) blocking the degradation of IκBα via enhanced synthesis of IL-10, (4) impairing the TNF-α-induced degradation of IκBα, and (5) competing for limited amounts of GR co-activators such as cAMP response element binding protein (CREB)-binding protein (CBP) and steroid receptor coactivator (SRC-)1. IκBα, in addition to holding NF-κB in an inactive cytoplasmic state, also translocates into the nucleus, where it binds activated NF-κB complexes to induce their export to the cytoplasm. GC-GRα may also decrease the stability of mRNA of several inflammatory cytokines and other molecules. The products of the genes that are stimulated by NF-κB activate this transcription factor. Thus, TNF-α and IL-1β both activate and are activated by NF-κB by forming a positive regulatory loop that amplifies and perpetuates inflammation. Reproduced with permission from Meduri, G. U., Muthiah, M. P., Carratu, P., et al. (2005), Nuclear factor-kappaB- and glucocorticoid receptor alpha-mediated mechanisms in the regulation of systemic and pulmonary inflammation during sepsis and acute respiratory distress syndrome: evidence for inflammation-induced target tissue resistance to glucocorticoids, *Neuroimmunomodulation* **12**(6), 321–338.

outcome. Patients failing to improve in the first week of mechanical ventilation (nonimprovers) have, compared to improvers, a persistent elevation in circulating and bronchoalveolar lavage (BAL) levels of inflammatory cytokines and chemokines, markers of alveolocapillary membrane (ACM) permeability and fibrogenesis. In sepsis and ARDS, the downregulation of inflammation is essential for the restoration of homeostasis and survival.

Systemic Inflammation-Associated Glucocorticoid Resistance

GCs as end effectors of the hypothalamic-pituitary-adrenal (HPA) axis are the most important physiological inhibitors of inflammation, affecting hundreds of genes involved in stress-related homeostasis. However, endogenous GCs are not always effective in suppressing life-threatening systemic inflammation,

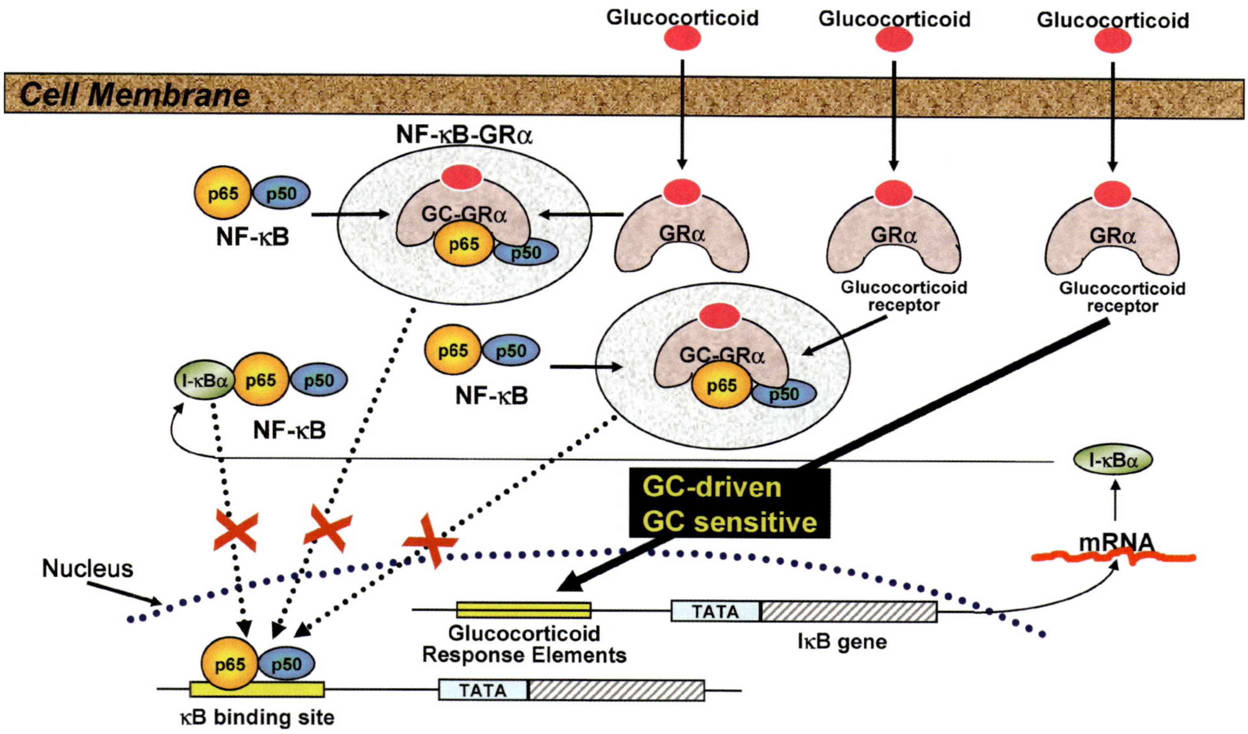

Figure 2 Regulated response interaction between NF-κB and the activated glucocorticoid receptor (GC-GRα). GC-GRα activation sufficient to maintain NF-κB levels in homeostasis and achieve a reduction in the transcription of inflammatory mediators over time is shown. In improvers, both GC-GRα binding to NF-κB and nuclear GC-GRα binding increased significantly over time, indicating an excess activation of GC-GRα compared to NF-κB (GC-GRα-driven response). Reproduced with permission from Meduri, G. U., Muthiah, M. P., Carratu, P., et al. (2005), Nuclear factor-kappaB- and glucocorticoid receptor alpha-mediated mechanisms in the regulation of systemic and pulmonary inflammation during sepsis and acute respiratory distress syndrome: evidence for inflammation-induced target tissue resistance to glucocorticoids, *Neuroimmunomodulation* **12**(6), 321–338.

and the degree of cortisolemia frequently correlates with the severity of illness and the mortality rate. Unquestionably, the elevation of GC secretion in nonsurvivors of sepsis and ARDS is inadequate to meet the needs of the concurrent inflammatory response and its adverse systemic effects. Its failure to suppress inflammation could be due to tissue resistance to GCs, the inadequacy of the level and duration of endogenous GC elevation to suppress a systemic inflammatory response gone awry, or both.

The concept of acquired GC resistance was first introduced by Kass and Finland in 1957. These investigators suggested that increased blood cortisol levels in nonsurvivors of sepsis might reflect a blocking of steroidal activity or transport as a consequence of the infection. In this situation, a small increase in blood levels with a low (equal to or less than physiological) dose of exogenous GCs was believed to be sufficient to facilitate the passage of steroids into host cells. GC resistance was originally described as a primary inherited familial syndrome and was recently recognized as an acquired condition. Among others, acquired immune tissue-specific GR resistance has been described in patients with asthma, acquired immunodeficiency syndrome (AIDS), severe sepsis, and sepsis-induced ARDS.

In vitro studies showed that cytokines may induce resistance to GCs by reducing GR binding affinity to cortisol and/or GC response elements (GREs). Such abnormalities of GR function were demonstrated in T cells incubated with a combination of interleukin (IL-)2 and IL-4, IL-1, IL-6, and interferon (IFN)-γ, or IL-13. GC resistance was induced in a cytokine concentration-dependent fashion and was reversed by the removal of cytokines. GR-mediated resistance in the presence of systemic inflammation was also studied in experimental models of sepsis and sepsis-induced ARDS. In a sheep model of sepsis-induced ARDS, the maximal binding capacity of GR decreased continuously after endotoxin infusion, whereas there was a marked elevation of cortisol levels. The reduced GR binding correlated negatively ($r = -0.87$, $p < 0.01$) with phospholipase A_2 (PLA_2) activity, a gene that is stimulated by NF-κB. In a rat model of septic shock, GR blockade by mifepristone (RU 486) exacerbated the physiological and pathological changes induced by endotoxemia. PLA_2 activity in rats with 80% GR blockade was more marked than in those with 50% GR blockade. The monocytes of patients with sepsis developed near-total GC resistance in vitro when cytokines, especially IL-2, were added.

Nuclear Factor κB and Glucocorticoid Receptor α Interaction

New evidence indicates that a primary pathogenetic mechanism explaining GC resistance or insensitivity in patients with life-threatening systemic inflammation is the imbalance between excessive NF-κB activation by inflammatory signals and deficient GRα activation by endogenous or exogenous glucocorticoids. Using an *ex vivo* model of systemic inflammation, our group investigated intracellular upstream and downstream events associated with DNA binding of NF-κB and GRα in naïve peripheral blood leukocytes (PBLs) stimulated with longitudinal plasma specimens obtained from 28 patients with sepsis-induced ARDS and correlated the physiological progression with laboratory findings. Exposure of naïve cells to longitudinal plasma samples led to divergent directions in NF-κB and GRα activation that reflected the severity of systemic inflammation (defined by plasma TNF-α and IL-1β levels). The activation of one transcription factor in excess of the other shifted cellular responses toward decreased (GRα-driven) or increased (NF-κB-driven) transcription of inflammatory mediators over time (**Figures 2–3**).

Plasma samples from patients with declining inflammatory cytokine levels over time elicited a progressive increase in all measured aspects of GC-GRα-mediated activity ($p = 0.0001$) and a corresponding reduction in NF-κB nuclear binding ($p = 0.0001$) and transcription of TNF-α and IL-1β (regulated, GRα-driven response; **Figure 2**). In contrast, plasma samples from patients with sustained elevations in inflammatory cytokine levels over time elicited only modest longitudinal increases in GC-GRα-mediated activity ($p = 0.04$) and a progressive increase in NF-κB nuclear binding over time ($p = 0.0001$) that was most striking in nonsurvivors (dysregulated, NF-κB-driven response; **Figure 3**). These findings demonstrate that insufficient GC-GRα-mediated activity is an important mechanism for early loss of autoregulation (i.e., downregulation of NF-κB activation) in nonimprovers. Deficient GRα activity in

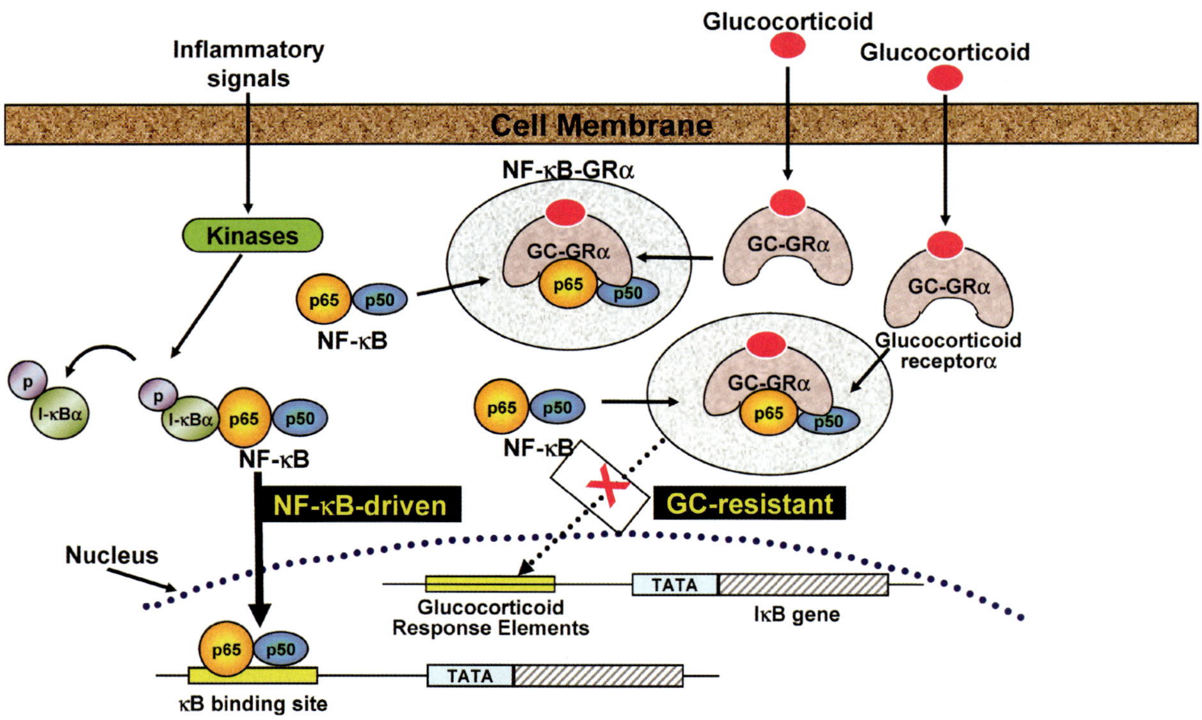

Figure 3 Dysregulated response interaction between NF-κB and the activated glucocorticoid receptor (GC-GRα). An excess of NF-κB activation is shown, leading to the protracted transcription of inflammatory mediators over time. In nonimprovers, GC-GRα binding to NF-κB was modestly increased, whereas nuclear NF-κB binding increased substantially over time and nuclear GC-GRα and cytoplasmic IκBα levels declined (NF-κB-driven response). Reproduced with permission from Meduri, G. U., Muthiah, M. P., Carratu, P., et al. (2005), Nuclear factor-kappaB- and glucocorticoid receptor alpha-mediated mechanisms in the regulation of systemic and pulmonary inflammation during sepsis and acute respiratory distress syndrome: evidence for inflammation-induced target tissue resistance to glucocorticoids, *Neuroimmunomodulation* **12**(6), 321–338.

naïve cells exposed to plasma from patients with dysregulated inflammation was observed despite elevated circulating cortisol and adrenocorticotropic hormone (ACTH) levels, implicating inflammatory cytokine-driven excess NF-κB activation as an important mechanism for target-organ insensitivity and/or resistance to cortisol.

Our findings are in agreement with two longitudinal studies that investigated NF-κB binding activity directly in the peripheral blood mononuclear cells of patients with sepsis or trauma. In both studies, nonsurvivors (compared to survivors) had a progressive increase in NF-κB activity over time. In one longitudinal study, nonsurvivors of septic shock had by days 2–6 a 200% increase in NF-κB activity compared to day 1. Similarly, using our *ex vivo* model we found that NF-κB binding activity on day 3 of ARDS clearly separated patients by outcome. In an immunohistochemistry analysis of lung tissue, areas with severe (vs. mild) ARDS had a higher nuclear uptake of NF-κB ($13 + 1.3$ vs. $7 + 2.9$; $p = 0.01$) and a lower ratio of GRα : NF-κB nuclear uptake (0.5 ± 0.2 vs.1.5 ± 0.2; $p = 0.007$). Thus, an uninhibited increase in NF-κB activation in circulating cells over time appears to be a significant premortem pathogenetic component of lethal sepsis and ARDS.

Systemic Inflammation-Induced Glucocorticoid Resistance Can Be Improved with Prolonged Glucocorticoid Supplementation

Our findings place GC-GRα-mediated downregulation of NF-κB activity as a critical factor for the reestablishment of homeostasis during the acute, life-threatening systemic inflammation that accompanies sepsis and ARDS. A subgroup of 11 patients with dysregulated inflammation and deficient GC-GRα activity were randomized to prolonged GC supplementation initiated on ARDS day 9 ± 3. Quantitatively adequate and prolonged hormonal supplementation restored GR anti-inflammatory function, decreasing the production of inflammatory cytokines, inflammatory cytokine-driven HPA axis activity, and inflammatory cytokine-driven organ dysfunction. Normal PBL exposed to plasma samples collected during GC versus placebo treatment exhibited rapid, progressive, and significant increases in GRα-mediated activities (GRα binding to NF-κB, GRα binding to GRE DNA, stimulation of inhibitory protein IκBα, and stimulation of IL-10 transcription) and significant reductions in NF-κB κb binding and transcription of TNF-α and IL-1β. During GC treatment, the relationship between NF-κB and GC-GRα signaling pathways changed from an initial NF-κB-driven and GC-GRα-resistant state to a GC-GRα-driven and GC-GRα-sensitive one. In aggregate, the findings indicate that systemic inflammation-induced GC resistance is an acquired generalized process mediated by excess NF-κB activation and potentially reversible by increasing GC-GRα activation with quantitatively adequate and prolonged GC supplementation.

Findings of Randomized Trials

At present, the administration of low-dose GCs is the only treatment shown in randomized trials to have a significant positive biological and physiological effect across the longitudinal spectrum of the severity of sepsis-associated systemic inflammation: severe sepsis, septic shock, early ARDS, and unresolving ARDS. All randomized studies showed significant physiological improvement and a reduction in the duration of stays in the intensive care unit. The overall effects on mortality are shown in **Table 1**.

In prolonged low-dose GC treatment, maximal benefits are obtained by (1) avoiding the premature removal of an effective drug, leading to rebound inflammation and physiological deterioration, and (2) preventing potential complications associated with GC treatment (infection surveillance and avoidance of paralysis). Uncontrolled studies have also shown a likely benefit in patients with viral pneumonia-induced ARDS, including SARS. The mortality rate in 849 cases of SARS treated with antiviral therapy and GC supplementation was only 7.7%. In hantavirus pulmonary syndrome, the mortality rate decreased from 47% in patients treated with antiviral therapy to 13% when GC supplementation was also included. The findings for severe viral pneumonia and the results of recent randomized controlled trials (RCTs) for ARDS indicate that prolonged methylprednisolone use might useful in the prevention of morbidity and mortality associated with avian influenza.

Conclusion

Dysregulated systemic inflammation has enormous health-care consequences. A new understanding of the cellular mechanisms responsible for inflammation-associated GC resistance provides a new rationale for investigating prolonged low-dose GC supplementation. The consistent positive results of small- to moderate-size randomized studies are very encouraging. Federal financial support is urgently needed to conduct additional RCTs investigating this inexpensive off-patent treatment in patients with life-threatening systemic inflammation.

Table 1 Prolonged glucocorticoid treatment in sepsis and ARDS: effect on mortality[a]

Severity of sepsis	*Number of RCTs*	*Number of patients (death of total)*			*Source*[b]
		Treated	*Control*	*p value*	
Severe sepsis	1	0 of 23 (0%)	7 of 23 (30%)	0.009	5
Septic shock	5	7 of 22	12 of 19		2
		3 of 20	4 of 20		3
		6 of 23	10 of 21		4
		82 of 151	91 of 149		1
		8 of 20	12 of 20		10
Total from meta-analysis		106 of 236 (45%)	129 of 229 (56%)	0.01	8
Early ARDS	1	50 of 63 (21%)	16 of 28 (43%)	0.03	6
Unresolving ARDS	2	2 of 16 (12%)	5 of 8 (62%)	0.03	7
		32 of 90 (36%)	31 of 90 (34%)	NS	9

[a]ARDS, acute respiratory distress; RCTs, randomized controlled trials.
[b]Data from:
1. Annane, D., Sebille, V., Charpentier, C., et al. (2002), Effect of treatment with low doses of hydrocortisone and fludrocortisone on mortality in patients with septic shock, *Journal of the American Medical Association* **288**(7), 62–871.
2. Bollaert, P. E., Charpentier, C., Levy, B., et al. (1998), Reversal of late septic shock with supraphysiologic doses of hydrocortisone, *Critical Care Medicine* **26**(4), 645–650.
3. Briegel, J., Forst, H., Haller, M., et al. (1999), Stress doses of hydrocortisone reverse hyperdynamic septic shock: a prospective, randomized, double-blind, single-center study, *Critical Care Medicine* **27**(4), 723–732.
4. Chawla, K., Kupfer, Y., Goldman, I., et al. (1999), Hydrocortisone reverses refractory septic shock, *Critical Care Medicine* **27**, A33.
5. Confalonieri, M., Urbino, R., Potena, A., et al. (2005), Hydrocortisone infusion for severe community-acquired pneumonia: a preliminary randomized study, *American Journal of Respiratory Critical Care Medicine* **171**(3), 242–248.
6. Meduri, G. U., Golden, E. , Freire, A. X., et al. (2005), Methylprednisolone infusion significantly improves lung function in patients with early acute respiratory distress syndrome: results of a randomized controlled trial, *Chest* **128**, S129.
7. Meduri, G. U., Headley, S., Golden, E., et al. (1998), Effect of prolonged methylprednisolone therapy in unresolving acute respiratory distress syndrome: a randomized controlled trial, *Journal of the American Medical Association* **280**, 159–165.
8. Minneci, P. C., Deans, K. J., Banks, S. M., et al. (2004), Meta-analysis: the effect of steroids on survival and shock during sepsis depends on the dose, *Annals of Internal Medicine* **141**(1), 47–56.
9. Steinberg, K. P., Hudson, L. D., Goodman, R. B., et al. (2006), Efficacy and safety of corticosteroids for persistent acute respiratory distress syndrome, *New England Journal of Medicine* **354**(16), 1671–1684.
10. Yildiz, O., Doganay, M., Aygen, B., et al. (2002), Physiological-dose steroid therapy in sepsis, *Critical Care* **6**(3), 251–259.

Acknowledgments

This work was supported by Grants from the Assisi Foundation of Memphis.

Further Reading

Annane, D., Sebille, V., Charpentier, C., et al. (2002). Effect of treatment with low doses of hydrocortisone and fludrocortisone on mortality in patients with septic shock. *Journal of the American Medical Association* 288(7), 62–871.

Annane, D., Sebille, V., Troche, G., et al. (2002). A 3-level prognostic classification in septic shock based on cortisol levels and cortisol response to corticotropin. *Journal of the American Medical Association* 283(8), 1038–1045.

Bollaert, P. E., Charpentier, C., Levy, B., et al. (1998). Reversal of late septic shock with supraphysiologic doses of hydrocortisone. *Critical Care Medicine* 26(4), 645–650.

Briegel, J., Forst, H., Haller, M., et al. (1999). Stress doses of hydrocortisone reverse hyperdynamic septic shock: a prospective, randomized, double-blind, single-center study. *Critical Care Medicine* 27(4), 723–732.

Chawla, K., Kupfer, Y., Goldman, I., et al. (1999). Hydrocortisone reverses refractory septic shock. *Critical Care Medicine* 27, A33.

Cheng, V. C., Tang, B. S., Wu, A. K., et al. (2004). Medical treatment of viral pneumonia including SARS in immunocompetent adult. *Journal of Infection* 49(4), 262–273.

Confalonieri, M., Urbino, R., Potena, A., et al. (2005). Hydrocortisone infusion for severe community-acquired pneumonia: a preliminary randomized study. *American Journal of Respiratory Critical Care Medicine* 171(3), 242–248.

Kass, E. H. and Finland, M. (1957). Adrenocortical hormones and the management of infection. *Annual Review of Medicine* 8, 1–18.

Meduri, G. U., Golden, E., Freire, A. X., et al. (2005). Methylprednisolone infusion significantly improves lung function in patients with early acute respiratory distress syndrome: results of a randomized controlled trial. *Chest* 128, S129.

Meduri, G. U., Headley, S., Golden, E., et al. (1998). Effect of prolonged methylprednisolone therapy in unresolving acute respiratory distress syndrome: a randomized controlled trial. *Journal of the American Medical Association* 280, 159–165.

Meduri, G. U., Muthiah, M. P., Carratu, P., et al. (2005). Nuclear factor-kappaB- and glucocorticoid receptor alpha-mediated mechanisms in the regulation of systemic and pulmonary inflammation during sepsis and acute respiratory distress syndrome: evidence for inflammation-induced target tissue resistance to glucocorticoids. *Neuroimmunomodulation* **12**(6), 321–338.

Meduri, G. U., Tolley, E. A., Chrousos, G. P., et al. (2002). Prolonged methylprednisolone treatment suppresses systemic inflammation in patients with unresolving acute respiratory distress syndrome: evidence for inadequate endogenous glucocorticoid secretion and inflammation-induced immune cell resistance to glucocorticoids. *American Journal of Respiratory Critical Care Medicine* **165**(7), 983–991.

Meduri, G. U. and Yates, C. R. (2004). Systemic inflammation-associated glucocorticoid resistance and outcome of ARDS. *Annals of the New York Academy of Sciences* **1024**, 24–53.

Minneci, P. C., Deans, K. J., Banks, S. M., et al. (2004). Meta-analysis: the effect of steroids on survival and shock during sepsis depends on the dose. *Annals of Internal Medicine* **141**(1), 47–56.

Rhen, T. and Cidlowski, J. A. (2005). Antiinflammatory action of glucocorticoids – new mechanisms for old drugs. *New England Journal of Medicine* **353**(16), 1711–1723.

Steinberg, K. P., Hudson, L. D., Goodman, R. B., et al. (2006). Efficacy and safety of corticosteroids for persistent acute respiratory distress syndrome. *New England Journal of Medicine* **354**(16), 1671–1684.

Yildiz, O., Doganay, M., Aygen, B., et al. (2002). Physiological-dose steroid therapy in sepsis. *Critical Care* **6**(3), 251–259.

B. Stress - Feeding - Obesity - Metabolic Syndrome

Obesity, Stress and

R Rosmond
Björndammsterrassen 41, Partille, Sweden

This is a revised version of the article by P Björntorp, R Rosmond and J Uddén, Encyclopedia of Stress, First edition, volume 3, pp 75–76, © 2000, Elsevier Inc.

Glossary

Hypothalamic-pituitary-adrenal axis — The hormonostatic endocrine axis that regulates cortisol production and secretion.

Leptin — An adipocyte-produced hormone that is involved in the regulation of satiety and energy expenditure.

The current understanding of the systems of the body and brain related to the control of energy intake, energy balance, and body weight has increased significantly since 2001. In the periphery, a variety of substances are believed to be involved in integrating physiological and behavioral systems directed towards energy homeostasis. The hormones insulin, leptin (secreted by adipocytes), and ghrelin (mainly secreted by the stomach) link the control of peripheral energy metabolism to the central nervous system (CNS) feeding behavior integrating unit by modulating short-term signals that determine meal initiation and termination as well as energy balance. The adrenal glucocorticoids (cortisol) predominantly influence the ingestion and metabolism of fat and carbohydrates. In addition to these hormones, the process of integrating metabolic information from the periphery in the CNS requires specialized functions of multiple brain areas. These include the lower brainstem, which integrates neural information between peripheral autonomic-endocrine organs and forebrain structures, the hypothalamus, which is closely linked to circulating metabolites and hormones, and the forebrain structures, such as the nucleus accumbens and amygdala, which integrate incoming information with various cognitive aspects of food.

The role of the hypothalamus in the process of relating hormones and metabolism to eating behavior has received considerable attention. A number of neuroendocrine systems have been identified in this structure and are believed to be involved in controlling appetite for the macronutrients, carbohydrate, fat, and protein. They also modulate metabolism and contribute ultimately to weight gain and obesity.

Stress-Eating

Many overweight people, particularly those with abdominal obesity, find that eating increases in situation of discomfort and also soothes their feelings of stress and anxiety. This phenomenon is usually called stress-eating or emotional-eating. While obese individuals may realize that in general they eat in response to stress/emotions, they are typically unable in the moment to stop themselves from eating. As will be discussed below, this type of stress-eating might be due to disruptions of central regulatory systems involved in the control of energy intake. In obese binge eaters, stress-eating occurs, and it is up to 100% specifically triggered by stress and negative moods (e.g., depression, anger, anxiety, etc.).

Stress-Eating and Obesity

It is not clear if stress-eating is secondary to being obese or vice versa, stress causing overeating, resulting in obesity. It is, however, clear that obese subjects have more body image distortion and distress about their weight than normal-weight subjects. Indeed, in our society being obese is so stigmatized that few individuals who are obese are able to feel good about their size. Negative body image and feelings of stress and anxiety about being obese may thus serve as a trigger for stress-eating. In addition, stress and anxiety about being obese may work indirectly, increasing negative emotions such as depression and thus rendering the individual more susceptible to eating in response to stress. However, no studies have been reported indicating that obese subjects overeat by stress mechanisms leading to a maintained or escalated obese state.

Our knowledge of human obesity has progressed beyond the simple generalization that obesity is fully explained by inappropriate eating. Still, in more than 80% of the cross-sectional studies linking intake data to degree of obesity, dietary fat intake was associated with obesity. It is, however, important to recognize that human obesity is not a single entity, and subgroups are clearly more or less afflicted by stress. Realizing this distinction, it may be possible to examine how stress may be directly associated with an increased energy intake, and eventually with obesity.

Obesity with an increased number of adipocytes (i.e., hypercellular obesity) typically begins in early or middle childhood. In contrast, obesity with enlarged adipocytes (i.e., hypertrophic obesity) tends to correlate with truncal fat distribution, which in turn is an important predictor of the health hazards of obesity. Certainly, differences in clinical symptomatology favor a separation of obesity into two broad categories: visceral and nonvisceral obesity. These two forms seem to have different associations to stress. Central, visceral obesity is often associated with psychosocial and socioeconomic handicaps and excess use of alcohol and tobacco, as well as traits of depression and anxiety. Psychosocial stressors might induce eating as comfort food that may directly result in reduction of the negative effects of the chronic stressor in the nucleus accumbens. In addition, socioeconomic difficulties may make it hard to purchase nutritionally healthy food.

Mechanism of Stress-Eating

The expression of appetite is underpinned by a complex set of peripherally generated signals. Key hormonal appetite factors include insulin, cortisol, and leptin. Leptin is a protein that is synthesized exclusively in adipose tissue and moderates the drive to consume food. Within the neural circuitry numerous neuropeptides, both orexogenic (e.g., neuropeptide Y and melanocortin), and anorexigenic (e.g., proopiomelanocortin and corticotropin-releasing hormone) have been identified which stimulate and inhibit food intake.

Resistance to the appetite-suppressing effects of leptin is associated with common forms of obesity. Is it possible that stress factors associated with central, visceral obesity might be interfering with the leptin system? The human body holds many effector systems including the hypothalamic-pituitary-adrenal (HPA) axis for maintaining homeostasis. The secretory end product of the HPA axis, cortisol, is kept within an optimal range through the feedback action of cortisol interacting with neural control mechanisms. Distressing events or situations evokes prominent HPA system activation, and after long-term exposure, the HPA axis will eventually become dishabituated, resulting in a disruption of central regulatory systems. Together with insulin, the cortisol stimulate drive for and ingestion of comfort foods that may directly result in reduction of the negative effects of the chronic stressor in the nucleus accumbens, through stimulation of the anterior, more pleasure-associated part of this cell group, thus reducing the weight of the stress-stimulated posterior, more defensive part. Studies in rats have indicated that cortisol is directly involved in the sensitivity of the leptin regulation of satiety. When rats are adrenalectomized, their leptin sensitivity becomes high and feeding is inhibited. When corticosterone is replaced in a dose-dependent manner, food intake and body weight follow in parallel, and with excess corticosterone, obesity due to overeating appears. Furthermore, most animal models of obesity have enlarged adrenals and overproduction of glucocorticoids. Upon adrenalectomy, the somatic feature of obesity disappears. In normal-weight subjects, cortisol induces a dose-dependent increase in plasma leptin concentrations. In obese humans, food intake is clearly elevated after glucocorticoid administration in spite of increased levels of circulating leptin, indicating the presence of leptin resistance. Taken together it seems reasonable to assume that stress-eating is primarily caused by interference of stress-related cortisol secretion, with the normal signaling of satiety by the leptin system. The resulting deficient satiety signal causes overeating and finally the appearance of overweight and obesity.

Further Reading

Björntorp, P. and Rosmond, R. (2000). Obesity and cortisol. *Nutrition* **16**, 924–936.

Dallman, M. F., Pecoraro, N. C. and la Fleur, S. E. (2005). Chronic stress and comfort foods: self-medication and abdominal obesity. *Brain, behavior, and immunity* **19**, 275–280.

Gautier, J. F., Chen, K., Salbe, A. D., et al. (2000). Differential brain responses to satiation in obese and lean men. *Diabetes* **49**, 838–846.

Mastorakos, G. and Zapanti, E. (2004). The hypothalamic-pituitary-adrenal axis in the neuroendocrine regulation of food intake and obesity: the role of corticotropin releasing hormone. *Nutritional Neuroscience* **7**, 271–280.

Rosmond, R., Dallman, M. F. and Björntorp, P. (1998). Stress-related cortisol secretion in men: relationships with abdominal obesity and endocrine, metabolic and hemodynamic abnormalities. *Journal of Clinical Endocrinology and Metabolism* **83**, 1853–1859.

Rosmond, R. (2005). Role of stress in the pathogenesis of the metabolic syndrome. *Psychoneuroendocrinology* **30**, 1–10.

Udden, J., Björntorp, P., Arner, P., et al. (2003). Effects of glucocorticoids on leptin levels and eating behaviour in women. *Journal of Internal Medicine* **253**, 225–231.

Zakrzewska, K. E., Cusin, I., Sainsbury, A., et al. (1997). Glucocorticoids as counterregulatory hormones of leptin: toward an understanding of leptin resistance. *Diabetes* **46**, 717–719.

Feeding Circuitry (and Neurochemistry)

S E La Fleur, J J G Hillebrand and R A H Adan
Rudolf Magnus Institute of Neuroscience, University Medical Centre Utrecht, Utrecht, The Netherlands

Glossary

Anorexigenic Inhibiting food intake (e.g., POMC (α-MSH), CART, leptin).

Arcuate nucleus A collection of neurons (nerve cells) in the hypothalamus.

Hypothalamus Region of the brain linking the nervous system to the endocrine system by synthesizing and secreting neurohormones and neuropeptides. The hypothalamus is also the area of the brain that controls hunger and thirst, body temperature, and circadian cycles.

Orexigenic Stimulating food intake (e.g., AgRP, NPY, ghrelin).

Neural Circuitry Involved in Food Intake

Food intake involves several aspects of different behaviors, such as hunting for food and decision making. The complexity of feeding behavior is reflected in the number of brain areas involved; several nuclei in the caudal brain stem, hypothalamus, and the corticolimbic area are part of the feeding circuitry. Despite the large number of brain areas involved in feeding behavior, the hypothalamus is regarded as the main center for regulation of homeostatic feeding in the brain. Within the hypothalamus, the arcuate nucleus is central to the regulation of food intake. The arcuate nucleus contains at least two distinct groups of neurons controlling food intake: neurons that contain the orexigenic neuropeptides agouti-related protein (AgRP) and neuropeptide Y (NPY) and neurons that contain the anorexigenic neuropeptides pro-opiomelanocortin (POMC) and cocaine- and amphetamine-regulated transcript (CART). These arcuate neurons contain different receptors of hormones that are secreted in the periphery by adipocytes, the pancreas, and the gut in response to nutrients passing or being stored. Leptin, for example, is secreted by adipocytes, reflecting the amount of fat stores in the body. When the body becomes fat, leptin will silence orexigenic neurons and trigger anorexigenic neurons in the arcuate nucleus to secrete α-melanocyte-stimulating hormone (α-MSH) (derived from POMC) and CART to decrease food intake. In contrast to leptin, the hormone ghrelin, which is released from the (empty) stomach and which has been associated with the anticipation of meals, activates NPY/AgRP neurons and inhibits POMC/CART neurons in the arcuate nucleus. The neurons of the arcuate nucleus project to several nuclei within the hypothalamus, such as the paraventricular (PVN) and the lateral hypothalamic (LHA) nuclei, which also receive and send information from and to the caudal brain stem and corticolimbic areas. In addition to the anorexigenic and orexigenic neuropeptides in the arcuate nucleus, within the PVN corticotropin-releasing hormone (CRH) and within the LHA melanin-concentrating hormone and orexin(s) are peptides also involved in food intake regulation. Within the brain stem, groups of catecholamine cell groups are localized that project to the hypothalamus and are important for the regulation of feeding behavior, for example, in response to a glucoprivation. In the brain stem, integration of signals from the periphery (such as cholecystokinin [CCK]) takes place, carrying information on gastrointestinal distention and presence of meals in the gastrointestinal tract and signals from the hypothalamus indicating long-term nutritional status. For instance, leptin and α-MSH affect meal size, probably by determining the sensitivity for CCK at the level of the brain stem, which is released when fat-containing foods reach the duodenum. Furthermore, within the corticolimbic area, the amygdala and nucleus accumbens are implicated in the evaluation of taste and rewarding aspects of food. Taken together, this complex neural circuitry holds many brain areas, in which neuropeptides and neurotransmitters convey information important for the regulation of feeding behavior.

The brain, however, does not function on its own. To maintain a stable body weight, food intake needs to be tuned to the needs of the peripheral body. This means that when fat stores are increasing or depleting, satiety or hunger factors (e.g., hormones) are produced by different organs to change feeding behavior. For example, leptin that is secreted from adipose tissue acts on its receptor in the arcuate nucleus to decrease food intake. In addition, glucocorticoids secreted by adrenals in response to fasting act as factors to adjust feeding behavior.

Interactions with the Stress Circuitry

During stress, several neuropeptides and hormones are affected that are part of the previously described neural circuitry involved in feeding behavior. CRH in the PVN plays an initiating role in hypothalamic-pituitary-adrenocortical (HPA) axis activity and is increased with acute stress and decreased with chronic stress (through feedback effects of released glucocorticoids). In addition, acute stress increases NPY mRNA in the arcuate nucleus. In the amygdala, which is also part of processing taste information, NPY mRNA will decrease whereas CRH mRNA will increase after a stressful event. Thus, during stress, depending on the anatomical site, anorexigenic (CRH) as well as orexigenic (NPY) signaling is increased. This might result in conflicting food intake signals. Interestingly, some eat more while others eat less following stressful experiences. The individual sensitivity and reactivity in these different neural circuits may underlie the response of food intake to a stressful situation. It has also been shown that NPY induces changes in the daily rhythm of circulating corticosterone (which shows a rhythm over the day–night cycle) when rats' food intake is restricted. Interestingly, AgRP, but not NPY, mRNA levels are reduced following a stressful event. Thus, although both orexigenic neuropeptides are colocalized in the arcuate nucleus and their expression appears similarly affected following fasting, their expression is differently regulated following a stressor. Also, α-MSH interacts with the stress circuitry; central administration of α-MSH stimulates grooming and the release of ACTH and corticosterone in rats, and this activation is further increased in stressed rats.

Another overlapping system for food intake and stress responsivity is the catecholaminergic pathway between the brain stem and the hypothalamus, which is involved in feeding behavior as well as in stress responsivity. Physiological evidence that these systems indeed interact is provided by data showing effects of stress on food intake and vice versa.

Effects of Stress on Food Intake

Human studies showed that the psychophysiological response to stress is related to greater food consumption. Stress is the main trigger for obese patients to start binge eating. Moreover, people that release more cortisol due to a stressor are consuming more calories and eat significantly more sweet foods across days. Stress eaters gain more weight and are at greater risk for cardiovascular disease and type II diabetes. In Cushing's disease as well as in patients treated with corticosteroids for longer periods, a typical visceral form of obesity is induced. Generally, adrenal insufficiency is accompanied by reduced food intake and body weight. Removal of the adrenal glands in rodents results in reduced food intake and body weight, which demonstrates that corticosteroids are essential for maintaining a normal body weight. More severe traumatic environmental stressors (e.g., the loss of a spouse) can have an opposite effect, decreasing food intake and fat stores. Stress is also thought to play a central role in anorexia nervosa. The neurodevelopmental model of anorexia nervosa proposes that chronic stress in predisposed individuals results in (maladaptive) hyperactivity of the HPA axis, resulting in a loss of nutritional homeostasis. Other models, however, state that the principles of anorexia nervosa are starvation and physical activity, and that the consequential activation of the HPA axis is rewarding for the patient.

In animal models, the influence of stress (ranging from physical stress to social stress) on food intake has been studied extensively. The typical response of rodents to a wide range of stressors is to decrease food intake. Only in Syrian hamsters has it been shown that social stress increases food intake and fat stores. Most experiments studying effects of stress on food intake in rats and mice have been done using normal lab chow, which is balanced, healthy, and high in carbohydrates. In daily society, however, humans have choices, and often have easy access to cheap foods with high fat and sugar content. Providing rats with a greater choice of food results in different food intake responses when animals are subjected to a chronic stressor. Rats were given access to normal lab chow, lard, and a bottle of 1 M sugar water and were repeatedly restrained for 5 days, 3 h/day. Rats increased their intake of the more palatable items, lard and sugar, and consumed more of those as compared to the nonstressed animals.

Effects of Feeding (or Fasting) on Stress Responses

Although stress alters food intake regulation, the absence of food (fasting or starvation) is itself a stressful event. For instance, stress hormones and CRH (anorexigenic) are chronically increased in anorexia nervosa patients, which may contribute to the difficulty these patients experience in trying to reverse their illness. Stress from absence of food is, however, different from stressors such as restraint stress. Glucocorticoid receptors (GRs) in the hypothalamus are downregulated following chronic, repeated restraint, thus decreasing negative feedback on CRH mRNA in the PVN. The decreased inhibition of CRH mRNA results in fewer anorexigenic effects of the PVN CRH during starvation. Furthermore, the ACTH response to stress is altered during fasting.

Not only does the absence of food change stress responsivity, but eating palatable (e.g., sugar- and fat-containing) food also changes the response to stress.

Rats that voluntarily choose the percentage of lard in their diets (composing their own high-fat diet) have reduced HPA responses to restraint stress; however, when forced to eat a high-fat diet the response of the HPA axis to restraint is high or similar compared to rats that consume only chow. Some controversy exists regarding the stress responsivity when animals are eating a high-fat diet. Although the choice to eat fat seems important for the response to stress, rats that were force-fed a high-fat diet for a longer time did have decreased responses in activity and body temperature when socially stressed (social defeat).

Concluding Remarks

Stress clearly affects the neural circuitry regulating food intake at several levels. Some people react to stress by overeating, which contributes to the development of obesity, whereas others (e.g., anorexia nervosa patients) reduce their food intake. Differences in these coping strategies may originate in subtle differences between individuals in the neural circuitry underlying food intake and stress. A better insight into how the stress system interacts with the food intake circuitry, as well as into the mechanism underlying individual responsiveness to stress, is necessary to find new strategies to treat eating disorders such as obesity and anorexia nervosa. The type of diet also affects the stress response. Future research is needed to understand the mechanisms underlying how palatable food interacts with the neural circuitry of the stress response.

See Also the Following Articles

Food Intake and Stress, Non-Human; Food Shift Effect; Leptin, Adiponectin, Resistin; Orexin.

Further Reading

Bergh, C. and Sodersten, P. (1996). Anorexia nervosa, self-starvation and the reward of stress. *Nature Medicine* **2**, 21–22.

Berthoud, H. R. (2004). Mind versus metabolism in the control of food intake and energy balance. *Physiology and Behavior* **81**, 781–793.

Buwalda, B., Blom, W. A., Koolhaas, J. M., et al. (2001). Behavioral and physiological responses to stress are affected by high-fat feeding in male rats. *Physiology and Behavior* **73**, 371–377.

Connan, H., Campbell, I. C., Katzman, M., et al. (2003). A neurodevelopmental model for anorexia nervosa. *Physiology and Behavior* **79**, 13–24.

Conrad, C. D. and McEwen, B. S. (2000). Acute stress increases neuropeptide Y mRNA within the arcuate nucleus and hilus of the dentate gyrus. *Molecular Brain Research* **79**, 102–109.

Dallman, M. F., Akana, S. F., Bhatnagar, S., et al. (2000). Bottomed out: metabolic significance of the circadian trough in glucocorticoid concentrations. *International Journal of Obesity and Related Metabolic Disorders* **24**(supplement 2), S40–S46.

Dallman, M. F., Pecoraro, N. C. and la Fleur, S. E. (2004). Chronic stress and comfort foods: self-medication and abdominal obesity. *Brain Behavior and Immunity* **19**, 275–280.

Donohoe, T. P. (1984). Stress-induced anorexia: implications for anorexia nervosa. *Life Science* **34**, 203–218.

Epel, E., Lapidus, R., McEwen, B., et al. (2001). Stress may add bite to appetite in women: a laboratory study of stress-induced cortisol and eating behavior. *Psychoneuroendocrinology* **26**, 37–49.

Foster, M. T., Solomon, M. B., Huhman, K. L. and Bartness, T. J. (2006). Social defeat increases food intake, body mass and adiposity in syrian hamsters. *American Journal of Physiology. Regulatory, Integrative and Comparative Physiology* **290**, R1284–R1293.

Hillebrand, J. J., De Wied, D. and Adan, R. A. (2002). Neuropeptides, food intake and body weight regulation: a hypothalamic focus. *Peptides* **23**, 2283–2306.

Inui, A. (2001). Eating behavior in anorexia nervosa – an excess of both orexigenic and anorexigenic signaling? *Molecular Psychiatry* **6**, 620–624.

Kas, M. J., Bruijnzeel, A. W., Haanstra, J. R., et al. (2005). Differential regulation of agouti-related protein and neuropeptide Y in hypothalamic neurons following a stressful event. *Journal of Molecular Endocrinology* **35**, 159–164.

la Fleur, S. E., Houshyar, H., Roy, M., et al. (2005). Choice of lard, but not total lard calories, damps adrenocorticotropin responses to restraint. *Endocrinology* **146**, 2193–2199.

Makino, S., Kaneda, T., Nishiyama, M., et al. (2001). Lack of decrease in hypothalamic and hippocampal glucocorticoid receptor mRNA during starvation. *Neuroendocrinology* **74**, 120–128.

Solomon, M. R. (2001). Eating as both coping and stressor in overweight control. *Journal of Advanced Nursing* **36**, 563–572.

Von Frijtag, J. C., Croiset, G., Gispen, W. H., et al. (1998). The role of central melanocortin receptors in the activation of the hypothalamus-pituitary-adrenal-axis and the induction of excessive grooming. *British Journal of Pharmacology* **123**, 1503–1508.

Leptin, Adiponectin, Resistin, Ghrelin

A Gavrila, D Barb and C S Mantzoros
Beth Israel Deaconess Medical Center, Boston, MA, USA

Glossary

Adipocytokine Cytokines secreted by adipose tissue (i.e., leptin, adiponectin, and resistin).

Adiponectin Hormone secreted by fat cells that modulates several physiological processes, such as glucose and fatty acid metabolism. Decreased plasma adiponectin levels are associated with obesity, insulin resistance, type 2 diabetes mellitus, and atherosclerosis.

Adipose tissue Specialized connective tissue composed of fat cells (adipocytes), which store droplets of fat in the form of triglycerides and have many other important metabolic roles.

Adipostatic peptide An agent that prevents adipocyte/fat cell accumulation.

Anorexia nervosa An eating disorder that occurs most frequently in adolescent females and is characterized by the lack or loss of appetite, known as anorexia. Other features include excessive fear of becoming overweight, body image disturbance, significant weight loss, refusal to maintain minimal normal weight, and amenorrhea.

Anorexigenic peptide An agent that transiently depresses food intake.

Cachexia Extreme weight loss, usually associated with chronic disease.

Cytokine A protein secreted by inflammatory leukocytes but also by nonleukocytic cells; cytokines act as intercellular mediators and differ from classic hormones in that they are produced by a number of tissues or cell types rather than by specialized glands.

Ghrelin A peptide produced and secreted from stomach that stimulates growth hormone release and, in addition, increases appetite and food intake.

Insulin A protein hormone secreted by the pancreas that plays a major role in the regulation of glucose metabolism, promoting the cellular use of glucose; also an important regulator of protein and lipid metabolism.

Leptin A hormone secreted by fat cells and implicated in the regulation of food intake and energy balance, depressing appetite and increasing energy expenditure.

Orexigenic peptide An agent that stimulates food intake.

Resistin A hormone secreted by fat cells that may play a role in insulin resistance and inflammation associated with obesity.

Introduction

Obesity has become a public health problem due to its increasing prevalence and associated morbidity and mortality, mainly from cardiovascular disease, type 2 diabetes, and certain malignancies. In addition to a genetic predisposition, environmental factors, physical inactivity, a high-energy high-fat diet, smoking, and stress (which results in dysregulation of endogenous hormones) strongly contribute to the development of this multifcatorial disorder.

Obesity is known to be associated with insulin resistance and development of the metabolic syndrome. However, not all obese patients are insulin-resistant and total fat mass *per se* is not the most important factor contributing to insulin resistance but, rather, the presence of central or visceral obesity. Central obesity has been associated with the dysregulation of the hypothalamic-pituitary-adrenal (HPA) axis and the sympathetic nervous system. The stress hormones of the HPA axis (i.e., cortisol) and the sympathetic system (catecholamines) oppose the effects of insulin, and this may promote insulin resistance. A chronically stressed HPA axis leads to decreased circadian variations in circulating cortisol levels, and chronic glucocorticoid exposure may lead to increased food intake and obesity.

In parallel with the increasing prevalence of obesity, there has been a tremendous increase in research activity in a global effort to better understand energy balance and the regulation of metabolism and body weight. Although a biological basis for body fat regulation was first proposed more than 50 years ago, the hypothesis of an endocrine feedback loop regulating body weight remained elusive until the discovery of the adipocyte-secreted hormone leptin in 1994. This discovery has dramatically changed our understanding of adipose tissue from an inert depot of energy storage to an active organ producing and secreting various molecules that regulate metabolism and energy homeostasis, such as leptin, adiponectin, and resistin (see **Table 1**). In addition, it has recently been recognized that other peripheral organs, such as the gastrointestinal tract, secrete molecules that also convey information on energy intake and balance. For example, ghrelin, a novel gastrointestinal tract-secreted

Table 1 Adipocytokines and ghrelin: effects on energy homeostasis[a]

Molecule	*Site of production*	*Circulating levels*	*Target organ/tissue*	*Effect on insulin sensitivity*	*Effect on energy expenditure*	*Stress interaction*	*Other effects*
Adiponectin	Adipose tissue (primary) Cardiomyocytes[b] Placenta[b]	Decreased in obesity, type 2 DM, CVD, malignancies	Muscle Liver Hypothalamus (PVN nucleus)	Increases insulin sensitivity Stimulates glucose uptake Stimulates fatty acid oxidation Decreases gluconeogenesis	Increases energy expenditure Decreases body weight without affecting food intake (ICV administration)	Exo- or endogenous glucocorticoids inhibit adiponectin secretion	Anti-inflammatory Anti-atherogenic Anti-carcinogenic
Ghrelin	GI tract: stomach (enterochromaffin cells) (primary)	Increased acutely before each meal	Pituitary (GH-releasing cells)	May reduce insulin sensitivity	Decreases energy expenditure	Ghrelin stimulates ACTH release and activates HPA	Increases gastric motility and acid secretion
	Hypothalamus (ARC nucleus)	Decreased in obesity	Hypothalamus (NPY and AgRP neurons)	Decreased glucose disposal rate during ghrelin infusion	Increases appetite and stimulates food intake	Acute psychological stress raises plasma ghrelin in rodents	Reduces locomotor activity
		Elevated in anorexia nervosa or cachexia		Increases GH release Enhances the use of carbohydrates and reduces fat use	Reduces thermogenesis	Activation of gut sympathetic nerves stimulate ghrelin secretion	
Leptin	Adipose tissue (primary) Hypothalamus[b] Pituitary[b] Placenta[b] Skeletal muscle[b] Gastric and mammary epithelia[b]	Increased in proportion to body fat	Hypothalamus (ARC) Brain stem	Increases insulin sensitivity Stimulates glucose uptake Stimulates free fatty acid oxidation	Increases energy expenditure Decreases appetite, food intake, and body weight Increases sympathetic activity Stimulates thermogenesis	Suppresses the activity of the HPA axis (CRH, ACTH, cortisol) Glucocorticoids stimulate leptin secretion, but excess may contribute to leptin resistance	Stimulates reproductive and thyroid functions Stimulates immunity Inhibits bone formation
Resistin	Adipose tissue Mononuclear leukocytes Macrophages	Variable in obesity	Liver ? Muscle ? Hypothalamus ?	Decreases insulin sensitivity in rodents (impairs insulin action on hepatic glucose production and may decrease fatty acid oxidation) Controversial in humans	May decrease energy expenditure in rodents Controversial in humans	Unknown	Inhibits adipocyte differentiation in rodents May have pro-inflammatory effects

[a]ACTH, adrenocorticotropic hormone; AgRP, agouti-related protein; ARC, arcuate nucleus; CRH, corticotropin releasing hormone; CVD, cardiovascular disease; DM, diabetes mellitus; GH, growth hormone; GI, gastrointestinal; HPA, hypothalamic-pituitary-adrenal; ICV, intracerebroventricular; NPY, neuropeptide Y; PVN, paraventricular nucleus.
[b]At low levels.

peptide, not only stimulates the secretion of growth hormone (GH) from the pituitary but also plays an important role in energy homeostasis, causing a positive energy balance by stimulating food intake.

The currently accepted model of energy homeostasis proposes that peripheral signals, such as molecules secreted into the circulation from the gut and the adipose tissue, are received and integrated by the central nervous system together with other signals/modulators of food intake and energy homeostasis, such as visual stimuli, smell, the presence of food, social habits or social behavior, and stress, with the final purpose to match food intake with energy expenditure. Signals from both adipose tissue and other peripheral organs not only are processed centrally in the brain to control body metabolism and energy but may also influence other physiological functions, such as the neuroendocrine and reproductive systems.

Various central and peripheral factors involved in energy homeostasis are being continuously discovered, and it is expected that a better understanding of these mechanisms will lead to effective treatments for the control of metabolism and obesity. This review discusses the potential role of four recently discovered molecules involved in metabolism and energy homeostasis: leptin, adiponectin, resistin, and ghrelin.

Adipose Tissue

The adipose tissue is considered today to be a very active and complex endocrine organ. Adipocytes produce and secrete a variety of bioactive molecules, including adipokines, which act at both the local (paracrine/autocrine) and systemic (endocrine) levels to exert diverse metabolic functions. These adipokines include leptin, tumor necrosis factor (TNF)-α, and interleukin (IL)-6, which have already been intensively studied, as well as newer molecules, such as adiponectin and resistin, which may prove to have important roles in controlling metabolism and energy homeostasis.

Leptin

Leptin (from Greek *leptos*, thin) is a 167-amino-acid protein discovered in 1994 as the product of the obese (*ob*) gene. Although known to have numerous other physiological functions in mice and humans, leptin is primarily involved in the control of the neuroendocrine and immune response to energy deprivation. Leptin is produced predominantly by adipose tissue and is secreted into the circulation at levels that are directly proportional to fat mass. Leptin is also expressed at low levels in the hypothalamus, pituitary, placenta, skeletal muscle, and gastric and mammary epithelia. Leptin is found in the peripheral circulation in both a free and a bound form; the free form crosses the blood–brain barrier, binds to the long isoform of a specific leptin class 1 cytokine receptor (also known as ObRb) and activates mainly the janus kinase (JAK)–signal transducer and activator of transcription (STAT) and phosphatidylinositol 3 (PI3)–AKT pathways to convey information to the central nervous system regarding the amount of energy stored in adipose tissue and acute changes in caloric intake. Leptin receptors are predominantly found in the hypothalamus, mainly in the arcuate nucleus but also in the brain stem and other regions of the central nervous system. The activation of hypothalamic receptors stimulates the production of anorectic peptides, such as α-melanin-stimulating hormone (α-MSH) and cocaine and amphetamine-regulated transcript (CART), and inhibits the production of orexigenic peptides, such as neuropeptide Y (NPY) and agouti-related peptide (AgRP), resulting in the inhibition of appetite. In addition, leptin binding to hypothalamic receptors results in increased sympathetic activity, which stimulates free fatty acid oxidation and thermogenesis in brown adipose tissue, thus favoring energy expenditure in mice.

Leptin expression is mainly controlled by the amount of body fat mass; caloric restriction and weight loss results in decreased circulating leptin levels, whereas overfeeding and increasing adipose tissue mass results in increased leptin levels. Leptin production and secretion is also increased by insulin, glucocorticoids, TNF-α, and estrogens; it is decreased by β_3-adrenergic activity, androgens, free fatty acids, growth hormone, and peroxisome proliferator activated receptor (PPAR)-γ agonists.

The direct involvement of leptin in the regulation of energy intake and expenditure (by signaling the adequacy of energy stores to the brain) was initially demonstrated in studies in mice. Mutations in the obese (*ob*) gene (leptin gene) and the diabetes (*db*) gene (leptin receptor gene) result in morbid obesity and diabetes, whereas the administration of leptin to leptin deficient (*ob/ob*) and normal rodents results in significant weight loss. However, diet-induced obese mice, the mouse model of obesity that most closely corresponds to garden-variety obesity in humans, are not able to lose weight significantly after leptin administration, indicating that these hyperleptinemic mice are leptin resistant, probably due to receptor or postreceptor defects.

Similarly, only a distinct minority of morbidly obese human subjects have congenital leptin deficiency due to mutations of the *ob* gene, which result in hyperphagia and early-onset, rapid weight gain. The administration of exogenous leptin to these patients results in the normalization of their hyperphagia, decreased caloric intake, and a significant loss of fat mass. Rare inactivating mutations of the leptin receptor gene have also been reported, which, similar to leptin gene defects, manifest clinically with hyperphagia and extreme obesity, as well as hypogonadotropic hypogonadism, but they are also associated with growth delay and secondary hypothyroidism. Our studies have shown that increasing leptin levels precede the onset of puberty, suggesting that leptin may be a permissive factor for the onset of puberty in humans.

Although exogeneous leptin administration is an effective treatment, resulting in significant weight loss in obese leptin-deficient subjects, the majority of the cases of human obesity do not respond to leptin therapy. It is now known that most obese individuals have increased leptin production and secretion from adipocytes as well as high circulating leptin levels, features that are consistent with a state of leptin resistance. Several mechanisms are involved in the leptin resistance of obese individuals, including defective transport of leptin across the blood–brain barrier into the brain and/or reduced hypothalamic leptin signaling, in part due to the upregulation of specific inhibitors of leptin signaling. A complete understanding of the pathogenesis of leptin resistance in humans may open new pathways for the treatment of obesity.

Interestingly, a small study reported that exogenous leptin administration to replace leptin levels to pre-weight-loss levels, prevented the regaining of weight, and promoted the loss of fat mass in a small group of subjects participating in a weight loss program. These findings need to be confirmed by larger studies.

There is accumulating evidence that leptin has complex neuroendocrine functions, regulating the activity of the HPA and also the hypothalamic-pituitary-gonadal and -thyroid axes. It has been reported that leptin suppresses the activity of the HPA; that is, decreased leptin levels during fasting/starvation are associated with increased activation of the HPA and cortisol secretion. In accordance with this, in critically ill patients the nocturnal fall in leptin levels is associated with a paradoxical increase of nocturnal adrenocorticotropic hormone (ACTH) and cortisol levels. Leptin-deficient mice and humans fail to go through puberty, and leptin administration reverses this abnormality. We have shown that the decreased leptin levels found in food deprivation are responsible for the starvation-induced suppression of the hypothalamic-pituitary-gonadal axis as well as changes in the function of other neuroendocrine axes in humans. In addition, extremely thin women with hypothalamic amenorrhea have low leptin levels and exogenous leptin administration normalizes their neuroendocrine and reproductive functions. Thus, it seems that leptin may act as the critical link between adipose tissue and not only hypothalamic centers regulating energy homeostasis but also the reproductive system, indicating whether adequate energy reserves are present for normal reproductive function. Further larger trials are needed to conclusively prove whether leptin replacement treatment can ameliorate or treat the neuroendocrine dysfunction and also the immune abnormalities, osteoporosis, and infertility in women with hypothalamic amenorrhea.

In addition to signaling in the central nervous system, leptin also acts in the periphery and has important roles in regulating insulin action and lipid metabolism. Other peripheral endocrine effects include the direct regulation of immune function, hematopoesis, angiogenesis, and direct and indirect effects on bone metabolism.

Taken together, these findings suggest that leptin plays a significant role in the central regulation of energy balance and that leptin is a critical signal for neuroendocrine function in humans; this raises the possibility that leptin is indeed not only an adipostatic hormone but also a stress-related hormone crucial for survival.

Adiponectin

Adiponectin (Acrp30, apM1 protein, adipoQ, or GBP28) is a 247-amino-acid protein discovered simultaneously by four different research groups in the mid-1990s. Adiponectin is produced and secreted exclusively by differentiated adipocytes and represents one of the most abundant serum proteins that circulates in tightly associated trimers and higher-order oligomers. Eight adiponectin isoforms with variable potency have been isolated, which bind and activate at least two adiponectin receptors. Adiponectin receptor 1 (AdipoR1) is expressed ubiquitously but most abundantly in skeletal muscle and has a high affinity for globular adiponectin and a very low affinity for full-length adiponectin; adiponectin receptor 2 (AdipoR2) is found predominantly in the liver and has an intermediate affinity for both forms.

Adiponectin decreases with increasing overall and central adiposity and increases with prolonged weight reduction. In humans, although short-term fasting does not influence circulating levels of adiponectin, prolonged caloric restriction results in weight loss and increased adiponectin levels. In addition, daily caloric intake, macronutrient intake, and high fat intake do not correlate with and do not affect circulating adiponectin levels in humans, except possibly in obese individuals, but a Mediterranean-type diet, which has beneficial effects on morbidity and mortality, increases adiponectin levels. Interestingly, studies in rodents have revealed that central and peripheral adiponectin administration increases energy expenditure by stimulating free fatty acid oxidation and glucose uptake, thus reducing body weight and visceral adiposity without affecting energy intake.

Although its role has not been definitively established, there is accumulating evidence that adiponectin regulates insulin sensitivity and is also involved in inflammation and atherosclerosis. Initial animal studies showed that adiponectin-knockout mice develop insulin resistance either independently of diet or only after high-fat and high-sucrose diet, whereas adiponectin treatment improves their insulin resistance. In addition, lipoatrophic and obese mice have low adiponectin levels and insulin resistance, which improve partially after exogenous adiponectin administration. Moreover, the decrease in circulating adiponectin levels parallels the development of insulin resistance and type 2 diabetes in a longitudinal study of rhesus monkeys.

Studies in humans showed that there is a negative correlation of adiponectin levels with fasting glucose, insulin, and insulin resistance and a positive correlation with insulin sensitivity, independent of body–mass index (BMI). We also know that the adiponectin gene has the same location as one of the diabetes susceptibility genes on chromosome 3q27, and several longitudinal studies showed that human subjects with lower baseline adiponectin levels are more likely to develop type 2 diabetes, independent of adiposity. In contrast, type 1 diabetic patients may have elevated adiponectin levels compared to nondiabetic individuals, whereas chronically administered insulin does not have an effect on adiponectin levels.

Taken together, all these findings show that adiponectin levels are low in states of insulin resistance, such as obesity and type 2 diabetes, and adiponectin levels increase with improved insulin sensitivity after weight reduction or treatment with insulin-sensitizing drugs (thiazolidindiones). It is currently thought that adiponectin represents a link among obesity, insulin resistance, and various other metabolic abnormalities associated with obesity.

Adiponectin improves insulin sensitivity through multiple cellular and molecular mechanisms that are not entirely known at present. An important enzyme stimulated by adiponectin is AMP-activated protein kinase (AMPK), which, in turn, phosphorylates several intracellular proteins to alter various cellular functions, including the enhancement of insulin-stimulated glucose uptake into fat and skeletal muscle as well as the suppression of hepatic glucose production and stimulation of fatty acid oxidation. By increasing fatty acid oxidation through AMPK activation, adiponectin decreases circulating free fatty acids, resulting thus in improved insulin action. Adiponectin may also improve insulin sensitivity by inducing the activation of the insulin signaling system. Moreover, by stimulating nitric oxide (NO) formation, adiponectin may augment vascular blood flow to promote glucose uptake.

In addition to its insulin-sensitizing effects, adiponectin is also related to the lipid profile, another independent risk factor for cardiovascular disease. Previous studies reported a strong positive association between adiponectin and high-density lipoprotein (HDL) cholesterol and a negative association with serum triglyceride levels. However, there is no independent relationship between adiponectin and low-density lipoprotein (LDL) or total cholesterol. Adiponectin may lead to a favorable lipid profile by stimulating fatty acid oxidation, an effect probably mediated by AMPK. However, one study reported increased fatty acid oxidation in muscle cells in adiponectin-knockout mice, and a cross-sectional study of humans found that plasma adiponectin levels did not correlate with lipid oxidation, as measured by energy expenditure and respiratory quotient. Thus, further studies are needed to understand adiponectin's effects on fatty acid oxidation.

Adiponectin may also exert important anti-inflammatory and atheroprotective effects. It inhibits the production and action of several inflammatory factors involved in atherosclerosis, including TNF-α, and also suppresses monocyte adhesion and macrophage transformation to foam cells within the vascular wall. In addition, adiponectin inhibits smooth muscle cell proliferation in the vascular wall by inhibiting growth factors that promote hyperplasia and promotes vasodilation and angiogenesis by increasing NO production in endothelial cells through AMPK activation. In conclusion, adiponectin's involvement in cardiovascular disease is probably multifactorial, including its effects on risk factors such as insulin resistance and dyslipidemia but also a direct effect on the vascular system.

Furthermore, there is emerging mechanistic and epidemiological evidence supporting a protective role of adiponectin in malignancies. *In vitro* treatment of acute myelomonocytic leukemia cell lines with adiponectin suppressed the growth of myelomonocyte cells, induced apoptosis, and downregulated *Bcl-2* gene expression. More recently, adiponectin has been shown to be a direct inhibitor of angiogenesis *in vivo* and *in vitro* through the activation of caspases in endothelial cells. Consistent with the *in vitro* studies, which suggest that adiponectin is an important negative regulator of hematopoesis and the immune system, *in vivo* intratumoral administration of murine adiponectin resulted in significant suppression of T241 fibrosarcoma tumor growth. Adiponectin receptors are expressed by prostate, hepatocellular carcinoma, and various other cancer cell types (breast, endometrial, colon, and neuroblastoma cell lines). Recent experiments suggest that adiponectin may act on tumor cells directly through the activation of c-jun NH_2-terminal kinase, a mammalian MAPK family involved in the regulation of cell proliferation and apoptosis, and also through the suppression of the transcription factor signal transducer and activator of transcription (STAT)3, which also regulates cell proliferation, differentiation, survival, and apoptosis. Therefore, given its antiangiogenesis properties and the inactivation of STAT3 reported in obesity and associated malignancies, adiponectin may prove to be an effective novel anticancer agent.

Epidemiological evidence also suggests that adiponectin plays an important role in the insulin-related pathways of carcinogenesis, independently of other known risk factors for cancers. We and others have recently reported that circulating adiponectin levels are inversely associated with risk for endometrial, breast, prostate, gastric, and colorectal cancer. In two recent case–control studies, we reported that women with high BMI and low plasma adiponectin had a 6.5-fold increased risk of endometrial cancer, independent of the possible effects of insulin-like growth factor (IGF-)1, IGF-2, IGF binding protein (IGFBP-)3, leptin, BMI, and other known risk factors of the disease. We also found in a prospective study in men that individuals in the highest quintile of adiponectin levels had an approximately 60% reduced risk for colorectal cancer compared to the lowest quintile. Significantly, these associations were also independent of body size and physical activity.

In addition, adiponectin levels may also correlate inversely with tumor size, histological grade, and disease stage in gastric and prostate cancer. Large association and prospective studies to prove adiponectin's role in the development of malignancies as well as mechanistic studies to address potential roles of adiponectin in cancer pathogenesis are needed.

Resistin

Resistin (adipose-tissue-specific secretory factor or FIZZ3) is a 94-amino-acid polypeptide with 11 cysteine residues. Resistin is almost entirely expressed and excreted from white adipose tissue in mice and circulates as a dimer. A single dicysteine residue is required for dimerization, whereas the remaining 10 cysteine residues are involved in determining the structure of the resistin monomeric unit.

Similar to adiponectin, resistin has been postulated to link obesity with insulin resistance, but these two molecules probably have opposite functions. In 2001, Steppan and colleagues reported that resistin secretion is decreased by the antidiabetic drug rosiglitazone and is increased in diet-induced and genetic mouse models of obesity. Moreover, the administration of antiresistin antibody improves blood sugar and insulin action in obese mice, and the administration of recombinant resistin impairs glucose tolerance and insulin action in normal mice. More recent studies have shown that resistin may increase hepatic insulin resistance by inhibiting AMPK and may also increase hepatic glucose production, thus controlling glucose and lipid metabolism. In addition, resistin has been postulated to regulate adipose tissue mass by inhibiting adipocyte differentiation and thus limit adipose tissue formation in response to increased energy intake. These observations have not been confirmed by other studies, however; thus, the role of resistin in mice remains controversial.

Human data are even more conflicting. Although resistin is expressed at very low levels in human adipose cells, high levels are expressed in circulating mononuclear leukocytes and macrophages. Similar to its distribution in rodents, resistin is found in human sera, and several studies (but not all) reported increased levels in obese and diabetic patients and a positive association with insulin resistance. One study showed that human resistin expression, but not serum levels, is proportional to insulin resistance, and several studies failed to show an association with insulin resistance. Resistin may have pro-inflammatory effects because recent *in vitro* studies found that resistin induces the expression of adhesion molecules such as vascular cell adhesion molecule (VCAM)-1 and intercellular adhesion molecule (ICAM)-1 in human endothelial cells.

Further studies are required to determine whether stress influences resistin levels and to elucidate the role of resistin in regulating insulin sensitivity. In addition, whether resistin influences obesity either directly or indirectly by altering glucose and insulin levels and whether resistin plays a role in inflammation associated with obesity warrant further investigation.

Gastrointestinal Tract: Ghrelin

Ghrelin, a 28-amino-acid lipophilic peptide with a labile octanoyl fatty acid side chain at the serine residue 3, was originally discovered by Kojima and coworkers during their search for an endogenous growth hormone secretagogue. This hormone is expressed primarily in specialized enterochromaffin cells (called X/A-like cells), which are located mainly in the mucosa of the fundus of the stomach. In addition, ghrelin-immunoreactive cells are also found in the intestine, with their concentration gradually decreasing from duodenum to colon; they are also found in the pancreatic islets, brain, and kidney. Ghrelin-producing neurons are located in the hypothalamus, more specifically in the hypothalamic arcuate nucleus, an important region controlling appetite, but also in previously uncharacterized neurons adjacent to the third ventricle, which send efferent fibers to NPY and AgRP neurons, stimulating the release of these orexigenic peptides.

Ghrelin binds to the growth hormone secretagogue receptor (GHS-R), a typical G-protein-coupled receptor, the activation of which by ghrelin results in increased intracellular calcium via the activation of the phospholipase C pathway. GHS-Rs are expressed in various regions of the brain, predominantly in the growth hormone-releasing somatotroph cells of the pituitary gland. Ghrelin stimulates the release of growth hormone from the pituitary in a dose-dependent manner and acts synergistically with growth hormone-releasing hormone (GHRH). In addition, ghrelin has a weak prolactin (PRL) and ACTH-releasing activity, but more important ghrelin can modulate gonadotropin-releasing hormone (GnRH) pulses, possibly being one of the signals that turns off the gonadal axis during starvation. The expression of ghrelin in the pituitary is high after birth and declines with puberty.

In addition to being a potent growth hormone secretagogue, ghrelin is a potent appetite stimulant. Ghrelin administration by intracerebroventricular, intravenous, or subcutaneous injection increases food intake and body weight, decreases fat use, and increases gastric acid output in a dose-dependent manner. Administered to rats by intracerebroventricular injections, ghrelin induces Fos protein expression, a marker of neuronal activation, in regions of primary importance in the regulation of feeding, including NPY neurons and AgRP neurons, but also in the neurons of the solitary tract nucleus and the dorsomotor nucleus of vagus. The latter may sustain a role for ghrelin in the central regulation of gastric acid secretion and gastric motility via vagal cholinergic pathways.

Ghrelin circulates in the bloodstream in two forms, acylated and desaclyl ghrelin, with the acylated form being the biologically active form of ghrelin. Serum levels of ghrelin depend on the state of nutrition and are negatively correlated with the BMI. Accordingly, circulating ghrelin levels are decreased in obesity but elevated during fasting and in anorexia nervosa and cachexia, a finding that may reflect a compensatory mechanism. Acute psychological stress raises plasma ghrelin in the rat, and the activation of gut sympathetic nerves directly stimulate ghrelin secretion. Also, an increase in plasma ghrelin leads to the release of ACTH and the activation of the HPA axis. Recent human data demonstrated an inverse correlation between ghrelin and leptin that is independent of adiposity, but there is no regulation of ghrelin by leptin administration over the short term (a few hours to a few days).

In normal humans, plasma ghrelin levels rise immediately before each meal and in response to diet-induced weight loss and fall to minimum levels 1 h after feeding. This fall in ghrelin levels after a meal is correlated with insulin peak, suggesting that insulin may be a negative regulator of ghrelin secretion in the postprandial state. This fall in ghrelin levels after a meal is absent or blunted in obese humans, a fact that, researchers propose, may contribute to the development of their obesity. Significantly, obese patients who undergo gastric bypass surgery have significantly lowered ghrelin levels after surgery, which, on the basis of observational studies, has been proposed to contribute to maintaining decreased weight after bypass surgery.

Finally, what are potential clinical applications of ghrelin? It has been suggested that blocking or neutralizing ghrelin action may prove to be a reasonable pharmacological approach to reverse a chronically positive energy balance, such as in obesity. However, in contrast to predictions made from the pharmacology of ghrelin, studies in ghrelin-null mice showed that the deletion of ghrelin impairs neither growth nor appetite. In fact, ghrelin-null mice are neither anorexic nor dwarfs and display normal responses to starvation and diet-induced obesity, strongly suggesting that ghrelin is not critically required for viability, fertility, growth, appetite, or fat deposition. Thus, antagonists of ghrelin may not prove to be very successful antiobesity agents. In contrast, exploring its orexigenic activity for the treatment of eating disorders such as anorexia nervosa or the replacement of ghrelin in ghrelin-deficient states such as cachexia or other catabolic states seems to be a more reasonable approach.

Conclusion

This brief review has covered recent advances in the area of molecules regulating energy homeostasis and metabolism – leptin, adiponectin, resistin, and ghrelin. Most probably, we can expect other related hormones to be added to this list in the near future. In addition, synthetic analogs, agonists, or antagonists are expected to be developed by the pharmaceutical industry for the management of states of energy excess, such as obesity and type 2 diabetes, and states of energy deficiency, such as anorexia nervosa and hypothalamic amenorrhea.

See Also the Following Articles

Feeding Circuitry (and Neurochemistry); Food Intake and Stress, Non-Human; Gleucocorticoid Negative Feedback; Obesity, Stress and; Orexin.

Further Reading

Ahima, R. S. (2005). Central actions of adipocyte hormones. *Trends in Endocrinology and Metabolism* **16**, 307–313.

Barb, D., Pazaitou-Panayiotou, K. and Mantzoros, C. S. (2006). Adiponectin: a link between obesity and cancer. *Expert Opinions on Investigational Drugs* **15**, 917–931.

Bjorbaek, C. and Kahn, B. B. (2004). Leptin signaling in the central nervous system and the periphery. *Recent Progress in Hormone Research* **59**, 305–331.

Bluher, S. and Mantzoros, C. S. (2004). The role of leptin in regulating neuroendocrine function in humans. *Journal of Nutrition* **134**, 2469S–2474S.

Brennan, A. M. and Mantzoros, C. S. (2006). Drug insight: the role of leptin in human physiology and pathophysiology-emerging clinical applications. *Nature Clinical Practice: Endocrinology & Metabolism* **2**(6), 318–324.

Buren, J. and Eriksson, J. W. (2005). Is insulin resistance caused by defects in insulin's target cells or by a stressed mind? *Diabetes/Metabolism Research and Reviews* **21**(6), 487–494.

Chan, J. L. and Mantzoros, C. S. (2005). Role of leptin in energy-deprivation states: normal human physiology and clinical implications for hypothalamic amenorrhoea and anorexia nervosa. *Lancet* **366**, 74–85.

Gale, S. M., Castracane, V. D. and Mantzoros, C. S. (2004). Energy homeostasis, obesity and eating disorders: recent advances in endocrinology. *Journal of Nutrition* **134**, 295–298.

Haslam, D. W. and James, W. P. (2005). Obesity. *Lancet* **366**, 1197–1209.

Havel, P. J. (2004). Update on adipocyte hormones: regulation of energy balance and carbohydrate/lipid metabolism. *Diabetes* **53**(supplement 1), S143–S151.

Kadowaki, T. and Yamauchi, T. (2005). Adiponectin and adiponectin receptors. *Endocrine Review* **26**, 439–451.

Kojima, M. and Kangawa, K. (2005). Ghrelin: structure and function. *Physiological Reviews* **85**, 495–522.

Munzberg, H., Bjornholm, M., Bates, S. H., et al. (2005). Leptin receptor action and mechanisms of leptin resistance. *Cellular and Molecular Life Sciences* **62**, 642–652.

Shetty, G. K., Barb, D. and Mantzoros, C. S. (2006). Nutrients and peripherally secreted molecules in regulation of energy homeostasis. In: Mantzoros, C. S. (ed.) *Obesity and diabetes*, pp. 69–86. Totowa, NJ: Humana Press.

Steppan, C. M. and Lazar, M. A. (2004). The current biology of resistin. *Journal of Internal Medicine* **255**, 439–447.

Orexin

W K Samson and M M White
St. Louis University, St. Louis, MO, USA
A V Ferguson
Queen's University, Kingston, ON, Canada

Glossary

Adrenocorticotropic hormone (ACTH)	A stress hormone that activates hormone secretion from the adrenal gland.
Cerebroventricles	Fluid-filled cavities in the brain where test compounds often are injected *in vivo*.
Circumventricular organs	Sites in the brain where there is no blood–brain barrier.
Corticosterone	A steroid hormone released from the adrenal gland during stress that facilitates energy delivery to the nervous system and stimulates the production of new glucose.
Hypothalamus	A brain region responsible for coordinating the appropriate endocrine, cardiovascular, and behavioral responses to stress.
Prolactin (PRL)	A hormone released from the anterior pituitary gland in stress that exerts multiple tissue-specific effects.
Rostral ventrolateral medulla	An important site in the hindbrain where neurons organize and control sympathetic efferent activity.
Stress hormones	Chemical messengers released from the anterior pituitary gland during physical or emotional stimuli.

Discovery of the Orexins

The lateral hypothalamic area (LHA) has long been considered to be an important site for the regulation of feeding behavior. In 1998, two groups independently identified the production of novel peptides in this region. deLecea and colleagues named these peptides hypocretins because of their apparent production in the hypothalamus and their structural homology to the members of the secretin family of peptides. Sakurai and collaborators named these peptides orexins on the basis of their ability when administered intracebroventricularly (ICV) to stimulate food intake. It is now recognized that the peptides exert many physiologically relevant actions in brain, the majority of which are seemingly related to behavioral, endocrine, and cardiovascular responses to stress.

For convenience we use here the nomenclature advanced by Sakurai. Orexin A and orexin B are postranslational products of the same prohormone (**Figure 1**). Two receptor proteins have been identified, the orexin type 1 receptor (OX_1R), which binds both peptides but prefers orexin A as a ligand, and the orexin type 2 receptor (OX_2R), which binds both peptides with approximately equal affinity. The two receptors are differentially distributed, as listed in **Table 1**.

The distribution of the orexin receptors predicted more biological actions than simply those related to food intake. Indeed, receptor localization in the dorsal raphe, tuberomammillary nuclei, and locus ceruleus (LC), areas known to be important in arousal state and sleep/wakefulness, predicted the eventual finding that the orexins are important determinants of sleep/wakefulness. The absence of the receptors in dogs and degeneration of orexin-expressing neurons in animal models and humans results in the syndrome narcolepsy/cataplexy. Thus, the major role recognized at this time for these peptides is one of arousal. Aspects of the narcolepsy/cataplexy syndrome highlight other reported biological actions of the orexins, particularly those related to stress.

Orexins and the Stress Response

Orexins and Cardiovascular Function

Soon after their discovery, the orexins were demonstrated by several groups to act in the brain to elevate blood pressure and heart rate. The effects are mediated via the activation of the sympathetic nervous system, as demonstrated by the use of α-adrenergic antagonist blockade (phentolamine) and the demonstration of increased sympathetic nerve activity. Increased cardiovascular function was observed following the ICV or direct tissue-specific administration of the peptides into the area postrema, rostral ventrolateral medulla, and medial nucleus tractus solitarius; the direct effects on preganglionic sympathetic neurons in the intermediolateral cell column (IMDL); and the ability of intrathecal administration of orexin to activate these neurons. In addition, orexin has been shown to influence the excitability of paraventricular nucleus (PVN) parvocellular and nucleus tractus solitarius (NTS) neurons. This does not rule out the potential contribution of vagal withdrawal to the observed increased heart rate following

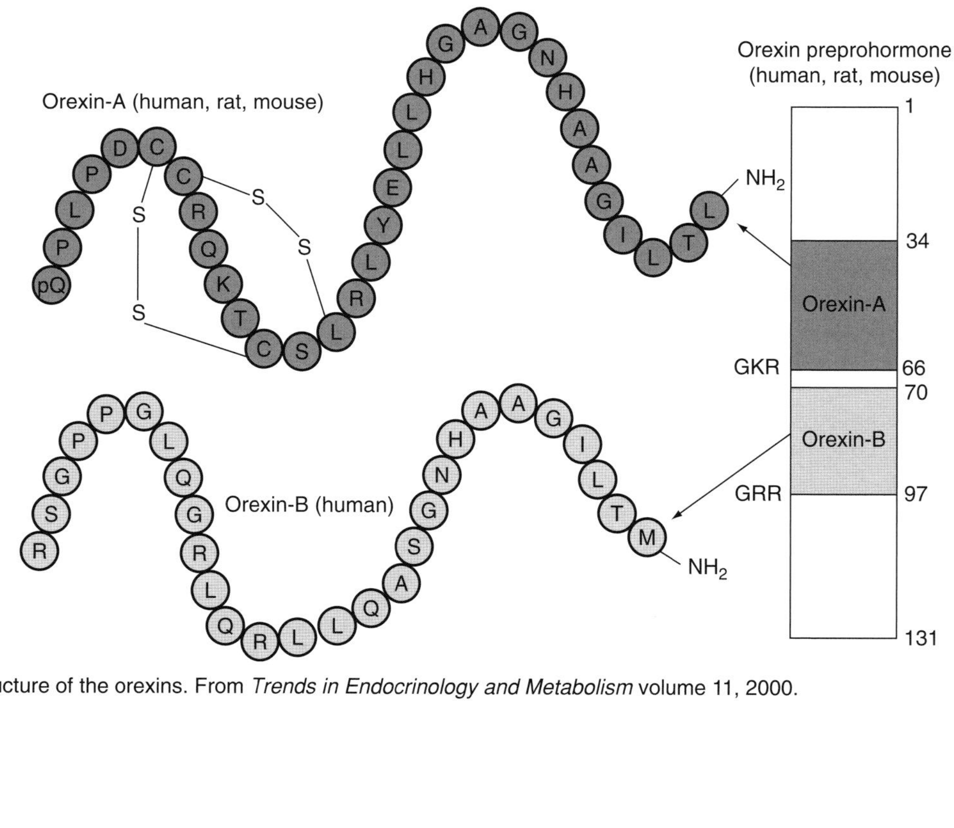

Figure 1 Structure of the orexins. From *Trends in Endocrinology and Metabolism* volume 11, 2000.

Table 1 Distribution of orexin receptor subtypes in brain regions important to the stress response[a]

Brain site	*OX_1R mRNA*	*OX_2R mRNA*
Bed nucleus, stria terminalis	High	Moderate
Medial amygdala (nucleus)	Moderate	Low
Cortical amygdala (nucleus)	Low	Moderate
Periventricular thalamus (nucleus)	High	Moderate
Medial preoptic hypothalamus (area)	Absent	Moderate
Medial preoptic hypothalamus (nucleus)	Moderate	Moderate
Organum vasculosum lamina terminalis	Low	Moderate
Median preoptic area	Low	Moderate
Anterior hypothalamic nucleus	High	Low
Hypothalamic arcuate nucleus	Absent	High
Lateral hypothalamus (area)	Low	High
Medial paraventricular nucleus (parvocellular)	Absent	High
Lateral paraventricular nucleus (parvocellular)	Absent	Low
Posterior paraventricular nucleus (magnocellular)	Absent	Absent
Tuberomammillary nuclei	Absent	High
Ventromedial hypothalamus (nucleus)	High	Moderate
Dorsomedial hypothalamus (nucleus)	Absent / low	Moderate
Midbrain A4, A5, and A7 cell groups	High	Absent
Dorsal motor nucleus of vagus	Moderate	Moderate
Dorsal raphe nucleus	Moderate	Moderate
Locus coeruleus	High	Low
Nucleus of the solitary tract	Moderate	Low
Parabrachial nucleus	Absent	Low
Periaqueductal grey	Moderate	Moderate
Sensory and spinal trigeminal nuclei	Absent	Moderate
Substantia nigra (pars compacta)	Moderate	Moderate
Ventral tegmental area	Moderate	Moderate
Zona incerta	Moderate	Moderate

[a]As determined by *in situ* hybridization histochemistry. Density of the histochemical signal detected is indicated as high, moderate, low, or absent (at background).

central orexin administration. In fact, direct effects of orexin on neurons in the dorsal motor nucleus of the vagus also have been reported.

Cellular mechanisms of action In an attempt to determine the cellular mechanism of action of orexin to raise blood pressure and heart rate by an action in the NTS, experiments were conducted in medullary slice preparations. Whole-cell recordings from NTS neurons in current clamp mode revealed that the depolarizing effect of orexin was maintained in the presence of tetrodotoxin, demonstrating direct post-synaptic actions of the peptide. In voltage clamp mode, orexin was observed to inhibit a specific potassium conductance (the sustained K^+ current) and to activate a nonselective cation conductance, leading to depolarization. Later a G-protein signaling mechanism was demonstrated to activate phospholipase C and protein kinase C but not protein kinase A (PKA).

The cellular effects of orexin also have been characterized in the area postrema (AP), a circumventricular organ located adjacent to the NTS. In dissociated AP neurons, orexin similarly activated a nonselective cation conductance, leading to depolarization. In these cells, however, no effects on potassium currents were observed. The activation of a nonselective cation conductance also has been demonstrated in parvocellular PVN neurons, which may in fact have been preautonomic cells projecting to sympathetic centers in the rostral ventrolateral medulla. As in the AP, there did not appear to be any action of orexin on potassium currents in neurons in parvocellular PVN.

In sympathetic preganglionic neurons in spinal cord, orexin's depolarizing effects are blocked by pertussis toxin, indicating a G-protein signaling mechanism. In these neurons, a PKA-mediated inhibition of potassium channels has been demonstrated. The direct effects of orexin to depolarize noradrenergic neurons in the LC occur due to decreased potassium conductance and the activation of an inward current. The exact receptor subtype responsible for these depolarizing actions of orexin in the NTS, AP, PVN, LC, or IMDL has not been identified; however, the similar (and in some cases diverse) signaling mechanisms described predict heterogeneity of receptor subtypes depending on tissue localization.

Physiological relevance of the pharmacological effects of orexin on cardiovascular function Mice in which the gene for orexin has been deleted (embryonic knockouts) and mice and rats engineered to suffer age-related loss of orexin neurons (orexin-ataxin 3 transgenes) display lower mean arterial blood pressures than their wild-type littermates under resting conditions and fail to mount a sympathetic response (increased heart rate or increased blood pressure) in the resident/intruder stress model. The reason for the lower resting blood pressures in these transgenic animals was established to be due to a loss of vasoconstrictor sympathetic tone because prazocin (α-adrenergic blockade) or hexamethonium (ganglionic blockade) failed to alter the already low pressures in these animals but brought pressures in wild-type littermates to levels similar to the transgenic animals. This was not accomplished by treatment with captopril (angiotensin-converting enzyme inhibitor) or a V_1 (vasopressin antagonist).

Does the syndrome narcolepsy/cataplexy in humans demonstrate compromised sympathetic function? Autonomic dysfunction has been reported in these patients, including the attenuation of cardiovascular reflexes to muscle contraction and the Valsalva maneuver. Frequent occurrences of orthostatic hypotension have been reported as well.

Neuroendocrine Actions of the Orexins

Orexin and the hypothlamic-pituitary-adrenal axis The presence of orexin receptors (**Table 1**) and broad distribution of orexin-positive nerve fibers in the hypothalamus suggested actions of the peptides on neuroendocrine centers in the diencephalon or the pituitary gland itself. Initial attention was drawn to potential actions in anterior pituitary gland because orexin receptors are abundant in the gland and the peptide appears to be delivered to the median eminence, where it could gain access to the hypophysial portal circulation. Although no significant effect of the orexins on prolactin (PRL) release were observed in dispersed anterior pituitary cell cultures, the release of the other major anterior lobe stress hormone, adrenocorticotropic hormone (ACTH), was significantly affected by the concentrations of peptide in the nanomolar range. Basal ACTH release was not affected by orexin; however, corticotropin releasing hormone (CRH)-stimulated ACTH release was inhibited in a concentration-related fashion. The effect appeared to be mediated by the OX_1R because the median effective concentration (EC_{50}) for orexin A was at least 1 log lower than that for orexin B and because the inhibitory action of orexin was absent when the production of the OX_1R (but not the OX_2R) was compromised by antisense oligonucleotide treatment. Recently, the selective OX_1R antagonist has been demonstrated to also block the action of orexin A on CRH-induced ACTH release *in vitro*. Furthermore, the relatively selective OX_2R agonist (Ala^{11}, Leu^{14}) orexin B did not exert actions similar to orexin A or orexin B. Orexin's action on the corticotroph appear to require the activation of a non-pertussis toxin-(non-PTX-) sensitive G-protein-coupled receptor to phospholipase C activation and the formation of inositol trisphosphate. In addition, the activation of PKC seems to be a necessary step in transduction of the inhibitory signal.

In the hypothalamus, orexin acts to stimulate the hypothalamic-pituitary-adrenal (HPA) axis by activating CRH-producing neurons. This was demonstrated by several groups using pretreatment with CRH antiserum or antagonists prior to the ICV administration of orexin. Whether this is a direct or indirect action of orexin on CRH-producing neurons in the parvocellular PVN is currently unknown, although single-cell the reverse transcription polymerase chain reaction (RT-PCR) approaches now employed in the authors' laboratories promise a future definitive answer to this question. Neurons in the PVN express both receptor subtypes, although the OX_2R appears more abundant. In addition, orexin-producing neurons that project to the PVN express glucocorticoid receptors, and thus the closed feedback loop of the HPA axis appears to include orexinergic neurons in the LHA (direct effects of orexin, of unknown origin, on adrenal steroid production and release have also been reported). As previously mentioned, direct postsynaptic effects of orexin on PVN neurons have been reported. The orexin effects on parvocellular PVN neurons, those projecting to median eminence or other brain sites (e.g., sympathetic centers in the brain stem) are direct (i.e., postsynaptic) and are mediated by the activation of nonselective cation conductances. In magnocellular PVN, the depolarizing effects of orexin are indirect (i.e., tetrodotoxin blockable), involving a glutamatergic interneuron. Because high concentrations of arginine vasopressin (AVP) are capable of stimulating ACTH release from cultured pituitary cells *in vitro* and under at least some *in vivo* conditions the compromise of AVP action reduces stress-induced ACTH release, it is possible that the ACTH response to the ICV administration of orexin may be mediated by AVP release into the median eminence. The central administration of orexin has been reported to increase both CRH and AVP mRNA levels in the PVN; however, in hypothalamic explant cultures, orexin did not stimulate AVP release. Thus, it appears that the hypothalamic action of orexin to stimulate the HPA axis is mediated primarily by CRH release into the median eminence.

Orexin and prolactin secretion Controversy exists over the potential action of orexin on PRL secretion. Orexin, in log molar concentrations ranging from 1.0 pM to 100 nM, did not alter basal or thyrotropin-releasing hormone (TRH)-stimulated PRL release from dispersed anterior pituitary cells *in vitro*. However, when it was administered ICV some groups observed stimulatory and others inhibitory effects on PRL levels in plasma. The suppressive effects of orexin on *in vivo* PRL secretion were reported to be the result of increased dopamine turnover in male, but not female, rats. Evidence for a stimulatory role for orexin on PRL and luteinizing hormone (LH) releases come from fasting studies in which the preovulatory PRL and LH surges, absent during fasting, were restored by central orexin administration. Even more support for the stimulatory actions of orexins comes from steroid-priming studies in ovariectomized rats, in which the PRL and LH surges were blocked by pretreatment with anti-orexin antibodies. Whether any of these pharmacological effects of orexin on PRL or LH secretion are physiologically relevant is unclear and may not be likely because orexin knockout mice are fertile and can nurse their pups. It is possible that physiologically relevant actions of the orexins on at least PRL secretion may not be related to reproductive function but instead to stress-induced hormone release. Thus, the actions of the peptide on tuberoinfundibular dopamine neurons of the arcuate nucleus, where the OX_2R is abundantly expressed, may be observed only in models of acute stress such as restraint (physical) or novel environment (anticipatory). The expression of early response genes in neurons of the LHA has been described in several experimental models of stress.

Orexin and Stress-Related Behaviors

The presence of orexin receptors and orexin-positive nerve fibers in central nervous system (CNS) sites known to be important in the arousal state, such as the LC and raphe nuclei, forms the anatomical basis for the effects of pharmacological doses of orexin on motivated and spontaneous behaviors. Several groups have described effects of orexin on locomotor behavior and general arousal state, and the obligatory role for endogenous orexin in sleep/wakefulness is well established. In our hands, the effects of orexin on general locomotor behavior and stereotypic behaviors parallel in dose relationship and time course the actions on sympathetic activity (i.e., blood pressure elevation). In addition, some of the feeding responses to orexin may be related to the peptide's ability to stimulate arousal, as well as exploratory and reward behaviors. These behaviors, observed following central orexin administration, mirror behaviors observed during stress; however, they differ from those observed following CRH administration, which are more anxiogenic in nature. There may be an important interplay between orexin neurons in the LHA and CRH neurons in the PVN. As already detailed, orexin appears to activate CRH neurons (resulting in ACTH release), and it has been reported that CRH receptors are present on orexin neurons in the LHA, where CRH itself exerts depolarizing effects. Thus, at least some of the behavioral arousal stimulated by CRH may be mediated by the effects of the peptide on endogenous orexin release.

The pharmacological actions of orexin on locomotor activity and arousal state are mirrored by determinations of orexin neuronal activity in these behaviors. Indeed, c-FOS expression correlates directly with wakefulness and locomotor activity, and the spontaneous activity of these neurons during such states has been characterized as well. One site of orexin action related to spontaneous locomotor activity is the PVN. In addition to stimulating feeding in the early light phase, orexin injection into the PVN increased spontaneous locomotor activity at all the times examined, and this was accompanied by increased oxygen consumption. The effect of orexin on spontaneous locomotor activity was antagonized by pretreatment with SB-334867 (an OX_1R antagonist). Those results suggest that physical activity independent of feeding is due to the actions of orexin in the hypothalamus. Indeed in recent studies, we observed that many, but not all, of the behavioral actions of exogenous orexin could be antagonized by pretreatment with the OX_1R antagonist, whereas some of the similar behavioral actions of the selective OX_2R agonist remain unaffected by OX_1R antagonist pretreatment. Thus, both receptors may be responsible for differing behavioral modalities elicited by orexin administration. It will be important to determine the receptor subtype selectivity of the individual behaviors so that the roles played by each receptor in not only locomotor but also stress-related behaviors can be elucidated.

Non-Central Nervous System Sites of Orexin Action Related to Stress

Orexin receptors have been identified in non-CNS tissues, and significantly, the adrenal gland expresses both receptors but the OX_2R more abundantly. Orexin acts both *in vitro* and *in vivo* to stimulate corticosterone release, with orexin A being more potent than orexin B. This suggests a role for the OX_1R in the control of adrenal cortical function. The effect is selective (aldosterone secretion was unaffected) and is blocked by H-89 pretreatment *in vitro*, suggesting a signaling pathway involving adenylyl cyclase. Because the major site of orexin production was the LHA and plasma levels of the peptide are extremely low, it remained unclear that these pharmacological effects of orexin in the adrenal gland had any physiological correlate. However, it is now known that the orexins are also produced in the adrenal gland and thus may exert autocrine or paracrine actions in the gland. It should be remembered that the direction of blood flow in the adrenal gland is from the outer cortex to the inner medulla, and thus orexin produced in the adrenal cortex might bathe the medulla in relatively high concentrations, similar to the situation with corticosterone. At least in human pheochromocytomas, orexins act via the OX_2R to stimulate epinephrine and norepinephrine release, suggesting an action of orexin to regulate catecholamine release from the normal adrenal gland. Whether orexin production and/or release from cortex increases during stress is at this point unknown; however, it is tempting to speculate that the adrenal actions of orexin complement the peptide's actions in brain related to metabolism and stress.

Summary and Conclusion

Abundant evidence support a role for endogenous orexins in the regulation of sleep/wakefulness and metabolic state. Central to all the actions of the orexins is the consistent finding that multiple indicators of stress are revealed following orexin administration and some are absent when orexin production or action is compromised. Remarkable progress has been made in understanding the importance of the endogenous orexin system, largely due to the development of transgenic models of orexin peptide or receptor compromise. In particular, the development of the orexin-ataxin-3 transgenic mice and rats has been a landmark in our ability to understand the broad impact of these peptides on multiple behavioral, endocrine, and cardiovascular systems. Now, with the availability of selective OX_1R antagonists and at least a relatively selective OX_2R agonist, additional elucidation of the sites and mechanisms of orexin actions in the brain can be accomplished. Because the replacement of the peptide restores normal sleep/wakefulness patterns in transgenic animals, the use of orexin or orexin analogs for the treatment of human narcolepsy/cataplexy holds much promise. Critical to the development of those potential therapeutic strategies is the recognition of the receptor subtypes responsible for the effects of orexin on cardiovascular and neuroendocrine function. Clearly, potential side effects related to cardiovascular control and hormone release are possible and should be monitored if orexin is to be tested for its therapeutic effect in humans.

See Also the Following Articles

Feeding Circuitry (and Neurochemistry).

Further Reading

de Lecea, L., Kilduff, T. S., Peyron, C., et al. (1998). The hypocretins: hypothalamus-specific peptides with neuroexcitatory activity. *Proceedings of the National Academy of Sciences USA* **95**, 322–327.

de Lecea, L. and Sutcliffe, J. G. (eds.) (2005). *Hypocretins: integrators of physiological functions.* New York: Springer.

Ferguson, A. V. and Samson, W. K. (2003). The orexin/hypocretin system: a critical regulator of neuroendocrine and autonomic function. *Frontiers in Neuroendocrinology* **24**, 141–150.

Hara, J., Beuckmann, C. T., Nambu, T., et al. (2001). Genetic ablation of orexin neurons in mice results in narcolepsy, hypophagia, and obesity. *Neuron* **30**, 345–354.

Kayaba, Y., Nakamura, A., Kasuya, Y., et al. (2003). Attenuated defense response and low blood pressure in orexin knockout mice. *American Journal of Physiology* **285**, R581–R593.

Kilduff, T. S. (2005). Hypocretin/orexin: maintenance of wakefulness and a multiplicity of other roles. *Sleep Medicine Reviews* **9**, 227–230.

Kiwaki, K., Kotz, C. M., Wang, C., et al. (2004). Orexin A (hypocretin 1) injected into hypothalamic paraventricular nucleus and spontaneous activity in acts. *American Journal of Physiology* **286**, E551–E559.

Marcus, J. N., Aschkenasi, C. J., Lee, C. E., et al. (2001). Differential expression of orexin receptors 1 and 2 in rat brain. *Journal of Comparative Neurology* **435**, 6–25.

Mieda, M., Willie, J. T., Hara, J., et al. (2004). Orexin peptides prevent cataplexy and improve wakefulness in an orexin-ablated model of narcolepsy in mice. *Proceedings of the National Academy of Sciences USA* **101**, 4649–4654.

Mileykoviskiy, B. Y., Kiyaschenko, L. I. and Siegel, J. M. (2005). Behavioral correlates of activity in identified hypocretin/orexin neurons. *Neuron* **46**, 787–798.

Peyron, C., Tighe, D. K., van den Pol, A. N., et al. (1998). Neurons containing hypocretin (orexin) project to multiple neuronal systems. *Journal of Neurosciences* **18**, 9996–10015.

Sakurai, T., Amemiya, A., Ishii, A., et al. (1998). Orexins and orexin receptors: a family of hypothalamic neuropeptides and G protein-coupled receptors that regulate feeding behavior. *Cell* **92**, 573–585.

Samson, W. K., Taylor, M. M. and Ferguson, A. V. (2005). Non-sleep effects of hypocretin/orexin. *Sleep Medicine Reviews* **9**, 243–252.

Willie, J. T., Chemelli, R. M., Sinton, C. M., et al. (2001). To eat or sleep?: orexin in the regulation of feeding and wakefulness. *Annual Reviews of Neuroscience* **24**, 429–458.

Food Intake and Stress, Non-Human

Belinda A Henry and Iain J Clarke
Monash University, Melbourne, Australia

This is a revised version of the article by I J Clarke, Encyclopedia of Stress, First edition, volume 2, pp 162–166, © 2000, Elsevier Inc.

Glossary

Basal metabolic rate	The rate of oxygen consumption, or calculated equivalent heat production, of an awake individual lying at rest who has had no food for at least 12 h.
Gluconeogenesis	The formation of glucose from non-carbohydrate sources such as lactate or fatty acids.
Nutritional stress	A physiological, environmental, or metabolic stress that is imposed on an organism to disrupt metabolic homeostasis, thus causing a neural and/or endocrine response.
Orexigenic factor	A factor that acts to increase appetite and stimulate food intake.
Satiety factor	A factor that acts on the appetite-regulating regions of the brain to indicate satiety or to reduce food intake.

Introduction

Nutritional stress is, in some cases, an environmental stress and, in all cases, a metabolic stress. In particular cases, such as pregnancy and lactation, it could be construed that the nutritional demands of these states impose a physiological stress demanding increased food intake. In nonhuman species, nutritional stress occurs with a reduction in the availability of food or increased metabolic demand, but obesity is also associated with increased levels of stress hormones. In humans, a nutritional stress may be voluntarily imposed or due to psychogenic factors that have poorly defined etiology. The degree of impact varies among species depending on the type of metabolism of the organism (monogastric versus ruminant, for example) and also on the amount of body reserves of the organism.

Nutritional stress causes an alteration in the metabolic status of the animal and leads to altered concentrations of circulating metabolic substrates and metabolic hormones such as insulin and leptin. It is clear that blood-borne substances signal the metabolic status of the animal to the brain and that this leads to the alteration of hormonal output. These are responses of the organism to the stressor, but it is unlikely that a single factor that fulfils this signaling role. The neuroendocrine response to such a stress is probably the result of integrated effects of a composite of blood-borne substances. The gut may also signal directly to the brain by a neural route and through the altered secretion of ghrelin to regulate brain function and hormonal status.

Nonhormonal Responses to Nutritional Stress

Stress due to undernutrition produces a catabolic state, typified by changes in the levels of various substances in the bloodstream. Changes in metabolic factors, however, can be influenced by other physiological stimuli, so variations in the concentrations of singular components do not often reflect metabolic state. For example, fat is metabolized during a fast to produce nonesterified fatty acids (NEFA) that are used to synthesize carbohydrates via gluconeogenesis. Accordingly, plasma NEFA levels are elevated during a fast. On the other hand, prolonged undernutrition decreases body fat, leading to reduced NEFA levels, and obese subjects have increased NEFA levels, due to increased body fat. Thus, plasma NEFA concentrations are increased in both fasting and obese states. Other changes indicative of a catabolic state include reduced plasma insulin and leptin levels and increased plasma urea concentrations (due to the breakdown of muscle tissue in an effort to mobilize amino acids for the production of carbohydrates via gluconeogenesis). Chronic undernutrition (and a reduction in gluconeogenic substrates such as NEFA and amino acids) is typically associated with a reduction in plasma glucose concentrations. Plasma levels of these metabolic factors are a reflection of nutritional state (undernutrition versus obesity) and also the extent of catabolic stress (fasting versus prolonged undernutrition).

Hormonal Responses to Nutritional Stress

Endocrine changes occur during food deprivation or food restriction and the effects of fasting are summarized in **Table 1**.

Nutritional Stress and the Hypothalamic-Pituitary-Adrenal Axis

General Considerations

The hypothalamic-pituitary-adrenal (HPA) axis is commonly activated by nutritional stress, which results in the increased secretion of glucocorticoids

Table 1 Endocrine changes occur during food deprivation or food restriction[a]

Hormone	*Change*	*Comments*
Small monogastric animals (e.g., laboratory rat)		
Catecholamines	↑	Reflects the output of adrenalin from the adrenal medulla; catecholamines are lipolytic, mobilizing fat stores in response to reduced energy substrate
Insulin	↓	Insulin facilitates the uptake of sugar from the bloodstream
Growth hormone	↓	Response is opposite to that seen in large animals and also opposite to the response seen in humans
Gonadotropins (LH and FSH)	↓	Fasting for a period of 1–2 days can prevent the preovulatory LH surge in rats
Gonadal steroids (estrogen, testosterone, progesterone)	↓	
Prolactin	↓	With extended period of undernutrition
ACTH	↑	
Cortisol	↑	
TSH	↓	
T_3	↓	Through reduced conversion of T_4 to T_3
Nonhuman primates		
Insulin	↓	
Catecholamines	Not known	
Growth hormone	↑	
Gonadotropins (LH and FSH)	↓	LH is decreased, but there is a slower response in terms of FSH
Prolactin	Not known	
ACTH	Not known	
Cortisol	↑	
TSH	Not changed in the short term	
T_3	↓	
Ruminants		
Catecholamines	Not known	
Growth hormone	↑	
Gonadotropins (LH and FSH)	↓	LH is decreased, but there is a slower response in terms of FSH
Prolactin	Not changed	
Adrenocorticotropin	Not known	
Cortisol	↑	Morning levels only

[a]ACTH, adrenocorticotropic hormone; FSH, follicle stimulating hormone; LH, luteinizing hormone; T_3, triiodothyronine; T_4, thyroxine; TSH, thyroid stimulating hormone.

from the adrenal cortex. Most information to date has been derived from the laboratory rodent. The degree of activation of the HPA axis is dependent on a variety of factors, including:

- The species studied (monogastric small mammals such as rodents versus larger ruminant mammals such as sheep).
- The degree of intensity of undernutrition.
- The duration of undernutrition.
- The nutritional state of the animal prior to onset of catabolic state.
- The time of day; there is a diurnal pattern of glucocorticoid secretion.

Plasma glucocorticoids are elevated in states of undernutrition and in obese subjects, so both conditions might be regarded as stressors. The degree of change in body condition is an important factor. With undernutrition, the rapidity of change may also be a determinant of the stress response because animals can adapt over time to reduced energy stores. In obesity, the impact on the stress axis (glucocorticoid levels) depends on the obesity phenotype (where fat is distributed in the body).

There are species differences in the stress response to changing nutritional status and effects on plasma glucocorticoid levels are summarized in **Table 2**. It is important to note that the major glucocorticoid in rodents is corticosterone, whereas larger species including humans produce cortisol. Small monogastric mammals such as rodents exhibit robust activation of the HPA axis in response to fasting, but the same is not true for ruminants, in which digestion of nutrients is slower. Ruminants have a dynamic digestive system, with four stomach compartments (rumen, reticulum, omasum, and abomasum), which enables them to digest their primary dietary component, cellulose. Ruminant digestion takes a considerable time, so there is a delayed response to fasting. Furthermore, ruminants stringently maintain blood glucose levels

Table 2 Species differences in glucocorticoid responses to nutritional stressors

	Laboratory rodent	*Sheep*	*Nonhuman primate*	*Human*
Fasting	↑ Corticosterone within 24–48 h	↑ Cortisol within 48–72 h	↑ Cortisol within 24 h	↑ Cortisol within 24 h
Food restriction	↑ Corticosterone	No change	Unknown	↑ Cortisol
Obesity	↑ Corticosterone in genetic models of obesity such as the fatty Zucker rat and the *ob/ob* mouse	No change in basal cortisol concentrations ↑ Cortisol response to stress	Unknown	↑ Cortisol (particularly in abdominal obesity)

by the mobilization of NEFA from fat stores. Small animals have higher basal metabolic rates, which impacts fuel utility. Small animals (rodents) also have very low fat stores (approximately 10%) in comparison to larger species, including both sheep and humans (approximately 20%).

The Effect of Fasting versus Food Restriction on Hypothalamic-Pituitary-Adrenal Axis Activity

The effect of nutritional stress on the HPA axis is dependent on the duration and the intensity of undernutrition. Fasting is often used in the laboratory as a nutritional stressor, and in rodents plasma corticosterone levels are elevated within 24 h. In sheep, the response takes longer and cortisol secretion is increased 48–72 h after the commencement of fasting. In rodents, chronic food restriction (animals fed a 50% maintenance diet) for 4 weeks increases plasma levels of corticosterone, but basal cortisol levels are minimally changed in sheep made lean by long-term food restriction. There is a perturbation of the diurnal pattern of cortisol secretion in fasting sheep, with higher morning levels.

Pregnancy and Lactation

Pregnancy and lactation can be considered physiological conditions that induce nutritional stress by virtue of the high energy demands consigned to the mother. In small mammals, it has been calculated that the energy demands of lactation are four times greater than those of nonpregnant females. The high metabolic demands of lactation are met by profoundly increased food intake, driven by changes in appetite-regulating systems in the brain. Unlike other typical nutritional stressors, however, lactation is associated with hyporesponsivity of the HPA axis; neuroendocrine responses to stress are blunted in lactating animals. adrenocorticotropic hormone (ACTH) and cortisol levels are maintained during pregnancy, whereas corticotropin releasing hormone (CRH) levels are elevated due to peripheral synthesis and secretion by the placenta. This increase in CRH production is counteracted by increased circulating levels of CRH-binding protein (which sequesters CRH), thus preventing inappropriate secretion of ACTH. This phenomenon, however, occurs only in mammals that produce placental CRH.

Nutritional Stress and Negative Feedback Mechanisms of the Hypothalamic-Pituitary-Adrenal Axis

The HPA axis is tightly regulated by glucocorticoid (and mineralocorticoid) feedback to the hypothalamus and the anterior pituitary gland to regulate the secretion of hypophysiotropic hormones (CRH and arginine vasopressin, AVP) from the hypothalamus and ACTH from the pituitary corticotrophs. It has been hypothesized that abdominal obesity in humans and other species leads to dysfunction of the negative feedback actions of glucocorticoids, causing upregulation of the HPA axis and increased plasma levels of cortisol. In rodents, it has been hypothesized that decreased negative feedback actions within the brain actually precedes the obese state; animals susceptible to diet-induced obesity have decreased levels of glucocorticoid receptor mRNA within the hippocampus compared to diet-resistant animals.

Some work suggests that the sensitivity of the HPA axis to the negative feedback effects of glucocorticoids depends on carbohydrate ingestion. Adrenalectomized rodents suffer various abnormalities within the HPA axis, including increased expression of CRH mRNA in the paraventricular nucleus of the hypothalamus and decreased expression of CRH mRNA in the central nucleus of the amygdala. Interestingly, these perturbations in the adrenalectomized animal can be ameliorated by the ingestion of sucrose. Similarly, feeding animals a diet high in fat content also impacts on the HPA axis. For example, feeding rats a diet containing 20% fat (control diet, 4% fat) increases both basal and stress-induced secretion of ACTH and corticosterone. In contrast, feeding rats a diet very high (60%) in fat can decrease hormonal responses to stress. Thus, in animals, as in humans, the macronutrient dietary content impacts the reactivity of the HPA axis.

Nonadrenal Production of Glucocorticoids in Obesity

Peripheral tissues, other than the adrenal cortex, are able to produce glucocorticoids. This occurs by conversion of inert 11-keto steroids (11-dehydrocorticosterone in rodents and cortisone in humans) to active 11-hydroxy steroids (corticosterone in rodents and cortisol in humans). This process is regulated by the 11β-hydroxysteroid dehydrogenase (11β-HSD) enzymes; 11β-HSD-1 catalyzes the synthesis of active 11-hydroxy steroids, and 11β-HSD-2 catalyzes the synthesis of the inactive 11-keto steroids. The 11β-HSD-1 enzyme is predominantly expressed in white adipose tissue, the liver, and the central nervous system (particularly the paraventricular nucleus of the hypothalamus and the hippocampus). In genetic models of obesity such as the *ob/ob* mice (a naturally occurring mutation in the gene that encodes leptin) and the fatty Zucker rat (a mutation in the gene that encodes the leptin receptor), the expression of 11β-HSD-1 mRNA and 11β-HSD-1 enzymatic activity is increased within adipose tissue, whereas expression is reduced in the liver. Furthermore, overexpressing 11β-HSD-1 mRNA within the adipose tissue of transgenic mice specifically increases local concentrations of corticosterone. Such animals have an obese phenotype, but this is not associated with increased plasma levels of corticosterone.

The Role of the Hypothalamic-Pituitary-Adrenal Axis in the Predisposition to Obesity

In rodents, genetic obesity (the *ob/ob* mouse and the fatty Zucker rat) causes elevated concentrations of corticosterone. Adrenalectomy attenuates (or completely reverses) the obese phenotype in these animals. Furthermore, in nonmutated rodents, adrenalectomy reduces food intake, and corticosterone replacement restores normal feeding behavior. The stimulatory effect of glucocorticoids on food intake, however, cannot be displayed in an adrenal-intact rodent.

In rodents, mild pain induced by tail pinch initially increases food intake, but this effect is abolished by repeated experience; chronic exposure to tail pinch reduces food intake and body weight. Similarly, in rats repeated restraint stress reduces food intake and body weight, and this effect can be mimicked by chronic treatment with corticosterone. This decrease, however, is in comparison to rats fed *ad libitum*. In contrast, animals pair-fed to a similar (and lower) plane of nutrition tend to have lower body weights and reduced fat deposition compared to animals exposed to either repeated restraint stress or glucocorticoid treatment.

Neuronal Systems Underlying Endocrine Perturbations Induced by Nutritional Stress

There are numerous neuropeptides and neurotransmitters that are involved in both the regulation of appetite and neuroendocrine functions. Within the hypothalamus, this involves a number of interconnected nuclei. The arcuate nucleus is essential to the regulation of food intake and body weight and produces a number of neuropeptides, including the appetite stimulators neuropeptide Y (NPY) and agouti-related protein (AGRP) as well as the appetite inhibitors α-melanocyte stimulating hormone (α-MSH: derived from the proopiomelanocortin, POMC, gene) and urocortin 2. Other regions of the hypothalamus involved in regulating food intake and neuroendocrine function include the paraventricular nucleus, which produces the appetite inhibitors CRH, urocortin 1, urocortin 2 and urocortin 3; the lateral hypothalamic area, which contains the appetite stimulators melanin-concentrating hormone (MCH) and the orexin; and the ventromedial hypothalamic nucleus. Various appetite-regulating peptides impact on the HPA axis and these are summarized in **Table 3**.

In addition to the hypothalamus, several nuclei in the brain stem also regulate feeding behavior and the HPA axis. Brain stem nuclei can regulate HPA function by ascending projections to the forebrain or via descending spinal projections to the adrenal gland. For example, noradrenergic input from the locus ceruleus to the paraventricular nucleus of the hypothalamus is involved in the regulation of HPA function as well as food intake. In sheep and rats, various studies document the effects of nutritional stress on the expression of genes that encode appetite-regulating peptides. For example, in sheep made lean by chronic food restriction, the expression of genes encoding NPY, AGRP, and MCH is increased, indicative of increased hunger drive; these animals, however, have normal basal cortisol secretion. On the other hand, in fasted rodents, the expression of the same genes (NPY, AGRP, and MCH) is increased and there is activation of the HPA axis. Species differences in neuronal circuitry regulating the HPA axis may be relevant to the way that alteration in body weight affects the stress axis.

Possible Hormonal Signals Involved in Mediating Nutritional Stress

Various hormonal signals relay information about nutritional state to the appetite-regulating and neuroendocrine centers of the brain. Three hormones that play an important role are leptin, ghrelin, and insulin.

Table 3 The effect of hypothalamic appetite-regulating peptides on the HPA axis[a]

	Neuropeptide	*Effect on food intake*	*Effect on HPA axis activity*
Arcuate nucleus	NPY	↑	↑
	AGRP	↑	↑
	α-MSH	↓	↑ Basal ACTH and corticosterone ↓ IL-1-induced HPA axis activity
	CART	↓	↑
	Urocortin 2	↓	No effect
Paraventricular nucleus	CRH	↓	↑
	Urocortin 1	↓	↑
	Urocortin 2	↓	No effect
	Urocortin 3	↓	No effect
Lateral hypothalamic area	MCH	↑	↑
	Orexins	↑	↑
	Urocortin 1	↓	↑

[a]ACTH, adrenocorticotropic hormone; AGRP, agouti-related protein; CART, cocaine and amphetamine regulated transcript; CRH, corticotropin releasing hormone; HPA, hypothalamic-pituitary-adrenal; IL, interleukin; MCH, melanin-concentrating hormone; MSH, melanocyte stimulating hormone; NPY, neuropeptide Y.

Leptin

Leptin is primarily produced by white fat tissue, and its plasma levels reflect the level of adiposity. In rodents, there is a tight negative correlation between the plasma levels of leptin and corticosterone. In rodents and sheep, the fasting-induced activation of the HPA axis is ameliorated by leptin treatment. Leptin also attenuates the ACTH and corticosterone responses to a physical stressor (hind-limb restraint) in rats. This suggests that leptin may in fact influence the neuroendocrine stress axis under conditions not associated with either nutritional or metabolic perturbations. The mechanisms by which leptin exerts such an effect are most likely to be centrally mediated. *In vitro* studies show that leptin can influence CRH secretion from isolated rat hypothalami but not ACTH secretion from cultured rat pituitary cells. A subpopulation of CRH-containing cells in the hypothalamus expresses the leptin receptor, allowing for direct action at this level of the HPA axis. Leptin receptors are also found in many cell types in the brain that provide afferents to the paraventricular nucleus, so there is likely to be relayed effects as well. Such cell types include those that produce NPY, MCH, and POMC.

Ghrelin

Ghrelin is primarily secreted from the stomach and has been shown to potently stimulate the secretion of growth hormone. In some species, ghrelin also acts within the brain to stimulate food intake. Studies in sheep show that a preprandial rise in ghrelin levels stimulates a postprandial rise in growth hormone levels. Plasma levels of ghrelin fall postprandially and are increased by fasting or reduction in body weight; levels are lower in obese individuals. In addition to the stimulation of growth hormone, ghrelin activates the HPA axis, although not in all species. Ghrelin mRNA levels are increased after both physical (tail pinch) and nutritional (fasting) stress. Thus, ghrelin may be an additional factor involved in the regulation of the HPA axis under stressful stimuli. Ghrelin acts via the growth hormone secretagogue receptor, which is present in both the central nervous system and the pituitary gland. In rodents, the *in vivo* action of ghrelin on the HPA axis is exerted centrally, via cells such as those that produce NPY and AGRP in the arcuate nucleus. The orexin system in the lateral hypothalamus has also been linked to ghrelin-induced corticosterone secretion.

Insulin

The role of insulin in the regulation of food intake and neuroendocrine function is sometimes confused with the confounding effects of insulin-induced hypoglycemia. The latter increases food intake due to glucose deprivation, whereas in other circumstances insulin acts to decrease food intake. In rodents, diabetes causes increased basal concentrations of ACTH and corticosterone but reduced responsiveness to stress. Streptozotocin-induced diabetes impacts various neuronal systems, which in turn may influence the HPA axis. For example, streptozotocin-induced diabetes increases the concentration of norepinephrine within the paraventricular nucleus of the hypothalamus, and this parallels increasing levels of corticosterone. This effect is dependent on insulin concentrations because insulin replacement restores levels of norepinephrine within the paraventricular nucleus and the peripheral concentrations of corticosterone. Interestingly leptin treatment, in the absence of insulin replacement, also corrects these streptozotocin-induced perturbations. In addition to effects on catecholaminergic systems, diabetes-associated changes in HPA axis function may be mediated via hypothalamic peptides such as NPY. In the rat, the arcuate nucleus contains insulin receptors and insulin decreases NPY mRNA expression in this region.

Further Reading

Bronson, F. H. (1985). Mammalian reproduction: an ecological perspective. *Biology of Reproduction* **32**, 1–26.
Cameron, J. L. (1996). Regulation of the reproductive hormone secretion in primates by short-term changes in nutrition. *Reviews of Reproduction* **1**, 117–126.
Dallman, M. F., Pecoraro, N., Akana, S. F., et al. (2003). Chronic stress and obesity: a new view of "comfort food." *Proceedings of the National Academy of Sciences USA* **100**, 11695–11701.
Friedman, J. M. and Halaas, J. L. (1998). Leptin and the regulation of body weight in mammals. *Nature* **395**, 763–770.
Henry, B. A. (2003). Links between appetite regulating systems and the neuroendocrine hypothalamus: lessons from the sheep. *Journal of Neuroendocrinology* **15**, 697–709.
Horvath, T. L. and Diano, S. (2004). The floating blueprint of hypothalamic feeding circuits. *Nature Reviews Neuroscience* **5**, 662–667.
Krysiak, R., Obuchowicz, E. and Herman, Z. S. (1999). Interactions between the neuropeptide Y system and the hypothalamic-pituitary-adrenal axis. *European Journal of Endocrinology* **140**, 130–136.
Seckl, J. R. and Walker, B. R. (2004). 11β-hydroxysteroid dehydrogenase type 1 as a modulator of glucocorticoid action: from metabolism to memory. *Trends in Endocrinology and Metabolism* **15**, 418–424.
Smith, M. S. and Grove, K. L. (2002). Integration of the regulation of reproduction function and energy balance: lactation as a model. *Frontiers in Neuroendocrinology* **23**, 225–256.
van der Lely, A. J., Tschop, M., Heiman, M. L., et al. (2004). Biological, physiological, pathophysiological and pharmacological aspects of ghrelin. *Endocrine Reviews* **25**, 426–457.

Cholesterol and Lipoproteins

C M Stoney
National Center for Complementary and Alternative Medicine, National Institutes of Health, Bethesda, MD, USA

This is a revised version of the article by C M Stoney and M Finney, Encyclopedia of Stress, First edition, volume 1, pp 454–459, © 2000, Elsevier Inc.

Glossary

Apolipoprotein	Proteins located on the surface of lipoproteins that transport proteins and bind to specialized enzymes.
Cholesterol	A fat-soluble molecule in the body used to form cholic acid in the liver, steroid hormones in the gonads and adrenals, and used in the formation of cell membranes.
Hemoconcentration	The generally transient and reversible filtration of fluid from the intravascular space.
Lipids	Chemical compounds in the body that are miscible with each other and which provide energy and a variety of intracellular functions. They include triglycerides, phospholipids, and cholesterol.
Lipoprotein	Large complexes of molecules that circulate and transport triglycerides, phospholipids, cholesterol, and proteins in the blood.
Lipid reactivity	Response of one or more of the lipids circulating in the blood to an external stimulus.

Structure and Function of Cholesterol and Lipoproteins

Lipoproteins are large, complex structures circulating in the blood that contain triglycerides, phospholipids, cholesterol, and proteins. Triglycerides are synthesized in the liver and adipose tissue, and are utilized as energy sources. Phospholipids are transported in lipoproteins, are formed in all cells of the body, and are particularly important in the formation of cellular membranes. Cholesterol, both exogenous and endogenous forms, also circulates in the lipoproteins and is used to form cholic acid in the liver. As with phospholipids, the most important function of cholesterol is the formation and permeability of cell membranes. High circulating concentrations of low-density lipoprotein-cholesterol (LDLC) and low circulating concentrations of high-density lipoprotein-cholesterol (HDLC) are associated with an increased risk of coronary heart disease (CHD).

Until recently, there has been a widely held understanding that blood cholesterol concentrations were relatively stable, showing only moderate elevations with aging, and transient but predictable elevations in triglycerides and related lipids postprandially, i.e. period of time after a meal. It is well documented that there are large inter- and intra-individual variations and fluctuations in plasma cholesterol, triglycerides, and LDLC concentrations. The variability within individuals is in the order of 10–20% over the course of a day or a week, and the degree of variability remains high even under reasonably standardized conditions.

Investigations of the factors responsible for such fluctuations are clinically relevant, because in order to make reasonable clinical decisions regarding assessment and treatment of hypercholesterolemia (condition describing a high concentration of cholesterol in the blood), an understanding of normal, biologically based variations in cholesterol concentrations are essential. As importantly, however, is the understanding of the causes of this variability in order to better understand the process of cholesterol regulation.

Environmental Influences on Lipid Concentrations and Lipid Variability

A variety of stimuli alter the blood concentrations of lipids. For example, numerous investigations have demonstrated that psychological stress reliably influences blood concentrations of cholesterol and lipoproteins. A separate and smaller literature has shown that individuals differ in their lipid responses to dietary challenge. Importantly, exaggerated lipid responsivity to diet is associated with an increased risk of CHD. To the extent that exaggerated lipid responses to environmental stimuli are atherogenic, investigation of the role of stress on lipid concentrations is of potential clinical importance. The task among behavioral scientists dedicated to investigating the phenomenon of stress-associated lipid changes is to delineate the potential mechanisms responsible for the effects, which will ultimately lead to either a confirmation or refutation of the notion that stress-associated lipid changes are atherogenic.

Several models have been proposed as potential pathways by which stress alters lipid concentrations in the blood; one such model is presented in **Figure 1**. Although the pathways are not mutually exclusive and are likely to be different under varying conditions of psychological stress, models such as these suggest ways of considering the current literature and point to obvious avenues for future research endeavors.

Chronic Stress Mechanisms of Lipid Variability

During chronically or pervasively stressful situations, cholesterol concentrations are elevated. A number of naturalistic studies have demonstrated that the stress associated with a major disaster or major stressor, such as the experience of earthquake, loss of job and income, and bereavement, can result in substantial increases in total cholesterol, LDLC, and triglycerides. Among better controlled laboratory studies of chronic stress, generally similar associations are noted between chronically stressful situations and elevated atherogenic lipids. Although there is not complete agreement, the preponderance of studies supports the notion that stress changes, or in some way is associated with, lipid concentrations in the blood. A meta-analysis of the bulk of the literature examining chronic or pervasive stressor effects on lipids demonstrates overall support for the notion that chronic stress is associated with elevated total cholesterol and LDLC concentrations (**Table 1**). Several prospective studies have further substantiated the notion that even when cholesterol concentrations are not elevated during periods of increased workload, there are still positive and significant associations between increased perceived stress and total cholesterol.

Behavioral Influences

Although it has been tempting to suggest that lipid changes are a result of stress-associated behavioral changes, such as diet and exercise modifications, which in turn increase lipid concentrations, data have not confirmed this as an adequate explanation. For example, a very early series of single case studies examined individuals while residing in a metabolic ward for periods of time ranging from 1 to 5 months. Diet, physical activity, exercise, and medication use were not only monitored, but actually closely regulated, and total cholesterol concentrations were measured frequently. Simultaneously, diaries were maintained periodically by both patients and the nursing staff, reporting on mood and perceived stress experiences. Total cholesterol levels were quite variable over time, despite the tightly controlled conditions and behaviors of the patients while in the ward. Moreover, total cholesterol fluctuations upwards were more prominent during times of self-reported perceived stress.

More contemporary studies of much larger groups of men and women similarly found that the chronic stress-associated lipid elevations were maintained even after rigidly controlling variations in diet, exercise, sleep, medication use, and physical activity. For example, healthy men and women undergoing several weeks of predictable but potent work stress had elevated blood total cholesterol, LDLC, and triglycerides relative to lower work stress periods, independent of changes in diet, exercise, physical activity, medication use, and sleep patterns.

That said, in certain circumstances and for certain vulnerable individuals, stress is associated with changes in behavioral risk factors that can have important effects on cholesterol concentrations. For example,

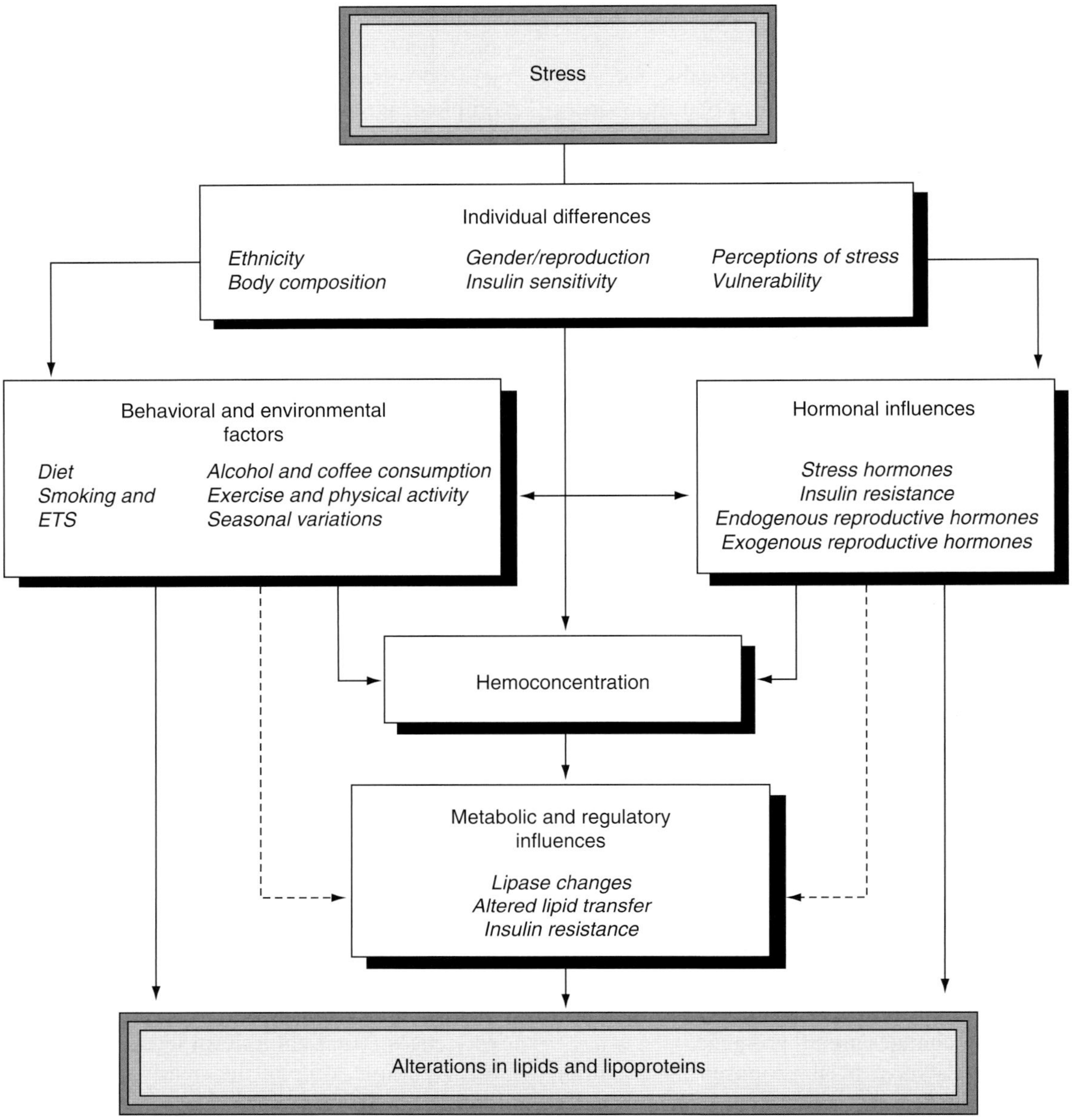

Figure 1 Potential pathways by which stress alters lipid concentrations in the blood (reprinted from Stoney & West (1997) Lipids, personality and stress: Mechanisms and Modulators. In: Hillbrand & Revben (eds) *Lipids, Health, and Behavior*, pp. 47–66. Washington, DC: American Psychological Association, with permission of the American Psychological Association). ETS, environemntal tobacco smoke Solid lines indicate that there is evidence for these pathways. Hashed lines indicate incomplete evidence for these hypothesized pathways.

Table 1 Meta-analysis on the effects of chronic stressors on lipid concentrations

Lipid variable	*Number of studies*	*Unweighted effect size estimates (d)*	*P value*
Total cholesterol	14	0.406	0.0001
LDLC	9	0.358	0.0001
Triglycerides	3	−0.014	0.05
Free fatty acids	5	0.071	0.05

LDLC, low-density lipoprotein-cholesterol.

both chronically and acutely stressful situations cause some people to eat more, while others eat less. Among those who are so-called 'stress eaters', the increased eating may be, in part, a consequence of higher stress-related cortisol elevations. Importantly, at least one study has reported that those who report increasing caloric intake during stress have higher total cholesterol/HDLC during stress. However, even among this subset of vulnerable individuals, the increased lipid concentrations are small. Thus, although there may be a portion of individuals for whom lipid alterations during chronic stress are an indirect consequence of stress-induced changes in eating patterns, this mechanism likely does not explain the larger total cholesterol elevations that occur during stress among the majority of individuals.

Hormonal Influences

One way that stress might influence lipid concentrations is through stress-induced hormonal changes that affect lipid metabolism. For example, stress-induced sympathetic nervous system activity leads to concomitant increases in catecholamines (epinephrine and norepinephrine), glucocorticoids (cortisol), and free fatty acids. These increases have resultant effects on metabolism of the lipoproteins. For example, catecholamines can directly stimulate adipose tissue to release free fatty acids into circulation through the process of lypolysis. In particular, epinephrine induces the release of free fatty acids; during epinephrine infusion and mental stress, free fatty acid concentrations increase concomitantly. Epinephrine-induced increase in free fatty acids may be the result of increased blood flow through adipose tissue or stimulation of adipose-β2 adrenoreceptors. In either case, the accumulation of circulating free fatty acids can trigger the production of triglyceride-rich, very low-density lipoprotein (VLDL) catabolism, which in turn will eventually result in increased concentrations of circulating LDLC. Further, epinephrine will decrease VLDL secretion and increase LDLC uptake by stimulating α1 adrenoreceptors.

Like epinephrine, norepinephrine influences lipoprotein metabolism. Increased norepinephrine activity stimulates adipose β adrenergic receptors. This may result in diminished lipoprotein lipase activity, a subsequent decline in triglyceride clearance, lower concentrations of HDL, and increasing levels of VLDL, intermediate-density lipoproteins (IDL) and LDL. Norepinephrine also decreases hepatic triglyceride lipase activity, which can increase plasma concentrations of both HDLC and triglyceride-risk lipoproteins.

Cortisol also has profound influences on the mobilization of lipids and lipid metabolism through activation of the hypothalamic-pituitary-adrenocortical (HPA) axis. Cortisol sensitizes adipose tissue to the lipolytic effects of catecholamines and increases concentrations of free fatty acids. Moreover, cortisol and free fatty acids stimulate the secretion of VLDL, increase the synthesis, of hepatic triglycerides, inhibit insulin secretion, and increase insulin insensitivity in the tissues. Insulin regulates triglyceride synthesis and hepatic production of VLDL. Thus, the decreased activity of insulin during stress inhibits the regulation of triglycerides and the production of VLDL. Further, insulin resistance and increased levels of cortisol suppress hepatic LDL receptors and catabolism, thereby delaying LDL clearance. Cortisol also stimulates apolipoprotein B (apo B) secretion from cultured rat hepatocytes.

This pathway of stress-related, epinephrine-induced free fatty acid release from adipose tissue, enhanced hepatic cholesterol secretion, cortisol-associated lypolysis, and increased circulating LDLC concentrations has some empirical support. Chronic epinephrine infusions into cynomolgus monkeys produce significant total cholesterol concentration increases, and the same pattern has been noted among humans. Additional data regarding the effects of cortisol are also available. For example, several types of stressors simultaneously elevate LDLC, total cholesterol, apo B, insulin, and plasma cortisol. In some studies, the changes in cortisol positively predict changes in lipids. For example, a recent study reported that individuals with high cortisol stress recovery (reflecting higher cortisol stress responses) also had the highest LDLC and total cholesterol/HDLC ratios. Thus, the sympathetic-adrenal-medullary axis and the HPA axis are likely to play a key role in modulating lipid and lipoprotein metabolism during times of pervasive psychological stress. There are continuing efforts to delineate these pathways more definitively.

Acute Stress Mechanisms of Lipid Variability

The hypothesis that chronic stress affects lipids due to stress-induced hormonal changes has considerable appeal, but it is unlikely to account for the abundant additional data demonstrating rapid and transient increases in plasma cholesterol concentrations during acute psychological stress. For example, many laboratory-based investigations have shown that very short-term stressors, such as those that might occur over a period of several minutes to 1–2 h, can induce

Table 2 Meta-analysis on the effects of acute stressors on lipid concentrations

Lipid variable	*Number of studies*	*Unweighted effect size estimate (d)*	*P value*
Total cholesterol	25	0.306	0.0001
LDLC	14	0.291	0.0002
Triglycerides	24	0.341	0.0001
Free fatty acids	37	0.717	0.0001

LDLC, low-density lipoprotein-cholesterol.

rapid and transient increases in blood concentrations of total cholesterol, LDLC, apo B, and triglycerides. A meta-analysis of these investigations has supported the notion that short-term stress reliably elevates total cholesterol, LDLC, triglycerides, and free fatty acids (**Table 2**). These elevations are clearly not a function of hormonally induced increased synthesis of lipids because the enhanced rate of lipoprotein entry into the circulation would simply take longer than the time period represented in these studies. Kinetic studies document that the manufacture of VLDL from fatty acids and subsequent conversion of LDL requires several hours to days to accomplish. Investigations of acute stress effects have also demonstrated little concordance between catecholamine and cortisol responses and acute changes in blood lipid concentrations. The effects of acute psychological stress on lipid concentrations are therefore likely to operate through a different mechanism or set of mechanisms.

Hemoconcentration Influences

Psychological stress causes a generally transient and rapid decline in the volume of blood plasma, with a resultant mild hemoconcentration of blood cells. This phenomenon is similar to the acute decreases in intravascular plasma volume that occur with postural changes, with a resultant posture-induced hemoconcentration of serum lipids. These plasma volume shifts can occur by increased red blood cell mass, alterations in kidney functioning, and/or through hemodynamically induced fluid shifts. Whatever the exact mechanism of the fluid volume shifts, it is clear that the resultant hemoconcentration leads to higher lipid concentrations in the blood. Thus, the increased lipid concentrations in the blood during acute stress are likely to be partially, but not fully, accounted for by hemoconcentration. Generally speaking, during mild stressors that induce no hemodynamic or hormonal (e.g., catecholamine and blood pressure) changes, a significant portion of the generally small lipid increases might reasonably be accounted for by plasma volume shifts. However, during more substantial psychological stressors that are accompanied by alterations in catecholamines, blood pressure, and cortisol, increases in cholesterol and LDLC are generally more substantial. In some, but not all investigations, the lipid (generally total cholesterol and triglyceride) and lipoprotein (LDLC) elevations remain significant even after correction for transvascular plasma volume shifts. For those investigations that do not show significant lipid elevations after correction for plasma volume shifts, it is possible that the failure to retain significance is related to decreased power in combination with modest effect sizes. The fact that some lipoproteins are consistently elevated during stress (e.g., LDLC) and others are not (e.g., HDLC) suggests that transvascular shifts cannot account for all of the stress-related changes observed, because otherwise all lipid particles would show the same pattern of response.

Metabolic Influences

This state of affairs has led to the speculation that there may be a metabolic explanation for the acute stress-induced elevation in blood lipid concentrations. For example, stress-associated elevations in lipids and lipoproteins may be due to metabolic effects of sympathetic activation. Pharmacologic blockade of sympathetic activation with a nonselective adrenoceptor antagonist among men completing several acutely challenging tasks blocked stress-associated increases in free fatty acids and triglycerides, but not total cholesterol or LDLC. These data add support to the notion that different lipids are likely influenced by environmental and psychological factors through different mechanisms.

Stoney et al. have reasoned that if stress does have a direct influence on certain blood lipid levels, that this may be reflected in the efficiency with which individuals metabolize a high-fat meal during stress. In a test of this hypothesis, a standard intravenous load of intralipid (a triglyceride-rich product) was administered to a group of middle-aged men and women under a condition of psychological stress, and then again during a condition of no psychological stress. In this test, which is similar conceptually to a glucose tolerance test, a triglyceride determination was made and then a standard bolus of intralipid was administered. Serial triglyceride determinations were then made over time, and the disappearance rate constant (K_2) was calculated. Thus, K_2 defines the clearance rate of the exogenous fat solution, with a higher K_2 value indicating a more efficient clearance of triglycerides from the circulation. When administering this test to a group of healthy individuals, Stoney et al. found that K_2 values declined significantly during stress, in relation to a nonstress period, showing that the increases in lipids during acute stress were due to altered clearance rates. They also found that individuals who were slow to clear a triglyceride load were more hostile than those who were more efficient at clearing the triglyceride load imposed. These data are the most compelling to date to indicate that blood lipid concentrations are altered during psychological stress because of altered triglyceride metabolism and that this may be related to an increased risk of CHD.

Interventions to Reduce Stress-Related Increases in Lipids

Outside of altering health behaviors or broad lifestyle changes, very few clinical interventions have been tested as potential means to reduce the stress-associated elevations in lipids. Stress reduction techniques such as relaxation, meditation, and self-monitoring likely have effects on both behavioral risk factors and lipid levels. For example, individuals with highly demanding jobs and who spent 3 weeks away from their job responsibilities and in a spa had more substantial decreases in LDLC and LDL/HDL ratio than did those who also spent time in a spa but who had less demanding occupations. However, no studies have explicitly tested the mechanisms by which reductions in perceived stress related to reductions in lipid and lipoprotein concentrations.

Clinical Implications of Variations in Lipids

There is little doubt about the presence of a direct relationship between blood cholesterol concentrations and the development and initiation of cardiovascular disease. For example, chronically elevated LDLC is associated with an elevated incidence of coronary artery disease (CAD), and lowering LDLC concentrations produces a regression of coronary atherosclerosis and coronary artery events in some individuals. Elevations in triglycerides and low levels of HDLC are also correlated positively with both CAD and CHD although it is not clear to what degree lowering triglyceride or raising HDLC levels also results in a diminished risk for cardiovascular disease.

Although there are no prospective investigations of the clinical relevance of stress-associated elevations in lipids, data from several cross-sectional investigations are informative. A number of investigations have demonstrated that healthy individuals at an elevated risk for the future development of cardiovascular disease have more profound short-term elevations in blood lipid concentrations during stress, relative to a nonstress period. For example, men, postmenopausal women, and healthy young offspring of parents with documented myocardial infarction all have greater elevations in total cholesterol and LDLC during acute psychological stress, relative to women, age-matched premenopausal women, and healthy offspring of parents with no cardiovascular disease, respectively. Additionally, psychosocial factors that have been shown to be related independently to CHD risk, such as hostility and anxiety, are also associated with total cholesterol and LDLC concentrations. Future cross-sectional and prospective investigations examining the extent to which stress-induced elevations in lipid concentrations are atherogenic are warranted.

Further Reading

Brennan, F. X., Cobb, C. L., Silbert, L. H., et al. (1997). Peripheral β adrenoreceptors and stress-induced hypercholesterolemia in rats. *Physiology and Behavior* **60**, 1307–1310.

Brindley, D. N., McCann, B. S., Niaura, R. S., et al. (1993). Stress and lipoprotein metabolism: modulators and mechanisms. *Metabolism* **42**(Suppl 1), 3–15.

Stoney, C. M. and West, S. (1997). Lipids, personality, and stress: Mechanisms and modulators. In: Hillbrand, M. & Spitz, R. T. (eds.) *Lipids, Health, and Behavior*, pp. 47–66. Washington, D.C.: American Psychological Association.

Stoney, C. M., Niaura, R., Bausserman, L., et al. (1999). Lipid reactivity to stress: I. Comparison of chronic and acute stress responses in middle-aged airline pilots. *Health Psychology* **18**, 241–250.

Stoney, C. M., West, S. G., Hughes, J. W., et al. (2002). Acute psychological stress reduces plasma triglyceride clearance. *Psychophysiology* **39**, 80–85.

Strass-Blasche, G., Ekmekcioglu, C. and Marktl, W. (2003). Serum lipid responses to a respite from occupational and domestic demands in subjects with varying levels of stress. *Journal of Psychosomatic Research* **55**, 521–524.

Stress, Insulin Resistance, and Type II Diabetes

C Tsigos and I Kyrou
Evgenidion Hospital, Athens University Medical School, Athens, Greece

Glossary

Adipokines Cytokine-like molecules produced and secreted by the adipose tissue (e.g., leptin, adiponectin, resistin, tumor necrosis factor α [TNF-α], interleukin-6 [IL-6]).

Insulin resistance Decreased ability of insulin to act on its target tissues, resulting in compensatory hyperinsulinemia. Considered to be the earlier abnormality in the natural history of type II diabetes.

Metabolic syndrome Syndrome characterized by the combination of central obesity, insulin resistance, dyslipidemia, and hypertension and correlated with high mortality rates due to cardiovascular complications, which aptly justify the description of the syndrome as the deadly quartet.

Visceral obesity Obesity characterized by fat accumulation predominantly in the abdominal area, also called central or abdominal obesity.

The Stress Response

Stress is defined as a state of disharmony or threatened homeostasis. The concepts of stress and homeostasis can be traced back to ancient Greek history; however, the integration of these notions with related physiological and pathophysiological mechanisms and their association with specific illnesses are much more recent.

When faced with excessive stress, whether biological, physical, or psychological, a subject's adaptive responses attain a stereotypic nonspecific nature, referred to by Selye as the general adaptation syndrome. During stress, attention is enhanced and the brain focuses on the perceived threat. Cardiac output and respiration are accelerated, catabolism is increased, and blood flow is redirected to provide the highest perfusion and fuel to the aroused brain, heart, and muscles.

The central control stations of the stress system are located in the hypothalamus and the brain stem and include the parvocellular corticotropin-releasing hormone (CRH) and arginine-vasopressin (AVP) neurons of the paraventricular nuclei of the hypothalamus and the locus ceruleus-norepinephrine system (central sympathetic system) (**Figure 1**). The hypothalamic-pituitary-adrenal (HPA) axis, together with the efferent sympathetic/adrenomedulary system, represent the effector limbs, via which the brain influences all body organs during exposure to threatening stimuli.

The Hypothalamic-Pituitary-Adrenal (HPA) Axis

The hypothalamus controls the secretion of adrenocorticotropic hormone (ACTH) from the anterior pituitary, which, in turn, stimulates the secretion by the adrenal cortex of glucocorticoids, mainly cortisol in humans. The principal hypothalamic stimulus to the pituitary-adrenal axis is CRH. AVP is a potent synergistic factor with CRH in stimulating ACTH secretion.

In nonstressful situations, both CRH and AVP are secreted into the hypophysial portal system in a circadian, pulsatile fashion, with a frequency of about two to three secretory episodes per hour. Under resting conditions, the amplitude of the CRH and AVP pulses increases in the early morning hours, resulting in ACTH and cortisol secretory bursts in the general circulation. These diurnal variations are perturbed by changes in lighting, feeding schedules, and activity and are disrupted by stress.

Circulating ACTH is the key regulator of glucocorticoid secretion by the adrenal cortex. Glucocorticoids are the final effectors of the HPA axis and participate in the control of whole body homeostasis and the organism's response to stress. They play a key regulatory role in the basal activity of the HPA axis and in the termination of the stress response by acting at the hypothalamus and the pituitary gland and at higher brain centers. Glucocorticoids exert these actions via their glucocorticoid receptors and the rigorous regulation of a plethora of genes that are directly or indirectly implicated in several metabolic pathways, either activating them through positive glucocorticoid responsive elements (GREs) (e.g., genes encoding enzymes of glucose, lipid and amino acid metabolism, lipoprotein receptors, leptin) or repressing them through negative GREs (e.g., CRH, proopiomelanocortin, various cytokines).

The Sympathetic Nervous System

The autonomic nervous system provides a rapidly responding mechanism to control a wide range of functions. Cardiovascular, respiratory, gastrointestinal, renal, endocrine, and other systems are regulated by the sympathetic nervous system, the parasympathetic system, or both. Sympathetic innervation of

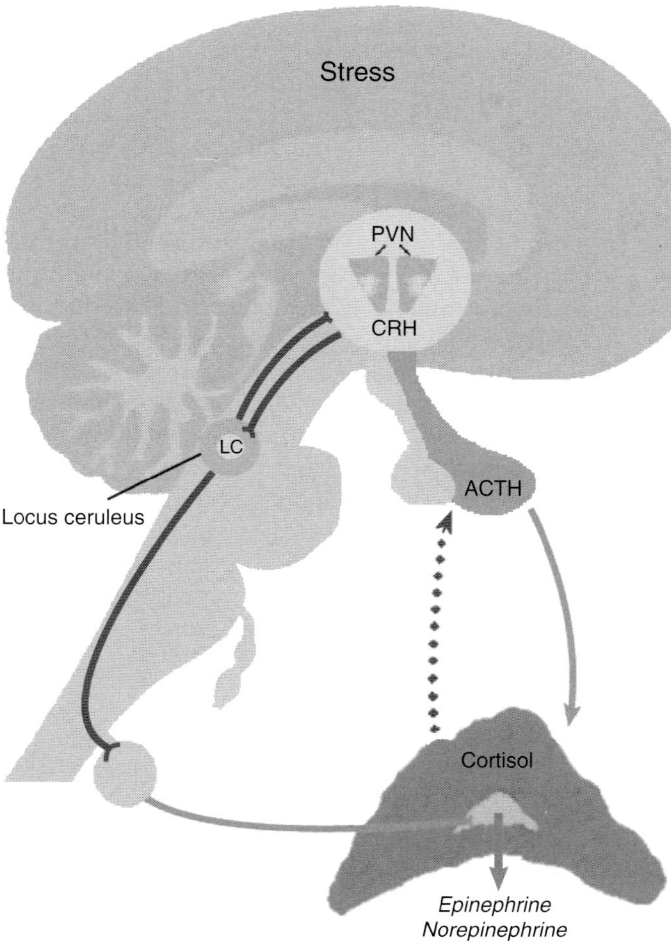

Figure 1 Schematic representation of the stress system, highlighting the major central and peripheral components involved in the stress response. PVN, paraventricular nucleus; CRH, corticotropin-releasing hormone; LC, locus ceruleus/norepinephrine-sympathetic system; ACTH, adrenocorticotropic hormone. Activation is represented by solid lines and inhibition by dashed lines.

peripheral organs is derived from the efferent preganglionic fibers, whose cell bodies lie in the intermediolateral column of the spinal cord. These nerves synapse in the bilateral chains of sympathetic ganglia, with postganglionic sympathetic neurons that richly innervate the smooth muscle of the vasculature, the heart, skeletal muscles, kidney, gut, fat, and many other organs. The sympathetic system also has a humoral contribution, providing most of the circulating epinephrine and some of the norepinephrine from the adrenal medulla (**Figure 1**).

Consequences of Chronic Stress

Generally, the stress response with the resultant activation of the HPA and the sympathetic nervous system axes is meant to be acute or at least of a limited duration. The time-limited nature of this process renders its accompanying antireproductive, antigrowth, catabolic, and immunosuppressive effects temporarily beneficial rather than damaging. In contrast, chronicity of stress system activation would lead to the syndromal state that Selye described in 1936.

The prototypic example of chronic hyperactivation of the stress system is manifested in melancholic depression. Owing to a chronically hyperactive stress system, patients with melancholic depression may sustain several severe somatic sequelae, such as osteoporosis, features of the metabolic syndrome (e.g., visceral fat accumulation, dyslipidemia, increased blood pressure, impaired glucose tolerance), varying degrees of atherosclerosis, immunosuppression, and certain infectious and neoplastic diseases. When not treated, these patients have a compromised life expectancy curtailed by 15–20 years after excluding suicides.

In addition to melancholic depression, a spectrum of other conditions may be associated with increased and prolonged activation of the HPA axis, including childhood sexual abuse, anorexia nervosa with or without malnutrition, obsessive-compulsive disorder, panic anxiety, chronic active alcoholism, and alcohol and narcotic withdrawal.

More specifically, in the context of a mobilized adaptive stress response, glucocorticoids exert a broad spectrum of primarily catabolic effects as part of a generalized effort to utilize every available energy resource against the challenge enforced by the stressors. Thus, glucocorticoids increase hepatic gluconeogenesis and elevate plasma glucose concentrations, induce lipolysis (although they favor abdominal and dorsocervical fat accumulation), and cause protein degradation at multiple tissues (e.g., muscle, bone, skin) to provide amino acids that would be used as an additional substrate for oxidative pathways. In addition to their direct catabolic actions, glucocorticoids also antagonize the beneficial anabolic actions of growth and thyroid hormones, insulin, and sex steroids on their target tissues (**Figure 2**). This stress-related shift of the metabolism toward a catabolic state normally reverses upon retraction of the posed stressor. Chronic exposure to stress and HPA axis activation, however, is expected to progressively increase visceral adiposity, decrease lean body (muscle and bone) mass, and cause insulin resistance (**Figure 2**). Interestingly, the phenotype of Cushing's syndrome, characterized by abdominal and trunk fat accumulation and decreased lean body mass, in combination with various other manifestations of the metabolic syndrome (insulin resistance, dyslipidemia, hypertension, hypercoagulability, and hypercytokinemia), is present in a variety of pathophysiological conditions, categorized as pseudo-Cushing's states. This cushingoid phenotype, under certain conditions of chronic stress, could be attributed to stress-induced mild hypercortisolism, possibly combined with increased peripheral tissue sensitivity to glucocorticoids, the latter depending on the tissue-specific concentration and activity of glucocorticoid receptors, cortisol-binding protein (CBG), and 11β-hydroxysteroid

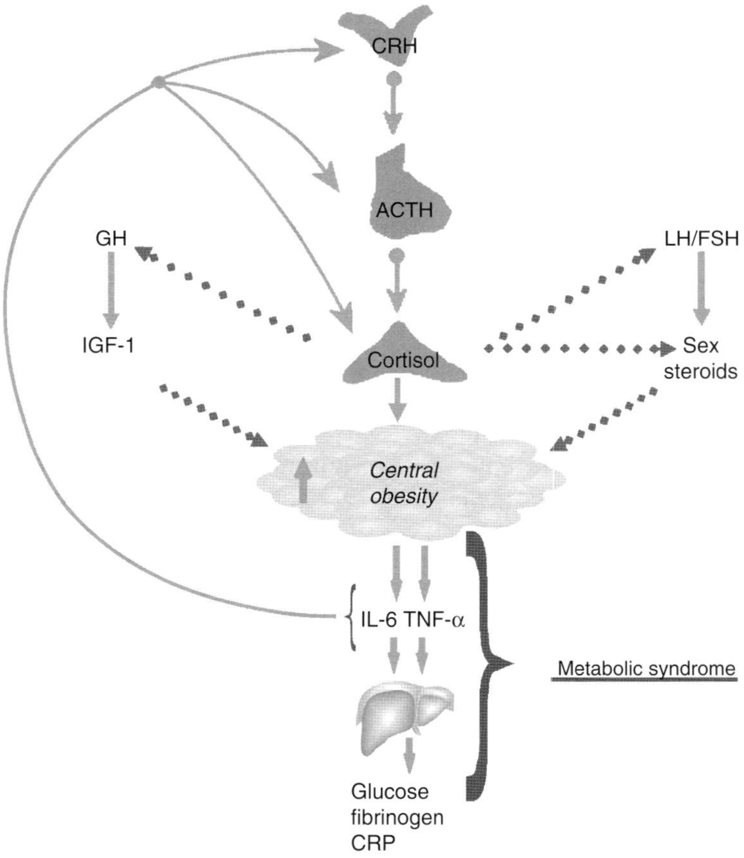

Figure 2 Schematic representation of the detrimental effects of chronic stress on adipose tissue that may lead to clinical manifestations of the metabolic syndrome. Chronic HPA axis activation favors visceral obesity, with cortisol suppressing the beneficial effects of both the gonadal and growth hormone axis and directly stimulating adipocyte proliferation. Hypersecretion of TNF-α and IL-6 is proportional to the cytokines further stimulate the HPA axis activation, thus forming a deleterious vicious cycle. CRH, corticotropin-releasing hormone; ACTH, adrenocorticotropic hormone; TNF-α, tumor necrosis factor α; IL-6, interleukin-6; CRP, C-reactive protein. Stimulatory effects are represented by solid arrows and inhibitory effects by dashed arrows.

dehydrogenase type 1 (11β-HSD1). Interestingly, 11β-HSD1 is an isoform expressed primarily in the liver, adipose tissue, kidneys, and brain that catalyzes the conversion of the inactive cortisone to active cortisol in humans and, thus, locally augments the concentration of the bioactive hormone. This tissue-specific amplification of the cortisol action, mediated by 11β-HSD1, appears to be very important for determining the tissue sensitivity to glucocorticoids and hence to the HPA axis hyperactivation, especially under conditions that potentiate 11β-HSD1 activity, such as visceral obesity.

Depression and Diabetes

Until very recently, the attention of the scientific community had been focused on the emotional consequences of diabetes mellitus, rather than on the emotional causes of the disease. Depression rates are roughly twice as high among persons with diabetes as among persons without diabetes and are higher than those for most other chronic physical illnesses. A meta-analysis of 42 eligible studies showed that the presence of diabetes doubles the odds of comorbid depression, a stable finding in both controlled and uncontrolled studies not affected by sex, subject source, assessment method, or type of diabetes. Yet most of these findings are based on cross-sectional data, so they actually tell us very little about causal relationships.

Recently, however, significant evidence from population-based prospective studies in the United States and Japan shows that being depressed at baseline doubles the risk of subsequently developing type II diabetes and that this association is not explained by other risk factors for type II diabetes, including obesity, activity level, smoking, alcohol consumption, and family history of type II diabetes. Thus, in some circumstances, depression may precede the onset of type II diabetes and may play an important role in its development. As described previously, depressive disorders are accompanied by increased sympathetic and sympatho-adrenal system activity, which is known to be associated with increased blood glucose and impaired glucose tolerance. Depressive disorders have also been associated with increased activity of the HPA axis, which results in an increased release of glucocorticoids, decreased glucose uptake, and elevated glucose levels. Depression may impair the ability to handle a carbohydrate load and then increase the risk of developing type II diabetes through a greater release of the counterregulatory hormones. More importantly, depression is associated with visceral fat accumulation, which is considered the key abnormality underlying the development of insulin resistance and the increased risk for type II diabetes and atherosclerosis. Changes in diet (e.g., unhealthy eating, alcohol consumption) and physical activity associated with chronic depression may also contribute to the glucose abnormalities that may develop.

Interestingly, effective treatment of depression in diabetic patients appears to produce a better glycemic control that is not due to differential effects of treatment on weight. Moreover, in controlled trials of cognitive-behavioral therapy, related improvements in depression produced significant improvements in glycemic control.

Stressful Life Events and Diabetes

Several studies have demonstrated a relationship of stress to glycemic control in samples of patients with type II diabetes. Stress can be managed through the use of behavioral stress management programs or through the administration of anxiolytic medications, both of which have been reported to improve long-term glycemic control in patients with type II diabetes. It is of note that staff-intensive individual training is not always required for a successful behavioral intervention, as group programs in a real-world setting can also result in clinically significant benefits for patients with type II diabetes.

A large recent study (the Hoorn Study) showed that a high number of rather common major life events, consistent with chronic psychological stress, during the past 5 years was indeed related to a higher prevalence of previously unknown type II diabetes, as well as to increased levels of visceral fat accumulation. These associations were independent of family history of diabetes, physical activity, heavy alcohol use, or low level of education. Furthermore, behavioral stress management programs, whether individualized or in groups, usually help.

Inflammation and Diabetes

It has been known for several decades that inflammatory stress is associated with concurrent activation of the HPA axis. Indeed, cytokines and other humoral mediators of inflammation are potent activators of the central stress response, constituting the afferent limb of the feedback loop through which the immune/inflammatory system and the central nervous system communicate (**Figure 3**).

All three inflammatory cytokines tumor necrosis factor α (TNF-α), interleukin-1β, and interleukin-6 (IL-6) can cause stimulation of the HPA axis alone, or in synergy with each other. There is evidence to suggest that IL-6, the main endocrine cytokine, plays the major role in the immune stimulation of the axis.

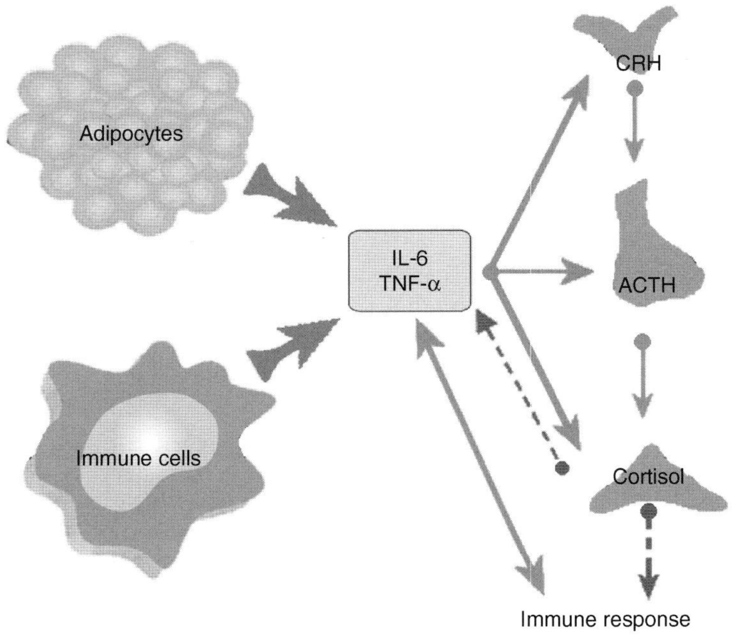

Figure 3 Schematic representation of the interactions between the pro-inflammatory cytokines, the HPA axis, and the immune system response. TNF-α and IL-6 secretion by the adipocytes is continuous and proportional to body mass index (BMI). TNF-α and IL-6 secretion by the immune cells at inflammatory sites occurs in a cascade-like fashion, with TNF-α appearing first followed by IL-6. TNF-α, tumor necrosis factor α; IL-6, interleukin-6; CRH, corticotropin-releasing hormone; ACTH, adrenocorticotropic hormone. Stimulatory effects are represented by solid arrows and inhibitory effects by dashed arrows.

Some of the activating effects of cytokines on the HPA axis may be exerted indirectly by stimulation of the central catecholaminergic pathways. Also, activation of peripheral nociceptive, somatosensory, and visceral afferent fibers would lead to stimulation of both the catecholaminergic and CRH neuronal systems via ascending spinal pathways.

In addition, TNF-α interferes directly with insulin signaling causing insulin resistance, and, together with the other inflammatory cytokines, has direct actions on the endothelium promoting the atherogenic process. Interestingly, TNF-α is overproduced by adipose tissue in obesity and appears to be one of the molecular links between obesity insulin resistance/diabetes and atherosclerosis. Increased production of other adipokines, such as resistin, visfatin, and leptin, and decreased production of adiponectin with expanding obesity, further increase the inflammatory load and the risk for insulin resistance and atherosclerosis.

Indeed, an increasing body of evidence supports a possible role for inflammation in the pathogenesis of type II diabetes. Thus, in the Women's Health Study, an ongoing U.S. primary prevention randomized clinical trial initiated in 1992, elevated levels of C-reactive protein (CRP) and IL-6 predicted the development of type II diabetes. Other common markers of inflammation (fibrinogen, haptoglobin, white-cell count, sialic acid) are also associated prospectively with the development of diabetes in adults. Furthermore, chronic subclinical inflammation relates independently to insulin resistance, even in nondiabetic subjects. It is therefore likely that anti-inflammatory therapy may be beneficial in improving insulin resistance and preventing the development of type II diabetes. Interestingly, thiazolidinediones, a new class of insulin sensitizers, also have anti-inflammatory properties, reducing CRP and TNF-α levels. Moreover, the observed significant reductions in the hazard of becoming diabetic with statins may be attributed at least partly to the anti-inflammatory properties of these drugs.

Conclusion

Chronic stress seems to contribute to the development of visceral obesity and, hence, of type II diabetes and atherosclerosis, and, conversely, the accumulation of visceral adipose tissue constitutes a chronic stressful state. The mechanisms that mediate this documented reciprocal relation and cause the derangement of the metabolic homeostasis are the subject of many recent research efforts, and their characterization will hopefully provide novel insights into the pathogenesis of type II diabetes and cardiometabolic complications and help the quest for more specific and effective therapeutic interventions. Moreover, treating depression in and providing effective stress management programs for people predisposed to diabetes may add a new dimension of primary prevention of type II diabetes to the treatment of traditional risk factors such as obesity, diet, and physical inactivity.

See Also the Following Articles

11ß-Hydroxysteroid Dehydrogenases; Inflammation; Metabolic Syndrome.

Further Reading

Anderson, R. J., Freedland, K. E., Clouse, R. E. and Lustman, P. J. (2001). The prevalence of comorbid depression in adults with diabetes. A meta-analysis. *Diabetes Care* **24**, 1069–1078.

Barzilay, J. I., Abraham, L., Heckbert, S. R., et al. (2001). The relation of markers of inflammation to the development of glucose disorders in the elderly. The Cardiovascular Health Study. *Diabetes* **50**, 2384–2389.

Bjorntorp, P., Holm, G. and Rosmond, R. (1999). Hypothalamic arousal, insulin resistance and type 2 diabetes mellitus. *Diabetic Medicine* **16**, 373–383.

Buren, J. and Eriksson, J. W. (2005). Is insulin resistance caused by defects in insulin's target cells or by a stressed mind? *Diabetes/Metabolism Research and Reviews* **21**, 487–494.

Chrousos, G. P. (1995). The hypothalamic-pituitary-adrenal axis and immune-mediated inflammation. *New England Journal of Medicine* **332**, 1351–1362.

Chrousos, G. P. (2000). The role of stress and the hypothalamic-pituitary-adrenal axis in the pathogenesis of the metabolic syndrome: neuro-endocrine and target tissue-related causes. *International Journal of Obesity* **24**(Supplement 2), S50–55.

Chrousos, G. P. and Gold, P. W. (1992). The concepts of stress system disorders: overview of behavioral and physical homeostasis. *Journal of the American Medical Association* **267**, 1244–1252.

Moller, D. E. and Kaufman, K. D. (2005). Metabolic syndrome: a clinical and molecular perspective. *Annual Reviews in Medicine* **56**, 45–62.

Rubin, R. R. and Peyrot, M. (2002). Was Willis right? Thoughts on the interaction of depression and diabetes. *Diabetes/Metabolism Research and Reviews* **18**, 173–175.

Schmidt, M. I., Duncan, B. B., Sharrett, A. R., et al. for the ARIC Investigators (1999). Markers of inflammation and prediction of diabetes mellitus in adults (Atherosclerosis Risk in Communities study): a cohort study. *Lancet* **353**, 1649–1652.

Seckl, J. R., Morton, N. M. and Chapman, K. E. (2004). Glucocorticoids and 11beta-hydroxysteroid dehydrogenase in adipose tissue. *Recent Progress in Hormone Research* **59**, 359–393.

Surwit, R. S., van Tilburg, M. A. L., Zucker, N., et al. (2002). Stress management improves long-term glycemic control in type 2 diabetes. *Diabetes Care* **25**, 30–34.

Tsigos, C. and Chrousos, G. P. (2002). Hypothalamic-pituitary-adrenal axis, neuroendocrine factors and stress. *Journal of Psychosomatic Research* **53**, 865–871.

Tsigos, C. and Kyrou, I. (2006). Hypothalamic-pituitary-adrenal axis, cytokines and the metabolic syndrome. *Obesity and Metabolism* **2**, 116–126.

Tsigos, C., Kyrou, I. and Chrousos, G. P. (2005). Stress, endocrine manifestations, and diseases. In: Cooper, C. L. (ed.) *Handbook of stress, medicine, and health* (2nd edn., pp. 101–131). Boca Raton, FL: CRC Press.

Metabolic Syndrome

L Keltikangas-Järvinen
University of Helsinki, Helsinki, Finland

Glossary

Innate temperament	A biologically rooted behavioral disposition that is stable across time and situations.
Metabolic syndrome (MetS)	A constellation of physiological and metabolic abnormalities.

What Is Metabolic Syndrome?

Metabolic syndrome (MetS), also called insulin resistance syndrome, is a cluster of various physiological and metabolic abnormalities including hyperinsulinemia, hyperglycemia, hypertension, a decreased plasma concentration of high-density lipoprotein (HDL) cholesterol, an increased plasma concentration of very low density lipoprotein (VLDL) triglyceride, glucose intolerance, and abdominal obesity. Insulin resistance is the primary metabolic defect of this syndrome, with compensatory hyperinsulinemia being the common denominator ultimately responsible for other changes of this constellation. In addition to insulin resistance, abdominal obesity is a key contributor to the development of MetS (see **Figure 1**).

MetS is a huge public health problem worldwide that is responsible for a growing number of premature deaths throughout the world. Its prevalence is approximately 16% among Caucasians. However,

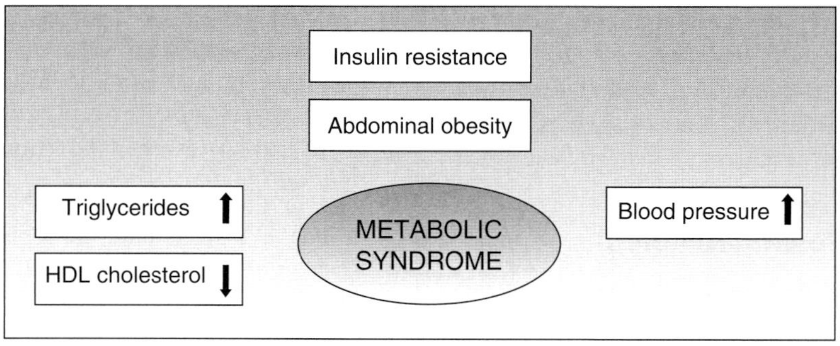

Figure 1 Contributing factors of metabolic syndrome.

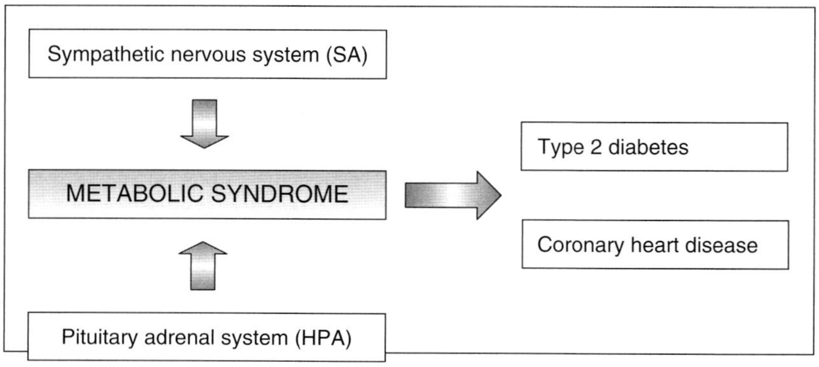

Figure 2 Stress contributes to the development of diabetes and coronary heart disease through metabolic syndrome.

comparison across different countries is difficult as there are different age structures of the population, and even though a World Health Organization (WHO) expert committee published a definition of MetS, there are other, differing definitions available.

MetS is significant because it plays an important role in the etiology of coronary heart disease (CHD) and non-insulin-dependent diabetes mellitus (type II diabetes). Type II diabetes is one of the most prevalent and serious metabolic diseases in the world, and among middle-aged men, CHD is still the leading cause of mortality in Western countries.

Origins of MetS

The exact cause of MetS is not known. It is generally accepted that a genetic predisposition, possibly an interaction of several genes, is an essential factor in the genesis of this disorder. In addition to a genetic predisposition, lifestyle factors such as physical inactivity, habitual alcohol drinking, and smoking play a role in the development of MetS. There is also compelling evidence that stress of diverse origins has a significant role in the development of MetS. It is well established that the development of MetS is indisputably related to activity and/or dysregulation in the two major physiological and neuroendocrine stress systems, the sympathetic-adrenomedullary (SA) system and the hypothalamic-pituitary-adrenomedullary (HPA) system, a key component being the activation of the HPA axis.

The primary role of SA and HPA systems is increasing the energy available for action; activity of these systems is needed in everyday performance. The label of stress systems is based on the fact that they are very sensitive to physical and mental stress. Stress usually refers to overactivity or dysregulation of those systems, not to their ordinary functioning.

SA and HPA systems are both known to exert marked insulin resistance. This is especially true with responses of serum cortisol, as it regulates glucose levels in the blood, with all of the accompanying consequences. To summarize, mental stress might contribute to the development of MetS and subsequently increase the risk of CHD and diabetes via the SA and HPA axes, with increased cortisol secretion being of basic importance (see **Figure 2**).

MetS and Environmental Stress

Evidence of the contribution of environmental stress to MetS via increased reactivity of the stress axis was first derived from animal experiments. It was shown that in standardized experimental stress situations, macaque monkeys reacted with helplessness and loss of control (i.e., with a behavioral stress reaction) and responded with an increased level of cortisol and detached MetS symptoms, especially body fat. Comparable findings have been reported with rats exposed to chronic, uncontrollable environmental stress.

In line with animal studies, it was shown in laboratory experiments with human beings that persons with a high level of MetS symptoms were likely to express elevated responses of serum cortisol during task-induced mental stress.

Research has predominantly emphasized the role of the HPA axis when searching for the mechanism mediating the relationship between stress and MetS. Enhanced sympathetic activity (SA activity) is, however, important as well because chronic sympathetic overactivity with hemodynamic consequences (increased heart rate and pulse pressure) may have pathogenic importance in the development of MetS.

It is also known that long-lasting stress predisposes a person to stronger acute stress reactions, both mental and physical; that is, chronically stressed individuals are likely to show greater reactivity to and prolonged recovery from short-term challenging tasks.

Evidence of the influence of stress on MetS has mostly been based on laboratory experiments, whereas real-life situations, that is, the influence of everyday mental stress, especially long-lasting stress, have not been well studied. The risk characteristic that has been systematically shown to be related to both reactivity of the HPA axis and MetS is vital exhaustion. Vital exhaustion is seen as an indicator of long-lasting mental stress and is characterized by feelings of excessive fatigue, loss of energy, increased irritability, and demoralization. It is also well established that vital exhaustion is a risk factor for CHD, especially for myocardial infarction. The highest risk here, however, is not related to a high level of cortisol but to hypocortisolemia, a state in which both mental and physiological reservoirs are unavailable. This questions the common argument that high risk would be related to high cortisol secretion.

We also know that several coronary-prone personality characteristics, such as type A behavior (i.e., a behavior pattern consisting of aggression, impatience, high striving for achievement, ambitiousness, competitiveness), hostility, and anger, are related to perceived stress and reactivity of SA and the HPA axis. They are also related to components of MetS, even though the empirical findings have not been consistent.

If environmental stress is likely to increase the level of MetS, there is also an inverse effect: environmental support is able to decrease the level of MetS. It is known that changes in perceived social support are associated inversely with changes in the MetS level; that is, increasing support decreases the level of MetS and vice versa. The effect of social support in stress and diseases is widely documented. It increases the overall positive effect, feelings of self-worth and acceptance. It may exert stress-buffering effects by affecting the appraisal of potential stressors or by bolstering coping efforts.

Development of MetS in Childhood

It is generally accepted that atherosclerosis, the underlying process of CHD, originates in childhood and adolescence and that CHD risk factors are already present then. In addition, fasting insulin levels in early adolescence have been shown to predict type II diabetes in young adulthood.

The MetS precursors also appear to be present as early as childhood. It has been shown that the essential parameters of MetS express strong clustering and high tracking, even in healthy children and adolescents. Consequently, the potential effect of stress on the parameters of MetS even in childhood and adolescence has evoked interest. Until recently, the studies were few in number. There are, however, findings that suggest that a stress-prone and inappropriate childhood environment predisposes a child to a high level and early tracking of the parameters of MetS. Sources of environmental childhood stress are, of course, likely to stem from the family environment, especially from parental child-rearing practices. It is well established that a mother's hostile child rearing, consisting of a strict disciplinary style, a tendency to emotionally reject the child, and a feeling that the child is a burden on her, preventing her self-fulfillment, indicates an environmental stress that, in some studies, has been shown to be correlated with an elevated level of a child's MetS parameters.

With regard to the child's own characteristics, some components of type A behavior in adolescence predict changes in the level of MetS, with aggressive competitiveness being especially associated with an increase of that syndrome. In addition, some findings suggest that childhood temperament, especially hyperactivity and negative emotionality, is associated with and predict a later elevated level of MetS (see **Figure 3**).

MetS and Inherited Temperament

The findings previously described are related to the question of whether inherited temperament could play a role as a stress buffer or make a person vulnerable to stress and consequently explain a variance of

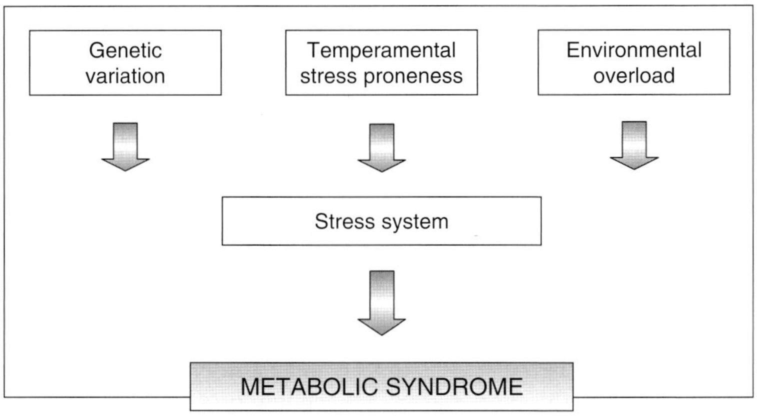

Figure 3 Origins of metabolic syndrome.

MetS. Temperament refers to biologically rooted individual differences in behavioral reactions and dispositions that are present early in life and are relatively stable across time and situations. Temperament is an inherited core of personality; personality is developed by the interaction of inherited temperament and environment, mostly parental child-rearing practices.

Temperament has its origins in brain structures, and individual differences in temperament reflect innate differences in neuroendocrine and autonomic nervous system functions. Therefore, a biologically determined temperament has been viewed as one of the sources responsible for individual differences in stress proneness. It has been suggested to explain the variance in events that are experienced as stressful, and especially why daily troubles have greater health consequences for some individuals than others. There is, indeed, increasing evidence that differences in SA and HPA systems, i.e., differences in major stress systems, are attributable to different temperament profiles.

Findings suggest that childhood temperament plays a direct and indirect role in a development of MetS; that is, it interacts with the environment, meaning that some childhood temperamental factors (e.g., hyperactivity and negative emotionality) are related to an adulthood risk for MetS. In addition, childhood temperament also has an indirect effect. It has been suggested that the influence of hostile maternal child-rearing practices on the child's MetS level may be mediated by the child's temperament. Children with a difficult temperament, conceptualized in terms of negative emotionality (aggression and anger proneness), high activity, and low sociability, are especially vulnerable. Children with this type of temperament are especially prone to high levels of MetS when faced with hostile child rearing.

Interest in the role of adulthood temperament in individual stress reactions has been increasing of late. Findings have conflicted slightly with previous opinions on risk personality. A coronary-prone personality has traditionally been described in terms of hostility, depression, social aloneness, and type A behavior. In contrast, risk temperament is not primarily related to these kind of features; the most vulnerable individuals (i.e., persons who expressed systematically high levels of MetS) are those dealing with oversocialization and overresponsibility. These persons are highly sensitive to social cues of approval or the praise of others, have a strong tendency to conform to peer pressures, and are sensitive to the rejection of others, leading to excessive reward-seeking behaviors such as overworking in response to social rejection or frustration. As workers, they are persistent overachievers who frequently push themselves to exhaustion.

Issues concerning the role of temperament in physiological and neuroendocrine stress reactivity are still new and thus in process. The findings, however, have been promising for explaining the complicated relationship between mental stress and MetS. The findings also suggest that psychological and physiological stress symptoms might have the same source – it may be possible in the future to find a solid neurobiological basis for both psychological and physiological stress reactions.

See Also the Following Articles

Stress, Insulin Resistance, and Type II Diabetes.

Further Reading

Björntorp, P. (1991). Metabolic implications of body fat distribution. *Diabetes Care* **14**, 1132.

Björntorp, P. (1992). Regional fat distribution: implications for type II diabetes. *International Journal of Obesity* **16** (supplement 4), S19–S27.

Björntorp, P. and Rosmond, R. (2000). The metabolic syndrome – a neuroendocrine disorder? *British Journal of Nutrition* **83**(supplement 1), S49–S57.

Black, P. H. (2003). The inflammatory response is an integral part of the stress response: implications for atherosclerosis, insulin resistance, type II diabetes and metabolic syndrome X. *Brain, Behavior, and Immunity* **17**, 350–364.

DeFronzo, R. A. and Ferrannini, E. (1991). Insulin resistance: a multifaceted syndrome responsible for NIDDM, obesity, hypertension, dyslipidemia, and atherosclerotic vascular disease. *Diabetes Care* **14**, 173–194.

Hansel, B., Giral, P., Nobecourt, E., et al. (2004). Metabolic syndrome is associated with elevated oxidative stress and dysfunctional dense high-density lipoprotein particles displaying impaired antioxidative activity. *The Journal of Clinical Endocrinology and Metabolism* **89**, 4963–4971.

Hjemdahl, P. (2002). Stress and the metabolic syndrome: an interesting but enigmatic association. *Circulation* **106**, 2634–2636.

Julius, S. and Gudbrandsson, T. (1992). Early association of sympathetic overactivity, hypertension, insulin resistance, and coronary risk. *Journal of Cardiovascular Pharmacology* **20**, S40–S48.

Keltikangas-Järvinen, L., Räikkonen, K., Hautanen, A., et al. (1996). Vital exhaustion, anger expression, and pituitary and adrenocortical hormones. *Arteriosclerosis, Thrombosis, and Vascular Biology* **16**, 275–280.

Lteif, A. and Mather, K. (2004). Insulin resistance, metabolic syndrome and vascular diseases: update on mechanistic linkages. *Canadian Journal of Cardiology* **20**(supplement B), 66B–76B.

Ravaja, N. and Keltikangas-Järvinen, L. (1995). Temperament and metabolic syndrome precursors in children: a three-year follow up. *Preventive Medicine* **24**, 518–527.

Rosmond, R. (2005). Role of stress in the pathogenesis of the metabolic syndrome. *Psychoneuroendocrinology* **30**, 1–10.

Räikkönen, K., Matthews, K. A. and Kuller, L. H. (2002). The relationship between psychological risk attributes and the metabolic syndrome in healthy women: antecedent or consequence? *Metabolism* **51**, 1573–1577.

Seematter, G., Binnert, C., Martin, J. L., et al. (2004). Relationship between stress, inflammation and metabolism. *Current Opinion in Clinical Nutrition and Metabolic Care* **7**, 169–173.

Circadian Metabolic Rhythms Regulated by the Suprachiasmatic Nucleus

R M Buijs
Universidad Nacional Autónoma de México, Mexico City, Mexico
C Escobar
Universidad Nacional Autónoma de México, Mexico City, Mexico
A Kalsbeek
Netherlands Institute for Neuroscience, Amsterdam, The Netherlands

Organisms Exhibit Metabolic Rhythms: Daily and Annual Rhythms

Humans as well as animals exhibit daily rhythms in the sleep–wake cycle and in feeding and drinking behavior. In addition to these clearly visible behavioral rhythms, there are many physiological rhythms that serve to support behavioral rhythms; for example, several hormones and body temperature have a clear daily rhythm, as well as blood glucose and liver enzymes, which control glycogenesis and glycolysis. Diurnal metabolic rhythms are characterized by their dependence on the suprachiasmatic nucleus (SCN) and are independent of food intake; that is, some metabolic rhythms are expressed both during fasting and with a regular feeding schedule. Other metabolic parameters show fluctuations directly related to feeding events. For example, there is a rise in blood concentration of insulin after each meal. Some species exhibit annual fluctuations in metabolic functions, something that is especially observed in organisms that migrate, hibernate, or accumulate fat for winter. In these species, there are certain periods during the year in which they increase food storage, food ingestion, and fat storage.

The SCN Generates Metabolic Rhythms

The SCN is the master circadian clock, strongly entrained by the light–dark (LD) cycle. The daily changes in activity and sleep of the animal are mainly organized by the SCN and are synchronized to the daily change of the light to dark and vice versa via the light information that reaches the SCN through the optic nerve. There is experimental evidence that SCN lesions abolish the expression of daily rhythms involving glucose and corticosterone, body temperature, locomotor activity, and food intake. Because food intake is driven by the SCN, one might conclude that the other metabolic rhythms are derived from SCN-driven food intake rhythms. However, protocols that force animals into arrhythmic food intake and do not alter the SCN do not abolish glucose rhythmicity in the blood or the rhythmicity in liver enzymes. Such is the case with a protocol during which the animal eats every 4 h 6 times a day: under these conditions, the glucose rhythm in the blood is still maintained (**Figure 1**). In addition, when animals are fasting, the rise in plasma glucose still occurs in anticipation of the coming activity period. The mechanisms behind this daily peak in plasma glucose concentrations were examined by small bolus injections of glucose at different moments of the day. At the

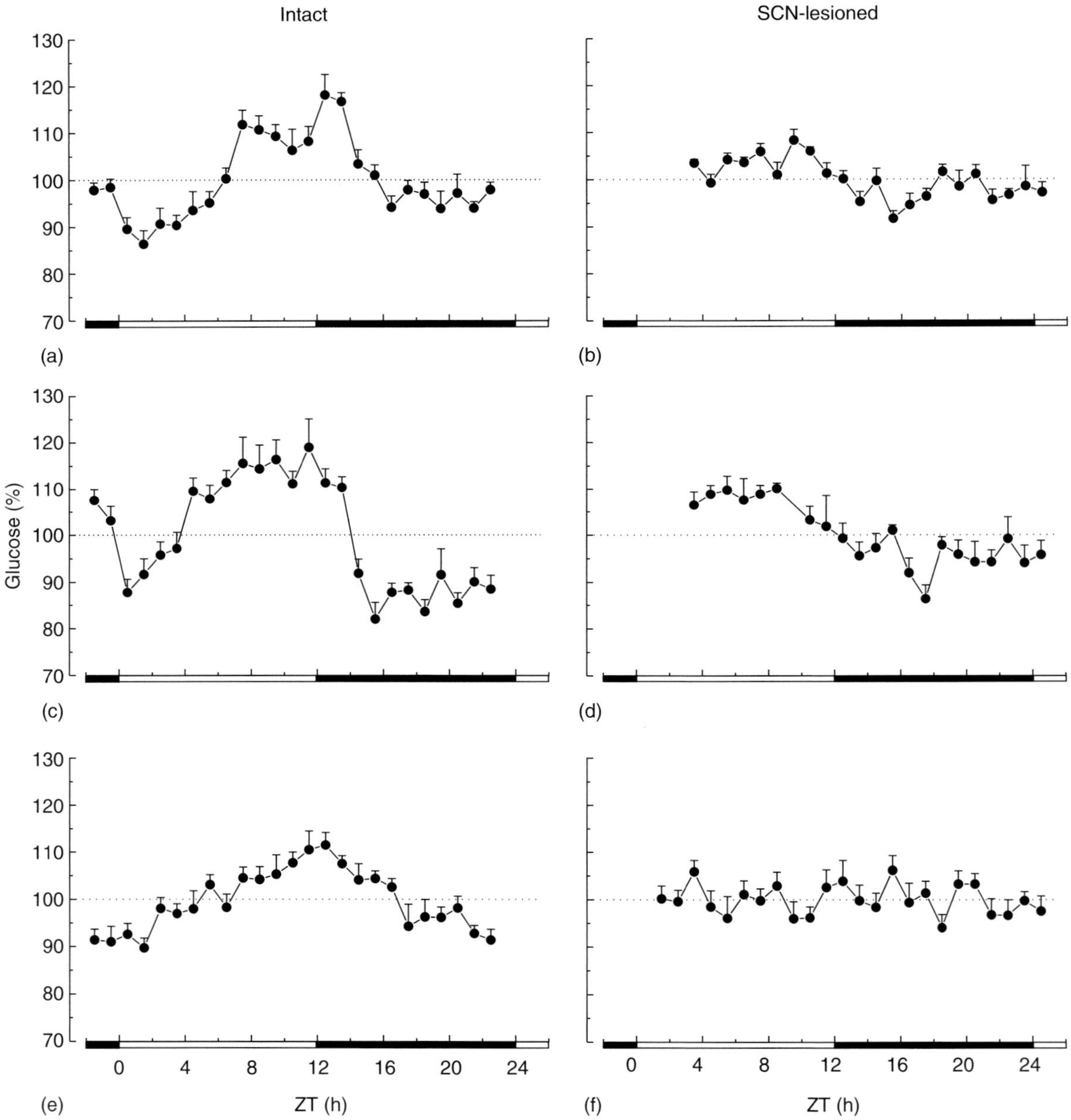

Figure 1 Basal glucose concentrations (values are percentages of the 24 h mean ± SEM) across the LD cycle, in intact rats (left panels; $n=8$) and in SCN-lesioned rats (right panels; $n=7$) under *ad libitum* feeding conditions (a, b), during fasting conditions (started at ZT = −12; c, d), and after having been subjected to a scheduled feeding regimen for at least 2 weeks (e, f). The scheduled feeding regimen consisted of a 10 to 12 min feeding opportunity provided every 4 h. Within 2 weeks, the animals learned to use each opportunity, that is, six every day, and consumed a meal of ±3.5 g at every occasion. The black areas indicate the dark period.

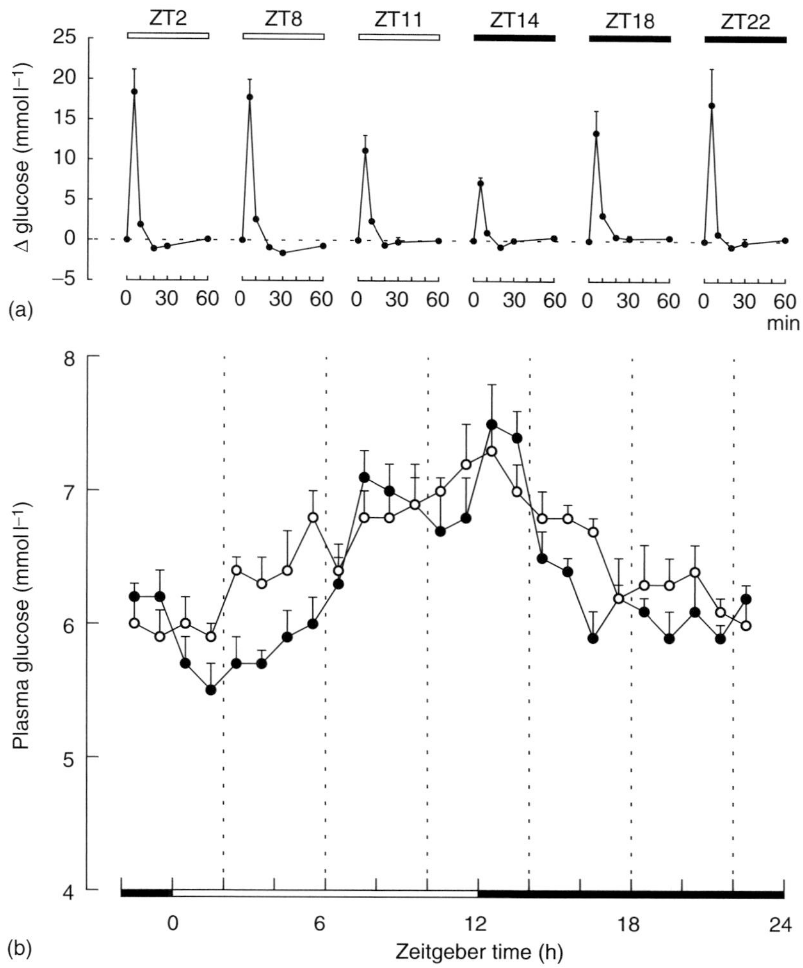

Figure 2 Plasma glucose concentrations after injection of a glucose bolus at different times of the light/dark-cycle (a) and 24 h plasma glucose concentrations during *ad libitum* feeding (closed circles) or during a scheduled-feeding regimen (open circles) (b). Responses in (a) are expressed as the difference with their respective $t = 0$ values. The smaller responses at ZT11 and ZT14 indicate an increased and more rapid uptake of glucose at these times of the LD cycle. The comparable plasma glucose curves of *ad libitum*-fed and scheduled-feeding animals in (b) indicate that the daily rise in plasma glucose concentrations before the dark period is not caused by a day/night rhythm in food intake. In addition, a comparison of the daily plasma glucose curves in (b) with the glucose uptake data in (a) evidences that the daily rise in plasma glucose concentrations is not the consequence of a decrease in peripheral glucose uptake. The black bars in (a) and (b) indicate the dark period.

moment of the highest glucose concentrations in the blood, the lowest induced peak with injected glucose was also seen, indicating that at that moment not only the 'production' of glucose is the highest but also its 'uptake' (**Figure 2**). These observations indicate that the organization of the 'simple' glucose peak in the blood that precedes the activity is a complex event that requires an organization at different levels.

How Does the SCN Induce Rhythms in Metabolic Systems?

Hormonal and autonomic pathways are the two main pathways used by the SCN to transmit its rhythmicity to the body (**Figure 3**).

The Endocrine System

Since a high dose of corticosterone increases glucose output, it has been suggested that the daily corticosterone peak causes the peak in glucose concentrations at the end of the light period. However, in humans, the rise in glucose at the end of the light period is intact after cortisol action has been blocked. Also, no relationship is found between the blood levels of growth hormone (GH) and adrenalin over the 24 h of the day and the daily rhythm of plasma glucose. The 24 h rhythm in GH in rats, for example, is completely different from that in humans, that is, male rats do not display a clear circadian rhythm in GH concentrations, but a strong ultradian rhythm of 3 h. Although there is less and less evidence that links the

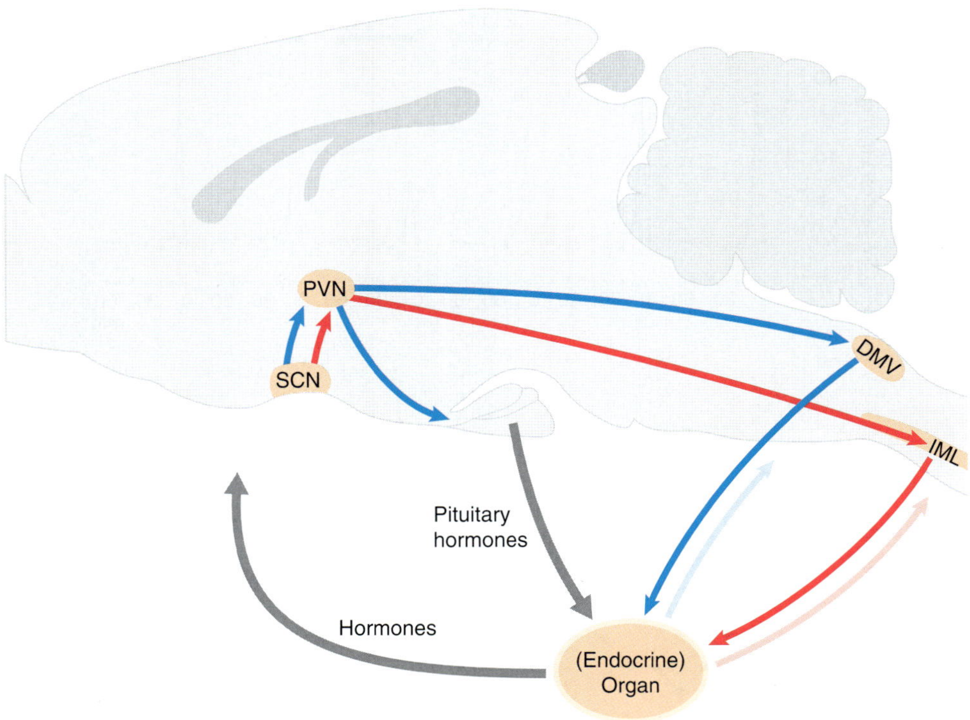

Figure 3 Sagittal scheme of the rat brain illustrates the main pathways by which the SCN communicates its circadian message to the body. Via its connections with the PVN of the hypothalamus (PVN), three different output systems are affected: (1) the neuroendocrine neurons of the PVN responsible for the control of pituitary hormones, (2) parasympathetically projecting neurons in the PVN that specifically target the dorsal motor nucleus of the vagus nerve (DMV), and (3) sympathetically projecting neurons in the PVN that specifically target the spinal cord preganglionic neurons located in the intermediolateral column (IML). The neuronal message prepares and sets the sensitivity of the (endocrine) organs for the arrival of the (pituitary) hormones. In return, the neuronal and hormonal message of the organs will feed back to the CNS (including the SCN), as indicated by the three arrows directed toward the brain.

circadian changes in corticosteroid levels in the blood to the production and release of glucose by the liver, corticosteroids are still assumed to play an important role in the circadian uptake of glucose by the cells of the body. There are several examples that show that glucocorticoids play an important role in preparing the animal for activity. For example, corticosteroids are increased when animals show food anticipatory activity. Moreover, when an animal shows two peaks of activity in 24 h, two anticipatory peaks in corticosterone are also observed.

The exact mechanism by which the SCN controls plasma glucose concentrations is still being explored. The finding, however, of a simultaneous rise in blood glucose concentration and glucose uptake toward the activity period (**Figure 2**) suggests that glucose output to the general circulation must be so powerful that it compensates for increased glucose uptake. Of course, it makes perfect sense functionally to prepare an individual for upcoming activity: at the same time that glucose production is increased, the uptake of glucose increases as well. Moreover, it shows that the SCN is able to organize two completely different processes at the same time. The main source for glucose production is the liver. Hepatic glucose production can be stimulated by the sympathetic nervous system either indirectly, via adrenal hormones and glucagon, or directly, by sympathetic innervation of the liver. However, the evidence for the involvement of glucagon and adrenalin for the SCN-regulated anticipatory increase in plasma glucose concentrations toward the beginning of the activity period is very weak. There is no daily variation in plasma insulin or glucagon levels during a six-meals-a-day schedule; whereas insulin declines after fasting, glucose, in spite of the fast, still increases in anticipation of the activity period. Moreover, the diurnal increase in adrenalin was also shown to be more related to activity than to the anticipatory peak in glucose.

Interestingly, in addition to the 'spontaneous' circadian changes, also in situations of an acute glucose challenge, the SCN sets the response of the endocrine system and autonomic nervous system (ANS). For example, when confronted with a hypoglycemic event in the early activity period, the low glucose level results in enormous changes in corticosterone secretion, while the same hypoglycemic event in the early sleep period results in hardly any changes in corticosterone.

Recently, the role of the arcuate nucleus has been investigated more closely, especially with respect to the control of metabolism. The arcuate nucleus, which lacks a blood–brain barrier and can be seen as a circumventricular organ (CVO), has intense reciprocal connections with the SCN. It is proposed that the SCN may control the sensitivity of the arcuate for circulating metabolites in a daily manner by means of this interaction. Moreover, several studies have also implicated the arcuate nucleus in the control of seasonal metabolic functions. For example, in hamsters, an increase in VGF protein/mRNA content in the arcuate nucleus precedes the photoperiod-induced increase in food intake and body fat. VGF is a protein involved in the control of food intake and has a widespread distribution in the central nervous system (CNS), including the SCN. Interestingly, in the hamster, the region of the arcuate is an important target for melatonin. This hormone, whose nightly secretion is organized by the SCN, has important seasonal functions. Since the arcuate nucleus is also an important target for SCN neurons, the organization of annual metabolic rhythms can be seen to be tightly linked to daily and seasonal metabolic functions.

Autonomic Output

The output of the SCN to the preautonomic neurons in the hypothalamus (mainly paraventricular nucleus (PVN)) is responsible for sending the circadian signal directly to our organs by the autonomic nerves (**Figure 3**). The PVN has extensive projections to sympathetic and parasympathetic motor neurons in the spinal cord and in the brain stem, respectively. Early studies using electric stimulation of the hypothalamus combined with blocking the output of the ANS showed that the effects of electrical stimulation on glucose metabolism were mainly reached by the ANS. Interestingly, at that time, it was also shown that exposure to bright light resulted in an increase in sympathetic nerve activity to the adrenal gland, liver, and pancreas, and in a decrease in vagal nerve activity to the pancreas and the liver. This effect disappeared after SCN lesioning, suggesting that light via the retinal terminals in the SCN was able to reach the target organs by the ANS. Recent studies have shown that the dorsomedial hypothalamus (DMH)/PVN area is essential for transmitting the circadian signal to the liver, pancreas, and fat tissue via the ANS. Later anatomical studies showed that after retrograde transneuronal tracer injection in the liver, pancreas, and fat tissue, separate sympathetic and parasympathetic pathways could be made visible that originate in different cells of the SCN. Consequently, the SCN contains neurons that are either preautonomic to the parasympathetic system or preautonomic to the sympathetic system, which projects to the pancreas, liver, or visceral fat. These SCN neurons transmit their message to the PVN, from which separate parasympathetic and sympathetic pathways target the respective autonomic motor neurons. Recent experiments have shown that the sympathetic innervation to the liver plays a major role in liberating glucose from the liver. Removing GABAergic blockade (γ-aminobutylic acid (GABA) from SCN terminals?) within the PVN by means of Bicucullin (a GABA-A antagonist) infusion showed that the resulting glucose peak was mainly induced via the sympathetic innervation of the liver and not by increases in corticosterone and glucagon.

The control by the SCN of glucose tolerance is more likely to be at the level of the muscle, where the major (insulin-mediated) glucose uptake occurs. The mechanisms by which the SCN affects glucose uptake are still not known.

Integration of Glucose Rhythms and Energy Balance

Interaction of the SCN with Hypothalamic Nuclei Involved in Energy Balance

Sensing energy stores The brain depends entirely on glucose as fuel for its energy, while other organs, such as the heart, kidney, and skeletal muscle, may also rely on free fatty acids (FFAs) or other metabolites. In addition, the brain can actively take up glucose via glucose transporters, independent of insulin, which assures that, when insulin levels are low (fasting), the brain acquires sufficient glucose preferentially, because other tissues are dependent on insulin for glucose uptake. Thus sufficient glucose is always available to the brain.

Of course, in order to be able to balance and direct energy fluxes, the brain needs a precise and clear view of the metabolic state of the body. Circulating humoral factors provide an average signal of the whole body status, while sensory information from specific body regions provides detailed information. Sensory information from tissues important for energy storage, such as the liver (short-term storage) and fat tissue (long-term storage), must be available; recent studies have shown that both liver and fat tissue do provide such sensory information to the brain. In addition, tissues that use up a great deal of energy, such as muscles (skeletal and heart) and kidney, also need to transmit their energy level (and requirements!) to the brain.

Consequently, the brain plays a crucial role in sensing circulating metabolites and hormones; the CVOs, which lack the blood–brain barrier, such as the ventromedial arcuate nucleus (vmARC), area postrema (AP), subfornical organ (SFO), and organum vasculosum of the lamina terminalis (OVLT), likely play an important role in this regard. At present, it seems likely that especially the AP and vmARC play a major role in metabolic sensing and signaling, while the OVLT and SFO functions are more adapted for maintaining the osmolarity and salt levels of the blood. Recently, reciprocal connections between the SCN and vmARC were described, indicating that not only is the SCN kept informed about circulating metabolites, but that it might also be able to gate this information at the vmARC, depending on the time of the day (**Figure 4**). This hypothalamic integration of peripheral metabolic information results in an immediate modulation of metabolism. For instance, fatty acids and insulin are sensed in the vmARC, which leads to a change in autonomic output, affecting endogenous glucose production by the liver, glycogen synthesis in muscle, and food intake. Also, leptin and glucose are sensed in the vmARC, and their increase leads to inhibition of food intake and activation of anabolic functions, such as promotion of glycogen synthesis and lipid storage.

Interaction with Other Hypothalamic Nuclei

For a better understanding of how the SCN affects metabolism, it is also necessary to have a view on how the different hypothalamic structures influence metabolism. Each hypothalamic structure has its own role and interacts and influences the other structures within the hypothalamus in a specific manner. Clearly, there are main food intake stimulatory centers such as the neuropeptide Y (NPY) and agouti-related peptide (AGRP)-containing neurons of the medial arcuate nucleus, while the food inhibitory centers (the pro-opiomelanocortin (POMC)-containing neurons) are in the lateral arcuate nucleus. In addition to these (according to the current views) main structures for controlling food intake, the ventromedial hypothalamus (VMH), the lateral hypothalamus, and the DMH are essential for integrating and transmitting visceral and hypothalamic information; the PVN

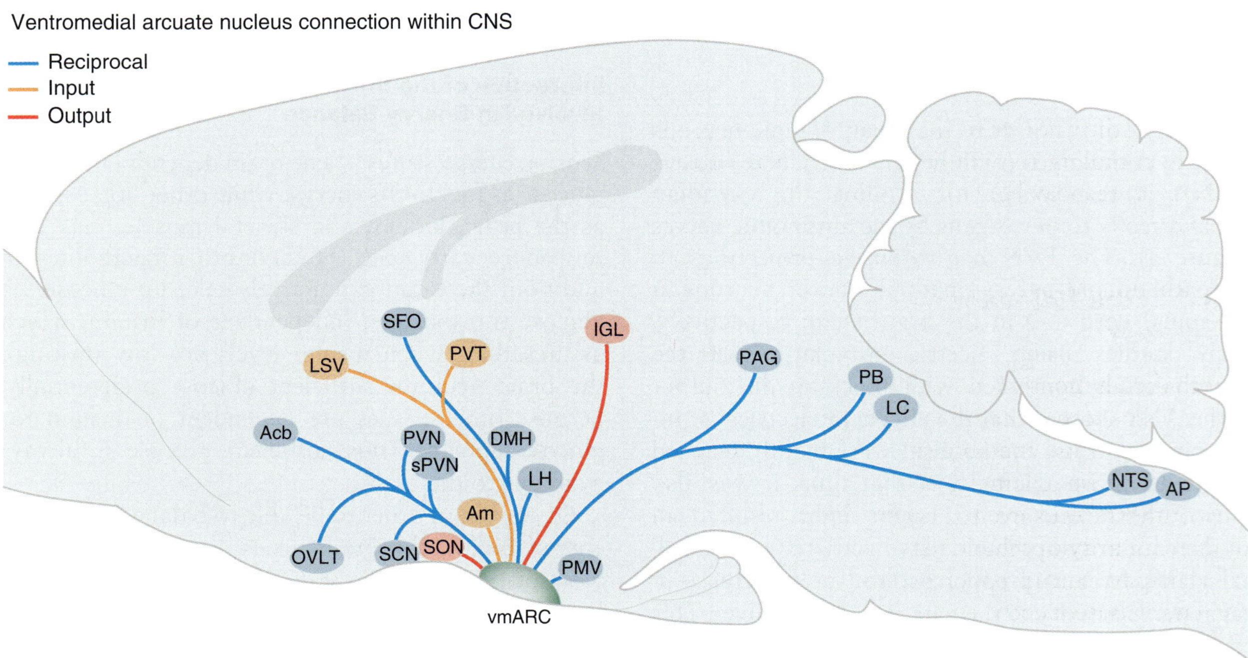

Figure 4 Sagittal scheme of the rat brain to illustrate the main connections of the ventromedial arcuate nucleus (vmARC) within the CNS. Brain areas that have reciprocal connections with the vmARC are indicated in blue. Brain areas with a significant input to the vmARC (i.e., PVT, LSV, and Am) are indicated in orange. Red areas (i.e., IGL and SON) represent those brain areas that receive a significant output from the vmARC. Acb, nucleus accumbens; LSV, lateral septal nucleus ventral part; OVLT, organum vasculosum lamina terminalis; SFO, subfornical organ; LH, lateral hypothalamus; SCN, suprachiasmatic nucleus; SON, supraoptic nucleus; PVN, paraventricular nucleus; sPVN, sub paraventricular nucleus; Am, amygdaloid complex; DMH, dorsomedial hypothalamic nucleus; PVT, paraventricular nucleus of the thalamus; PMV, premammilary nuceus ventral part; IGL, intergeniculate leaflet; PAG, periaquaductal grey; NTS, nucleus tract solitarius, LC, locus coeruleus; AP, area postrema; PB, parabrachial nucleus.

seems to play a role mainly as integration and output center (hormonal and autonomic) of the hypothalamus. In addition to these structures that are directly involved in the control of food intake, there are also structures that are involved in related functions, which are also very important for metabolism, such as the medial preoptic area (MPO), which is essential for the control of thermoregulation. The importance of this interaction becomes clear when one evaluates the consequences of fasting for the physiological organization of the body. Fasting results in a diminishment in temperature, but only during the sleep period; it lowers the heart rate, during the day as well as at night; and it increases running wheel activity in rats in spite of the diminishing energy stores. At the same level, induced obesity in rats also affects the organization of hypothalamic functions; it diminishes the amplitude of the circadian activity and decreases nighttime body temperature. On the other hand, infection also has a large impact on hypothalamic function; it increases corticosterone secretion, diminishes activity, increases temperature, and induces sleep. These observations emphasize the interactions between the different hypothalamic structures and how they affect the functioning of the biological clock. In order to understand these mechanisms, it is important to consider that, in addition to light information that reaches the SCN, mainly in the ventral part, also (metabolic) information from the circulation may reach the SCN via CVOs such as the arcuate nucleus. This site of integration in the SCN (i.e., light and metabolic data target the same area) may allow metabolic information to modify the activity of the SCN similar or contrary to the way light affects the SCN.

What is the Relevance of Metabolic Rhythms?

Metabolic rhythms allow adaptation to daily activities and to annual geographical fluctuations in temperature and food availability, thus allowing animals to adjust their energy balance according to the environment. And even more importantly, because of the regularity of these rhythms, they allow animals to anticipate and prepare for those environmental changes. Consequently, the coherence of endogenous metabolic oscillations with the external cycles of the environment is very important for health and homeostasis. When endogenous rhythms uncouple from the external cycles, individuals cannot exhibit the adequate response at the moment when it is needed and they develop health problems and disease. Such is the case in shift workers who work regularly during the normal sleeping period.

Anticipation of Changes in Energy Requirement

In order to maintain homeostasis, the body needs to anticipate changes in the environment. One of the clearest examples is the anticipation of seasonal changes. Here the SCN–pineal axis is essential for preparing the animal for the upcoming change in food supply, which forces profound changes in reproduction and metabolism. Day length influences the duration of melatonin secretion, and when the period of melatonin secretion is increased or decreased for some time, the reproductive axis, food intake, and fat storage are simultaneously affected. A number of species (especially humans) are not (notably) influenced by the change in seasons, but in all mammals the biological clock, the SCN, has a special role, in that it takes care of anticipating change in metabolism prior to a period of activity. This anticipatory role of the SCN is characteristic of its involvement in the organization of the physiology in animals, and its influence on metabolism can be seen, for example, in the rise in glucose, corticosterone, and body temperature just before awaking (**Figure 1**). The appropriate organization of the metabolism is essential for the life of an organism: this may be the reason why, in addition to the circadian system, a number of other physiological systems and/or functions also influence metabolic functions, such as body temperature, fluid balance, the immune system, and reproduction. These functions are all organized within the hypothalamus, where the main tasks of the body are controlled and transmitted to the body by hormones and the autonomic nervous system. Clearly, the organization of metabolic functions takes place within this circuit of brain–body interaction, and a change anywhere in this circuit has repercussions for both brain and body. For example, the metabolic syndrome is a metabolic disease which is characterized by hyperlipidemia, visceral obesity, hypertension, or diabetes. Disturbed circadian rhythms are a prominent feature of the metabolic syndrome.

Metabolic Rhythms without the SCN; Food Entrainment

Under special conditions, when food is restricted to a short daily event, animals show metabolic adjustments that enable them to deal with such a restricted feeding schedule. Also, animals modify their behavioral patterns in order to be active and anticipate meal time. Animals show increased arousal, foraging, and locomotion 2–3 h before expected food access, a preparatory behavior known as 'food anticipatory activity.' This anticipatory behavior appears independent of the SCN-driven nocturnal activity characteristic of most rodents, which remains, although with decreased amplitude. In order to adjust to the feeding schedule, metabolic rhythms show phase shifts and exhibit peaks related to meal time; some of them, like the corticosterone rhythm, exhibit a peak during meal time anticipation, while the largest part of the SCN cellular activity and metabolism remains adjusted to the LD cycle. Metabolic rhythms persist independent of the SCN and continue to oscillate with a 24 h period, probably driven by food-entrained oscillators. This conclusion is based on the observation that food entrainment is also visible in SCN-lesioned animals, indicating that the SCN is not essential for food entrainment. Due to this latter fact, for approximately 30 years, there has been a search for a different biological clock, the food-entrained oscillator, which is thought to drive food-entrained rhythms when food access is uncoupled from the LD cycle. The functional and anatomical identity of this clock remains unknown to date. Recent studies have evidenced that under restricted feeding schedules, food becomes a powerful entraining signal for most of the peripheral organs in which diverse cellular functions exhibit food-entrained rhythms. In both peripheral organs and in brain structures, feeding schedules entrain daily oscillations of clock genes. Thus it has become clear that food, when restricted to a few hours a day, can override the signals of the LD cycle-driven clock and can uncouple the metabolic oscillations from the SCN. However, this does not imply that, under normal circumstances, the SCN is not involved in food entrainment, because in such conditions animals organize their meals according to their activity phase.

In order to approach phenomena of internal desynchronization resulting from jet lag, shift work, or nocturnal activities, it is important to keep in mind that food can exert a powerful influence as an entraining signal to the peripheral organs and metabolic processes. Such circadian disorders can be approached by tightly controlling the feeding schedules in order to shift metabolic rhythms to the expected phases. Also, it remains to be established whether disorganized feeding schedules can be linked to metabolic problems due to uncoupling of peripheral oscillators from the SCN.

The Metabolic Syndrome: A Brain Disease?

Ignoring the Signal of the Clock

The background of the mechanisms causing the metabolic syndrome is incompletely understood. In general, there is agreement that the cause for this outbreak of obesity must lie in the abundance of food in modern societies and the fact that evolution has shaped us for periods of scarcity rather than surplus. In addition, our evolutionary-shaped homeostatic systems have 'learned' to adapt to the everchanging LD cycle, in such a way that the body anticipates the upcoming sleep and activity periods. During the past century, life has changed dramatically in industrialized countries. Food has become abundant and snacking frequency has increased and shifted toward the end of the day, while at the same time the necessity for physical effort has become considerably reduced. Also, physical activity no longer necessarily coincides with the light period. We hypothesize that in such conditions the susceptible brain loses its feeling for internal and external rhythm. As a result, the environment sensed by the brain has become metabolically flattened and arrhythmic. Since the brain uses the ANS to implement the internal rhythmicity, we propose an unbalanced and arrhythmic ANS as a major cause of the metabolic syndrome.

The organization of the output of the SCN via the ANS forms the basis for this proposal. For a long time, fat tissue has been assumed to be targeted by hormones or to be innervated by the sympathetic nervous system only. Recently, it was demonstrated that parasympathetic input from the vagal motor nucleus to fat tissue clearly modulates insulin sensitivity and glucose and fat metabolism in fat tissue in an anabolic way. This allows the brain to stimulate either the burning of fat (sympathetic) or the accumulation of fat (parasympathetic). Moreover, we demonstrated that the brain has an astonishing capacity with respect to the specialization of neurons in the hypothalamus and SCN. For example, preautonomic neurons are present in the SCN and other hypothalamic areas that project either to the intra-abdominal or the subcutaneous body compartment. The significance of this is that the intra-abdominal organs, for example, visceral fat, liver, and pancreas, receive input from the same neurons (**Figure 5**). Since consuming a meal stimulates the parasympathetic output to the pancreas and results in insulin secretion, the consequence of this hard ANS wiring is that the same stimulus will also increase the insulin sensitivity of the liver and of the visceral fat. Since meals consumed in the evening are known to lead to enhanced insulin secretion, a more efficient uptake of glucose in visceral fat will accordingly result in easier accumulation of intra-abdominal fat. These facts, taken together, indicate that as a consequence of the changed lifestyle in industrialized countries, the metabolic syndrome is on the rise as well, not necessarily because too much food is consumed, but because food is eaten at the wrong time!

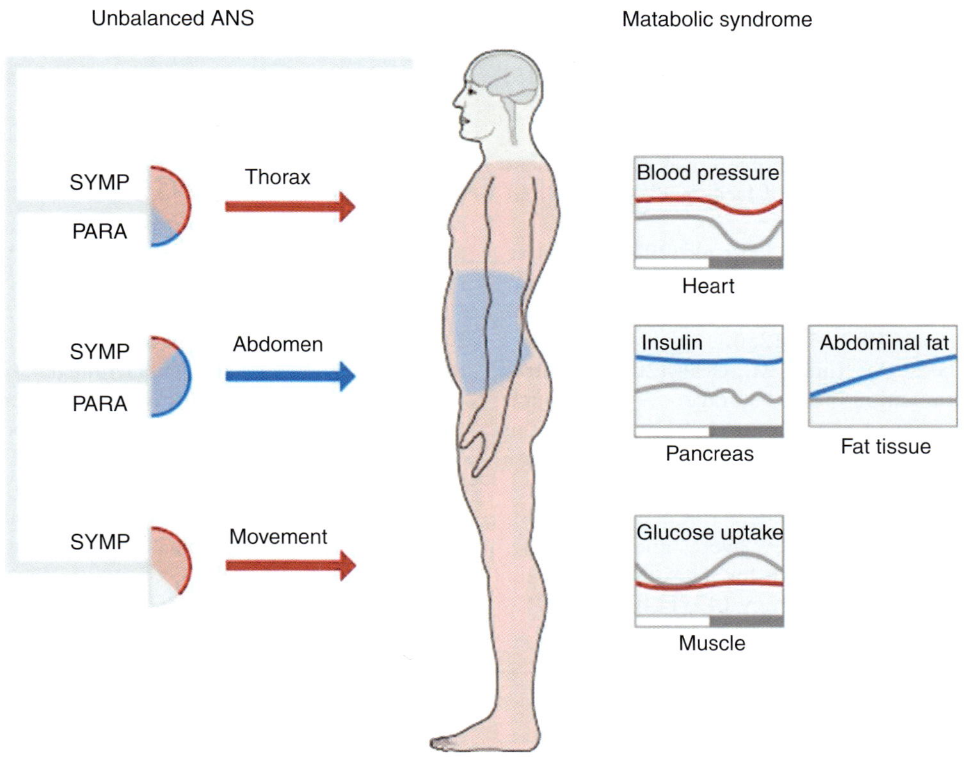

Figure 5 Model of the metabolic syndrome caused by a central nervous deregulation. The disturbed output of the biological clock affects the selective balance of the autonomic nervous system (ANS) in different parts of the body. In the intra-abdominal compartment, the ANS is shifted in favor of the parasympathetic branch, resulting in high insulin secretion, growth of intra-abdominal fat tissue, and fatty liver. Contrarily, in the thorax and movement compartment, the sympathetic branch prevails, leading to high blood pressure and impaired glucose uptake by the muscle. In this model, the symptoms of the metabolic syndrome are result and not cause of the disease.

Further Reading

Buijs, R. M., Chun, S. J., Niijima, A., et al. (2001). Parasympathetic and sympathetic control of the pancreas: A role for the suprachiasmatic nucleus and other hypothalamic centers that are involved in the regulation of food intake. *Journal of Comparative Neurology* **431**, 405–423.

Buijs, R. M. and Kalsbeek, A. (2001). The day–night balance of everyday life: Central and peripheral clocks interacting in the hypothalamus. *Nature Reviews Neuroscience* **2**, 521–526.

Buijs, R. M., La Fleur, S. E., Van Heijningen, C., et al. (2003). The suprachiasmatic nucleus balances sympathetic and parasympathetic output to peripheral organs through separate preautonomic neurons. *Journal of Comparative Neurology* **464**, 36–48.

Buijs, R. M., Wortel, J., Van Heerikhuize, J. J., et al. (1999). Anatomical and functional demonstration of a multisynaptic suprachiasmatic nucleus adrenal (cortex) pathway. *European Journal of Neuroscience* **11**, 1535–1544.

Cailotto, C., La Fleur, S. E., Van Heijningen, C., et al. (2005). The suprachiasmatic nucleus controls the daily variation of plasma glucose via its autonomic output to the liver: Are the clock genes involved? *European Journal of Neuroscience* **22**, 2531–2540.

Damiola, F., Le Minh, N., Preitner, N., et al. (2000). Restricted feeding uncouples circadian oscillators in peripheral tissues from the central pacemaker in the suprachiasmatic nucleus. *Genes and Development* **14**, 2950–2961.

Fleur la, S. E., Kalsbeek, A., Wortel, J., et al. (1999). A suprachiasmatic nucleus generated rhythm in basal glucose concentrations. *Journal of Neuroendocrinology* **11**, 643–652.

Fleur la, S. E., Kalsbeek, A., Wortel, J., et al. (2000). Polysynaptic neural pathways between the hypothalamus, including the suprachiasmatic nucleus, and the liver. *Brain Research* **871**, 50–56.

Kalsbeek, A. and Buijs, R. M. (2002). Output pathways of the mammalian suprachiasmatic nucleus: Coding circadian time by transmitter selection and specific targeting. *Cell Tissue Research* **309**, 109–118.

Kalsbeek, A., Fliers, E., Romijn, J. A., et al. (2001). The suprachiasmatic nucleus directly generates the diurnal changes in plasma leptin levels. *Endocrinology* **142**, 2677–2685.

Kalsbeek, A., La Fleur, S. E., Van Heijningen, C., et al. (2004). Suprachiasmatic GABAergic inputs to the PVN control plasma glucose concentrations in the rat via sympathetic innervation of the liver. *Journal of Neuroscience* **24**, 7604–7613.

Kalsbeek, A., Ruiter, M., La Fleur, S. E., et al. (2003). The diurnal modulation of hormonal responses in the rat varies with stimuli. *Journal of Neuroendocrinology* **15**, 1144–1155.
Kalsbeek, A. and Strubbe, J. H. (1998). Circadian control of insulin secretion and glucose homeostasis is independent of the temporal distribution of feeding. *Physiology and Behavior* **63**, 553–560.
Kreier, F., Fliers, E., Voshol, P. J., et al. (2002). Selective parasympathetic innervation of subcutaneous and intra-abdominal fat – functional implications. *Journal of Clinical Investigation* **110**, 1243–1250.
Kreier, F., Kalsbeek, A., Ruiter, M., et al. (2003). Central nervous determination of food storage – A daily switch from conservation to expenditure. Implications for the metabolic syndrome. *European Journal of Pharmacology* **480**, 51–65.
Kreier, F., Kap, Y. S., Mettenleiter, T. C., et al. (2006). Tracing from fat tissue, liver and pancreas: A neuroanatomical framework for the role of the brain in type 2 diabetes. *Endocrinology* **147**, 1140–1147.
Kreier, F., Yilmaz, A., Kalsbeek, A., et al. (2003). Hypothesis: Shifting the equilibrium from activity to food leads to autonomic unbalance and the metabolic syndrome. *Diabetes* **52**, 2652–2656.
La Fleur, S. E., Kalsbeek, A., Wortel, J., et al. (2001). A daily rhythm in glucose tolerance. A role for the suprachiasmatic nucleus. *Diabetes* **50**, 1237–1243.
Niijima, A., Nagai, K., Nagai, N., et al. (1999). Light enhances sympathetic and suppresses vagal outflows and lesions including the suprachiasmatic nucleus eliminate these changes in rats. *Journal of the Autonomic Nervous System* **40**, 155–160.
Ruiter, M., La Fleur, S. E., Van Heijningen, C., et al. (2003). The daily rhythm in plasma glucagon concentrations in the rat is modulated by the biological clock and by feeding behaviour. *Diabetes* **52**, 1709–1715.
Yi, C., Van Der Vliet, J., Dai, J., et al. (2006). Ventromedial arcuate nucleus communicates peripheral metabolic information to the suprachiasmatic nucleus. *Endocrinology* **147**, 283–294.

Metabolic Syndrome and Sleep

F W Turek
Northwestern University, Evanston, IL, USA

Introduction

Simply observing people – at the beach, at a shopping mall, walking down a crowded street, at a sports stadium, or in the workplace – will lead the observant individual to the inescapable conclusion that there is a major medical problem in the United States: obesity. Obesity is a disease that in just the past few decades has been increasing dramatically in developed countries, and it has reached epidemic levels in the United States. Color maps of the United States provided by the US Centers for Disease Control and Prevention, depicting the prevalence of overweight people in individual states, reveal in a dramatic fashion just how rapidly the 'obesity invasion' has occurred and the enormity of the epidemic. ('Overweight' refers to a body mass index, or BMI, between 25 and 30, and obesity is a BMI >30; this measure of obesity is calculated as weight in kilograms divided by the square of height in meters.) The obesity epidemic is not limited to adults, as there are numerous epidemiological studies demonstrating an alarming increase in obesity in children. This increase is even leading diabetologists to rethink the term 'adult-onset diabetes,' to differentiate adult-onset (type 2) from juvenile-onset (type 1) diabetes, as many juveniles are now being diagnosed with insulin resistance and type 2 diabetes. Furthermore, this epidemic of obesity is not limited to the developed, food-rich countries of the world, as increased signs of obesity and diabetes are being found in less developed countries, including the two most populous countries, China and India.

Besides the social stigma attached to obesity, the upward trends in BMI are cause for concern because of risks of secondary complications, including signs of what has been referred to as the 'metabolic syndrome' (formerly referred to as syndrome X), including insulin resistance, hyperglycemia, dyslipidemia, hypertension, inflammation, and coagulation disorders. Obesity and the metabolic syndrome have been linked to heart attack, stroke, diabetes, cancer, and arthritis, all of which are responsible in part for some of the major health problems facing the industrialized world today.

While less easy to observe by just watching people walk down the street, in the United States there has been a parallel epidemic – an epidemic many have attributed to the fast pace of our '24/7' industrial societies – involving chronic partial sleep loss. Voluntary chronic sleep loss represents an increasingly common condition in industrialized societies and is due primarily to socioeconomic and cultural pressures.

The incidence of symptoms of insufficient sleep has been increasing since about 1950. Around-the-clock operations imply chronic partial sleep loss for the large population of shift workers, and schedules compressing the workweek by the use of extended work shifts (for example, 12 h workdays) and unscheduled overtime have become routine in a number of industries.

The relationship between the rise in obesity and the loss of sleep, hypothesized to be 'interacting epidemics,' is depicted in **Figure 1**. However, are these epidemics interacting or are they simply correlated, with no cause-and-effect relationship to one another? The following discussions provide both epidemiological and clinical research results which indicate that long-term partial chronic sleep loss is indeed an underlying cause of obesity, diabetes, and the metabolic changes associated with the metabolic syndrome. In addition, data from animal models supporting the connection between sleep loss and metabolic dysfunction are provided, in addition to a discussion of how the two interacting epidemics could be connected on a mechanistic level. It should be noted that we are at an early stage in our understanding of how the obesity and chronic sleep loss epidemics are linked to one another, as their possible dependency on one another has only emerged in the past few years.

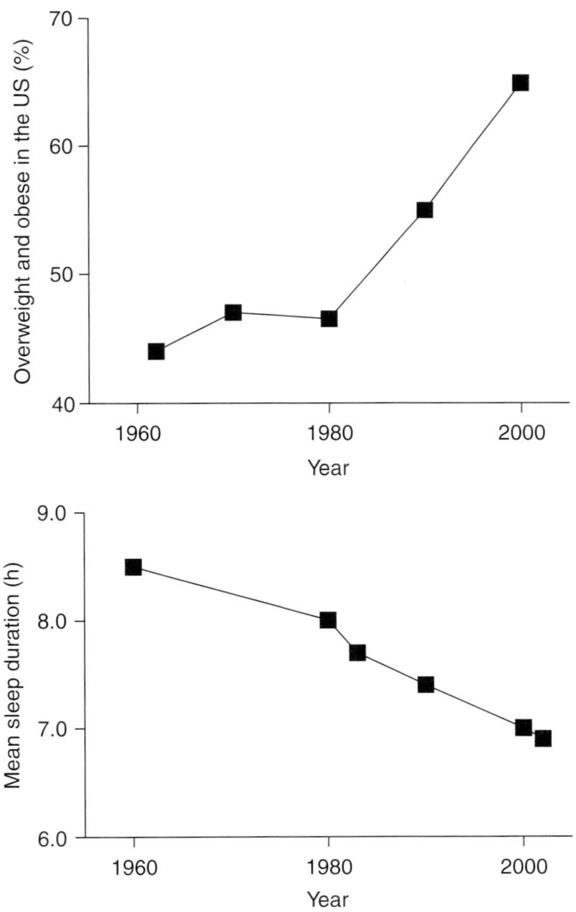

Figure 1 Time lines for the epidemics of obesity and sleep loss in the United States. The figures have been redrawn from data collected for the Centers for Disease Control and Prevention National Health and Nutrition Examination Study (obesity) and from National Sleep Foundation polls (sleep duration).

Sleep Loss and Metabolic Syndrome: Interacting Epidemics – Epidemiological Studies

There are now numerous epidemiologic surveys indicating a strong association between sleep disturbances, or shortened sleep durations, and cardiovascular disease, diabetes mellitus, and respiratory disorders. Indeed, as of 2006, there were at least 35 epidemiological studies linking short sleep periods with adverse health outcomes, including obesity, diabetes, and cardiovascular disease. For example, individuals who sleep less than 5 h a night have a threefold increased risk of heart attacks, and patients with coronary heart disease had more complaints of disturbed sleep than did patients without coronary heart disease. Another example is sleep apnea, which has been shown to increase the risk of cardiovascular disease and diabetes mellitus. In turn, cardiovascular and metabolic disorders, most notably hypertension, congestive heart failure, coronary heart disease, and diabetes mellitus, are associated with a higher prevalence of sleep apnea. Recent studies indicate that the relationship between short sleep duration and obesity extends beyond urban settings to rural populations, for whom lifestyle factors, nutrition, physical activity levels, and work hours are often different than for city dwellers.

For individuals with type 2 diabetes mellitus, sleep disturbances may be related to obesity and sleep apnea, and recent studies have also demonstrated a strong association between obesity, impaired glucose tolerance, insulin resistance, and sleep apnea. Results from both short-term physiological and epidemiologic studies consistently suggest that decreased sleep duration or quality may increase the risk for diabetes mellitus. Indeed, in patients with type 2 diabetes mellitus, decreased subjective sleep duration and quality are predictive of poorer glycemic control. These are notable findings for health care professionals and patients because they indicate not only that voluntary chronic partial sleep deprivation may increase the risk for diabetes mellitus, but also that continuing this pattern renders it more difficult to treat the condition.

In another study that analyzed 924 patients from four primary care practices in Virginia, a reduced amount of sleep was associated with overweight and obese status, with patients in the obese group showing a near inverse linear relationship between weight and reported sleep time. Findings from the Amsterdam Growth and Health Longitudinal Study, which began collecting data on study participants at 13 years of age, on factors such as fatness, fitness, and lifestyle, revealed these factors to be important determinants of the metabolic syndrome in 10% of the studied population by the age of 36 years – an indication that the obesity epidemic in young people is not confined to the United States. An alarming statistic defines a major problem among North American youth: between 1980 and 2000, the percentage of obese young people has risen from 5% to 15%, and another 15% has moved into that classification in young adulthood. While this epidemic in such a young population has received national attention, less well known is the finding that children of all ages in the United States are sleeping 1–2 h less per night than they need, according to a recent poll taken by the National Sleep Foundation. While insufficient sleep has often been associated with the elderly population, the increasing demands and lifestyles of modern society have imposed restricted sleep regimens on youth as well. It is now critical to determine the importance of a lack of sufficient sleep during the early formative years, and how that may be involved in putting the young on a trajectory toward obesity and the metabolic syndrome – a trajectory that could be altered in some cases, if sleep loss is indeed playing a role in this epidemic.

Sleep Loss and Obesity and the Metabolic Syndrome: Interacting Epidemics – Clinical Research Studies

Van Cauter and colleagues published a pivotal study in 1995 that demonstrated in humans that sleep loss has clear negative consequences for the body, beyond the brain. In this laboratory experiment, 6 days of restricted time (4 h per night) in bed in young men was associated with alterations in glucose metabolism that, over the long term, could increase the risk of developing diabetes. A similar study demonstrated that even short-term chronic sleep loss was associated with alterations in the levels of two hormones involved in appetite regulation: leptin and ghrelin. These alterations led to increased appetite, raising the possibility that such changes could ultimately increase the risk of weight gain. Similar associations between sleep duration and leptin and ghrelin were observed in a larger sample from the Wisconsin Sleep Cohort Study, providing further evidence for the link between sleep and appetite regulation. Such studies in chronically sleep-deprived humans has renewed interest in the role of insufficient sleep as a cause of many of the metabolic abnormalities associated with sleep apnea. However, while there is a growing awareness among some sleep, metabolic, cardiovascular, and diabetes researchers that insufficient sleep could be leading to a cascade of disorders, few in the general medical profession or in the lay public have yet made the connection.

Sleep Loss and Obesity and the Metabolic Syndrome: Interacting Epidemics – Evidence from Animal Studies

Unfortunately, most of the weight-conscious public, and even many in the health care professional community, still view weight control as a biological black box and ascribe obesity to laziness and a lack of will. However, the experience of those whose body weight is 'defended,' even though they are dieting and trying to lose weight, suggests that body weight regulation is more complex than just will power. Indeed, it is controlled much like a thermostat, with fluctuation around a programmed set point that can be altered after weight gain. The magic bullet for preventing obesity has proved elusive because, like other complex diseases (e.g., hypertension, hyperlipidemia, and cancer), multiple genetic and environmental factors contribute to body weight dysregulation and its secondary complications. An important goal in developing new therapies for obesity and the metabolic syndrome is to elucidate the elaborate pathways that regulate appetite, food intake, and energy expenditure, and to determine how interactions between behavior, metabolism, and the environment contribute to long-term energy balance. It is of particular interest to determine the cellular and neural mechanisms that underlie the effects of acute and/or chronic sleep loss on metabolism.

Genetic and clinical observations both point to interconnections between sleep and metabolic regulation. A major finding that set the stage for investigating neural interconnections linking sleep and metabolic homeostasis was the discovery of the orexins (also called hypocretins). These neuropeptides are part of signaling pathways within the energy center of the brain. A major discovery by Mignot and colleagues was the identification of the orexin receptor as the causative genetic defect in the most common form of canine narcolepsy. While these two fundamental systems appear to have distinct functions in human physiology, the discovery of overlapping molecular components suggests a co-regulation that may have coordinated the alternance between periods of fasting and sleep and periods of wakefulness, food seeking, and energy storage. A lack of sleep may perturb the homeostatic coordination of these pathways, activating metabolic pathways that trigger energy conservation (increased food intake and decreased expenditure) in excess of the energy cost of increased wakefulness. Indeed, our recent analysis of leptin-deficient animals suggests that leptin *per se* may be necessary for consolidated sleep, since animals with a genetic absence of leptin display markedly increased sleep fragmentation and experience increased periods of microsleep during the active period. In view of observations, from experimental models and human clinical studies, on the relationship between the sleep–wake cycle and fuel homeostasis, it may well be that interventions to improve sleep may ameliorate some of the metabolic deficits associated with overweight and obesity.

Recent genetic studies in mice have also provided strong evidence for there being important linkages between the sleep and body weight regulatory systems. We have recently discovered that homozygous *Clock* mutant mice have a greatly attenuated diurnal feeding rhythm, are hyperphagic and obese, and develop a metabolic syndrome of hyperleptinemia, hyperlipidemia, hepatic steatosis, and hyperglycemia, with insufficient compensatory insulin production, a hallmark of type 2 diabetes mellitus. In addition, levels in the expression of hypothalamic peptides associated with energy balance were greatly attenuated in the *Clock* mutant animals. The *Clock* gene is a major component in the transcriptional–translational feedback loops that make up the molecular circadian clock in mammals. Taken together, these results indicate that the circadian clock gene network plays an important role in mammalian energy balance involving a number of central and peripheral tissues, and that disruption of this network can lead to obesity and the metabolic syndrome in mice.

Chronic sleep loss is often associated with disrupted circadian rhythms. This is particularly true in shift workers, who not only have disturbed circadian rhythms as they continually shift their sleep and wake times to different times of the 24 h day, but who also do not obtain sufficient sleep often over the course of many years. In view of recent findings indicating that disrupted rhythms can lead to metabolic dysfunction in animal models, and that at the molecular level circadian clock genes also interact with other genes that regulate glucose and lipid metabolism, adverse effects on metabolism may in some cases be due to a combination of sleep loss and disrupted rhythms. Distinguishing between adverse metabolic outcomes as a function of sleep loss as opposed to disturbed rhythms can be problematic, since for many animal models both sleep loss and circadian disruption occur simultaneously. For example, while we concluded that decreased longevity in cardiomyopathic hamsters exposed to a light–dark cycle that was reversed on a weekly basis was due to the chronic disruption of the normal circadian organization, it could be expected that such forced re-entrainment on a weekly basis would have adverse effects as well on the quantity and/or quality of sleep. Similarly, while the development of obesity and signs of the metabolic syndrome in the *Clock* mutant animal have been attributed to circadian dysfunction at the organismal and/or molecular levels, *Clock* mutant animals show reduced sleep of 1–2 h per day; such chronic loss of sleep could also be contributing to the adverse metabolic events. While it will be important to determine the underlying links between disturbed rhythms and/or sleep loss on metabolic function from a mechanistic point of view, from a health perspective, the finding that loss of sleep and/or circadian disruption on a chronic basis, for whatever reason, can have severe adverse metabolic consequences, has important health implications that need to be addressed as our society faces an unprecedented epidemic in obesity, diabetes, and associated diseases.

Summary

Many fingers are being pointed at the possible multitude of causes for the obesity epidemic: not enough exercise, high-fat foods, poor eating habits, watching too much television, genetics, family history, fast-food hysteria, or exposure to advertising luring us to eat unhealthy foods. Even our early prenatal and postnatal environments may be putting us on a trajectory for an unhealthy metabolic state later in life, as many studies have now demonstrated that nutritional state early in life predicts how one will respond to dietary inputs later in life. Our genes evolved in humans engaged in high levels of physical activity (much of it chasing and looking for food), with eating habits requiring them to eat as much as possible (and as much meat and fat as possible) when a meal became available (i.e., rarely); today, many humans have food available all of the time, and this modern 'food everywhere' environment is a reality that may predispose modern humans to obesity.

It is hoped that the book by Kiess and colleagues, *Obesity in Childhood and Adolescence,* has raised the clinical community's awareness of the causes, consequences, and therapies of obesity in the young. However, it is noteworthy that none of the 21 chapter titles in that book contain the word 'sleep,' indicating that the connection between sleep loss and obesity is still not a major consideration in the war on obesity. The Institute of Medicine recently published a report titled *Sleep Disorders and Sleep Deprivation: An Unmet Public Health Problem*, in which it was stated, "The cumulative effects of sleep loss and sleep disorders represent an under-recognized public health problem and have been associated with a wide range of health consequences." Thus the alarm has been sounded – will people and health care professionals wake up?

Further Reading

Ayas, N. T., White, D. P., Manson, J. E., et al. (2003). A prospective study of sleep duration and coronary heart disease in women. *Archives of Internal Medicine* **163**, 205–209.

Gangwisch, J. E., Heymsfield, S. B., Boden-Albala, B., et al. (2006). Short sleep duration as a risk factor for hypertension: Analyses of the first National Health and Nutrition Examination Survey. *Hypertension* **47**, 833–839.

Gluckman, P. D. and Hanson, M. A. (2004). The developmental origins of the metabolic syndrome. *Trends in Endocrinology Metabolism* **15**, 183–187.

Laposky, A., Shelton, J., Bass, J., Dugouic, C., Perrino, N. and Turek, F. W. (2006). Altered sleep regulation in leptin-deficient mice. *American Journal of physiology regulation Integrative and Comparative phsiology* **290**, R1–R10.

Liu, Y. and Tanaka, H. (2002). Overtime work, insufficient sleep, and risk of non-fatal acute myocardial infarction in Japanese men. *Occupational and Environmental Medicine* **59**, 447–451.

Newman, A. B., Spiekerman, C. F., Enright, P., et al. (2000). Daytime sleepiness predicts mortality and cardiovascular disease in older adults. The Cardiovascular Health Study Research Group. *Journal of the American Geriatrics Society* **48**, 115–123.

Punjabi, N. M., Shahar, E., Redline, S., et al. (2004). Sleep-disordered breathing, glucose intolerance, and insulin resistance: The Sleep Heart Health Study. *American Journal of Epidemiology* **160**, 521–530.

Resnick, H. E., Redline, S., Shahar, E., et al. (2003). Diabetes and sleep disturbances: Findings from the Sleep Heart Health Study. *Diabetes Care* **26**, 702–709.

Rosa, R. R. (1995). Extended workshifts and excessive fatigue. *Journal of Sleep Research* **4**, 51–56.

Sanders, M. H., Newman, A. B., Haggerty, C. L., et al. (2003). Sleep and sleep-disordered breathing in adults with predominantly mild obstructive airway disease. *American Journal of Respiratory and Critical Care Medicine* **167**, 7–14.

Schwartz, S. W., Cornoni-Huntley, J., Cole, S. R., et al. (1998). Are sleep complaints an independent risk factor for myocardial infarction? *Annals of Epidemiology* **8**, 384–392.

Shahar, E., Whitney, C. W., Redline, S., et al. (2001). Sleep-disordered breathing and cardiovascular disease: Cross-sectional results of the Sleep Heart Health Study. *American Journal of Respiratory and Critical Care Medicine* **163**, 19–25.

Spiegel, K., Leproult, R., L'Hermite-Baleriaux, M., et al. (2004). Leptin levels are dependent on sleep duration: Relationships with sympathovagal balance, carbohydrate regulation, cortisol, and thyrotropin. *Journal of Clinical Endocrinology and Metabolism* **89**, 5762–5771.

Spiegel, K., Tasali, E., Penev, P., et al. (2004). Brief communication: Sleep curtailment in healthy young men is associated with decreased leptin levels, elevated ghrelin levels, and increased hunger and appetite. *Annals of Internal Medicine* **141**, 846–850.

Taheri, S., Lin, L., Austin, D., et al. (2004). Short sleep duration is associated with reduced leptin, elevated ghrelin, and increased body mass index. *PLoS Medicine* **1**, 62.

Turek, F. W., Joshu, C., Kohsaka, A., et al. (2005). Obesity and metabolic syndrome in circadian clock mutant mice. *Science* **308**, 1043–1045.

Van Cauter, E., Copinschi, G. and Turek, F. W. (2001). Endocrine and other biological rhythms. In: DeGroot, L. J. & Jameson, J. L. (eds.) *Endocrinology* (4th edn.,) (vol. 1)), pp. 235–256. W.B. Saunders: New York.

Vorona, R. D., Winn, M. P., Babineau, T. W., et al. (2005). Overweight and obese patients in a primary care population report less sleep than patients with a normal body mass index. *Archives of Internal Medicine* **165**, 25–30.

Wehr, T. A., Moul, D. E., Barbato, G., et al. (2005). Conservation of photoperiod-responsive mechanisms in humans. *American Journal of Physiology* **265**, R846–R857.

Yaggi, H. K., Araujo, A. B. and McKinlay, J. B. (2005). Sleep duration as a risk factor for the development of type 2 diabetes. *Diabetes Care* **29**, 657–661.

Young, J. B. and Landsberg, L. (2005). Stimulation of the sympathetic nervous system during sucrose feeding. *Nature* **269**, 615–617.

Young, J. B. and Landsberg, L. (2005). Suppression of sympathetic nervous system during fasting. *Science* **196**, 1473–1475.

Relevant Websites

http://www.cdc.gov – Centers for Disease Control and Prevention (United States).

http://www.sleepfoundation.org – National Sleep Foundation (United States and Territories, and International).

Fetal Stress

M Eleftheriades, P Pervanidou and G P Chrousos
Athens University Medical School, Athens, Greece

Glossary

Biophysical profile A noninvasive test that identifies a compromised fetus. It integrates five parameters to determine the biophysical profile score: the nonstress test, ultrasound measurement of the amniotic fluid volume, observation of the presence or absence of fetal breathing movements, gross body movements, and fetal tone.

Cardiotocography (CTG) A method of monitoring fetal heart rate using either an abdominal transducer or a probe on the fetal scalp; in addition, another transducer placed over the uterine fundus monitors uterine activity (contractions).

Cordocentesis An invasive procedure that involves the aspiration of fetal blood from the umbilical cord under sonographic guidance for diagnostic (fetal-karyotyping) or therapeutic (blood/platelet-transfusion) purposes.

Doppler ultrasound A noninvasive technique of blood-flow velocity measurement. The Doppler effect (named after Christian Andreas Doppler) is the apparent change in frequency and wavelength of a wave that is perceived by an observer moving relative to the source of the waves; the total Doppler effect may result from either the motion of the source or motion of the observer. For the velocity measurement of blood, ultrasound is transmitted into a vessel and the sound that is reflected from the blood is detected.

Preeclampsia A pregnancy-specific multisystem disorder that is characterized by the development of hypertension of 140 mmHg or higher systolic or 90 mmHg or higher diastolic after 20 weeks of gestation in a woman with previously normal blood pressure and proteinuria of 0.3 g or more of protein in a 24-h urine collection (usually corresponds to 1+ or greater on a urine dipstick test).

Programming The process whereby a stimulus or insult, when applied during a critical or sensitive period of development, results in a long-term or permanent effect on the structure or function of the organism.

Fetal Programming and Fetal Origins of Adult Disease

Experimental and clinical studies have highlighted the importance of the fetal environment in the subsequent growth and development of an individual. Indeed, a poor *in utero* environment elicited by maternal malnutrition or placental insufficiency may increase the susceptibility of the fetus to the later development of metabolic and cardiovascular disease. The fetal origins of adult disease hypothesis originated from the epidemiological research of Barker and colleagues, which demonstrated an association between low birth weight and cardiovascular disease, hypertension, insulin resistance, and dyslipidaemia later in life. In an attempt to explain this association, Hales and Barker proposed the thrifty phenotype hypothesis, according to which the fetus in a poor intrauterine environment maximizes the uptake and conservation of fuel resources by altering its metabolism. This alteration is adaptive in a deprived environment but maladaptive in an environment of plentiful resources.

The fetal programming response to environmental stressors, predictive adaptive response (PAR), however, is much broader that the one suggested by Barker and colleagues, extending well beyond energy use and conservation. PAR uses developmentally plastic processes to set a postnatal physiological and behavioral phenotype that the fetus predicts will offer an optimal chance for survival and reproduction during adulthood. The prediction of an adverse, deprived, risky, and hence stressful environment leads to adaptive changes in body size, body composition, organ size, neurohormonal activity, and many aspects of behavior. These predictive adjustments could be advantageous in a deprived environment but are maladaptive under abundant conditions.

Mediators of the Predictive Adaptive Response

The fetal adaptive response to stressors is mediated largely by the stress system. The hypothalamic-pituitary-adrenal (HPA) axis and the locus ceruleus–norepinephrine–sympathetic nervous system (LC-NE-SNS) and their mediators corticotropin releasing hormone (CRH), arginine vasopressin (AVP), norepinephrine (NE), epinephrine (E), and cortisol are responsible for both the concurrent adaptive response to the stressor and for causing the long-term organizational changes in the brain and periphery that constitute the PAR. Indeed, CRH and cortisol have been shown to have strong activating and organizational effects.

Fetal Distress – Clinical Evaluation

In perinatology practice, the term fetal distress has been employed as the condition in which the fetal heart rate (FHR) pattern detected by cardiotocography (CTG) is abnormal during antepartum surveillance. The generation of reactive FHR patterns constitutes a complex process involving appropriately for gestational age mature brain-stem centres, normally functioning sympathetic and parasympathetic system, intact electrical pathways to conduct the contractile stimulus, appropriately functioning cardiomyocytes' neurohormone receptors, and normal cardiac partitioning and development.

CTG tracing patterns indicative of fetal hypoxemia and/or acidemia are characterized by fixed FHR baselines, loss of FHR variability, absence of accelerations and are described as 'non-reassuring'. Documentation of spontaneous late decelerations is associated with a significant risk of fetal compromise. CTG patterns can be influenced by constitutional and environmental parameters, such as fetal congenital abnormalities, fetal maturation (depending mainly on gestational age) and movements. Moreover, maternal emotional or physical stress and the use of medication can also generate abnormal FHR patterns. Fetuses exhibit restricted central nervous system maturation and therefore cerebral activity before 28 weeks of gestation. Thus, CTG monitoring before this gestational age usually demonstrates reduced variability and benign spontaneous decelerations. Fetal sleep cycles are frequent and longer monitoring is required to record reactivity.

In addition FHR patterns are correlated to the nature of the hypoxic insult. Acute hypoxemia generates abrupt and profound declines in FHR baseline and variability and fetal activity. Chronic hypoxemia is associated with a more gradual deterioration in these parameters and therefore may remain undiagnosed by CTG monitoring for days to weeks.

Numerous studies have assessed CTG sensitivity, specificity, and predictive values. Most of them have documented relatively high specificity (>90%) but much lower sensitivity (averaging 50%). Positive and negative predictive values are less than 50% and more than 90%, respectively, suggesting that the non stress test (NTS) is better at excluding than diagnosing fetal compromise.

Despite extensive research, the association between a compromised fetus (invasively traceable by altered biochemical parameters) and a nonreassuring CTG pattern remains an unresolved issue. In addition, the correlation between an acute or chronic intrauterine adversity and the extent of fetal compromise caused by it, is not clearly defined regarding stressor's threshold level, intensity and duration required to impair fetal developmental, physiological and metabolic mechanisms. Furthermore, fetal capability to sustain a stressor is characterized by a wide range of adaptive mechanisms whose efficacy depends on gestational age and other only partially elucidated factors.

Fetal hypoxemia can be categorized, depending on the severity and duration of the *in utero* adversity, as acute or chronic. Acute hypoxemia as a stressor activates the fetal stress system. There is evidence from experimental studies that acute hypoxemia is associated with bradycardia and compensatory tachycardia, elevated blood pressure, reduced fetal breathing and reduced gross body movements, and increased cerebral blood flow, indicating cardiac redistribution. The fetal ovine HPA axis responds to acute hypoxemia with elevated arterial plasma concentrations of ACTH and cortisol. Furthermore, catecholamines and vasopressin concentrations are elevated in the hypoxic ovine fetus. In the sheep fetus during late gestation, episodes of acute stress induce endocrine responses that promote fetal adaptation and survival during the period of adversity.

Chronic hypoxemia is associated with the progressive return of fetal body movements, heart rate, and blood pressure to normal. However, cardiac output redistribution is maintained, as documented by increased cerebral blood flow. In fetal sheep, the partial compression of the umbilical cord for a period of three days causing a 30% reduction in umbilical blood flow can produce reversible mild fetal asphyxia, a transient increase in fetal plasma ACTH concentration, and a progressive and sustained increase in fetal plasma cortisol. Chronic hypoxemia is associated with increased NE concentrations. On the contrary epinephrine concentrations are restored to control levels during the course of hypoxemic period.

Hypoxia can activate a sequence of systemic, cellular, and metabolic responses, allowing tissue adaptation to the adverse effect of the lack of oxygen. Furthermore, hypoxia can induce altered gene expression with long-term detrimental outcome. The underlying molecular mechanisms that determine fetal development in response to hypoxia are not clearly defined, and it is suggested that placental gene upregulation is associated with the inflammatory response after the hypoxic exposure. Hypoxia may cause placental insufficiency or may induce preeclampsia through an inflammatory response, leading to FGR or even to *in utero* demise. Additionally pro-inflammatory molecules, such as cytokines, are considered responsible for the systemic maternal inflammatory response observed in pregnancies complicated with preeclampsia.

Current research suggests that exposure to inflammatory stressors during the critical developmental windows may induce altered gene expression of the neuroendocrine–immune axis. Evidence of HPA axis and autonomic nervous system (ANS) activation during inflammation supports the hypothesis that inflammatory stress during fetal development induces the programming of both the neuroendocrine and immune systems, influencing vulnerability to disease development later in life. Moreover, both clinical and experimental studies suggest that low-grade systemic inflammation is present in the metabolic syndrome participating in the development of atherosclerosis and cardiovascular disease.

Fetal Growth Restriction (FGR)

Genetically predetermined fetal growth potential influenced by environmental parameters determines fetal growth and birth weight. These parameters can be physiological (fetal and maternal health and placental function), behavioral (maternal emotional stress), social (socioeconomic status, life-style and malnutrition), and ecological (starvation/famine). The interaction between genome and environment in the regulation of fetal growth and development constitutes a complex process. Intrauterine adversities challenge the growing fetus, forcing it to reallocate its energy resources between the adaptation to the challenge and growth in order to ensure survival, reproduction enhancement and genome preservation. Thus, FGR is the evolutionary result of adaptation to a suboptimal intrauterine milieu.

FGR occurs in approximately 5% of all human pregnancies and is associated with a substantially increased risk of perinatal mortality and long-term morbidity. The definition of FGR excludes small for gestational age (SGA) fetuses that are constitutionally small. Based on growth curves, growth-restricted fetuses are considered to be those with estimated weights below the 10th percentile for gestational age, below the 5th percentile for gestational age, or two standard deviations (<3%) below the mean for gestational age. Approximately 80% of fetuses with estimated weights below the 10th percentile for gestational age are constitutionally small (normal small), 15% are starved small due to placental insufficiency, and 5% are abnormal small. The lower the percentile that defines SGA, the higher the likelihood of FGR.

FGR is further categorized as symmetric or asymmetric. Symmetric FGR is characterized by proportional reduction in growth velocity of both the fetal head circumference (HC) and abdominal circumference (AC), indicating a constitutionally small fetus. Symmetric FGR can also be indicative of *in utero* adversities such as chromosomal abnormalities, genetic syndromes, congenital infections, use of medication or teratogenic agents. Asymmetric FGR is characterized by a disproportional reduction in growth velocity of the fetal HC to AC and is mainly associated with placental insufficiency. However, body proportionality does not always specify the causes of FGR. Snijders et al. performed fetal blood karyotyping on 458 fetuses between 17 and 39 weeks gestation who had been referred for evaluation of intrauterine growth restriction (IUGR) and they demonstrated that the relative shortening of the femur can be found in both chromosomally normal and abnormal fetuses. In the same study, fetuses with triploidy had been found to have severe, early-onset, asymmetric FGR, whereas fetuses with chromosomal abnormalities other than triploidy were symmetrically growth retarded at <30 weeks. Chromosomally abnormal IUGR fetuses diagnosed after 30 weeks are usually asymmetrically growth restricted. The authors suggested that the asymmetry results from superimposed starvation due to placental insufficiency.

Placental insufficiency and fetal abnormalities (chromosomal, structural and congenital infections) are responsible for the majority of FGR cases in singleton pregnancies. According to histopathological studies, placental insufficiency is associated with abnormal trophoblast invasion and villous development that impairs placental vascular function, restricting nutrient and oxygen transfer to the fetus. The severity of placental insufficiency can be manifested in both maternal and fetal vascular compartments, (uterine and umbilical arteries respectively). The discrepancy between fetal growth demands and environmental conditions, mainly defined by placental vascular dysfunction, determines the severity of the compromised growth velocity that may manifest as FGR or even as fetal demise.

Clinical studies have documented the correlation between increased blood flow impedance in the uterine arteries and the subsequent development of preeclampsia, and FGR. Abnormal Doppler waveform in the uterine arteries is associated with a 70% chance of developing preeclampsia and an approximately 30% chance of developing growth restriction. In FGR pregnancies increased Doppler indices in the umbilical arteries are associated with fetal hypoxemia and acidemia correlated to the severity of the impedance of the umbilical flow. Fetal cardiovascular adaptations to placental insufficiency result in the redistribution of cardiac output. As a consequence, there is an increase in the blood supply to the brain, myocardium, and the adrenal glands at the expense of the kidneys, gastrointestinal tract, and lower extremities. The aforementioned redistribution of cardiac output can be documented by the reduced impedance of the blood flow in the middle cerebral artery. Fetuses exhibiting blood flow redistribution are usually hypoxemic, while acidemia may still not be clinically apparent. Further deterioration of fetal circulatory status is manifested by cardiac decompensation due to the exhaustion of adaptive mechanisms to hypoxia, indicated by right heart failure and abnormal organ autoregulation.

Elegant studies investigating the metabolic status of growth-restricted fetuses by cordocentesis have documented fetal compromise by hypoxemia, hypercapnia, hyperlacticemia, and acidosis. Growth-restricted fetuses are deprived of glucose and amino acids and are hypertriglyceridemic. In addition, some of these fetuses are hypoinsulinemic and their degree of hypoinsulinemia is disproportional to the degree of hypoglycemia, suggesting pancreatic dysfunction. In growth-restricted fetuses, the plasma cortisol concentration is increased and inversely correlated to fetal hypoglycemia. There is evidence of a significant correlation between umbilical cord plasma CRH and both ACTH and cortisol concentrations, as well as a significant negative correlation between CRH and dehydroepiandrosterone sulfate (DHEAS) levels in the growth-restricted fetuses. The umbilical cord plasma CRH level is extremely elevated compared to that of normal fetuses.

Placental CRH synthesis and release, in contrast to hypothalamic CRH, appears to be stimulated by glucocorticoids. In pregnancies complicated by uteroplacental insufficiency, placental CRH production may be enhanced by increased fetal glucocorticoids. In turn, placental CRH may modulate fetal pituitary-adrenal steroidogenesis to favor increased cortisol secretion. Conditions of chronic stress may stimulate hypothalamic as well as placental CRH, modulating fetal pituitary-adrenal function and consequently fetal response to a compromised intrauterine environment.

In FGR fetuses there is delayed maturation of biophysical parameters is apparent in IUGR fetuses. Fetal behavioral responses to placental insufficiency can affect heart-rate control by delaying the physiological decline of the baseline heart rate and maturation of reactivity and by decreasing short- and long-term variability.

Diagnostic Approach to Fetal Growth Restriction

The best method to diagnose the growth-restricted fetus and determine its growth velocity is ultrasound evaluation. The diagnostic approach to the FGR fetus is based on a detailed biometric and anatomic assessment evaluating for growth, chromosomal and structural defects, and congenital infections. Compared to other fetal biometric parameters, the AC is regarded as the most accurate measurement with the highest sensitivity and negative predictive value for identifying FGR. However, assessment of the estimated fetal weight (EFW) requires additional measurement of the HC and femur length.

The assessment of fetal growth velocity by serial ultrasound evaluation of AC and EFW is superior to single estimates of AC and EFW in the prediction of FGR. Moreover, it is important to assess the amniotic fluid volume. Placental insufficiency and fetal hypoxemia cause fetal oliguria and consequently oligohydramnios. Decreased amniotic fluid volume is regarded as an early sign of IUGR and oligohydramnios is defined as the presence of a largest vertical pocket of amniotic fluid less than 2 cm or amniotic fluid index (AFI) less than 5 cm.

The next essential step in the diagnostic process of FGR is based on Doppler blood-flow studies. It is well established that Doppler ultrasound assessment of the uterine and umbilical arteries helps to distinguish growth restricted fetuses due to impaired placentation from constitutionally small fetuses. In FGR fetuses, abnormal blood flow in the umbilical artery usually precedes other cardiovascular adaptations. Abnormal Doppler findings indicative of uteroplacental insufficiency include increased impendance with absent or reversed end-diastolic flow in the umbilical artery.

The further evaluation of the fetal cardiovascular system involves the assessment of the middle cerebral artery and the ductus venosus. When redistribution occurs, ductus venosus blood flow is usually normal and biophysical abnormalities are generally not clinically apparent. Abnormal ductus venosus blood flow indicates a decompensation of the cardiovascular system, which is followed by abnormalities in biophysical parameters. The biophysical profile consists of fetal tone, breathing movements, gross body movements, amniotic fluid volume assessment, and CTG monitoring, and it reflects the fetal behavioral status. The deterioration of the fetal biophysical profile associated with Doppler evidence of right heart failure indicates intrauterine fetal jeopardy. Optimizing the time of delivery, in which iatrogenic intervention should be delayed to avoid the risks of premature birth without increasing the risks of exposure to an adverse intrauterine environment, remains a challenge for perinatologists.

Perinatal mortality and long-term morbidity, including neurodevelopmental delay, is considerably increased in FGR fetuses with evidence of abnormal ductus venosus blood flow. The delivery decision should not be based merely on the umbilical artery waveform alone but mainly on the combination of abnormal venous Doppler indices and abnormal biophysical profile parameters. Furthermore, if early delivery is required, the gestation- and birth weight-specific charts produced by a study by Draper et al. should be used to determine the likelihood of survival.

Preterm Birth

Stress experienced during pregnancy increases the risk of preterm labor. Preterm birth, i.e. delivery before 37 weeks of gestation, occurs in approximately 10% of all pregnancies constituting the leading cause of neonatal morbidity and mortality. It is noteworthy that the incidence of premature labor remains unaffected by improvements in social health care and socioeconomic level observed in Western countries during the last 50 years. A substantial body of evidence has emphasized the role of stress as a major risk factor for preterm delivery. Furthermore, a correlation has been documented between maternal stress, either physical or emotional and premature delivery and it is proposed that the earlier in pregnancy the adversity is experienced, the earlier parturition occurs.

It has been suggested that premature activation of placental CRH gene expression in response to stressors induces early fetal neuroendocrine maturation and premature labor. Indeed, maternal and placental endocrine dysfunction triggered by a variety of stressors and the consequent occurrence of fetal stress may generate the process leading to preterm delivery. Although the early expulsion of the stressed FGR fetus from an adverse intrauterine environment carries the evolutionary advantage of genome maintenance it has the cost of increased risk of perinatal morbidity and mortality as well as the development of dysmetabolic syndrome in adulthood.

Further Reading

Barker, D. J. (2002). Fetal programming of coronary heart disease. *Trends in Endocrinology and Metabolism* **13**(9), 364–368.

Barker, D. J. P., Osmond, C., Forsen, T. J., et al. (2005). Trajectories of growth among children who have coronary events as adults. *New England Journal of Medicine* **353**, 1802–1809.

Baschat, A. A. (2004). Pathophysiology of fetal growth restriction: implications for diagnosis and surveillance. *Obstetrical and Gynecological Survey* **59**(8), 617–627.

Baschat, A. A., Gembruch, U. and Harman, C. R. (2001). The sequence of changes in Doppler and biophysical parameters as severe fetal growth restriction worsens. *Ultrasound in Obstetrics and Gynecology* **18**(6), 571–577.

Challis, J. R. G., Sloboda, D., Matthews, S. G., et al. (2001). The fetal placental hypothalamic-pituitary-adrenal (HPA) axis, parturition and post natal health. *Molecular and Cellular Endocrinology* **185**(1–2), 135–144.

Chrousos, G. P. and Gold, P. W. (1992). The concepts and stress and stress systems disorders. *Journal of the American Medical Association* **267**, 1244–1252.

Devoe, L. D. and Jones, C. R. (2002). Nonstress test: evidence-based use in high-risk pregnancy. *Clinical Obstetrics and Gynecology* **45**(4), 986–992.

Dole, N., Savitz, D. A., Hertz-Picciotto, I., et al. (2003). Maternal stress and preterm birth. *American Journal of Epidemiology* **157**, 14–24.

Draper, E. S., Manktelow, B., Field, D. J., et al. (1999). Prediction of survival for preterm births by weight and gestational age: retrospective population based study. *British Medical Journal* **319**(7217), 1093–1097.

Gluckman, P. D. and Hanson, M. A. (2006). The consequences of being born small – an adaptive perspective. *Hormone Research* **65**(supplement 3), 5–14.

Gluckman, P. D., Hanson, M. A. and Spencer, H. G. (2005). Predictive adaptive responses and human evolution. *Trends in Ecology and Evolution* **20**(10), 527–533.

Hales, C. N. and Barker, D. J. P. (2001). The thrifty phenotype hypothesis. *British Medical Bulletin* **60**, 5–20.

Huang, S.-T. J., Vo, K. C. T., Lyell, D. J., et al. (2004). Developmental response to hypoxia. *FASEB Journal* **18**(12), 1348–1365.

Kofman, O. (2002). The role of prenatal stress in the etiology of developmental behavioural disorders. *Neuroscience and Biobehavioral Reviews* **26**(4), 457–470.

Laplante, D. P., Barr, R. G. and Brunet, A. (2004). Stress during pregnancy affects general intellectual and language functioning in human toddlers. *Pediatric Research* **56**(3), 400–410.

Latini, G., De Mitri, B., Del Vecchio, A., et al. (2004). Foetal growth of kidneys, liver and spleen in intrauterine growth restriction: "programming" causing "metabolic syndrome" in adult age. *Acta Paediatrrica* **93**(12), 1635–1639.

McMillen, I. C. and Robinson, J. S. (2000). Developmental origins of the metabolic syndrome: prediction, plasticity and programming. *Physiological Reviews* **85**, 571–633.

Nicolaides, K. H., Bilardo, C. M., Soothill, P. W., et al. (1988). Absence of end diastolic frequencies in umbilical artery: a sign of fetal hypoxia and acidosis. *British Medical Journal* **297**(6655), 1026–1027.

Ozanne, S. E. and Hales, C. N. (2002). Early programming of glucose-insulin metabolism,. *Trends in Endocrinology and Metabolism* **13**(9), 368–373.

Phillips, D. (2002). Endocrine programming and fetal origins of adult disease. *Trends in Endocrinology and Metabolism* **13**(9), 363.

Seckl, J. R. (2001). Glucocorticoid programming of the fetus; adult phenotypes and molecular mechanisms. *Molecular and Cellular Endocrinology* **185**(1–2), 61–71.

Snijders, R. J. M., Sherrod, C., Gosden, C. M., et al. (1993). Fetal growth retardation: associated malformations and chromosome abnormalities. *American Journal of Obstetrics and Gynecology* **168**(2), 547–555.

Smith, J. F., Jr. and Onstad, J. H. (2005). Assessment of the fetus: intermittent auscultation, electronic fetal heart rate tracing, and fetal pulse oximetry. *Obstetrics and Gynecology Clinics of North America* **32**(2), 245–254.

Soothill, P. W., Nicolaides, K. H. and Campbell, S. (1987). Prenatal asphyxia, hyperlacticaemia, hypoglycaemia, and erythroblastosis in growth retarded fetuses. *British Medical Journal Clinical Research Edition* **294**(6579), 1051–1053.

Ward, A. M., Syddall, H. E., Wood, P. J., et al. (2004). Fetal programming of the hypothalamic-pituitary-adrenal (HPA) axis: low birth weight and central HPA regulation. *Journal of Clinical Endocrinology and Metabolism* **89**(3), 1227–1233.

C. Cardiovascular System and Disorders

Cardiovascular System and Stress

P Hjemdahl
Karolinska Institute and University Hospital, Stockholm, Sweden

This is a revised version of the article by P Hjemdahl, Encyclopedia of Stress, First edition, volume 1, pp 389–403, © 2000, Elsevier Inc.

Glossary

Epinephrine (EPI) — The hormonal link of the sympathoadrenal system; epinephrine is released into the bloodstream from the adrenal glands.

Norepinephrine — The principal neurotransmitter (chemical signaling substance) released from the sympathetic nerves. A neurotransmitter acts locally where it is released.

Rapid eye movement (REM) sleep — Dream sleep.

Receptors — Molecular structures that carry messages into cells from biological substances (e.g., neurotransmitters and hormones) outside of the cells that they influence. Sympathetic receptors are also termed adrenoceptors.

Renin-angiotensin system — Renin is released from the kidney and regulates the formation of angiotensin II, which is a potent vasoconstrictor and has many other functions. β-Adrenoceptor stimulation increases renin release.

Stroke volume — The volume of blood pumped into the vascular system by one heart beat.

Sympathetic neuroeffector mechanisms — The regulation of sympathetic nerve function (i.e., nerve activity), the release of norepinephrine, and its effects on the cells that it influences via the stimulation of specific receptors (α- or β-adrenoceptors).

Sympathetic system — One of the two classic autonomic systems of nerves that regulate bodily functions. Sympathetic nerves to the heart increase heart rate and contractility via β-adrenoceptor stimulation by norepinephrine, whereas the parasympathetic vagal nerve slows the heart rate via release of its neurotransmitter acetylcholine.

Tachycardia — A rapid heart rate.

Thrombosis — Blood clotting that blocks the flow of blood.

Vasoconstriction — The narrowing of a blood vessel to decrease blood flow.

Vasodilatation — The widening of a blood vessel to increase blood flow.

Background

The cardiovascular system adapts to stress by changes that, from a teleological perspective, are meant to improve the chances of survival when the organism is threatened. The response pattern has been called the defense reaction and serves, in its simplest form, to prepare the organism for fight or flight. Animal experiments by Hilton, Folkow, and others have established a typical pattern of cardiovascular responses to stress, which may be elicited by the electrical stimulation of certain regions of the brain as well as by environmental stimuli in awake animals. The defense reaction involves elevations of cardiac output and blood pressure and a redirection of blood flow from the kidneys and splanchnic organs to skeletal muscle. A similar response pattern is elicited by mental stress in humans. The short-term survival benefits of the changes associated with the defense reaction may not be paralleled by beneficial consequences in the long term, when elicited repeatedly in individuals living in an urban society with everyday stresses.

Research on the importance of psychosocial factors and stress in cardiovascular disease has been rather intense. There is consensus that stress is of importance, but its exact role in cardiovascular pathophysiology has been somewhat illusive for many reasons: what is stress? how do positive and negative stresses differ? how can stress be quantitated? is laboratory stress testing relevant for the everyday situation? and how do personality factors influence cardiovascular responses to stress and for consequences of these responses? Despite this complexity, it is clear that stress (in terms of stimuli that influence the cardiovascular system in a certain direction) is involved in cardiovascular disease and its consequences. This presentation focuses on the effects of mental stress on the cardiovascular system and the mechanisms probably involved, with a few comparisons with the effects of physical exercise and other stressors.

Historical Perspective

From a cardiovascular point of view, it is pertinent to mention the work of Walter B. Cannon, who, in the first decades of the twentieth century, studied the responses of animals to stress. He described the fight-or-flight reaction and a homeostatic theory of how organisms adapt to threatening environmental influences. Cannon recognized the importance of the sympathetic system and proposed that the adrenal glands secreted sympathin, which mediated the responses to stress. However, von Euler could later show that sympathetic nerves use the neurotransmitter norepinephrine, whereas the circulating hormone secreted by the adrenal glands was a related substance, epinephrine. Later, adrenocorticotropic hormone (ACTH) and glucocorticoids secreted from the adrenal cortex were added to the list of stress hormones. Goldstein reviewed the homeostatic mechanisms in relation to research on stress and distress from Darwin and Bernard to 1995. He noted the lack of a unifying concept of stress and that this reflects the complexity with which the organism may respond to stress due to feedback regulation and the multiplicity of systems involved in the control of homeostasis.

Methodological Comments

In cardiovascular stress research, the conditions for resting measurements are most important because any expression of cardiovascular reactivity to stress depends on the basal value with which the stress value is compared. In fact, the basality of resting measurements (as reflected by, e.g., heart rate and plasma epinephrine levels) may be the most important determinant of study results. The stress test used should, of course, be standardized when comparing stress reactivity in individuals or between groups. Responses should be of sufficient amplitude to allow the discrimination between different conditions and be reasonably reproducible. Many factors, including personality factors, modulate the perception of stress and the degree of arousal caused by the stressor, as well as cardiovascular responses elicited by it (**Figure 1**).

What Is a Relevant Stressor?

For a cardiologist, stress testing means evaluating whether myocardial ischemia can be provoked by a stimulus that increases myocardial oxygen demand, such as physical exercise. However, mental stress may also provoke ischemia. Any increase in mental activity – even quiet speaking and REM periods (dreaming) during sleep – evokes cardiovascular changes. In fact, REM sleep may even precipitate myocardial infarction. Interviews on sensitive personal issues may be most relevant when studying the cardiovascular risks of stress, but they cannot be standardized for comparing individuals or groups. The question is whether laboratory stress tests mimic responses elicited by mental stimuli normally encountered. Herd used an operational definition of relevant stressors whereby "a psychological stressor is one that causes a predictable stress response in a predictable percentage of index subjects" and went on to define the cardiovascular stress response as changes seen in the defense reaction (1991). Various standardized stress tests have been developed that fit this definition.

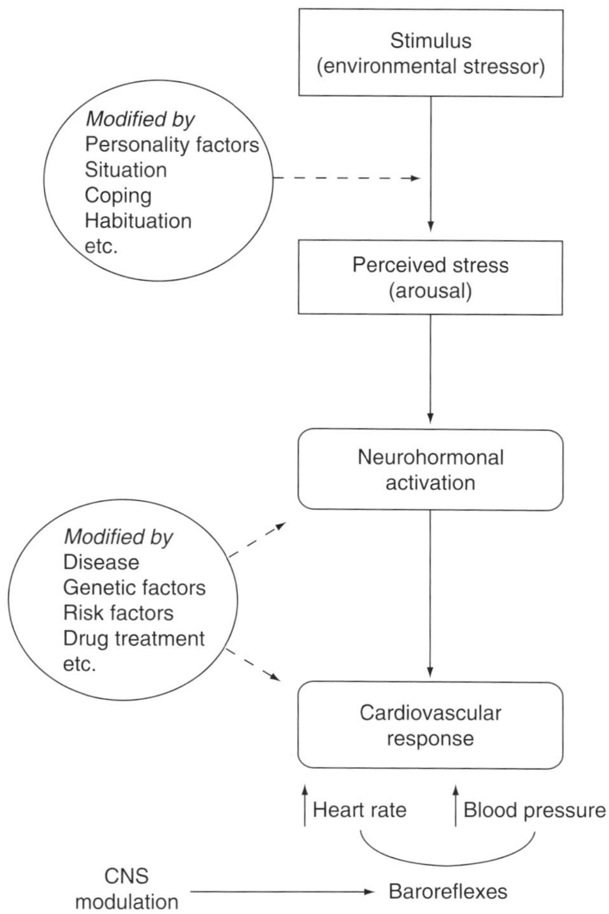

Figure 1 Stimulus–response scheme for cardiovascular responses to psychological stress. The perception of stress is modified by multiple factors, which reinforce or attenuate the arousal evoked by the stimulus. The cardiovascular response is mediated by neurohormonal activation. Several factors may modify the neurohormonal activation, as well as responses to the mediating neurohormones. Finally, the cardiovascular responses may be buffered by baroreflexes aiming at maintaining blood pressure at prestimulus levels, but the efficiency of the baroreflex is attenuated during stress. CNS, central nervous system.

Among the most common mental stress tests for cardiovascular research are mental arithmetic (MA) and Stroop's color word conflict test (CWT). Tests may also be based on auditory feedback or video games. MA is simple to administer, but the test results are influenced by the speed of the test and by the (variable?) harassment of the subject; individuals may also have very different abilities for coping with mathematics. MA produces substantial responses in some studies (e.g., those of Brod and coworkers), but weak responses in other studies. CWT is administered in different ways, and the magnitudes of responses depend on the version used (how color words are presented, how responses are made, and whether there is auditory interference). We have used MA (in various versions, with or without external pacing) and CWT in a modification with auditory interference developed by Frankenhaeuser in the 1960s and have found the latter to be particularly useful.

Adaptation to the same stressor occurs on repeated administration, whereas responses to a novel stressor are either intact or enhanced. Such adaptation involves information processing (coping, etc.) rather than the desensitization of the target organs. Animal experiments suggest that chronic stress can even result in enhanced responses to a novel stressor due to increased synthesis, storage, and release of neurotransmitters.

In clinical research, it may be difficult to find newly diagnosed patients who have not received any treatment. When drug treatment is discontinued, the researcher should minimize carryover effects or rebound phenomena by allowing sufficient time for the treatment effects to disappear. For example, diuretics may have long-lasting effects on sodium and fluid balance, and the withdrawal of a β-blocker may lead to rebound phenomena with increased β-adrenoceptor sensitivity. Such aftereffects may persist longer than is appreciated by many authors and should be taken into account.

Neurohormonal Mechanisms

Before describing the cardiovascular responses to mental stress, I briefly comment on the neurohormonal systems that may be involved and that are discussed in relation to these responses. In general, neurogenic control is suited for fine-tuned influences on individual organs or cells, whereas hormonal influences are diffuse.

The Sympathoadrenal System

The sympathoadrenal system is involved in short-term (phasic) responses to stress. Epinephrine (adrenaline), which is often considered to be *the* stress hormone, is secreted during stress, and epinephrine levels in plasma or urine reflect the degree of arousal experienced.

The sympathetic nerves may operate in a differentiated fashion, with varying levels of activity and varying responses to stress in different organs. Muscle sympathetic nerve activity during stress may even differ in different parts of the body. Thus, the common term sympathetic tone, which indicates synchronized activity throughout the body, is not appropriate. If possible, sympathetic activity should be studied locally, in the organ of interest.

Norepinephrine is the principal neurotransmitter of sympathetic nerves, although the cotransmitter neuropeptide Y may contribute to vasoconstrictor responses when sympathetic nerves fire at high frequencies. Norepinephrine stimulates α- and β_1-adrenoceptors. Catecholamines are rapidly cleared from plasma, with half-lives of 1–2 min, but the effect of a sympathetic nerve impulse is much shorter than that, due to local inactivating mechanisms such as the reuptake of norepinephrine into the nerve. Norepinephrine may also function as a circulating hormone when the plasma levels of norepinephrine are markedly elevated, such as during physical exercise. Resting levels of norepinephrine in plasma are ≈ 1 nmol l^{-1}, and threshold levels for hormonal effects are 3–4 nmol l^{-1}. Sympathetic nerve activity may be monitored in humans by:

- Direct recordings of impulse activity in nerves supplying skeletal muscle and skin but not in organs of perhaps greater interest in the context of mental stress.
- Analyses of heart rate variability (for cardiac sympathetic activity).
- Measurements of norepinephrine levels in plasma and norepinephrine release from various organs. Measurements of norepinephrine release and spillover into plasma can be refined by the use of an isotope dilution method involving infusions of radiolabeled norepinephrine, which was developed by Esler and coworkers.

These techniques all have their technical difficulties and limitations. They complement one another because the release of norepinephrine from the sympathetic nerves is influenced by prejunctional regulation (i.e., variable release per nerve impulse) and the sensitivity of the receptors involved may vary when measuring functional responses, such as heart rate.

Epinephrine may, as a circulating hormone, stimulate α- and β-adrenoceptors in all organs. Under certain circumstances, epinephrine can be taken up into and re-released from sympathetic nerves in such quantities that a role as a co-transmitter is possible, but this is normally not important. Thus, epinephrine is the classic hormonal link of the sympathoadrenal system.

There is functional differentiation of sympathetic neuroeffector mechanisms; β_1-adrenoceptors appear to be innervated receptors, and β_2-adrenoceptors appear to be noninnervated or humoral receptors. This leads to epinephrine being functionally β_2-selective at physiological concentrations in blood plasma (even though it is also an effective β_1-agonist in *in vitro* systems) and provides a possibility of studying the importance of epinephrine for physiological responses to stress by examining the β-adrenoceptor subtype involved in the response. Similarly, α_1-adrenoceptors appear to be innervated and α_2-adrenoceptors non-innervated in the cardiovascular system, which has therapeutic implications and allows the separation of neurogenic and humoral influences.

Cholinergic Mechanisms

The heart is under dual autonomic control, with excitatory sympathetic nerves (stimulating β_1-adrenoceptors) and inhibitory vagal nerves (releasing acetylcholine and stimulating muscarinic receptors). Acetylcholine is very rapidly inactivated after its release, allowing beat-to-beat control of the heart rate. The intrinsic rate of the sinus node is ≈90–100 beats/min. Thus, the resting heart rate (usually 60–80 beats/min) is controlled to a large extent by vagal activity. Increased physical fitness reduces the resting heart rate by increasing vagal activity. Stress may thus increase heart rate by activating sympathetic nerves and/or by inhibiting the parasympathetic vagus nerve.

Animal research on vasodilator responses in skeletal muscle has demonstrated sympathetic vasodilator nerves that release acetylcholine. Work by Hilton suggested that such vasodilator nerves did not exist in primates, but early studies in humans suggested that it indeed was possible to elicit cholinergic vasodilatation in the forearm with certain stressors. However, the literature on cholinergic vasodilatation in human skeletal muscle is divided, and it cannot be definitely stated that this mechanism is of importance or under which conditions it may contribute.

Other Mediators and Mechanisms

The renin–angiotensin system may be activated by stress. Renin release from the kidney is under the influence of several factors, one of which is sympathetic nerve activity and β_1-adrenoceptor stimulation. Salt deprivation increases renin secretion, and salt loading decreases it. Renin catalyzes the formation of angiotensin II, which is a potent vasoconstrictor peptide with several other biological actions, including the enhancement of aldosterone secretion. Thus, the system is salt-conserving. The relative importance of angiotensin II and norepinephrine as mediators of vasoconstriction during stress may vary. High sodium intake tends to enhance cardiovascular responses to mental stress, but this is most likely independent of the renin–angiotensin system, which should be downregulated under such conditions.

There are several neuropeptides (e.g., neuropeptide Y and calcitonin gene-related peptide), and other peptides (e.g., atrial natriuretic factor and endothelin) that may be involved in cardiovascular responses to stress. Their roles during stress have not been sufficiently elucidated, in part due to the lack of good antagonists for human use.

Platelets store serotonin (5-hydroxytryptamine), which is released when the cells are activated, and activated platelets synthesize thromboxane A2. Both of these substances may stimulate platelets (positive feedback) and cause vasoconstriction, especially when the vascular endothelium is not functioning normally. Stress may activate platelets.

Flow-mediated vasodilatation has been recognized for a long time. Furchgott showed the importance of endothelial cells for vasodilator responses and proposed the existence of an endothelium-derived relaxing factor (EDRF). Nitric oxide (NO) was shown by others to be an important component, if not the only EDRF. NO released from the vascular endothelium serves both as a vasodilator and an inhibitor of platelet adhesion and aggregation, and the inhibition of NO synthesis or defective NO production by the endothelial cells may increase vascular tone and the risk of thrombosis. NO appears to be a rather ubiquitous substance in the body, which may be involved in neurogenic mechanisms and influence cardiac function as well. However, the importance of this for stress responses of the cardiovascular system is unknown. Flow-mediated vasodilatation (i.e., NO) is probably important for vasodilator responses to stress in some organs.

Baroreflexes and Blood Pressure Regulation

The cardiovascular system is regulated in a complex manner, with compensatory adjustments when changes are elicited by various stimuli. Normally this fine-tuned system strives to maintain a certain blood pressure (which may be either normal or high, if the individual has hypertension) via arterial baroreflexes, which serve to dampen the change. If the blood pressure rises, there is a reflexogenic inhibition of the heart and reduced vasocontrictor nerve activity; conversely, if the blood pressure decreases there is a reflexogenic stimulation of the heart with increases in heart rate and cardiac output and a compensatory increase in vasoconstrictor nerve activity. If cardiac output is lowered (e.g., by drug treatment), peripheral blood flow will decrease to maintain the blood pressure. In the long term, baroreflexes are reset to the new blood pressure level if, for example, a patient with hypertension is treated with a blood pressure lowering drug.

There are also receptors that sense venous pressure and participate in volume regulation. If venous pressure decreases, reflexogenic and hormonal changes occur that serve to conserve salt and water (i.e., renal responses) and to maintain blood pressure by increasing venous tone and reducing peripheral blood flow. The kidney is intimately involved in the regulation of blood pressure according to the Guyton's classic theory of cardiovascular homeostasis. However, there are also indications that blood pressure is a regulated variable and that neurogenic mechanisms are important for both short- and long-term levels of blood pressure.

During stress, the influence of baroreflex regulation of the circulation diminishes, and centrally elicited pressor mechanisms may operate under less influence of reflexogenic modulation than if blood pressure is increased by other maneuvers (**Figure 1**). As discussed by Julius, there seems to be some blood pressure-sensing mechanism that regulates the blood pressure during stress because interference with one pressor mechanism often leads to another one taking over and the pressor response to the stimulus remaining intact.

Human Studies of Cardiovascular Responses to Mental Stress

Figure 2 illustrates schematically how mental stress elevates blood pressure in humans, based on results from a number of studies. Pressor responses to mental stress generally depend on the increase in cardiac output because systemic vascular resistance decreases. In an early series of investigations, Brod and coworkers studied the cardiovascular responses to mental stress, mainly forced MA (using procedures creating substantial hemodynamic responses), in normotensive and hypertensive subjects. An example is given in **Figure 3**, which shows that arousal caused by the suggestion of exercise elicited responses that were qualitatively similar to those from mental arithmetic. A few examples of responses to CWT, from our work, are mentioned next.

Cardiac Responses

The increase in cardiac output is caused mainly by an increase in heart rate, but an increase in stroke volume also contributes (**Figures 2**). Tachycardia may be elicited by both increased sympathetic nerve activity and vagal withdrawal. Increases in stroke volume are related to increased contractility (which can be demonstrated by, e.g., echocardiography), as well as an increase in venous return, which supports the filling of the heart in diastole. Thus, work by Brod and coworkers has demonstrated that stress causes venoconstriction, which results in the centralization of the blood volume and supports cardiac filling. Studies with pacing alone showed that an isolated increase in heart rate does not efficiently elevate cardiac output – an increase in contractility and an adequate distension of the heart in diastole contribute to the stress response.

The effects of β-blockade by metoprolol (β1-selective) or propranolol (nonselective) on some invasive hemodynamic variables are illustrated in **Figure 4**. Healthy volunteers were subjected to CWT (the Frankenhaeuser version), which was found to elicit clear-cut and rather reproducible (see control group) responses. The two β-blockers inhibited the heart rate response similarly, indicating that the sympathetic component was β_1-mediated (neurogenic). The vagal component in the tachycardia elicited by mental stress is reflected in the persisting, although blunted, tachycardia seen after β-blockade in sufficient doses to eliminate the increase in stroke volume during stress (**Figure 4**). The stroke volume response was attenuated by metoprolol and abolished by propranolol, suggesting contributions of both neurogenic (norepinephrine) and hormonal (epinephrine) effects. However, stroke volume is also sensitive to afterload, and the effects of β-blockade on systemic vascular resistance may have influenced the stroke volume response to stress.

The coronary circulation is to a large extent regulated by cardiac metabolism, and it is difficult to separate β-adrenoceptor-mediated coronary vasodilatation from that induced by increased cardiac metabolism and flow-mediated vasodilatation. However, α-adrenergic coronary vasoconstriction may occur when the endothelium is dysfunctional or when cardiac metabolism is inhibited.

Peripheral Vascular Responses

The decrease in systemic vascular resistance during mental stress is related to vasodilatation in skeletal muscle and adipose tissue, whereas there is vasoconstriction in the kidneys, splanchnic organs, and skin (**Figure 2**). The experiment of Brod and coworkers (**Figure 3**) illustrates marked vasodilatation in the forearm simultaneously with reduced renal clearance of para-aminohippurate (i.e., renal vasoconstriction) and a decrease in skin temperature (i.e., vasoconstriction in skin); other experiments have show splanchnic vasoconstriction.

Limb blood flow The decrease in systemic vascular resistance in the experiments illustrated in **Figure 4** was attenuated by β_1-blockade and abolished by propranolol. These effects of β-blockade may reflect blockade of vascular β-adrenoceptors (which are of the β_2 subtype) and/or peripheral vascular adaptation to the effects of β-blockade on the cardiac response to stress. The increase in blood pressure during mental stress was little influenced by β-blockade (data not shown), which is in agreement with the results of several other studies. If, as discussed

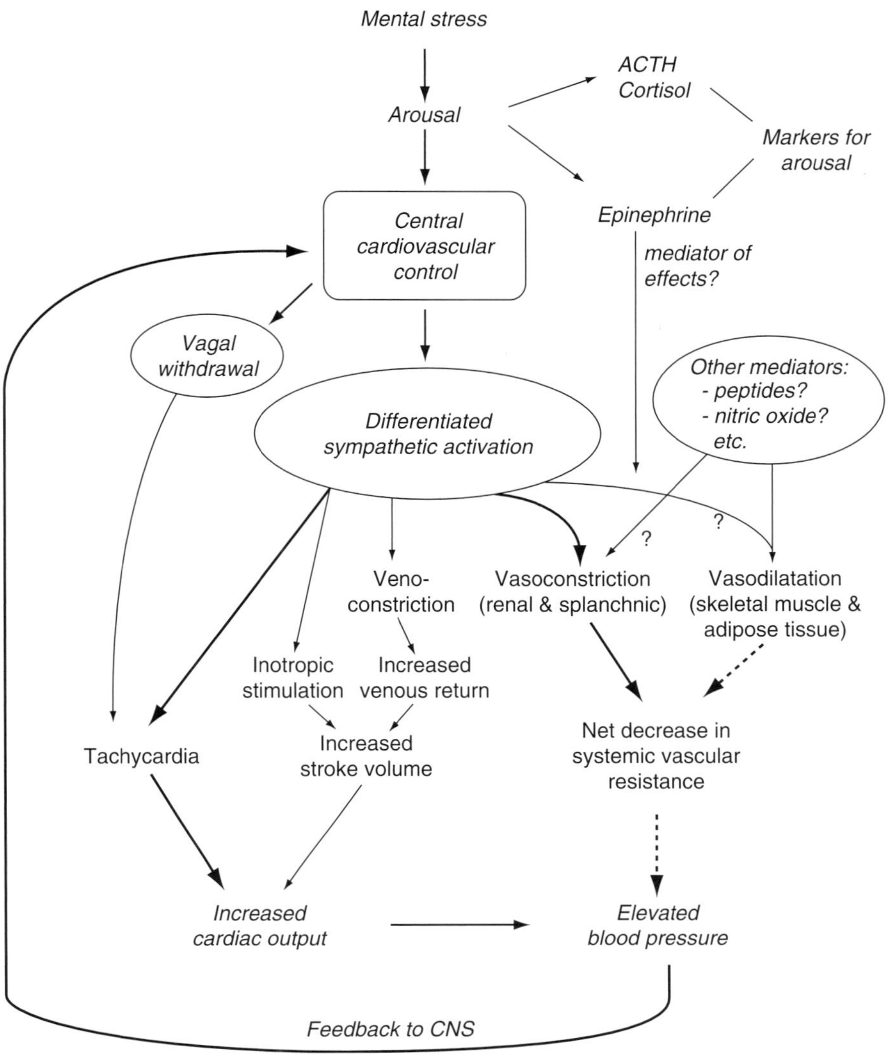

Figure 2 Schematic representation of the cardiovascular response pattern of the defense reaction. The pressor response is mainly cardiac output-dependent, and the increase in cardiac output depends mainly on an increase in heart rate. The vascular response is a net reduction of systemic vascular resistance, but responses of individual organs vary considerably. ACTH, cortisol, and epinephrine are markers of the arousal evoked by the stressor. Established and possible mediators of the cardiovascular responses are indicated. ACTH, adrenocorticotropic hormone; CNS, central nervous system. Modified from Hjemdahl, P. (1993), Plasma catecholamines – analytical challenges and physiological limitations, *Baillère's Clinical Endocrinology and Metabolism* **7**, 307–353.

by Julius, blood pressure is the primarily regulated variable, the attenutation of the increase in cardiac output results in compensatory changes in vascular responses in order to achieve the same level of blood pressure during stress as would be obtained without such attenuation. Vasodilator responses are then secondary to, and governed by, cardiac responses. Further support for this idea was obtained in studies of systemic NO synthesis inhibition, which increased vascular resistance and blood pressure at rest but did not influence the blood pressure level achieved during stress.

These experiments included measurements of calf blood flow (by plethysmography) and of adipose tissue and skeletal muscle blood flow (by isotope clearance methods). **Figure 5** shows similar vasodilatation in adipose tissue, skeletal muscle (the gastrocnemius muscle) and the entire calf in response to CWT. β-Blockade inhibited these local vasodilator responses similarly, as previously shown for systemic vascular resistance. In other studies, even greater vasodilator responses than those seen in the leg were found in the human forearm with the same stress test (**Figure 6**). Of interest are findings by Rusch and coworkers that blood flow responses of the arm and leg to different stimuli (including MA) differed and that vasodilatation was more prominent in the arm than in the leg. Others have found that differences in the baroreceptor mediated the control of limb blood flow in the leg and the forearm. Recordings of muscle sympathetic nerve activity by Anderson and coworkers showed

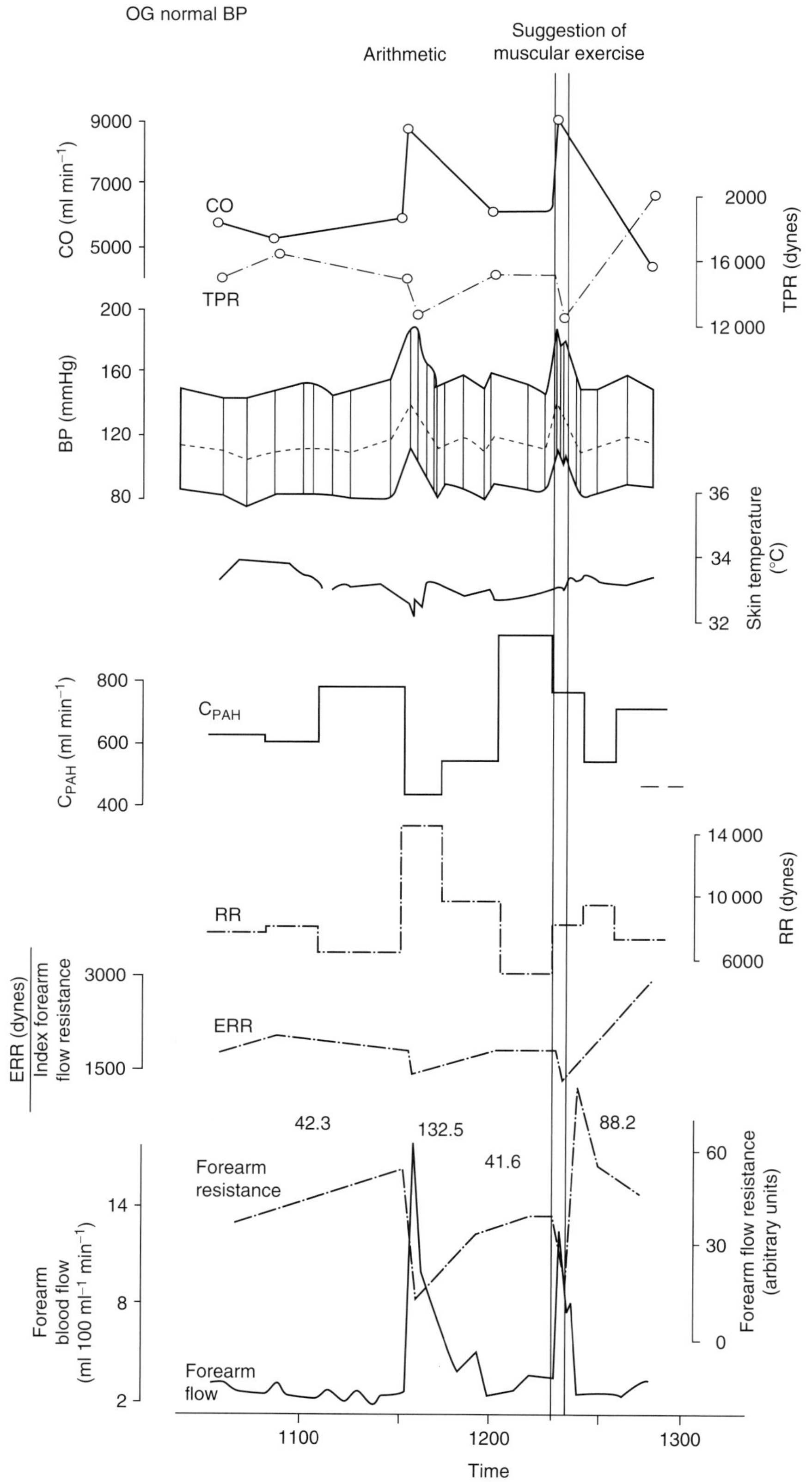

Figure 3 Comparison of general and regional hemodynamic responses to mental arithmetic stress and suggestion of heavy muscular exercise in a healthy subject from the studies of Brod and coworkers. Mental stress and the anticipation of physical stress elicited similar cardiovascular responses, both of which resemble the defense reaction. Illustrated are cardiac output (CO), systemic vascular resistance (TPR), blood pressure (BP), skin temperature, renal paraaminohippurate clearance (C_{PAH}), renal vascular resistance (RR), extrarenal vascular resistance (ERR), forearm vascular resistance, and forearm blood flow . From Brod, J. (1963), Haemodynamic basis of acute pressor reactions and hypertension, *British Heart Journal* **25**, 227–245, with permission from the BMJ Publishing Group.

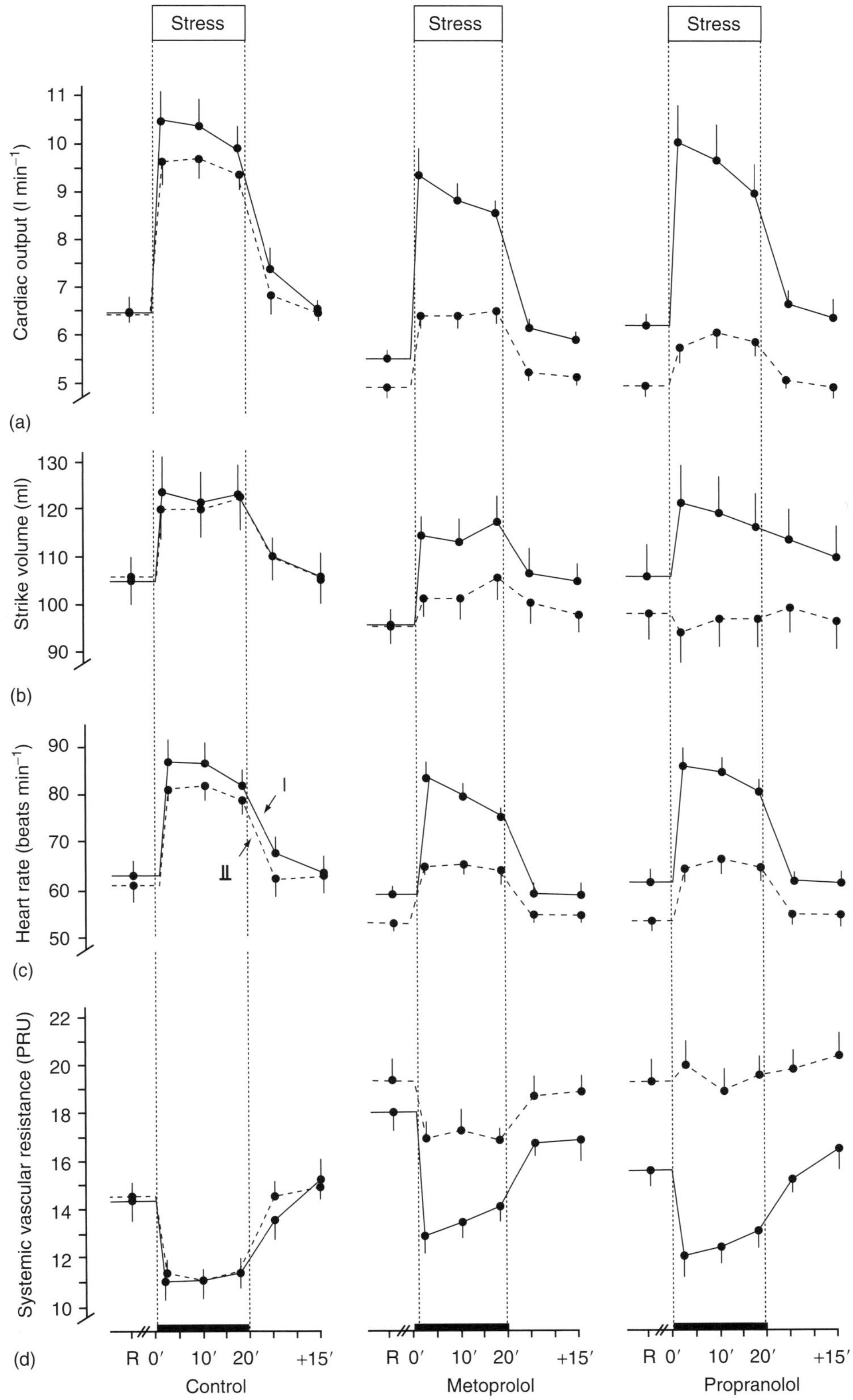

Figure 4 Cardiac and systremic vascular responses to mental stress induced by Stroop's color word conflict test (CWT; the Frankenhaeuser version) in healthy male volunteers. a, Cardiac output (measured by thermodilution); b, stroke volume; c, heart rate; d, systemic vascular resistance. Thirty subjects were divided into three groups, in which CWT (stress) was repeated without treatment (control) or after intravenous injection of the β_1-blocker metoprolol or the nonselective β-blocker propranolol. The mean arterial pressure response to stress ($\approx$20 mmHg) was little affected by the treatments given. PRU, peripheral resistance units. From Freyschuss et al. (1988), *American Journal of Physiology* **255**, H443–H451, with permission from the American Physiological Society.

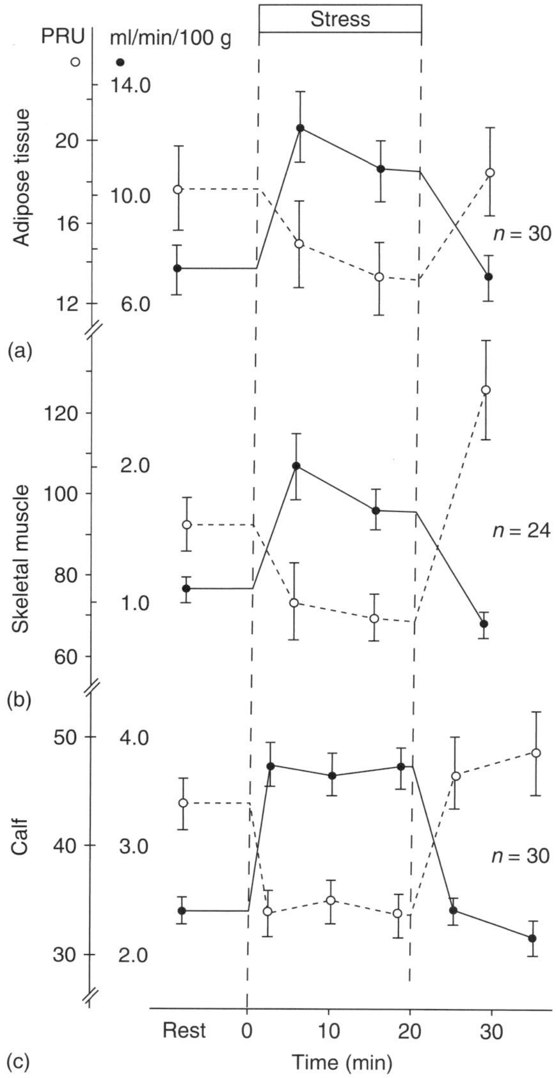

Figure 5 Peripheral vascular responses to mental stress (Stroop's color word conflict test, CWT) in the experiments illustrated in **Figure 4**. a, Adipose tissue; b, skeletal muscle; c, calf. CWT elicited similar vasodilatation in adipose tissue of the abdomen (similar responses were found in adipose tissue on the thigh), skeletal muscle (gastrocnemius muscle), and the calf. Tissue blood flows were determined by the local clearance of ^{133}Xenon; and calf blood flow was measured by venous occlusion plethysmography. PRU, peripheral resistance units. From Linde et al. (1989), *American Journal of Physiology* **256**, E12–E18, with permission from the American Physiological Society.

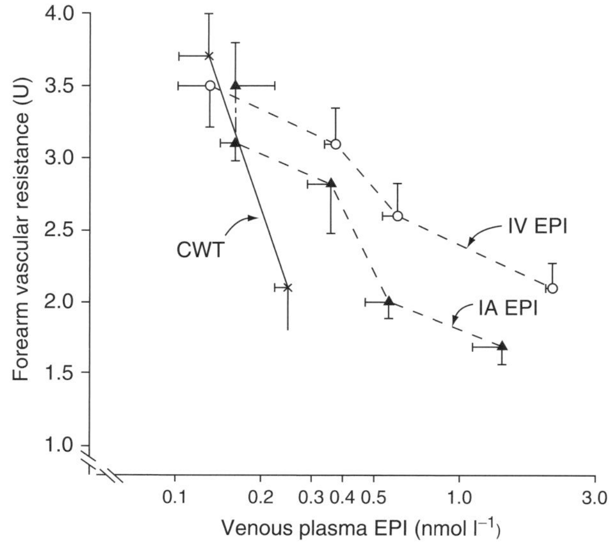

Figure 6 Forearm vascular responses to Stroop's color word conflict test (CWT) and to intravenous (IV) and intra-arterial (IA) infusions of epinephrine (EPI), in relation to epinephrine concentrations before and during interventions. CWT elicited a marked forearm vasodilator response with a small increase in venous plasma epinephrine. Responses to IA epinephrine were greater than those to IV epinephrine, suggesting reflexogenic buffering of the forearm vasodilator response to systemic epinephrine. Interpolation of vasodilator responses to the epinephrine concentration achieved by the same individual during CWT showed that epinephrine may have contributed 10–30% of the vasodilator response to stress. From Lindqvist et al. (1996), *American Journal of Physiology* **270**, E393–E399, with permission from the American Physiological Society.

that MA increased muscle sympathetic activity in the leg but not in the arm, when they were simultaneously recorded (**Figure 7**). Thus, the sympathetic response to mental stress is so differentiated that differences in muscle sympathetic nerve activity can be seen even between the upper and lower limbs. Increases in muscle sympathetic nerve activity may serve to buffer the vasodilator response to stress.

NO release and flow-mediated vasodilatation may be involved in the blood flow response of skeletal muscle to mental stress. Other possible mediators are acetylcholine (although we found no neurogenic component in the sustained forearm vasodilator response to CWT), vasodilating peptides, and epinephrine. Of interest is that the forearm vasodilator response to CWT (a 50% decrease of local vascular resistance) was not altered by systemic NO synthesis inhibition, even though previous studies had shown attenuation of stress-induced forearm vasodilatation with local inhibition of NO synthesis. Thus, systemic (centrally mediated?) influences on muscle blood flow may override locally acting influences by, for example, NO released from the endothelium.

Thus, it is well established from work by several groups and with several different stress tests that limb blood flow increases due to vasodilatation in the skeletal muscle and adipose tissue, whereas there is vasoconstriction in the skin. Interestingly, skeletal muscle vasodilatation appears to differ in different regions of the body. The mechanisms involved are not entirely clear.

Renal blood flow The kidneys, which receive ≈20% of the cardiac output, are important in the regulation of blood pressure – both in the short term, and in the

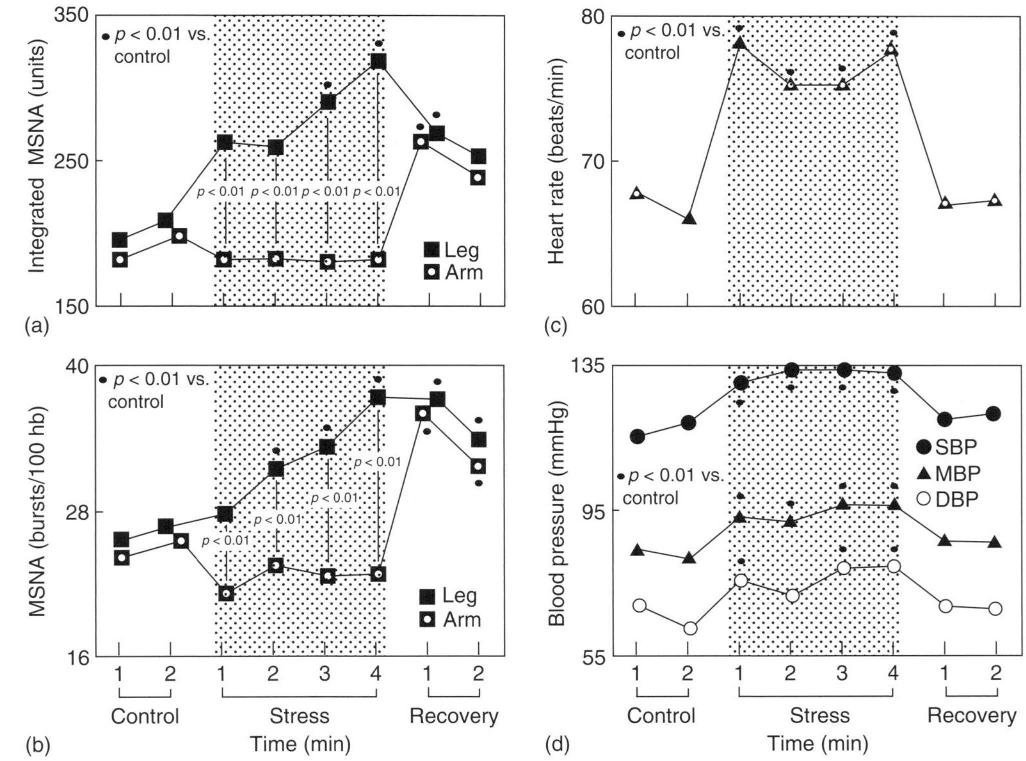

Figure 7 Simultaneously recorded activity in the arm and leg in healthy individuals during mental arithmetic. a, Integrated muscle sympathetic nerve activity (MSNA); b, MSNA (bursts/100 heart beats); c, heart rate; d, blood pressure. MSNA increased in the leg but not in the arm in response to mental stress, indicating that skeletal muscle blood flow is under different neurogenic modulation in different regions of the body during stress.
DBP, diastolic blood pressure; MBP, mean blood pressure; SBP, systolic blood pressure;
From Anderson, Wallin and Mark (1987), *Hypertension* **9**(supplement. 3), 114–119, with permission from Lippincott, Williams & Wilkins.

long term – and appear to be a target for stress effects. Several groups have shown renal vasoconstriction, renin release, and/or altered renal function in response to mental stress. Examples are shown in **Figure 3** for the work of Brod and coworkers and in **Table 1** for our work. Of particular interest is that renal vascular responses to mental stress may be enhanced in hypertension. Thus, Hollenberg and coworkers found that very mild stress induced by a nonverbal IQ test (which did not increase blood pressure) elicited clear-cut renal vasoconstriction among hypertensives but not among normotensives without a family history of hypertension; those with a family history of hypertension had an intermediate response. Renin release was similarly differentiated among individuals in the Hollenberg study.

Tidgren and coworkers performed a series of investigations of renal vascular responses to different stimuli, based on a renal venous thermodilution technique that allowed rapid measurements of renal blood flow. **Table 1** lists some of these results. It may be seen that mental stress (CWT) increased renal vascular resistance by 50% and increased the renal overflows of renin and norepinephrine markedly. Isometric handgrip exercise was less efficient, especially regarding renin release, despite a similar increase in mean arterial pressure (approximately 20 mmHg with both stimuli). The renal vasoconstrictor response to mental stress was similar to that elicited by dynamic exercise of moderate intensity (60% of maximum effort). Heart rate and arterial plasma epinephrine increased more with CWT than with isometric handgrip, whereas dynamic exercise increased heart rate still more, with a smaller increase in epinephrine at a similar level of renal vasoconstriction. Thus, the patterns of responses differ among these three stimuli. The renal vasoconstrictor and renin responses to mental stress were correlated to the renal norepinephrine overflow response (i.e., sympathetic nerve activity). The possible importance of epinephrine is discussed next.

Animal studies by di Bona, Koepke, Thorén and others have shown that renal vasoconstriction, as well as decreases in renal sodium excretion and increases in renin release, elicited by mental stress are sympathetically mediated and that these responses are enhanced in spontaneously hypertensive animals. Thus, the sympathetic nerves are important for renal responses to stress. Work in humans is less extensive, but the results discussed here tend to support the

Table 1 A comparison of responses to mental stress, isometric handgrip exercise, and dynamic exercise in healthy male volunteers[a]

Condition	*Renal vascular resistance (PRU)*	*Renal renin release (units min^{-1})*	*Arterial (nmol l^{-1})*	*Norepinephrine Renal venous (nmol l^{-1})*	*Renal overflow (pmol min^{-1})*	*Epinephrine arterial (nmol l^{-1})*	*Heart rate (beats min^{-1})*	*Source*[b]
Rest	0.15 ± 0.01	75[c]	0.78 ± 0.06	1.09 ± 0.10	252 ± 29	0.26 ± 0.04	59 ± 2	1
Mental stress	0.22 ± 0.02***	247***	1.34 ± 0.11***	2.93 ± 0.54***	708 ± 79***	0.68 ± 0.11***	81 ± 5***	
Rest	0.16 ± 0.02	54 ± 17	0.98 ± 0.13	1.24 ± 0.14	228 ± 34	0.24 ± 0.03	56 ± 2	2
Isometric handgrip	0.20 ± 0.03*	≈60 (n.s.)[c]	1.49 ± 0.16***	2.36 ± 0.29***	508 ± 73***	0.38 ± 0.04***	68 ± 3***	
Rest	0.14 ± 0.02	69 ± 28	0.87 ± 0.08	1.05 ± 0.11	201 ± 33	0.32 ± 0.07	67 ± 3	3
Exercise (60%)[d]	≈0.22**	≈200**	≈3**	≈5**	≈1000**	≈0.5**	≈140***	
(maximum effort)	0.33 ± 0.03***	825 ± 302***	11.4 ± 2.45***	19.8 ± 5.69***	3039 ± 806***	2.12 ± 0.54***	175 ± 6***	

[a]Mental stress was induced by Stroop's color word conflict test (CWT; Frankenhaueser Version), isometric handgrip exercise used maximum effort, and dynamic exercise used graded supine exercise (levels 2 and 3). Renal blood flow was measured by a renal venous thermodilution technique and renal vascular resistance was calculated on the basis of intra-arterially determined blood pressures. For transformation of catecholamine values, 1 nmol l^{-1} = 169 pg ml^{-1} (norepinephrine) or 183 pg ml^{-1} (epinephrine). Mean values ±SEM (or median) for resting and peak values are shown ($n = 8$–12). * indicates $p < 0.05$; ** indicates $p < 0.01$; *** indicates $p < 0.001$; n.s., not significant; PRU, peripheral resistance units.
[b]Data from:1. Tidgren and Hjemdahl (1989), *American Journal of Physiology* **257,** F682–F689.

2. Tidgren and Hjemdahl (1988), *Acta Physiologica Scandinavia* **134,** 23–34.

3. Tidgren et al. (1991), *Journal of Applied Physiology* **70,** 2279–2286.

[c]Median values reported, due to skewed distribution of renin release.
[d]Estimated from graphs.

conclusion that the kidney is a target organ for stress and that sympathetic nerve activity is involved.

Is Epinephrine an Important Stress Hormone?

When given intravenously, epinephrine increases cardiac output mainly by increasing stroke volume. This is perceived as tachycardia (or the heart is pumping harder), even though the heart rate is relatively little influenced unless the dosage of epinephrine is high. The increase in stroke volume is related to an increase in cardiac contractility as well as a reduction of afterload due to the systemic vasodilatation elicited by epinephrine. During stress, however, the increase in cardiac output is mainly related to an increase in heart rate, due to increased cardiac sympathetic nerve activity and vagal withdrawal. Even though the human heart is endowed with epinephrine sensitive β_2-adrenoceptors, the cardiac response to stress is thus mainly neurogenic.

Epinephrine is a potent vasodilator when infused intravenously or intra-arterially. The vasodilator response is elicited by β_2-adrenoceptor stimulation, and the α agonistic effects of epinephrine become apparent only after blockade of vascular β_2-adrenoceptors or at supraphysiological concentrations of epinephrine. In the absence of β-blockade, intravenously infused epinephrine does not change mean arterial pressure within the physiological range, but concentration-dependent decreases in diastolic blood pressure (reflecting systemic vasodilatation) and increases in systolic blood pressure (reflecting increased stroke volume) are elicited. The importance of epinephrine for vascular responses to stress may be deduced from comparisons of the plasma concentrations achieved during stress and those required for physiological responses, as well as by effects of β-blockade. **Figure 6** illustrates intraindividual comparisons of responses to CWT and infused epinephrine with regard to the forearm circulation; similar comparisons were made in our kidney studies.

Intravenously infused epinephrine may elicit reflexogenic increases in muscle sympathetic nerve activity. This is seen in **Figure 6**, which illustrates that epinephrine is more efficient when infused locally (intra-arterially) than intravenously. When vasodilator responses to CWT and epinephrine were compared, we found that epinephrine contributed to only a small extent (10–30%, on average). Data on local infusions of propranolol support this contention. Thus, epinephrine does not explain the vasodilatation in human skeletal muscle during mental stress.

In the kidney study of mental stress (**Table 1**), there was no vasoconstrictor (or vasodilator) response to intravenously infused epinephrine, even at plasma concentrations as high as 6 nmol l^{-1}. Renal norepinephrine overflow was little influenced, but there was a concentration-dependent increase in renin release from the kidney. Epinephrine might thus contribute slightly ($\approx$20%) to renin release but not to renal vasoconstriction during mental stress.

In summary, the cardiovascular responses to mental stress in humans cannot be explained by epinephrine, but this hormonal link of the sympathoadrenal system may contribute to certain responses. The conception that epinephrine is the stress hormone is not correct from a functional point of view. However, the epinephrine response to stress does reflect the stress perceived and the arousal of the individual, and it is a good marker for the stimulus intensity of a stressor.

Pathophysiological Aspects

Stress is considered to be involved in the pathogenesis of several cardiovascular disease states, and stress may provoke acute cardiovascular complications, such as myocardial infarction and sudden death in individuals with symptomatic or asymptomatic atherosclerosis. However, for reasons already discussed, it is difficult to define the exact role of stress in cardiovascular disease.

Animal studies have shown that repeated mild activation of the defense reaction (by stress or by electrical stimulation of certain brain regions) may contribute to the development of hypertension. In addition, animals and humans with a genetic predisposition for hypertension often show enhanced cardiovascular and neurogenic reactivity to stress. Animal studies have also shown that stress may accelerate the development of atherosclerosis, as illustrated by elegant experiments by Clarkson, Kaplan, and Manuck in cynomolgus monkeys showing increased atherosclerosis and by Henry in mice. In humans, it has been more difficult to link stress to atherosclerosis, but there are indications that stress, anxiety, and personality factors are involved. Furthermore, biobehavioral modifications may alter the course of coronary artery disease. Metabolic disturbances, such as diabetes and the metabolic syndrome (a cluster of risk factors with disturbed glucose regulation and often hypertension), are increasingly being linked to atherosclerotic disease. It is of interest that stress may accelerate these processes via the activation of the hypothalamic-pituitary-adrenal axis and release of cortisol. Thus, stress may indeed be involved in the pathogenesis of atherosclerosis, in agreement with popular views on the subject.

Various everyday stresses may trigger serious cardiovascular events, such as myocardial infarction, stroke, and sudden death (due to arrhythmia or myocardial infarction). Work by Mittleman, Muller, Willich, and others has shown diurnal variation in the incidence of myocardial infarction and that physical or mental stress precedes myocardial infarction or sudden death more frequently than would be expected by chance.

Acute myocardial infarction involves thrombosis in the coronary arteries, which may be triggered by many factors, including stress. The hemodynamic changes associated with mental or physical stress increase the risk of atherosclerotic plaque rupture, which is a potent stimulus for local thrombus formation. The mechanisms involved in thrombosis are complex and involve platelets and the coagulation system, as well as factors that oppose coagulation and dissolve blood clots (fibrinolysis). Stress-induced platelet activation may lead to the release of vasoactive substances, which promote ischemia and thrombus formation. Platelet activation may be enhanced by endothelial dysfunction (reduced release of NO and prostacyclin), increased shear stress in an atherosclerotic vessel, and other platelet-activating effects of stress that operate also among healthy individuals. Endothelial dysfunction also promotes vasoconstrictor responses to stress in the coronary arteries and may contribute to imbalances between blood flow and metabolic demands (i.e., myocardial ischemia). Mental stress has indeed been shown to elicit abnormal coronary vasoconstriction and myocardial ischemia among patients with coronary artery disease. The ischemic myocardium is vulnerable to life-threatening arrhythmias, especially when sympathetic activity is increased and vagal activity is reduced, as is the case during stress. Thus, stress elicits cardiovascular and neurohormonal changes that are beneficial to the healthy subject but detrimental to patients with coronary artery disease. In addition, stress produces prothrombotic alterations that may further increase the risk of myocardial infarction.

Further Reading

Anderson, E. A., Wallin, B. G. and Mark, A. L. (1987). *Hypertension* **9** (supplement 3), 114–119.

Bennet, T. and Gardiner, S. M. (eds.) (1996). *Nervous control of blood vessels.* Amsterdam: Harwood Academic.

Brod, J. (1963). Haemodynamic basis of acute pressor reactions and hypertension. *British Heart Journal* **25**, 227–245.

Byrne, D. G. and Rosenman, R. H. (eds.) (1990). *Anxiety and the heart.* New York: Hemisphere.

Folkow, B. (1982). Physiological aspects of primary hypertension. *Physiological Reviews* **62**, 347–504.

Fuster, V., Badimon, L., Badimon, J. J., et al. (1992). The pathogenesis of coronary artery disease and the acute coronary syndromes. *New England Journal of Medicine* **326**, 242–250, 310–318.

Goldstein, D. S. (1995). Clinical assessment of sympathetic responses to stress. *Annals of the New York Academy of Sciences* 771, 570–593.

Goldstein, D. S. (1995). Stress as a scientific idea – a homeostatic theory of stress and distress. *Homeostasis* **36**, 177–215.

Hemingway, H. and Marmot, M. (1998). Psychosocial factors in the primary and secondary prevention of coronary heart disease: a systematic review. In: Yusuf, S., Cairns, J. A., Camm, A. J., Fallen, E. L. & Gersh, B. J. (eds.) *Evidence based cardiology*, pp. 269–285. London: BMJ Books.

Freyschuss, U., Hjemdah, P., Juhlin-Dannefelt, A. and Linde, B. (1988). Cardiovascular and sympatho-adrenal responses to mental stress – influence of beta-blockade. *American Journal of Physiology* **255**, H1443–H1451.

Herd, J. A. (1991). Cardiovascular responses to stress. *Physiological Reviews* **71**, 305–330.

Hjemdahl, P. (1993). Plasma catecholamines – analytical challenges and physiological limitations. *Baillère's Clinical Endocrinology and Metabolism* **7**, 307–353.

Hjemdahl, P. (2002). Stress and the metabolic syndrome – an interesting but enigmatic association. *Circulation* **106**, 2534–2536.

Hjemdahl, P., Larsson, P. T. and Wallén, H. (1991). Effects of stress and β-blockade on platelet function. *Circulation* **84**, VI-44–VI-61.

Julius, S. (1988). The blood pressure seeking properties of the central nervous system. *Journal of Hypertension* **6**, 177–185.

Linde, B., Freyschuss, U., Hjemdahl, P. and Juhlin-Dannefelt, A. (1989). Adipose tissue and skeletal muscle responses to mental stress. *American Journal of Physiology* **256**, E12–E18.

Lindqvist, M., Melcher, A. and Hjemdahl, P. (2004). Hemodynamic and sympatho-adrenal responses to mental stress during nitric oxide synthesis blockade. *American Journal of Physiology: Heart Circulatory Physiology* **287**, H2309–H2315.

Lindqvist, M., Kahan, T., Melcher, A., Bie, P. and Hjemdahl, P. (1996). Forearm vasodilator mechanisms during mental stress – possible roles of epinephrine and ANP. *American Journal of Physiology* **270**, E393–E399.

McCarty, R., Horwatt, K. and Konarska, M. (1988). Chronic stress and sympathetic-adrenal medullary responsiveness. *Social Science & Medicine* **26**, 333–341.

Rosmond, R. (2005). Role of stress in the pathogenesis of the metabolic syndrome. *Psychoneuroendocrinology* **30**, 1–10.

Shepherd, J. T. and Weiss, S. M. (eds.) (1987). *Special issue on behavioral medicine and cardiovascular disease. Circulation*, **76** (Part 2).

Steptoe, A. and Vögele, C. (1991). Methodology of mental stress testing in cardiovascular research. *Circulation* **83**, II-14–II-24.

Strike, P. C. and Steptoe, A. (2003). Systematic review of mental stress-induced myocardial ischemia. *European Heart Journal* **24**, 690–703.

Tidgren, B. and Hjemdahl, P. (1988). Reflex activation of renal nerves in humans: effects on norepinephrine, dopamine and renin overflow to renal venous plasma. *Acta Physiologica Scandinavia* **134**, 23–34.

Tidgren, B. and Hjemdahl, P. (1989). Renal responses to mental stress and epinephrine in man. *American Journal of Physiology* **257**, F682–F689.

Tidgren, B., Hjemdahl, P., Theodorsson, E. and Nussberger, J. (1991). Renal neurohormonal and vascular responses to dynamic exercise in man. *Journal of Applied Physiology* 70, 2279–2286.
Vane, J. R., Änggård, E. E. and Botting, R. M. (1990). Regulatory functions of the vascular endothelium. *New England Journal of Medicine* 323, 27–36.
Verrier, R. L. and Mittleman, M. A. (1996). Life-threatening cardiovascular consequences of anger in patients with coronary heart disease. *Cardiology Clinics* 14, 289–307.
Willerson, J. T., Golino, P., Eidt, J., et al. (1989). Specific platelet mediators and unstable coronary artery lesions: experimental evidence and potential clinical implications. *Circulation* 80, 198–205.
Willich, S. N. and Muller, J. E. (eds.) (1996). *Triggering of acute coronary syndromes – implications for prevention.* Dordrecht: Kluwer Academic.

Autonomic Nervous System: Central Cardiovascular Control

M C Andresen
Oregon Health & Science University, Portland, OR, USA
D Mendelowitz
George Washington University, Washington, DC, USA

Introduction

Vital nourishment of all tissues is assured by a properly regulated cardiovascular system. Consistent and coordinated contractions of the heart provide pressure for the circulation system and vessel conduits distribute the blood to flow throughout the body. Thus, the goal of cardiovascular control is to maintain and allocate blood flow that meets tissue demands over a diverse range of circumstances. Cardiac contractions are normally initiated by electrical pacemaker activity within the sinus node of the right atrium, and without external stimuli, intrinsic pacemaking automatically maintains rates that are fairly constant. However, the autonomic nervous system is responsible for adjustments that meet changing circulatory demands such as exercise or postural challenges. Thus, the nervous system orchestrates optimal adjustments in the pump function of the heart. Both rate and the timing of events between atria and ventricles are altered by released neurotransmitters to facilitate efficient pumping. Neurotransmitter activation of smooth muscle in blood vessels adjusts vessel caliber and thus flow patterns. These cardiovascular adjustments are accomplished by neurotransmitters released by autonomic nerves. Overall, the level of arterial blood pressure at all times is a dominant factor in driving the circulation of blood. Multiple neural reflexes rapidly control blood pressure to accommodate a wide range of systemic and regional demands and priorities. Acute postural change, for example, can require changes in pump rate at the very next heart beat, and such rapid adjustments use the autonomic nervous system to quickly fine-tune the heart and the vascular distribution of blood.

The organization of the central nervous system (CNS), directed toward control of the cardiovascular system, follows a general, prototypic pattern for these reflex pathways. Afferent information arises from a network of afferent neurons distributed within key portions of the cardiovascular system. The peripheral endings of cardiovascular afferent neurons are unequally distributed and are particularly concentrated in the centralmost portions of the vascular tree (aorta, common carotid artery, vena cava, and jugular vein) and within the heart. Mechanosensitive afferent neurons (e.g., arterial baroreceptors) transduce local vessel and chamber stretch as an index of filling or local pressure. This 'filling' information plays a key role in rapid cardiovascular adjustments on a beat-to-beat basis. Afferent neurons arising from the heart as with many other visceral organs have cell bodies in cervical ganglia associated with the IX and X cranial nerves (nodose, jugular, and petrosal ganglia). Additional cardiovascular afferents arise from neurons of the dorsal root ganglia and often these spinal afferent neurons send axons that travel via the sympathetic nerve trunks and have been termed sympathetic afferents in the literature. Visceral afferents dominate reflexes that adjust the autonomic outflow back to the organ of origin, but often additionally contribute to the control of entirely different organs (e.g., respiratory afferents that alter cardiac control). Both cardiac and arterial mechanosensory neurons initiate rapidly responding, relatively short pathways for parasympathetic efferent adjustments as well as longer latency reflexes via the spinal cord that modulate sympathetic efferent neurons. Cardiovascular reflex pathways predominantly involve networks of neurons in the brain stem and spinal cord. Control of heart rate and arterial pressure is the primary focus of this overview.

The arterial baroreceptor reflex (baroreflex) control of heart rate is perhaps one of the most basic autonomic regulatory reflexes and serves as a central pathway prototype for reflexes arising from many other cranial visceral afferents. The parasympathetic reflex control of the heart is fundamentally better understood than control of arterial pressure or venous capacitance. The consensus view of the core circuit for the cardiac parasympathetic control suggests that this reflex arc relies on structures confined to the medulla. Baroreceptor afferents project to brain stem neurons in the nucleus of the solitary tract (NTS). NTS neurons, in turn, contact output neurons within the nucleus ambiguus (NA) that exit the brain stem to contact final parasympathetic motor neurons within the heart itself. While this constitutes the simplest pathway of cardiovascular control, additional, more convoluted, brain stem pathways exist as well as indirect contributions arising from ascending spinal viscerosensory pathways.

Medulla Oblongata

The arterial baroreflex is organized as a classic negative feedback system in which increases in arterial blood pressure activate mechanosensitive arterial baroreceptors (**Figure 1**) that trigger reflex responses that ultimately reduce arterial blood pressure. The discharge of arterial baroreceptors is conducted along cranial nerve axons (IX and X) projecting directly into the brain stem to neurons in the NTS where they make the first synapse in the baroreflex pathway (**Figure 2**). Processed afferent signals exit NTS to activate vagal preganglionic neurons located primarily in NA that project to cardioinhibitory parasympathetic postganglionic neurons in the heart. NTS neurons also activate sympathoinhibitory neurons located in the caudal ventrolateral medulla (CVLM). Thus, activity along dual, cardiac directed autonomic pathways is oppositely regulated to produce negative feedback control of cardiac pumping by (1) increased release of acetylcholine by parasympathetic postganglionic neurons and (2) decreased release of norepinephrine by sympathetic postganglionic neurons.

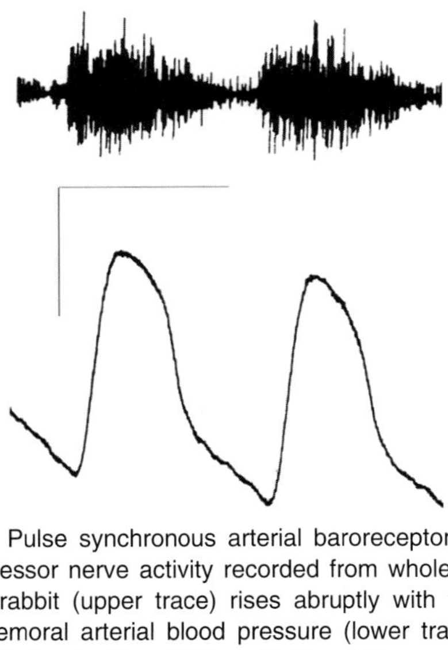

Figure 1 Pulse synchronous arterial baroreceptor discharge. Aortic depressor nerve activity recorded from whole nerve in a conscious rabbit (upper trace) rises abruptly with the systolic phase of femoral arterial blood pressure (lower trace). Scales are 20 mmHg (vertical) and 500 ms (horizontal).

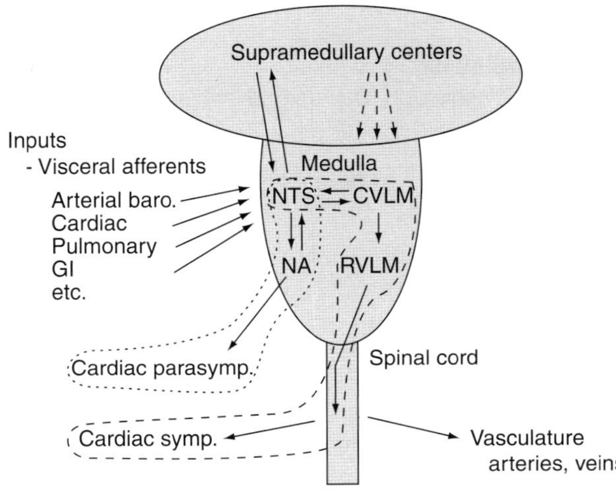

Figure 2 Schematic of core baroreflex pathways for cardiovascular control. Reflex responses are initiated from visceral primary afferent neurons such as cardiac afferent and arterial baroreceptor neurons (left) that converge on initial central neurons (second-order neurons) within the nucleus of the solitary tract (NTS). From there, information diverges to two key autonomic centers along the parasympathetic pathway to nucleus ambiguus (NA) and along the sympathetic pathway to the caudal ventrolateral medulla (CVLM). The parasympathetic pathway (dotted outline) leaves NA to target the intrinsic cardiac network including postganglionic neurons at the heart. The sympathetic regulatory pathway (dashed outline) goes on to neurons in the rostral ventrolateral medulla (RVLM) before descending to the spinal cord at the intermediolateral cell column and out to the sympathetic postganglionic neurons. NTS is reciprocally connected to a wide range of CNS regions (bidirectional arrows) including many supramedullary regions that modulate reflex function but are not part of the essential core circuit. Forebrain regions, for example, often act to modify activity within the core brain stem circuits. A wide range of pathways (excitatory and inhibitory) contacts neurons of the core baroreflex pathway. Note that the negative feedback and slowing of the heart rate occurs peripherally in the parasympathetic pathway by actions of the postganglionic neurotransmitter acetylcholine, but centrally in the sympathetic pathway as CVLM-released GABA inhibits RVLM neurons (and sympathetic activity).

In the resting, conscious state, midcollicular decerebration does not alter the gain (sensitivity) of this heart rate baroreflex, suggesting that brain stem mechanisms are sufficient for reflex function. Although brain structures above the medulla are not required, information from the forebrain and other higher CNS sites modulate the baroreflex during various behaviors including stressful emotional responses. Thus, the core baroreflex circuit appears to reside below the pons and contains both short and longer latency pathways. The shortest anatomical pathway activates cardiac parasympathetic efferent neurons by engaging, at a minimum, (1) primary afferent neurons associated with cardiovascular mechanoreceptors, (2) second-order NTS neurons, (3) cardiac parasympathetic preganglionic motor neurons located primarily in the NA, and (4) parasympathetic postganglionic neurons intrinsic to the heart. Such a parasympathetic pathway is responsible for relatively short-latency (<100 ms) cardiovascular-cardiac reflexes that adjust heart rate within one cardiac cycle (**Figure 2**).

Primary Afferent Neurons of the Arterial Baroreflex

Cardiovascular regulation depends on the constant monitoring of arterial pressure, central venous pressure, and cardiac rate and force. Populations of cardiovascular-selective sensory neurons supply a constant stream of information and these viscerosensory neurons belong to cellular/molecular phenotypic classes based on axon myelination that are broadly similar to sensory neurons of the skin (somatic afferents). Baroreceptors are concentrated near the bifurcation of the common carotid artery (carotid sinus) and just outside the left ventricle in the arch of the thoracic aorta. Neurites from arterial baroreceptors lie within the adventitia, the outermost layer of the artery wall. This position within the artery wall means that they are stretched with each expansion of the artery wall that accompanies each expulsion of blood from the heart. A-type baroreceptors rapidly conduct responses via myelinated fibers (2.5–25 m s^{-1}) in brief bursts of activity during each pressure pulse (**Figure 1**). A-type baroreceptors discharge within the normal range of blood pressures even at rest and their discharge activity is quite regular and encodes mean arterial pressure, as well as the rate of rise and amplitude of the pressure pulse. A much larger number of arterial baroreceptors are C-type and conduct more irregular discharge patterns along slowly conducting (<1 m s^{-1}), unmyelinated axons. C-type baroreceptors are often silent at resting blood pressures and become active with sparse, intermittent discharge only at higher pressures than the A-type baroreceptors. A minority of C-type baroreceptors is activated at normal arterial pressures. The relationship between the amplitude of sensory terminal stretch and the frequency of evoked discharge defines the 'baroreceptor sensitivity.' This is not a fixed relationship, but displays 'plastic' changes both acutely and chronically in the face of sustained blood pressure changes. Under physiological and pathological conditions, the roles played by specific afferent neuronal populations can become 'reset' and change along with changes in cardiovascular regulation.

Solitary Tract Nucleus – Arterial Baroreflex Second-Order Neurons

Neurons within dorsal medial portions of the caudal NTS mark the central first step of the medullary baroreceptor reflex. Sensory inputs from baroreceptor afferent neurons release glutamate as their primary neurotransmitter to activate non-*N*-methyl-D-aspartate (NMDA) receptors on second-order NTS neurons. Inhibitory transmission via γ-aminobutyric acid (GABA) is prominent at second-order neurons in the medial NTS with inhibitory postsynaptic potentials arriving shortly after visceral afferent glutamatergic excitatory synaptic potentials. Since a majority of these GABAergic neurons are themselves directly coupled to viscerosensory afferent inputs, this organization provides effective short-latency feedback inhibition within this cardiovascular-cardiac reflex. These two amino acid transmitters activate ionotropic (ion channel coupled) receptors to convey fast transmission but both glutamate and GABA, in addition, activate metabotropic receptors that are coupled to intracellular second messengers. Thus, heterosynaptic cross talk between neurotransmitters is common and provides afferent-linked mechanisms that are very sensitive to the frequency content of afferent patterns of discharge. A wide range of accessory transmitters such as peptides like ATP, substance P, and calcitonin gene-related peptide are also involved in such transmission, although their precise roles are less certain.

Cardiac Parasympathetic Neurons

Cardiac parasympathetic motor neurons exert powerful control on cardiodynamics. Heart rate is dominated by the activity of the cardioinhibitory parasympathetic nervous system (**Figure 2**). Cardiac parasympathetic neurons are tonically active at rest but little, if any, cardiac sympathetic activity is commonly present under normal conditions. Preganglionic cardiac vagal neurons have cell bodies located mostly in the NA and, to a lesser extent, in the dorsal motor nucleus of the vagus. These parasympathetic preganglionic neurons send axons that exit the brain stem via the vagus nerves to contact postganglionic neurons located in cardiac ganglia. These cardiac ganglia are found within the connective and fatty tissue that surround the right atrium and vena cava. Parasympathetic postganglionic fibers emerge from these ganglia to make extensive synaptic contacts with the nearby sinoatrial and atrioventricular nodes of the heart where they release the neurotransmitter acetylcholine.

Activity within the arterial baroreflex is a major determinant of the tonic activity of the parasympathetic efferent preganglionic neurons that target the heart. During normal states, parasympathetic efferent preganglionic neuronal activity occurs during specific phases of the cardiac cycle initiated by this fast-responding reflex. Heart rate is dominated by the activity of the cardioinhibitory parasympathetic nervous system. Measures of these ongoing, tonic, and rapid adjustments in parasympathetic activity (e.g., heart rate variability) are indicators of cardiac health and, when absent, can predict an important risk of cardiac sudden death. During increases in arterial pressure, the initial reflex-induced slowing of the heart (bradycardia) is caused primarily, if not exclusively, by increases in cardiac vagal nerve activity. During decreases in arterial pressure, the baroreflex-induced cardiac acceleration (tachycardia) is caused mostly by decreases in parasympathetic along with somewhat later-arriving increases in sympathetic nerve activity. When both parasympathetic and sympathetic activities are present, parasympathetic activity generally dominates the control of heart rate. Increases in parasympathetic activity evoke a cardiac slowing that is more pronounced when there is a high level of sympathetic firing. When there is a moderate or high level of parasympathetic activity, changes in sympathetic firing elicit negligible changes in heart rate.

The CNS system normally controls the parasympathetic activity reaching the heart. Preganglionic cardiac vagal fibers tonically fire with a cardiac pulse synchronous pattern that is reduced during inspiration. Interruption of links to the CNS by cutting the cardiac vagal preganglionic fibers leads to an increase in heart rate demonstrating that the remaining, intact cardiac parasympathetic postganglionic neurons by themselves cannot sustain normal cardiac rates. Similarly, synaptic blockade silences parasympathetic neurons within the brain stem indicating an absence of pacemaker-like activity such as repetitive or phasic depolarizations or action potential. However, even small depolarizing currents (100 pA) evoke sustained, repetitive firing in cardiac vagal neurons with minimal spike frequency adaptation. The voltage-gated currents and firing characteristics of cardiac vagal neurons enable them to closely follow fast synaptic drive as well as to integrate long-lasting modulatory influences. Together, the characteristics of both these preganglionic and postganglionic cardiac parasympathetic neurons suggest that heart rate at rest is determined by activity within the parasympathetic pathways that arises from the integration of afferent and other drives to produce normal levels of cardiac vagal tone.

The activity of cardiac vagal preganglionic neurons is controlled by three major classes of synaptic inputs: glutamatergic, GABAergic, and glycinergic. NTS neurons provide a major glutamatergic input pathway that activates both NMDA and non-NMDA postsynaptic currents in cardiac vagal neurons. Owing to baroreceptor activation of NTS neurons, this glutamatergic pathway to cardiac vagal neurons likely constitutes the essential link between increases in blood pressure and the parasympathetic component of the arterial baroreceptor reflex. Additionally, NTS activation triggers GABAergic inputs to cardiac vagal neurons. Electrical stimulation of afferents in the vagus nerve evokes both GABAergic and glutamatergic responses in cardiac vagal neurons. In addition, the pungent active ingredient in hot peppers, capsaicin, can chemically activate and then, with prolonged exposure, inactivate visceral sensory C-type afferents including baroreceptors. Blockade of C-type afferents by capsaicin increases the latency of the GABAergic response without changing the latency of the glutamatergic responses. Such findings suggest that an inhibitory GABAergic pathway is involved in patterning of cardiac vagal activity to produce bursting synchronous with the cardiac cycle.

Cardiac vagal nerve activity also has pronounced respiratory modulation that mediates respiratory sinus arrhythmia, a pattern of slowing and accelerating heart rate in phase with lung inflation and deflation. Cardiac vagal fibers fire most rapidly in the postinspiration period, and often fall silent during inspiration. A form of this firing activity of cardiac vagal neurons during the phases of respiration persists in slices of the medulla that contain cardiac vagal neurons, pre-Bötzinger complex, and local circuits for motor output generation, and inspiratory motor discharge patterns can be recorded in hypoglossal cranial nerves (**Figure 3**). The firing of cardiac vagal neurons is inhibited during inspiratory activity.

Nicotinic cholinergic mechanisms have important actions on cardiac vagal neurons. During inspiration, the frequency of both GABAergic and glycinergic synaptic events increases substantially (**Figure 4**). A nicotinic antagonist, selective for a specific subset of nicotinic receptors ($\alpha 4\beta 2$), abolishes this respiratory-evoked increase in GABAergic events supporting the critical role of cholinergic inputs in shaping cardiac parasympathetic control. This is a highly specific interaction since this intervention has no effect on

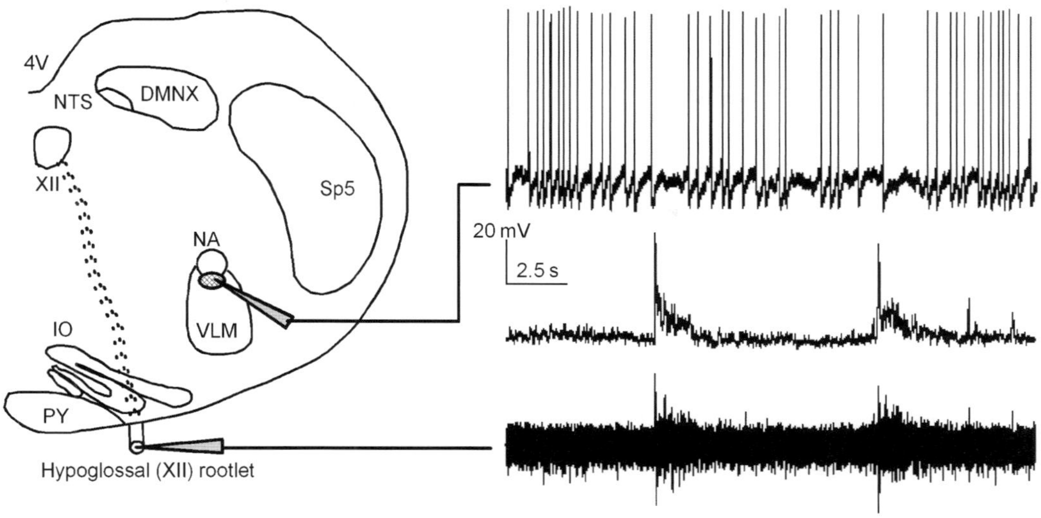

Figure 3 The medullary slice preparation that contains the cardiac vagal neurons, pre-Bötzinger complex, and respiratory hypoglossal motor neurons with intact hypoglossal cranial nerves is illustrated. Inspiratory activity recorded from the hypoglossal rootlet is shown bottom trace, right, and integrated, middle trace, right. The firing activity of a cardiac vagal neuron, induced to fire repetitively with a constant injection of inward current (~50 pA), top right, is inhibited during each inspiratory burst.

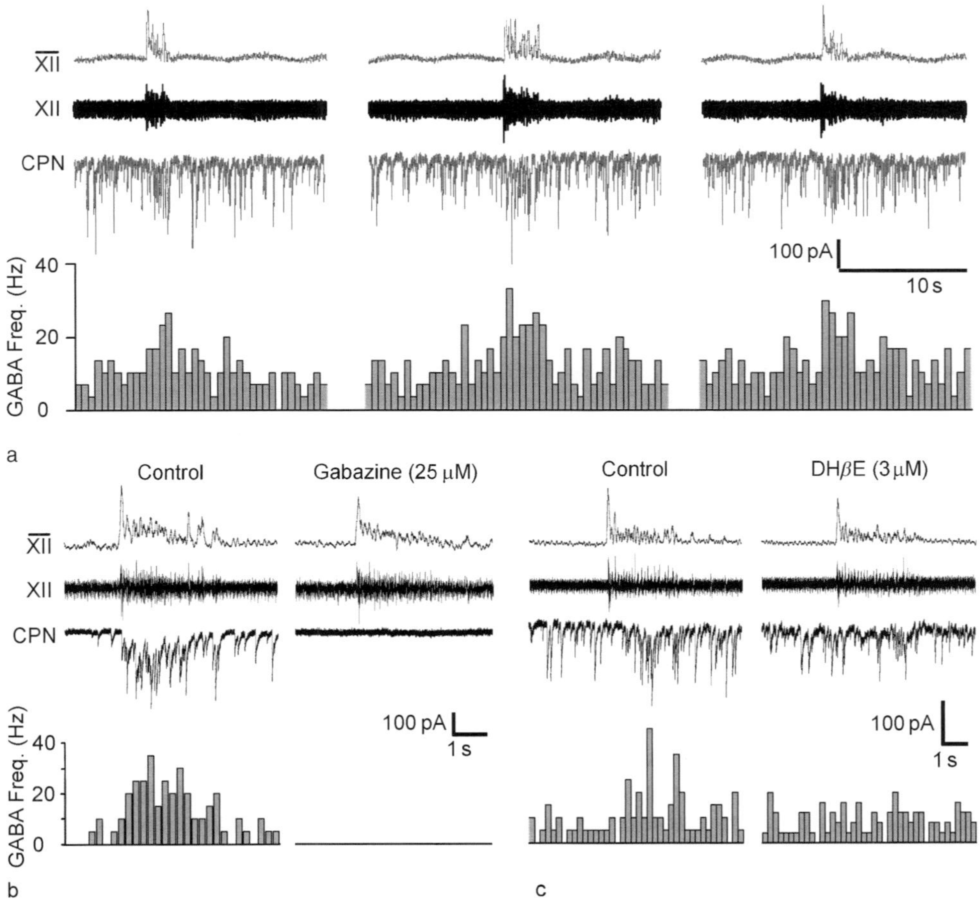

Figure 4 Inspiratory-related bursting activity was recorded from the hypoglossal rootlet (XII) and rectified and adjacent averaged ($\overline{\text{XII}}$). GABAergic inhibitory postsynaptic currents (IPSCs) were isolated by focal application of the NMDA, non-NMDA, and glycine receptor antagonists AP-5 (50 μM), CNQX (50 μM), and strychnine (1 mM), respectively. (a) During inspiratory activity, the frequency of GABAergic IPSCs in cardiac vagal neurons was significantly increased ($p < 0.05$). (b) The $GABA_A$ antagonist gabazine blocked all IPSCs. (c) This inspiratory-related increase in GABA synaptic frequency was abolished by focal application of the nicotinic receptor antagonist dihydro-β-erithroidine (DhβE) at a concentration selective for the $\alpha4\beta2$ receptor subtype DHβE did not significantly change GABA synaptic frequency between inspiratory bursts.

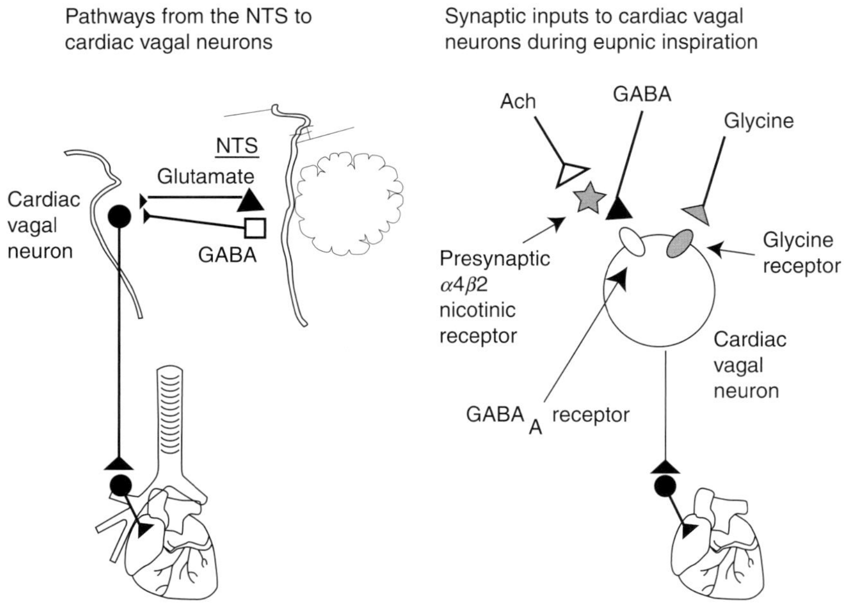

Figure 5 Neurotransmitter actions in the core reflex pathway in the control of cardiac parasympathetic neurons. NTS sends glutamatergic and GABAergic but not glycinergic pathways to cardiac vagal neurons (left). Inspiratory activity increases both GABAergic and glycinergic inputs to cardiac vagal neurons (right). Nicotinic $\alpha4\beta2$ receptors presynaptically facilitate GABAergic, but not glycinergic, neurotransmission.

the increase in glycinergic synaptic events during inspiration. Together, such findings provide a basic outline of interactions between glutamate, glycine, and acetylcholine in the control of heart rate in this core NTS–NA pathway (**Figure 5**).

Spinal Cord

Sympathetic preganglionic neurons related to the cardiovascular system are located within the intermediolateral cell column of the spinal cord and constitute a second major autonomic effector pathway. These sympathetic preganglionic neurons send processes from the spinal cord to activate postganglionic neurons within peripheral ganglia. The postganglionic sympathetic neurons themselves send axons to contact visceral organs and blood vessels where they release the neurotransmitter norepinephrine. Activity in these sympathetic neurons influences all aspects of cardiac function including heart rate, cardiac conduction, the strength of cardiac contraction, and ventricular stroke volume. Many sympathetic motor neurons are directed to blood vessels resulting in activation of smooth muscle and changes in vessel diameter and local arterial resistance or venous capacitance.

Although reflexes within the medulla exert substantial influence on cardiovascular sympathetic efferent neurons, at present these reflexes are incompletely defined. Sympathetic premotor neurons within the rostral ventrolateral medulla (**Figure 2**) send axons to modulate spinal cord cardiovascular sympathetic preganglionic neurons. An important determinant of cardiovascular sympathetic regulation arises from sympathoinhibitory neurons lying within the CVLM that secrete GABA onto sympathetic premotor neurons within the rostral ventrolateral medulla. The full range of mechanisms of the control of sympathetic premotor neurons remains to be established. However, baroreflex pathways provide substantial sympathoinhibitory input and thus remain part of a functionally negative feedback system that, for example, reduces heart rate by inhibiting (i.e., withdrawing) ongoing norepinephrine release. Thus, NTS neurons that receive tonic inputs from cardiovascular afferent neurons activate sympathoinhibitory neurons that, in turn, phasically depress sympathetic premotor neuronal activity. These premotor neurons, in turn, project to sympathetic efferent preganglionic neurons in the intermediolateral cell column of the spinal cord. The cranial thoracic spinal cord preganglionic neurons project to cardiac sympathetic efferent postganglionic neurons distributed throughout the intrathoracic and superior cervical ganglia. Interestingly, such spinal cord sympathetic motor neurons also receive inputs from cardiac afferent neurons in dorsal root ganglia. Unlike the medullary cardiovascular reflexes depicted above, activation of spinal cardiac afferent neurons results in the activation of spinal cord sympathetic premotor neurons involved in enhancing cardiac rate and contractile force – a positive feedback mechanism. Spinal cord sympathetic preganglionic motor neurons also innervate peripheral blood vessels and influence arterial vascular resistance and venous capacitance. The interrelationship between positive and negative feedback pathways controlling cardiovascular sympathetic motor neurons is poorly understood, although often suspected to be involved during pathophysiological circumstances.

Higher Centers

Under many normal and pathophysiological conditions, the gain or sensitivity of the heart rate baroreflex can be altered by influences arising from supramedullary brain structures such as the hypothalamus or amygdala. Under stress and even during physiological states, these supramedullary inputs transform the operation of the baroreflex to accommodate integrative responses for exercise or strong emotional behaviors. Thus, cardiovascular regulation including the major baroreflex pathways is often an integral component of major homeostatic and highly complex patterned responses. These descending inputs from higher center neurons modulate both the fast-responding parasympathetic reflexes that provide beat-to-beat adjustments in cardiac performance as well as the longer latency cardio-cardiac reflexes involving spinal cord (sympathetic) neurons.

Clinical Implications

As a powerful, classic negative feedback system, the baroreflex provides rapid cardiovascular adjustments to the changing demands on the heart and great vessels. Cardiovascular feedback is constantly responding and remodeling to altered physiological status such as occurs during prolonged bed rest or zero gravity conditions. Substantial remodeling and reshaping of these reflex pathways also occurs in pathological states such as essential hypertension or heart failure. Prominent alterations in neuronal structures and neurotransmitter density within the NTS are associated with cases of sudden infant death syndrome, for example. The quantitative performance characteristics of the cardiac baroreflex have been linked to postmyocardial infarction survival as well as risk of sudden death from lethal cardiac arrhythmias. The sensitivity of the multiple reflexes involved in blood pressure regulation is reshaped at all stages of the cardiovascular neuroaxis during development of hypertension. The mechanisms for integration of all of the central neuronal reflexes involved in the maintenance of normal arterial pressure are not fully understood but presumably neural system remodels during the evolution of diseases hold keys to understanding essential hypertension as well as the development of novel and optimally effectively targeted therapies to treat such syndromes.

Further Reading

Andresen, M. C. and Kunze, D. L. (1994). Nucleus tractus solitarius: Gateway to neural circulatory control. *Annual Review of Physiology* **56**, 93–116.

Andresen, M. C., Kunze, D. L. and Mendelowitz, D. (2004). Central nervous system regulation of the heart. In: Armour, J. A. & Ardell, J. L. (eds.) *Basic and Clinical Neurocardiology* (2nd edn., pp. 187–219). New York: Oxford University Press.

Armour, J. A. (1976). Instant to instant reflex cardiac regulation. *Cardiology* **61**, 309–328.

Cole, C. R., Blackstone, E. H., Pashkow, F. J., Snader, C. E. and Lauer, M. S. (1999). Heart-rate recovery immediately after exercise as a predictor of mortality. *New England Journal of Medicine* **341**, 1351–1357.

Kinney, H. C., Filiano, J. J. and Harper, R. M. (1992). The neuropathology of the sudden infant death syndrome. A review. *Journal of Neuropathology and Experimental Neurology* **51**, 115–126.

Kunze, D. L. and Andresen, M. C. (1991). Arterial baroreceptors. In: Zucker, I. H. & Gilmore, J. P. (eds.) *Excitation and Modulation, Reflex Control of the Circulation*, pp. 141–166. Boca Raton: CRC Press.

LaRovere, M. T., Pinna, G. D., Hohnloser, S. H., et al. (2001). ATRAMI investigators: Baroreflex sensitivity and heart rate variability in the identification of patients at risk for life-threatening arrhythmias: Implications for clinical trials. *Circulation* **103**, 2072–2077.

Loewy, A. D. (1990). Central autonomic pathways. In: Loewy, A. D. & Spyer, K. M. (eds.) *Central Regulation of Autonomic Functions*, pp. 88–103. New York: Oxford University Press.

Mayr, U. and Keele, S. (2000) Changing internal constraints on action: The role of backward inhibition. *Journal of Experimental Psychology: General* 129: 4–26.

Mendelowitz, D. (1999). Advances in parasympathetic control of heart rate and cardiac function. *News in Physiological Sciences* **14**, 155–161.

Spooner, P. M., Albert, C., Benjamin, E. J., et al. (2001). Sudden cardiac death, genes, and arrhythmogenesis: Consideration of new population and mechanistic approaches from a national heart, lung, and blood institute workshop. Part I & II. *Circulation* **103**, 2447–2452.

Circadian Rhythm Effects on Cardiovascular and Other Stress-Related Events

R Manfredini, B Boari, R Salmi, A M Malagoni and F Manfredini
Vascular Diseases Center, University of Ferrara, Italy

Glossary

Aortic aneurysm	Dilatation or ballooning of the wall of thoracic or abdominal aorta.
Chronobiology	The study of biological systems as affected by time.
Circadian rhythm	Biological rhythm with regular recurrence in cycles of about 24 h.
Coagulation	Process of interaction of blood coagulation factors to form a fibrin clot.
Hypertension	Persistently high systemic arterial blood pressure.
Myocardial infarction	Necrosis of the myocardium, as a result of interruption of blood supply.
Stroke	Sudden and severe cerebral attack, ischemic or hemorrhagic.

Chronobiology and Circadian Rhythms

Chronobiology is a branch of biomedical sciences devoted to the study of biological rhythms. Biological rhythms exist at any level of living organisms and, according to their cycle length, may be divided into three main types: (1) circadian rhythms (from the Latin *circa diem*, characterized by a period of approximately 24 h), (2) ultradian rhythms (period shorter than 24 h, e.g., hours, minutes or even seconds), and (3) infradian rhythms (period longer than 24 h, e.g., days, weeks, months). Circadian rhythms are the most commonly and widely studied biological rhythms.

The cardiovascular system is organized according to a specific temporal order that is oscillatory in nature, and most cardiovascular functions exhibit circadian changes. Such predictable-in-time differences in the physiological status of the cardiovascular system give rise to rhythmic variations in the susceptibility of human beings to morbid and mortal events. On the other hand, the pathological mechanisms of cardiovascular disease themselves exhibit temporal changes in both their manifestation and severity, leading to predictable-in-time differences in their ability to precipitate and graduate the overt expression of disease. A growing body of evidence suggests that the occurrence of cardiovascular events is not evenly distributed in time, but shows peculiar temporal patterns that vary with time of the day, the day of the week, and the month of the year. These patterns coincide with the temporal variation in the pathophysiological mechanisms that trigger cardiovascular events and the physiological changes in the body rhythms. These contribute to the definition of the new concept of chronorisk, in which several factors, not harmful if taken alone, are capable of triggering unfavorable events when presenting all together within the same temporal window.

Circadian Rhythm of Cardiovascular Events

Myocardial Ischemia and Infarction

Coronary heart disease (CHD) is the number one cause of death worldwide, leading to more than 7 million deaths annually. CHD occurs when the coronary arteries are unable to supply adequate oxygenated blood to myocardial tissue, leading to myocardial ischemia and possible acute myocardial infarction (AMI). A reversible injury to myocardial tissue leads to ischemia, while AMI represents cell death after prolonged ischemia. The development of AMI is based on two major components. The first is vascular injury and/or dysfunction with loss of a nonthrombogenic endothelial surface, most frequently due to atherosclerotic plaques. In response to intraluminal stress, for example, the circadian periodic or incidental rise in blood pressure, plaques may rupture and release thrombogenic factors into the bloodstream. The second is activation of the blood-clotting mechanism beyond the capacity of the simultaneously activated fibrinolytic mechanisms to remove the fibrin formed and prevent the formation of a clot, thus leading to occlusion of the vessel.

As for circadian variation in onset, both stable coronary disease and ischemic attacks with ST segment elevation show a peak in the morning hours, particularly in the first few hours after waking and commencing activity. Myocardial infarction shows an evident circadian rhythm as well, characterized by a higher frequency of onset during morning hours. It has been estimated that the incidence rate of AMI onset is 40% higher in the morning period than throughout the rest of the day, and nearly 28% of morning infarctions and 22% of sudden cardiac deaths (accounting for approximately 9% and 7% of all AMIs and sudden deaths, respectively) are attributable to the morning excess. Compared with all other times of the day, morning shows a relative risk of AMI of

1.4, rising to a threefold increase in the first 3 h after waking, when almost 25% of all AMIs occur. A series of studies has indicated that this circadian pattern in the incidence of AMI was similar in different subgroups of patients and was independent of gender, age, and clinical characteristics, for example, lower or higher ejection fraction, presence of one-, two-, or three-vessel disease, type of infarction (Q-wave or non-Q-wave), and site of infarction (anterior or inferior). Diabetes mellitus, however, represents a peculiar entity. Diabetic subjects, who are more at risk of AMI compared with nondiabetics, show attenuation of morning peak or, in some cases, the absence of a significant circadian variation of AMI onset. It is thus possible that diabetic subjects are exposed to a steady and high risk of myocardial infarction during the 24 h, maybe due to a marked diminution of parasympathetic activation during sleep.

Drugs may also suppress diurnal variation. Specifically, an absence or attenuation of the morning peak of AMI has been observed in patients taking β-blockers. Additionally, in those taking aspirin, the primary morning peak of infarction was attenuated: there was an additional 25% protective effect associated with aspirin specifically between 4 and 10 a.m., the hours of awakening from sleep and assuming the upright posture.

Stroke

Stroke is the end result of a heterogeneous group of vascular diseases that are manifested by ischemia or hemorrhage of one or more vessels of the brain. Worldwide, stroke is the second leading cause of death and the leading cause of disability and long-term care costs. Although the frequency of and mortality from stroke have declined in the United States and many other industrialized countries during the past 30 years, in the United States stroke continues to affect ~700 000 persons and to cause ~165 000 deaths per year, and a similar or even higher incidence of stroke is reported in other countries. A number of studies have indicated that the incidence of all subtypes of stroke (e.g., lacunar, thrombotic, embolic, and hemorrhagic) shows a significant circadian rhythm, characterized by a higher frequency during morning hours. A comprehensive meta-analysis of 31 separate studies in which the clock time of events was verifiable confirmed the prominent 24-h pattern of cerebrovascular events. Thus, for example, the incidence of transient ischemic attack (TIA) and hemorrhagic and ischemic stroke reaches a peak between 6 and 12 a.m. Approximately 55% of all ischemic strokes, 34% of all hemorrhagic strokes, and 50% of all TIAs occurred during this temporal window.

Rupture/Dissection of Aortic Aneurysm

Acute aortic dissection and rupture of aortic aneurysms are serious, life-threatening cardiovascular emergencies that carry high fatality rates. In fact, many patients with either an acute aortic dissection or rupture of an aortic aneurysm die before hospitalization, and data from the large population enrolled in the International Registry of Acute Aortic Dissection (IRAD) show a 24% mortality rate in patients reaching hospitals even in centers with advanced technology and considerable expertise. Also, several studies have found a circadian variation for aortic aneurysm, characterized by an increased risk of both aortic rupture as well as aortic dissection during early hours of morning. Analysis of the IRAD registry showed that this morning peak (around 8–9 a.m.) was independent of gender, type A or B dissection, age $<$ or $\geq$ 70 years, and presence or absence of hypertension.

Circadian Rhythm of Underlying Risk and Triggering Factors

Several variables indicative of cardiovascular and cerebrovascular status exhibit prominent circadian rhythms and may contribute to the circadian pattern of cardiovascular events (**Figure 1**).

Vascular Tone and Arterial Blood Pressure

Sympathetic activity is circadian rhythmic, reaching peak level in the morning when vascular receptors exhibit greatest sensitivity, and this can play a role in the sharp morning rise in arterial blood pressure (BP) and heart rate (HR). The morning rise in BP is significantly amplified by biological responses to events that occur upon awakening from nighttime sleep, that is, assumption of upright posture, commencement of physical activity, and exposure to emotional stress, all of which further elevate catecholamine secretion and sympathetic tone. The circadian variation in BP, characterized by a double peak in the early morning and in the early evening, plays an important role in the onset of cardiovascular and cerebrovascular events. Moreover, night BP levels are important as well. In normotension and in uncomplicated essential hypertension, in fact, systolic BP (SBP) and diastolic BP (DBP) normally decline during nocturnal sleep by 10–20% relative to the respective daytime mean levels. Some persons exhibit a so-called non-dipping pattern, that is, a less than 10% decline (or even rise) in SBP and/or DBP during nighttime sleep relative to their daytime levels. The cumulative effect over time of abnormally elevated nighttime BP load on target organs, for example, heart, brain, and kidney, may lead to deleterious effects.

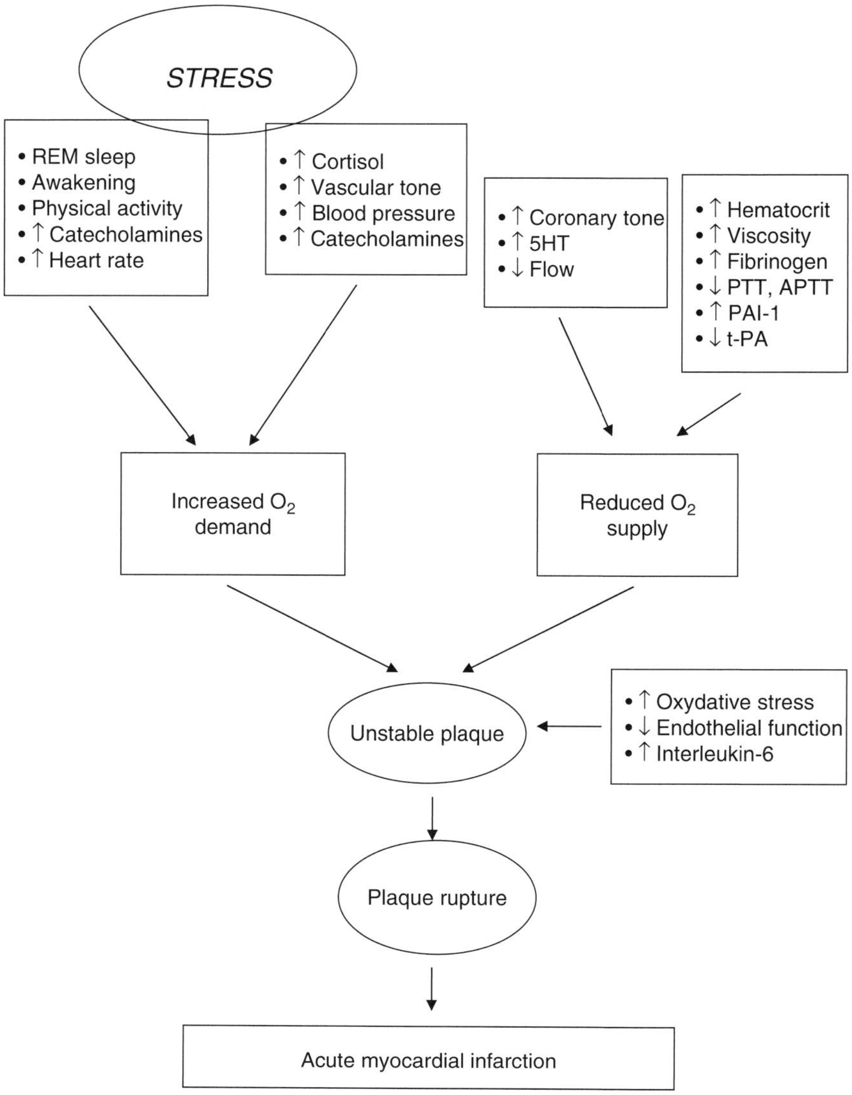

Figure 1 Schematic outline of the way in which several concurring risk factors might contribute to trigger the onset of acute myocardial infarction during morning hours. Abbreviations: REM, rapid eye movement; 5HT, 5-hydroxytryptamine; PTT, partial thromboplastin time; APTT, activated partial thromboplastin time; PAI-1, plasminogen activator inhibitor-1; t-PA, tissue plasminogen activator.

Blood Coagulation and Fibrinolysis

Circadian rhythms in blood coagulation and fibrinolysis are also key components of the multifactor pathogenesis of cardiovascular and cerebrovascular events and their 24-h patterns. The *in vitro* aggregation response of platelets to stimulants such as ADP and epinephrine is circadian rhythmic, and each of these rhythms peaks during the late night or morning hours and declines to the trough in the afternoon. Activation of platelet aggregation is brought about by the increased secretion of catecholamines, which is initiated by the activation of the sympathetic nervous system during nocturnal episodes of rapid eye movement (REM) sleep. Since REM episodes are more frequent during final hours of nighttime rest in normal sleepers, the rise in catecholamine concentration commences at that time, and increases further in the morning due to baroreflex with the change from supine to upright posture upon awakening and the commencement of physical activity and exposure to emotional stress. Moreover, circadian rhythms have been found in several factors of the coagulation cascade, on the intrinsic as well as the extrinsic and common pathways of blood coagulation. Circadian rhythms in factors II (thrombin), VII (tissue thromboplastin), VIII, and IX, with peak activity in the morning hours, were observed in clinically healthy human subjects.

As a result of these rhythms, the global screening tests of different steps in the coagulation cascade, such as prothrombin time (PT) and activated partial thromboplastin time (aPTT), show the lowest values (indicative of blood hypercoagulability) in the morning. The extent of the differences in PT, aPTT, and thrombin time (TT) was found to be about 10% of the respective means.

Activation of the coagulation cascade is followed in healthy subjects by an increase in fibrinolytic activity, which serves to limit the coagulation process and avoid vascular occlusion. Fibrinolysis also shows an evident circadian rhythmic variation. The circadian rhythm in fibrinolysis, although dependent on multiple influences, is to a large extent determined by the interaction between tissue plasminogen activator (t-PA) and its potent inhibitor, tissue plasminogen activator inhibitor-1 (PAI-1). Both t-PA antigen and PAI-1 antigen are circadian rhythmic, showing peak concentrations in the morning, but the circadian rhythm of t-PA activity is almost 12 h out of phase with the circadian rhythm in t-PA antigen concentration. Thus, PAI-1, the activity of which parallels its concentration, suppresses t-PA activity during the late night and early morning hours when thromboembolic events are most frequent. The circadian rhythm in PAI-1 is of large amplitude, showing excursions as great as 250%, thereby contributing in diurnally active subjects to the relative hypercoagulability of the blood in the morning and relative hypocoagulability of the blood in the evening.

Stress and Circadian Rhythms

At least two major physiological systems play a crucial role in the adaptation of the organism to environmental challenges: the circadian system and the stress response system, which are tightly coupled.

Activation of the hypothalamic-pituitary-adrenocortical (HPA) axis in response to stressful stimuli is a crucial mechanism that allows an organism to maintain homeostasis and adapt to environmental conditions. It is known that HPA has a circadian activity in basal activity, and the rhythmicity in secretory activity is controlled by the suprachiasmatic nucleus (SCN) of the hypothalamus. However, the SCN is not the only biological clock. In fact, cloning of the clock genes in the late 1990s revealed that clock genes are expressed and oscillate with a circadian rhythm in each organ or cell, suggesting that each of them has its own internal clock. Thus, this clock system has been denominated as a peripheral clock in comparison with the central clock in SCN. It seems that the SCN-based central clock is capable of synchronizing peripheral clock systems.

Stress-induced secretion of corticotropin-releasing factor (CRF) from the paraventricular nucleus (PVN) of the hypothalamus triggers the synthesis and release of ACTH and, ultimately, glucocorticoids. Thus, the hypothalamic PVN receives convergent information from both stress and the circadian clock, and it has been demonstrated that, at least in mice, the mammalian orthologs *Per1*, *Per2*, and *Per3* of the *Drosophila melanogaster* clock gene *Period* are expressed in different areas of the central nervous system (e.g., PVN) and peripheral tissue.

Stress is capable of exerting major effects upon the circulatory system of coronary patients, particularly in the morning. Stress acts on the cardiovascular system in multiple ways, and a direct link has been demonstrated in both laboratory and ambulatory studies between emotional stress and changes in HR, systolic and diastolic BP, left ventricular stroke work, cardiac output, blood viscosity, and coagulation. These and other stress-related changes can trigger angina in coronary syndrome patients and are perceived to act in a primary or secondary way in the triggering cerebrovascular events through the sudden increase in BP and blood coagulation. Acute coronary syndromes may also be triggered by emotional stress, and studies demonstrated that emotional stress preceded the onset of AMI in 11% of men and 16% of women. Anger is important as well, and it has been reported that there is a twofold increased relative risk of acute coronary syndromes in the 2 h after an emotional burst of anger. Mental stress has also been shown to inhibit flow-mediated brachial artery vasodilatation, a validated indicator of endothelial function, and the hemodynamic response to mental stimuli, consisting of the combination of a reduction in blood supply and an increase in cardiac demand, might explain the role of mental stress in the onset of myocardial ischemia. Indeed, the effect of stress on human cardiac, vascular, and hemostatic status appears to be circadian rhythmic, with the effects being greater in the morning. Experimental studies on rats showed the molecular mechanisms of stress-induced heart attacks, with a rapid activation of the p44/p42 mitogen-activated protein kinase, followed by transient upregulation of the immediate early genes of the smooth muscle cells of the coronary arteries, endothelial cells, and myocardium. It is interesting to observe that the 24-h pattern of acute cardiovascular and cerebrovascular events is tightly coupled in time, suggesting that they share numerous risk factors. An exaggerated cardiovascular response to behavioral challenges has been suggested as a potential factor that enhances the risk of hypertension and CHD. Thus, individuals who exhibit large increases in BP during acute psychological stress are at risk for atherosclerosis, probably secondary to endothelial damage by BP surge, via increased flow turbulence and subsequent release of inflammatory and pro-atherogenic cytokines.

Emotional stress can also play a role in the triggering of stroke. In patients with acute ischemic stroke, the finding that salivary cortisol levels are positively correlated with 24-h and nighttime BP suggests that stress may induce endocrine changes that result in BP increase. In asymptomatic older adults, stress-induced BP reactivity is enhanced in those diagnosed with silent cerebrovascular disease, independently of the resting BP levels, suggesting that mental stress at the start of the day can intensify the morning BP surge and contribute to the higher frequency of strokes at this time.

Circadian Rhythms and Possible Implications for Treatment of Cardiovascular Diseases

In conclusion, it seems that the temporal rhythmic organization of the vascular functions is such that the defense mechanisms against disease are incapable of providing the same degree of protection at all times of the day. A point of interest is the possible influence on chronobiologic rhythms and outcome of cardiovascular events. At present, only a limited amount of data is available on the prognostic implications of the concept of chronorisk. For example, the clock time of onset seems to affect the clinical course and outcome of patients with AMI. Moreover, the concept of chronorisk implies that the delivery of protective or preventive medications should be synchronized in time in proportion to need as determined by established rhythmic patterns in cardiovascular risk, during the 24 h and in a manner that will avert or minimize undesired side effects. A chronotherapeutic approach to cardiovascular diseases has been suggested. For example, a growing interest is given to morning BP surge as an important risk factor. It is known that some drugs have different effects when administered in the morning compared to in the evening. In fact, it should not be assumed that a long-acting, once-daily antihypertensive drug administered in the morning will have the same antihypertensive effect as when administered in the evening. Thus, the effects of time of drug administration on the pharmacodynamics of antihypertensive drugs are an important consideration for antihypertensive therapeutics. Improved control of the morning BP surge by means of a tailored antihypertensive therapy might provide maximal benefit during the particularly vulnerable time periods.

See Also the Following Articles

Circadian Clock Genes as Modulators of Sensitivity to Genotoxic Stress; Circadian Rhythms, Genetics of.

Further Reading

Andreotti, F., Davies, G. J., Hackett, D. R., et al. (1988). Major circadian fluctuations in fibrinolytic factors and possible relevance to time of onset of myocardial infarction, sudden cardiac death and stroke. *American Journal of Cardiology* **62**, 635–637.

Elliott, W. J. (1998). Circadian variation in the time of stroke onset: a meta-analysis. *Stroke* **29**, 992–996.

Haus, E., Cusulos, M., Sackett-Lundeen, L. and Swoyer, J. (1990). Circadian variations in blood coagulation parameters, alpha-antitrypsin antigen and platelet aggregation. *Chronobiology International* **7**, 203–216.

Lemmer, B. (2005). Chronopharmacology and controlled drug release. *Expert Opinion on Drug Delivery* **2**, 667–681.

Manfredini, R., Gallerani, M., Portaluppi, F. and Fersini, C. (1996). Relationships of the circadian rhythms of thrombotic, ischemic, hemorrhagic, and arrhythmic events to blood pressure rhythms. *Annals of the New York Academy of Science* **783**, 141–158.

Manfredini, R., Gallerani, M., Portaluppi, F., Salmi, R. and Fersini, C. (1997). Chronobiological patterns of onset of acute cerebrovascular diseases. *Thrombosis Research* **88**, 451–465.

Manfredini, R., Boari, B., Gallerani, M., et al. (2004). Chronobiology of rupture and dissection of aortic aneurysms. *Journal of Vascular Surgery* **40**, 382–388.

Manfredini, R., Boari, B., Smolensky, M. H., et al. (2005). Circadian variation in stroke onset: identical temporal pattern in ischemic and hemorrhagic events. *Chronobiology International* **22**, 417–453.

Manfredini, R., Boari, B., Smolensky, M. H., et al. (2005). Seasonal variation in onset of myocardial infarction – a 7-year single-center study in Italy. *Chronobiology International* **22**, 1121–1135.

Muller, J. E. (1999). Circadian variation and triggering of acute coronary events. *American Heart Journal* **137** (4 Pt 2), S1–S8.

Portaluppi, F., Manfredini, R. and Fersini, C. (1999). From a static to a dynamic concept of risk: the circadian epidemiology of cardiovascular events. *Chronobiology International* **16**, 33–49.

Stone, P. H. (2004). Triggering myocardial infarction. *New England Journal of Medicine* **351**, 1716–1718.

Heart Failure, Stress Effects

M Alevizaki
Evgenidion Hospital and Alexandra Hospital, Athens University School of Medicine, Athens, Greece
G P Chrousos
Evgenidion Hospital and Athens University School of Medicine, Athens, Greece

Glossary

Apoptosis	(From the Greek words *apo* = from and *ptosis* = falling); one of the main types of programmed cell death.
Atrial natriuretic peptide (ANP)	Released by atrial cardiomyocytes and has a direct diuretic, natriuretic and vasodilator effect.
Cardiomyocytes	Striated muscle cells of the heart, deriving from cardiac myoblasts; they participate in the contraction of the heart.
Catecholamines	Biogenic amines produced mainly from the adrenal medulla and the postganglionic neurons of the sympathetic nervous system; they participate in the stress system, influencing heart rate, blood pressure and various metabolic parameters.
Cytokines	Polypeptides produced in a variety of tissues; mediators of the inflammatory and immune responses.
Nitric oxide synthase (NOS)	Enzyme responsible for the synthesis of nitric oxide (NO).
Norepinephrine (noradrenaline)	A catecholamine, released both from noradrenergic neurons of the sympathetic nervous system and from the medulla of adrenal glands.
Pheochromocytoma	Tumor arising from cells of neural rest origin of the medulla of the adrenal gland.
Renin–angiotensin–aldosterone system	Participates in the regulation of the extracellular fluid volume and the long-term arterial pressure, as well as in the maintenance of Na and K blood concentrations.

Heart failure is the end result of declining pumping capacity of the heart; it follows some initial injury to the heart, which may be of either an acute or progressive nature. In recent years, neurohormonal mechanisms that may be involved in the progression of heart failure have been proposed. These represent compensatory physiological responses activated to assist the heart and to slow down the deterioration of its pumping function. The increased secretion of catecholamines; release of various peptides with vasodilatory effects, such as the atrial natriuretic peptides; and production of the gas hormone nitric oxide all contribute in the assistance of the heart. Several cells from within the heart, however, produce other hormones, such as endothelin, with vasoconstrictive effects, which, when present at increased levels or when administered in excess, are able to partially reproduce the syndrome of heart failure in experimental animal models. These effects are generally reversible.

Stress is classically linked to elevated adrenergic activity. In the failing heart the original increase in adrenergic activity is beneficial because it facilitates an increase in the heart rate and contractility. However, in the progress of heart failure, further increases in circulating norepinephrine occur, which may be detrimental to the myocardium. Elevated norepinephrine concentrations are positively correlated with the severity of heart failure, with the more elevated levels linked to a worse prognosis and higher mortality. Chronically elevated catecholamines may be cardiotoxic, and heart failure associated with pheochromocytoma is a well-recognized entity. Prolonged and excessive β-adrenergic receptor stimulation may result in intracellular calcium overload, which may promote cardiomyocyte apoptosis. Therefore, the effects of increased adrenergic stimulation are paradoxical and change as the disease progresses, starting as beneficial and ending as detrimental. Slowly, the failing heart may lose its ability to respond to catecholamines.

The use of antagonists of neurohormonal factors may reverse heart failure progression to some extent; thus, the use of both β-adrenergic blockade and of angiotensin-converting enzyme inhibitors partially reverse the progression of heart failure.

Stress is also associated with the production of pro-inflammatory cytokines. Recently, an important role of pro-inflammatory cytokines in the pathophysiology and progression of heart failure has been recognized. These cytokines may be produced under the influence of stress by cardiac myocytes independently of the activation of the immune system and have direct adverse effects on the cardiovascular system. Studies have specifically shown that tumor necrosis factor (TNF-)α, interleukin (IL)-2, and IL-6 exert immediate negative inotropic effects on the heart and, thus, aggravate heart failure. Increased circulating TNF-α levels are associated with more severe degrees of heart failure. It also appears that these molecules may have adverse effects on the remodeling of the cardiac cells and left ventricular structure through effects on apoptosis, as well as on the endothelium, by influencing the transcription of the NO synthase.

This knowledge has led to clinical trials studying the effects of TNF-α blockade on the progression of heart failure; these studies, however, have not shown encouraging results. Interestingly, the blockade of nuclear factor (NF-) κB activity, which is a ubiquitous transcription factor involved in the transcription of the pro-inflammatory cytokine genes, has also been associated with an improvement in heart failure. It has thus been suggested that NF-κB might be a promising target for future drug development for the treatment of heart failure. The current general view is that there is an interplay among catecholamines, the renin–angiotensin system, and pro-inflammatory cytokines that is involved in the pathophysiology of heart failure. Thus, many conventional therapeutic modalities may be acting through their effects on the pro-inflammatory cytokines. One example is that angiotensin type I receptor antagonists reduce the level of circulating inflammatory mediators in patients with heart failure.

Another interesting observation linking hormones that help the body adapt to stress with heart failure was recently published. It was shown that corticotropin releasing hormone receptor 2 (CRH-R2)- and urocortin 2-deficiencies were associated with heart failure in an animal model and that the reversal of this abnormality was associated with improvement in cardiovascular function.

Finally, it was recently suggested that certain cases of cardiovascular disease may be linked to posttraumatic stress disorder (PTSD). This is not surprising because these conditions are characterized by increased sympathetic activity and elevated concentrations of circulating cytokines such as IL-6. PTSD has, indeed, been associated with heart-rate abnormalities and increased incidence of coronary artery disease; thus, although direct links of PTSD with heart failure have not been shown, the association of this disorder with coronary artery disease points in that direction.

See Also the Following Articles

Primate Models, Cardiovascular Disease.

Further Reading

Bale, T. L., Hoshijima, M., Gu, Y., et al. (2004). The cardiovascular physiologic actions of urocortin II: acute effects in murine heart failure. *Proceedings of the National Academy of Sciences USA* **101**, 2697–3702.

Bozkurt, B., Kribbs, S., Clubb, F. J., Jr., et al. (1998). Pathophysiologically relevant concentrations of TNFα promote progressive left ventricular dysfunction and remodeling in rats. *Circulation* **97**, 1382–1391.

Cotter, G., Milo-Cotter, O., Rubinstein, D., et al. (2006). Posttraumatic stress disorder: a missed link between psychiatric and cardiovascular morbidity? *CNS Spectrums* **11**, 129–136.

Deswal, A., Petersen, N. J., Feldman, A. M., et al. (2001). Cytokines and cytokine receptors in advanced heart failure: an analysis of the cytokine database from the versarinone trial (VEST). *Circulation* **103**, 2055–2059.

Gurlek, A., Kilickap, M., Dincer, I., et al. (2001). Effect of losartan on circulating TNF alpha levels and left ventricular systolic performance in patients with heart failure. *Journal of Cardiovascular Risk* **8**, 279–282.

Kapadia, S., Dibbs, Z., Kurrelmeyer, K., et al. (1998). The role of cytokines in the failing human heart. *Cardiology Clinics* **16**, 645–656.

Levine, B., Kalman, J., Mayer, L., et al. (1990). Elevated circulating levels of TNF in severe chronic heart failure. *New England Journal of Medicine* **223**, 236–241.

Mann, D. L. (2004). Activation of inflammatory mediators in heart failure. In: Mann, U. (ed.) *Heart failure: a companion to Brownwald's Heart Disease*, pp. 159–180. Philadelphia: Saunders.

Port, J. D., Linseman, J. V. and Bristow, M. R. (2004). Adrenergic receptor signaling in chronic heart failure. In: Mann, U. (ed.) *Heart failure: a companion to Brownwald's Heart Disease*, pp. 145–158. Philadelphia: Saunders.

Brain Natriuretic Peptide (BNP)

P Pervanidou and G P Chrousos
University of Athens, Aghia Sophia Children's Hospital, Athens, Greece

Glossary

Amygdala	Brain region involved in the central regulation of the stress response.
Body mass index (BMI)	The weight in kilograms divided by the square of height in meters.
Cardiac myocyte	A cell of myocardial origin.
Dual-energy X-ray absorptiometry (DEXA)	Imaging study assessing body composition and bone mineral density. A useful method for measuring body fat.
Hypothalamic nuclei	Neuron collections in the brain regulating a variety of hormonal secretions and functions.
Prohormone	The initial molecule (peptide in this case) from which the active hormone is derived.
Renin-angiotensin-aldosterone system	Endocrine system that regulates water homeostasis and blood pressure.

Brain natriuretic peptide (BNP) is a hormone of cardiac origin, secreted from the heart ventricles in response to pressure overload. It was isolated originally from porcine brain extracts, but it was soon discovered that heart was its main source. Natriuretic peptides (atrial natriuretic peptide, ANP; BNP; and C-type natriuretic peptide, CNP), deriving from three different genes, comprise a peptide family of high structural homology, as they share a 17-amino acid internal ring. Cardiac ANP and BNP act on the same peripheral receptors, causing diuresis, vasodilatation, and antagonism of the actions of renin and aldosterone. The source of CNP is kidney endothelium and its main action is the regulation of the vascular tone.

BNP is derived from a prohormone, an intracellular 108 amino acid precursor, which is cleaved into two fragments, a 76-amino-acid N-terminal fragment (NT-proBNP) and BNP. Both BNP and the NT-proBNP, have emerged as strong biological markers of cardiac dysfunction: levels of circulating BNP positively correlate with the severity of heart failure (HF) and BNP can improve cardiac disease diagnosis and management. Recombinant human BNP ("Natrecor", Scios Inc) has proved useful in the treatment of some forms of cardiac failure, especially in advance of cardiac surgery. BNP and NT-proBNP have the same diagnostic and prognostic value. Gender, body mass index (BMI) and age (through cardiac and renal function) may influence natriuretic peptide concentrations, but the underlying mechanisms for this are not well known.

Cardiac myocyte stretch, hormones (catecholamines, angiotensin II, and endothelin) and myocardial hypoxia are the main factors causing the observed changes in the plasma concentrations of these peptides. Stretching of cardiac myocytes is followed by the activation of proBNP gene and *de novo* myocyte peptide synthesis and secretion and there is a positive correlation between the amount of stretch and the resulting increase in BNP and NT-proBNP concentrations. In the normal state, the atrium is the main cardiac production site, but as HF develops, there is a profound activation of ventricular BNP synthesis.

Brain Natriuretic Peptide and Stress Physiology

Besides their peripheral circulation and actions in water and blood pressure regulation, natriuretic peptides and their receptors (NPR-A, NPR-B, and NPR-C), are distributed throughout the central nervous system (CNS) of different species. In the CNS, they represent an important neuromodulatory system, which directly influences the secretion of stress hormones and behavioral manifestations such as arousal and anxiety.

In the CNS of the rat, BNP has a distribution that is different from that of ANP. Furthermore, high-affinity binding sites for BNP and ANP have been found in various brain regions of rats, such as area postrema and certain hypothalamic nuclei. In the CNS of humans and rodents NPR-A is located in the cortex and hippocampus, NPR-B in the amygdala and several brainstem sites, while NPR-C is found in many areas such as the neocortex, limbic cortex, hippocampus and amygdala.

In humans and rodents, ANP has an inhibitory effect on the hypothalamic-pituitary-adrenal (HPA) axis at the pituitary and hypothalamic levels, while CNP induces the opposite effect by stimulating the release of cortisol.

In rats, BNP administration into the cerebral ventricles did not modify the basal plasma corticosterone secretion (which is used as a measure of HPA activity). When rats were subjected to three different stressors (stress, electric shock, and restraint), BNP inhibited stress-induced elevation in plasma corticosterone in a dose-dependent manner. While there is evidence for the inhibitory role of BNP in the HPA axis, the effect of CNP is greater and more stress specific than that of BNP, perhaps due to the different distributions of NPRs in the CNS.

Brain Natriuretic Peptide and the Exercise-Stressed Myocardium in Healthy Individuals

BNP and NT-proBNP are elevated in healthy subjects after prolonged and strenuous exercise. Although these peptides have been established as strong biological markers of heart disease, the underlying mechanisms that lead to exercise-induced elevation of BNP and NT-proBNP in healthy individuals are not well known.

Myocardial stress, expressed as increased ventricular pressure or cardiac output during exercise, may lead to increased synthesis of BNP and NT-proBNP concentrations in order to lower cardiac afterload by peripheral vasodilatation and diuresis. This relation between exercise and BNP levels seems to be time-dependent.

BNP is a well-known antagonist of the renin-angiotensin-aldosterone system. BNP is elevated in situations of increased central blood volume (fluid overload), such as edematous situations, HF, and exhaustive exercise. Ventricular wall stress is greatly increased in strenuous long-term exercise, as plasma volume increases by up to 22%. BNP is released into the circulation as a counterregulatory homeostatic response, and induces diuresis and vasodilatation and reduces pulmonary and systemic vascular resistance, resulting in reduction of left ventricular (LV) end-diastolic pressure. BNP increases immediately at the onset of, stays elevated during, and decreases with the termination of exercise. BNP is a good marker of volume regulatory response of the hemodynamically stressed myocardium.

Age and cardiac function influence BNP secretion. Thus, older and less trained individuals have higher levels of NT-proBNP. It should be noted that this elevation represents cardiac fatigue, which is different from that resulting from irreversible subclinical cardiac injury.

Brain Natriuretic Peptide and the Failing Heart

The value of cardiac peptides has been recognized by their inclusion in the recent European Guidelines for the diagnosis of chronic HF.

HF is characterized by progressive fatigue and dyspnea and leads to reduced tolerance to efforts. Increased wall stress and neurohormonal (adrenergic, renin-angiotensin-aldosterone, endothelin, and vasopressin) activation stimulate BNP and NT-proBNP secretion and these peptides negatively correlate to LV systolic function.

The majority of studies has proved the relationship between cardiac peptides and cardiac disease: BNP levels are higher in patients with LV hypertrophy and in patients with LV diastolic dysfunction and the specificity of BNP in detecting these situations has been well established. Additionally, BNP correlates with systolic blood pressure (SBP) and pulse pressure (PP) and PP increase has been recognized as an independent risk factor of cardiovascular disease.

BNP and NT-proBNP have become an important addition to the diagnostic tools of heart diseases. They were the first biomarkers to prove their value in screening for LV dysfunction, assessing the prognosis while monitoring patients, decision making during therapy, and predicting adverse cardiac events and readmissions in HF patients.

Brain Natriuretic Peptide and Myocardial Ischemia

BNP concentrations are elevated in individuals with stress-induced myocardial ischemia and the rise in BNP levels are related to the degree of ischemia induced. Additionally, baseline BNP levels before stress testing are higher in those who subsequently develop stress-induced ischemia.

The combination of exercise electrocardiography (ECG) with baseline or peak BNP concentrations increases diagnostic accuracy compared with ECG only. The exact mechanism underlying the association between myocardial ischemia and the release of BNP are not well known. It is possible that the ischemia-induced decrease in LV function and/or ischemia-induced neurohormonal activation may increase ventricular wall stress and BNP secretion.

NT-Pro BNP in Relation to Metabolic Risk Factors

BNP and NT-proBNP levels correlate negatively with BNP and increased expression of clearence receptors by adipose tissue was initially hypothesized to be responsible for the rapid degradation of BNP in obese individuals. In a recent study using dual-energy X-ray absorptiometry (DEXA) instead of BMI as a measure of obesity, lean body mass and not fat mass was responsible for the association between higher BMI and lower BNP and NT-proBNP levels. A substance produced by lean mass that suppresses BNP synthesis or release was then hypothesized to be the underlying cause of this association.

Furthermore, an inverse association between serum NT-proBNP and other risk factors, such as fasting serum insulin, cholesterol and triglycerides and metabolic syndrome itself, has been found independently of age and gender in the adult population. Indeed, NT-proBNP concentrations correlate with PP and the response curve is shifted to the right in adults with the metabolic syndrome.

Brain Natriuretic Peptide and NT-ProBNP in Pediatrics

Reference values of NT-proBNP serum concentrations in umbilical cord and in healthy neonates and children show a significant increase in the first days of life followed by a rapid decrease during the first year and a gradual decrease throughout infancy. This change may reflect an adaptive mechanism to extra-uterine physiology.

Similarly to adults, NT-proBNP and BNP concentrations are elevated in children with LV dysfunction. Children with congenital or acquired heart diseases, such as dilated cardiomyopathy and myocarditis have elevated NT-proBNP levels, depending on the type and the severity of the disease. Furthermore, NT-proBNP levels are higher in children with HF and are negatively correlated with ejection fraction and positively correlated with New York Heart Association clinical score. There is also a correlation between BNP levels and left-to-right shunt, ventricular volume, and pulmonary-to-systemic pressure ratio in high-pressure lesions.

In conclusion, despite its name brain natriuretic peptide seems to be the least of the three natriuretic peptides involved in CNS regulation of stress. In contrast, it is an established biological marker, extremely useful in the diagnosis and management of acute cardiac incidents as well as the evaluation of exercise-induced myocardial stress in healthy individuals and cardiac patients.

Further Reading

Das, S. R., Drazner, M. H., Dries, D. L., et al. (2005). Impact of body mass and body composition on circulating levels of natriuretic peptides: results from the Dallas Heart Study. *Circulation* **112**, 2163–2168.

Grandi, A. M., Laurita, E., Selva, E., et al. (2004). Natriuretic peptides as markers of preclinical cardiac disease in obesity. *European Journal of Clinical Investigation* **34**, 342–348.

Hall, C. (2005). NT-ProBNP: the mechanism behind the marker. *Journal of Cardiac Failure* **11**, 81–83.

Horwich, T. B., Fonarow, G. C., Hamilton, M. A., et al. (2001). The relationship between obesity and mortality in patients with heart failure. *Journal of the American College of Cardiology* **38**, 789–795.

Jaszberenyi, M., Bujdoso, E. and Telegdy, G. (2000). Effects of brain natriuretic peptide on pituitary-adrenal activation in rats. *Life Sciences* **66**, 1655–1661.

Lavie, C. J., Osman, A. F., Milani, R. V., et al. (2003). Body composition and prognosis in chronic systolic heart failure: the obesity paradox. *American Journal of Cardiology* **91**, 891–894.

Leers, M. P., Schepers, R. and Baumgarten, R. (2006). Effects of a long distance run on cardiac markers in healthy athletes. *Clinical Chemistry and Laboratory Medicine* **44**, 999–1003.

Maeda, K., Tsutamota, T., Wada, A., et al. (1998). Plasma brain natriuretic peptide as a biochemical marker of high left ventricular end-diastolic pressure in patients with symptomatic left ventricular dysfunction. *American Heart Journal* **135**, 825–832.

McCord, J., Mundy, B. J., Hudson, M. P., et al. (2004). Relationship between obesity and B-type natriuretic peptide levels. *Archives of Internal Medicine* **164**, 2247–2252.

Mehra, M. R., Uber, P. A., Park, M. H., et al. (2004). Obesity and suppressed B-type natriuretic peptide levels in heart failure. *Journal of the American College of Cardiology* **43**, 1590–1595.

Mir, T. S., Flato, M., Falkenberg, J., et al. (2006). Plasma concentrations of N-terminal brain natriuretic peptide in healthy children, adolescents and young adults: effect of age and gender. *Pediatric Cardiology* **27**, 73–77.

Mosterd, A., Cost, B., Hoes, A. W., et al. (2001). The prognosis of heart failure in the general population: the Rotterdam Study. *European Heart Journal* **22**, 1318–1327.

Nir, A. and Nasser, N. (2005). Clinical value of NT-ProBNP and BNP in pediatric cardiology. *Journal of Cardiac Failure* **11**, S76–S80.

Nir, A., Bar-Oz, B., Perles, Z., et al. (2004). N-terminal pro-B-type natriuretic peptide: reference plasma levels from birth to adolescence. Elevated levels at birth and in infants and children with heart diseases. *Acta Paediatrica* **93**, 603–607.

Olsen, M. H., Hansen, T. W., Christensen, M. K., et al. (2005). N-terminal pro brain natriuretic peptide is inversely related to metabolic cardiovascular risk factors and the metabolic syndrome. *Hypertension* **46**, 660–666.

Passino, C., Poletti, R., Bramanti, F., et al. (2006). Neuro-hormonal activation predicts ventilatory response to exercise and functional capacity in patients with heart failure. *European Journal of Heart Failure* **8**, 46–53.

Passino, C., Severino, S., Poletti, R., et al. (2006). Aerobic training decreases b-type natriuretic peptide expression and adrenergic activation in patients with heart failure. *Journal of the American College of Cardiology* **7**, 1835–1839.

Sabatine, M. S., Morrow, D. A., de Lemos, J. A., et al. (2004). Acute changes in circulating natriuretic peptide levels in relation to myocardial ischemia. *Journal of the American College of Cardiology* **44**, 1988–1995.

Sarzani, R., Dessi-Fulgheri, P., Paci, V. M., et al. (1996). Expression of natriuretic peptide receptors in human adipose and other tissues. *Journal of Endocrinological Investigation* **19**, 581–585.

Scharhag, J., Herrmann, M., Urhausen, A., et al. (2005). Independent elevations of N-terminal pro-brain natriuretic peptide and cardiac troponins in endurance athletes after prolonged strenuous exercise. *American Heart Journal* **150**, 1128–1134.

Schwachtgen, L., Hermann, M., Georg, T., et al. (2005). Reference values of NT-proBNP serum concentrations in the umbilical cord blood and in healthy neonates and children. *Journal of Cardiology* **94**, 399–404.
Sengenes, C., Berlan, M., De Glisezinski, I., et al. (2000). Natriuretic peptides: a new lipolytic pathway in human adipocytes. *FASEB Journal* **14**, 1345–1351.
Silver, M. A., Maisel, A., Yancy, C. W., et al. (2004). BNP Consensus Panel 2004: a clinical approach for the diagnostic, prognostic, screening, treatment monitoring, and therapeutic roles of natriuretic peptides in cardiovascular diseases. *Congestive Heart Failure* **10**, 1–30.
Staub, M. D., Nusbaumer, C., Zellweger, M. J., et al. (2006). Use of B-type natriuretic peptide in the detection of myocardial ischemia. *American Heart Journal* **151**, 1223–1230.
Wang, T. J., Larson, M. G., Levy, D., et al. (2004). Impact of obesity on plasma natriuretic peptide levels. *Circulation* **109**, 594–600.
Wiedemann, K., Jahn, H. and Kellner, M. (2000). Effects of natriuretic peptides upon hypothalamic-pituitary-adrenocortical system activity and anxiety behavior. *Experimental and Clinical Endocrinology & Diabetes* **108**, 5–13.
Yoshibavashi, M., Kamiva, T., Saito, Y., et al. (1995). Plasma brain natriuretic peptide concentrations in healthy children from birth to adolescence: marked and rapid increase after birth. *European Journal of Endocrinology* **133**, 207–209.

Vasoactive Peptides

W K Samson and M M White
Saint Louis University School of Medicine, St. Louis, MO, USA

This is a revised version of the article by Z T Resch and W K Samson, Encyclopedia of Stress, First edition, volume 3, pp 643–649, © 2000, Elsevier Inc.

Glossary

Calcitonin gene-related peptide (CGRP)	A peptide homologous in structure and function to AM.
Chronotropism	The rate of cardiac muscle contraction.
Diuresis	The excretion of water in urine.
Inotropism	The strength of cardiac muscle contraction.
Intermedin	The recently discovered member of the adrenomedullin-calcitonin gene-related peptide (AM-CGRP) family of peptides.
Natriuresis	The excretion of sodium in urine.
Natriuretic peptides	A family of three homologous mammalian peptides, encoded by three distinct genes, that are produced in heart and the vasculature and that were initially discovered on the basis of their renal actions to stimulate sodium excretion.
Preproadrenomedullin-derived peptides	One mammalian gene encodes a prohormone that is posttranslationally modified to yield two vasoactive peptides: adrenomedullin (AM) and proadrenomedullin N-terminal 20 peptide (PAMP).
Receptor activity modifying proteins (RAMPs)	Receptor proteins that provide selectivity for the actions of adrenomedullin and calcitonin gene-related peptide.
Salt appetite	The behavior of selective ingestion of osmotically active solute.

Regardless of the operant definition, stress elicits significant, physiologically relevant changes in not only emotional behaviors, but also endocrine and cardiovascular function. Poised appropriately between the perception of a stressor and the integrative response to that insult are vasoactive peptides, factors that exert potent physiological effects in brain, pituitary gland, and the periphery. In many ways, these hormones serve to integrate the responses of multiple tissue systems in a manner parallel and complementary to the autonomic nervous system. Indeed, vasoactive peptides act in brain to modulate sympathetic efferent activity, fluid and electrolyte balance, and neuroendocrine responses to stress. In the pituitary gland, they significantly contribute to the regulation of corticotroph function. In the periphery, these hormones determine vascular tone, cardiac pumping efficiency, adrenal hormone production and release, and, importantly, renal handling of fluid and electrolytes. Two families of vasoactive hormones, known to be released in response to numerous stressors, provide excellent examples of the integrative biology of the stress response. The natriuretic peptides and members of the adrenomedullin-calcitonin gene-related peptide (AM-CGRP) family of peptides are produced in brain and pituitary gland, as well as in the peripheral vasculature, heart, and kidney. They act both locally as autocrine factors and after release into the circulation as classic hormones to in some cases initiate and in others modify stress responses at the cellular and whole organ level.

Vasoactive Peptides

The simplest definition of a vasoactive peptide is a small protein that exerts either prorelaxant or procontractile effects in intact blood vessels. These effects may be endothelium dependent, requiring the recruitment of additional peptides, prostaglandins, or diffusable gases from the endothelial cell, or they may be endothelium independent, reflecting a direct effect on the vascular smooth muscle itself. Vascular tone is determined primarily by neurogenic mechanisms, largely mandated by the level of sympathetic activation. Circulating and locally produced factors also play important roles in the selective activation of distinct vascular beds and in the overall maintenance of vascular pressure, the single most important determinant of adequate perfusion of the vital organs in stress. Local factors not only directly affect vascular reactivity, but also, via presynaptic mechanisms, modify sympathetic tone. These factors also contribute to the maintenance of adequate perfusion pressures by altering cardiac performance and adjusting vascular volume.

Natriuretic Peptides

Originally discovered in extracts of cardiac atrium, the prototype of natriuretic peptides was originally named atrial natriuretic peptide (ANP) due to its isolation site, biological action, and protein structure. A second member of the family, originally thought to be produced in brain, but now known to be of almost exclusively myocyte (indeed, ventricular myocytes) origin, is B-type natriuretic peptide (BNP). Both ANP and BNP are released in response to volume overload, sensed by the myocardium as excess stretch. They share major actions to stimulate sodium and water excretion in the urine (**Figure 1**). ANP appears more relevant under physiological conditions, and BNP seems to be recruited in more chronic conditions of volume/pressure overload. Production of at least ANP also occurs in brain and pituitary gland, and actions there related to stress are numerous and diverse. The third member of this family of peptides, all products of unique genes, is C-type natriuretic peptide (CNP). Produced predominantly in brain and vasculature, very little, if any, CNP is produced in the myocardium. Although CNP is a poor natriuretic and diuretic agent, it is a profound vasodilator and can exert apparently paradoxical effects on sympathetic tone via central nervous system (CNS) actions. Much is known of the molecular biology, pharmacology, physiology, and pathophysiology of the natriuretic peptides.

Preproadrenomedullin-Derived Peptides and Their Homologs

Surprisingly, vasodilatory activities were isolated from extracts of a pheochromocytoma, and these peptides were later discovered to be posttranslational products of the same messenger RNA. Produced not only in adrenal medulla, but even more widely in the blood vessels, brain, and pituitary gland, these two vasodilatory factors exert complementary actions via unique signaling mechanisms (**Figure 2**). Adrenomedullin (AM), a 52-amino-acid peptide from the C-terminal portion of the proadrenomedullin precursor, exerts its vasorelaxant effects by stimulating nitric oxide synthase activity in endothelial cells of the vasculature. Proadrenomedullin N-terminal 20 peptide (PAMP), however, is a potent vasorelaxant due to its ability to exert presynaptic inhibition on sympathetic fibers innervating the vessel and to negatively modulate cholinergic activation of the chromaffin cells of the adrenal medulla and therefore reduce the level of epinephrine released in stress. Not all the actions of AM and PAMP are shared. For example, AM is a potent natriuretic and diuretic agent but does not affect catecholamine release significantly. A role for PAMP in sodium homeostasis also exists, however, as even in the absence of renotropic actions PAMP can stimulate sodium excretion due to its profound inhibitory effects on aldosterone secretion.

CGRP is a 37-amino-acid homolog of AM, and both are members of a larger family of peptides that includes calcitonin, amylin, and the recently described 47-amino-acid peptide intermedin (IMD; also named adrenomedullin-2). There is some evidence that these peptides may share an ancestral gene, and in addition to their structural similarities, they exert many shared biological activities (and perhaps receptors). CGRP, like AM, is a potent vasodilator when administered intravenously and has been demonstrated to inhibit aldosterone secretion *in vitro*. When given into the CNS, like AM, it activates sympathetic tone, thus raising blood pressure. IMD exerts these same peripheral and central actions related to cardiovascular function and, like AM, exerts direct effects in the heart to increase contractility (inotropism) and beating frequency (chronotropism). Renal effects of IMD may parallel those of AM as well. It is not surprising that these homologous peptides exert similar actions (although unique effects may exist for each) since they share a common family of biological receptors. Those receptors are actually a complex of at least two proteins, the calcitonin receptor-like receptor (CRLR) and one of three possible receptor activity modifying proteins (RAMP1, RAMP2, or RAMP3). The relative combination of the respective

RAMPs with the CRLR defines the specificity of the binding of each ligand. The CRLR–RAMP1 complex binds CGRP preferentially, while CRLRs in association with either RAMP2 or RAMP3 are the AM receptors. IMD binds promiscuously with all three CRLR–RAMP complexes, and thus it is not surprising that the hypotensive effects of IMD are at least partially blocked by relatively selective CGRP and/or AM antagonists.

Vasoactive Peptides and the Pituitary Response to Stress

Conventionally, the pituitary response to stress is considered to be the release of the hormone adrenocorticotropin (ACTH). The release of ACTH is controlled mainly by corticotropin-releasing hormone (CRH) levels in the hypophysial portal plasma; however, stimulation by vasopressin and oxytocin, as well as epinephrine, has been demonstrated. Thus, the effect of CRH can be modulated physiologically by factors also present in the portal circulation or by factors produced locally in the pituitary gland itself.

Natriuretic Peptides

ANP is produced in the hypothalamus, where it exerts inhibitory effects on the releases of vasopressin and CRH. These effects may have physiological relevance, as stress-induced ACTH secretion is accentuated in rats pretreated centrally with anti-ANP antiserum, and glucocorticoid negative feedback is reduced when endogenous, brain-derived ANP is neutralized with the same antibodies. The effects are not limited only to ANP, as central administration of CNP also inhibits the stress response.

In addition to production in neurons projecting to stress centers in the hypothalamus (the paraventricular nucleus in particular), ANP and CNP are produced in cells of the anterior pituitary gland, where again CNP appears to be the most abundant gene product. Indeed, both the natriuretic peptide A receptor (NPR-A), which binds ANP preferentially, and the natriuretic peptide B receptor (NPR-B), which prefers CNP, are present. Even the third natriuretic peptide receptor (NPR-C), the clearance receptor, is found in the gland, although to a much lesser degree. Importantly, the NPR-A and NPR-B receptors have been localized to the corticotrophs, lactotrophs, and gonadotrophs. Both the NPR-A and the NPR-B are particulate guanylyl cyclase-linked receptors, activation of which results in elevated cellular levels of cGMP. ANP, but not CNP, potently stimulates the accumulation of cGMP levels in dispersed anterior pituitary cells. Activation of guanylyl cyclase is known in many cells to result in the stimulation of cGMP-dependent phoshodiesterases, which limit the activity of preformed cAMP. Because CRH stimulates ACTH secretion by activating adenylyl cyclase with the cAMP formed then stimulating protein kinase A activity, it is was not surprising that ANP, but not CNP, could inhibit CRH-induced ACTH secretion in cultured pituitary cells.

What pool of ANP could act in this fashion *in vivo*? ANP not only is produced in the pituitary gland, but also is delivered in the portal blood. Thus, the peptide could be acting to circumscribe ACTH secretion via a local paracrine mechanism or via a more classical neuroendocrine fashion. Are these pharmacological effects of ANP in cell culture physiologically relevant? While one group failed to observe any significant effects of physiological doses of ANP on CRH-stimulated ACTH secretion in humans, two other human trials did reveal a significant inhibitory effect of intravenously administered ANP on ACTH release.

Preproadrenomedullin-Derived Peptides

The adrenomedullin gene is transcribed in the hypothalamus, and AM-immunoreactive positive neurons projecting to neuroendocrine centers related to stress have been identified. Indeed, direct application of AM caused depolarization of parvocellular neurons of the paraventricular nucleus (PVN) in brain slices. Although the chemical phenotype of those AM-responsive parvocellular PVN neurons was not identified, they are composed of at least two classes of neurons, both playing a role in the hypothalamic control of the stress response. One subset projects to median eminence and delivers releasing factors, including CRH, to the hypophysial portal vessels for transport to the anterior pituitary gland. The other subset, also including some CRH-producing neurons, projects to autonomic centers in brain stem and thus may coordinate the cardiovascular stress response with that of the hypothalamic-pituitary-adrenocortical (HPA) axis. In fact, AM administration has been reported to increase Fos expression in CRH-positive hypothalamic neurons and to activate the HPA axis. Convincing evidence for a direct action of AM on CRH-producing neurons that project to median eminence comes from studies in which the ability of centrally administered AM to stimulate ACTH release was abrogated by pretreatment with a neutralizing anti-CRH antibody. The central action of CGRP to stimulate the HPA axis similarly was blocked by pretreatment with an anti-CRH antibody, and recently IMD was demonstrated to activate the HPA axis by stimulating CRH release into the median eminence.

While AM immunoreactivity is not abundant in the external layer of the median eminence, and thus a neuroendocrine role for AM or PAMP in the regulation of ACTH secretion cannot be predicted, AM gene products are widely distributed in the anterior lobe of the pituitary gland and binding for AM has been demonstrated. On the basis of the ability of AM and PAMP to inhibit angiotensin II and potassium-stimulated aldosterone secretion from zona glomerulosa cells *in vitro*, it was predicted that the peptides might also inhibit ACTH release from corticotrophs in culture. Basal and CRH-stimulated ACTH secretion *in vitro* is inhibited significantly by doses of AM, which approximate those present in the gland *in vivo*. The effects are dose and time dependent and are not related to the well-known ability of the peptide to activate adenylyl cyclase in peripheral tissues. In fact, the mechanism of the inhibitory effect of AM on ACTH remains unknown, as the peptide did not stimulate adenylyl or guanylyl cyclase activity in these cell cultures and similarly did not alter the levels of nitric oxide present during the incubations. A direct effect on the membrane polarization state could be hypothesized; however, a potassium channel blocker, glybenclamide, did not alter the action of AM to inhibit ACTH secretion under basal conditions.

The second posttranslational product of prepro-adrenomedullin (PAMP) also inhibits basal ACTH in a time- and dose-dependent fashion. It too exerts this effect at physiological concentrations and, like AM, does not directly alter adenylyl or guanylyl cyclase activity *in vitro*. Unlike AM, PAMP does not affect CRH-stimulated ACTH secretion. The ability of PAMP to reduce basal, but not stimulated, hormone secretion suggested an effect on the membrane polarization state. Because PAMP has been reported to act in other cell lines via an ATP-sensitive potassium channel, the pituitary effect was hypothesized to be due to opening of such a channel and hyperpolarization of the corticotroph membrane. Indeed, the ATP-sensitive potassium channel blocker glybenclamide completely blocked the inhibitory action of PAMP on ACTH secretion.

It remains to be determined whether these *in vitro* findings reflect physiological relevance in the *in vivo* setting. However, evidence for an *in vivo* effect of at least AM on ACTH secretion comes from studies in conscious sheep where the intravenous, but not intracerebroventricular, administration of AM lowered plasma levels of ACTH. It will be important to determine how the endogenous production of AM and PAMP in the pituitary gland is regulated. In the periphery, inflammatory stimuli such as interleukins and tumor necrosis factor-α are potent stimulators of AM gene transcription and peptide release. Thus, proinflammatory signals may also regulate pituitary production of the peptides as well, and proinflammatory cytokines are known effectors of ACTH secretion.

It is in the pituitary gland that the biological actions of the members of the AM-CGRP-IMD family of peptides diverge. Unlike the inhibitory effects of AM on ACTH release, CGRP has been reported to stimulate hormone secretion via a cAMP-protein kinase A-dependent pathway. On the other hand, IMD has been reported to lack significant effects on basal or CRH-stimulated ACTH release. Furthermore, IMD inhibits releasing factor-stimulated growth hormone (GH) secretion *in vitro*, which is quite the opposite of the reported actions of AM and CGRP to stimulate GH secretion. The effect of IMD on somatotroph function suggests the existence of an IMD receptor unique from the CRLR-RAMP receptor complexes. This *in vitro* action of IMD may be physiologically relevant since in rodents stress results in inhibition of GH release and this peptide acts both centrally and at the level of the pituitary gland to decrease GH release. The actual source of the IMD that may be exerting these actions is unknown; however, the gastrointestinal tract is a prime candidate, since the highest levels of the peptide have been detected in stomach, as well as in kidney and brain.

All three members of the AM-CGRP-IMD family of peptides exert behavioral effects that may reflect a response to stress. The peptides inhibit food appetite and water drinking when administered into the brain, and at least in the case of AM, the effects on water drinking and salt appetite have been shown to be physiologically relevant. It appears that the actions of AM are more related to fluid and electrolyte homeostasis and those of CGRP to energy intake. Intermedin exerts anorexigenic effects similar to those of CGRP; however, the actions of IMD on thirst more closely parallel those of AM.

Integration of Central and Peripheral Responses to Stress

The integrative response to stress requires a coordination of multiple organ systems. Because of their diverse sites and mechanisms of action, vasoactive peptides are excellent candidates for physiological regulators of these integrative responses. Natriuretic peptides provide the best example of factors that exert complementary actions in multiple tissue sites. Their ability to unload excess vascular volume via direct natriuretic and diuretic actions in kidney is matched by inhibitory actions on releases of the volume conservatory hormones vasopressin, renin, and aldosterone. Behavioral actions within brain also complement these renal effects. ANP not only stimu-

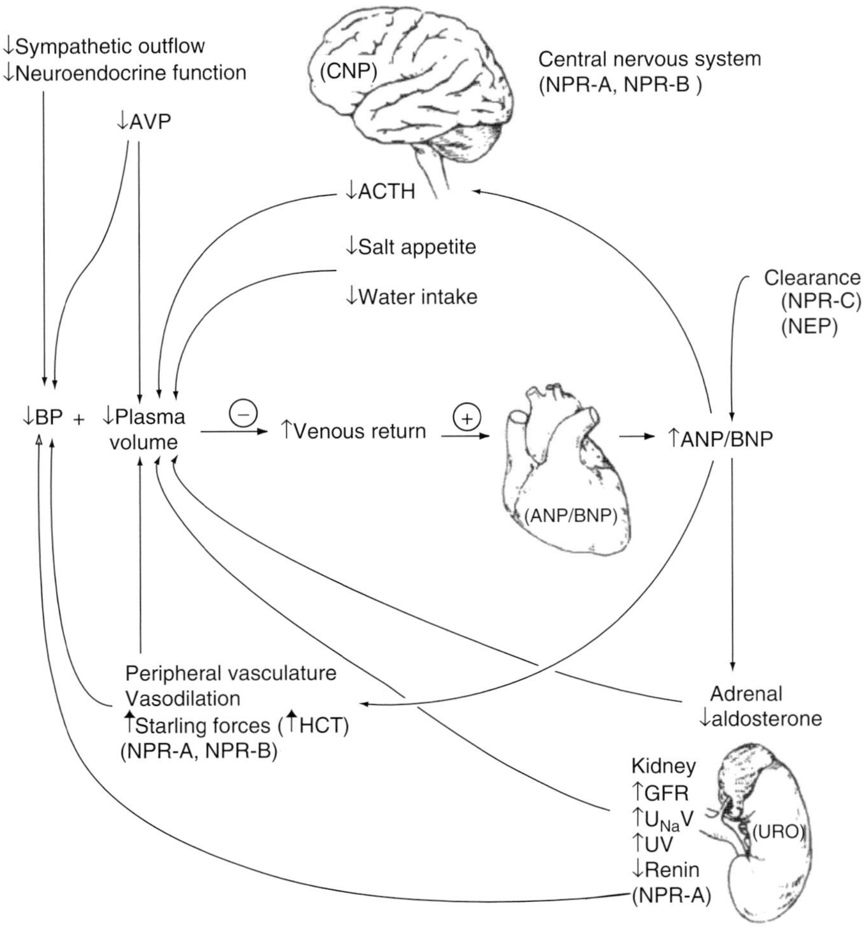

Figure 1 Pharmacological actions of the atrial natriuretic peptide (ANP) and B-type natriuretic peptide (BNP). AVP, vasopressin release; ACTH, adrenocorticotropin release; VR, venous return; BP, blood pressure, HCT, hematocrit; NPR-A, guanylyl cyclase A receptor; NPR-B, guanylyl cyclase B receptor; GFR, glomerular filtration; $U_{Na}V$, urinary sodium excretion; UV, urine volume. Also indicated is the production of C-type natriuretic peptide (CNP) in brain and urodilatin (URO), an N-terminally extended form of ANP in kidney. ANP and BNP are removed from the circulation by binding to the clearance receptor (NPR-C) and via degradation by neutral endopeptidase (NEP). Modified from the original and reprinted from Samson (1995), with permission of Humana Press.

lates fluid and electrolyte excretion, but also, in what is now known to be a physiologically relevant manner, inhibits water drinking and salt intake, thus allowing time for the renal mechanisms to compensate before the addition of new fluid volume to the already taxed vascular tree. In states of volume depletion, these mechanisms are inhibited, thus permitting sodium and water retention and additional intakes to replenish lost volume. The blood pressure-lowering effects of the natriuretic peptides are not remarkable, but they can be demonstrated at pharmacological doses *in vivo*, and data from ANP and NPR-A knockout mice suggest an important role for the peptide in blood pressure regulation.

In times of excess secretion, such as during cardiac overload states, endogenous natriuretic peptides may unload the heart by a vasodilatory mechanism that is complemented by increases in vascular permeability. One group has demonstrated a sympatholytic effect of ANP in the brain stem, which would also lower vascular pressure. Thus, the actions of natriuretic peptides seem well coordinated to facilitate fluid and electrolyte balance and the response to volume stress. Whether the peptides play any role in psychogenic stress remains to be seen. However, the ability of both ANP and CNP to inhibit the hypothalamic drive for gonadotropin secretion suggests that some stress-induced infertility may involve the hypothalamic actions of these peptides. Evidence for the physiological relevance of this effect has been provided in studies employing selective cell targeting of NPR-B receptive neurons in hypothalamus.

Adrenomedullin gene products provide a very different example of the potential importance of vasoactive peptides in the body's response to stress. Because of its profound effects on brain, pituitary, vascular, adrenal, and renal mechanisms related to fluid and electrolyte homeostasis, overexposure of the body

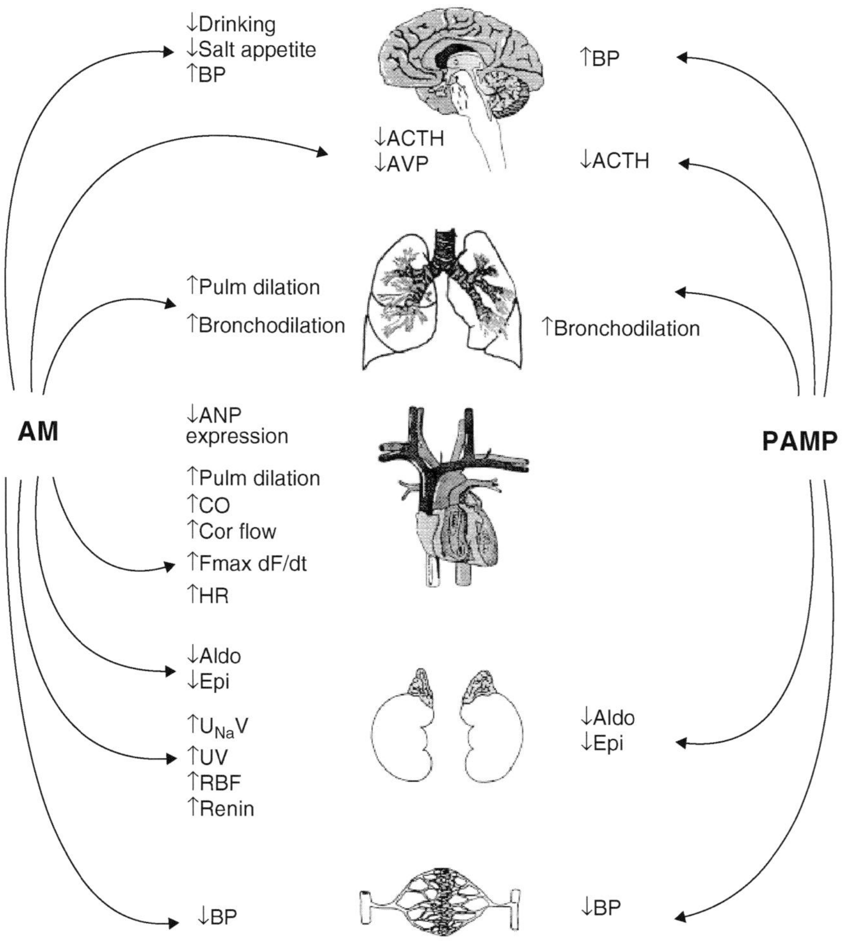

Figure 2 Pharmacological actions of adrenomedullin (AM) and proadrenomedullin N-terminal 20 peptide (PAMP). BP, blood pressure; ACTH, adrenocorticotropin secretion; AVP, vasopressin release; Pulm dilation, pulmonary dilation; ANP, atrial natriuretic peptide; CO, cardiac output, Cor Flow, coronary blood flow; Fmax dF/dt; maximum force of contraction; HR, heart rate; Aldo, aldosterone secretion, Epi, epinephrine release; $U_{Na}V$, urinary sodium excretion; UV, urine volume, RBF, renal blood flow, ET, endothelin production. Reproduced from Samson (1999), with permission from the *Annual Review of Physiology*, Volume 61, © 1999, by Annual Reviews.

to high levels of AM could have disastrous consequences. AM potently inhibits water drinking and sodium appetite, ACTH secretion, aldosterone release, vascular tone, and renal fluid reabsorption. Thus, when released in large amounts, as in sepsis, potentially fatal hypotension and the resultant underperfusion of vital organ systems could result. Fortunately, the actions of AM, and to some degree PAMP, include compensatory effects that protect against cardiac collapse. Indeed, in clinical studies the levels of AM attained in plasma during sepsis predict survival, probably due to the cardioprotective effects of those high levels of peptide. Furthermore, transgenic overexpression of the AM gene in mice results in enhanced survival outcomes during experimentally induced septic shock.

How is this accomplished? In brain, AM and PAMP are sympathostimulatory. This may seem a paradox in light of the profound hypotensive effects of the peptide in the periphery. However, their action in brain may compensate for not only the vasorelaxant effects of the peptides, but also the ability of AM to dampen baroreflexes and thus the perception of volume depletion. This central activation of sympathetic efferents may assure adequate perfusion of vital tissues. Similarly, direct effects of AM on cardiac contractility have been documented. While decreasing venous return by peripheral vasodilation, AM also exerts positive inotropic and chronotropic effects in heart, which can maintain ejection fraction and stroke volume, again protecting against cardiac collapse. At least one additional protective effect of AM has been demonstrated. Even in the face of profound hypotension, renal perfusion pressure is maintained due to the dilatory effects of the peptide on both afferent and efferent renal arterioles. Thus, AM and PAMP exert protective effects that assure perfusion of the vital organ systems during hypotension, and these mechanisms must be considered important for the response of an individual to stress.

A Question of Physiological Relevance

With the exceptions of CNS actions of both ANP and AM to inhibit thirst and salt appetite, of AM to stimulate vasopressin release, of CNP to inhibit GnRH release, and of ANP to contribute to blood pressure regulation during sodium excess, much of the current knowledge of the physiological relevance of the vasoactive peptides remains based solely on pharmacological evidences. Only recently have combinations of methodologies been attempted to identify and confirm physiological relevance. For example, the salt appetite-suppressive effect of AM was suggested to have physiological relevance by studies employing selective antibodies that neutralized endogenous brain-derived AM. These initial findings were then confirmed by the antisense oligonucleotide approach in studies in which excessive salt appetite occurred when the endogenous production of AM was interrupted.

Why is it important to establish the physiological relevance of any peptide's pharmacological effects? The obvious answer is the potential use of an exogenous peptide in a therapeutic setting. Less obvious is the importance of elucidating the potential involvement of a given peptide in the genesis of a pathological state. Because of their pleuripotent biological activities, vasoactive peptides hold promise for both therapeutic use and the diagnosis of evolving pathology. In particular, plasma BNP levels are now accepted as diagnostic of the progression of cardiac overload in congestive heart failure in humans, and ANP is a clinical tool employed to unload excessive vascular volume in this disease. The ACTH-inhibiting effect of ANP during such treatment would certainly provide an extra therapeutic advantage. This again points to the significance of multiple sites and mechanisms of actions of vasoactive peptides during challenges to normal homeostasis, which by any definition mean stress.

Further Reading

John, S. W. M., Krege, J. H., Oliver, P., et al. (1995). Genetically decreased levels of atrial natriuretic peptide and salt-sensitive hypertension. *Science* **267**, 679–681.

Samson, W. K. (1995). Cardiovascular hormones. In: Conn, P. M. & Melmed, S. (eds.) *Endocrinology: bsic a& clinical principles*, pp. 361–376. Totowa, NJ: Humana Press.

Samson, W. K. and Taylor, M. M. (2005). Cardiovascular hormones. In: Conn, P. M. & Melmed, S. (eds.) *Endocrinology: bsic a& clinical principles* (2nd edn., pp. 321–335). Totowa, NJ: Humana Press.

Taylor, M. M. and Samson, W. K. (2002). Adrenomedullin and the integrative physiology of fluid and electrolyte balance. *Microscopy Research and Techniques* **57**, 105–109.

Taylor, M. M., Bagley, S. L. and Samson, W. K. (2004). A possible mechanism for the action of adrenomedullin in brain to stimulate stress hormone secretion. *Endocrinology* **145**, 4890–4896.

Taylor, M. M., Bagley, S. L. and Samson, W. K. (2005). Intermedin /adrenomedullin-2 acts within central nervous system to elevate blood pressure and inhibit food and water intake. *American Journal of Physiology* **288**, R919–R927.

Taylor, M. M., Bagley, S. L. and Samson, W. K. (2005). Stress hormone secretion is altered by central administration of intermedin/adrenomedullin-2. *Brain Research* **1045**, 199–205.

Taylor, M. M., Bagley, S. L. and Samson, W. K. (2006). Intermedin /adrenomedullin-2 inhibits growth hormone release from cultured, primary anterior pituitary cells. *Endocrinology* **147**, 859–864.

Heart Rate

J R Jennings
University of Pittsburgh School of Medicine, Pittsburgh, PA, USA

This is a revised version of the article by J R Jennings, Encyclopedia of Stress, First edition, volume 2, pp 333–337, © 2000, Elsevier Inc.

Glossary

Baseline A condition to which responses are compared. This can be a resting condition with no stimulation or a condition that has all the elements of the task or stressor condition except for the critical task or stress element.

Electrocardiogram A changing voltage over time collected from the chest of a person using surface electrodes. The electrocardiogram's changing voltages show atrial contraction (p wave) followed by ventricular contraction (qrs wave) and then ventricular recovery (t wave). Because of its relatively large amplitude, the qrs wave is typically used as the marker for the computation of heart rate or interbeat interval, although the heartbeat is initiated by the atrial contraction (p wave).

Heart rate The number of contractions (beats) of the heart expressed per unit time, typically the number of heartbeats per minute.

Interbeat interval The time, typically expressed in milliseconds, between contractions of the heart.

Phasic response A transient change in the rate of the heart (or other index) induced by an environmental or physiological stimulus. Phasic responses are typically compared to a baseline and last for a second or more but less than a minute.

Stressor/task Any event that poses a challenge to an individual. Conditions that threaten to induce harm or pain or frustrate achievement of positive rewards are termed stressors. Conditions that pose a requirement to mentally or physically manipulate objects are typically termed tasks; these may or may not also be stressors.

Tonic response A sustained change in the rate of the heart (or other index) induced by an environmental or physiological condition. Tonic responses are typically compared to a baseline and last for a minute or more.

Forms of Heart Rate Measurement

Clinical

The pulse, obtained by palpitation over an artery, is the basic means of obtaining heart rate in the medical clinic. The contractions of the heart are counted based on the mechanical sensation in the thumb or finger of the observer induced by the expansion of the artery due to cardiac contraction. The experience of the pulse during stress probably arises from a similar mechanism: mechanical sensations from the viscera induced by cardiac contraction – contractions that increase in force during stress. Collection of heart rate via palpitation requires the presence of another person and physical contact. The person must accurately sense the heartbeats and time the interval over which the counts are made. Use of palpated heart rate in studies of stress has been reduced due to the possibility of error in judgments of timing and beat occurrence as well as the likelihood that the presence of a person may alter any laboratory-induced stress. Heart rate derived by this technique is typically expressed as beats per minute.

Physiological

Heart rate in physiological studies is typically derived from measurements taken from the electrocardiogram. The number of qrs waves per unit time are counted or the time between these waves is measured. Time between waves (interbeat interval) can be translated to the rate of the heart for any pair of beats. For example, if the time between heartbeats is 1000 ms (1 s), then the corresponding heart rate would be 60 beats/min; that is, 60 of these intervals of 1000 ms would equal 60 000 ms, 60 s, or 1 min. Such detailed measurements permit the tracking of how the heart is reacting beat by beat (or second by second) to environmental and physiological stimuli.

Heart rate arises from the integration of an individual's intrinsic rate with the influences of the sympathetic and parasympathetic branch of the nervous system. The heartbeat is initiated in the sinus node of the heart, which is a patch of spontaneously active neural tissue located in the cardiac atrium. The sinus node discharge rate depends on a basic intrinsic or constitutional rate for that person as modulated by the speeding influences of sympathetic nervous system firing and the slowing influences of parasympathetic system (vagus nerve) firing upon the sinus node. Thus, a second-by-second recording of heart rate provides a second-by-second record of a balance between sympathetic and parasympathetic nervous system influences on the heart.

Psychological

The sensitivity of heart rate to nervous system activation provides the justification for its use as an index of psychological stress. Stress is typically assumed to activate the sympathetic nervous system and deactivate the parasympathetic nervous system. Direct influences of the sympathetic nervous system on the sinus node as well as indirect influences via circulating catecholamines (derived primarily from the endocrine gland, the adrenal medulla) will activate β-adrenergic receptors, resulting in a speeding of the heart rate and an increase in cardiac contractility. Both nervous and endocrine reactions are transient responses to stressors. Some individuals report being in stressful circumstances lasting a year or more; such circumstances are unlikely to be directly reflected in heightened heart rate or even adrenomedullary reactions because these are reactions that return to baseline values after a brief period. Specific stressors arising from stressful circumstances can induce tonic reactions or phasic reactions of heart rate. Reactions to stressor lasting minutes to hours can be detected by examining tonic reactions in which the average heart rate over periods of minutes can be demonstrated to be elevated relative to a baseline period. Acute reactions to specific stressors may induce transient nervous system responses lasting seconds rather than minutes. Such phasic responses are typically assessed by comparing heart rate (or interbeat interval) for the seconds after the stressor to that of the seconds just before the stressor. The rapidity with which heart rate returns to baseline can also be informative. Increased vagal activation or decreased sympathetic activation will return heart rate to baseline values. Psychological factors, such as rumination over the stressful incident, may prolong heart rate speeding in some individuals. Concurrently, physiological factors may play a role in the recovery of heart rate, e.g., some individuals may have rapid vagal activation after a stressor with consequently brief heart rate reactions to stress. In short, the measurement of heart rate as an index of stress must be gauged to the type of stress, most particularly its temporal duration.

Heart Rate Assessment in Behavioral Medicine

Cardiovascular Reactivity

Because of its influence on the cardiovascular system, stress may influence the course of cardiovascular disease. A general hypothesis, the reactivity hypothesis, states that the cardiovascular reactivity resulting from repeated stressful events might contribute to the development of hypertension, myocardial infarction, and stroke. Presumably certain individuals are predisposed to show consistent and large cardiovascular reactions to stress, or are placed in an environment in which stressors are frequent and repetitive, or both. This hypothesis has been widely investigated using both laboratory challenges to assess reactivity and the ambulatory monitoring of heart rate and blood pressure as individuals perform their usual activities. The consistency within an individual over time of heart rate responses to laboratory stress has been established. Heart rate also changes in response to daily events in ambulatory recordings.

The number and size of heart rate responses do not seem, however, to predict cardiovascular disease onset and course; blood pressure increases in response to stressors have proven more predictive. The extensive parasympathetic influence on heart rate may explain this difference in the predictive utility of heart rate and blood pressure.

Heart Rate Variability

Derived measures of heart rate related to nervous system function have been found to correlate positively with cardiovascular health. Parasympathetic influences on heart rate are exerted via the vagus nerve, which innervates the heart (along with innervation by the cardiac sympathetic nerves). The vagus is more important than the sympathetic nerves for most transient changes in heart rate. Vagal firing influencing the heart waxes and wanes with respiration; this results in heart rate increasing during inspiration and decreasing during expiration. The rhythmic changes in heart rate over time, heart rate variability, can then be used to measure vagal influence on the heart. Heart rate has been found to show rhythmic changes with lower frequencies than respiration as well. For example, a frequency of 0.1 Hz has been related in part to sympathetic activity related to blood pressure, and heart rate shows a 24-h rhythm related to the sleep–wake cycle. Variability at the respiratory rate has been shown to be due almost completely to vagal/parasympathetic activity. Variability at other frequencies is not as well defined. Relatively greater variability has in general, however, been associated with cardiovascular health. A related measure positively associated with cardiovascular health is baroreceptor sensitivity. The baroreceptors are sense organs in major arteries that sense pressure change and transmit this to the brain, which then alters sympathetic and parasympathetic control to return blood pressure to normal. Pressure increases induce a vagal activation reducing heart rate. Greater heart rate change per unit of heart rate change (baroreceptor sensitivity) is correlated with better cardiovascular health. The associations of cardiac variability and baroreceptor sensitivity with cardiovascular health have led to the hypothesis that cardiac variability, most specifically parasympathetically induced variability, may act to buffer the influence of stress on the cardiovascular system.

Heart Rate Assessment in Psychological Science

Motivation/Affect

A psychological analysis of stress typically suggests that the threat or stressor induces an affective reaction as well as influences a person's motivational state. Subsequently, coping with the stressor may require other psychological processes. Behavioral medicine investigations have not typically attempted to separate the different processes influenced by stress, but the psychological analysis raises the question of whether heart rate reactions are controlled by one or more of the different psychological processes. The inference of a psychological process that is not directly observable is difficult, and this difficulty is compounded when the processes are as complex and conceptually overlapping as categories of affect and motivation. Studies do show that heart rate increases with the induction of most emotions, with the exception of disgust. Similarly, cues for reward or punishment can induce heart rate increases, perhaps with stronger increases related to cues for reward. Interpretation is further complicated by the possibility that coping with the affect or acting upon the motivational cue may elicit other processes controlling heart rate. For example, the induction of affect with an imaged scenario that contains an action element appears to induce greater heart rate change than induction with a more passive scenario.

Attention/Cognition

Coping refers to a set of action and mental processes that permit the person to redefine the threat and/or develop a means of neutralizing the threat. Thus, a multitude of cognitions and actions may be elicited as coping. If heart rate responds to processes such as attention and memory processes, then the involvement of these processes in coping, or even in the initial evaluation of the stressor, may be the source of phasic heart rate changes after a stressor. Muscle activation is a strong metabolic stimulus that induces rapid increases in heart rate. Similarly, change in breathing patterns, e.g., breath holding, have rapid, large effects on heart rate. These changes can readily be demonstrated in the absence of a stressor, while it is difficult to ensure that reactions to a stressor do not include muscle tension changes or changes in breathing pattern. Of greater psychological interest is attentive waiting, which induces clear phasic changes in heart rate. Heart rate decreases during the anticipation of any significant task or task element. Conceptually, heart rate seems to decrease whenever an action must be chosen at a specific point in time and potentially competing actions must be inhibited. The heart slows reliably prior to a signal to respond, even when that signal is accompanied by an electrical shock. This slowing of the heart rate does not appear to be due to respiratory changes or the inhibition of the peripheral musculature. The relevance of this observation to behavioral medicine studies of reactivity is clear. Many studies have used as their stressor/challenge computer games with periods of anticipatory attention.

Interpretive Issues

Heart rate can serve as an index of stress, but its utility and validity can be increased by a few simple precautions. First, stress and stress reactions should be conceptualized. Should heart rate in response to an increase in muscle tension be considered a stress reaction or a muscle artifact? Second, the stressor and overall conditions of eliciting the stress reaction should be controlled or assessed so it is possible to separate heart rate changes due to motor activity, respiration, transient attention, and affect/motivation. If a tonic response is of greatest interest, than scoring of the heart rate should occur after transient changes related to attention, breath holding, and muscle tensing. Fortunately, many of these phasic changes disappear after the initial few seconds of a task or stimulus presentation. Care must be taken in interpretation to recognize all the possible sources – other than those defined as stress – of the observed change in heart rate.

Summary

Heart rate increases rapidly during stress. The response may be initiated by motivational threat, affect, or the thoughts and actions induced by the stressor. Separation of the cause of the heart rate change is difficult in both the laboratory and real life. The degree of heart rate increase in response to stress or psychological challenge has been less predictive of medically significant cardiovascular disease than degree of change of blood pressure. The degree of variability of heart rate over time has, however, been associated with relatively better cardiovascular health.

Acknowledgment

The author acknowledges the assistance in writing this article from the support of NIH grant HL57529.

See Also the Following Articles

Blood Pressure; Sympathetic Nervous System.

Further Reading

Bernston, G. G. and Cacioppo, J. T. (2000). Homestasic to allodynamic regulation. In: Cacioppo, J. T., Tassinary, L. G. & Bernston, G. G. (eds.) *Handbook of psychophysiology* (2nd edn., pp. 459–490). Cambridge, UK: Cambridge University Press.

Dekker, J. M., Crow, R. S., Folsom, A. R., et al. (2000). Low heart rate variability in a 2-minute rhythm strip predicts risk of coronary heart disease and mortality from several causes: the ARIC Study. Atherosclerosis risk in communities. *Circulation* **102**, 1239–1244.

Huikuri, H. V., Jokinen, V., Syvanne, M., et al. (1999). Heart rate variability and progression of coronary atherosclerosis. *Arteriosclerosis, Thrombosis, and Vascular Biology* **19**(8), 1979–1985.

Jennings, J. R., Berg, W. K., Hutcheson, J. S., et al. (1981). Publication guidelines for the heart rate studies in man. *Psychophysiology* **19**, 226–231.

Jennings, J. R., van der Molen, M. W., Somsen, R. J., et al. (2002). Vagal function in health and disease: studies in Pittsburgh. *Physiology and Behavior* 77(4–5), 693–698.

Jennings, J. R., Kamarck, T. W., Everson-Rose, S. A., et al. (2004). Exaggerated blood pressure responses during mental stress are prospectively related to enhanced carotid atherosclerosis in middle-aged Finnish men. *Circulation* **110**(15), 2198–2203.

Kamarck, T. W., Jennings, J. R., Debski, T. T., et al. (1992). Reliable measures of behaviorally-evoked cardiovascular reactivity from a PC-based test battery: results from student and community samples. *Psychophysiology* **29**, 17–28.

Krantz, D. S. and Manuck, S. B. (1984). Acute psychophysiologic reactivity and risk of cardiovascular disease: a review and methodologic critique. *Psychological Bulletin* **96**, 435–464.

Lovallo, W. R. (2005). *Stress and health: biological and psychological interactions* (2nd edn.). Thousand Oaks, CA: Sage.

Noble, D. (1979). *The initiation of the heart beat.* Oxford, UK: Clarendon Press.

Task Force. (1996). Heart rate variability: standards of measurement, physiological interpretation, and clinical use. *Circulation* **93**, 1043–1065.

Kidney Function

W J Welch
Georgetown University, Washington, D.C., USA

Glossary

Renal sympathetic nerve activity	Net activity (measured in Hz) of renal nerve bundles supplying the kidney.
Renal vascular resistance	Vascular resistance of blood flow through the kidney, calculated as systemic mean arterial blood pressure factored by renal blood flow.
Sodium retention	Excess reabsorption of Na^+ from various segments of the nephron, resulting in increased extracellular volume.

Introduction

The kidney's primary function is to maintain homeostasis by the efficient elimination of excess fluid and solute. This key function is regulated by both extrarenal and intrarenal mechanisms that control the kidney's ability to maintain proper fluid and electrolyte balance.

The sympathetic nervous system (SNS) is an integral part of the homeostatic control system that maintains normal kidney function, with an extensive network of nerves identified in most renal tissues. The SNS modulates short-term regulation of renal function, and under normal conditions renal sympathetic nerve activity is low. During acute stress, however, elevated renal sympathetic activity depresses renal function. Chronic stress studies have been less conclusive and are difficult to design due to additional pathologies induced by stress, such as hypertension and cardiovascular complications. Major renal effects of mental stress include increased renal vasoconstriction, causing greater renal vascular resistance (RVR), and increased Na^+ transport, causing greater Na^+ retention. Both of these effects may contribute to the development of hypertension, and some investigators propose that this may be the primary mechanism of human essential hypertension. Therefore, most studies on the renal effects of stress have focused on its relationship to hypertension. Though the effects of stress are more pronounced in hypertensive humans and animals, stress increases renal vasoconstriction and Na^+ retention in normal subjects and animals, as well.

Renal Vascular Resistance (RVR)

The systemic blood pressure determines the renal perfusion pressure (RPP) and is a major determinant of RVR. The kidney has a unique ability to autoregulate its own blood flow that is efficient over a wide range of RPPs. Renal blood flow (RBF) changes very little over a large range of RPPs, therefore maintaining a stable RVR. This is due to the exquisite control of vascular tone in the primary renal resistance vessels, the preglomerular afferent arterioles and the postglomerular efferent arterioles. However, many hormonal and neural disturbances can alter autoregulation, often targeting these arterioles, leading to inappropriate increases in RVR. Increased sympathetic activity increases arteriolar resistance and RVR. Increased RVR exacerbates hypertension via its contribution to overall increased total peripheral resistance (since RBF is 20–25% of cardiac output) and its ability to promote Na^+ reabsorption. Stress can induce both neural and hormonal changes that affect RVR.

Renal Sympathetic Nerve Activity (RSNA) and RVR

Multiple studies using several types of acute stress in rats have shown that RBF is reduced and blood pressure (BP) and RVR over the period of stress are elevated. Renal sympathetic nerve activity (RSNA) when measured is increased and is now associated with the stress-induced changes in RVR. Renal sympathetic nerves act primarily by release of norepinephrine (NE), and nerve endings extend to most renal structures, including arterioles and tubules. In studies designed to test the effects of RSNA alone, higher RSNA frequencies within the range observed during stress increased RVR. The mechanism of RSNA stimulation on vascular tone is linked to increased release of NE and higher circulating epinephrine, acting on α- and β-adrenergic receptors, modulated by Ang II.

Experiments that stimulated RSNA show that there are at least three renal neuroeffector targets: renin-containing juxtaglomerular cells, the tubule, and the arterial vascular resistance. The sequence of RSNA input shows that renin is released at lower levels of RNSA, tubular reabsorption is increased at slightly higher intensities, and renal vasoconstriction occurs at even higher intensities. Each system appears to be regulated differently over a range of RSNA. Nonetheless, it appears that only moderate stress is sufficient to increase RSNA to levels that can alter major renal effectors. The role of RSNA on the renal contribution to hypertension is less clear. In studies in which periodic or prolonged periods of stress increased RSNA, there are only short-term effects on BP.

Many of the RSNA pacing studies have been limited to anesthetized rats, which may have altered basal RSNA. However, recent radiotelemetry techniques developed to measure RSNA in conscious rabbits exposed to stress have confirmed the role of renal nerves on increased RVR and have been used to explore the mechanisms. In response to air jet or white noise stress, RSNA was increased by 55 and 40%, respectively, within 1–2 min, and returned to normal by 9 min in conscious rabbits. Following treatment with rilmenidine, an imidazoline I (1) receptor agonist that reduces sympathetic-induced vascular tone, basal RSNA was reduced. However, the early response to air jet stress was reduced by 35%, whereas rilmenidine had no effect on white noise stress. Therefore, stress stimulates RSNA, but different stressor pathways may involve different central processing.

Increased RSNA impairs renal autoregulation, but the effects appear to be greater in hypertensive animals, suggesting a critical interaction with BP and RPP. However, stress also increases RSNA and BP in normotensive animals. WKY rats exposed to two different strategies of territorial stress (TS) developed higher BP over 5 months compared to control, unstressed rats. There was no evidence that changes in renal function contributed to the hypertension. Indeed, renal function in spontaneously hypertensive rats (SHR) in which higher BP correlates to RSNA is not different from normotensive WKY. However, in this study TS rats had higher levels of serum corticosterone and catecholamines early in the study, but the values were similar to unstressed rats after 10–12 weeks. This suggested that early exposure to stress might have long-term effects. To test this idea, young normotensive rats were exposed to acute injection of the α-1 adrenoreceptor agonist phenylephrine, which transiently increased BP and decreased glomerular filtration rate (GFR). After recovery, the animals were normotensive, but developed hypertension with reduced GFR when exposed to a high-salt (HS) diet, 8–10 weeks later. Together, these studies suggest that stress-induced surges in catecholamines, rather than constant stress, may enhance the susceptibility to other environmental stimuli, such as HS intake, and lead to hypertension and renal injury.

Based on the results from rat denervation studies, chronic increases in RSNA impact renal function. Under normal conditions, RSNA is low and renal denervation does not lead to changes in RBF or RVR. However, when RSNA is high, such as in the SHR or in heart failure rats, renal denervation increases RBF and decreases RVR. This occurs despite the similar RBF measured in intact SHR and WKY rats. Denervation does not alter RBF in WKY. This shows that chronic stress/increased RSNA tends to suppress RBF and increase RVR in SHR. However, it is not clear whether this effect contributes to the development of hypertension in SHR.

The role of stress on RVR has also been studied in human models, where stress-induced renal vasoconstriction also increases RSNA. RSNA is determined by measuring plasma or renal outflow of NE. In healthy volunteers, a short period of mental stress was accompanied by increased renal release of NE and epinephrine (Epi) and renin release, which led to a 48% increase in RVR. Renal arteries also appear to be more sensitive than other visceral vessels to stress in humans. Renal artery (RA) and small mesenteric artery (SMA) resistance and blood velocity were measured by simultaneous pulse and echo Doppler ultrasound flowmetry in 16 young female volunteers for 3 min before and 3 min during a mental stress test. RA vascular resistance was increased and RA blood velocity was decreased during the first minute of stress. SMA resistance was modestly increased, but velocity was unaffected by stress. This suggests that renal blood flow is exquisitely sensitive to mental stress and the accompanying increase in RSNA.

Hormonal Modulators

In addition to direct actions of renal nerves and activation of α-adrenergic receptors, multiple vasoactive hormones may contribute to stress-induced RVR. Endothelin is a peptide hormone that acts on receptors in endothelial cells and on vascular smooth muscle cells, generating vasoconstriction. In a series of human trials in elderly and young women, acute mental stress (30 min) increased BP, heart rate (HR), plasma NE, effective renal plasma flow, and RVR, but its effect on RVR was more prolonged in the elderly group. Urinary excretion of endothelin-1 was elevated in both groups, whereas excretion of vasodilating prostaglandins and nitric oxide (NO) was high only during the mental stress period in elderly subjects but was sustained at a higher excretion levels in young subjects. The balance between these opposing vasoactive hormones may therefore determine the level of stress-induced RVR. These studies provide good evidence that the balance between renal vasoconstrictors and vasodilators is invoked in the kidney's ability to autoregulate blood flow during mental stress. However, studies that evaluate the direct effects of endothelin infusion do not support a major role for endothelin as a potent vasoconstrictor during stress.

Several studies have shown that renin is released into the renal circulation during various forms of stress. However, it is not clear whether the levels of renin and locally produced Ang II are sufficient to contribute to the increased vasoconstriction that accompanies increased sympathetic activity. One report suggests that Ang II modulates the effects of catecholamine activation of adrenergic receptors, but the interaction has not been carefully investigated.

The role of NO was examined in adult borderline hypertensive rats (offspring of SHR and Wistar rats) during 5 weeks of crowding stress. Compared to unstressed controls, BP, HR, and nitric oxide synthase (NOS) activity in the aorta were higher. However, NOS activity in the heart, adrenal gland, and kidney was not affected. Superoxide (O_2^-), which scavenges NO, may contribute to RSNA. The higher RSNA activity in SHR compared to WKY was normalized by tempol, a powerful antioxidant, which reduced BP and RSNA to a greater extent in SHR than in WKY. However, the effect of reactive oxygen species on other influences on renal function could not be ruled out in this study.

The renal levels of neuropeptide Y (NPY) and calcitonin gene-related peptide (CGRP) were measured following a period of mental stress (word conflict test) or after low-dose adrenalin infusion in 12 healthy volunteers. Mental stress caused a threefold increase in NE renal overflow but had no effect on NPY or CGRP, whereas Epi infusion increased levels of all neurotransmitters.

The pro-inflammatory transcription factor nuclear factor-κB (NF-κB) has been linked to psychosocial stress as a possible mediator of organ damage, specifically in the kidney. NF-κB activation in renal tissue was greater in tissue from patients with renal complications. NF-κB in peripheral blood mononuclear cells (PBMC), which can be easily measured, correlated with the degree of albuminuria in diabetic nephropathy patients and was reduced by antioxidant therapy. Similar levels of NF-κB activation in PBMC were observed in healthy volunteers during a 15-min psychosocial stress test. The activation of NF-κB in PBMC correlated with the stress-induced increases in catecholamines and cortisol. Though the long-term effects of stress on NF-κB have not been tested, these acute studies provide a possible mechanism of kidney damage caused by stress.

Sodium Reabsorption

A major hypothesis for the development of hypertension invokes the role of the kidney in the inappropriate retention of solute and fluid resulting in increased fluid volume. In order to maintain homeostatic control of body fluids during periods of hypertension, the kidney excretes greater levels of urine and solute, resetting a lower extracellular fluid volume.

However, the increases in BP seen during periodic stress does not always generate this pressure-natriuresis response, partially due to the increased RSNA, which simultaneously increases Na^+ reabsorption. As some studies suggest, the inability to excrete more solute and fluid during periods of increased BP may predispose those individuals to hypertension. The observation that acute stress can cause Na^+ retention has led to the popular theory that human essential hypertension is primarily due to chronic stress mediating excess extracellular fluid volume via a renal mechanism. Acute stress clearly increases RSNA, and several animal models of hypertension show increased renal sympathetic activity. However, RSNA is determined by postganglionic fibers and is controlled by the arterial baroreceptor reflex, which is not associated with long-term BP control. Though recent evidence shows a stronger correlation of RSNA and long-term control, RSNA generated by stress provides primarily acute regulation of renal function-induced hypertension.

Animal studies show that acute stress consistently increases RSNA and decreases Na^+ excretion in normotensive rats and dogs and does so to an even greater extent in hypertensive rats. The neurohormonal regulation of these effects has been the focus of several studies. In conscious rats, a 10-min air jet stress increased BP and RSNA and reduced urine volume and Na^+ excretion by three- to fourfold (**Figure 2**). After denervation, urine volume and Na^+ excretion were not affected by stress, demonstrating the dependency of neural activity. Treatment with an AT1-R antagonist also prevented a decrease in urine flow or Na^+ excretion after stress, though RSNA was not affected. This suggests that Ang II mediates the antidiuresis and antinatriuresis induced by stress without affecting nerve activity. Previous studies showed that increases in RSNA led to greater Na^+ reabsorption, which was mediated by α-2 receptors. Inhibition of Ang II also decreased the RSNA effect, suggesting that Ang II interacts with α-2 receptors to regulate Na^+ reabsorption. Therefore, changes in RSNA induced by mental stress may have similar regulation by Ang II and α-2 receptors.

Results from human studies are less consistent but do show the effects of stress, and the associated increases in sympathetic activity on Na^+ retention are more closely associated with hypertension than in normotensive humans. In a well-controlled human subject trial, two 20-min periods of stress increased BP and decreased Na^+ excretion in 10 normotensive adult males, without altering GFR, measured by the clearance of inulin, or renal plasma flow (RPF), measured by the clearance of para-aminohippurate (PAH). Fractional Na^+ reabsorption was increased by stress and was primarily due to increases in reabsorption in the proximal tubule (PT), based on fractional lithium clearance measurements. Rilminedine, an imidazoline-I1 receptor antagonist, lowered basal BP but did not alter the effects of stress.

In a study that tested the interaction of hypertension and stress on renal function, three groups were evaluated: normotensive offspring of hypertensives (HP), hypertensive subjects (HT), and normotensive offspring of normotensives (NP). Basal BP, which differed between groups, was elevated by stress in all groups. However, the BP increased more in HP than in the other groups (**Figure 1**). Basal GFR and RBF were higher in HP than in the other groups. However, GFR was reduced by stress in HP and HT but not in NP, and RBF was reduced in HT and NP but not in HP. More interesting, however, were the responses to stress in normal subjects. Stress

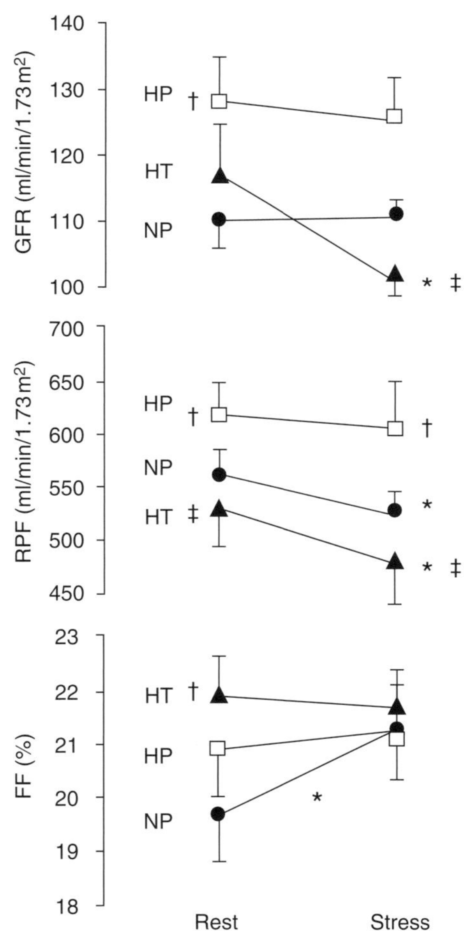

Figure 1 The effect of stress on GFR, RPF, and filtration fraction (FF) in normotensive (NP), normotensive with hypertensive parents (HP), and hypertensive (HT) subjects. From Ducher, M., et al. (2002). *American Journal of Hypertension* **15**, 346–350. © 2002 American Journal of Hypertension, Ltd.

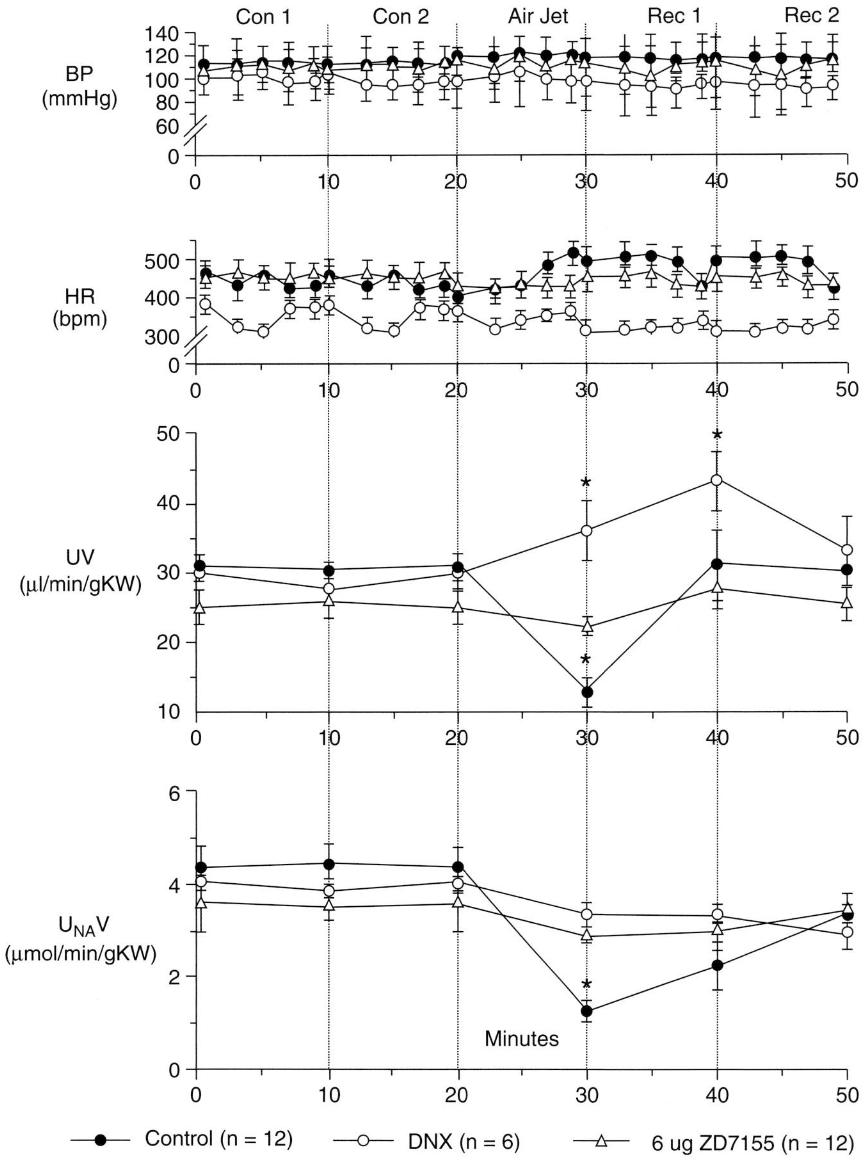

Figure 2 Effects of 10-min air-jet stress on BP, HR, urine flow rate (UV), and Na^+ excretion rate ($U_{NA}V$). UV and $U_{NA}V$ are reduced during stress in conscious control rats. This effect is blocked by either denervation (DNX) or by Ang II, type 1 receptor blocker (ZD7155). From Veelken, R., et al. (1996). *Hypertension* **28**, 825–832.

increased the filtration fraction, which suggests that efferent arteriolar resistance was elevated. There was also a paradoxical decrease in Na^+ excretion given that BP was higher. Again, the decrease in Na^+ reabsorption was attributed to increased PT reabsorption, based on the changes in lithium clearance.

However, Na^+ retention induced by stress is not always observed in normal subjects. In three groups designed to test the potential for the development of hypertension, the effects of mental stress on Na^+ excretion were evaluated in normotensive young males with and without a family of hypertension and compared to hypertensive males. Each subject was studied with or without 1 week of therapy with an angiotensin converting enzyme inhibitor (cilazapril). A 30-min period of mental stress led to increased BP, HR, and GFR and decreased RBF in all groups. However, Na^+ excretion was increased in both normotensive groups, eliciting the appropriate pressure-natriuresis response, whereas the hypertensive group failed to change. Angiotensin converting enzyme therapy restored the increased Na^+ excretion in the hypertensive group, suggesting that the failed natriuretic response is due to the observed elevation of Ang II in hypertensive subjects. Together, these studies suggest that individuals who respond to stress by decreasing Na^+ excretion are predisposed to Na^+ retention and hypertension, whereas normotensive humans with the appropriate natriuresis response to stress are less likely to progress to hypertension via stress.

Does Chronic Stress Cause Hypertension by a Renal Mechanism?

As discussed previously, most of the studies that have shown increased RSNA, RVR, and Na^+ reabsorption to stress were observed during acute stress. Under these acute conditions the increased RVR and renin release may contribute to the acute rise in BP. However, it is difficult to assign a role for Na^+ retention in acute hypertension, which occurs almost immediately. Therefore, caution should be observed when using acute studies to interpret chronic stress-induced hypertension. Studies in normotensive rats and mice have shown that prolonged stress for as much as 4–5 months increases BP during this period. Mice have shown progressive arteriosclerosis, myocardial hypertrophy, increased catecholamine levels, and greater angiotensin sensitivity, since Ang II blockade prevented hypertension. However, there were no measurements of Na^+ balance during the development of hypertension to evaluate the kidney's role. In hypertensive models, such as SHR, renal function and volume status also rarely differ. The use of prehypertensive models has suggested a stronger role for the kidney in the development of hypertension but has not controlled adequately for the genetic backgrounds of these models. A more valuable set of data has been made in renal denervation studies, which have indicated that antinatriuresis and renal vasoconstriction may be due to the elevated RSNA in SHR.

Another issue of concern is that stress in rodents and humans may differ substantially. Human studies have not always found renal dysfunction in acute stress in normal subjects. This would be expected, since genetic predisposition appears to be necessary for the failure of the kidneys to adjust to high BP with appropriate natriuresis. It is possible that some normotensive subjects used in these studies had unknown genetic predisposition. Rodent studies have consistently shown the lack of renal compensation to acute stress, which is surprising but may not relate to the kidney's role, if any, in chronic stress. Indeed, chronic stress in rodents has been associated with cardiac and vascular remodeling.

The proper resolution of this question, at least in animals, will require a reproducible chronic stress model in rodents with noninvasive measurements of BP and renal function that can measure the critical components of renal influences on the development of hypertension over a chronic period. Lacking this type of information, the current evidence does not strongly support a role for changes in renal function contributing significantly to chronic stress-induced hypertension.

Summary

In summary, acute mental stress increases RSNA, BP, RVR, and Na^+ reabsorption in both animal and human studies. These effects are exaggerated in borderline hypertensive or hypertensive subjects, and many effects are blocked by Ang II inhibition, though multiple hormonal systems may be involved. The effects of chronic mental stress are more controversial, with few consistent observations. Though RSNA and general sympathetic activity is increased in SHR, there are rarely any reports of renal dysfunction that would be expected if stress had permanent effects on renal function. The concept of mental stress altering renal function that leads to hypertension needs further experimental evidence.

See Also the Following Articles

Angiotensin; Blood Pressure; Vasoactive Peptides.

Further Reading

Barrett, C. J., Ramchandra, R., Guild, S. J., et al. (2003). What sets the long-term level of renal sympathetic nerve activity: a role for angiotensin II and baroreflexes? *Circulation Research* **92**, 1330–1336.

Bierhaus, A., Wolf, J., Andrassy, M., et al. (2003). A mechanism converting psychosocial stress into mononuclear cell activation. *Proceedings of the National Academy of Science USA* **100**, 1920–1925.

Castellani, S., Ungar, A., Cantini, C., et al. (1999). Impaired renal adaptation to stress in the elderly with isolated systolic hypertension. *Hypertension* **34**, 1106–1111.

Di Bona, G. F. (2004). The sympathetic nervous system and hypertension: recent developments. *Hypertension* **43**, 147–150.

Di Bona, G. F. and Kopp, U. C. (1997). Neural control of renal function. *Physiological Reviews* **77**, 75–197.

Ducher, M., Bertram, D., Pozet, N., et al. (2002). Stress-induced renal alterations in normotensive offspring of hypertensives and in hypertensives. *American Journal of Hypertension* **15**, 346–350.

Schmeider, R. E., Veelken, R., Schobel, H., et al. (1997). Glomerular hypertension during sympathetic nervous system activation in early essential hypertension. *Journal of the American Society of Nephrologists* **8**, 893–900.

Schneider, M. P., Klingbeil, A. U., Schlaich, M. P., et al. (2001). Impaired sodium excretion during mental stress in mild essential hypertension. *Hypertension* **37**, 923–927.

Veelken, R., Hilgers, K. F., Stetter, A., et al. (1996). Nerve-mediated antidiuresis and antinatriuresis after air-jet stress is modulate by angiotensin II. *Hypertension* **28**, 825–832.

Blood Pressure

A Sherwood and R A Carels
Duke University Medical Center

This is a revised version of the article by A Sherwood and R A Carels, Encyclopedia of Stress, First edition, volume 1, pp 331–338, © 2000, Elsevier Inc.

Glossary

Ambulatory blood pressure	Measurements recorded during the course of normal daily activities, using a wearable blood pressure monitor.
Cardiac output	The volume flow rate (l/min) of blood ejected from the left ventricle of the heart into the systemic circulation.
Diastolic blood pressure	The lowest pressure (mmHg) in the arterial system, occurring during cardiac diastole.
Hemo-dynamics	Assessment of the circulation in terms of blood pressure, cardiac output, and systemic vascular resistance.
Hypertension	Resting blood pressure that is higher than 140/90 mmHg.
Reactivity	A psychophysiological trait expressed as cardiovascular response to one or more psychological stressors.
Sympathetic nervous system	A division of the autonomic nervous system that is activated in association with psychological stress and is involved in cardiovascular regulation.
Systemic vascular resistance	The total peripheral resistance of the systemic vasculature (dynes s cm^{-5}).
Systolic blood pressure	The highest pressure (mmHg) in the arterial system, occurring during cardiac systole.

Blood Pressure Measurement

When the left ventricle of the heart contracts, a bolus of blood is ejected into the systemic circulation, creating a pulse pressure waveform that propagates through the arterial tree. The peak pressure reached in the arterial system is referred to as systolic pressure, since it occurs in association with cardiac systole, or the heart's contraction phase. Once systolic pressure is reached, pulsatile pressure falls as the heart relaxes during diastole, with the lowest pressure, referred to as diastolic pressure, occurring just prior to the onset of the next systolic phase. Pulse pressure is defined as the difference between systolic and diastolic pressure. Mean arterial pressure refers to the average pressure in the arterial system. All blood pressure measurements are recorded in millimeters of mercury (mmHg).

Systolic and diastolic pressure are the most commonly measured aspects of arterial blood pressure. The emphasis on these parameters in medicine is partly a reflection of their relative ease of measurement using noninvasive techniques. Although arterial blood pressure varies according to where it is measured in the arterial tree, it is most commonly assessed in the brachial artery, which runs through the upper region of the arm. Two commonly employed measurement techniques, auscultatory and oscillometric, employ an occlusion cuff that contains an inflatable bladder applying pressure through the arm to first interrupt and then progressively restore blood flow through the brachial artery.

With the ausculatory method, a stethoscope or microphone is positioned over the brachial artery, distal to the occlusion cuff. When the pressure in the occlusion cuff is above systolic pressure, the brachial artery is compressed and no sounds are detected distal to the cuff. When the slowly deflating occlusion cuff drops below the systolic pressure, the compressed artery opens momentarily and the brief episode of turbulent blood flow distal to the cuff is detected as a faint tapping sound; the first phase I Korotkoff sound is used to indicate systolic blood pressure. As the cuff pressure continues to fall, the Korotkoff sounds increase in intensity and quality, followed by a muffling of the sound (phase IV) and ultimately their disappearance (phase V). Diastolic pressure is usually defined as phase V in adults, while in children phase IV may be a closer approximation. With the ausculatatory technique, mean arterial pressure cannot be measured directly, but may be estimated as diastolic pressure plus one-third of the pulse pressure.

The oscillometric method also employs the occlusion cuff in a manner similar to that for ausculatory measurement. However, with the oscillometric technique, cuff pressure oscillations coincident with pulsatile pressure variations in the artery form the basis of blood pressure measurement. As the occlusion cuff is deflated, systolic pressure is indicated by a sharp rise in cuff pressure oscillations. The lowest pressure at which the cuff oscillations are at their greatest amplitude identifies mean arterial pressure. Diastolic pressure is recorded as the point at which the cuff pressure oscillations decrease no further in amplitude.

The ausculatatory and oscillometric methods are by far the most widely utilized methods for measuring blood pressure. One of their limitations is that because they use a slowly deflating occlusion cuff, blood pressure measurements are limited in frequency to approximately once per minute. Other techniques include direct arterial pressure recording via a pressure transducer on the tip of an intra-arterial catheter, a method often employed to monitor vital signs during major surgery. One advantage of this invasive method is that it provides a continuous measurement of blood pressure on a beat-by-beat basis. A number of research-orientated techniques, including cuff tracking, vascular unloading, arterial tonometry, and pulse transit time, provide methods to assess blood pressure beat by beat, yet nonivasively, each offering specific strengths and limitations. All of the methods described above have been employed in studies examining the effects of stress on blood pressure.

Hypertension

Hypertension is defined as systolic blood pressure of 140 mmHg or greater, and/or diastolic blood pressure of 90 mmHg or greater. These criteria, based on seated clinic blood pressure measurements, are recognized by the World Health Organization/International Society of Hypertension and the United States Joint National Committee on Prevention, Detection, Evaluation, and Treatment of High Blood Pressure (JNC). Pressures in excess of 140/90 mmHg are further categorized in terms of severity of hypertension, currently defined as stages 1 and 2 (JNC VII). While blood pressures less than 140/90 mmHg were once considered normal, the JNC VII report now classifies blood pressures in the range 120–139/80–89 mmHg as prehypertension. This new category reflects a growing recognition that the clinical criteria for hypertension are somewhat arbitrary, and that cardiovascular morbidity associated with high blood pressure is more of a progressive phenomenon than one associated with a specific pressure threshold that engenders a sudden rise in health risk. The term prehypertension also signifies that individuals with pressures in this range are at greater risk of developing hypertension than individuals with lower pressures. Only pressures below 120/80 mmHg are considered optimal.

Prevalence of hypertension is related to age, race, and gender. Hypertension incidence is higher in Blacks than in Whites, particularly in the United States. In young to middle-aged adults, prevalence is much greater in males than females, while incidence increases quite dramatically in women after menopause. Though hypertension is defined by elevation of arterial blood pressure, its clinical significance is derived from morbid events affecting the heart, brain, and kidneys. Complications such as myocardial infarction and stroke are not directly due to elevated pressures, but to the resulting structural changes in the heart and blood vessels. One of the structural consequences of hypertension, hypertrophy of the left ventricle (LVH), is the strongest known predictor, other than advancing age, of cardiovascular morbidity and mortality.

Hypertension is a disease that typically develops over years or decades, and in approximately 90% of cases it is diagnosed as primary (or essential) hypertension, indicating nonspecific etiology. The natural history of hypertension not only is characterized by a progressive increase in blood pressure, but also is accompanied by a progressive rise in systemic vascular resistance (SVR). The structural autoregulation theory of hypertension, originated by Folkow, helps explain why hypertension becomes a disease of elevated SVR. Arterial resistance vessels (arterioles) serve to regulate blood flow in accordance with local tissue demands. Vascular smooth muscle hypertrophy occurs as a physiological adaptation to increased blood pressure, which allows the vessel to maintain its ability to regulate blood flow at higher pressures. However, a consequence of this restructuring of the vessel is that it creates a rise in SVR, which increasingly provides the basis for the hypertension. Thus, structural autoregulation is a cascading pathophysiological adaptation. However, the unresolved question is what causes an individual's pressure to initially rise from normotensive levels, allowing the onset of pathophysiological processes. The answer to this question is likely multiple interacting factors, which vary across individuals, as reflected in Page's Mosaic Theory of hypertension. However, there is overwhelming evidence that the sympathetic nervous system is frequently implicated in the early stages of hypertension. In some, though not all, instances, this may give rise to a hyperkinetic circulatory state in which blood pressure elevations are due to abnormally high cardiac output (CO) levels. It is the potentially pathophysiological effects of the sympathetic nervous system that suggest that stress may be implicated in the etiology of hypertension.

Stress and Blood Pressure

Psychophysiology of Stress

The impact of emotions and stress on blood pressure were recognized as early as the seventeenth century, as reflected in William Harvey's studies of the circulation. However, it was not until the twentieth century that the psychophysiological mechanisms by which stress influenced blood pressure became better understood. In 1915, Walter Cannon proposed that the sympathetic nervous system served to mobilize the cardiovascular system in preparation for fight or flight by engendering an increase in blood pressure and blood flow to the skeletal muscle vasculature. In the 1940s, the work of Hess identified the defense response, which was characterized by an integrative behavioral and cardiovascular activation pattern in response to electrical stimulation of the hypothalamus. This early animal research set the groundwork for our conception of the stress response as a psychophysiological phenomenon that primes the body in anticipation of recourse to sudden physical exertion.

In the latter half of the twentieth century, human research on the effects of stress on blood pressure was dominated by what has been termed cardiovascular reactivity studies, in which a variety of cardiovascular measures are recorded while volunteers are subjected to psychologically challenging tasks in a research laboratory setting. One of the earliest human studies was reported by Brod and colleagues in 1959, describing detailed cardiovascular response patterns observed while participants performed a stressful mental arithmetic task. Responses typically paralleled those of the animal defense response, with increased blood pressure and circulatory mobilization that occurred in the absence of significant metabolic demands. Essentially the same approach used by Brod has since been utilized extensively, and has led to the documentation of responses to a wide variety of laboratory stressors, including reaction time tasks, Stroop color–word conflict tasks, cold pressor tasks, simulated public speaking, and a variety of psychomotor tasks. One of the consistently striking observations from these studies is the individual differences in the magnitude of blood pressure responses: while at one extreme some individuals may show essentially no change in blood pressure, others may respond with an increase of 50 mmHg or more to exactly the same laboratory stressor. There is compelling evidence that these individual differences in blood pressure reactivity to stress are relatively robust, exhibiting consistency across a variety of laboratory tasks, and showing stability over time.

Blood pressure alone provides a limited picture of the hemodynamic pattern of changes elicited by stress. Hemodynamic studies emphasize the interrelationships among blood pressure, CO, and SVR. Since blood pressure is the product of CO and SVR, the concurrent measurement of blood pressure and CO permits the derivation of SVR, providing a more complete description of the hemodynamic response. Two very early stress studies conducted in the 1940s used invasive procedures to measure CO and, moreover, considered the measurement procedures themselves as presenting the source of psychological stress. These studies demonstrated how the stress response associated with anxiety was characterized by a mobilization of the cardiovascular system, leading to blood pressure increases due to an increase in CO. The same response pattern to a mental arithmetic task was observed over a decade later by Brod. In this classic study, CO was measured invasively using dye dilution, and forearm blood flow was also measured, leading to the demonstration that the increased CO during psychological stress appeared to be distributed to the skeletal muscle vasculature. These studies demonstrated that the fight-or-flight response, previously observed in animals, could be elicited in humans by psychological stressors.

With the development of noninvasive methods to measure cardiac output unobtrusively, in the past two decades there has been a resurgence of laboratory studies of the hemodynamic aspects of the stress response. These studies have consistently illustrated that there are dramatic individual differences in the hemodynamic patterns underlying blood pressure increases during stress. Thus, apparently similar cardiovascular responses to a stressor in terms of blood pressure change may belie very different underlying hemodynamic mechanisms. While some individuals exhibit blood pressure increases during stress due to an increase in CO and a decrease in SVR (fight-or-flight response), others may vasoconstrict, leading to an increase in blood pressure due entirely to increased SVR. Observations of this kind have led to an extension of descriptive categories in cardiovascular reactivity research, from high vs. low or hot vs. cold reactors, referring to the magnitude of blood pressure responses, to myocardial and vascular reactors, referring to the hemodynamic mechanism producing the blood pressure response. The mechanisms and potential health consequences of these individual differences are currently under exploration.

Stress and Hypertension

Although acute stress can indisputably raise blood pressure for brief periods into the range defining hypertension, its role in the etiology of sustained hypertension remains controversial.

Observational studies of stress reactivity There is some evidence that risk of hypertension development may be related to stress reactivity. Hypertensive individuals have been found to show greater blood pressure reactivity than normotensives. Individuals with normal blood pressure who have hypertensive parents also typically exhibit greater blood pressure reactivity to laboratory stressors than normotensives with no family history. Whereas studies describing only observations of the magnitude of blood pressure responses have reported inconsistent findings for the effects of race, a number of studies have reported that Black men, who are at increased risk for hypertension, appear to exhibit abnormally elevated vascular tone, indexed by SVR, during exposure to a variety of laboratory stressors. Gender differences in reactivity have also been observed, with men exhibiting greater systolic blood pressure and SVR increases than premenopausal women. These gender differences in SVR response are consistent with those observed for race in that men are more likely to develop hypertension than premenopausal women.

Since hypertension is a disease whose natural history involves progressively increasing blood pressure, which in turn is secondary to progressively increasing SVR, the tendency for individuals at greater risk for developing hypertension to exhibit pronounced stress-induced blood pressure and/or SVR reactivity is provocative. Reactivity studies have also demonstrated that stress can modify renal function, leading to sodium and fluid retention in some individuals, which may heighten and prolong stress-induced blood pressure elevations; altered renal function may be one of the target organ effects of stress that could impact long-term blood regulation. Additionally, several recent studies have reported an association between blood pressure reactivity and LVH, whereby the magnitude of blood pressure response during stress is directly related to LV mass.

Prospective studies of stress reactivity Although correlational evidence of the kind described previously is provocative, it is inconclusive since it does not rule out the possibility that associations of stress reactivity to hypertension risk and/or end organ damage may simply be a manifestation of underlying pathophysiology; the stress response may be a marker rather than a mechanism of disease. Prospective studies should help resolve these cause–effect limitations by focusing on the temporal relationship of the correlated observations. As previously noted, hypertensive individuals are characterized by blood pressure hyperreactivity, but is blood pressure hyperactivity in normotensives associated with the subsequent development of hypertension? Evidence relating to this question comes both from human and animal studies.

Animal studies In 1969, Forsyth described the effects of prolonged daily exposure to unsignaled shock avoidance schedules in rhesus monkeys. After several months, three of four animals developed hypertension. However, these findings were not replicated in other species. Beginning in the 1970s, a series of elegant studies was reported by Henry and colleagues on the effects of chronic social conflict in mice. When reared in isolation and subsequently transferred to colonies that made social conflict unavoidable, hypertension developed after several months, suggesting that chronic social stress could be a cause of hypertension. However, subsequent studies in other species were again less definitive. The importance of genetic susceptibility was demonstrated by Lawler's 1980s studies of borderline hypertensive rats, which developed hypertension when exposed to prolonged aversive reinforcement contingencies, whereas control animals typically remained normotensive. Other studies have suggested that the development of hypertension in salt-sensitive strains of animals of various species is exacerbated by exposure to stressful behavioral paradigms. In summary, the animal studies suggest that stress may play a role in the development of hypertension, but its impact is only likely to be important in the context of a pre-existing disposition to develop the disease.

Human studies There has been much interest in the possibility that individuals characterized by unusually large magnitude blood pressure reactivity may be at increased risk for the development of hypertension. Several studies have generated indirect support for the so-called stress reactivity hypothesis. In an early study of White males, blood pressure reactivity in response to a hand cold pressor task was examined as a predictor of the development of hypertension at 20- and 36-year follow-up. The study revealed that subjects in the top quartile of systolic blood pressure reactivity had a greater incidence of hypertension from age 40 onward, compared to the less reactive subjects. Other relatively long-term follow-up studies have shown the cold pressor task to predict the development of elevated blood pressure. One criticism of these studies is that the cold pressor may not be a purely behavioral stressor, since it is a painful stimulus for most individuals; although, in common with other laboratory behavioral stress tasks, its cardiovascular effects are mediated primarily by sympathetic nervous system activation.

Blood pressure reactivity to a reaction time task involving threat of shock was found by Light and colleagues to predict increases in blood pressure 10 to 15 years later. High levels of systolic blood pressure during the reaction time task were associated with higher clinic and ambulatory systolic pressure at follow-up, even after controlling for parental history of hypertension and baseline resting systolic and diastolic blood pressure. Several studies in adolescents and young adults examining reactivity to mental arithmetic as a predictor of hypertension have also found evidence that high blood pressure reactivity and/or delayed recovery of the stress-induced blood pressure response predicts the development of hypertension at follow-up 1–5 years later. Other studies have made similar observations based on initial reactivity assessments using video games, Stropp color–word conflict, and mirror trace tasks. The studies reported to date are inconsistent in whether systolic blood pressure reactivity, diastolic blood pressure reactivity, or both is predictive of hypertension development. This discrepancy may also reflect differences in the population sample being studied, as well as differences in the nature of the blood pressure response associated with the specific stressor employed in a given study. It is also of note that the degree to which reactivity has predicted the development of high pressure or hypertension has been generally modest. As suggested by the animal studies, genetic susceptibility (i.e., family history of hypertension) is likely to be an important determinant of hypertension development, but was not considered in all of the reactivity studies. Furthermore, if stress reactivity is viewed as a disease mechanism, then the predictive value of high reactivity is likely to be largely moderated by the extent to which repeated acute stress responses occur in the time interval from assessment to follow-up. Assessing the frequency of stress responses over the long term presents a methodological challenge that has yet to be met in reactivity studies.

Psychosocial factors and hypertension Relatively few prospective studies have examined the relationship of psychosocial factors to the subsequent development of hypertension. The Framingham Heart Study examined the role of anxiety, anger intensity, and anger suppression in normotensive men. After controlling for biological risk factors, anxiety at baseline remained an independent predictor of hypertension in middle-aged men. The National Health and Nutrition Examination Survey I Epidemiologic Follow-up Study also followed several thousand initially normotensive individuals for 7 to 16 years to test the hypothesis that symptoms of anxiety and depression increased the risk of developing hypertension. High anxiety and depression were independent predictors of incident hypertension ($\geq$160/95 mmHg) in White men aged 45 to 64 years and Black men aged 25 to 64 years. In a large prospective study in Alameda County, California, unemployment, job insecurity, and concerns over job performance in men and low-status work in women were associated with increased likelihood of developing hypertension, after controlling for demographic and behavioral risk factors. Finally, several smaller correlational and prospective studies have found a significant relationship between the personality trait defensiveness and hypertension.

Studies of chronic stress Studies of environments that may engender chronic states of stress also provide a test of the effects of stress on blood pressure. In a study of individuals residing near the Three Mile Island nuclear power plant, blood pressure was found to rise shortly after the 1979 accident in which part of the facility was destroyed. Blood pressure remained elevated for 5 years and was associated with increased sympathetic nervous system activity compared to individuals residing further from the nuclear plant. Studies of prisoners also suggest that living in overcrowded conditions is associated with elevated blood pressure. Occupations considered to be associated with chronic stress include air traffic controllers, who have been found to show a much greater incidence of hypertension than workers in comparable, but less stressful, occupations. A relationship between occupational stress and elevated blood pressure and/or hypertension is supported by other studies, including those utilizing ambulatory blood pressure measurement technology to measure blood pressure in the working environment.

Ambulatory Blood Pressure

Methodology

Advances in computer and miniaturization technology over the past 25 years have aided the development of wearable ambulatory blood pressure (ABP) monitors. ABP monitors are able to capture the normal activities and environmental interactions during the course of an individual's day. Utilizing common blood pressure measurement techniques, ABP monitors permit frequent noninvasive blood pressure recordings based upon auscultatory and/or oscillometric measurement principles. ABP monitors are typically programmed to take blood pressure measurements several times per hour, at variable intervals, throughout the workday, evening, and overnight. Individuals are ordinarily instructed to follow a normal schedule during waking hours and to complete a brief diary immediately following each reading indicating factors such as time, posture, activity, location, and current emotional/cognitive state. Factors such as posture and physical activity have been shown to systematically influence blood pressure. Location and emotional state have also been found to affect blood pressure, but the magnitude of their effects varies greatly from individual to individual. Finally, recent research suggests that the degree of familiarity with a conversant as well as the positiveness or negativeness of the interpersonal interaction affects ABP levels.

White Coat Hypertension

Because morbid events are often associated with hypertension, blood pressure is routinely measured during visits to a physician's office. However, psychological stress associated with visiting a doctor's office can spuriously inflate clinic blood pressures in some patients. Individuals whose blood pressures are in the hypertensive range when measured in the clinic but are normal in other contexts, as indicated by ABP measurements and/or automated home measurements, are classified as white coat hypertensives. Studies suggest that when compared to sustained hypertensives, white coat hypertensives are more likely to be younger female nonsmokers with a lower body mass index. Although most studies have found no association between psychological factors and white coat hypertension, there is some evidence that anxiety may be a related characteristic. Multiple ABP measurements throughout the day are thought to be more representative than clinic measures of the overall load that is placed on the cardiovascular system. Thus, 24-h ABP recordings can provide important supplementation of clinic readings in the accurate diagnosis of hypertension and are more closely correlated with end organ damage, including left ventricular mass, than clinic blood pressure.

Emotional States, Psychosocial Characteristics, and ABP

ABP monitoring is particularly well suited for capturing acute affective states that occur in response to daily stress. Several studies have indicated that emotions, as indicated by diary ratings of moods, influence ABP levels. Both negative and positive moods have been found to be associated with increased ABP. However, a great deal of individual variability in the reporting of diary-rated moods has been observed, suggesting that certain individuals may be more susceptible to experiencing emotional upset throughout the day. Similarly, the effects of emotions on ABP are more pronounced in some individuals than in others. Nonetheless, studies indicate that for diary ratings of negative emotions, including stress, frustration, and tension, greater emotional intensity is accompanied by higher ABP.

There is some evidence that psychosocial characteristics that are risk factors for cardiovascular disease, including anxiety, depression, and lack of social support, are associated with greater fluctuations in diary ratings of negative moods; these individuals have also been found to exhibit a greater impact of emotion on ABP. There is also evidence to suggest that negative emotional dispositions, such as hostility, may have an impact on ABP, but only in certain social contexts. While recent studies indicate that dispositional characteristics (e.g., defensiveness and pessimism), coping responses (e.g., religious coping), and reactions to racial inequality (e.g., perceived racism) may be associated with ABP levels, these preliminary findings would benefit from further replication.

ABP and Location

Work If a 24-h day is divided into work, home, and overnight periods, most people's blood pressure will be highest during work, lower while at home, and lowest during the overnight period. However, these locational effects on blood pressure vary greatly from one individual to the next. This suggests that location per se is not directly associated with blood pressure, but rather that location is associated with a variety of behavioral factors (e.g., activity level, posture) and psychosocial factors (e.g., mood, social support, negative interpersonal exchanges, stress) that under certain circumstances may influence blood pressure. ABP studies conducted on individuals across a variety of occupations (e.g., paramedics, physicians, clerical personnel) indicate that perceived or actual occupational stress does, in fact, increase ABP levels. These associations have prompted researchers to examine specific job characteristics that might contribute to elevations in blood pressure across a variety of occupations. One model of job characteristics that contributes to work-related stress is Karasek and Theorell's job strain model. Karasek and Theorell maintain that a deleterious combination of high psychological job demands and low decision latitude at work results in a condition of job strain. Numerous studies have found that higher levels of job strain are associated with higher blood pressure, particularly in men. There is also evidence that job strain is associated with increased LV mass, which may be a consequence of ABP effects.

Home Behavioral and psychosocial influences on ABP at home are likely to be very different from behavioral and psychosocial influences at work. The home environment may be influenced by factors such as the quality of familial relationships and their ability to provide social support, the level of domestic and family responsibilities, and the existence of role conflict or dissatisfaction. Although research on the home environment and ABP is sparse, one study that examined blood pressure in working women found that married working women had higher ABP than unmarried working women. These findings suggest that, compared to unmarried working women, the higher ABP levels found in married working women may reflect their greater combined work and home responsibilities, possibly suggesting a total greater workload. Elevated ABP in the home environment may also be associated with home stress, making it more difficult to unwind, both psychologically and physiologically, after work.

Sleep Blood pressure typically falls during nighttime sleep. Most individuals are characterized by >10% fall in nighttime blood pressure and are referred to as dippers, in contrast to non-dippers, who exhibit <10% nighttime blood pressure fall. Sleep blood pressures may be influenced, at least in part, by events that occur during waking hours. Studies have found that the daily experience of negative moods on blood pressure appears to carry over from daytime waking to nighttime sleep. Individuals that frequently report anger during the day tend to have higher levels of blood pressure, especially during sleep. There has been some speculation that unresolved stressful experiences and negative mood states that occur during the day might contribute to disrupted sleep patterns, a diminished quality of sleep, or somatic tension that influences blood pressure levels. In addition, a positive family history of hypertension, low socioeconomic status, and African American ethnicity have been associated with blunted nocturnal blood pressure dipping. Dietary factors, including high sodium consumption and low potassium consumption, also have been related to blunted nighttime blood pressure dipping. Sympathetic nervous system activity also appears to be an important factor, with nighttime catecholamine levels and vascular adrenergic receptor activity also appearing to play a role in nocturnal blood pressure dipping. The magnitude of nocturnal decline in blood pressure has been found to relate to LV mass,with non-dippersexhibiting elevated LV mass and higher likelihood of LVH compared to dippers. This evidence underscores the importance of studying nighttime blood pressures and its possibly complex biopsychosocial determinants.

See Also the Following Articles

Cardiovascular System and Stress; Sympathetic Nervous System.

Further Reading

Joint National Committee on Prevention, Detection, Evaluation Treatment of High Blood Pressure. (2003). The seventh report of the joint national committee on prevention, detection, evaluation and treatment of high blood pressure. *Journal of the American Medical Association* **289**, 2560–2572.

Lloyd-Jones, D. M., Evans, J. C. and Levy, D. (2005). Hypertension in adults across the age spectrum: current outcomes and control in the community. *JAMA* **294**, 466–472.

Manuck, S. B., Kasprowicz, A. L. and Muldoon, M. F. (1990). Behaviorally-evoked cardiovascular reactivity and hypertension: conceptual issues and potential associations. *Annals of Behavioral Medicine* **12**, 17–29.

O'Rourke, M. F., Kelly, R. and Avolio, A. (1992). *The arterial pulse.* Malvern, PA: Lea & Febiger.

Pickering, T. (1997). The effects of occupational stress on blood pressure in men and women. *Acta Physiologica Scandinavica* **640**(supplement), 125–128.

Pickering, T. G., Shimbo, D. and Haas, D. (2006). Current concepts: Ambulatory blood-pressure monitoring. *New England Journal of Medicine* **354**, 2368–2374.

Shapiro, D., Jamner, L. D., Lane, J. D., et al. (1996). Blood pressure publication guidelines. *Pychophysiology* **33**, 1–12.

Steptoe, A. (1997). Behavior and blood pressure: implications for hypertension. In: Zanchettii, A. & Mancia, G. (eds.) *Handbook of hypertension, Vol. 17: Pathophysiology of hypertension*, pp. 674–708. Amsterdam, The Netherlands: Elsevier.

Angiotensin

O Baltatu
Max-Delbrück-Center for Molecular Medicine, Berlin-Buch, Germany, and Sultan Qaboos University, Muscat, Sultanate of Oman
M Bader
Max-Delbrück-Center for Molecular Medicine, Berlin-Buch, Germany

This is a revised version of the article by O Baltatu, M Bader, and D Ganten, Encyclopedia of Stress, First edition, volume 1, pp 195–199, © 2000, Elsevier Inc.

Glossary

Blood–brain barrier — A term for the impermeability of the endothelial cells of cerebral capillaries to components of the blood, due *inter alia* to tight junctions, so that endo- and transcytotic transport across the capillary wall occurs in a highly specific and regulated manner.

Cardiovascular control — Control of cardiovascular homeostasis by neural and local mechanisms.

Cardiovascular homeostasis — The maintenance of the cardiovascular parameters, especially blood pressure and blood volume at levels optimal for blood supply to all organs.

Components of the Renin–Angiotensin System

Angiotensinogen

Angiotensinogen (AOGEN) is the only known precursor molecule to be converted by the renin–angiotensin system (RAS) into active angiotensins.

It is a glycoprotein with a molecular weight between 61 and 65 kDa, and it shows close structural similarities to the serine protease inhibitor family. Originally found to be synthesized in the liver, AOGEN is known to be present in several other organs, especially in glial cells of the brain.

Renin

Renin is a very specific aspartyl proteinase whose only known substrate is AOGEN. Renin cleaves the decapeptide angiotensin I (Ang I) from the N-terminus of mature AOGEN. Renin is produced primarily by the kidney and released into the circulation, but is also produced in other tissues. Renin synthesis is stimulated by the sympathetic nervous system and by loss of volume and sodium.

Angiotensin Converting Enzyme

Angiotensin converting enzyme (ACE) is a dipeptidyl-carboxypeptidase that cleaves the C-terminal histidine-leucine of Ang I to generate angiotensin II (Ang II). It is found in high concentrations in the lung, kidney, and heart and is distributed throughout the brain. High amounts are detected in areas lacking the blood–brain barrier such as the diencephalon, pituitary, and pineal gland. ACE is also able to hydrolyze other substrates, such as bradykinin, opioid peptides, and substance P. Thus, ACE is additionally involved in physiological mechanisms beyond the RAS.

Active Angiotensins

The best studied peptide of the system is Ang II, and the functions of the RAS are largely attributed to this active metabolite. Besides Ang II, additional peptides of the RAS have been found to be biologically active, such as Ang III, Ang IV, and Ang II(1–7). In fact, Ang III may be even more potent than Ang II in the brain when acting on a common receptor. Ang II(1–7) can be formed via an ACE-independent mechanism and has the same potency as Ang II in vasopressin release. Studies on Ang IV suggest a biological role for this peptide as well.

There is evidence that proteases other than renin and ACE can produce bioactive angiotensin species. Such proteases include ACE 2, cathepsin G, tonin, tissue plasminogen activator, chymase, and other neutral peptidases.

Receptors

The use of highly specific ligands has led to the description and cloning of two main Ang II receptors, namely AT_1 and AT_2. Most of the known classical cardiovascular effects of Ang II are attributed to the AT_1 receptor. In contrast to humans, two different subtypes have been found for this receptor in rodents: AT_{1a} and AT_{1b}. Whereas AT_{1a} has been localized in blood vessels, kidney, lung, liver, and specific brain areas that are involved in the control of blood pressure and fluid homeostasis, AT_{1b} receptors were originally described in glandular tissues, such as the anterior pituitary and adrenal gland.

Endocrine Plasma Renin-Angiotensin System

The endocrine RAS is dependent on renin released by the kidney into the blood, so that AOGEN is cleaved

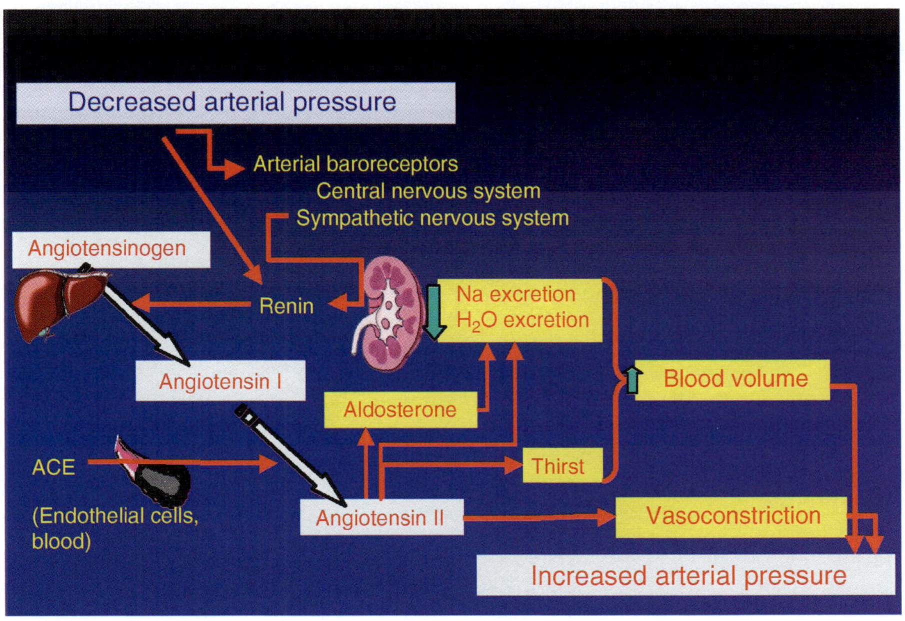

Figure 1 Roles of the renin–angiotensin system in cardiovascular and fluid–electrolyte regulation.

in the circulation to liberate the inactive decapeptide Ang I. ACE then cleaves Ang I to yield the octapeptide Ang II, the active molecule of the system. Circulating Ang II is one of the most potent vasoconstrictors and acts on specific receptors to elicit the following localized effects:

- constriction of the vasculature
- reabsorption of sodium and water in the kidney
- release of aldosterone from the adrenal glands
- induction of inotropic and arrythmogenic effects in the heart
- incitement of thirst at specific brain areas outside the blood–brain barrier

Figure 1 summarizes the roles of the RAS in cardiovascular and fluid–electrolyte regulation.

Paracrine Tissue Renin–Angiotensin System

In addition to the circulating RAS, a local formation and action of Ang II has been observed at the level of various organs. The components of the RAS have been detected in several tissues including the heart, vasculature, kidney, adrenal glands, and brain. The local formation and action of Ang II in peripheral organs can therefore occur independent from the circulating RAS. However, RAS components required for angiotensin synthesis, such as renin and AOGEN, can be also taken up from the circulating blood. The latter is possible only for organs accessible to blood proteins, such as the kidney, heart, adrenal glands, and brain areas situated outside the blood–brain

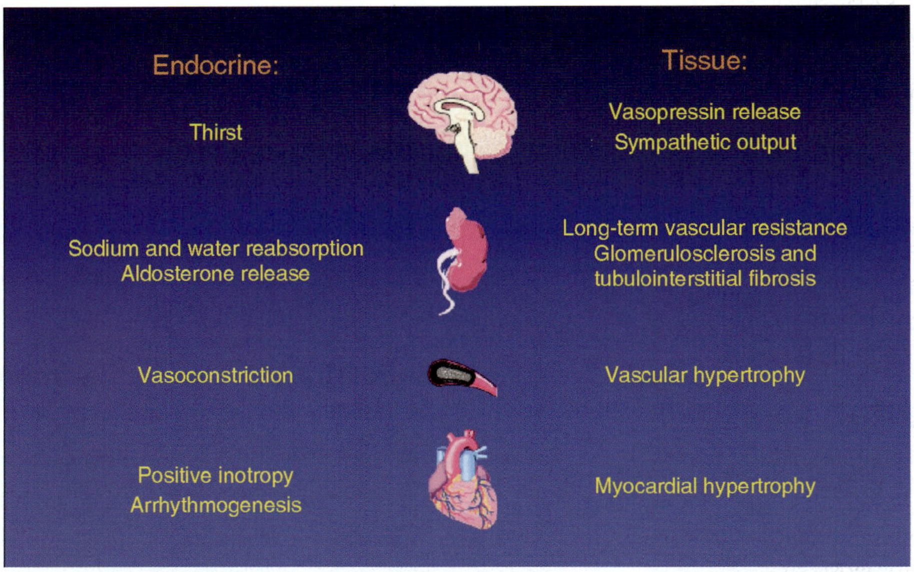

Figure 2 Functions of the endocrine and tissue renin–angiotensin systems.

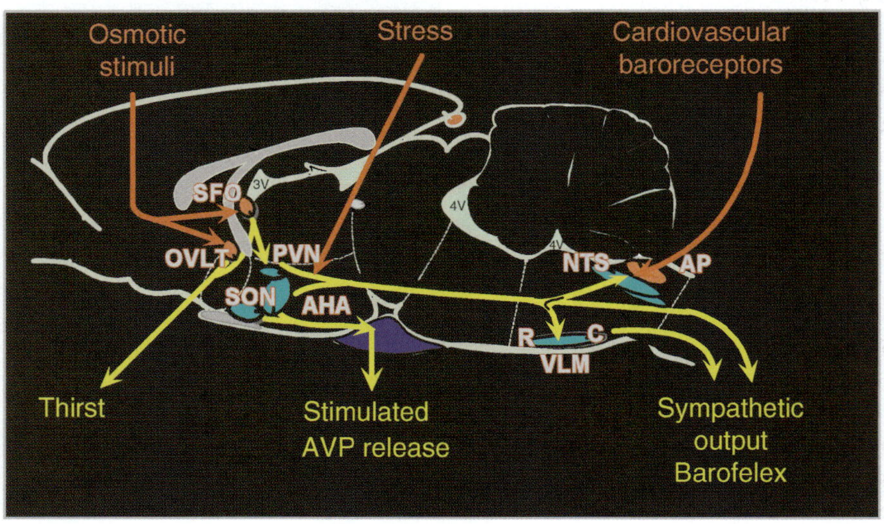

Figure 3 Angiotensin sites involved in the central control of homeostasis.

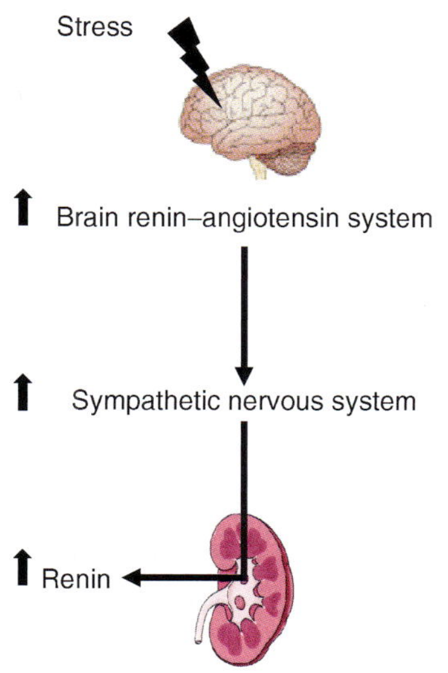

Figure 4 Stress-induced brain RAS activation may induce renin release from the kidney, possibly through sympathetic pathways.

barrier. Nevertheless, there are areas in the brain that are inaccessible to the circulating Ang II because of the blood–brain barrier but that express functional angiotensin receptors. In these brain regions, only locally formed angiotensins can act.

The tissue RASs seem to regulate long-term organ function and may be responsible for pathological structural changes. **Figure 2** illustrates the functions of the endocrine and tissue RASs.

Renin–Angiotensin System and Stress

Both physical and emotional stressors induce peripheral and central responses designed to preserve cardiovascular homeostasis. As one of the main regulators of cardiovascular homeostasis, the RAS is stimulated by stressors that lead to a lowering in the blood pressure, such as hemorrhage, loss of blood volume and sodium, or increased activity of the sympathetic nervous system. The RAS acts synergistically with the sympathetic nervous system, increasing blood pressure and maintaining organ perfusion, and electrolyte and volume balance. Recently, it has been demonstrated that Ang II is also an important mediator of inflammation by stimulating oxidative stress.

The physical and behavioral responses to stress are integrated at the level of the central nervous system, including areas known to regulate the homeostasis of the *milieu interieur.* AOGEN and the angiotensin receptors are present in areas responsible for the maintenance of homeostasis, such as the hypothalamic and brain-stem nuclei (**Figure 3**), and participate in the stress response.

The sympathetic nervous system, the component of the autonomic nervous system that is essentially involved in the fight-or-flight reaction, is modulated by the RAS not only in the periphery but also in central areas of autonomic control. During the reaction to stress, there is an increase in blood levels of renin in addition to epinephrine. In the central nervous system, an interrelationship between the activity of the brain RAS and the sympathetic system and other central autonomic pathways has also been shown. Stress-induced brain RAS activation may induce renin release from the kidney, possibly through sympathetic pathways (**Figure 4**).

Various stressor agents activate the hypothalamic-pituitary axis. Ang II, together with other neurotransmitters and neuromodulators, modulates the activity of the hypothalamic–pituitary axis and stimulates the release of vasopressin and corticotropin-releasing factor (CRF). In addition, it has been proposed that the brain RAS is involved in behavioral responses, such as cognition, memory, and central analgesia.

Prolonged overactivation of the RAS may lead to a disease state. Drugs that block the actions of the RAS, such as ACE or renin inhibitors and AT1 antagonists, are widely used for the treatment of various cardiovascular diseases, and their effectiveness may be partially due to the inhibition of the brain RAS and thereby the attenuation of the sympathetic output and the stress response.

See Also the Following Articles

Angiotensin Receptors; Blood Pressure.

Further Reading

Bader, M., Peters, J., Baltatu, O., et al. (2001). Tissue renin-angiotensin systems: new insights from experimental animal models in hypertension research. *Journal of Molecular Medicine* 79, 76–102.

Baltatu, O., Bader, M. and Ganten, D. (1998). Brain and renin-angiotensin system. In: Nicholls, M. G., Ikram, H., Brunner, H. & Sweet, C. (eds.) *100 Years of Renin-Angiotensin System*, pp. 167–170. Oxford: Hughes Associates.

Baltatu, O., Bader, M. and Ganten, D. (1998). Functional testing of components of the brain renin-angiotensin system in transgenic animals. In: Ulfendahl, H. & Aurell, M. (eds.) *Renin-Angiotensin*, pp. 105–114. London: Portland Press.

Baltatu, O. and Bader, M. (2003). Brain renin-angiotensin system – lessons from functional genomics. *Neuroendocrinology* 78, 253–259.

Baltatu, O., Campos, L. A. and Bader, M. (2004). Genetic targeting of the brain renin-angiotensin system in transgenic rats: impact on stress-induced renin release. *Acta Physiologica Scandinavia* 181, 579–584.

de Gasparo, M., Catt, K. J., Inagami, T., et al. (2000). International union of pharmacology, XXIII. The angiotensin II receptors. *Pharmacology Reviews* 52, 415–472.

Fink, G. D. (1997). Long-term sympatho-excitatory effect of angiotensin II: a mechanism of spontaneous and renovascular hypertension. *Clinical and Experimental Pharmacology and Physiology* **24**, 91–95.
Henry, J. P. (1992). Biological basis of the stress response. *Integrative Physiological and Behavioral Science* **27**, 66–83.
Leckie, B. J. (2005). Targeting the renin-angiotensin system: what's new? *Current Medical and Chemical Cardiovascular Hematology Agents* **3**, 23–32.
Morgan, L., Broughton, P. F. and Kalsheker, N. (1996). Angiotensinogen: molecular biology, biochemistry and physiology. *International Journal of Biochemistry and Cell Biology* **28**, 1211–1222.
Saavedra, J. M., Ando, H., Armando, I., et al. (2004). Brain angiotensin II, an important stress hormone: regulatory sites and therapeutic opportunities. *Annals of the New York Academy of Sciences* **1018**, 76–84.
Touyz, R. M. (2005). Molecular and cellular mechanisms in vascular injury in hypertension: role of angiotensin II – editorial review. *Current Opinions in Nephrology and Hypertension* **14**, 125–131.

Angiotensin Receptors

T A Jenkins and F A O Mendelsohn
University of Melbourne, Parkville, Victoria, Australia

Glossary

Angiotensin-converting enzyme (ACE)	Enzyme that converts angiotensin I to angiotensin II.
Angiotensin II receptors	The two classes of Ang II receptors, AT_1 and AT_2, occur in a variety of tissues, including brain, adrenal, heart, vessel wall, and kidney.
Angiotensin II (Ang II)	Octapeptide; a major active mediator of the renin-angiotensin cascade.
Cardiovascular disease	Disease of the heart and blood vessels.
Hypertension	High arterial blood pressure.
Renin-angiotensin system (RAS)	Hormone system that plays an important role in regulating body fluid balance, blood volume, arterial pressure, and cardiac, vascular, and renal function.

The physiological roles of the renin-angiotensin system (RAS) include regulation of blood pressure, fluid and electrolyte homeostasis, and aldosterone and pituitary hormone release. The octapeptide angiotensin II (Ang II) is the major active component of the RAS and is generated by cleavage of the substrate, angiotensinogen, through the successive actions of two proteolytic enzymes, renin and angiotensin-converting enzyme (ACE). Ang II acts via two receptors, AT_1 and AT_2. Although originally viewed solely as a circulating system, all components of the RAS have been found in a variety of tissues, including brain, adrenal, heart, vessel wall, and kidney, suggesting the presence of tissue-specific systems participating in physiological and pathophysiological effects of the RAS (**Figure 1**).

Recently, the classical view of the RAS was changed by the discovery of the enzyme ACE2, a human homolog of ACE, and awareness that other angiotensin peptides, such as Ang IV and Ang 1–7, may have physiological actions.

Angiotensin Receptors

AT_1 Receptor

The AT_1 receptor mediates most of the classical actions of Ang II. It displays a seven transmembrane domain topology and is a member of the G-protein-coupled receptor family, with signaling predominantly via $G_{q/11}$, phosphoinositides, and calcium. In addition, AT_1 activation is linked to vascular and cardiac hypertrophy through transactivation of the epidermal growth factor (EGRF) and its signaling pathways, primarily through mitogen-activated protein (MAP) kinase activation. In rodents, two subtypes exist, AT_{1A} and AT_{1B}, which have 95% homology.

Many of the functions of Ang II are paralleled by the distribution of AT_1 receptors in cardiovascular, nervous, renal, endocrine, and reproductive tissues. In the central nervous system, AT_1 receptors are found in the circumventricular organs, including the subfornical organ (SFO) and vascular organ of the laminar terminalis (OVLT), and regions of the hypothalamus such as the paraventricular nucleus and median eminence, which regulate body fluid homeostasis. AT_1 receptors in the nucleus of the solitary tract and ventrolateral medulla reflect important roles of Ang II in cardiovascular control. In the periphery, AT_1 receptors occur in high levels in the zona glomerulosa of the adrenal cortex and adrenal medulla. In the

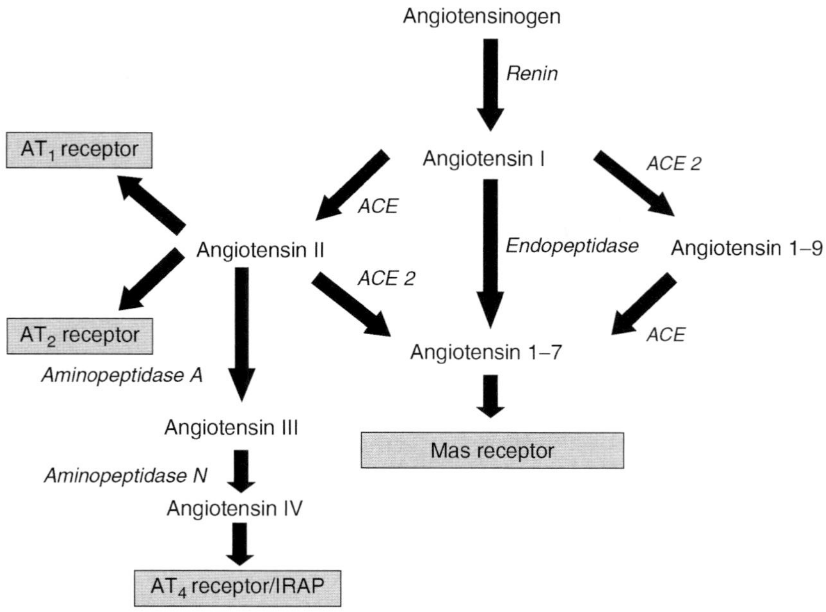

Figure 1 The renin-angiotensin system.

kidney, AT_1 receptors occur in glomeruli, proximal tubule, and medullary interstitial cells. AT_1 receptors occur on vascular smooth muscle cells and in the conduction system and vagal ganglia of the heart.

The antagonists losartan and candesartan are AT_1 selective and are used clinically to treat hypertension and cardiovascular disease.

AT_2 Receptor

The function and characteristics of the AT_2 receptor are less well understood. While it is also a seven transmembrane receptor, it shares only 34% homology with the AT_1 receptor. The signaling mechanisms are distinct from the AT_1 receptor and include stimulation of tyrosine or serine/threonine phosphatases, which inactivate MAP kinases, and potassium channel activation. AT_2 receptor stimulation may inhibit growth and promote apoptosis, thereby opposing actions at the AT_1 receptor.

The AT_2 receptor is highly expressed during fetal development and rapidly declines at birth. In the adult brain, AT_2 receptors are constrained to the molecular layer of the cerebellum, thalamus, and superior colliculus. In neurons, AT_2 receptor activation may result in hyperpolarization and decreased excitability via enhanced K^+ channel activity. In the periphery, it is found within the adrenal medulla, cardiac fibroblasts, and the non-pregnant uterus. Expression of the AT_2 receptor is upregulated in pathological conditions such as heart failure, renal failure, vascular injury, and wound healing. AT_2 receptor stimulation also induces vasodilation mediated by bradykinin, nitric oxide, and cyclic GMP. The AT_2 receptor also binds directly to the AT_1 receptor, and may antagonize its function via this heterodimerization.

The AT_2 receptor is selectively inhibited by the nonpeptide compound PD 123319 while the peptide analog CGP 42112A acts as a partial agonist.

AT_4 Receptor

The hexapeptide fragment of angiotensin (3–8) (Ang IV) has actions distinct from Ang II and binds to a novel binding site distinct from the AT_1 and AT_2 receptors. The AT_4 receptor is a type II integral membrane protein identical to the insulin-regulated aminopeptidase (IRAP), a zinc metallopeptidase of the M1 family that translocates rapidly to the cell surface after insulin stimulation.

The AT_4/IRAP receptor occurs abundantly in the brain within in the neocortex, CA1 to CA3 regions of the hippocampus and motor nuclei, where it is closely associated with cholinergic neurons, consistent with the memory-enhancing properties of Ang IV. In the periphery, it is found in blood vessels, cortex, and outer stripe of the outer medulla of the kidney and adrenal medulla and cortex. Its main peripheral physiological effect is vasodilation.

Two N-terminally modified analogs of Ang IV have high affinities for the AT_4 receptor: Nle^1-Ang IV and norleucinal Ang IV and exhibit agonist properties along with a structurally distinct peptide, LVV-hemorphin 7.

Ang 1–7 Receptor

A possible role for Ang 1–7 as a cardioprotective peptide with vasodilator, diuretic, and antiproliferative effects has recently been suggested. The Ang 1–7 receptor may be the G-protein-coupled receptor Mas, encoded by the Mas1 proto-oncogene.

Actions of Angiotensin

Fluid and Electrolyte Balance

Ang II rapidly induces drinking, whether administered peripherally, where it acts on AT_1 receptors within the circumventricular organs, or centrally, where the lamina terminalis encompassing the median preoptic nucleus is the principal site of action.

Centrally administered Ang II also stimulates salt appetite. This action is blocked by centrally administered AT_1 and AT_2 receptor antagonists; however, the central sites of action of Ang II-induced salt appetite have yet to be determined. Mineralocorticoids have a major influence over this stimulus and are believed to have a concomitant action with the RAS in initiating salt appetite.

Blood Pressure Regulation

Infusion of Ang II into the periphery or brain raises blood pressure. Peripheral administration of Ang II increases arterial pressure via increased vascular resistance, a consequence of both direct action on vascular smooth muscle and central actions resulting in activation of the sympathetic nervous system and stimulation of vasopressin release.

In a genetic animal model, the spontaneous hypertensive rat (SHR), the brain Ang II system is overactive. Higher levels of Ang II and angiotensin receptors have been observed, and the SHR exhibits an exaggerated pressor response to central Ang II.

Hormone Release

Ang II has several roles as a neuropeptide. Central infusion of Ang II is a potent stimulant for the release of vasopressin. Ang II may also participate in cyclic regulation of reproductive hormones. Plasma Ang II is raised in the luteal phase of the menstrual cycle, and administered Ang II elevates plasma levels of luteinizing hormone during this phase.

Behavior

The RAS, either acting directly or through the modulation of various neurotransmitters, has been implicated in a range of behavioral and cognitive processes. While there is conflicting evidence of the role of Ang II in memory and learning, it is clear that central infusions of Ang IV facilitate memory retention and retrieval in rats. Ang IV promotes learning in passive avoidance and spatial memory tasks, and reverses memory deficits induced by scopolamine-induced amnesia and bilateral perforant pathway lesions. The mechanisms of how AT_4 ligands mediate their effects are unclear, but may involve interactions with brain cholinergic systems, modulation of neural glucose metabolism, or inhibition of neuropeptide metabolism by IRAP.

Pathophysiology of the RAS

The local tissue RAS has important effects on the pathological changes of organ structure that are mediated by altered modulated gene expression, growth, fibrosis, and the inflammatory response.

Hypertension

The RAS regulates blood pressure, and inhibitors of the system have important therapeutic actions in treating hypertension. ACE inhibitors are widely used in hypertension and cardiovascular and renal disorders. AT_1 antagonists, such as losartan and candesartan, are increasingly used in hypertension and are well tolerated.

Cardiac Hypertrophy

Cardiac hypertrophy is characterized by increased deposition of extracellular matrix (ECM) constituents, proliferation of cardiac fibroblasts, and hypertrophic growth of cardiac myocytes, which alter the contractile properties of the heart.

The RAS is a key mediator of cardiac adaptations to hemodynamic overload. Ang II directly induces cellular responses in myocardial cells. In cultured cardiac fibroblasts, Ang II stimulates fibroblast proliferation, collagen synthesis, and the expression of ECM proteins such as fibronectin via activation of the AT_1 receptor. In cardiac myocytes, Ang II exerts a direct growth-promoting effect on only neonatal cells, and thus may act indirectly by inducing the expression of growth factors such as TGF-β_1.

Both clinical and experimental studies demonstrate a favorable impact of AT_1 antagonists and ACE inhibitor therapy on the progressive remodeling and ventricular dysfunction of cardiac hypertrophy by reducing the action of Ang II. In addition, the beneficial effect of ACE inhibition might be related to local accumulation of bradykinin.

Microvascular Injury

Kidney Both ACE inhibitors and AT_1 antagonists exert protective effects in chronic renal disease by improving glomerular filtration, preventing glomerular and tubulointerstitial toxicity of ultrafiltered proteins, and limiting the direct nephrotoxic effects of Ang II, especially in diabetes.

Eye Neovascularization in the retina of diabetic patients is a major cause of visual loss. There is a large body of evidence for a local RAS within the eye that is activated in diabetes. This appears to be directly responsible for an increase in vascular endothelial growth factor (VEGF) that is implicated in the pathogenesis of diabetic retinopathy. Inhibition of ACE appears to reduce concentrations of VEGF, with a concurrent antiproliferative effect independent of systemic VEGF levels or blood pressure. AT_1 receptor blockade has been shown to reduce neovascularization independent of VEGF levels in animal models. This may be due to antagonism of activation of MAP kinase, which is a potent cellular proliferation stimulator, by Ang II.

Brain Circulating and locally formed Ang II controls cerebral blood flow by AT_1 receptor stimulation in cerebral vessels and sympathetic nerves. The Perindopril Protection against Recurrent Stroke Study (PROGRESS) has shown that ACE inhibitor therapy combined with diuretics can decrease recurrence of stroke by 44% in hypertensive patients and by 42% in nonhypertensive patients. Chronic AT_1 blockade inhibits brain and cerebral artery AT_1 receptor and reduces cortical ischemia and tissue swelling produced by middle cerebral artery occlusion with reperfusion.

Atherosclerosis

Ang II plays a critical role in the initiation and progression of atherosclerosis via promotion of superoxide production and acting as a pro-inflammatory molecule, with resultant local inflammation and tissue damage. Treatment with ACE inhibitors or AT_1 antagonists may slow progression of atherosclerosis. This is in part associated with decreased expression of inflammatory mediators and improved endothelial function.

The RAS and Stress

Both brain and peripheral Ang II participate in the stress response. In response to stress, AT_1 receptor expression increases in the hypothalamic paraventricular nucleus and median eminence, key sites controlling the hypothalamic-pituitary-adrenal (HPA) axis. Concurrently, there is increased synthesis and release of corticotropin-releasing factor (CRF) from the median eminence and adrenocorticotropic hormone (ACTH) from the anterior pituitary and consequently adrenal glucocorticoid responses (**Figure 2**). Associated with this are central actions that contribute to enhanced peripheral sympathetic activity.

The increase in sympathetic stimulation leads to enhanced renin release, increased circulating Ang II, and, consequently, fluid retention and vasoconstriction, with increased blood pressure and heart rate.

The RAS has been implicated in a number of experimental models of stress. Restraint stress in rats increases AT_1 receptor levels in the hypothalamic paraventricular nucleus, SFO, and median eminence, consistent with roles in HPA activation. Concurrent changes in Ang II receptor number in the anterior pituitary and adrenal zona glomerulosa and medulla parallel the peripheral influences of the RAS on the

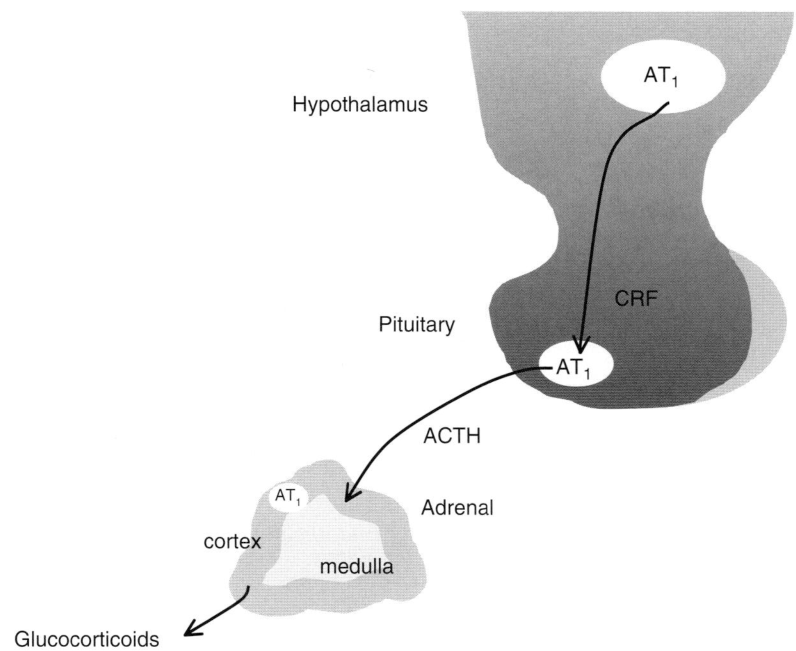

Figure 2 Angiotensin II and the stress response.

HPA axis. Isolation stress enhances brain Ang II receptor numbers, which can be suppressed by AT_1 receptor antagonists. Conversely, central AT_1 receptor antagonism attenuates stress-induced sympathetic nervous and adrenomedullary responses.

The SHR is more susceptible to stress than normotensive Wistar-Kyoto (WKY) rats, and has an overactive central RAS. Differential expression of AT_{1A}:AT_{1B} receptors is observed in the HPA of SHR, and Ang II produces an exaggerated response of ACTH and corticosterone.

See Also the Following Articles

Adrenal Cortex; Adrenal Medulla; Angiotensin; Kidney Function.

Further Reading

Albiston, A. L., Mustafa, T., McDowall, S. G., et al. (2003). AT4 receptor is insulin-regulated membrane aminopeptidase: potential mechanisms of memory enhancement. *Trends in Endocrinology and Metabolism* **14**, 72–77.

Ferrario, C. M. and Chappell, M. C. (2004). Novel angiotensin peptides. *Cellular and Molecular Life Sciences* **61**, 2720–2727.

Gallinat, S., Busche, S., Raizada, M. K. and Sumners, C. (2000). The angiotensin II type 2 receptor: an enigma with multiple variations. *American Journal of Physiology, Endocrinology and Metabolism* **278**, E357–E374.

Gard, P. R. (2004). Angiotensin as a target for the treatment of Alzheimer's disease, anxiety and depression. *Expert Opinion on Therapeutic Targets* **8**, 1–8.

Kaschina, E. and Unger, T. (2003). Angiotensin AT1/AT2 receptors: regulation, signalling and function. *Blood Pressure* **12**, 70–88.

Kim, S. and Iwao, H. (2000). Molecular and cellular mechanisms of angiotensin II-mediated cardiovascular and renal diseases. *Pharmacological Reviews* **52**, 11–34.

McKinley, M. J., Albiston, A. L., Allen, A. M., et al. (2003). The brain renin-angiotensin system: location and physiological roles. *International Journal of Biochemistry and Cell Biology* **35**, 901–918.

Saavedra, J. M., Ando, H., Armando, I., et al. (2004). Brain angiotensin II, an important stress hormone: regulatory sites and therapeutic opportunities. *Annals of the New York Academy of Sciences* **1018**, 76–84.

Saavedra, J. M. J., Ando, H., Armando, I., et al. (2005). Anti-stress and anti-anxiety effects of centrally acting angiotensin II AT1 receptor antagonists. *Regulatory Peptides* **128**, 227–238.

Unger, T. (2002). The role of the renin-angiotensin system in the development of cardiovascular disease. *American Journal of Cardiology* **89**(2A), 3–9.

Watanabe, T., Fujioka, T., Hashimoto, M. and Nakamura, S. (1998). Stress and brain angiotensin II receptors. *Critical Reviews of Neurobiology* **12**, 305–317.

Wright, J. W. and Harding, J. W. (2004). The brain angiotensin system and extracellular matrix molecules in neural plasticity, learning, and memory. *Progress in Neurobiology* **72**, 263–293.

Primate Models, Cardiovascular Disease

J R Kaplan
Wake Forest University School of Medicine, Winston Salem, NC, USA

This is a revised version of the article by J R Kaplan, Encyclopedia of Stress, First edition, volume 3, pp 230–235, © 2000, Elsevier Inc.

Glossary

Abnormal coronary vascular reactivity — The tendency for coronary arteries to lose their ability to dilate rather than constrict as demand for blood is increased.

Atherosclerosis — A gruel-like accumulation of fatty substance in the intima (inner layer) of the large muscular and elastic arteries of the body.

Beta-blocker — A class of drugs that inhibits the activation of the sympathetic nervous system (i.e., heart rate, blood pressure, and cardiac output) by blocking the response of β-adrenergic receptors in the arteries and heart.

Coronary heart disease (CHD) — A disease spectrum subsuming myocardial infarction (heart attack), angina pectoris (ischemic chest pain), and disruptions to the rhythm and electrical activity of the heart.

Dominant/subordinate social status — The position that an animal occupies in a pecking order. High-status animals (dominants) predictably defeat low-status animals (subordinates) in competitive encounters. Subordinate animals generally exhibit signs of stress (e.g., exaggerated release of cortisol from the adrenal cortex and behavioral withdrawal).

Endothelium — The inner wall of the artery; a normally functioning endothelium causes the artery to dilate and constrict appropriately in response to blood flow.

Heart rate reactivity — The degree to which an individual's heart rate increases in response to stressful situations. High heart rate reactivity is probably due to excessive activation of the sympathetic nervous system, and it is associated with the increased development of atherosclerosis in people and monkeys.

Hypertension A sustained increase in blood pressure.

Ischemia A reduction in blood flow to an organ or tissue, due to obstruction (e.g., a blood clot), arterial constriction, atherosclerosis, or a combination of factors.

Plasma lipids Fats or fatlike substances (insoluble in water) that include total plasma cholesterol (TPC), high-density lipoprotein cholesterol (HDLC), and low-density lipoprotein cholesterol (LDLC). In general, TPC = HDLC + LDLC. Elevations in plasma levels of LDLC (and the resulting increases in TPC) are highly atherogenic. High plasma concentrations of HDLC (the good cholesterol) are protective.

Quantitative coronary angiography An imaging procedure in which an opaque dye is infused into the coronary arteries, allowing them to be visualized radiographically and measured.

Sympathetic nervous system (SNS) That part of the involuntary or self-regulating nervous system that controls responses (e.g., heart rate and blood pressure increases) to stressful situations.

Cardiovascular disease is manifested most prominently in human beings as coronary heart disease (CHD) and stroke. Atherosclerosis in the coronary arteries is a usual cause of CHD, whereas atherosclerosis in the cerebral arteries contributes to both transient ischemic attacks and ischemic stroke. Epidemiological and clinical studies have provided considerable evidence that behavioral factors influence the development of cardiovascular disease and the underlying atherosclerosis. However, logistical and ethical considerations prevent many questions regarding risk factors and mechanisms from being addressed directly in people. Animal models offer an alternative means of answering such questions.

Nonhuman Primates as Animal Models

The ideal animal for evaluating behavioral influences on cardiovascular disease would respond to a fat- and cholesterol-containing diet by exhibiting both an intimal accumulation of atherosclerosis in the large proximal coronary arteries and a susceptibility to infarction and ischemia. Furthermore, this animal would resemble human beings in cardiovascular and reproductive physiology and in neurobiology. Finally, the animal's behavioral responses and characteristics would vary along dimensions (e.g., aggressiveness and competitiveness, social support) analogous to those thought important in the epidemiology of atherosclerosis and CHD in human beings. Of all animal models, the nonhuman primates best approximate the foregoing characteristics.

Numerous investigators have used primates to explore one facet or another of the hypothesis that behaviorally evoked, excessive perturbations of the body's principal axes of neuroendocrine response (i.e., the adrenal cortex or the SNS) may produce pathophysiological consequences. Some of these studies provide data regarding the influence of stress on the risk factors for cardiovascular disease (e.g., elevations in plasma lipids and blood pressure) or on mediating factors (circulating concentrations of immune or inflammatory markers), whereas others have focused primarily on the characteristics of atherosclerotic lesions or abnormalities in vascular reactivity to changes in blood flow. Taken together, existing studies present a clear and convincing case that behavioral factors (either stressful environments or particular characteristics of temperament) influence both atherosclerosis and clinical events in ways that have relevance for human beings.

Behavioral Influences on Risk Factors for Cardiovascular Disease

Plasma Lipids

Elevations in plasma lipids (e.g., total plasma cholesterol, TPC; low-density lipoprotein cholesterol, LDLC) are associated with the exacerbation of atherosclerosis and increased risk of CHD and ischemic stroke. Thus, behavioral factors may contribute to cardiovascular disease through a mechanism involving adverse changes in plasma lipids. Among primates, the lipids of squirrel monkeys (*Saimiri sciurius*, a New World primate) seem particularly susceptible to behavioral influences. In one study, for example, there was an increase in plasma lipids as animals were transported from South America to a laboratory in the United States. Interestingly, both TPC and LDLC declined in these animals after they were put in a secluded environment, but increased again following exposure to a busy laboratory. All of these changes occurred in the absence of any cholesterol in the diet and are attributed most reasonably to the influence of psychic stress. Cholesterol-fed squirrel monkeys are similarly responsive to experimental manipulations; exposure to either a shock-avoidance paradigm (in which the animal presses a lever to avoid a shock) or a restraint box leads to a significant and sustained increase in TPC and LDLC.

Among the Old World monkeys, adverse serum lipid profiles have been observed in relation to individual differences in social status and individual differences in heart rate reactivity to stress. In both baboons (*Papio hamadrayas*) and cynomolgus macaques (*Macaca fascicularis*), for example, subordinate social status is associated with suppressed plasma concentrations of high-density lipoprotein cholesterol (HDLC), which is a risk factor for atherosclerosis. Notably, cynomolgus macaques that reliably exhibit exaggerated heart rate responses to psychological stress (e.g., exposure to a threatening object) also tend to have suppressed plasma concentrations of HDLC.

Data from Old and New World monkeys suggest that stressful environments, low social status, and exaggerated SNS responsivity to challenge are all associated with potentially harmful plasma lipid profiles. Among human beings, there are also numerous observations relating either elevations in LDLC or reductions in HDLC to stressful circumstances or particular personality characteristics.

Blood Pressure

Elevated blood pressure (hypertension) is associated with increased risk of CHD and stroke. High blood pressure also exacerbates atherosclerosis in the coronary and cerebral arteries. Numerous studies indicate that behavioral stress can lead to sustained, potentially pathogenic increases in both systolic and diastolic blood pressure. For example, squirrel monkeys trained to avoid a shock by pressing a lever ultimately exhibit increases in blood pressure that persist across experimental sessions. Rhesus monkeys (*M. mulatta*) exposed to a similar manipulation also develop a steady elevation in blood pressure. Further, rhesus monkeys as well as baboons experience sustained increases in blood pressure when light signals and shock are paired and combined with a bar press for the delivery of food (called conflict manipulation). Chronic exposure to loud noise also produces elevated blood pressure in cynomolgus and rhesus macaques. Notably, adult male baboons that typically live together with a number of females in a harem develop hypertension when they are separated from their harems and forced to watch the females feed first. Males also exhibit a hypertensive response when they are separated from their harems and are forced to observe a new male being introduced to these females. These latter manipulations are purely social and more closely model the kind of stress most likely to affect human beings.

Behavioral Influences on Atherosclerosis

Atherosclerosis in Males

Primates typically do not develop atherosclerosis to any significant degree unless they are fed a diet relatively high in saturated fat and cholesterol, similar to the diet often consumed by people living in industrialized nations. Early investigations used physical restraint or exposure to a shock-avoidance manipulation to provide evidence that psychic stress, in combination with an atherogenic diet, could potentiate atherosclerosis in monkeys. However, social manipulations also influence the development of atherosclerosis in monkeys. For example, when cynomolgus males are housed in groups that either remain stable in composition or that are perturbed (by distributing members across groups), dominant and subordinate animals tend to retain their relative rankings irrespective of social condition (i.e., stable or unstable groups). A quantitative evaluation of the coronary arteries of such animals revealed that monkeys housed in an unstable condition had significantly more coronary artery atherosclerosis than animals in a stable environment but only if they were dominant in their groups. This finding suggests that the behavioral demands of retaining dominant social status in an unstable social setting potentiate atherosclerosis, at least in males of this species consuming an atherogenic diet. A similar pattern was obtained (although with markedly smaller lesions), among animals that consumed a diet modeled on the recommendations of the American Heart Association. Thus, behavioral factors might, even in the absence of dietary provocation, cause damage that could initiate the earliest lesions of atherosclerosis. Subsequent investigations have shown that exposure to the stress of social perturbation for as little as 72 h can cause the degeneration and death of endothelial cells, thus marking the first stage of atherosclerosis progression.

Mediating Role of Sympathetic Nervous System Activation in the Atherosclerosis of Males

Significantly, behavioral effects observed in the social manipulation experiments were independent of variation in serum lipid concentrations and resting blood pressure. Numerous investigators have proposed that recurrent SNS activation in response to behavioral stimulation could promote the development of atherosclerosis and its clinical sequelae. Testing the hypothesis that excessive SNS activation might have potentiated atherogenesis among dominant animals in the foregoing studies, male monkeys in a subsequent investigation were all housed in unstable social groups and fed an atherogenic diet; here, half of the monkeys also received a beta-blocker, propranolol, throughout the 2-year study. Untreated dominant monkeys again had twice the amount of atherosclerosis of their subordinate counterparts, replicating the results from the unstable treatment condition of earlier experiments. Dominant monkeys treated with propranolol, however, developed less than half the coronary atherosclerosis of untreated dominants and had roughly the same extent of lesion as both treated and untreated subordinate animals. Hence, the more pronounced atherosclerosis characteristic of untreated (i.e., autonomically intact) dominant monkeys, when housed in groups of rotating membership and fed a cholesterol containing diet, can be prevented by the long-term administration of a beta-blocker and is therefore dependent on concomitant SNS activation. Furthermore, the monkey studies also provide evidence that behaviorally induced SNS activation initiates atherogenesis independently of the presence of a high-fat diet. Hence, the endothelial cell death associated with the short-term (72-h) perturbation previously described occurs in the absence of elevated plasma lipids and can be inhibited by pretreatment with a beta-blocker.

Other data from this species further support the speculation that a heightened SNS responsivity to behavioral stimuli increases the risk for atherosclerosis. Specifically, cynomolgus macaques display reliable and significant individual differences in heart rate response (assessed via radiotelemetry) to a standardized social stressor (exposure to an unknown human). Animals can thus be characterized as either high or low in heart rate reactivity to stress. Notably, the atherosclerotic lesions of high heart rate reactors are twice as large as those of their low-reactive counterparts. Taken together, the results of the macaque experiments indicate that some individuals (e.g., high heart rate reactors) may be susceptible to the development of atherosclerosis because of an intrinsic SNS hyperresponsivity to behavioral stimuli, whereas others (dominant individuals in unstable social environments) may be at increased risk because of frequent elicitation of such responses in stressful environments. SNS activation, provoked in either of two ways, may thus provide the common pathway by which pathogenesis is mediated in male monkeys.

Summary for Male Monkeys

The studies of male monkeys relate a behavioral predisposition (social dominance, i.e., successful aggression) and excessive SNS stimulation to the exacerbation of atherosclerosis. Both domains appear to have analogs among human beings. There are other behavioral risk factors, however, about which the studies in male monkeys provide little data or insight. Such factors include depression, sleep disturbances, and a propensity to anxiety or panic, all of which have been associated reliably with elevated risk of CHD in human beings. Moreover, social support is often believed to be cardioprotective. Although several measures of social support have been evaluated in the foregoing studies of male monkeys, there is no evidence that animals differing by these measures vary in their extent of atherosclerosis.

Sex Differences in Atherosclerosis

The relative sparing of premenopausal women compared to men of similar ages is a prominent feature of CHD, ischemic stroke, and atherosclerosis. Although this phenomenon is sometimes referred to as female protection, it is characterized more accurately as a delay in disease onset, with the incidence curve for women lagging behind that of men by approximately 10 years. The various effects of estrogen are believed to account for most of this sex difference, at least with respect to CHD incidence and underlying atherosclerosis. Not only are premenopausal women protected from CHD, but the provision of estrogen replacement to women immediately prior to or immediately following menopause is associated with a significant reduction in CHD risk (it must be noted that such protection is not apparent when hormone therapy is initiated in women with preexisting disease or who are 10 or more years postmenopausal).

Because atherosclerosis progresses over decades, it is likely that the clinical events occurring in postmenopausal women have their beginnings in the premenopausal years. This conclusion is supported by autopsy assessments showing that by 34 years of age, at least one-third of all women (regardless of race) have raised lesions in their coronary arteries. *In vivo* arterial imaging also demonstrates the presence of relatively extensive focal atherosclerosis in premenopausal women. The observations that atherosclerosis begins premenopausally raises the question of whether there are particular risk factors that place some women on a higher-risk trajectory than others. Considerable effort has been focused on this question in studies employing premenopausal monkeys as a model of reproductive-age women. The major results of these studies are described next.

Social Stress and Female Protection from Atherosclerosis in Monkeys

Investigations using socially housed female cynomolgus monkeys provide evidence that stress-induced ovarian dysfunction eliminates premenopausal protection from atherosclerosis. For example, in one 2-year experiment contrasting the atherosclerosis of socially housed males and females, the females were divided into groups of five. Each of these groups contained a vasectomized male; additional males were placed together in groups of five. All animals consumed an atherogenic diet. Quantitative evaluation of the coronary arteries at the end of this experiment demonstrated that female protection with regard to atherosclerosis extended only to the dominant animals (i.e., those ranking first or second in their social groups); subordinate females (ranking third or below) were indistinguishable from males. Subordinate females also had five times as many anovulatory cycles and three times as many cycles characterized by luteal-phase progesterone deficiencies as did their dominant counterparts. Notably, females with the most extensive atherosclerosis were all subordinate, and all had marked ovarian endocrine dysfunction. These data suggest that the stress of social subordination may increase the risk of atherosclerosis in females by inducing a relative ovarian endocrine deficiency state similar to that observed in postmenopausal women. Interestingly, investigations in premenopausal women also have also linked stress-induced estrogen deficiency to severity of angiographically documented CHD.

In a further study, ovariectomized females were placed in social groups for the same amount of time and fed the same diet as the reproductively intact females just described. The ovariectomized females as a group had significantly more extensive coronary artery atherosclerosis than the intact females. This effect was due entirely to the loss of protection experienced by the ovariectomized dominant animals compared with their intact counterparts. The subordinates, intact and ovariectomized, were affected equally with atherosclerosis. Additional studies have extended these findings by showing that the treatment of premenopausal females with either an oral contraceptive or unopposed estrogen treatment eliminates the difference between dominant and subordinate individuals. Parenthetically, it should be noted that subordinate females tended to be hypercortisolemic compared to dominants, leading some scientists to suggest that the atherosclerosis distinctions between such animals may be mediated in part by the excessive activation of the hypothalamic-pituitary-adrenocortical axis. The fact that dominant and subordinate animals continue to differ in adrenocortical activation – but not atherosclerosis extent – following ovariectomy argues against this hypothesis.

Finally, a recent life-course study demonstrated that premenopausal behavioral and hormonal status predict postmenopausal atherosclerosis outcomes independently of any postmenopausal hormone exposure. Specifically, females that were subordinate in their social groups – and thus were ovarian-suppressed and estrogen-deficient – developed more atherosclerosis premenopausally and postmenopausally than did their dominant, ovarian-normal counterparts. Significantly, the worsened atherosclerosis of the subordinate, socially stressed individuals could be mitigated by premenopausal treatment with exogenous estrogen in the form of an oral contraceptive. This important set of observations implies for women that premenopausal behavioral and associated hormonal (estrogenic) characteristics establish the trajectory of atherosclerosis progression that ultimately culminates in postmenopausal CHD events. The monkey research thus emphasizes the importance of early pathogenesis and early intervention, a perspective supported by recent reevaluations of clinical trial data.

The different patterns in which social status influences atherosclerosis in male and female monkeys deserves comment. Subordinate female primates, like subordinate and stressed females of many other mammalian species, tend to experience impaired ovarian function. This impairment eliminates female protection from atherosclerosis in monkeys and, by implication, women. Subordinate male monkeys also experience stress, possibly including impaired reproductive activity; however, the physiological sequelae of social subordination among males do not seem to affect the coronary arteries. Instead, dominant males in unstable settings are predisposed to atherosclerosis because they experience marked elevations in artery-damaging SNS activity as they attempt to maintain behavioral preeminence in the face of challenge.

Social Isolation, Depression, and Atherosclerosis in Females

The exacerbation of atherosclerosis in female monkeys is also observed in conjunction with single-cage housing (i.e., social separation). Specifically, females housed in single cages have significantly more coronary artery atherosclerosis than comparably treated animals housed in social groups. Single-caged animals are most similar in atherosclerosis extent to socially housed subordinates. Interestingly, this worsening of atherosclerosis among single-caged females is not related to ovarian impairment; rather, such animals exhibit elevations in heart rate. This latter observation suggests that, at least in female monkeys, social separation exacerbates coronary artery atherosclerosis via exaggerated SNS activity. No similar studies have been done in male monkeys. This outcome in females is, however, consistent with extensive literature documenting the cardioprotective effects of social support and the detrimental impact on CHD of social isolation in human beings.

Epidemiological studies have linked depression to CHD, and it is well known that women suffer from a higher incidence of depression than men. The role of depression in the coronary artery atherosclerosis of female monkeys has not been systematically evaluated, in part because primate depression usually has been studied with respect to developmental abnormalities caused by early separation of infants from their mothers. Recently, however, it has been shown that a proportion of socially housed, premenopausal cynomolgus monkeys exhibited behavioral and physiological characteristics that model adult human depression. This model offers for the first time the possibility of determining experimentally whether depression is causally associated with the development of atherosclerosis, the primary underlying cause of CHD.

Behaviorally Induced Abnormalities in Vascular Reactivity

Evaluation of Abnormalities in Vascular Reactivity

Numerous investigators have proposed that behavioral stress contributes to the occurrence of myocardial ischemia by causing the arteries to constrict inappropriately, thus cutting off the flow of blood to the heart. The potential for ischemia is evaluated by assessing the responses of coronary arteries to the infusion of vasoactive substances in the context of behavioral investigations. The normal endothelium, for example, dilates in response to acetylcholine. In contrast, endothelial damage causes a paradoxical constriction in response to acetylcholine. Nitroglycerine, an endothelium-independent dilator, reliably causes arterial dilation irrespective of the condition of the endothelium. Using such vasoactive substances and appropriate imaging techniques, it is now possible to visualize and quantitate the responsivity of the coronary arteries of monkeys exposed to various kinds of stress. Such functional assessments have markedly extended the usefulness of monkeys in cardiovascular research.

Studies in Male Monkeys

In one such study, quantitative coronary angiography was used to evaluate arterial responses to acetylcholine and nitroglycerine in male cynomolgus monkeys that either were or were not exposed to the stress of repeated reorganization of social-group membership (i.e., social instability). The coronary arteries of animals living in unstable groups constricted in response to acetylcholine, whereas those of monkeys from stable groups dilated. Significantly, the degree of constriction observed in this experiment was independent of the extent of the underlying atherosclerosis; animals with little atherosclerosis but living in unstable groups had a degree of constriction equivalent to unstable monkeys that had extensive atherosclerosis. In contrast, monkeys living in stable groups dilated, irrespective of the amount of atherosclerosis.

The previous study, and others like it, demonstrate that chronic social stress impairs endothelium-dependent vascular responses, an effect that is not necessarily dependent on the extent of atherosclerosis. It should be noted that none of these investigations revealed an influence of dominance status on vascular reactivity. Hence, the pattern of behavioral influences on blood flow (and thus on ischemia) differs somewhat from that observed with respect to atherosclerosis, at least among socially housed cynomolgus males.

Studies in Female Monkeys

As with atherosclerosis, behavioral influences on vascular reactivity among females are apparently mediated by social subordination and ovarian dysfunction. Hence, the coronary arteries of socially subordinate female cynomolgus monkeys, compared to dominants, constrict in response to acetylcholine. In contrast, nitroglycerine dilates the arteries of all monkeys, irrespective of status. As in the other studies, subordinates here were characterized by ovarian dysfunction (low plasma estradiol and luteal-phase abnormalities in progesterone). Notably, the extent of vascular constriction in response to acetylcholine was directly related to the degree of ovarian impairment as indicated by plasma estradiol concentrations on the day of testing. These observations not only demonstrate the role of behavioral factors on coronary vascular reactivity among females, they emphasize again the cardioprotective significance of normal ovarian function.

Summary

Systematic studies in nonhuman primates have shown that stress, both social and nonsocial, consistently affects the risk factors for CHD and the underlying atherosclerosis. Studies involving socially housed individuals are probably of most relevance to human beings; such investigations have focused primarily on the development of coronary artery atherosclerosis in macaque monkeys. Stress clearly exacerbates atherosclerosis in these animals, albeit differently in males and females.

Among males, dominant individuals in unstable settings and those who exhibit exaggerated heart rate reactivity to challenge are at greatest risk. These outcomes are most likely mediated by excessive SNS activation. These findings are reminiscent of observations in men linking excessive hostility and high heart rate reactivity to increased CHD risk. The monkey results imply that the pathogenicity of hostility (approximated in the animals by social dominance) is most prominent under stressful disrupted social conditions. Notably, indices of social support have not been found to predict patterns of atherosclerosis among male monkeys.

The situation among females is different. Normal ovarian function seems critical for the premenopausal inhibition of atherosclerosis among animals consuming a diet relatively high in fat and cholesterol. Notably, among groups of females, animals occupying the lower status positions are stressed and experience ovarian impairment and relative estrogen deficiency. Such individuals are characterized by a rapid acceleration of premenopausal atherosclerosis, which can be inhibited by exogenous estrogen. A novel observation is that the atherosclerosis trajectory established by premenopausal behavioral and hormonal conditions predicts the postmenopausal atherosclerosis extent. These findings suggest that primary prevention of CHD in women should begin prior to or immediately at menopause. The studies in female monkeys also identify social isolation and social support as potential factors affecting disease risk. Systematic studies of the role played by depression in the development of atherosclerosis have not yet been conducted, but they hold promise for the future.

Further Reading

Bairey Merz, C. N., Johnson, B. D., Sharaf, B. L., et al. (2003). Hypoestrogenemia of hypothalamic origin and coronary artery disease in premenopausal women: a report from the NHLBI-sponsored WISE study. *Journal of the American College of Cardiology* **41**, 413–419.

Cohen, S., Kaplan, J. R. and Manuck, S. B. (1994). Social support and coronary heart disease: underlying psychologic and biologic mechanisms. In: Schumaker, S. & Czajkowski, S. M. (eds.) *Social support and cardiovascular disease*, pp. 195–221. New York: Plenum Press.

Henry, J. P. and Stephens, P. M. (1977). *Stress, health and the social environment: a sociobiologic approach to medicine*. New York: Springer-Verlag.

Kaplan, J. R. and Manuck, S. B. (1999). Status, stress, and atherosclerosis: the role of environment and individual behavior. *Annals of the New York Academy of Sciences* **896**, 145–161.

Kaplan, J. R. and Manuck, S. B. (2004). Ovarian dysfunction, stress, and disease: a primate continuum. *ILAR Journal* **45**, 89–115.

Kaplan, J. R., Manuck, S. B., Anthony, M. S., et al. (2002). Premenopausal social status and hormone exposure predict postmenopausal atherosclerosis in female monkeys. *Obstetrics and Gynecology* **99**(3), 381–388.

Kaplan, J. R., Manuck, S. B., Clarkson, T. B., et al. (1985). Animal models of behavioral influences on atherogenesis. *Advances in Behavioral Medicine* **1**, 115–163.

Klaiber, E. L., Vogel, W. and Rako, S. (2005). A critique of the Women's Health Initiative hormone therapy study. *Fertility and Sterility* **84**, 1589–1601.

Mikkola, T. S. and Clarkson, T. B. (2006). Coronary heart disease and postmenopausal therapy: conundrum explained by timing? *Journal of Women's Health* **15**, 51–53.

Rozanski, A., Blumenthal, J. A. and Kaplan, J. R. (1999). Impact of psychological factors on the pathogenesis of cardiovascular disease and implications for therapy. *Circulation* **99**, 2192–2217.

Schneiderman, N. (1987). Psychophysiologic factors in atherogenesis and coronary artery disease. *Circulation* **76**(supplement I), I41–I47.

Shively, C. S., Register, T. C., Friedman, D. P., et al. (2005). Social stress-associated depression in adult female cynomolgus monkeys (*Macaca fascicularis*). *Biological Psychology* **69**, 67–84.

Skantze, H. B., Kaplan, J., Pettersson, K., et al. (1998). Psychosocial stress causes endothelial injury in cynomolgus monkeys via α_1-adrenoceptor activation. *Atherosclerosis* **136**, 153–161.

D. Reproduction, Effects on

Gender and Stress

R J Handa and W C J Chung
Colorado State University, Fort Collins, CO, USA

This is a revised version of the article by R J Handa and R F McGivern, Encyclopedia of Stress, First edition, volume 2, pp 196–204, © 2000, Elsevier Inc.

Glossary

5α-Dihydrotestosterone (DHT) Androgen responsible for the masculinization of the genitalia during development. It is metabolized from testosterone by the enzymatic actions of 5α-reductase.

α-Fetoprotein A protein produced by the liver. α-Fetoprotein can bind circulating estrogen and sequester it from the brain.

Activational actions of sex steroids The actions of estrogens and androgens that occur transiently, in direct response to the presence of hormone. Activational effects can occur at any time during life.

Aromatase An enzyme belonging to the P450 family of enzymes. Aromatase is primarily responsible for the metabolism of testosterone to estrogen.

Critical period of sexual differentiation The period of time when the central nervous system is most sensitive to the organizing actions of sex steroids. The timing and length of the critical period can vary depending on the species, parameter, and hormone examined.

Estrogen The main class of sex steroid hormones found in females. Estrogen is produced predominantly in the ovary; however, it can be produced *de novo* in other tissues and even in brain tissue in both women and men.

Organizational actions of sex steroids The actions of estrogen and androgen that result in permanent changes in the structure or function of the brain. Organizational effects result from exposure during development or during a period of high sensitivity to the hormone in question.

Testosterone The main class of sex steroid hormone found in males. Testosterone is produced predominantly by the testis; however, circulating testosterone is also found in females. Testosterone is metabolized to estrogenic as well as androgenic products.

Evidence Supporting Gender Differences in Stress Responses

Gender Differences in Adrenal Function

The early work of Hans Selye described adrenal gland function and its role in homeostasis. This work also provided the first compelling evidence for potential sex differences in stress responses. In supporting the observations of Selye, many studies showed that the adrenal gland is larger in females than in males, even when corrected for sex differences in body weight. Correspondingly, the rate of hormone secretion by the adrenal gland differs between males and females. Moreover, some studies in rodents reported that females show a greater diurnal fluctuation in corticosterone or cortisol, the main steroid hormone secreted by the adrenal cortex (corticosterone in the mouse and rat, cortisol in the hamster and human; **Figure 1**). Similarly, the adrenal response in secreting these glucocorticoid hormones following stressful, or perceived stressful, situations such as exposure to noxious fumes, exposure to a novel environment, immobilization, or a brief electric shock (see **Gleucocorticoid Negative Feedback, Glucocorticoids, Effects of Stress on, Glucocorticoids – Adverse Effects on the Nervous System,**) resulted in peak elevations in adrenal glucocorticoid hormone levels that were 1.5–2 times greater in females than in males.

In adult animal models, sex differences in adrenal function appear to be relatively confined to glucocorticoids because gender differences in other adrenal cortex-derived steroid hormones, such as progesterone and androgen, have not been reported in the literature. Androgen and progesterone are secreted predominantly by the gonads at relatively high levels. Therefore, gonad-derived steroids may mask any sex differences in adrenal-derived steroids, which may underlie the absence of these types of studies in the literature.

Sex Differences in Neuroendocrine Function

Pituitary hormone secretion The sex difference in adrenal function is in part due to sex differences in the neuroendocrine axis that regulates adrenal hormone secretion. This axis has been termed the hypothalamic-pituitary-adrenal (HPA) axis because of the interaction of each of these tissues in regulating one another's secretory activity (**Figure 1**). Similar to sex differences in the adrenal glucocorticoid release, adrenocorticotropic hormone (ACTH) is also released in a sexually dimorphic fashion. ACTH is a hormone secreted by the anterior pituitary gland into the general circulation, which in turn stimulates adrenal synthesis and secretion of glucocorticoids. Animal studies also demonstrated that the increases in circulating ACTH levels following physical or psychological stressors are greater and more prolonged in females than in males. An enhanced ACTH response in female rodents seems to depend on the hypothalamic peptide called corticotropin releasing hormone (CRH), suggesting that the sex difference in ACTH response

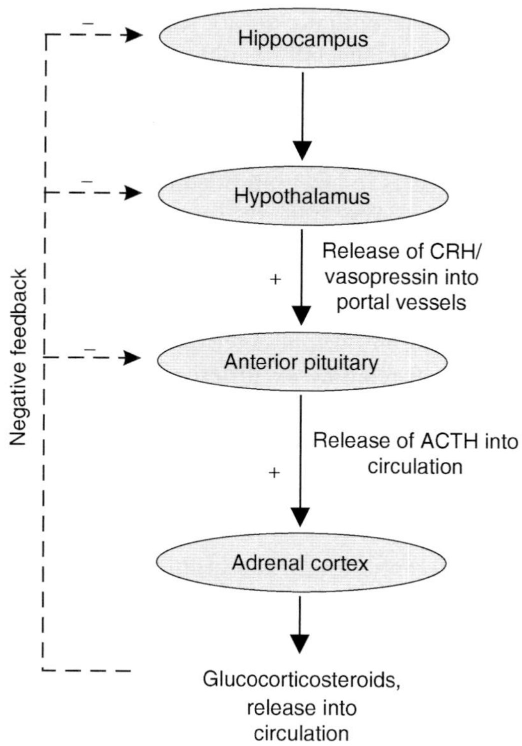

Figure 1 Schematic representation of the hypothalamic-pituitary-adrenal (HPA) axis. The positive feedback portion of the HPA starts at the level of the paraventricular nucleus of the hypothalamus. Neurons residing in this nucleus release corticotropin releasing hormone (CRH) and vasopressin into the hypophysial portal vessels to the anterior pituitary to stimulate the synthesis and release of ACTH. This in turn stimulates both synthesis and release of adrenal glucocorticoids into the general circulation to elicit an appropriate stress response. The presence of increased levels of glucocorticosteroids in turn induces an inhibitory effect (i.e., negative feedback) on the HPA axis, which is thought to be mainly mediated through glucocorticoid-responsive neurons in the hippocampus.

may, in part, be the result of a sex difference in anterior pituitary responsiveness to CRH.

Hypothalamic function The secretion of ACTH from the anterior pituitary is controlled by hormones that are synthesized in neurons residing in the paraventricular nucleus of the hypothalamus (PVN). These hormones are released into the hypophysial portal vasculature via the median eminence (**Figure 1**). The most important releasing factors for ACTH appear to be CRH and vasopressin. Both CRH and vasopressin are potent ACTH secretagogues, and vasopressin potentiates the ACTH-releasing activity of CRH several-fold. Animal studies have shown that the PVN in females contains more CRH neurons than in males. Moreover, females exhibited a more pronounced diurnal variation in hypothalamic CRH immunoreactivity than males. These data are consistent with physiological data demonstrating a greater activation of the HPA axis in females.

Studies have demonstrated sex differences in the release of vasopressin following a stressor. Indeed, vasopressin was released in female rats following immobilization stress, whereas this was not the case in male rats. Although, vasopressin immunoreactivity in the PVN is not sexually dimorphic, the presence of a sex difference in the functional sensitivity of vasopressin cells in the PVN to stressors may help explain sex differences in neuroendocrine responses.

Negative feedback regulation The stimulatory limb of the HPA axis (CRH, vasopressin, and ACTH) is kept in check by continuous feedback inhibition by circulating glucocorticoid hormones. Thus, it has been hypothesized that the intensity of this negative feedback action may be an underlying factor in the sexually dimorphic secretion of adrenal glucocorticoid hormones. The negative feedback glucocorticoids is mediated by two receptor types – mineralocorticoid receptor (MR) and glucocorticoid receptor (GR) – that reside in target neurons in the hypothalamus, hippocampus, and anterior pituitary gland, as well as other brain areas. Both receptors appear to be involved in differing aspects of the negative feedback regulation. Because of their high affinity for glucocorticoids, MRs are thought to regulate basal hormone secretion, whereas GRs, which exhibit a lower affinity for glucocorticoids, are thought to return stress-responsive elevations in glucocorticoids back to baseline. Assuming that the number of receptors accurately reflects the sensitivity of a tissue for a hormone, it is logical to conclude that sex differences in the HPA axis may result from a sex difference in the number of receptors in a given cell. A greater negative-feedback sensitivity would be indicated by more receptors and consequently result in lower basal and stress-activated hormone secretion. On the other hand, lower levels of receptors would indicate weaker negative feedback and thus result in higher basal and stress-responsive hormone secretion. This hypothesis has been supported by sex differences in the concentration and function of MRs and GRs. Overall, females tend to have lower levels of MRs and GRs in many brain regions, including the hypothalamus and hippocampus, which is consistent with the pattern found in other tissues, such as the thymus and liver. Given similar levels of hormone, GR- or MR-mediated functions (e.g., autoregulation of the receptors) was reported to be less sensitive to glucocorticosteroid modulation in females than in males.

Sex Differences in Behavioral Responses to Stress

Sex differences in behavioral responses to stress have been well-documented in humans and animals.

Laboratory animals have provided much of what we know regarding gender differences in response to stress. When placed in a given stressful situation, animals undergo a series of well-described behaviors that have been interpreted to indicate the degree of fear or anxiety that is being experienced. Freezing, defecation, and vocalization are a few good examples of these behaviors. Females appear to be less sensitive to stress-associated novel or aversive environments. For example, when placed into a novel environment or an elevated plus maze, female animals show less freezing and defecation than males. Females also enter a compartment in which they have been previously shocked more readily. In these behavioral paradigms, females also show more activity and exploration, behaviors that have been interpreted as signifying a lesser expression of fear and anxiety. However, when exposed to a variety of chronic stress paradigms, females are found to habituate significantly less than males.

In a well-studied animal model of chronic stress known as learned helplessness, animals are subjected to a repeated inescapable stressor, such as an intermittent tail shock. Subsequently, when allowed to escape, male rats are impaired in their escape performance, whereas female rats do not show this deficit to the same extent. However, when stressed repeatedly over a long period of time, it appears that males adapt more readily (eventually do not show reduced activity), whereas females fail to adapt over the same time period. It appears that this sex difference in adaptability may be dependent on levels of glucocorticoids because the reduction of the poststress glucocorticoid levels in females to levels attained in males allows the adaptation to repeated restraint. However, these effects are not always observed across studies. One reason may be related findings from studies showing that both strain and stress exposure during early development are important determinants in the expression of stress-related sex differences in behavior in adulthood.

Basic Mechanisms of Sexual Differentiation of Neural Function

Sexual differentiation of the brain occurs as a result of the presence of gonadal steroid hormones acting during either development or adulthood (**Figure 2**). The actions of gonadal steroid hormones on the brain have been classified as being either organizational or activational. Organizational actions are permanent changes in brain structure or function that occur during development. Generally, these permanent effects of gonadal steroid hormones are greatest during a defined critical window of opportunity,

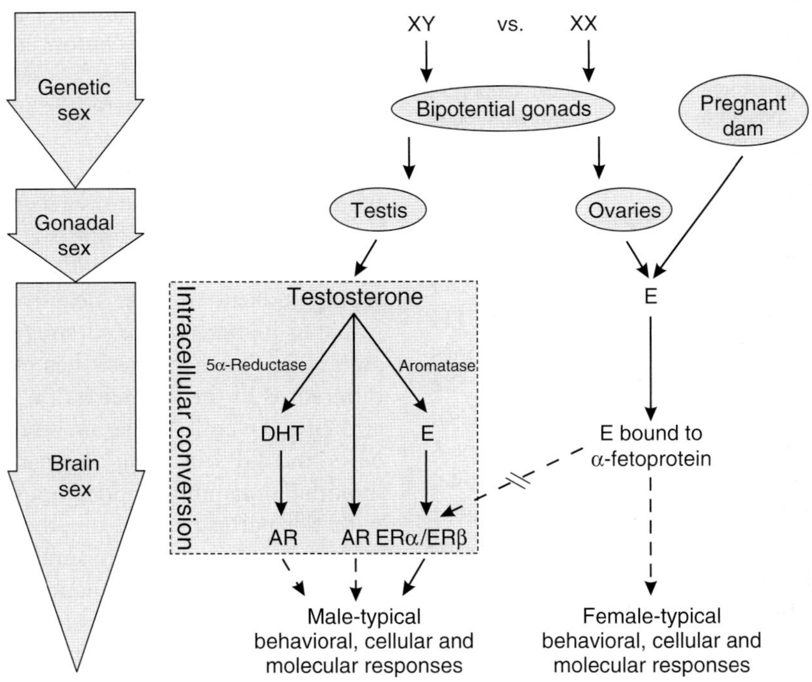

Figure 2 Schematic representation of the gonadal steroid hormones involved in the sexual differentiation of the vertebrate brain during development. According to this scheme, α-fetoprotein sequesters circulating estrogen, thereby preventing the defeminization (or masculinization) of the male or female brain. Therefore, the brain is thought to be initially programmed to develop in the female direction. However, α-fetoprotein is bypassed in the male brain because circulating testosterone is converted intraneuronally into estrogen by the enzyme aromatase, thus enabling estrogen to defemininize (or masculinize) the male brain, which is mediated through estrogen receptors. AR, androgen receptor; DHT, 5α-dihydrotestosterone; E, estrogen; ER, estrogen receptor.

usually during gestation or early postnatal life. The removal of gonadal steroid hormones after this critical period does not alter the organization or function of the brain appreciably. In contrast, the activational effects of gonadal steroid hormones are those that occur transiently, in direct response to the presence of a gonadal steroid hormone. Indeed, the removal of gonadal steroid hormones from the circulation, through castration or ovariectomy, results in a loss of effect. The activational effects of gonadal steroid hormones can occur throughout life, but are generally thought to have a maximal influence on gender differences during adulthood.

The literature regarding sexual differentiation of the brain suggests that the mammalian brain is an undifferentiated or perhaps neutral state and that, in response to normal circulating levels of testosterone (from the fetal male gonad), it develops toward the male direction. In contrast, if testosterone is low or absent, the brain develops toward the default mode, which is female (see **Figure 2**).

Although testosterone or its androgenic metabolite DHT may play a role in the masculinization of the brain, through their intracellular androgen receptor, in rodent models the functional gonadal steroid hormone for the organizational sexual differentiation of the brain is considered to be estrogen (**Figure 2**). This steroid hormone is produced intracellularly as a metabolite of testosterone due to the actions of the enzyme aromatase. The defeminizing effects of estrogen on the developing brain are mediated by estrogen receptors (ERs), although the exact role of each of the two forms of ERs, ERα and ERβ, is not known. Circulating estrogen from the mother or the developing ovary of the female is bound to a liver-derived protein called α-fetoprotein, which is present in high levels during perinatal development. Consequently, circulating estrogens are sequestered and cannot defeminize (or masculinize) the developing male or female brain. In contrast, defeminization (or masculinization) by estrogen can occur in the male brain because the estrogen-sequestering abilities of α-fetoprotein are circumvented due to its intracellular origin through the aromatization of testosterone. In rodents, the high levels of α-fetoprotein decrease during the second and third weeks of life, which coincides with increasing levels of unbound estrogens in the circulating, thus allowing the organizational and activational effects of estrogens to occur at puberty and in adulthood.

Organizational Effects of Gonadal Steroid Hormones on Stress Responses

Gonadal steroid hormones may act during early development to permanently organize adult responses to stress. This is best illustrated by examining the effects of perinatal hormone removal and replacement on the development of the adult pattern of behavior in response to stress. An example is the earlier described sex difference in the performance of the elevated plus maze and open-field test, in which female rats showed more activity and were less anxious than male rats. Indeed, the activity of an adult male rat that was castrated postnatally (a procedure that removes circulating levels of testosterone and its associated metabolites, such as estrogen) is similar to that of a female rat. The castration of male rats up to 21 days after birth prevents the development of the sex difference in activity. In contrast, neither the castration of adult males nor estrogen or testosterone replacement affects the sex difference in the level of activity. Similarly, the treatment of female rats with testosterone or estrogen up through 4 weeks after birth, but not in adulthood, results in a more malelike activity pattern. These studies indicate a critical period of sensitivity for the organizing actions of gonadal steroid hormones; moreover, they also show that sex differences in the activity level do not arise until after puberty.

Few studies have examined the occurrence of similar organizational effects of sex steroids on neuroendocrine responses to stress. The neonatal gonadectomy of male rats produces a more female-like hormonal response to stress in adulthood, but much of this may be due to the absence of hormones in adulthood because adult gonadectomy has a similar effect. On balance, it appears that the predominant effects of gonadal steroid hormones on neuroendocrine stress responses are activational in nature, with organizational influences contributing a much more modest amount to the overall sex difference.

Activational Effects of Gonadal Steroid Hormones on Stress Responses

The activational effects of gonadal steroid hormones on stress responses can be demonstrated easily by the gonadectomy of males and females in adulthood. The castration of male rats results in an increase in stress-responsive ACTH and corticosterone secretion. Similarly, the ovariectomy of female rats results in a decrease in stress-responsive HPA axis activity. These are gonadal steroid hormone-specific effects because they were reversed by the replacement of gonadal steroid hormones to gonadectomized animals. Moreover, androgen and estrogen have opposing actions in regulating stress-responsive hormone secretion. The treatment of gonadectomized male and female rats with estrogen augments subsequent ACTH and corticosterone responses to stress, whereas treatment with testosterone, or the nonaromatizable androgen, DHT, effectively inhibits HPA axis responses to stress. These studies provide a good mechanistic understanding as to why the stress-responsive hormone secretion is greatest in female rats during proestrus, when estrogen levels are highest.

Testosterone and estrogen can limit or augment the ACTH and corticosterone response to stress at several sites. These include the adrenal gland, anterior pituitary, hypothalamus, and higher brain centers such as the hippocampus. Receptors for androgen and estrogen exist in all these tissues, and the effects of estrogen and androgen on cellular parameters relevant to HPA activation have been demonstrated in all tissues.

At the level of the adrenal gland, estrogen has been shown to increase the adrenal secretory response to ACTH administration. Similarly, some studies showed that in the presence of estrogen the anterior pituitary gland responds to CRH with a greater secretion of ACTH than in the absence of estrogen. Increases in CRH immunoreactivity and mRNA have also been demonstrated in the hypothalamus in response to estrogen treatment. Whether these are direct actions on CRH neurons or mediated transsynaptically is currently in question. However, studies have demonstrated that the promoter sequence of the human CRH gene contains sequences (estrogen response elements) that respond to occupied estrogen receptors by increasing gene transcription, suggesting a direct action on the CRH gene. More recently, studies in rodents and humans showed the presence of ERs in some populations of CRH neurons of the PVN.

Similarly, androgen also appears to act at several sites. Castration increases adrenal enzyme activity and the synthesis of corticosterone by the adrenal gland *in vitro*, suggesting that testosterone acts to inhibit adrenal activity. Although testosterone does not appear to alter the anterior pituitary ACTH response to CRH administration, it does decrease CRH immunoreactivity in the hypothalamus of castrated rats. A direct action of testosterone on CRH synthesis or secretion does not seem to be the case because CRH neurons do not contain androgen receptors; thus upstream sites containing androgen receptors and projecting to CRH cells in the hypothalamus have been implicated, including the medial preoptic area, septum, and bed nucleus of the stria terminalis.

Sex differences in circulating estrogen and testosterone are also responsible for the sex differences in brain GR and MR levels or function. These effects underlie the reported sex differences in the negative feedback modulation of the HPA axis. Estrogen decreases GR and MR levels and their respective mRNAs in some brain areas and interferes with the ability of GR to autoregulate gene expression following changes in circulating glucocorticoids. These effects of estrogen could arise secondarily as a result of estrogen-induced increases in corticosteroid-binding globulin (CBG). In response to estrogen exposure, increased levels of CBG can sequester circulating glucocorticoid hormones from the brain, resulting in a decrease in negative feedback. However, estrogen has also been reported to increase GR in some tissues, such as the pituitary gland, and decrease the efficacy of corticosteroid receptor agonists that are not bound by CBG. Thus, it is likely that the actions of estrogen on the negative feedback are not solely mediated by an increase in CBG.

At the molecular level, interactions between ERs and GRs have been demonstrated with each modulating the functional response of the other. Testosterone also appears to interact with glucocorticoids in the regulation of GRs, but not MRs; however, a clear role for androgen receptors in altering negative feedback mechanisms has yet to be demonstrated.

Clinical Implications for Gender Differences in Stress Responses

Hans Selye's work in the 1940s also introduced the concept that stress accelerates the onset of disease through pathophysiological changes in endocrine and autonomic regulatory systems. Stress alone does not cause disease, but it is hypothesized to increase an individual's susceptibility to disease. In the past quarter century, this concept has been supported by results from numerous clinical and epidemiological studies related to cardiovascular disease, affective disorders, gastrointestinal disorders, diabetes, and physiological disorders associated with normal aging.

The mechanisms linking stress to disease states in humans are not fully understood, but hormonal changes, induced by the stress response, are recognized as a major influence. Glucocorticoids have a primary role but one that is modulated by gonadal steroid hormones. Androgen receptors, ERs, and GRs are found in many tissues that are stress-responsive. Some of these include the heart muscle, blood vessels, and immune tissues such as the spleen, thymus, and bone marrow. Gonadal steroid hormone receptors are also found in brain regions that mediate emotional and autonomic responses to stress, such as the hippocampus, hypothalamus, and amygdala. Thus gender differences in stress-related disease susceptibility appear to involve an interaction between glucocorticoid and gonadal hormones.

The role of stress in psychological and physiological disorders is complex. Animal studies have demonstrated that adult stress responsiveness is influenced developmentally by both genetics and the early environment. This bidirectional influence of both factors makes it difficult to predict the stress-related susceptibility to disease in individuals. However, physiological gender differences are still evident in humans regardless of early environment.

Many of these differences parallel sex differences in animals. For instance, the unstressed basal heart rate in women is greater than in men. Women also exhibit a larger exercise-induced increase in heart rate. However, in response to anger and psychological stress, men exhibit greater emotional and cardiovascular lability with respect to both heart rate and blood pressure. This lability, resulting in larger increases in systolic pressure, is thought to contribute significantly to the greater risk in men for cardiovascular morbidity. Protection from heart disease in women is also related to estrogen, which provides protection against arteriosclerosis until menopause. The anti-atherosclerotic effects of estrogen also appear to involve the presence of ERs in cardiovascular tissue.

Physical or psychologically stressful stimuli also produce a greater stimulation of the HPA axis in women than in men, similar to the stress effects observed in other mammals. Administering CRH to women induces a greater release of ACTH and a prolonged elevation of cortisol than administering it to men, indicating that these gender differences probably involve processes directly under the regulation of the central nervous system. However, unlike animals, gender differences in the human HPA axis responsiveness to psychological stressors appear to be much more dependent on the type of psychological stress and the environmental circumstances in which it occurs. Studies suggest that psychological factors associated with social stress, such as taking care of an elderly parent, have more impact on HPA reactivity in women than in men, perhaps placing women's health at greater risk under such circumstances.

A primary factor underlying gender differences in the HPA response to stress appears to be higher estrogen levels in women. During the normal menstrual cycle, HPA activity is enhanced during the follicular phase, when estrogen levels peak, and is reduced during the luteal phase, when progesterone levels are elevated. The removal of the ovaries prior to menopause reduces the HPA sensitivity to CRH stimulation. The effect of estrogen on HPA reactivity is not gender-specific because normal men who were administered a short-term regimen of estrogen also exhibited increased HPA activity. One possible explanation for such effects of estrogen is provided by observations that estrogen therapy increases circulating levels of CBG in women. Although not yet shown to be the case, such increases in CBG, and the resulting decreases in free cortisol, could play a role in the elevated HPA activity in response to stress reported in women (due to a decrease in cortisol bioavailability). Similarly, it remains to be determined whether men and women are equally sensitive to the influence of estrogen on the HPA and whether organizational influences of gonadal steroids confer a differential sensitivity to the later hormonal modulation of HPA activity.

The incidence of autoimmune disease is also sexually dimorphic, and the severity and onset are exacerbated by life stress. The overall incidence in women is approximately 2.5-fold greater then in men. In contrast to the protective role estrogen plays in cardiovascular disease, it appears to be a major contributory factor to the gender difference observed in autoimmune diseases such as multiple sclerosis, rheumatoid arthritis, and lupus. Estrogen can regulate immune responses through ERs present on thymocytes, macrophages, and endothelial cells, all of which also express GRs. The interaction between estrogen and glucocorticoids on immunomodulation is a rapidly expanding area of research interest and one that is likely to underlie the gender difference in autoimmune disease susceptibility.

Numerous clinical studies have reported a greater incidence of depression in women. The reasons underlying this gender difference are controversial, but both hormonal status and stress may be involved. Women have been reported to be more susceptible to depression during periods of fluctuations in estrogen and progesterone levels. However, although such changes have often been cited as causes of mood disorders in women, the literature does not provide strong support for a direct causal relationship between gonadal hormone status and depression or anxiety disorders. An additional mediating factor may be life stress. The onset of clinical depression is well known to be exacerbated by life stress, and data suggest that a link to a gender bias in mood disorders involves an increased susceptibility in some women to the combined effects of stress and hormonal status. Thus, fluctuations in estrogen and progesterone during the menstrual cycle have been proposed to confer a susceptibility to depression in women that can be exacerbated by life stress.

A gender difference is also observed in the incidence of posttraumatic stress disorder (PTSD), which is a stress-induced pathological condition that is clinically distinct from depression or other affective disorders. Long-term physiological changes are observed in PTSD patients that involve increased adrenergic tone and alterations in HPA function. Following exposure to prolonged psychological trauma, women exhibit PTSD symptoms twice as frequently as men, even when the type of trauma is equivalent. The organizational effects of hormones may also play a role in gender differences in the incidence of PTSD. This stems from findings showing that experiencing psychologically traumatizing events prior to puberty greatly increases the susceptibility to PTSD in adulthood in females compared to males. This increased susceptibility appears to relate specifically to experiencing childhood psychological trauma because accidents or injury during this period do not increase the risk for PTSD in either gender when later psychological trauma is experienced.

In summary, current research studying the interrelationships among gender, stress, and pathophysiology strongly implicate a role for gonadal hormones in predicting gender differences related to disease or psychopathology. However, a definitive understanding of the role of gender in the elicitation of stress-induced pathophysiology awaits a better understanding of the complex relationship among the environment, steroid hormones, and other stress-induced biochemical factors.

See Also the Following Articles

Adrenal Cortex; Autoimmunity; Gleucocorticoid Negative Feedback; Glucocorticoids – Adverse Effects on the Nervous System; Glucocorticoids, Effects of Stress on.

Further Reading

Beatty, W. W. (1979). Gonadal hormones and sex differences in nonreproductive behaviors in rodents: organizational and activational influences. *Hormones and Behavior* **12**, 112–163.

Breslau, N., Glenn, C., Andreski, P., et al. (1997). Sex differences in posttraumatic stress disorder. *Archives of General Psychiatry* **54**, 1044–1048.

Chrousos, G. P., Torpy, D. J. and Gold, P. W. (1998). Interactions between the hypothalamic-pituitary-adrenal axis and the female reproductive system: clinical implications. *Annals of Internal Medicine* **129**, 229.

Gorski, R. A. (1985). The 13th J. A. F. Stevenson memorial lecture: sexual differentiation of the brain: possible mechanisms and implications. *Canadian Journal of Physiology and Pharmacology* **63**, 577–594.

Handa, R. J., Burgess, L. H., Kerr, J. E., et al. (1994). Gonadal steroid hormone receptors and sex differences in the hypothalamo-pituitary-adrenal axis. *Hormones and Behavior* **28**, 464–476.

Handa, R. J., Price, R. H., Jr. and Wilson, M. E. (1998). Steroid hormone receptors and the assessment of feedback sensitivity. In: VandeKar, L. (ed.) *Methods in neuroendocrinology: the cellular and molecular neuropharmacology series*, pp. 49–68. Boca Raton, FL: CRC Press.

Seeman, M. V. (1997). Psychopathology in women and men: focus on female hormones. *American Journal of Psychiatry* **154**, 1641–1647.

Turner, B. B. (1997). Influence of gonadal steroids on brain corticosteroid receptors: a minireview. *Neurochemical Research* **22**, 1375–1385.

Vogele, C., Jarvis, A. and Cheeseman, K. (1997). Anger suppression, reactivity and hypertension risk: gender makes a difference. *Annals of Behavioral Medicine* **19**, 61–69.

Wilder, R. L. (1995). Neuroendocrine-immune system interactions and autoimmunity. *Annual Review of Immunology* **13**, 307–338.

Gonadotropin Secretion, Effects of Stress on

M Ferin
Columbia University, New York NY, USA

This is a revised version of the article by M Ferin, Encyclopedia of Stress, First edition, volume 2, pp 283–288, © 2000, Elsevier Inc.

Glossary

Amenorrhea — The absence of menstruation, denoting a silent hypothalamic-pituitary-ovarian endocrine axis.

Arginine vasopressin (AVP) — An adjunct neurohormone in control of the hypothalamic-pituitary-adrenal endocrine axis. It is colocated with and released together with CRH in response to stressors.

Corticotropin releasing hormone (CRH) — The main neurohormone in control of the hypothalamic-pituitary-adrenal endocrine axis. Its release from the hypothalamic paraventricular nucleus is activated by stressors. It stimulates the pituitary to secrete adrenocorticotropic hormone.

Estradiol — The main sex steroid secreted by the ovarian follicle.

Follicular phase — The first stage of the menstrual cycle, during which the process of folliculogenesis is completed through the maturation of the soon-to-be-ovulated dominant follicle.

Follicle stimulating hormone (FSH) — A gonadotropin that promotes the recruitment of a new cohort of follicles at the start of each follicular phase.

Gonadotropin releasing hormone (GnRH) pulse generator — The hypothalamic structure responsible for the pulsatile release of GnRH, in a process that is essential for the normal function of the reproductive process.

Gonadotropin — Two hormones, follicle stimulating hormone and luteinizing hormone, released by the anterior pituitary following stimulation by GnRH.

Luteal phase — The second stage of the menstrual cycle, when the ovulated follicle is transformed into a new structure, the corpus

	luteum, which secretes both estradiol and progesterone.
Luteinizing hormone (LH)	A gonadotropin that stimulates the release of estradiol from the maturing follicle and of progesterone from the corpus luteum.
Progesterone	The main sex steroid secreted by the corpus luteum. It prepares the uterus for the implantation of the fertilized egg.
Proopiomelanocortin (POMC)	The common precursor molecule to β-endorphin (an endogenous opioid peptide) and to α-melanocyte stimulating hormone. Both peptides modulate the gonadotropin response to stressors.

Control of Normal Gonadotropin Secretion

Hypothalamic Control: The Gonadotropin Releasing Hormone Pulse Generator

The hypothalamic-pituitary-gonadal (HPG) axis, which governs the reproductive system, is driven by the brain. Gonadotropin (FSH and LH) secretion by the anterior pituitary gland is controlled by the hypothalamus through the release of GnRH. GnRH, a 10-amino-acid peptide, is synthesized within several hypothalamic nuclei and released into the hypophysial portal circulation to stimulate the release of both gonadotropins. This direct vascular connection between the hypothalamus and the anterior pituitary allows for the rapid and undiluted transport of minute amounts of GnRH to its target, the pituitary gonadotroph. Gonadotropins, in turn, act on the gonads, the ovaries or testes, to induce specific morphological changes and to stimulate the release of gonadal steroids, such as testosterone, estradiol, and progesterone. Constant communication between the several levels of the HPG axis through the negative feedback loop is essential for normal function; estradiol or testosterone secreted by the ovaries or testes continuously feeds back to the hypothalamus and pituitary to adjust GnRH, LH, and FSH secretion. The interruption of this negative feedback loop, for instance, following castration, results in an increase of GnRH, FSH, and LH release.

Significantly, GnRH is released from the hypothalamus in a pulsatile fashion (the GnRH pulse generator), and thus tonic secretion of gonadotropins is pulsatile in nature. Each pulse of LH consists of an abrupt and brief release of the hormone followed by an exponential decrease according to its half-life. A pulsatile GnRH stimulus is required to increase the transcription of the gonadotropin subunit genes. Pathological events that interfere with the function of the GnRH pulse generator disrupt the pituitary-gonadal axis. For example, the complete absence of GnRH pulsatility results in a dormant reproductive axis, whereas lesser abnormalities, such as a decrease in GnRH pulse frequency, may interfere with proper reproductive function.

Gonadotropins and the Reproductive Cycle

The reproductive cycle, estrous cycle (in rodent and sheep) or menstrual cycle (in nonhuman primate and human) involves a remarkable coordination of hormonal secretion and morphological changes within the HPG axis. In the primate, a rise in FSH at the start of the follicular phase promotes the recruitment of a cohort of antral follicles from which the dominant follicle destined for ovulation will be selected. Stimulated by the pulsatile release of the gonadotropins, the dominant follicle grows exponentially and releases estradiol in amounts proportional to its size. The maturity of the dominant follicle is marked by a high estradiol release, which when a threshold is reached activates the positive estradiol feedback loop; this induces the ovulatory LH surge and ovulation. After ovulation, the dominant follicle is transformed into the corpus luteum, which secretes both estradiol and progesterone when stimulated by LH. Substantial progesterone secretion promotes uterine differentiation in preparation for implantation of the fertilized egg.

A proper pattern of GnRH and gonadotropin pulsatile release is required for the normal reproductive cycle to occur. In the human, for example, an optimal GnRH–LH pulse frequency of approximately one pulse every 90 min is required for normal folliculogenesis to occur during the follicular phase. A pulse frequency that is too low may fail to bring the recruited follicle to a timely maturation, and a too rapid pulse frequency may result in pathology (such as polycystic ovary syndrome).

The Gonadotropin Response to Stressors: Cross-Talk between the Hypothalamic-Pituitary-Adrenal and the Hypothalamic-Pituitary-Gonadal Axes

Effects of Stressors on Tonic Gonadotropin Release

The activation of the hypothalamic-pituitary-adrenal (HPA) axis by several types of stressors, such as immune/inflammatory challenges as simulated by the administration of endotoxin or cytokines, temporary restraint, or insulin-induced hypoglycemia, results in an inhibition of tonic pulsatile LH release, mainly in the form of a decrease in LH pulse frequency. In women, psychogenic stress has also been related to lower basal tonic levels of FSH, LH, and estradiol compared to normal cycling women; these patients have reduced integrated 24-h LH and FSH concentrations, reduced LH pulse frequency, and increased LH interpulse interval.

Overall evidence suggests that this decrease in tonic pulsatile LH release is primarily related to a central action of stressors exerted through an inhibitory action on the hypothalamic GnRH pulse generator; a decline in the generator's ability to properly stimulate the gonadotroph, mainly through a reduction in the frequency of pulsatile GnRH release, appears to be the main mechanism involved. In addition, there is experimental evidence that stressors may also subtly influence the gonadotroph's responsiveness to GnRH and thereby decrease the amplitude of the gonadotropin response. This effect may reflect a pituitary action of adrenal corticosteroids released in response to the activation of the HPA axis by the stressor.

Effects of Stressors on the Surge Mode of Luteinizing Hormone Release

Data in the rodent and ewe also suggest that an immune/inflammatory challenge or restraint (and possibly other stressors) can also suppress the estradiol-induced ovulatory LH surge. In the rodent, this effect appears to be exerted at the level of GnRH perikarya, where the percentage of GnRH neurons expressing the c-fos protein and the GnRH primary transcript are significantly reduced by these stressors. The administration of a GnRH agonist concomitantly with the stressor completely restores the LH surge. In the ewe, endotoxin was shown to prevent the GnRH surge into the hypophysial portal circulation, also suggesting a central effect of the challenge. Significantly, this inhibitory action is seen only if the stressor acts quite ahead of the expected time of the LH surge, primarily at the initial time of activation of the estradiol positive feedback signal.

Stressors and an Early Short-Term Rise in Gonadotropins

In addition to the previously mentioned inhibitory action of stressors on gonadotropin release, investigators have also reported a very transient rise in LH in rodents within the first hour of the response to various stressors, such as handling; restraint; exposure to ether or to a novel environment; or visual, audiogenic, and thermal stressors. This rapid and transient stimulatory effect of stressors on tonic LH release has been reported mostly in the intact, but generally not in the castrated, male rat, and in men but not women. The mechanisms behind this phenomenon and its role in the stress response remain to be elucidated.

Central Pathways Mediating the Stress Response

The Hypothalamic Paraventricular Nucleus

The paraventricular nucleus (PVN) plays a pivotal role in the response to stressors. The neuroendocrine activation of the HPA axis by stressors involves the release of two neuropeptides, corticotropin releasing hormone (CRH) and AVP, from discrete populations of hypophysiotrophic neurons in parvocellular areas of PVN. These two neuropeptides, which are colocalized within perikarya of PVN neurons and in secretory granules, play a complementary role in mediating the effects of stressors on the HPA axis (see **Figure 1**).

There is good experimental evidence for an active mediatory role by CRH in the inhibition of GnRH and gonadotropins that follow stressors. In the non-human primate, the administration of a CRH receptor antagonist or of a drug decreasing endogenous CRH activity prevents not only the cortisol increase but also the inhibition of pulsatile GnRH–LH release induced by stressors such as an immune/inflammatory challenge (**Figure 2a**) or insulin-induced hypoglycemia. Similar mediatory effects of a CRH antagonist or of CRH antiserum have been reported in the rodent after various stressors, except in the response

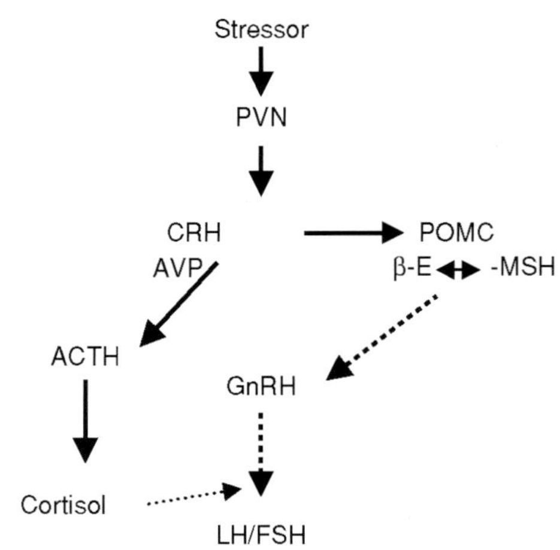

Figure 1 Main pathways mediating the inhibitory effects of stressors on pulsatile gonadotropin release. α-MSH, α-melanocyte stimulating hormone; β-E, β-endorphin; ACTH, adrenocorticotropic hormone; AVP, arginine vasopressin; CRH, corticotropin releasing hormone; FSH, follicle stimulating hormone; GnRH, gonadotropin releasing hormone; LH, luteinizing hormone; POMC, proopiomelanocortin; PVN, paraventricular nucleus.

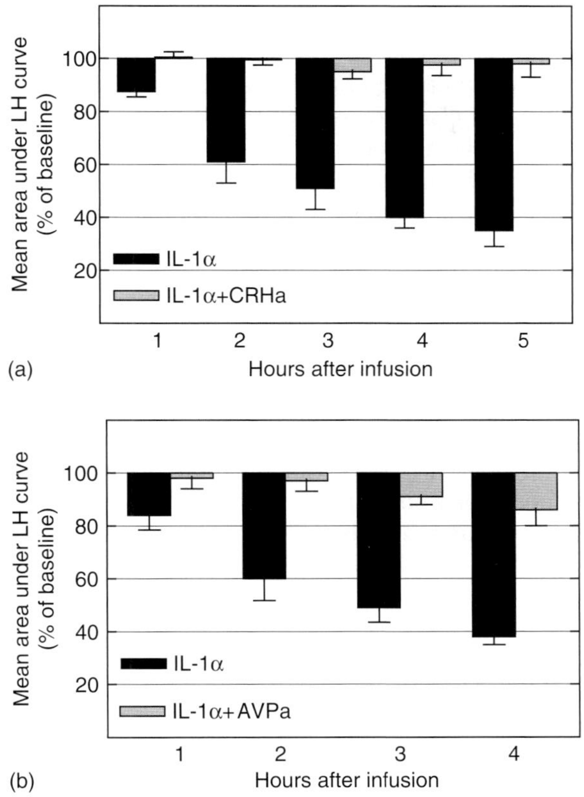

Figure 2 Reversal of the inhibitory effects of an intracerebroventricular infusion of interleukin (IL)-1 on luteinizing hormone (LH) release. a, By a CRH antagonist (CRHa); b, By a VP antagonist (AVPa). Reprinted with permission from (a) Feng, Y. J., Shalts, E., Xia, L., Rivier, J., Rivier, C., Vale, W., Ferin, M. (1991) An inhibitory effect of interleukin-1 on basal gonadotropin release in the ovariectomized rhesus monkey: reversal by a corticotropin-releasing factor antagonist, *Endocrinology* **128**, 2077–2082, Copyright 1991, The Endocrine Society; and (b) Shalts, E., Feng, Y. J., Ferin, M. (1992) Vasopressin mediates the interleukin-1α-indiced decrease in LH secretion in the ovariectomized rhesus monkey, *Endocrinology* **131**, 153–158, Copyright 1992, The Endocrine Society.

to an inflammatory challenge. The latter is in a marked difference with the primate. The administration of CRH also results in a rapid inhibition of pulsatile LH release and in a decrease in the frequency and duration of GnRH pulses. Data in the nonhuman primate suggest that this inhibitory action is not mediated by downstream activation of the pituitary-adrenal axis: indeed, the inhibitory effects of a CRH infusion on pulsatile LH release cannot be mimicked by adrenocorticotropic hormone (ACTH) infusion, are not reversed by treatment with metyrapone (an inhibitor of adrenal steroidogenesis), and persist following adrenalectomy.

Data in CRH-deficient male and female mice indicate that stressors such as restraint or food withdrawal can still inhibit tonic LH secretion or the proestrus LH surge, suggesting that molecules other than CRH may also play a role. Although there fewer data, AVP has also been shown to mediate the inhibitory action of certain stressors on the HPG axis and conceivably may take over in the CRH-deficient animal. In the ovx monkey, the inhibitory effects of a central infusion of interleukin (IL)-1 on pulsatile LH release are prevented by the co-administration of an AVP antagonist, even though the antagonist is without effect on the cortisol increase (**Figure 2b**). Some, but not all, investigators also report that the same antagonist prevents hypoglycemia-induced LH suppression in ovx and in male monkeys.

The Endogenous Opioid Peptides

There is substantial evidence to indicate that the inhibitory action of CRH and of most stressors on pulsatile GnRH–LH release occurs at suprapituitary sites that not only involve the neuroendocrine HPA axis but also mediation by endogenous opioid peptidergic pathways. Endogenous β-endorphin is known to be a powerful inhibitor of the GnRH pulse generator; for instance, during the luteal phase of the menstrual cycle of the human and nonhuman primate, there is a marked decreased in LH pulse frequency that parallels elevated endogenous β-endorphin activity and that is prevented by the administration of naloxone, a μ-opioid receptor antagonist. Hypothalamic β-endorphin activity is stimulated by CRH and by stressors. Naloxone administration also prevents the CRH- or AVP-mediated suppression of GnRH–gonadotropin release and restores pulsatile LH secretion (**Figure 3a**). This opioid antagonist also prevents the LH inhibition that follows several types of stressors, except for insulin-induced LH inhibition.

β-Endorphin derives from POMC, a large glycoprotein precursor molecule synthesized primarily in the hypothalamus and pituitary gland. Posttranslational processing of POMC is tissue-specific and in the hypothalamus yields not only β-endorphin but also α-melanocyte stimulating hormone (α-MSH). α-MSH has been shown to antagonize some of the actions of β-endorphin and may function as an endogenous opioid antagonist. In fact, α-MSH antagonizes the inhibitory action of exogenously administered β-endorphin on LH release and restores normal pulsatile LH release in ovx monkeys treated with CRH (**Figure 3b**) or subjected to an immune/inflammatory challenge. These data support the notion that post-translational processing of POMC may represent an important step in the response mechanisms to stressors and that the ratio of β-endorphin to α-MSH may be more significant than the absolute β-endorphin concentration in determining the ultimate effects of stressors on pulsatile LH release.

Stressors and the Reproductive Cycle

Stress and Amenorrhea

The reproductive cycle requires a remarkable coordination of hormonal secretion and morphological changes within all levels of the hypothalamic-pituitary-ovarian-uterine axis. Thus, it is not surprising that stressors can disrupt the normal estrous or

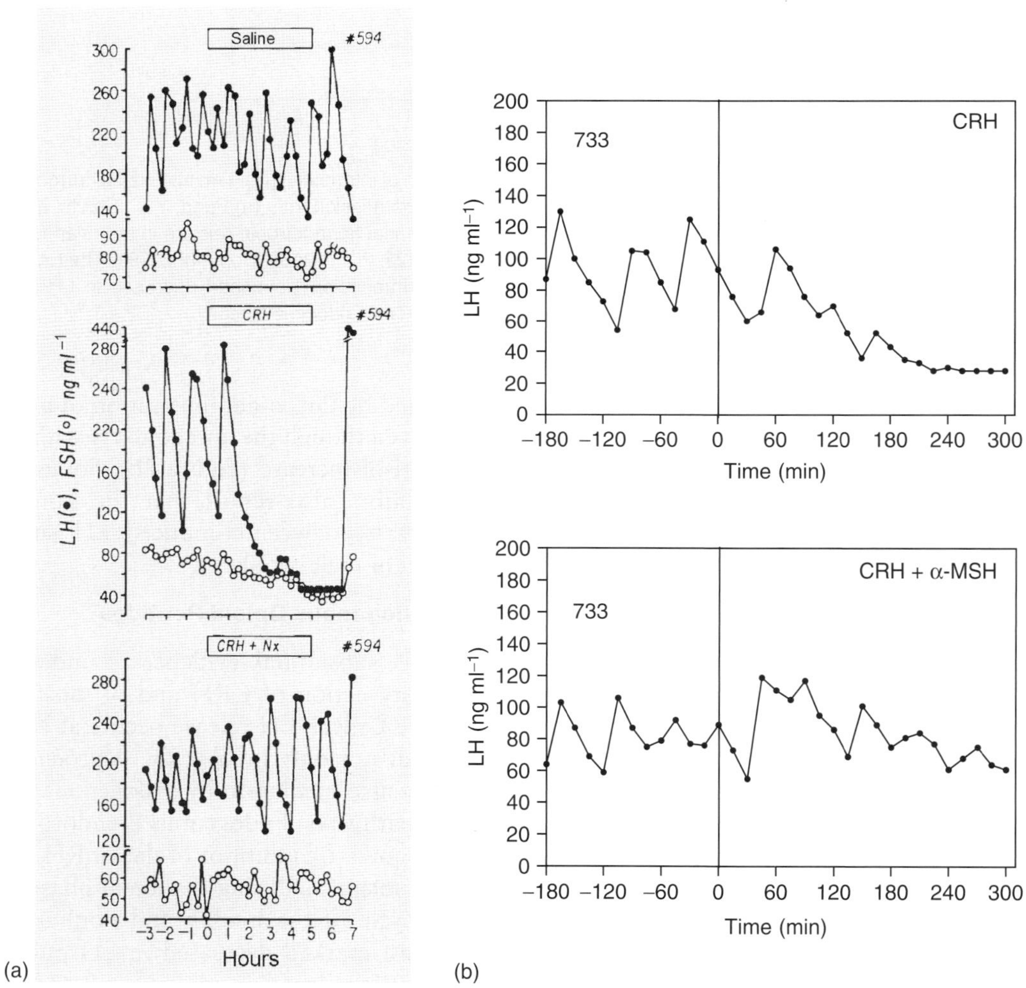

Figure 3 Reversal of the inhibitory effects of CRH on pulsatile LH release. a, By naloxone (Nx); b, By α-MSH. Reprinted with permission from (a) Gindoff, P. R., Ferin, M. (1987) Endogenous opioid peptides modulate the effect of corticotropin-releasing hormone (CRH) on gonadotropin release in the primate, *Endocrinology* **121**, 837–842, Copyright 1987, The Endocrine Society; and (b) Shalts, E., Feng, Y. J., Ferin, M., Wardlaw, S. L. (1992) α-Melanocyte-stimulating hormone antagonizes the neuroendocrine effects of corticotropin-releasing factor and interleukin-la in the primate, *Endocrinology* **131**, 132–138, Copyright 1992, The Endocrine Society.

menstrual cycle. If sufficiently intense or chronic, stressors can completely interrupt the cycle. In women, psychogenic stress, usually the result of overt or latent psychological disturbances, is known to interfere with normal reproductive function and thought to be a common cause of amenorrhea in a syndrome known as functional hypothalamic chronic anovulation (FHCA). When fully established, the syndrome is characterized by ovarian quiescence, amenorrhea, and infertility. Several studies in the human underscore the association among FHCA, increased HPA activity in the form of an amplified circadian cortisol excursion, and low basal tonic levels of FSH and LH coupled with reduced LH pulse frequency.

Stress and Menstrual Cycle Defects

Although the long-term consequences of chronic stress may include amenorrhea and infertility and result in the full-blown FHCA syndrome, more recent data also demonstrate that stressors that initially are of an insufficient intensity to induce amenorrhea may nevertheless produce temporary cyclic defects.

Prolongation of the follicular phase As shown in the ewe and monkey, endotoxin administration, mimicking an inflammatory/immune challenge, or exercise during the follicular phase results in a lengthening of the follicular phase and in the interruption of the normal follicular estradiol profile. The stressor prevents the development of high-frequency LH pulses that are the essential stimulus for the preovulatory increase in estradiol secretion; without these, the estradiol rise is curtailed and the preovulatory LH surge is delayed. Significantly, in the monkey, the delay in the resumption of a normal follicular phase greatly exceeds the duration of the stress challenge itself.

Inadequate luteal phase In the monkey, a short-term inflammatory/immune challenge or a psychogenic-like stress, whether confined to the follicular or luteal phase of the menstrual cycle, invariably result in reduced luteal function, as demonstrated by overall diminished progesterone and inhibin A secretion during the luteal phase (**Figure 4**). In many animals, these short-term stress challenges continue to interfere with normal luteal function through the first or two subsequent stressor-free cycles. The lower progesterone levels are related to the decrease in LH induced by the stressor. Inadequate luteal phases have also been reported during exercise, suggesting that this syndrome may well represent a general initial response to stressors and/or energy-related demands in the normal cyclic female.

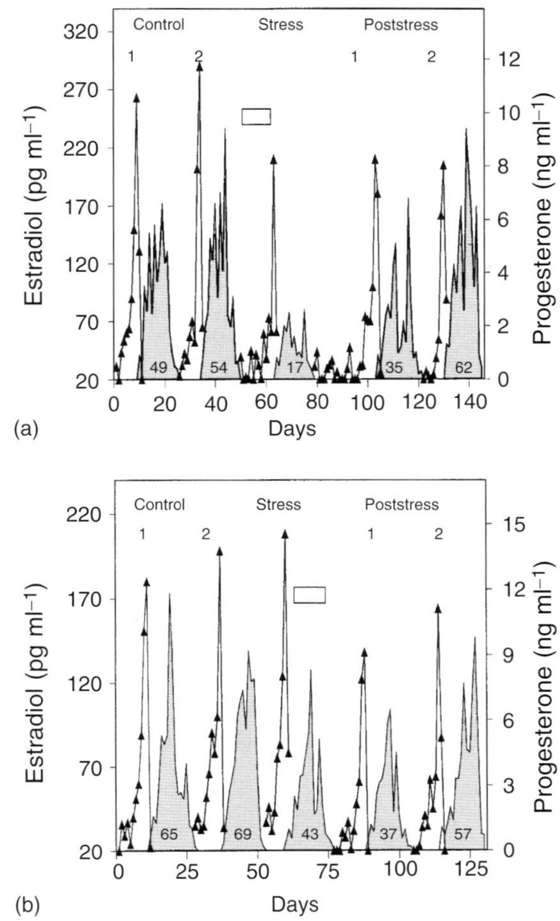

Figure 4 Inadequate luteal phase following a 10-day psychogenic-like stress. a, During the follicular phase; b, During the luteal phase. Illustrated are daily levels of estradiol during the follicular phase (triangles) and of progesterone during the luteal phase (shaded areas) throughout two control menstrual cycles, the stress cycle, and two poststress cycles. Luteal progesterone secretion is significantly decreased in the stress cycle and in the first of the two poststress cycles (numbers within the shaded areas are integrated luteal progesterone values). Reprinted with permission from Xiao, E., Xia-Zhang, L., Ferin, M. (2002) Inadequate luteal function is the initial clinical cyclic defect in a 12-day stress model that includes a psychogenic component in the Rhesus monkey, *Journal of Clinical Endocrinology & Metabolism* **87**, 2232–2237, Copyright 2002, The Endocrine Society.

Premature ovulatory luteinizing hormone surge Studies in the primate have shown that the activation of the HPA axis by endotoxin or IL-1 in the mid- to late follicular phase (but not at other stages of the cycle) results in a large release of LH. Data in the monkey suggest that progesterone, which is released in small amounts by the adrenals in response to the stressor, may be responsible for this acute release of LH because this effect is prevented by a progesterone or CRH antagonist. Smaller increases in LH have also been reported in women following exercise during the mid-follicular phase.

The precise physiopathological significance of these three cyclic defects in response to a stressor during the menstrual cycle remains to be further studied in patients. The data, however, suggest that the HPG axis is closely monitored by the brain and that a stress challenge, even one not sufficient or extended enough to interrupt the cycle and to result in amenorrhea, may well induce endocrine changes too subtle to be appreciated in the clinical environment but nonetheless substantial enough to temporarily impact on fertility or to provide a temporary suspension of pregnancy in suboptimal conditions. For instance, decreased luteal progesterone secretion in response to a stressor may interfere with the process of implantation of a fertilized egg and result in spontaneous abortion by delaying the endometrial changes required for proper implantation. Prematurely elevated LH concentrations in the follicular phase may damage the maturing follicle and/or oocyte and desynchronize the ovulatory signal from a timely follicular maturation process and thereby result in early pregnancy loss.

See Also the Following Article

Reproduction, Effects of Social Stress on.

Further Reading

Battaglia, D. F., Brown, M. E., Krasa, H. B., et al. (1998). Systemic challenge with endotoxin stimulates corticotropin-releasing hormone and arginine vasopressin secretion into hypophysial portal blood: coincidence with gonadotropin-releasing hormone suppression. *Endocrinology* **139**, 4175–4181.

Berga, S. L. (1996). Functional hypothalamic chronic anovulation. In: Adashi, E. Y., Rock, J. A. & Rosenwaks, Z. (eds.) *Reproductive endocrinology, surgery, and technology*, pp. 1061–1075. Philadelphia: Lippincott-Raven.

Chrousos, G. P., Torpy, D. J. and Gold, P. W. (1998). Interactions between the hypothalamic-pituitary-adrenal axis and the female reproductive system: clinical implications. *Annals of Internal Medicine* **129**, 229–240.

Feng, Y. J., Shalts, E., Xia, L., et al. (1991). An inhibitory effect of interleukin-1 on basal gonadotropin release in the ovariectomized rhesus monkey: reversal by a corticotropin-releasing factor antagonist. *Endocrinology* **128**, 2077–2082.

Ferin, M. (1999). Clinical review 105: stress and the reproductive cycle. *Journal of Clinical Endocrinology & Metabolism* **84**, 1768–1774.

Ferin M. (2006). Stress and the reproductive system. In: Knobil, E. & Neill, J. (eds.) *The physiology of reproduction* (3rd edn., pp. 2627–2696). San Diego, CA: Elsevier.

Gindoff, P. R. and Ferin, M. (1987). Endogenous opioid peptides modulate the effect of corticotropin-releasing hormone (CRH) on gonadotropin release in the primate. *Endocrinology* **121**, 837–842.

Karsch, F. J., Battaglia, D. F., Breen, K. M., et al. (2002). Mechanisms for ovarian cycle disruption by immune/inflammatory stress. *Stress* **5**, 101–112.

Rivest, S. and Rivier, C. (1995). The role of corticotropin-releasing factor and interleukin-1 in the regulation of neurons controlling reproductive functions. *Endocrine Review* **16**, 177–199.

Shalts, E., Feng, Y. J. and Ferin, M. (1992). Vasopressin mediates the interleukin-1 alpha-induced decrease in luteinizing hormone secretion in the ovariectomized rhesus monkey. *Endocrinology* **131**, 153–158.

Shalts, E., Feng, Y. J., Ferin, M., et al. (1992). α-Melanocyte-stimulating hormone antagonizes the neuroendocrine effects of corticotropin-releasing factor and interleukin-1 α in the primate. *Endocrinology* **131**, 132–138.

Xiao, E., Xia-Zhang, L., Barth, A., et al. (1998). Stress and the menstrual cycle: relevance of cycle quality in the short- and long-term response to a 5-day endotoxin challenge during the follicular phase in the rhesus monkey. *Journal of Clinical Endocrinology & Metabolism* **83**, 2454–2460.

Xiao, E., Xia-Zhang, L. and Ferin, M. (2002). Inadequate luteal function is the initial clinical cyclic defect in a 12-day stress model that includes a psychogenic component in the Rhesus monkey. *Journal of Clinical Endocrinology & Metabolism* **87**, 2232–2237.

Xiao, E., Xia-Zhang, L., Thornell, D., et al. (1996). Interleukin-1 stimulates luteinizing hormone release during the midfollicular phase in the rhesus monkey: a novel way in which stress may influence the menstrual cycle. *Journal of Clinical Endocrinology & Metabolism* **81**, 2136–2141.

Menstrual Cycles and Stress

R Suri
UCLA Neuropsychiatric Institute and Hospital, Los Angeles, CA, USA
L Altshuler
UCLA Neuropsychiatric Institute and Hospital and West LA Veterans Administration Medical Center, Los Angeles, CA, USA

This is a revised version of the article by R Suri and L Altshuler, Encyclopedia of Stress, First edition, volume 2, pp 736–741, © 2000, Elsevier Inc.

Glossary

Amenorrhea The absence of menses for 3 months or longer.

Anorexia nervosa An eating disorder characterized by the refusal to maintain a minimally normal body weight; symptoms also include the absence of at least three consecutive menstrual cycles.

Corticotropin releasing hormone (CRH) A 41-amino-acid peptide secreted by the paraventricular nucleus of the hypothalamus, which stimulates pituitary secretion of adrenocorticotropic hormone and, consequently, cortisol secretion by the adrenal cortex.

Functional hypothalamic amenorrhea Amenorrhea associated with factors such as psychogenic stressors, excessive exercise, or weight loss.

Gonadotropin-releasing hormone (GnRH) A decapeptide hormone that plays a significant role in reproductive physiology through stimulation of follicular stimulating hormone and luteinizing hormone by the pituitary. GnRH is secreted by neurons of the preoptic and arcuate nuclei of the hypothalamus in a pulsatile manner, with the amplitude and frequency of its secretions under the regulation of estrogen, progesterone, catecholamines, and neuropeptides.

Secondary amenorrhea Amenorrhea that occurs when the patient has menstruated in the past but has stopped for at least 3–6 months. Causes can include pregnancy, lesions of the hypothalamus or pituitary (from surgery, infection, irradiation, chemotherapy, infarction, or tumor), emotional stress, endocrine disease (e.g., thyroid, adrenal, or diabetes), or medications.

Stress can be conceptualized as a state of disharmony or threatened homeostasis, with the patient's adaptive response being specific to the stressor or being more generalized. Although the demands and complexity of society continue to increase, the physiological mechanisms for coping with adversity have not changed appreciably over the past thousands of years, and the physiological responses to social pressures, rapid changes, and increased information are often similar to responses to physical danger and threats to survival. The effects of stress can be profound, resulting in the mobilization of adaptive behaviors and peripheral functions and the inhibition of biologically costly behaviors such as reproduction. For many animals, environmental stress, or conditions of high population density, are associated with chronic anovulation and infertility. During unfavorable circumstances, the lack of reproduction allows females to focus scarce resources on survival, improvement in overall condition, and investment in existing offspring. Although animal studies have provided information on the hormonal pathways through which stressors impact reproductive function, these mechanisms are poorly understood in humans. Nevertheless, for women, psychosocial stressors such as bereavement or separation from family, in the absence of a psychiatric diagnosis, have been linked to abnormalities of the menstrual cycle. Rates of menstrual irregularities increase in proportion to chronic stress, which, if severe enough, can completely inhibit the female reproductive system. Although the nature of the actual stressor can be significant, the response of the individual to the stressor, as well as certain cognitive, behavioral, or personality traits, may cause some women to be more vulnerable to the stress of daily living than other women and may play a more significant role in affecting menstruation than the actual stressor itself. The impact of stress can range from a lack of menstrual cycles to persisting cycles of marginal quality.

The Menstrual Cycle

The menstrual cycle is defined by the regular, repetitive monthly occurrence of ovulation throughout a woman's reproductive life. Menarche, defined as the onset of the first menses, occurs in the United States between the ages of 9 and 12, with a mean of 12.6 years. The mean duration of the cycle is 28 days, and the cycle is divided into two functional phases: the follicular (or proliferative) phase and the luteal (or secretory) phase. Polymenorrhea refers to menstrual cycles that occur at intervals of less than 21 days, whereas oligomenorrhea describes menstrual cycles occuring at intervals greater than 35 days. Menstrual cycles tend to be most irregular in the first 2 years after menarche and in the 3–5 years before menopause (perimenopause).

The follicular phase of the menstrual cycles starts at the first day of menses, continues until ovulation, and is characterized by a variable length, low basal body temperature, development of ovarian follicles, vascular growth of the endometrium, and the secretion of estrogen from the ovary. The luteal phase begins with ovulation, continues until the beginning of menses, and is characterized by a relatively constant duration of 12–16 days, an elevated basal body temperature, the formation of the corpus luteum in the ovary with the secretion of progesterone and estrogen, and preparation of the endometrium for implantation of an embryo.

Regular menstrual cycles occur as a result of complex, coordinated interactions among the central nervous system, the hypothalamus, the pituitary, and the ovary. Specifically, menstrual cyclicity occurs as a result of the pulsatile secretion of gonadotropin-releasing hormone (GnRH) by neurons in the preoptic and arcuate nuclei of the hypothalamus. GnRH then acts on the pituitary to stimulate release of the gonadotropins luteinizing hormone (LH) and follicular stimulating hormone (FSH), which influence the selection and maturation of the follicle for ovulation as well as secretion of ovarian steroid hormones that act on the genital tract. GnRH is secreted in a pulsatile manner at approximately 1 pulse per h in the follicular phase and 1 pulse per 2–3 h in the luteal phase, and the amplitude and frequency of secretions are influenced by feedback from estrogen and progesterone as well as catecholamines, dopamine, and norepinephrine within the brain. Estrogen levels rise in the follicular phase, reaching a peak approximately 24–36 h before ovulation. LH increases steadily until the midcycle when there is a surge, and ovulation occurs approximately 10–12 h after the LH peak. In the absence of pregnancy, decreasing steroid levels result in the constriction of the arteries supplying the upper two-thirds of the endometrium, with subsequent shedding of the degraded endometrial tissue.

Biological Effects of Stress on Menstruation

Amenorrhea is defined by the absence of menses for 3 or more months. The failure of menarche to occur is referred to as primary amenorrhea; secondary amenorrhea refers to the discontinuation of menses after the onset of menarche. Prevalence rates for secondary amenorrhea range from 8.5% among women ages 13–18 years, 7.6% among women ages 15–24 years, and 3% among women ages 25–34 years.

Identifiable or organic causes of secondary amenorrhea and anovulation include a pituitary adenoma or hypothalamic tumor; however, the most common cause of amenorrhea is not the result of an identifiable organic source but is, rather, associated with psychological and lifestyle variables, including excessive exercise, low weight, affective and eating disorders, substance use, and stress. This condition is known as functional hypothalamic amenorrhea (FHA). The function of the hypothalamus is to maintain homeostasis and promote adaptation by regulating the neuroendocrine axis. It receives afferent neural information from other brain areas, as well as signals from the periphery that cross the blood–brain barrier, and then releases hormones that influence the synthesis and release of specific pituitary hormones in an integrated fashion, coordinating endocrine responses with internal and external demands. Changes in activity at one hypothalamic area can result in profound changes in the function of other areas. Psychophysiological factors, for instance, affect central neuroregulatory networks that subsequently disrupt the GnRH pulse generator and impact reproductivity. Specifically, stress can result in a decrease in GnRH drive, with the frequency and amplitude of the pulsatile release of GnRH falling out of the normal range. In general, catecholamines, epinephrine, and norepinephrine increase GnRH release, whereas β-endorphins decrease GnRH release. Although plasma concentrations of GnRH are too low to measure, LH levels correlate well with those of GnRH, and its secretory patterns can be used for information on hypothalamic-pituitary-gonadal (HPG) activity. LH pulses normally have a constant amplitude with a frequency of 2–6 h in the follicular phase and a more variable amplitude with a frequency of 2–6 h in the luteal phase. Studies have shown that, in women with the presence of both a stressful life event and a psychiatric diagnosis, spontaneous LH pulse frequency is inhibited. A study of 67 patients with hypothalamic secondary amenorrhea found that the onset of the menstrual disorder was correlated with a psychosocial stressor in close to half of the patients. When both a psychiatric diagnosis and a stressful life event are present, LH pulse frequency can be reduced by as much as 50% of that for normally menstruating women. Studies have also demonstrated that the presence of an anxiety or depressive disorder reduces pulse amplitude significantly. However, for women with amenorrhea without a psychiatric disorder or a stressful life event, the pulsatile release of LH is similar to that in normally menstruating women in the follicular phase. Thus psychogenic factors appear to influence LH release, reflecting effects on HPG activity and GnRH secretion. With significant declines in pulsatile GnRH secretion, the pituitary secretion of LH and FSH is reduced, compromising folliculogenesis and ovulation.

A possible mechanism that may link the GnRH pulse generator and stress involves the hypothalamic-pituitary-adrenal (HPA) axis, which is activated by stress. Women with secondary amenorrhea often display hypercortisolism, and in monkeys and rats, the administration of corticotropin releasing hormone (CRH) results in an acute decrease in pulsatile GnRH and gonadotropin release. CRH also inhibits LH by central effects, partially mediated by central endogenous opiates. Stress stimulates the expression of CRH and vasopressin. In monkeys, vasopressin has been shown to decrease LH secretion acutely when administered intracerebroventricularly.

Further evidence suggesting involvement of the HPA axis has been provided by Berga, who demonstrated that cortisol concentrations, which reflect HPA activity, are elevated in women with FHA. In women with other causes of anovulation, cortisol concentrations were found to be comparable to those observed in women who were eumenorrheic with biochemical evidence of ovulation. Women with FHA who resumed ovulation had cortisol concentrations similar to eumenorrheic women and lower than women with persistent FHA.

Anorexia Nervosa and Amenorrhea

Much of the literature on stress and menstruation focuses on women with anorexia nervosa. Anorexia nervosa is characterized by a refusal to maintain body weight at or above the minimally normal weight for age and height, an intense fear of gaining weight even though underweight, disturbance in the way in which one's body weight or shape is experienced, and the absence of at least three consecutive menstrual cycles. The disorder has a prevalence rate of 0.5–1.0% among females of late adolescence and early adulthood, although individuals with eating disorders that do not meet the full criteria for anorexia are more common. Anorexia accounts for 15–34.5% of patients with amenorrhea.

Clinical traits of anorexia often include an obsessive preoccupation with dieting, a desire to regress to prepubertal body habits to disguise femininity, and intense, obsessive-compulsive personality traits that result in hyperachievement. Mean age of onset for the disorder is 17 years, with possible bimodal peaks at ages 14 and 18. The onset of illness is often associated with a stressful life event, such as leaving home for college or the breakup of a relationship. The onset of dieting may be related to the stressor or may begin more insidiously, and amenorrhea can precede or be associated with weight loss. Unless the psychological stress is also addressed, menstrual cycles can remain abnormal, despite adequate weight gain. Follow-up studies at 2 years have found that psychological impairment persists in one-third to one-half of patients, with one-third of patients experiencing recurrent affective disorders and one-fourth of patients not regaining menses or attaining 75% of ideal body weight.

Females with anorexia nervosa demonstrate a pattern of 24-h gonadotropin secretion that is similar to prepubertal girls, with reversion to adult patterns following adequate weight gain and a change in behavior. Compared with normally menstruating women, the LH response to GnRH is diminished in the follicular phase. For women with secondary amenorrhea or infertility and weight loss, but without anorexia, similar but less severe changes in LH are seen.

Exercise, Stress, and the Menstrual Cycle

Strenuous, regular physical activity has also been associated with menstrual irregularities, oligomenorrhea, amenorrhea, or delayed menarche. Up to 50% of competitive runners, 25% of recreational runners, and 12% of cyclists and swimmers demonstrate amenorrhea. Both weight loss and stress have been implicated in the cause of exercise-associated amenorrhea through the disruption of GnRH secretion. Stress can be metabolic, psychological, or a combination of both, and its effects may be partly mediated by the increased β-endorphin levels that impact the amplitude and frequency of LH pulses. In addition, the release of CRH in endurance exercise can inhibit gonadotropin secretion and activate the release of corticosteroids and androgenic steroids. Although psychological stress may result in erratic menstrual cycles, its role in exercise-related amenorrhea appears to involve initiation more than continuation.

Effects of Menstrual Cycle on Stress, Mood, and Psychiatric Symptoms

In addition to the influence of stress on the menstrual cycle, monthly fluctuations of reproductive hormones can impact a woman's vulnerability to the experience of stress. Some studies, for example, reported a fourfold increase in the prevalence of suicide attempts and allergic bronchial asthma attacks in the late luteal phase of the menstrual cycle.

The levels of estrogen, progesterone, and their metabolites fall during the late luteal phase of the menstrual cycle and remain low during the early follicular phase. These gonadal steroids modulate the central neurotransmitter function of serotonin, dopamine, norepinephrine, and γ-aminobutyric acid and thus, as their levels vary across the menstrual cycle, may influence symptoms of irritability, anxiety, depression, and fatigue. For example, the progesterone metabolites allopregnanolone and pregnanolone may have anxiolytic properties through their barbiturate-like effect on γ-aminobutyric acid receptors, with decreased levels of these metabolites correlating with increased tension and anxiety.

Premenstrual asthma, or the worsening of asthma symptoms and pulmonary function in relation to menstruation, has been described in approximately one-third of women. A number of studies reported increases in asthma prior to menstruation and, to a lesser extent, during menstruation. Mirdal suggested a relationship among lowered resistance to stress, lowered resistance to infections, and increased bronchial hyperreactivity as background etiological factors for the occurrence of premenstrual asthma.

The premenstrual and menstrual phases of the menstrual cycle have been associated with an increased vulnerability to an exacerbation of psychiatric symptoms, as well as a peak in psychiatric admissions. Literature in this area is limited to case reports and small studies, which have found evidence of premenstrual exacerbation in schizophrenia, depression, bulimia nervosa, anxiety disorders, and substance abuse. For example, in a prospective study of 27 women with research diagnostic criteria for major, minor, or intermittent depression responding to treatment with imipramine or phenelzine, one-fourth of the women experienced premenstrual recurrence of symptoms of low mood, anhedonia, anxiety, increased appetite, and hypersomnia, which remitted following menses. For some women, an increased consumption of alcohol and marijuana occurs premenstrually. A study of 14 women with alcohol dependence found an association between alcohol intake and severity of premenstrual symptoms. Similar findings were reported in a prospective study of 21 women with a history of regular marijuana use. Smoking frequency has also been shown to vary across the menstrual cycle, with approximately 70% of women reporting an increase in the 7–10 days before their menstrual period. Researchers postulate that reproductive hormones may influence psychiatric symptoms by direct effects on central neurotransmitter function, as well as by causing the serum concentrations of medication to vary across the menstrual cycle.

Consequences of Amenorrhea

The hypoestrogenism associated with secondary amenorrhea can have long-term effects, the most significant of which is osteoporosis. Osteoporosis results from an imbalance between bone formation and bone resorption. Rapid increases in bone density are seen during puberty, with peak bone density of the spine and hip occurring by age 20. Females ages 14–18 with amenorrhea, especially if associated with weight changes, anorexia, or excessive exercise, risk decreased bone mineral density compared with normally menstruating young women. Amenorrheic athletes, for instance, have a significantly reduced spinal bone mineral content compared with controls with normal menstrual cycles. The peak bone density of premenopausal women influences the onset of osteoporosis later in life; thus, as life expectancy increases, the potential morbidity from osteoporosis also increases.

Treatment Issues

Stress can have a profound impact on menstruation and reproduction, ranging from cycles of marginal quality to chronic anovulation. Although mediated through biological actions on the hypothalamus, GnRH, and the HPA axis, these effects are potentially reversible. In managing women with functional hypothalamic amenorrhea, the psychological, behavioral, and psychiatric variables that influence hypothalamic function must be considered. Although pharmacological interventions can supply appropriate sex steroid exposure, restore hormonal balance, or induce ovulation, hormonal treatments can prevent the recognition of important emotional, behavioral, or psychiatric symptoms. Many women with FHA may have a potentially reversible condition that can be addressed with education, changes in lifestyle, psychotherapy, assistance in identifying and coping with stressors, or attention to a psychiatric condition. Cognitive-behavioral therapy, for instance, has been shown to result in the recovery of ovarian function for women with FHA who do not have a psychiatric disorder or engage in excessive exercise. Such interventions can help ameliorate the long-term consequences of stress and anovulation, as well as the health hazards associated with relative hypoestrogenism.

Finally, in evaluating a woman of reproductive age, the relationship between her symptoms and her menstrual cycle should be considered. Emotional symptoms can vary across the menstrual cycle because reproductive hormones can influence vulnerability to stress as well as mood changes and anxiety. With an awareness of these fluctuations, women may benefit from a greater sense of predictability and control over their symptoms. In addition, overmedication or undermedication with pharmacological agents can be avoided.

Further Reading

Barnea, E. R. and Tal, J. (1991). Stress-related reproductive failure. *Journal of In Vitro Fertilization and Embryo Transfer* **8**, 15–23.

Berga, S. L. (1996). Functional hypothalamic chronic ovulation. In: Adashi, E. Y., Rock, J. A. & Rosenwaks, Z. (eds.) *Reproductive endocrinology, surgery and technology* (vol. 1), pp. 1061–1075. Philadelphia: Lippincott-Raven.

Berga, S. L. (1996). Stress and ovarian function. *American Journal of Sports Medicine* **24**, S36–S37.

Berga, S. L., Daniels, T. L. and Giles, D. E. (1997). Women with functional hypothalamic amenorrhea but not other forms of anovulation display amplified cortisol concentrations. *Fertilization and Sterilization* **67**, 1024–1030.

Berga, S. L. and Girton, L. G. (1989). The psychoneuroendocrinology of functional hypothalamic amenorrhea. *Psychiatric Clinics of North America: Women's Disorders* **12**, 105–116.

Berga, S. L., Marcus, M. D., Loucks, T. L., et al. (2003). Recovery of ovarian activity in women with functional hypothalamic amenorrhea who were treated with cognitive behavioral therapy. *Fertilization and Sterilization* **80**, 976–981.

Buskirk, E. R., Mendez, J. and Durfee, S. (1985). Effects of exercise on the body composition of women. *Seminars in Reproductive Endocrinology* **3**, 9–16.

Carpenter, S. E. (1994). Psychosocial menstrual disorders: stress, exercise and diet's effect on the menstrual cycle. *Current Opinion in Obstetrics and Gynecology* **6**, 536–539.

Christia, J. S., Loyd, J. A. and Davis, D. E. (1965). The role of endocrines in the self regulation of mammalian population. *Recent Progress in Hormone Research* **21**, 501–578.

Chrousos, G. P. and Gold, P. W. (1992). The concepts of stress and stress system disorders. *Journal of the American Medical Association* **267**, 1244–1252.

Collins, A., Eneroth, P. and Landgren, B. M. (1985). Psychoneuroendocrine stress responses and mood as related to the menstrual cycle. *Psychosomatic Medicine* **47**, 512–527.

Dalton, K. (1964). The influence of menstruation on health and disease. *Proceedings of the Royal Society of Medicine* **57**, 18–20.

Drinkwater, B. L. (1984). Bone mineral content of amenorrheic athletes. *New England Journal of Medicine* **311**, 277–281.

Facchinetti, F., Fava, M., Fioroni, L., et al. (1993). Stressful life events and affective disorders inhibit pulsatile LH secretion in hypothalamic amenorrhea. *Psychoneuroendocrinology* **18**, 397–404.

Feingold, K. R., Gavin, L. A., Schambelan, M., et al. (1990). Female endocrinology. In: Andreoli, T. E., Carpenter, C. C., Plum, F. & Smith, L. H. (eds.) *Cecil essentials of medicine* (2nd edn., pp. 478–486). Philadelphia: Saunders.

Freeman, E. W., Purdy, R. H., Coutifaris, C., et al. (1993). Anxiolytic metabolites of progesterone: correlation with mood and performance measures following oral progesterone administration to healthy female volunteers. *Neuroendocrinology* **58**, 478–484.

Fries, H., Nillius, S. and Pettersson, F. (1974). Epidemiology of secondary amenorrhea. II: A retrospective evaluation of etiology with special regard to psychogenic factors and weight loss. *American Journal of Obstetrics and Gynecology* **118**, 473–479.

Glick, R., Harrison, W., Endicott, J., et al. (1991). Treatment of premenstrual dysphoric symptoms in depressed women. *Journal of the American Medical Women's Association* **46**, 182–185.

Hendrick, V., Altshuler, L. L. and Burt, V. K. (1996). Course of psychiatric disorders across the menstrual cycle. *Harvard Review of Psychiatry* **4**, 200–207.

Herzog, D. B. and Copeland, P. M. (1985). Eating disorders. *New England Journal of Medicine* **313**, 295–303.

Marshall, J. (1989). Regulation of gonadotropin secretion. In: Degroot, L., Besser, G., Marshal, J., et al. (eds.) *Endocrinology.* Philadelphia: Saunders.

Melo, N. K., Mendelson, J. H. and Lex, B. W. (1990). Alcohol use and premenstrual symptoms in social drinkers. *Psychopharmacology* **101**, 448–455.

Melo, N. K., Mendelson, J. H. and Palmieri, S. L. (1987). Cigarette smoking by women: interactions with alcohol use. *Psychopharmacology* **93**, 8–15.

Mirdal, G. M., Petersson, B., Weeke, B., et al. (1998). Asthma and menstruation: the relationship between psychological and bronchial hyperreactivity. *British Journal of Medicine and Psychology* **71**, 47–55.

Nepomnaschy, P. A., Welch, K., McConnell, D., et al. (2004). Stress and female reproductive function: a study of daily variations in cortisol, gonadotropins, and gonadal steroids in a rural Mayan population. *American Journal of Human Biology* **16**, 523–532.

Podolsky, E. (1963). The woman alcoholic and premenstrual tension. *Journal of the American Medical Women's Association* **18**, 816–818.

Reame, N., Sauder, S., Kelch, R., et al. (1984). Pulsatile gonadotropin secretion during the human menstrual cycle: evidence for altered frequency of gonadotropin-releasing hormone secretion. *Journal of Clinical Endocrinology and Metabolism* **59**, 328–337.

Rivier, C. and Vale, W. (1984). Influence of corticotropin releasing factor on reproductive function in the rat. *Endocrinology* **114**, 914–921.

Sapolsky, R. M., Romero, L. M. and Munck, A. U. (2000). How do glucocorticoids influence stress responses?: integrating permissive, suppressive, stimulatory, and preparative actions. *Endocrine Reviews* **21**, 55–89.

Schachter, M. and Shoham, Z. (1994). Amenorrhea during the reproductive years: is it safe? *Fertilization and Sterilization* **62**, 1–16.

Shalts, E., Xia, L., Xiao, E., et al. (1994). Inhibitory effects of arginine-vasopressin on LH secretion in the ovariectomized rhesus monkey. *Neuroendocrinology* **59**, 336–342.

Shangold, M. M. (1985). Exercise and amenorrhea. *Seminars in Reproductive Endocrinology* **3**, 35–43.

Taylor, J. W. (1974). The timing of menstrual-related symptoms assessed by a daily symptom rating scale. *Acta Psychiatrica Scandinavica* **60**, 87–105.
Tilbrook, A. J., Turner, A. I. and Clarke, I. J. (2000). Effects of stress on reproduction in non-rodent mammals: the role of glucocorticoids and sex differences. *Reviews of Reproduction* **5**, 105–113.
Tilbrook, A. J., Turner, A. I. and Clarke, I. J. (2002). Stress and reproduction: central mechanisms and sex differences in non-rodent species. *Stress* **5**, 83–100.
Warren, M. P. (1996). Clinical review 77: evaluation of secondary emenorrhea. *Journal of Clinical Endocrinology and Metabolism* **81**, 437–442.
Xiao, E. and Ferin, M. (1997). Stress-related disturbances of the menstrual cycle. *Annals of Medicine* **29**, 215–219.

Reproduction, Effects of Social Stress On

C A Shively
Wake Forest University School of Medicine, Winston-Salem, NC, USA

This is a revised version of the article by C A Shively, Encyclopedia of Stress, First edition, volume 3, pp 360–365, © 2000, Elsevier Inc.

Glossary

Functional hypothalamic chronic anovulation	Inhibition of ovulation due to stress.
Hypothalamic-pituitary-adrenocortical axis	A major stress reactive system in the body involving the hypothalamus, pituitary, and adrenal glands.
Hypothalamic-pituitary-gonadal axis	The pathway of the reproductive system that controls gonadal function.
Luteal phase deficiency	Abnormalities of the luteal phase of the menstrual cycle that may include reduced sex hormone concentrations and changes in phase length.
Stereotypy	A locomotor (e.g., pacing) or self-directed (e.g., biting) behavior that is performed precisely the same way, repeatedly in quick succession.

Reproductive failure rates are uniformly high across the mammalian order. From the perspective of human medicine, reproductive failure is often viewed as evidence of a disorder that requires treatment. However, mammologists and evolutionary biologists understandreproductive failure as an evolutionary safeguard against wasting energy on reproduction when the likelihood of a successful outcome is relatively low. From this perspective, it makes sense that the reproductive system would be especially sensitive to environmental variables that might influence the outcome of reproductive effort. Female mammals have a greater investment in reproduction than males, and the female reproductive system is particularly sensitive to environmental factors signaling adverse conditions for successful reproduction. Thus, there is less data available concerning stress effects on reproductive function of males than on that of females. For species that live in groups, social factors are key aspects of the environment. One type of social environmental influence to which the reproductive system of mammals appears quite sensitive is social stress. Social stress is defined here as a social environmental factor that perturbs homeostasis and elicits behavioral or physiological change. The purpose of this article is to examine the evidence of parental social stress on reproductive health, including fertility, pregnancy outcome, neonatal health, and the lifelong health of the offspring.

Social Stress and the Likelihood of Conception

Physiological Mechanisms

The mechanisms by which social stress may influence the likelihood of conception are not completely understood. However, stress-induced activation of the hypothalamic-pituitary-adrenocortical (HPA) axis inhibits the hypothalamic-pituitary-gonadal (HPG) axis at multiple levels. Corticotropin-releasing hormone (CRH) inhibits hypothalamic gonadotropin-releasing hormone (GnRH). CRH stimulates pituitary adrenocorticotropin (ACTH) secretion, which in turn increases adrenal glucocorticoid secretion. Glucocorticoids inhibit GnRH secretion, as well as pituitary luteinizing hormone and ovarian estrogen and progesterone secretion. CRH also stimulates β-endorphin, which in turn inhibits GnRH secretion. Gonadal dysfunction results from alterations in GnRH pulsatility from the hypothalamic pulse generator impairing ovulation. Other neurotransmitters that mediate stress effects on the GnRH pulse generator include dopamine, neuropeptide Y, norepinephrine, γ-aminobutyric acid (GABA), and endogenous opioid peptides.

Dopamine receptors appear to mediate stress-induced transcription of hypothalamic CRH and proopiomelanocortin, from which a number of peptides are derived, including ACTH and endogenous opioids. The results of a series of nonhuman primate studies suggest that dopamine is involved in the effect of one type of social stress on the reproductive system. A major social organizing mechanism of primate society is the social status hierarchy. Among group-living primates, low social status, or social subordination, appears stressful and is associated with lower reproductive output in females. Socially subordinate female cynomolgus monkeys (*Macaca fascicularis*) receive more aggression, maintain a high level of vigilance, are groomed less by conspecifics, and spend more time alone than their dominant counterparts. Their adrenal glands hypersecrete cortisol, and they are insensitive to glucocorticoid negative feedback. The central dopaminergic function of these females is also deranged, as evidenced by insensitivity to haloperidol, lower cerebrospinal fluid levels of homovanillic acid (HVA), a dopamine metabolite, and lower D_2 receptor binding potential in striatum observed by positron emission tomography. In males, the relationship between social subordination stress and reproductive output is less consistent than in females. Associations between social status and offspring sired are observed in some years but not others. Likewise, the relationship between low social status and activated HPA function is less apparent in male than in female Old World primates. However, central dopaminergic function of subordinate males is different than that of dominants, as evidenced by lower cerebral spinal fluid (CSF) HVA concentrations and lower striatal D_2 receptor binding potential. Thus, social subordination stress may alter central dopaminergic function, increase HPA activity, and inhibit HPG function.

Another mechanism that may mediate stress effects on conception involves reactive oxygen species (ROS). ROS can modify cell function and endanger cell survival. Because these are normal consequences of oxygen metabolism, ROS must be continuously deactivated by antioxidant defense mechanisms to avoid oxidative stress. There is some evidence that psychosocial stress may increase ROS, decrease DNA repair, and alter rates of apoptosis. Thus, oxidative damage may occur during stress. High levels of ROS are found in the semen of infertile men and the peritoneal and follicular fluid of infertile women.

Inhibition/Delay of Sexual Maturation

Two hypotheses address the relationship between social stress and sexual maturation. The social suppression hypothesis posits that stress suppresses sexual development. In support of this hypothesis, it has been widely observed in monkeys that low social status is associated with delayed sexual maturation and that dominant females reproduce at an earlier age than subordinate females. Likewise, girls from higher social classes enter puberty earlier than girls from lower social classes. Delayed sexual maturation following severe stress (e.g., war) has been documented in boys and girls, though is not well studied. In contrast, the psychosocial acceleration theory posits that under certain types of stressful conditions in which low-quality parental investment signals that parental investment does not promote reproductive success, sexual maturation may accelerate so that reproduction may occur earlier and more often. There is some evidence that family warmth and positivity may delay, and family conflict and coercion may accelerate, pubertal development. Thus, the nature of the psychosocial stressor may be critical in predicting effects on sexual development.

Inhibition/Delay of Ovulation

Low social status is associated with inhibition of ovulation in baboons and macaques (*Macaca* spp.). Female cynomolgus monkeys (*M. fascicularis*) have menstrual cycles that are very similar to those of women. Socially subordinate female cynomolgus monkeys have low luteal phase progesterone concentrations, low follicular phase estradiol concentrations, a greater proportion of menstrual cycles with impaired luteal function, and a greater proportion of anovulatory menstrual cycles. Furthermore, when female monkeys change social status, their menstrual cycle characteristics change also (**Table 1**), suggesting that the reproductive system of these females is exquisitely sensitive to their social environment.

Socially suppressed ovarian function in these monkeys is associated with deleterious effects on the skeletal and cardiovascular systems, suggesting that socially induced hormonal impairments unaccompanied by amenorrhea have far-reaching effects on health.

Social stress may also inhibit ovulation in women, a condition referred to as functional hypothalamic amenorrhea or functional hypothalamic chronic anovulation (FHCA). Diagnosis is by exclusion of all other potential organic causes. The best indicator that FHCA is stress related is that it is generally accompanied by hypercortisolemia. Note that socially subordinate female monkeys that are stressed do not necessarily have more anovulatory cycles than their nonstressed dominant counterparts. Thus, in extrapolating to women, it is important to consider that stress-induced suppression of reproductive function may not manifest as frank amenorrhea, complicating

Table 1 Effect of changing social status on menstrual cycles[a]

Initial status	*Subordinate*		*Dominant*		*Final status effect p* ≤
Final status	*Subordinate*	*Dominant*	*Subordinate*	*Dominant*	
Number of cycles	15.2 (0.94)	15.4 (1.03)	14.4 (1.52)	15.1 (1.1)	0.60
Percent ovulatory	68.1 (9.19)	91.4 (3.36)	81.6 (6.34)	88.4 (4.42)	0.03
Percent impaired	19.4 (5.21)	4.2 (1.65)	8.4 (2.8)	8.1 (2.60)	0.08
Percent anovulatory	12.5 (6.00)	4.5 (2.21)	9.9 (5.44)	3.5 (2.76)	0.17
Progesterone (ng/ml)	6.7 (0.96)	10.4 (1.72)	8.1 (0.98)	9.6 (0.97)	0.03

[a] Means and standard errors. Social status of 42 female cynomolgus monkeys living in small social groups was documented for 2 months. The constituency of the social groups was changed such that half of the subordinates became dominant and half of the dominants became subordinate, and social status and menstrual cycle characteristics were documented for 24 months.

diagnosis. In women, perturbations in GnRH pulsatility may result in ovarian dysfunction manifested as amenorrhea, polymenorrhea, oligomenorrhea, or luteal phase deficiency, the latter of which may go undetected unless infertility issues arise. FHCA also appears reversible in women. The prevalence of FHCA varies depending on the subpopulation considered. Estimates in the general population range from 2 to 7%, whereas in high-risk populations, such as women going to college or joining the armed forces and women with depression, the prevalence may be as high as 70%. Under these circumstances ovulatory impairment appears to coincide with psychosocial stress and precede nutritional stress. Women that develop FHCA are more likely to be anxious, be perfectionists, and have difficulty coping.

Impairment of Hypothalamic-Pituitary-Testicular Function

During periods of social instability, low social status and aggression received are both associated with suppressed plasma testosterone concentrations in male macaques and baboons. In men, stressful events (e.g., work stress, exams, or competitions) may decrease testosterone levels, which can lead to decreased libido, diminished muscle mass, change in hair growth, and decreased spermatogenesis. Decreased testosterone may be due to perturbations in GnRH pulsatility or to direct effects of cortisol on testicular Leydig cell testosterone production. Social stress (e.g., death of a close family member) can result in oligoasthenozoospermia, which may remain undetected unless infertility issues arise. Decreased sperm number and quality are associated with decreased fertility.

Social Stress and Pregnancy Outcome

Physiological Mechanisms

There are several ways in which neuroendocrine stress responsivity may affect pregnancy. CRH regulates the HPA responses to stress. During pregnancy it also coordinates and controls the physiology of parturition. CRH is produced in the placenta, and placental CRH is stress sensitive. Maternal pituitary-adrenal hormones stimulate placental CRH secretion. Maternal stress is positively associated with circulating ACTH concentrations, and maternal social support is negatively associated with circulating concentrations of ACTH, β-endorphin, and cortisol. Maternal β-endorphin secretion during the third trimester is associated with increased fetal heart rate reactivity and decreased uroplacental blood flow, the latter being consistent with fetal hypoxia. Elevated CRH levels are associated with preterm labor and preterm delivery. Onset of the birthing process also involves oxytocin, vasopressin, and prostaglandins, as well as HPA activation. Secretion of these hormones may be altered by stress, thus affecting the timing of birth. Indeed, uteri from preterm deliveries appear to be hypersensitive to oxytocin. Stress-induced catecholamine and oxytocin may reduce the threshold of uterine contractility, thus resulting in preterm labor.

There is substantial evidence that HPA axis peptides (including ACTH and β-endorphin) affect the development of fetal brain and behavior and that perinatal exposure to ACTH and its analogues permanently alters growth and behavior. Thus, maternal stress may alter the trajectory of development beginning *in utero*.

Neuroendocrine stress responses are known to suppress the immune system; however, these processes have been little studied during pregnancy. Pregnancy involves immunosuppression in order to avoid fetal rejection. Thus, stress-related immunosuppression may be superimposed on the normal physiological immunosuppression of pregnancy, potentially affecting pregnancy outcome. Stress-induced immunosuppression increases vulnerability to infection. Infection, in turn, may induce preterm delivery. Preeclampsia is also associated with altered immune function and thus may be affected by stress-induced immunosuppression. Preterm birth is associated with enhanced expression of pro-inflammatory cytokines. Pro-inflammatory cytokines stimulate prostaglandin and metalloprotease synthesis in gestational tissues, which promote spontaneous labor and rupture of membranes. They also stimulate fetal-placental production of steroids and CRH, which promote parturition.

Norepinephrine and epinephrine are stress-responsive catecholamines that decrease blood flow to the uterus. Decreased uterine blood flow may cause hypoxia, hypotension, bradycardia, and malformations in the fetus. Hypoxia may result in increased ROS production. Oxidative stress due to increased ROS and/or decreased antioxidant defense mechanisms has been implicated in miscarriage and preeclampsia.

Thus, maternal, placental, and fetal neuroendocrine, immune, and cardiovascular processes link maternal stress during pregnancy with adverse pregnancy outcomes.

Failure of Implantation

It is difficult to determine failure of implantation, especially to discriminate it from ovulatory difficulties. Both social status and current ecological conditions affect the likelihood of successful implantation in yellow baboons. Under poor environmental conditions, socially dominant females (with low social stress) are more likely to achieve successful implantation than their subordinate, stressed counterparts. Likewise, in an *in vitro* fertilization study, implantation rates were reportedly higher in women with relatively low cardiovascular reactivity to a standardized laboratory stressor.

Spontaneous Abortion

There is an association between spontaneous abortion and psychological stress in pigtail macaques (*M. nemestrina*). Low social status, psychological stress, low control, and low social support have been associated with spontaneous abortion in humans. In 192 women with recent spontaneous abortions, it was found that recent negative life events significantly increased the likelihood of spontaneous abortion of chromosomally normal conceptions. In perhaps one of the largest studies available ($n = 214{,}108$), adverse pregnancy outcomes, including spontaneous abortion, were most frequent in women working in jobs characterized by high demand and low control. In another study of several thousand women, stressful work increased spontaneous abortion by a factor of 2.45 (95% confidence interval [CI] 1.03–5.81) in older women, 2.96 (95% CI 1.16–7.52) in smokers, and 2.27 (95% CI 0.97–5.27) in primigravid women. Thus, stressful life events, work characterized by high demand and low control, and stressful work may increase rates of spontaneous abortion.

Maternal Stress and Neonatal Mortality

Associations of neonatal mortality and maternal social stress are well documented in nonhuman primates. Rhesus macaque infants born to socially dominant females have a higher rate of survival than those born to socially subordinate mothers. Higher mortality also has been observed among offspring of psychologically stressed pigtail macaques. Chimpanzee and gorilla offspring born to subordinate mothers are subject to greater neonatal mortality than those born to dominants, in part due to infanticide. Maternal psychological stress and low social status have been associated with neonatal mortality in humans. In a large study ($n = 214{,}108$), adverse pregnancy outcomes, including stillbirth, were most frequent in women working in jobs characterized by high demand and low control. Maternal risk factors for sudden infant death syndrome (SIDS) include low socioeconomic status (SES), unmarried status, teen age, less education, depression, drug use, and ethnicity. These characteristics are also risk factors for low birth weight, and low birth weight is a powerful predictor of SIDS. While it is difficult at this time to tease apart the relative contributions of these risk factors, all may involve increased maternal stress during gestation.

Maternal Stress and Neonatal Morbidity

The effects of maternal social stress during pregnancy on neonatal morbidity are more subtle and difficult to determine than neonatal mortality. Measures of neonatal morbidity include labor and delivery complications, gestational age, Apgar scores, birth weight, and neuromotor and neurobehavioral development during the first 30 days.

A series of studies in squirrel (*Saimiri boliviensis*) and rhesus monkeys demonstrated that mild maternal stress (e.g., removal from a home cage daily followed by 10 min of white noise during mid-late gestation) results in lower birth weight, impaired neuromotor development (as measured by a modified Brazelton Newborn Behavioral Assessment Scale), and impaired neurobehavioral development of attention and orienting. Early gestation stress was associated with more profound impairments to growth and neuromotor development during the first postnatal month than late gestation stress. These impairments are mimicked by administering ACTH to pregnant females for 2 weeks at mid-pregnancy, suggesting that activation of the HPA axis is instrumental in the deleterious effects of maternal prenatal stress on infant morbidity. Similar decrements in offspring development continue into adolescence (see later).

A large number of studies have been conducted to test the hypothesis that prenatal maternal stress causes infant morbidity in humans, and the balance of the literature supports this hypothesis. Birth weight and gestational age are the most commonly measured outcome variables. Low birth weight can be due to preterm delivery (less than 37 weeks gestation with an appropriate infant weight for gestational age) or to retarded fetal growth (inappropriate weight for gestational age). Maternal anxiety and depression result in low birth weight and perhaps smaller head size. The magnitude of the effect is comparable to that of smoking. Composite measures of maternal prenatal stress (including some combination of trait or state anxiety, depression, life events, social support, and self esteem) best predict preterm delivery/low gestational age. Likewise, the association between psychosocial stressors and birth weight is strongest when composite measures of maternal stress (e.g., exposure to stressors such as life event scales, social support, anxiety, health risk behaviors) were used. The timing of the stress is important. Low birth weight and shorter gestational age have been observed when the stressors occur in the first trimester, whereas preterm delivery is associated with third trimester stress. In one of the largest studies available ($n = 214{,}108$), adverse pregnancy outcomes, including light-for-date birth weight and full-term low birth weight, were most frequent in women working in jobs characterized by high demand and low control.

Long-Term Health of the Offspring

Maternal Stress and Offspring Central Nervous System (CNS) Function

The effects of maternal stress during gestation have been shown to affect CNS function of rhesus monkeys (*M. mulatta*) through adolescence (4 years of age). Six-month-old offspring from control mothers and mothers that experienced a daily mild stressor (three random white noise bursts over 10 min) were evaluated during the latter half of pregnancy. In a response to a novel environment, offspring of prenatally stressed mothers exhibited more disturbance behavior (e.g., clinging to attachment object, self-directed stereotypic behaviors) and lower levels of gross motor and exploratory behavior than those of nonstressed mothers. At 8 and 18 months, prenatal stress-derived monkeys had higher CSF concentrations of metabolites of dopamine and norepinephrine, suggesting altered CNS function. The behavioral responses of these monkeys to social separation stress were evaluated. Disturbances in exploratory, locomotor, and clinging behavior observed at 6 months of age continued, and disturbances in social play were also observed. The effects of prenatal stress on later behavioral responses to stress were more profound for social than for nonsocial behavior, and suggest that offspring from prenatally stressed mothers are behaviorally hyperresponsive to stress. Between 6 months and 1 year of age, male offspring of prenatally stressed mothers had smaller, and females had larger, corpus callosum. At 14–19 months of age, prenatal stress-derived monkeys had higher ACTH and cortisol levels at baseline and under anesthesia. Furthermore, in response to stress, prenatal stress-derived offspring had higher ACTH and similar cortisol responses as control offspring. These observations suggest that the HPA axis of offspring of primate mothers stressed during pregnancy hyperresponds to stress later in life, and that the components of this stress-responsive system are dysregulated. The behavior of these prenatal stress-derived offspring was characterized again at 4 years of age, a time corresponding to human adolescence. At this age, the behavioral pathology of the prenatal stress-derived offspring was profound and included greater locomotion, stereotypies (pathological repetitive behaviors such as rocking), clinging, and self-clasping. These monkeys explored less in a novel environment and engaged in less social interaction in a playroom environment. At 5–7 years of age, *in vivo* imaging studies revealed a perturbed striatal dopaminergic system, which is critically involved in drug abuse vulnerability and sensitive to adult social stresses. Taken together, these observations suggest that prenatal stress can have profound and long-term effects on the behavior and neurobiology of primate offspring that is particularly apparent in response to stress.

Similar data from human studies are difficult to acquire. However, the results of a number of studies suggest that prenatal stress may perturb CNS function of newborns. There are reports of increased fetal activity associated with maternal anxiety and catastrophic stress due to earthquake. Anxious, type A, or depressed mothers have newborns who cry more and are more difficult to soothe. First trimester maternal stress and anxiety have been associated with low scores on cognitive and psychomotor tests, poor adaptation to novel environments, and difficult behavior in infants 8 months of age. At 9 years of age, attention deficits and aggressiveness were more common in the offspring of mothers who were anxious during pregnancy. Maternal stress is also linked to offspring psychopathology. Schizophrenia, in particular, has been linked to prenatal stress. Maternal exposure to death of a loved one, influenza infection, or catastrophic stressors increase the risk of the offspring developing schizophrenia, the onset of which is most common between 16 and 30 years of age.

The Significance of Low Birth Weight to Health in Later Life

Cardiovascular disease (CVD) is the leading killer ofmen and women. Low birth weight has been associated with all-cause mortality, coronary heart disease, stroke, type II (non-insulin-dependent) diabetes mellitus, hypertension, and the metabolic syndrome. The metabolic syndrome is a cluster of characteristics (e.g., abdominal fat deposition, hyperglycemia, hyperinsulinemia, hypertension, and an atherogenic lipid profile) that greatly increase risk of CVD. Given the patterning of associations, it appears that low birth weight may be associated with lifelong derangement of the metabolic function of several major systems that culminates in increased risk of cardiovascular disease. Hypotheses currently being tested to explain fetal programming of adult health include the possibility that suboptimal environmental influences on fetal growth lead to permanent changes in organogenesis (i.e., particularly those involved with energy metabolism) that may serve to preserve the growth of certain organs, like the brain, to the expense of the function of other systems. Prenatal exposure to excess cortisol is considered a likely mechanism by which maternal stress during gestation may lead to fetal programming of cardiovascular, metabolic, and neuroendocrine disorders in adult life.

Exaggerated maternal stress responses can bathe the fetus in excessive glucocorticoids, resulting in an adult programmed for exaggerated HPA responses to stress. If this adult gestates young, she may also produce offspring with exaggerated stress responses, and thus intergenerational transmission of stress reactivity and subsequent ill health may be perpetuated. Indeed, low-birth-weight women are more likely to have low-birth-weight babies.

See Also the Following Articles

Social Stress, Animal Models of.

Further Reading

Amiel-Tison, C., Cabrol, D., Denver, R., et al. (2004). Fetal adaptation to stress: Part II. Evolutionary aspects; stress-induced hippocampal damage; long-term effects on behavior; consequences on adult health. *Early Human Development* **78**(2), 81–94.

Berga, S. L. (1997). Behaviorally induced reproductive compromise in women and men. *Seminars in Reproductive Endocrinology* **15**, 47–53.

Buitelaar, J. K., Huizink, A. C., Mulder, E. J., et al. (2003). Prenatal stress and cognitive development and temperament in infants. *Neurobiology of Aging* **24**(supplement 1), S53–S60.

Burton, G. J. and Jauniaux, E. (2004). Placental oxidative stress: from miscarriage to preeclampsia. *Journal of the Society for Gynecologic Investigation* **11**(6), 342–352.

Drake, A. J. and Walker, B. R. (2004). The intergenerational effects of fetal programming: non-genomic mechanisms for the inheritance of low birth weight and cardiovascular risk. *The Journal of Endocrinology* **180**(1), 1–16.

Federenko, I. S. and Wadhwa, P. D. (2004). Women's mental health during pregnancy influences fetal and infant developmental and health outcomes. *CNS Spectrum* **9**, 198–206.

Huizink, A. C., Mulder, E. J. and Buitelaar, J. K. (2004). Prenatal stress and risk for psychopathology: specific effects or induction of general susceptibility? *Psychological Bulletin* **130**, 115–142.

Kaplan, J. R. and Manuck, S. B. (2004). Ovarian dysfunction, stress, and disease: a primate continuum. *Institute of Laboratory Animal Resources Journal* **45**, 89–115.

Koenig, J. I., Kirkpatrick, B. and Lee, P. (2002). Glucocorticoid hormones and early brain development in schizophrenia. *Neuropsychopharmacology* **27**(2), 309–318.

Mulder, E. J., Robles de Medina, P. G. and Huizink, A. C. (2002). Prenatal maternal stress: effects on pregnancy and the (unborn) child. *Early Human Development* **70**(1-2), 3–14.

Roberts, A. D., Moore, C. F., DeJesus, O. T., et al. (2004). Prenatal stress, moderate fetal alcohol, and dopamine system function in rhesus monkeys. *Neurotoxicology and Teratology* **26**(2), 169–178.

Schneider, M. L., Roughton, E. C., Koehler, A. J., et al. (1999). Growth and development following prenatal stress exposure in primates: an examination of ontogenetic vulnerability. *Child Development* **70**(2), 263–274.

Seckl, J. R. (2004). Prenatal glucocorticoids and long-term programming. *European Journal of Endocrinology* **151**(supplement 3), U49–U62.

Sullivan, F. M. and Barlow, S. M. (2001). Review of risk factors for sudden infant death syndrome. *Paediatric and Perinatal Epidemiology* **15**(2), 144–200.

Wasser, S. K. and Barash, D. P. (1983). Reproductive suppression among female mammals: implications for biomedicine and sexual selection theory. *The Quarterly Review of Biology* **58**, 513–538.

Zitzmann, M. and Nieschlag, E. (2001). Testosterone levels in healthy men and the relation to behavioural and physical characteristics: facts and constructs. *European Journal of Endocrinology* **144**(3), 183–197.

Pheromones

A Kumar, C A Dudley, S Chakravarty and R L Moss
University of Texas Southwestern Medical Center, Dallas, TX, USA

This is a revised version of the article by C A Dudley, A Kumar and R L Moss, Encyclopedia of Stress, First edition, volume 3, pp 162–168, © 2000, Elsevier Inc.

Glossary

Accessory olfactory bulb (AOB)	A neural structure located at the dorsocaudal end of the main olfactory bulb but distinguished from the main olfactory bulb by the types of signals detected and by its central nervous system projection sites.
c-Fos immunocytochemistry	A method for measuring cellular activation by detecting the expression of the c-fos oncogene.
Chemo-architecture	The relationship between cellular topography and the cellular machinery used in signal detection and processing.
Chemosensory stimulation	An environmental stimulus detected by a sensory system via ligand–receptor binding.
Gonadotropin-releasing hormone (GnRH)	A decapeptide produced in the hypothalamus, responsible for stimulating the release of luteinizing hormone from the pituitary gland; also referred to as LHRH.
Sociogenic stress	A set of stresses caused by conspecific interactions.
Vomeronasal organ (VNO)	a specialized chemosensory structure for pheromone signaling.

Chemical Communication and Social Odors

Interorganism communication is an indispensable feature of species survival, and the signals employed for this purpose are quite diverse. Among the various senses employed, chemosensation (the detection and transduction of chemical environmental stimuli) is perhaps the most primitive. In addition to aiding in locating nutrition, chemosensory transduction allows an animal to find suitable mating partners and avoid dangerous predators. Pheromones are compounds used for intraspecies chemical communication that are secreted or excreted by one individual and elicit behavioral or physiological responses in the recipient. However, the great diversity of signals used in chemical communication by vertebrates suggests that this communication is not mediated exclusively by pheromones. A multiplicity of signals may be present in the same secretion, and it is unlikely that the response to this complex signal is mediated exclusively by a single sensory system. Johnston has recently suggested the term chemical signals for the wide array of odors regulating vertebrate behavior and physiology. Indeed, various chemosensory structures have been found in vertebrates that transduce chemosensory cues. Pheromones act on the recipient through olfaction, ingestion, or absorption; however, all mammalian pheromones studied so far act through olfactory pathways. Olfactory-mediated pheromonal communication in mammals is used to organize a wide range of social behaviors, such as mating, dominance, aggression, and maternal bonding, and hence these cues are also frequently referred to as social odors.

Mammalian pheromones elicit both long-lasting effects that bring about changes in the endocrine state of the recipient animal and short-term rapid effects on the recipient's behavior. For example, male mouse pheromones have been shown to induce advanced onset puberty in female counterparts (the Vandenbergh effect), the onset of estrus (the Whitten effect), and the termination of pregnancy (the Bruce effect) by an increase in luteinizing hormone (LH) and a decrease in prolactin. Female mouse pheromones cause a delay in the onset of puberty and a suppression of estrus in other female mice by increased release of prolactin. These delayed neuroendocrine effects on reproductive physiology and behavior have been termed the primer effect of mammalian pheromones.

The faster-acting releaser effects are elicited immediately, and these pheromones have been implicated in the regulation of intermale aggression, initiation of male ultrasonic vocalization and copulatory behavior, induction of lordosis (the receptive posture adopted by female rodents anticipating sexual intercourse), and parental care. Releaser effects are also modulated by the hormonal status of the animal, which is itself under pheromonal regulation. Gonadotropin-releasing hormone (GnRH) and LH play crucial roles in regulating these pheromone-induced fast behavioral responses.

The Vomeronasal Organ

Pheromone molecules are chemically unrelated and are contained in body fluids such as urine, sweat, and sebum. Pheromones are detected by peripheral sensory neurons sequestered in a tiny cigar-shaped bony capsule called the vomeronasal organ (VNO) or Jacobson's organ (**Figure 1a**). Located bilaterally on the posterodorsal aspect of the nasal septum, this tubular structure opens into the nasal or oral cavity via the vomeronasal duct, allowing chemical stimuli to reach VNO neurons from both the nose and mouth. In some mammals such as ungulates and felines, the males display a behavior called flehmen, which consists of curling of the upper lip and throwing the head up after investigating the female's genital area. This helps in facilitating the transport of the odorous compounds in female urine into the VNO of male, thus allowing the detection of the female's receptive state. In rodents, however, a pumping activity of the VNO associated with the autonomic afferent system appears to actively draw pheromone compounds into the lumen of the VNO, where they bind to receptors. These receptors lie on microvillous extensions of the dendrites of the vomeronasal receptor neurons (VNRNs). Patch clamp recordings from dissociated VNRNs reveal that they possess voltage-gated inward and outward currents consistent with the ability to generate action potentials. VNRNs from the mouse respond to putative pheromones from mouse urine with the generation of an outward current accompanied by a decrease in membrane conductance (**Figure 2**). In a current clamp mode, pheromone application causes hyperpolarization of the membrane. The binding of pheromone molecules to their specific membrane receptors activates an intracellular signaling cascade involving G-proteins ($G_{\alpha i2}$ in the apical neurons, $G_{\alpha o}$ in basal neurons), phospholipase C-β (PLC), and diacylglycerol (DAG). DAG, the second messenger, is the gating factor for a cation channel known as transient receptor potential channel 2 (TRPC2), whose opening leads to an influx of Na^+/Ca^{2+} that causes membrane depolarization. The spread of membrane depolarization along the dendrite leads to the activation of voltage-gated Na^+ and K^+ channels, with the consequent generation of an action potential. The propagation of impulse along the nerve fibers allows VNO neurons to communicate with the first central processing unit, the accessory olfactory bulb (AOB).

Much insight into the molecular and anatomical components of VNO-signal transduction has been gained from the study of mutant mice. Mice that lack a functional TRPC2 channel show normal olfactory function but fail to respond to urinary vomeronasal stimuli. These mice do not display male–male aggression and engage in sexual and courtship behaviors toward both males and females. They also have deficits in maternal aggression toward male intruders. This lack of aggressiveness in these mutant mice is in accordance with similar findings in mice following VNO lesions. The mouse VNO has two broad receptor gene families, V1Rs and V2Rs, comprising over 250 receptors genes. When the genes for 16 of the V1R family clustered together were deleted using chromosomal engineering (which amounted to 12%

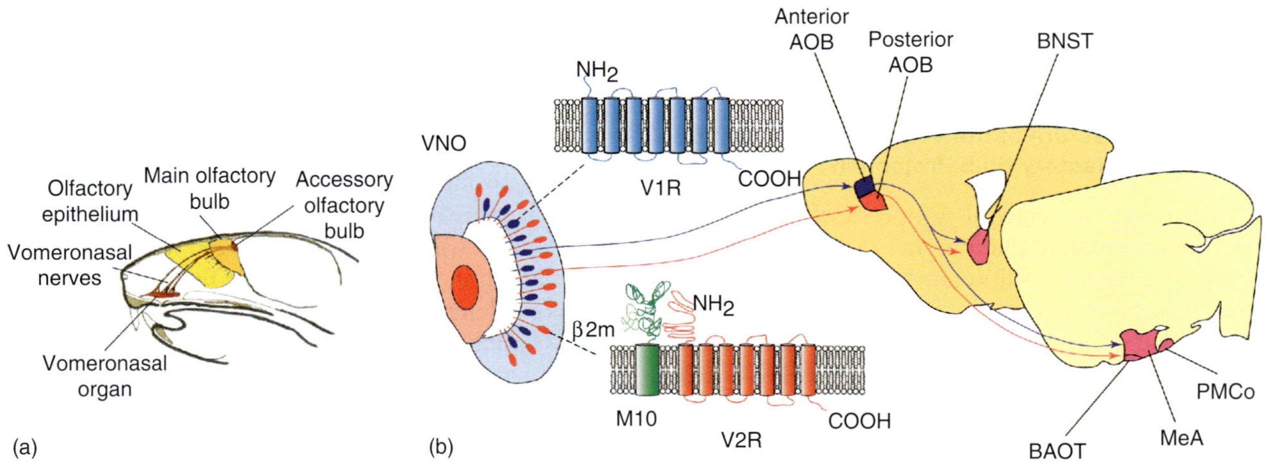

Figure 1 Rodent vomeronasal organ (VNO). a, Sagittal view showing the location in relation to the main olfactory epithelium; b, anatomy and central neural projections, with the sensory vomeronasal receptor neurons (VNRNs) shown in a coronal cross section of the VNO. Two discrete classes of VNRNs (V1Rs and V2Rs), G-protein-coupled receptors, project separately to the anterior and posterior accessory olfactory bulb (AOB), respectively. The V2Rs differ markedly from the V1Rs in that they have a large extracellular N-terminus and form a receptor complex with members of the M10 family of major histocompatibility complex (MHC) class Ib molecules and β_2-microglobulin (β2m). The information from the V1Rs and V2Rs are processed in the AOB and then converges in overlapping projections to the bed nucleus of the stria terminalis (BNST), bed nucleus of the accessory olfactory tract (BAOT), medial amygdala (MeA) and the posteromedial cortical nucleus (PMCo) of the amygdala. COOH, From Brennan, P. A. and Keverne, E. B. (2004), Something in the air?: new insights into mammalian pheromones, *Current Biology* **14**, R81–R89, with permission.

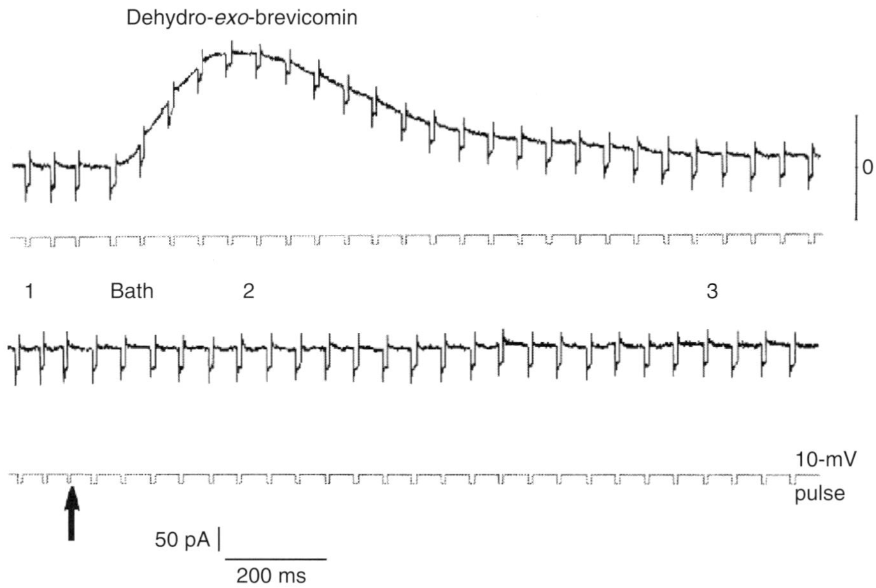

Figure 2 Application of the putative pheromone dehydro-*exo*-brevicomin (DHB) to a VNRN evoked an outward current accompanied by a decrease in conductance. Depolarizing pulses of 10 mV were applied continuously before (1), during (2), and after (3) DHB or bath. In the presence of DHB, the amplitude of the current pulses was decreased. From Moss, R. L., Flynn, R. E., Shen, X. M., et al. (1997), Urine-derived compound evokes membrane responses in mouse vomeronasal receptor neurons, *Journal of Neurophysiology* **77**, 2856–2862, with permission.

of the V1R population), male mice were impaired in their sexual behavior to females, with fewer males initiating sexual activity toward females than the genetically intact controls. These mice, too, fail to initiate maternal aggression toward intruder males, as was found in TrpC2-deficient mice, although there were no differences in the aggressive behavior of these V1R cluster-deficient males. These and other studies have yielded important insights into the functioning of the vomeronasal system and have helped researchers appreciate the complexities of this chemosensory system.

Chemoarchitecture of the Vomeronasal Organ to Accessory Olfactory Bulb Projection

The diversity in electrical responses of VN receptor neurons to putative pheromones, as well as the vast array of behaviors subjected to pheromone regulation, may be related to the fact that VNRNs appear to be divided into at least two chemoarchitecturally distinct populations: VNRNs located in layers close to the lumen of the VNO express $G_{\alpha i2}$ and project to the anterior portion of the AOB; VNRNs located more basally express $G_{\alpha o}$ and project to the posterior part of the AOB. The significance of this division has become more apparent with studies identifying two families of VNO receptor genes, with V1Rs and V2Rs expressed in $G_{\alpha i2}$ and $G_{\alpha o}$ VNRNs, respectively. This expression pattern suggests that there exist two functionally distinct processing units responsible for relaying signals from the VNO to the AOB.

Until now, the physiological basis for chemoarchitecturally segregated populations of VNO neurons was largely unexplored. Presuming that both populations of VNO cells are involved in pheromone detection, they may recognize separate categories of pheromones (volatile vs. nonvolatile, or primer vs. releasing) or may be involved in the mediation of separate behavioral responses. In the male mouse, the VNO is involved in at least two distinct behaviors: reproduction and aggression. Experiments have demonstrated that neurons in the anterior portion of the AOB of the male mouse are preferentially activated by exposure to female-soiled bedding, as opposed to familiar male-soiled bedding. The differential activation was dependent on an intact VNO and was not observed in the main olfactory bulb (MOB). These data indicate that the position of a vomeronasal receptor cell within the VNO is reflected at the level of the AOB by a functional division along the anterior–posterior axis. Recently, Katz's group performed the first recordings of pheromonal responses in the AOB of awake-behaving mice that demonstrated that responses of the AOB mitral cells are highly selective to strain and the sex of conspecifics. It is also possible that nuclei downstream of the AOB, such as the medial amygdale (mAMG), may also be preferentially activated. The nature of the information processing by V1Rs and V2Rs is yet to be understood, but the anterior and posterior AOB projections completely overlap at the level of amygdala, the bed nucleus of the accessory olfactory tract (nAOT), and the bed nucleus of the stria terminalis (BNST).

Central Neural Pathways of the Vomeronasal System

The anatomical pathway linking pheromone detection in the VNO to the hypothalamic centers controlling sexual and reproductive events has been well defined by studies using transsynaptic tracers. VNRNs project directly to the AOB, where they synapse onto mitral cell dendrites. The mitral cell axons project to the mAMYG, BNST, and nAOT. Connections between the mAMYG and the preoptic area (POA) and between the mAMYG and the ventromedial hypothalamus (VMH) complete the circuit by which pheromones may modulate the hypothalamic and/or limbic centers involved in reproductive behavior. Lesions of the VNO, AOB, mAMYG, or VMH significantly impair the ability of the female rat to display increases in sexual receptivity in response to male sexual contacts. The possibility of direct projections from the VNO to the POA and VMH has received some support and may provide an additional pathway for pheromonal control over GnRH-secreting neurons located in the hypothalamus. The surgical removal of the VNO adversely affects the copulatory behavior in males and lordosis behavior in female rodents. GnRH has been shown to facilitate mating behavior in the female rat, and GnRH has also been demonstrated to restore mating behavior in the female rat and male hamster after VNO removal.

Activation of Vomeronasal Neural Pathways

Studies employing c-fos-immunocytochemistry as a marker of cellular activation have revealed that vomeronasal neurons are activated by chemosensory stimulation. Following mating with a male, female rats exhibited a VNO-dependent increase in c-fos expression in all vomeronasal system nuclei. A particularly dense concentration of activated cells was observed in the mitral and granule layers of the AOB (**Figure 3a**) and in the mAMYG (**Figure 3b**), with increases in cellular activation also noted in the BNST, the nAOT, and the ventrolateral VMH. Female cervical stimulation or exposure of male rats to female-soiled bedding evoked a similar pattern of c-fos activation. In the male hamster, mating or exposure to vaginal discharge also produced activation of the vomeronasal system.

Activation of Gonadotropin-Releasing Hormone Neurons

During copulation, the female rat becomes more receptive over time and exhibits a release of LH (**Figure 4**). Because LH release is stimulated by GnRH, the chemosensory stimulation obtained during copulation is likely to activate GnRH neurons.

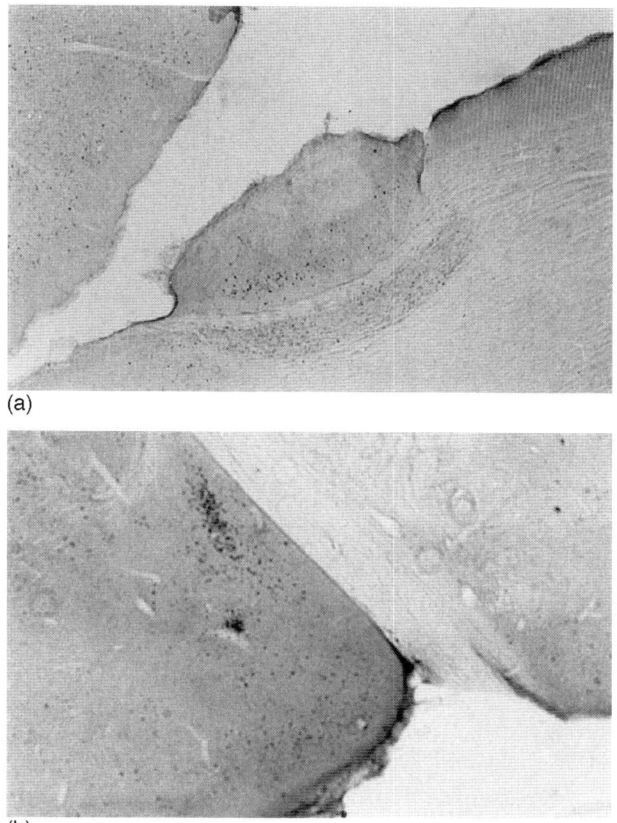

(a)

(b)

Figure 3 Samples from female rats exposed to 3 h of repetitive mating. a, the accessory olfactory bulb; b, the medial amygdala (mAMYG). c-Fos-immunopositive cells are indicated by small black dots. Note the cluster of c-fos-immunopositive cells parallel to the optic tract in the mAMYG. From Dudley, C. A., Sudderth, S. B. and Moss, R. L. (1992), LHRH neurons in the medial septal-diagonal band-preoptic area do not project directly to the hippocampus: a double-labeling immunohistochemical study, *Synapse* **12**, 139–146, with permission.

Indeed, double-labeling immunocytochemical studies demonstrated that mating activated approximately 80% of the GnRH neurons, whereas after VNO removal only approximately 38% of the GnRH neurons were activated (see **Figure 5**). Similar studies from other laboratories also revealed an increase in the activation of GnRH neurons in the female mouse during mating and in the female rat during vaginocervical stimulation. These observations provide firm evidence that chemosensory stimulation at the level of the VNO influences endocrine events at the hypothalamic level.

Vomeronasal Organ Response to Olfactory Stimuli and Olfactory System Response to Pheromonal Stimuli

Recent reports have indicated that cross-talk seems to exist between the vomeronasal system (VNS) and the main olfactory system. Although the VNO is mainly

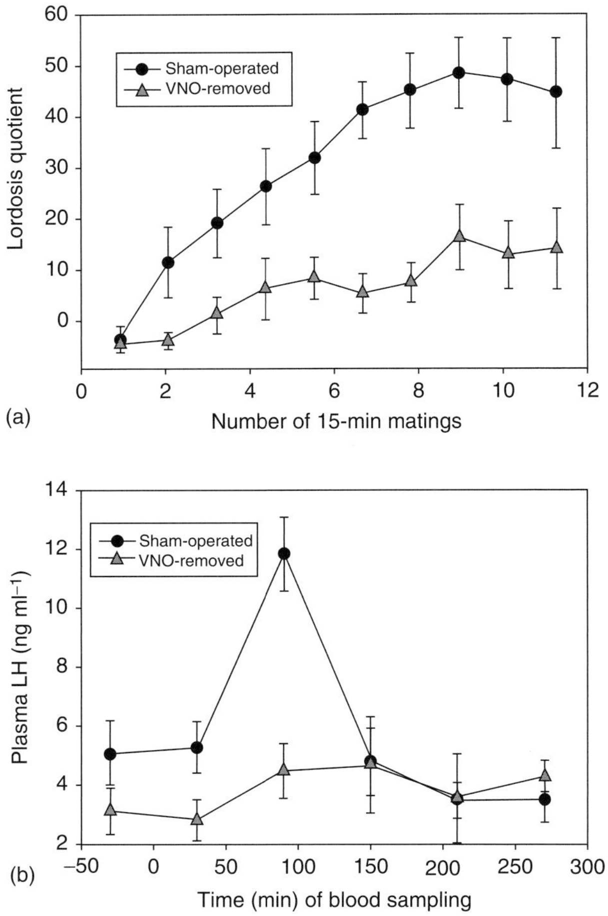

Figure 4 The effect of VNO removal in female rats. a, On lordotic responsiveness; b, on mating-induced luteinizing-hormone (LH) release. From Rajendren, G., Dudley, C. A. and Moss, R. L. (1990), Role of the vomeronasal organ in the male-induced enhancement of sexual receptivity in female rats, *Neuroendocrinology* **52**, 368–372, with permission.

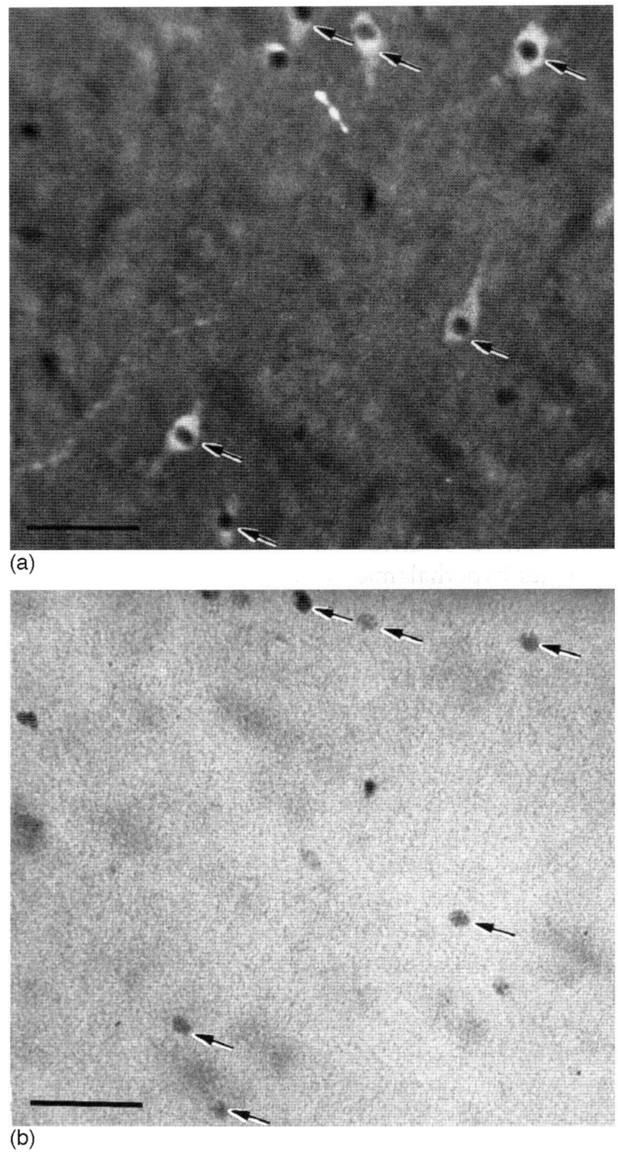

Figure 5 GnRH-containing neurons that were activated by 3 h of repetitive mating in the female rat. a, Arrows point to GnRH neurons labeled immunofluorescently with Texas Red; b, arrows point to c-fos-immunopositive nuclei. In a, the five GnRH-containing cells also contained the c-fos protein. From Rajendren, G., Dudley, C. A. and Moss, R. L. (1993), Influence of male rats on the luteinizing hormone-releasing hormone neuronal system in female rats: role of the vomeronasal organ, *Neuroendocrinology* **57**, 898–906, with permission.

dedicated to sensing pheromones and the main olfactory epithelium that lines the nasal cavity senses common odors, recent findings make us rethink how pheromones control hormonal responses. This is particularly relevant for humans, in which adults lack a functional VNO. In mammals, mating and the reproductive behavior of females are controlled by GnRH neurons in the hypothalamus. GnRH is secreted into the hypophysial portal system, through which it regulates the action of gonadotropin-secreting pituitary neurons. Recent findings have brought the main olfactory system into the limelight in the pheromone and behavior field, not only by showing its crucial role in sexual and aggressive behavior but also by revealing a direct anatomical projection from the main olfactory epithelium to luteinizing hormone-releasing hormone (LHRH) neurons in the hypothalamus, which regulate the gonadal hormone release. There is also evidence that the VNO in the sexually naïve male hamster is crucial for the female pheromone-induced mating behavior in male, but the main olfactory system takes over the functional role of the VNO in the context of sexual behavior. Thus, the traditional distinction that common odors are perceived through the olfactory pathway and pheromones by the vomeronasal pathway does not hold true; rather, the main olfactory system and vomeronasal system complement one another in chemosensory communication.

In the human fetus, a VNO develops and appears to guide the migration of GnRH neurons to the hypothalamus. However, the lack of a functional VNO in human adults does not imply that pheromone signaling does not occur in humans. Most of the vomeronasal receptor genes in the human genome are pseudogenes; however, four of these seem to be functional, of which one, hV1RL1, is expressed in olfactory mucosa and is likely to have a transducing function. At present, the only reproducible pheromonal effect in humans is the effectiveness of axillary secretions from women in different stages of their menstrual cycles to alter the cycle lengths of other women living in close proximity, thus causing menstrual synchronization. The recent findings in mice that the main olfactory pathway is required for reproductive behavior and that it projects to and activates hypothalamic GnRH/LHRH neurons might explain how organisms without a functional VNO, such as humans, use olfactory inputs in order to activate subcortical hard-wired circuits controlling innate sexual and reproductive behavior. Advances in neuroimaging have allowed us to visualize brain activity patterns in awake humans, and these techniques have shown that sex pheromones activate wide regions of the human brain, including areas traditionally thought to mediate cognition. These studies suggest that, as in the rodent, the pheromone-activated endocrine system is much more extensive than previously thought. Thus, it appears that we need to learn more about how intimately neuroendocrine functions, controlled by pheromones acting through our noses, might interact with other operations within the brain to control human behavior and cognition.

Stress and Reproduction

Social Interactions

Stresses of a social nature have the potential to exert negative effects on reproduction. The most common social stress in animals of the same species is caused by high population density. Crowded conditions give rise to complex emotional states that may interfere with reproductive function. In addition, pheromonal cues emitted and detected in crowded conditions contribute to a decline in endocrine function. Although the exact mechanisms are uncertain, a wide array of noxious physical stimuli and distressed emotional states, including those of social origin, can enhance the activity of the hypothalamic-pituitary-adrenal (HPA) axis. The enhanced activity of this system is correlated with the suppression of reproductive processes at many levels in the reproductive axis. This suppression appears to be brought about by several specific actions that affect the GnRH system of neurons. First, corticotropin releasing hormone (CRH) and the proopiomelanocortin (POMC)-derived peptides adrenocorticotropic hormone (ACTH) and β-endorphin can act in the brain to inhibit the release of GnRH. Second, corticosteroids themselves can decrease the responsiveness of the pituitary to GnRH. All these actions can interfere with the stimulatory effect of LH on steroidogenesis in the gonad. However, the extent of reproductive inhibition varies with social rank, sex, maturity, season, and some other factors.

The negative effect of emotional stress on reproduction is well illustrated in studies performed on cages of mice that are densely populated. Typically, a large cage is populated by a few pairs and the population is allowed to grow until it regulates itself. Maintaining this regulated population level often involves a marked inhibition of sexual maturation among young animals, as well as a cessation of reproduction by adults. In crowded deer mice, the effects of high population density on reproductive function are profound. When young deer mice are allowed to grow in pairs in small cages with adults of the opposite sex, they become fertile at 5–8 weeks of age. On rearing in dense populations, however, by 12–13 weeks of age, as many as 95% of these deer mice still are not fertile. According to Terman and colleagues, many die at well over 1 year of age without ever having achieved fertility. To some extent, pheromones can alleviate the negative effects of environmental stress on estrous cycling. Female mice housed in grouped, crowded conditions experience a lack of estrous cycling, which can be overcome by urinary cues from a conspecific male or by putative pheromones isolated from male mouse urine.

Agonistic Interactions

Intermale aggression in the form of fighting is common among densely populated animals. Losers of these fights as well as other social subordinates and most of the onlookers seem physiologically stressed. Male mice fight to establish dominance even when only two are brought together. Agonistic interactions have been shown to have a profound impact on the endocrine system. The defeated animal experiences an almost immediate inhibition of LH secretion, lowered testosterone levels, and a dramatic rise in the secretion of corticosterone. Moreover, the increase in corticosterone can be conditioned to occur in response to the mere presence of a dominant male. Thus, even without the occurrence of overt fighting, subordinate animals may have depressed LH secretion. Such alterations in hormone levels may have negative consequences for health and fertility because the long-term hyperactivation of the HPA axis is related to a decline in immune system activity and reduced gonadal activity may result in sterility.

In higher vertebrates, behavioral responses to unfamiliar conspecifics are dependent on the actual environmental situation as well as social experiences made during behavioral development. Sapolsky's studies of a population of wild African olive baboons found that high- and low-ranking baboons differ in levels of cortisol and testosterone during periods of social instability, when overt aggression is quite common. Dominant males tended to have the lowest levels of cortisol. During periods of relative stability in the colony, differences in cortisol and testosterone between dominant and subordinate males were no longer detectable. Differences in cortisol levels appear to be extremely important, not only in terms of reproductive success but also in terms of survival. Males with the lowest cortisol levels survived the longest. A strong relationship exists among environmental factors (the rearing conditions as well as the actual situation), aggressive behavior, endocrine responses, and health.

Recently, two synthetic pheromones, 2,3-dehydro-*exo*-brevicomin (DHB) and 2-*sec*-butyl-dihydrothiazole (SBT), the urinary constituents in male mice, have been shown to elicit aggression in mice. The level of two other urinary constituents from male mouse, α- and β-farnesene, were elevated in the excreted urine of dominant male mice even several days after establishing dominance. The farnesene, absent in bladder urine but abundant in the preputial gland, when mixed with water or bladder urine significantly reduced the amount of time subordinate males investigated the urine deposits of dominant males. Thus, these four different urinary constituents have been shown to contribute to male–male agonistic interactions in mice.

Nonsocial Interactions

Reproductive events are also affected by stress encountered in nonsocial situations. The endocrine system appears to be more susceptible to emotional stress than to physical stress. For example, immobilized female rats display an immediate loss of LH pulsatile activity, but no change in pulsing was observed after an experimenter administered limb fracture. The stressful nature of immobilization has also been observed in cattle restricted for the first time by a stanchion, haltered, and prepared surgically for sequential blood collection via jugular cannulae. In these conditions, greatly elevated plasma cortisol levels and no pulsatile release of LH were noticed. However, repeated exposure to this procedure resulted in low levels of plasma cortisol and a normal episodic pattern of LH release.

Stress Signaling Mediated by Pheromones

Pheromone detection is an important component in the animal's ability to respond appropriately to stressful cues in social and agonistic interactions. It is well documented in several mammalian species that animals experiencing stress and fear release chemical signals that induce behavioral, endocrinological, and immunological changes in the recipient animals of the same species. Aggressive behavior is displayed in many species in day-to-day social interactions. This behavior is elicited by the appropriate recognition of an adversary as a potential threat or sexual competitor, and this recognition involves the detection of social odors by the VNS and/or olfactory system. The involvement of the VNS in such recognition is clearly demonstrated by several studies. Genetic ablation of the TrpC2 channel results in the failure of the male mice to display aggression toward other males, similar to behavior shown by male mice after vomeronasalectomy, and also eliminates aggressive behavior of lactating female mice. However, in contrast, vomeronasalectomy does not reduce the maternal aggression of lactating female rats. Vomeronasalectomy also has been shown to decrease aggressive behavior in the male lesser mouse lemur, a prosimian.

In socially stressed crowded female rats, the removal of the VNO eliminates the resumption of estrous cycling induced by male rat urine. Mechanisms underlying the VNO-dependent responses to sociogenic stress are largely unknown at this time. Finding neural sites in which the stress-activated HPA axis interacts with the vomeronasal system seems a good strategy for determining where to begin research from a mechanistic point of view.

See Also the Following Articles

Reproduction, Effects of Social Stress on.

Further Reading

Boehm, U., Zou, Z. and Buck, L. B. (2005). Feedback loops link odor and pheromone signaling with reproduction. *Cell* **123**, 683–695.

Brennan, P. A. and Keverne, E. B. (2004). Something in the air?: new insights into mammalian pheromones. *Current Biology* **14**, R81–R89.

Bronson, F. H. (1988). Seasonal regulation of reproduction in mammals. In: Knobil, E. & Neill, J. D. (eds.) *The physiology of reproduction* (vol. 2), pp. 1831–1871. New York: Raven Press.

Bronson, F. H. (1995). Seasonal variation in human reproduction: environmental factors. *Quarterly Review of Biology* **70**, 141–164.

Calegro, A. E., Bagdy, G. and D'Agata, R. (1998). Mechanisms of stress on reproduction: evidence for complex intra-hypothalamic circuit. *Annals of the New York Academy of Sciences* **851**, 364–370.

Dudley, C. A., Rajendren, G. and Moss, R. L. (1996). Signal processing in the vomeronasal system: modulation of sexual behavior in the female rat. *Critical Review of Neurobiology* **10**, 265–290.

Dudley, C. A., Sudderth, S. B. and Moss, R. L. (1992). LHRH neurons in the medial septal-diagonal band-preoptic area do not project directly to the hippocampus: a double-labeling immunohistochemical study. *Synapse* **12**, 139–146.

Dulac, C. and Torello, T. A. (2003). Molecular detection of pheromone signals in mammals: from genes to behaviour. *Nature Reviews Neuroscience* **4**, 551–562.

Halpern, M. and Martinez-Marcos, A. (2003). Structure and function of the vomeronasal system: an update. *Progress in Neurobiology* **70**, 245–318.

Kumar, A., Dudley, C. A. and Moss, R. L. (1999). Functional dichotomy within the vomeronasal system: distinct zones of neuronal activity in the accessory olfactory bulb correlate with sex-specific behaviors. *Journal of Neuroscience* **19**(20), RC32.

Luo, M., Fee, M. S. and Katz, L. C. (2003). Encoding pheromonal signals in the accessory olfactory bulb of behaving mice. *Science* **299**, 1196–1201.

Marchlewska-Koj, A. (1997). Sociogenic stress and rodent reproduction. *Neuroscience and Biobehavioral Review* **21**, 669–703.

Meredith, M. and Fernandez-Fewell, G. (1994). Vomeronasal system, LHRH, and sex behaviour. *Psychoneuroendocrinology* **19**, 657–672.

Mombaerts, P. (2004). Genes and ligands for odorant, vomeronasal and taste receptors. *Nature Reviews Neuroscience* **5**, 263–278.

Moss, R. L., Flynn, R. E., Shen, X. M., et al. (1997). Urine-derived compound evokes membrane responses in mouse vomeronasal receptor neurons. *Journal of Neurophysiology* **77**, 2856–2862.

Przekop, F. and Tomaszewska, D. (1996). Responses in the hypothalamic monoaminergic system activity in ewes to beta-endorphin, CRF, and their antagonists. *Acta Neurobiologiae Experimentalis* **56**, 807–817.

Rajendren, G., Dudley, C. A. and Moss, R. L. (1990). Role of the vomeronasal organ in the male-induced enhancement of sexual receptivity in female rats. *Neuroendocrinology* **52**, 368–372.

Rajendren, G., Dudley, C. A. and Moss, R. L. (1993). Influence of male rats on the luteinizing hormone-releasing hormone neuronal system in female rats: role of the vomeronasal organ. *Neuroendocrinology* **57**, 898–906.

Yoon, H., Enquist, L. W. and Dulac, C. (2005). Olfactory inputs to hypothalamic neurons controlling reproduction and fertility. *Cell* **123**, 669–682.

SUBJECT INDEX

NOTES

Cross-reference terms in italics are general cross-references, or refer to subentry terms within the main entry (the main entry is not repeated to save space). Readers are also advised to refer to the end of each article for additional cross-references – not all of these cross-references have been included in the index cross-references.

The index is arranged in set-out style with a maximum of three levels of heading. Major discussion of a subject is indicated by bold page numbers. Page numbers suffixed by *t* and *f* refer to Tables and Figures respectively; *vs.* indicates a comparison.

Nomenclature used within the index reflects that used in the text.

This index is in letter-by-letter order, whereby hyphens and spaces within index headings are ignored in the alphabetization. Prefixes and terms in parentheses are excluded from the initial alphabetization.

Common abbreviations used in subentries:

ACTH – adrenocorticotropic hormone

ADHD – attention deficit hyperactivity disorder

CRF – corticotropin-releasing factor

CRH – corticotropin-releasing hormone

HPA axis – hypothalamic–pituitary–adrenal axis

HPG axis – hypothalamic–pituitary–gonadal axis

HPT axis – hypothalamic–pituitary–thyroid axis

PTSD – posttraumatic stress disorder

SNP – single nucleotide polymorphism

A

C

D

E

F

H

I

J

K

L

M

N

O

P

Q

R

S

U

V

W

Y

Z